Neuroscience Nursing

Evidence-Based Practice

Neuroscience Nursing
Evidence-Based Practice

Edited by

Sue Woodward
Lecturer, Florence Nightingale School of Nursing and Midwifery,
King's College London

and

Ann-Marie Mestecky
Lecturer, Florence Nightingale School of Nursing and Midwifery,
King's College London

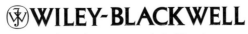
A John Wiley & Sons, Ltd., Publication

Library of Congress Cataloging-in-Publication Data
Neuroscience nursing : evidence-based practice / edited by Sue Woodward and Ann-Marie Mestecky.
    p. ; cm.
  Includes bibliographical references and index.
  ISBN 978-1-4051-6356-9 (pbk. : alk. paper)
1. Neurological nursing.   2. Evidence-based nursing.
I. Woodward, Sue (Susan Janet), 1965-   II. Mestecky, Ann-Marie.
  [DNLM: 1. Nervous System Diseases–nursing.
2. Evidence-Based Nursing.   WY 160.5]
  RC350.5.N4885 2011
  616.8′04231–dc22

                                        2010031661

A catalogue record for this book is available from the British Library.

Set in 9.5/12 pt Times by Toppan Best-set Premedia Limited
Printed and bound in Malaysia by Vivar Printing Sdn Bhd

1   2011

Contents

Contributor List

Thom Aird
Principal Lecturer, Faculty of Health of Health and Social Care, London South Bank University

Kirsty Andrews
Senior Lecturer, Faculty of Health of Health and Social Care, London South Bank University

David Ash
Urology Nurse practitioner & Research Nurse, Princess Royal Spinal Injuries Centre, Northern General Hospital, Sheffield

Beverley Bennett
Senior Lecturer, Faculty of Health & Wellbeing, Sheffield Hallam University

Iain Bowie
Lecturer, Florence Nightingale School of Nursing and Midwifery, King's College London (Retired)

Mary Braine
Lecturer, School of Nursing, Faculty of Health and Social Care, University of Salford

Chris Brunker
Clinical Nurse Specialist, Neuro ICU St.George's Healthcare NHS Trust, London

Kathryn Chappell
Highly Specialist Speech and Language Therapist, Surrey Community Health (East Locality), East Surrey Hospital

Maureen Coggrave
Clinical Nurse Specialist, The National Spinal Injuries Centre, Stoke Mandeville Hospital

Neal Cook
Lecturer in Nursing, School of Nursing, University of Ulster

Jane Dundas
Stroke Co-ordinator, Croydon Community Health Services

Ava Easton
Development Manager, The Encephalitis Society, Malton, North Yorkshire

Chris Eberhardie
Honorary Prinicipal Lecturer in Nursing, Faculty of Health and Social Care Sciences, Kingston University and St George's, University of London

Nikki Embrey
Clinical Nurse Specialist (MS), North Midland MS Service

Karen Harrison Dening
Consultant Admiral Nurse, Barnet Enfield and Haringey Mental Health NHS Trust

Paul Harrison
Clinical Development Officer, Princess Royal Spinal Injuries Centre, Northern General Hospital, Sheffield

Stuart Hibbins
Senior Lecturer, Faculty of Health and Social Care, London South Bank University

Alison Hobden
Lecturer, Department of Health Science, University of Liverpool

Saiju Jacob
Honorary Consultant Neurologist, Queen Elizabeth Neurosciences Centre, University Hospitals of Birmingham NHS Foundation Trust

Leann Johnson
Specialist Registrar, Infectious Diseases Research Dept., North Manchester General Hospital

Katy Judd
Consultant Nurse, Dementia Research Centre, National Hospital for Neurology and Neurosurgery, London

Ehsan Khan
Lecturer, Florence Nightingale School of Nursing and Midwifery, King's College London

Stephen Leyshon
Primary Care Lead, National Patient Safety Agency, UK

Anthony Linklater
Epilepsy Specialist Nurse, National Hospital for Neurology Neurosurgery, Queen Square London

Vicki Matthews
MS Specialist Nurse Advisor, MS Trust

Pauline McDonald
Parkinson's Disease Nurse Specialist, Imperial College Heathcare NHS Trust

Anne McLeod
Senior Lecturer in Critical Care, School of Community and Health Sciences, City University, London

Siobhan McLernon
Senior Lecturer, Faculty of Health and Social Care, London South Bank University

Ann-Marie Mestecky
Lecturer, Florence Nightingale School of Nursing and Midwifery, King's College London

Mary O'Brien
Senior Lecturer, Evidence-Based Practice Research Centre, Faculty of Health, Edge Hill University

Glynis Pellatt
Senior Lecturer, Faculty of Heath and Social Science, University of Bedfordshire

Stephen Pewter
School of Psychology, University of Exeter

Anne Preece
Professional Development Nurse, Neuroscience Critical Care Unit, University Hospitals Birmingham NHS Foundation Trust

Liz Scott
Parkinson's Disease Nurse Specialist, Buckinghamshire Hospitals NHS Trust

Julia Slark
Clinical Nurse Specialist Stroke, Imperial College Healthcare NHS Trust

Rachel Taylor
Nurse Consultant, Dept of Neurogenetics, The National Hospital for Neurology and Neurosurgery, London

Emma Townsley
Macmillan CNS Neuro-oncology The National Hospital for Neurology and Neurosurgery, UCLH

Colm Treacy
Lecturer, School of Community and Health Sciences, City University, London

Cath Waterhouse
Clinical Nurse Educator, Neuroscience Unit, Royal Hallamshire Hospital, Sheffield

Ian Weatherhead
Lead Nurse, Admiral Nursing Direct For Dementia

Mandy Wells
Consultant Nurse/Head of Dept, Bladder, Bowel and Pelvic Floor Dysfunction, NHS Devon

Ed Wilkins
Consultant and Clinical Director of Infectious Diseases,
North Manchester General Hospital

Huw Williams
School of Psychology, Washington Singer Labs,
University of Exeter

Sue Woodward
Lecturer, Florence Nightingale School of Nursing and
Midwifery, King's College London

Deborah Yarde
Senior Specialist Nurse Bladder and Bowel Care, NHS
Devon

Preface

This is the first evidence-based UK neuroscience nursing textbook for nurses working with people with neurological problems in a wide variety of settings including prevention, primary care, acute and critical care settings, rehabilitation and palliative care. It aims to inform the practice of neuroscience nursing through the report of current research, best available evidence, policy and education and reflects both the richness and the diversity of contemporary neuroscience nursing.

Authors of this edited text have been drawn from nurse specialists, nurse consultants, academics and subject experts from throughout the UK. Each chapter provides a critique of the available evidence underpinning practice, including reference to evidence-based guidelines where relevant. Throughout the text guidelines that have been developed by the National Institute for Health and Clinical Excellence have been referred to in the main. Nurses working in the NHS in Scotland should be mindful that they should also refer to Scottish Intercollegiate Guidelines Network (SIGN) guidelines where these exist.

The text is divided into several different sections covering anatomy and physiology, aspects of assessment, management of patients with a variety of common neurological conditions and other concepts that underpin neuroscience nursing practice. Uniquely, this text includes patients' perspectives of living with a variety of neurological conditions.

This book is aimed primarily at qualified nurses working specifically with people with neurological problems and has been written in an accessible style appropriate to a staff nurse audience. However, it also provides sufficient detail for more experienced practitioners as the core text underpinning practice and will also enable nursing students who have a particular interest in this field to develop a greater understanding of the specialist management of patients with neurological problems. It also furnishes practitioners in non-specialist areas with the specialist knowledge to enable them to meet the requirements for the National Service Framework for Long-term conditions. Many general, primary care and critical care nurses encounter patients with neurological problems as part of their everyday practice and yet very often they do not have the knowledge and skills to meet these patients' neurological needs. This book therefore also provides a key reference for non-specialist nurses faced with this situation.

Acknowledgements

We would like to express our thanks to all those who have contributed to the writing and production of this text. It has been a major undertaking and would not have been possible without the expert knowledge of the many contributors. They helped to bring our vision into being.

We would also like to thank the following, who generously gave of their time and expertise in undertaking peer review of the text: Maryanne Ampong, Aimee Aubeeluck, Gill Blackler, Emma Briggs, Chris Brunker, Shuna Colville, Bridgit Dimond, Maria Fitzpatrick, Alison Gallagher, Daiga Heisters, Victoria Hurwitz, Ehsan Khan, Louise Jarrett, Rachael Macarthur, Lindy May, Shanne McNamara, Jacky Powell, Cathy Queally, Tina Stephens, Ben Sullivan, Richard Warner and John Whitaker.

Furthermore we would like to thank all those who shared their experiences of living with a neurological condition or who have experienced injury to the CNS, Alison Wertheimer and Sarah Hill, Ben Edward and the Association for Spina Bifida and Hydrocephalus, amongst others. Their words will help nurses to understand the personal impact of living with a neurological condition. We are also grateful to all those patients and colleagues who agreed to be photographed for this edition.

We thank Sue Scullard for her time in designing a number of the figures.

Sue would like to thank her husband and children for their support and patience.

Ann-Marie would like to thank David, for his good humour, patience, support and above all encouragement, as well as Joseph, Mum and Dad.

Section I

Anatomy and Physiology of the Nervous System

1

Cells of the CNS and How They Communicate

Colm Treacy

INTRODUCTION

The neurone (or nerve cell) is the most important component of the nervous system. Its main function is to rapidly process and transmit information. The human nervous system contains about 300–500 billion neurones (approximately 80,000/mm^2), integrated into an intricate functional network by millions of connections with other neurones. Neurones communicate primarily via chemical synapses. The action potential is the fundamental process underlying synaptic transmission. It occurs as a result of waves of voltage that are generated by the electrically excitable membrane of the neurone.

This chapter will explore the histology of the nervous tissue and the physiology of neurotransmission.

COMPONENTS OF THE NEURONE AND THEIR FUNCTIONS

Neurones contain components and organelles that are crucial to normal cellular function and these generally resemble those of non-neuronal cells. Neurones of various types have different morphologies and functional features, depending on their location in the central nervous system (CNS). The prototypical neurone (Figure 1.1) consists of a stellate cell body (soma), a single axon that emerges from the soma, a number of thin processes called dendrites (the axon and dendrites are collectively known as neurites) and points of functional contact at the axon terminal with other cells, glands or organs, called synapses. The integrative functions of these unique structures are what differentiate neurones from non-neuronal cells and underlie the

generation and transmission of information, which is so unique and fundamental to nervous system activity.

Like other cells in the body, the neurone is enclosed by a bi-layered lipoprotein-rich cell membrane, called the neuronal membrane. This membrane is approximately 5–7.5 nm thick and separates the cytoplasmic contents from the extracellular environment.

As in non-neuronal cells, the soma, (or cell body, also known as the perikaryon), is roughly spherical in shape and measures around 20 μm in diameter. The soma of smaller neurones may measure as little as 5 μm, whereas in the case of large motor neurones, they can be as much as 135 μm in diameter. The soma is the site of routine cellular housekeeping functions, including the synthesis of all the neuronal proteins that are necessary for the upkeep of the axon and axon terminals (Longstaff, 2000). In common with non-neuronal cells, the soma also includes important cellular organelles, such as the nucleus, Golgi apparatus, endoplasmic reticulum (ER), ribosomes, lysosomes and mitochondria.

The nucleus

The nucleus is approximately 5–10 μm in diameter and is surrounded by a granular, double-layered membrane, known as the nuclear envelope, which is perforated by small pores measuring around 0.1 μm wide. These small pores act as passageways between the nucleoplasm (interior of the nucleus) and the surrounding cytoplasm. By comparison with non-neuronal cells, the nuclei of neurones tend to be larger, which is thought to be related to the high levels of protein synthesis within the neurone. The nucleus contains the genetic material, deoxyribonucleic acid (DNA), which is responsible for directing the metabolic activities of the cell. Messenger ribonucleic acid

Neuroscience Nursing: Evidence-Based Practice, 1st Edition.
Edited by Sue Woodward and Ann-Marie Mestecky
© 2011 Blackwell Publishing Ltd

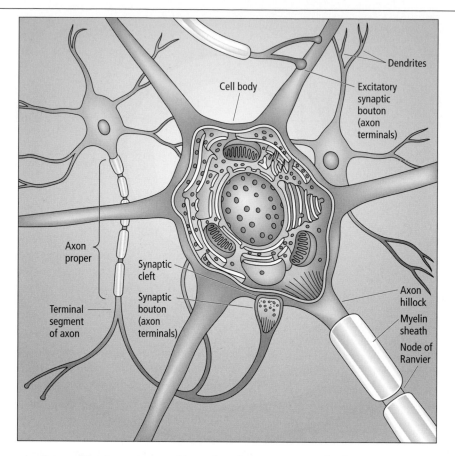

Figure 1.1 Diagram of a multipolar neurone. Note that the processes of other neurones make synaptic contacts with it. Synapses may be formed, as illustrated, with the soma or with the dendrites, although other types of synapses also occur. Reproduced from Maria A Patestas and Leslie P Gartner, *A Textbook of Neuroanatomy*, Wiley-Blackwell, with permission.

(mRNA) is also found within the nucleus. It is responsible for copying the specific genetic instructions from the DNA (transcription) for protein synthesis and carrying it to the site of protein production in the cytoplasm.

The rough endoplasmic reticulum (RER)

The RER is adjacent to the nucleus and is composed of rows of plate-like membranous sacs, which are covered in granular ribosomes. The RER synthesises the majority of protein needed to meet the functional demands of the neurone. It does this under the direction of mRNA. The ribosomes build proteins from amino acids delivered by transfer RNA from the genetic instructions held within messenger RNA. Rough ER is especially abundant in neurones, more so than in glia or other non-neuronal cells. It is densely packed within the soma and the shafts of dendrites, giving rise to distinct structures called *Nissl bodies*.

The smooth endoplasmic reticulum (SER)

The SER is made up of an extensive network of stacked membranous structures that are continuous with the nuclear membrane and RER. It is thought to be the main site of protein-folding. Smooth ER is heterogeneous in function and, depending on its location in the soma, it has important functions in several metabolic processes including protein synthesis, carbohydrate metabolism and regulation of calcium, hormones and lipids. It also serves as a temporary storage area for vesicles that transport proteins to various destinations throughout the neurone.

The Golgi apparatus

The Golgi apparatus is a highly specialised form of smooth endoplasmic reticulum that lies furthest away from the nucleus. In most neurones, the Golgi apparatus completely surrounds the nucleus and extends into the dendrites; however it does not extend into axons. It is composed of aggregated, smooth-surfaced cisternae that are perforated by circular openings to allow the two-way passage of proteins and other molecules. It is surrounded by a mixed group of smaller organelles, which includes mitochondria, lysosomes, multivesicular bodies and vacuoles. The primary function of the Golgi apparatus is to process and package large molecules, primarily proteins and lipids, that are destined for different parts of the neurone such as the axon or dendrites.

Lysosomes

Lysosomes are the principal organelles responsible for the degradation of cellular waste-products. They are membrane-bound vesicles that contain various enzymes (acid hydrolases) that catalyse the breakdown of large unwanted molecules (bacteria, toxins, etc.) within the neurone. Lysosomes are more numerous and conspicuous in injured or diseased neurones. For this reason, they are often used as biomarkers for ageing and neurodegeneration. *Multivesicular bodies* are derived from primary lysosomes and are made up of several tiny spherical vesicles that also contain acid hydrolases. They are small oval snaped, single membrane-bound sacs, approximately 0.5 μm in diameter and have also been noted in various forms of neurodegeneration.

Mitochondria

Mitochondria are the 'power houses' of cells. They are responsible for oxidative phosphorylation and cellular respiration – crucial for the function of all aerobic cells, including neurones. Measuring between 1 μm and 10 μm in length, these organelles are concentrated in the soma and the synaptic terminals, where they produce adenosine triphosphate (ATP), the cell's energy source (Hollenbeck and Saxton, 2005). In addition to energy production, mitochondria also perform a number of other essential functions within the neurone, which include buffering cytosolic calcium levels (Gunter *et al.*, 2004) and sequestering proteins involved in apoptosis (see Chapter 32) (Gulbins *et al.*, 2003). The complex folding of the cristae within mitochondria provides a large surface area to harbour a number of enzymes. These enzymes, which diffuse through the mitochondrial matrix, catalyse the critical metabolic steps involved in cellular respiration. Because of the high energy demands of cellular function and protein synthesis, the number of mitochondria correlates with the neurone's level of metabolic activity.

The cytoskeleton

The cytoskeleton provides a dynamically regulated 'scaffolding' that gives neurones their characteristic shape and facilitates the transport of newly synthesised proteins and organelles from one part of the neurone to another (Brown, 2001). The main components of the cytoskeleton include microfilaments, microtubules and neurofilaments.

Microfilaments

Microfilaments are particularly abundant in axons and dendrites (neurites), but they are also distributed throughout the neuronal cytoplasm. They are also abundant in the expanded tips of growing neurites, known as growth cones (Dent *et al.*, 2003; Kiernan, 2004). They are made from a polymer called actin, a contractile protein that is most commonly associated with muscle contraction. They are composed of two intertwined chains of actin, arranged to create double helix filaments, measuring around 4–6 nm in diameter and a few hundred nanometres in length. The main role of microfilaments is the movement of cytoskeletal and membrane proteins.

Microtubules

Microtubules measure 20–24 nm in diameter and can be several hundred nanometres in length. They are made of strands of globular protein, tubulin, arranged in a helix around a hollow core, to give the microtubule its characteristic thick-walled, tube-like appearance. Microtubules play an important role in maintaining neuronal structure and they also act as tracks for the two-way transport (see: Axonal transport) of cellular organelles.

Neurofilaments (NFs)

Neurofilaments are a type of intermediate filament (IF), seen almost exclusively in neuronal cells. Measuring about 10 nm in diameter, neurofilaments can be several micrometres long and they frequently occur in bundles (Raine, 1999). Like their IF counterparts in non-neuronal cells, they are assembled in a complex series of steps that give rise to solid, rod-like filaments. These filaments are made up of polypeptides that are coiled in a tight, spring-like configuration. They are sparsely distributed in dendrites but they are abundant in large axons, where they facilitate axonal movement and growth.

Axonal transport

Protein synthesis does not usually occur within the axon, therefore any protein requirements for the repair and upkeep of the neurone must be met by the soma. In the soma, various components (including organelles, lipids and proteins) are assembled and packaged into membranous vesicles and transported to their final cellular destination by a process known as *axonal transport* (axoplasmic transport). Axonal transport involves movement from the soma, towards the synapse, called *anterograde transport* and movement away from the axon, towards the soma, called *retrograde transport*.

Axonal transport can be further divided into fast and slow subtypes. *Fast anterograde transport* occurs at a rate of 100–400 mm/day and involves the movement of free elements including synaptic vesicles, neurotransmitters, mitochondria, and lipid and protein molecules (including receptor proteins) for insertion/repair of the plasma membrane. *Slow anterograde transport* on the other hand, occurs at a rate of 0.3–1 mm/day and involves the movement of soluble proteins (involved in neurotransmitter release at the synapse) and cytoskeletal elements (Snell, 2006). Both types of anterograde transport are mediated by a group of motor proteins called kinesins (Brown, 2001). Retrograde transport involves the movement of damaged membranes and organelles towards the soma, where they are eventually degraded by lysosomes (found only in the soma). It is mediated by a different kind of motor protein known as dynein.

The axon

The organelles and cellular components already discussed are not unique to neurones and may be found (with a few exceptions) in almost any cell in the body. However, the main feature that distinguishes neurones from other cells is the axon, the projection that emerges from the soma, and its associated elaborate process of dendrites. Under the microscope, it is hard to distinguish the axon from dendrites of some neurones, but in others it is easily identified on the basis of length. Whilst some neurones have no axons at all (e.g. the amacrine cell, found in the retina), most neurones have a single axon. The axons of some neurones branch to form axon collatcrals, along which the impulse splits and travels to signal several cells simultaneously.

Neurones can be broadly classified according to length of their axonal processes. *Golgi type I* neurones contain long-projecting axonal processes, whilst *Golgi type II* neurones have shorter axonal processes. Another way of classifying neurones is according to their location within the central nervous system, or on the basis of their morphological appearance. Examples of specific types of neurones include Basket, Betz, Medium spiny, Purkinje, Renshaw and Pyramidal cells. Neurones may also be classified according to the number of branches that originate from the soma (Figure 1.2):

- Unipolar or pseudounipolar neurones are characterised by a single neurite that emerges and branches or divides a short distance from the soma. Most sensory neurones of the peripheral nervous system are unipolar.

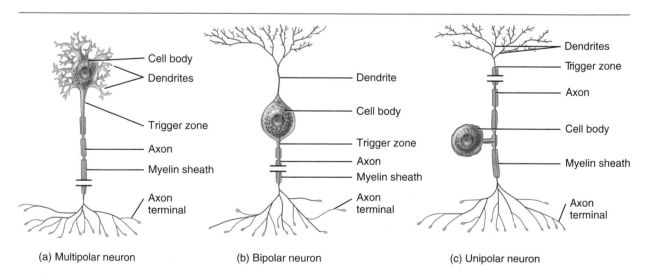

Figure 1.2 Structural classification of neurones. Breaks indicate that axons are longer than shown. (a) Multipolar neurone. (b) Bipolar neurone. (c) Unipolar neurone. Reproduced from *Principles of Anatomy and Physiology 12e* by Gerard Tortora and Bryan Derrickson. Copyright (2009, John Wiley & Sons). Reprinted with permission of John Wiley & Sons Inc.

- Bipolar neurones are characterised by a single axon and a single dendrite that emerge from opposite ends of an elongated soma. These types of neurones are found in the sensory ganglia of the cochlear and vestibular system and also in the retina.
- Multipolar neurones are characterised by a number of dendrites that arise and branch close to the soma. They make up the majority of neurones in the CNS.

The primary function of the axon is to transmit electrochemical signals to other neurones (sometimes over a considerable distance). Transmission occurs at rates that are appropriate to the type and function of the individual neurone. Because of this, the axonal length of a given neurone may vary from as little as a few micrometres, to over 1 metre in humans. For example, the sciatic nerve, which runs from the base of the spine to the foot, may extend a metre or even longer. Typical diameters can range from 0.2 to 20 μm for large myelinated axons.

The axon has four regions: the axon hillock (or trigger zone), the initial segment, the axon proper and the axon terminals. The *axon hillock* originates at the soma; adjacent to the axon hillock is the *initial segment*. The plasma membranes of these two regions contain large numbers of specialised, voltage sensitive ion channels and most action potentials originate in this area (see below: Action potentials). Beyond the initial segment, the *axon proper* maintains a relatively uniform, cylindrical shape, with little or no tapering. The consistent diameter of the axon (axon calibre) is maintained by components of the cytoskeleton and this feature also helps to maintain a uniform rate of conduction along the axon. In addition to the axon calibre, the rate of conduction along the axon is influenced by the presence of the myelin sheath, which begins near the axon hillock and ends short of the *axon terminals*.

Myelination

Myelin is a specialised protein, formed of closely apposed glial cells that wrap themselves several times around the axon (Kiernan, 2004). In the central nervous system, the glial cells making up the myelin sheath are called oligodendrocytes, whereas in the peripheral nervous system, they are known as Schwann cells (see: Neuroglia). Several axons may be surrounded simultaneously by a single glial cell.

The myelin sheath insulates the axon and prevents the passive movement of ions between the axoplasm and the extracellular compartment. Myelinated axons also contain gaps at evenly-spaced intervals along the axon, known as nodes of Ranvier (Figures 1.1 and 1.3). These nodes are

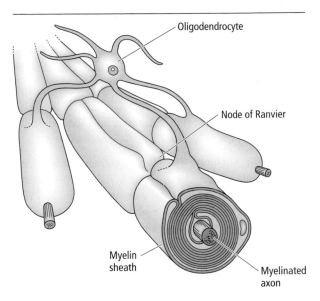

Figure 1.3 A single oligodendrocyte is capable of myelinating a single internode of numerous axons. Reproduced from Maria A Patestas and Leslie P Gartner, *A Textbook of Neuroanatomy*, Wiley-Blackwell, with permission.

the only points where the axonal membrane is in direct contact with the extracellular compartment and where ions can readily flow across the axonal membrane. Therefore, any electrical activity in the axon is confined to this part. In myelinated axons, the nodes of Ranvier contain clusters of voltage-gated sodium (Na^+) channels, whereas in unmyelinated axons, these voltage-gated Na^+ channels are distributed uniformly along the *whole* of the axon. This feature enables the axon to conduct action potentials over long distances, with high fidelity and a constant speed, and underlies the ability of the neurone to conduct impulses by a process known as saltatory conduction. Saltatory conduction (from the Latin *saltare*, to 'jump'), enables action potentials to literally jump from one node to the next, rather than travelling along the membrane (Ritchie, 1984). Saltation allows significantly faster conduction (between 10 and 100 metres per second) in myelinated axons, compared with the slower conduction rates seen in their unmyelinated counterparts.

The increased speed afforded by saltatory conduction therefore allows the organism to process information more quickly and to react faster, which confers a distinct advantage for survival. In addition to this, the high concentrations of ion channels at the nodal intervals conserve energy, as they reduce the requirements for sodium–potassium pumps throughout the axonal membrane. Multiple sclerosis (MS) is a demyelinating disease, characterised by patchy loss of myelin in the brain and spinal cord. As a result of the demyelinating process, plaques develop in the white matter, which result in a reduced concentration of sodium ion channels at the nodes of Ranvier and a slowing of action potentials (see Chapter 28).

The terminal portion of the axon is known as the axon terminal, where the axon arborises (or branches) and enlarges. This region goes by a variety of other names, including the terminal bouton, the synaptic knob or the axon foot. The axon terminal contains synaptic vesicles which contain neurotransmitters (see: Neurotransmitters).

Dendrites

Dendrites are the afferent components of neurones, i.e. they receive incoming information. The dendrites (together with the soma) provide the major site for synaptic contact made by the axon endings of other neurones. Dendrites are generally arranged around the soma of the neurone in a stellate (or star-shaped), configuration. In some neurones, dendrites arise from a single trunk, from which they branch out, giving rise to the notion of a dendritic tree (Raine, 1999). Under the microscope, it can be difficult to distinguish the terminal segments of axons from small dendrites, or small unmyelinated axons. However, unlike the diameters of axons, the main distinguishing feature of dendrites is that they taper, so that successive branches become narrower as they move further away from the soma. In addition, unlike axons, small branches of dendrites tend to lack any neurofilaments, although they may contain fragments of Nissl substance; however, large branches of dendrites proximal to the axon may contain small bundles of neurofilaments. The synaptic points of contact on dendrites occur either along the main stems or at small eminences known as dendritic spines – the axon terminals of other neurones adjoin these structures.

NEUROGLIA

Neuroglia (Figure 1.4), usually referred to simply as glia (from the Greek word meaning 'glue') or glial cells, are morphologically and functionally distinct from neurones. Neuroglia comprise almost half the total volume of the brain and spinal cord. They are smaller than neurones and more numerous – outnumbering them almost 10-fold (Snell, 2006). Although they have complex processes extending from their cell bodies, they lack any axons or dendritic processes.

Previously it was assumed that glia do not participate directly in any signalling or synaptic interactions with other neurones. However, recent studies have indicated that their supportive functions help to define synaptic contacts and that they are crucial facilitators of action potentials. Other roles attributed to neuroglia include: maintaining the ionic environment in the brain, modulating the rate of signal propagation, and having a synaptic action by controlling the uptake of neurotransmitters. They also provide a scaffold for some aspects of neural development, and play an important role in recovery from neuronal injury (or, in some instances, prevention). They also have an important nutritive role and release factors which modulate pre-synaptic function.

There are four main types of glial cells in the mature CNS: astrocytes, oligodendrocytes, microglial cells and ependymal cells – the description, location and function of these are summarised in Table 1.1.

COMMUNICATION BY NEURONES

The resting membrane potential

The neuronal membrane is about 8 nm thick and is made up of a hydrophobic lipid bi-layer, which acts as a selective barrier to the diffusion of ions between the cytoplasm (intracellular) and extracellular compartments. The unequal distribution of ions (positively or negatively charged atoms) either side of the cell membrane results in a difference of electrical charge (potential difference) between the inside and the outside of the cell membrane. The overall effect of this gives rise to the resting membrane potential. It is called the resting membrane potential because it occurs when the neurone is in an unstimulated state, i.e. not conducting an impulse. In this state, the neurone is said to be polarised, because there is a relative excess of positive electrical charge outside the cell membrane and a relative excess of negative charge inside. To maintain a steady resting membrane potential, the separation of charges across the membrane must be constant, so that any efflux of charge is balanced against any charge influx (Gilman and Winans Newman, 2003). By convention therefore, the charge outside the neuronal membrane is arbitrarily defined as zero, whilst the inside of the neurone (relative to the outside) is negatively charged ($-70\,mV$).

The extracellular fluid contains a dilute solution of sodium (Na^+) and chloride (Cl^-) ions. By contrast, the axoplasm contains high concentrations of potassium (K^+) ions and organic anions (large negatively charged organic acids, sulphates, amino acids and proteins) (Holmes, 1993). Two passive forces (diffusional and electrostatic) act simultaneously upon these ions to maintain the resting potential. Diffusional (chemical) forces drive Na^+ ions

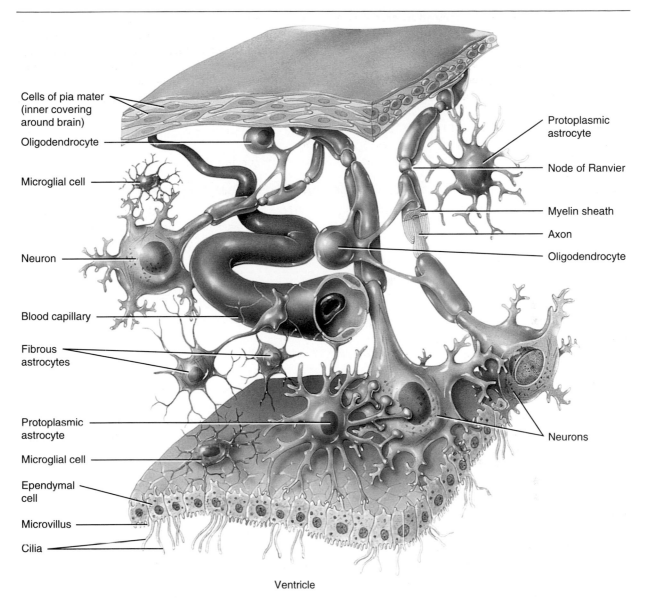

Cells of pia mater (inner covering around brain)

Oligodendrocyte

Microglial cell

Neuron

Blood capillary

Fibrous astrocytes

Protoplasmic astrocyte

Microglial cell

Ependymal cell

Microvillus

Cilia

Protoplasmic astrocyte

Node of Ranvier

Myelin sheath

Axon

Oligodendrocyte

Neurons

Ventricle

Figure 1.4 Neuroglia of the central nervous system (CNS). Reproduced from *Principles of Anatomy and Physiology 12e* by Gerard Tortora and Bryan Derrickson. Copyright (2009, John Wiley & Sons). Reprinted with permission of John Wiley & Sons Inc.

inwards and K^+ ions outwards, from areas of high concentration to areas of low concentration, i.e. down their respective chemical concentration gradients. Secondly, electrostatic forces (charge) move ions across the membrane, in a direction that depends on their electrical charge, so that the positively charged Na^+ and K^+ ions are attracted towards the negatively-charged cell interior (Waxman, 2000).

In addition to these diffusional and electrostatic forces, the resting potential is also influenced by the action of ion-specific membrane-spanning channels. These ion channels selectively allow the passage of certain ions, whilst excluding others. Two types of ion channels exist, which can be in an open or closed state: voltage gated and non-gated ion channels. Non-gated channels, which are primarily important in maintaining the resting potential are

Table 1.1 Description, location and function of specific neuroglia.

Neuroglial cell	Structural features	Location	Function
Astrocytes			
Fibrous astrocytes	Small cell bodies and long slender processes – contain cytoplasmic filaments and sparsely branched processes that extend between nerve fibres	White matter	• Maintain integrity of blood–brain barrier (BBB) • Structural support for mature neurones and migrating immature neurones during embryonic development • Cover synaptic contacts and act as insulators – preventing axon terminals from influencing neighbouring, unrelated neurones • Role in synaptic transmission – contributing to the reuptake of γ-aminobutyric acid (GABA) and glutamate from synaptic terminal & limiting influences of these neurotransmitters • Role in maintaining a favourable ionic environment (ionic homeostasis) & maintenance of K^+ ion concentration in the extracellular spaces
Protoplasmic astrocytes	Multiple, short branching processes – end as expansions on capillaries (perivascular feet)	Grey matter	• Produce substances that have a trophic influence on surrounding neurones • Nutritive role & glycogen storage in the cytoplasm • Role in phagocytosis – taking up degenerating/damaged synaptic axon terminals • Proliferate and occupy spaces previously left by disease /dead neurones – *replacement gliosis*
Oligodendrocytes	Small cell bodies with a few delicate processes. Do not contain any cytoplasmic filaments	Myelinated neurones of the CNS and PNS	• Myelination of neurones and formation of the myelin sheath in the CNS and PNS
Microglial cells	Smallest of the neuroglia, with long spiny processes – derived from haematopoietic stem cells	Found scattered throughout the CNS	• Release of growth factors during development • In collaboration with tissue macrophages, prominent role in phagocytosis and removal of cellular debris in response to normal cell turnover or brain injury

Table 1.1 *Continued*

Neuroglial cell	Structural features	Location	Function
Ependymal cells			
Ependymocytes	Cuboidal and columnar shape, with microvilli, cilia and gap junctions	Found lining the ventricles and the central canal of the spinal cord	• Cilia assist in circulation of CSF within brain cavities and central canal of the spinal cord • Role in absorption of CSF
Tanycytes	Long processes, with end feet on blood capillaries	Found lining floor of third ventricle and overlying the medial eminence of the hypothalamus	• Transport of blood-derived hormones and substances from the CSF into capillaries that supply medial eminence of the hypothalamus (hypophyseal-portal system)
Choroidal epithelial cells	Sides and bases tightly folded – held together by tight junctions to prevent leakage of CSF into underlying structures	Cover the surfaces of the choroid plexuses	• Production and secretion of CSF

CNS – central nervous system; PNS – peripheral nervous system; BBB – blood–brain barrier; CSF – cerebrospinal fluid.

always open and are not influenced significantly by extrinsic factors, these gates allow for the passive diffusion of K^+ and Na^+ ions. Gated channels, however, open and close in response to specific electrical, mechanical, or chemical signals and their conformational states (i.e. whether they are open or not) depend on the voltage across them (Longstaff, 2000). When the neurone is polarised (i.e. is at resting membrane potential) these gates are closed.

At resting membrane potential, the neuronal membrane is relatively permeable to K^+ ions, which passively diffuse out of the cell, through non-gated potassium channels. This causes a net increase in the negative charge on the inside of the cell membrane. In addition to the outward leakage of potassium, negatively charged anions (which cannot diffuse across the membrane because of their large size) add further to the overall negative intracellular charge. The majority of sodium channels are closed at resting membrane potential, so diffusion of Na^+ along its own ionic gradient is prevented. In addition, the *sodium–potassium pump* actively transports Na^+ ions out of the cell, while taking in K^+. The pump moves three sodium ions out of the cell for every two potassium ions that it

brings in. The sodium–potassium pump therefore moves Na^+ and K^+ *against* their net electrochemical gradients, which requires the use of energy (from the hydrolysis of ATP).

As long as the force of the K^+ ions diffusing outwards exceeds the oppositely oriented electrical charge, a net efflux of K^+ continues from inside the cell. But as more K^+ ions travel out (along the K^+ concentration gradient), the electrical force (negative charge) attracting K^+ ions into the cell, gradually increases (Wright, 2004; Barnett and Larkman, 2007). If a state was reached whereby the chemical and electrical forces balanced, (equilibrium potential of potassium) there would be no K^+ ion movement. This equilibrium potential for potassium occurs at $-90\,mV$. However an equilibrium potential for potassium is never quite reached due to the small continual leakage of sodium from the cell.

Changes in the resting membrane potential

Changes in the resting membrane potential will occur when a stimulus causes gated ion channels to open thereby changing the membrane's permeability to an ion. Depending on the type and strength of the stimulus, the change in the resting membrane potential will produce either a graded potential or an action potential. If the stimulus alters a local area of the membrane only and does not conduct far beyond the point of stimulation it is referred to as a graded potential (see below: Neurotransmitters). If the stimulus is of sufficient strength to cause a change in the entire membrane potential the response is referred to as an action potential.

An increase in the negativity of the resting membrane potential, e.g. −70 mV to −80 mV is referred to as hyperpolarisation. Conversely, any reduction in the negativity of the membrane potential, e.g. −70 mV to −65 mV, is referred to as depolarisation.

The action potential

An action potential (Figure 1.5) is initiated when a stimulus causes the voltage gated sodium channels to open. Sodium ions rapidly diffuse through the neuronal membrane down their electrochemical gradient attracted by the negative charge inside the neurone. The most common site of initiation of the action potential is the axon hillock (also called the trigger zone), where the highest concentration of voltage-gated ion channels is found (previously described).

The rush of Na^+ into the neurone briefly reverses the polarity of the membrane from a negative charge of −70 mV (resting membrane potential) typically to a positive charge of +30 mV (depolarisation). The influx of Na^+ and subsequent depolarisation of one section of the axonal membrane, i.e. the trigger zone, is the stimulus to open additional voltage gated sodium channels in the adjacent membrane, thus the depolarisation spreads forward along the axonal membrane. The voltage gated sodium channels are open only briefly, they become inactivated when the charge reaches +30 mV, stopping any further influx of Na^+ into the neurone. This brief alteration in charge lasts approximately 5 milliseconds.

Whilst the voltage gated sodium channels are closing, voltage-gated potassium channels open resulting in a huge efflux of K^+ ions (downward stroke) which continues until the cell has repolarised to its resting potential (from +30 mV to −70 mV). During repolarisation the voltage gated sodium channels remain inactivated.

Following repolarisation, the neurone is briefly unyielding to any further action potentials, a phase known as the recovery/relative refractory period. The absolute refractory period is the time during which a second action potential absolutely cannot be initiated (see Figure 1.5). The sodium–

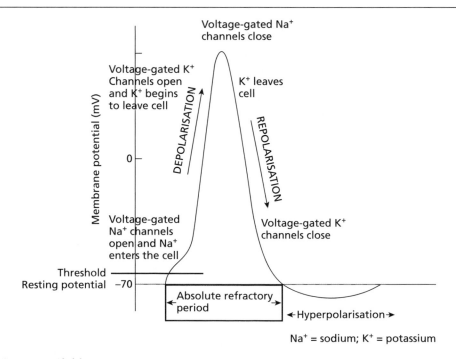

Figure 1.5 Action potential in a neurone.

potassium pump actively transports K$^+$ and Na$^+$ ions across the membrane, (against their respective chemical concentration gradients), to re-establish the resting potential.

Threshold stimulus and the all-or-none phenomenon

The stimulus must depolarise the membrane potential to a threshold value, which is typically to −55 mV for an action potential to occur. If the membrane does not reach the threshold value an action potential will not occur. If the threshold is reached the action potential will propagate forward at maximal strength regardless of the strength of the initial stimulus. Therefore the action potential will occur maximally or not at all. This is the 'all-or-none phenomenon'.

NEUROTRANSMISSION

Synapses

Once the action potential reaches the axon terminal it needs to transfer to another cell. The *synapse* (Figure 1.6)

is the location of signal transmission from one neurone to another or, in most cases, many other neurones. The synapse is typically between the axon terminal of a neurone (pre-synaptic) and the surface of a dendrite or cell body of another neurone (post-synaptic). The number of synaptic inputs to a typical neurone in the human nervous system ranges from 1 to about 100,000, with an average in the thousands.

Two types of synapse exist: electrical and chemical. In *electrical synapses*, ion channels (connections) arrange themselves around a central hollow core to form gap junctions. These gap junctions allow electrical coupling and the passage of water, small molecules (<1.2 nm diameter) and various ions between adjacent cells. Electrical synapses are predominantly associated with electrical activity in cardiac and smooth muscle. They are also found between astrocytes and are crucially involved in the coupling of horizontal cells found in the retina. Electrical signalling is bi-directional in electrical synapses.

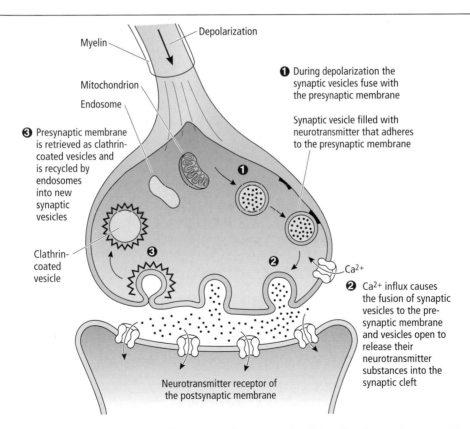

Figure 1.6 An example of an ionotropic effect occurring at a synapse indicating the events that occur before, during, and after the release of neurotransmitter substances. Reproduced from Maria A Patestas and Leslie P Gartner, *A Textbook of Neuroanatomy*, Wiley-Blackwell, with permission.

In humans, the majority of synapses are *chemical synapses* and therefore rely on the release of neurotransmitters and their binding with receptor proteins on the post-synaptic membrane of the target neurone. Typically, the pre-synaptic terminal is immediately adjacent to a post-synaptic region but there is no physical continuity between these regions. Instead, the components communicate by chemical neurotransmitters that cross the extracellular space known as the *synaptic cleft* to bind to receptors in the post-synaptic region.

Neurotransmitters

Neurotransmitters are the molecules responsible for chemical signalling in the nervous system. Neurotransmitters are synthesised in the soma and are transported to the terminal parts of the axon (near the synaptic region), where they are packaged into vesicles and stored in areas known as active zones, ready for release at the synapse. When an action potential reaches the axon terminal voltage gated calcium channels open, the influx of calcium ions cause the vesicles to fuse with the pre-synaptic membrane and vesicular contents are released in discreet packets or quanta, into the synaptic cleft, by a process of *exocytosis*. Each quantum represents the release of the contents of a single vesicle (around 4000 molecules of neurotransmitter) (Longstaff, 2000). Following exocytosis, the vesicular membrane proteins are recycled by a process known as *endocytosis* .

The first neurotransmitter to be described was *acetylcholine (ACh)*, by Loewi in 1926, following his extensive work on frog cardiac muscle. Subsequently, a wide range of other neurotransmitters have been described, each of which may be chemically differentiated on the basis their molecular structure, patterns of distribution, localisation to specific brain areas and their association with specific functions (Michael-Titus *et al.*, 2007).

The effects of the main neurotransmitters and their mode of action are summarised in Table 1.2.

In addition to the principal neurotransmitters, other chemicals can also *modulate* the impact of neurotransmitter on the post-synaptic neurone. They do this by enhancing, prolonging, inhibiting or limiting the effect of a particular neurotransmitter on the post-synaptic neurone, so that the response of metabotropic receptors (see below) may last several minutes or longer. These substances are called *neuromodulators*, because they modulate the response of the neurone to other inputs. It is widely accepted that some molecules can act simultaneously as a neurotransmitter or a neuromodulator (termed *co-transmission*) and classification largely depends on

whether its action occurs over a long range or is localised to the synapse.

Neurotransmitters exert their effects on post-synaptic receptors of target neurones. The action of a given neurotransmitter on a target neurone or indeed peripherally on a particular effector organ (see Chapter 5) largely depends on the types of receptors present on that target. Most types of neurotransmitters have a number of specific receptor subtypes that they can activate. These receptors can be classified according to their overall structure and function. The effects of neurotransmitters depend on the summation of responses at the post-synaptic membrane.

Two broad superfamilies of receptor have been described, which include ionotropic and metabotropic receptors. The *ionotropic*, or *ligand-gated ion channel* receptors, are made up of ion-selective channels that are integral to the receptor. Binding of neurotransmitter directly results in the selective opening or closure of the channel and directly increasing or decreasing its permeability to particular ions, as described above.

Ionotropic or ligand-gated ion channel receptors

The binding of a neurotransmitter to an ionotropic receptor will cause a change in the post-synaptic membrane potential by either bringing about the opening or closing of ion channels. When the neurotransmitter causes the opening of positive ion channels (e.g. Na^+ channels) in the post-synaptic membrane the net effect is to reduce the negativity of the membrane potential (e.g. from $-70\,mV$ to $-68\,mV$). This is known as an *excitatory post-synaptic potential* (EPSP). This is below the level required to lift the potential to threshold level for an action potential to occur. When the neurotransmitter causes the opening of potassium channels, thereby allowing positive ions to leave the neurone, or opens chloride (Cl^-) channels the effect is to reduce the resting potential i.e. make it more negative this is known as *inhibitory post-synaptic potential* (IPSP). The IPSP reduces the post-synaptic neurone's ability to generate an action potential. These small shifts are called graded potentials. Whether an action potential is generated or not depends on the summation of the graded potentials. Several EPSPs are needed to convert resting potential to an action potential. Summation may be temporal (the cumulative effect of repeated impulses from a single synapse) or spatial (the net effect of simultaneous impulses from different synapses along the membrane).

The second superfamily of receptors are known as the *metabotropic receptors*. Binding of neurotransmitters to these receptors has longer lasting effects on the post-synaptic cell. When a neurotransmitter binds to these

Table 1.2 Key central nervous system neurotransmitters.

Group	Neurotransmitter	Source	Action
Biogenic amines (classical)			
	Acetylcholine	• Found in many brain areas and large pyramidal cells • Some cells of basal ganglia • Motor neurones that innervate skeletal muscle • Pre-ganglionic neurones – autonomic nervous system • Postganglionic neurones of sympathetic and parasympathetic nervous system	• Usually excitatory • Inhibitory effect on parasympathetic organs (e.g. reduced heart rate, as a result of vagus nerve stimulation)
Catecholamines	**Dopamine**	• Neurones in substantia nigra and projections to basal ganglia that are involved in coordinated skeletal muscle activity	• Usually inhibitory
	Noradrenaline	• Neurones with cell bodies in brain stem and hypothalamus and postganglionic neurones of sympathetic nervous system	• Usually excitatory, occasionally inhibitory
	Adrenaline	• Synthesised and stored in chromaffin tissue in adrenal medulla	• Excitatory
	Serotonin (5-hydroxytryptamine; 5-HT)	• Median raphe nuclei of brain stem and projections to other areas, including hypothalamus and dorsal horns of spinal cord	• Inhibitory – modulates neurone voltage potentials to inhibit glutamate activity and neurotransmitter firing. Key role in control of mood and sleep
Amino acids (classical)	**Glutamate**	• Presynaptic terminals of sensory nerves and some cortical areas	• Excitatory – acts on ionotropic (kainite, AMPA and NMDA) receptors and metabotropic receptors
	Aspartate γ-aminobutyric acid (GABA)	• Brain stem and spinal cord • Nerve terminals of the spinal cord, cerebellum, basal ganglia and some cortical regions. Found in 30–40% of all synapses	• Excitatory • Inhibitory – the main inhibitory NT in the mammalian CNS. Regulates activity of glutamate and prevents overstimulation

Continued

Table 1.2 *Continued*

Group	Neurotransmitter	Source	Action
	Glycine	• Brain stem and spinal cord	• Inhibitory neuromodulator – regulates excitatory neurotransmission in much the same way as GABA
Opioids (peptides)	**Endorphins**	• Pituitary gland and other brain areas	• Excitatory to systems that inhibit pain and binds to opiate receptors in the brain and pituitary gland
	Encephalins	• Nerve terminals in the spinal cord, brain stem, thalamus and hypothalamus	• Excitatory to systems that inhibit pain and binds to opiate receptors
	Dynorphins	• Hypothalamus, hippocampus and spinal cord	• Inhibitory – opiate-like activity. Role in oxytocin secretion and control of appetite
Tachykinins (peptides)	**Substance P**	• Basal ganglia, hypothalamus and pain fibre terminals in dorsal horn of spinal cord	• Excitatory

receptors, small intracellular proteins called *G-proteins* are activated. G-proteins exert their effects on the post-synaptic membrane by binding ion channels directly, or by indirectly activating *second messengers*. Second messengers are molecules that are produced or released inside the cell; the most common being cyclic-adenosine monophosphate (cAMP). Second messengers can activate other enzymes in the cytosol that can regulate ion-channel function or alter the metabolic activities of the cell, hence the name metabotropic.

Inactivation and removal of neurotransmitters

Typically, neurotransmitter binding takes less than 5 μs, but not all neurotransmitter that has been released binds to the post-synaptic membrane of the target neurone. The distance between the pre- and post-synaptic membrane is as little as 12 nm across, but due to reuptake of neurotransmitter, passive diffusion away from the synaptic cleft and inactivation by various enzymes, the amount of transmitter available for binding is reduced. For example, enzymatic degradation of ACh (by *acetylcholinesterases*) takes place in the synaptic cleft at the neuromuscular junction or other cholinergic synapses. These enzymes cleave ACh into its inactive components, acetate and choline, which are recy-

cled and used to synthesise further ACh by combination with acetyl-coenzyme-A.

Other neurotransmitters are inactivated in a similar way, or they may be inactivated by direct removal from the synaptic cleft. Direct removal from the synaptic cleft is carried out by reuptake transporters, which actively transport unused neurotransmitter to surrounding neurones or glia. The importance of the mechanisms of reuptake is highlighted by the impact of certain drugs on brain function. Illicit drugs, such as ecstasy (3, 4-methylenedioxy-N-methamphetamine; MDMA), for example, block the reuptake of serotonin (5-hydroxytryptamine; 5HT). This results in an excess of serotonin in the synaptic cleft, which contributes to its euphoric effects (McCann *et al.*, 2005). Similarly, other illicit drugs such as cocaine inhibit the reuptake of dopamine, which is responsible for its euphoric and addictive effects (Mash *et al.*, 2002). Of course, neurotransmitter reuptake blockade can also have more useful, therapeutic applications, for example in the treatment of depression with selective serotonin reuptake inhibitors (SSRIs), which block the reuptake of serotonin. The therapeutic use of drugs that inhibit reuptake of neurotransmitters will be discussed in the relevant chapters on specific diseases.

SUMMARY

The nervous system is vital for maintaining the homeostasis of the body. It continuously receives information which it must process and rapidly respond to. These vital functions are made possible by the generation of action potentials and chemical synapses. Neurotransmitters released at a synapse can have either excitatory or inhibitory effects whereas neuromodulators prolong, inhibit, or limit the effect of a particular neurotransmitter on the post-synaptic neurone.

REFERENCES

Barnett MW, Larkman PM (2007) The action potential. *Practical Neurology* 7(3): 192–197.

Brown AG (2001) Introduction to nerve cells and nervous systems. In: *Nerve Cells and Nervous Systems: an introduction to neuroscience.* (2nd edition). London and New York: Springer.

Dent EW, Tang F, Kalil K (2003) Axon guidance by growth cones and branches: common cytoskeletal and signaling mechanisms. *Neuroscientist* 9(5):343–353.

Gilman S, Winans Newman S (2003) Physiology of nerve cells. In *Manter and Gatz's Essentials of Clinical Neuroanatomy and Neurophysiology.* (10th edition). John Tinkham Manter, Arthur John Gatz, Sarah Winans Newman eds. Philadelphia: FA Davis.

Gulbins E, Dreschers S, Bock J (2003) Role of mitochondria in apoptosis. *Experimental Physiology* 88(1):85–90.

Gunter TE, Yule D I, Gunter KK *et al.* (2004) Calcium and mitochondria. *FEBS Letters* 567(1):96–102.

Hollenbeck PJ, Saxton WM (2005) The axonal transport of mitochondria. *Journal of Cell Science* 118(23): 5411–5419.

Holmes O (1993) *Nerve.* (2nd edition). London, Chapman and Hall.

Kiernan JA (2004) *Barr's The Human Nervous System: an anatomical viewpoint.* Baltimore: Lippincott Williams and Wilkins.

Longstaff A (2000) *Neuroscience.* Oxford, BIOS Scientific Publishers Limited.

Mash DC, Pablo J, Ouyang Q (2002) Dopamine transport function is elevated in cocaine users. *Journal of Neurochemistry* 81(2):292–300

McCann UD, Szabo Z, Seckin E *et al.* (2005) Quantitative PET studies of the serotonin transporter in MDMA users and controls using [11C]McN5652 and [11C]DASB. *Neuropsychopharmacology* 30(9):1741–1750.

Michael-Titus A, Revest P, Shortland P (2007) Elements of cellular and molecular neuroscience. In: Michael-Titus A, Revest P, Shortland P (eds). *Nervous System.* Edinburgh: hurchill Livingstone.

Raine CS (1999) Neurocellular anatomy. In *Basic Neurochemistry: Molecular, cellular and medical aspects.* (6th edition). George J. Siegel *et al.* eds. Philadelphia: Lippincott-Raven Publishers.

Ritchie JM (1984) Physiological basis of conduction in myelinated nerve fibres. In: *Myelin.* Pierre Morell ed. New York: Plenum Press pp 117–146.

Snell R (2006) The neurobiology of the neuron and the neuroglia. In: *Clinical Neuroanatomy.* (6th edition). Baltimore: Lippincott, Williams and Wilkins pp 31–67.

Waxman SG (2000) Signaling in the nervous system In: *Correlative Neuroanatomy.* (24th edition). John Butler and Harriet Lebowitz eds. New York: McGraw-Hill pp 20–34.

Wright SH (2004) Generation of resting membrane potential. *Advances in Physiology Education* 28(1–4):139–142.

2

The Structural and Biochemical Defences of the CNS

Ehsan Khan

INTRODUCTION

The central nervous system (CNS) is one of the most delicate structures within the body. It is a vital part of the body that needs to function continuously to maintain life. The tissue that comprises the CNS is extremely delicate, and the CNS is consequently extremely susceptible to both mechanical and chemical insult. To reduce the risk of mechano-chemical injury, protection of this delicate system comprises structural as well as biochemical defences. This chapter will describe the defensive features of the CNS, providing the reader with a conceptual and functional understanding of these structures and processes. This information will help the reader to understand the clinical consequences of failure of these structures and processes.

The defences of the central nervous system include the following.

Structural defences:

* Bony encasement
* Membranes – meninges and the blood–brain barrier (BBB)
* Cerebrospinal fluid (CSF)

Biochemical defences:

* Enzymes
* Efflux proteins
* Metabolic enzymes

Neuroscience Nursing: Evidence-Based Practice, 1st Edition.
Edited by Sue Woodward and Ann-Marie Mestecky
© 2011 Blackwell Publishing Ltd

BONY ENCASEMENT

The skull

The skull is made up of a number of flat bones that are joined together by serrated junctions known as sutures (Figure 2.1). The skull comprises the cranial and facial bones. The cranial bones include the brain casing or the skull cap (the calvaria) and the bones of the cranial cavity floor. The sinusoidal flat bones of the skull have a spongy diploe centre that is sandwiched between the hard external and internal compact layers of the skull bone. This arrangement affords the skull considerable strength and resistance to trauma while maintaining a low weight. It provides protection together with support and ease of movement of the head.

The calvaria

The skull cap or calvaria is formed by the frontal bone, two parietal bones and the occipital bone.

The fontal bone

The frontal bone is the anterior segment of the calvaria which joins with the anterior two halves of the parietal bones by the coronal suture. The frontal bone can be divided into the flat anterior section the squamous frontalis (forehead) and the horizontal inferior portion (pars orbitalis) that forms the superior borders of the orbits and nasal cavity.

Internally the frontal bone has a longitudinal protuberance that runs anterior–posteriorly. The initial portion of this protuberance is known as the frontal crest and gives rise to a swollen rough surface (the crista galli) which serves as a point of attachment for the falx cerebri, the fold of dura matter that sagittally divides the two cerebral hemispheres. The frontal crest travels posteriorly forming

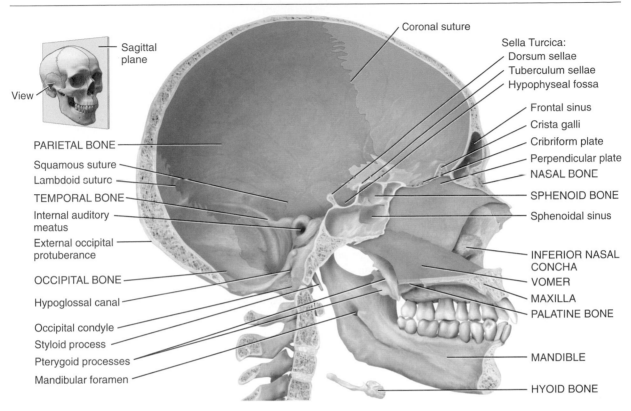

Figure 2.1 Medial view of sagittal section of skull. Although the hyoid bone is not part of the skull, it is included in the illustration for reference. Reproduced from *Principles of Anatomy and Physiology 12e* by Gerard Tortora and Bryan Derrickson. Copyright (2009, John Wiley & Sons). Reprinted with permission of John Wiley & Sons Inc.

a shallow groove the sagittal sulcus which houses the superior sagittal sinus.

The parietal bones

The parietal bones make up the lateral surfaces and superior surface of the calvaria and are joined by the sagittal suture. The parietal bones join inferiorly with the temporal bone by the squamous suture and posteriorly to the occipital bone by the lambdoid suture. Internally there are bilateral grooves for the middle meningeal arteries and a larger groove, the sagittal sulcus that extends from the frontal bone and houses the superior sagittal sinus.

The occipital bone

The occipital bones form the posterior surface of the calvaria covering the occipital lobes of the brain. The occipital bone is trapezoid in shape and curved to form the posterior and posterior-inferior wall (squamous occipita-

lis) of the cranial cavity floor. It joins the two temporal bones by the occipito-mastoid sutures. There is a large opening in the inferior part of the bone called the foramen magnum, which provides a passage for the spinal cord from the cranium into the vertebral column.

Internally the occipital crest provides posterior attachment for the falx cerebri. There is a bilateral groove for the posterior meningeal arteries. There is a sloping depression above the anterior margin of the foramen magnum known as the clivus which provides space for the pons. Towards the anterior portion of the foramen magnum is a small opening, the hypoglossal canal, which as its names suggests provides passage for the XII cranial nerve (hypoglossal) to the tongue.

Floor of the cranial cavity

The floor of the cranial cavity is formed by the temporal, sphenoid and ethmoid bones.

Temporal bones

Below the parietal bone is the temporal bone. Due to its association with many other structures, i.e. the ears, pharynx and cranial nerves, it has a complex structure and comprises five parts:

• Squamous
• Mastoid
• Petrous
• Tympanic
• Styloid process

The squamous part of the temporal bone

This bone forms a border superiorly with the parietal bone via the squamousal suture. Externally the squamous bone provides attachment for the temporal muscle and fascia via a marked line, the temporal line. Continuing from this line is a thick process that projects from the inferior part of the temporal bone called the zygomatic process which forms the beginnings of the cheek bone. Internally there is a groove for the middle meningeal arteries.

The mastoid portion of the temporal bone

This bone has a number of borders. Posteriorly it joins with the occipital bone via the occipitomastoid suture and the parietal bone via the parietomastoid suture. Superiorly it is continuous with the squamous part of the temporal bones. Anteriorly the mastoid contributes to the formation of the external auditory meatus and the auditory cavity. The mastoid process provides attachment to the large sternocliedomastoid muscle. Internally the mastoid presents a deep groove, the sigmoid sulcus that supports the transverse sinus. The sigmoid sulcus has an opening, the mastoid foramen, that provides passage for blood vessels to the transverse sinus and occipital dura mater.

The petrous part of the temporal bone

This bone is located anterior to the mastoid process, and inferior and medial to the temporal line, which it joins via the petrosquamous suture, forming and housing structures essential for hearing. It is an extremely dense and hard bone.

The tympanic part of the temporal bone

This bone is found lateral to the petrous part, inferio-posterior to the squamous part and anterior to the mastoid part of the temporal bone. This part of the temporal bone surrounds the external auditory meatus (external ear canal).

The styloid process of the temporal bone

The styloid process serves as attachment for several tongue and neck muscles.

Sphenoid bone

The sphenoid bone is located in the middle of the base of the skull (Figure 2.2). The sphenoid bone is made up of a cuboidal central portion from which two bony plates radiate on each side. Together these structures provide surfaces for particular brain structures and openings for a number of cranial nerves and blood vessels.

The superior surface of the main body of the sphenoid bone is divided sagittally by the ethmoid spine that articulates with the cribriform plate of the ethmoid bone, behind which on either side is an area for the olfactory bulbs. Posterior to this is a groove, the pre-chiasmatic groove, which terminates bilaterally with the optic foramen that allows the optic nerve and ophthalmic artery to enter the orbital cavity. The pre-chiasmatic groove is bordered posteriorly by a ridge, the tuberculum sellae, which continues into a deep depression, the sella turcica. The deepest part of this, the hypophyseal fossa, provides space for the pituitary gland.

Posterior to the hypophyseal fossa is a bony plate known as the dorsum sallae, which has small processes on either side to attach the tentorium cerebri, a sheet of dura mater that separates the cerebellum from the occipital lobes.

Running laterally either side the body of the sphenoid bone is a series of openings. On the level of the hypophyseal fossa is a bilateral fissure, the superior orbital fissure, that divides the two radiating plates of the sphenoid bone into the anterior lesser wings and posterior greater wings. This fissure is of great importance as it acts as a passage for a number of structures including the oculomotor [III], trochlear [IV], ophthalmic branch of the trigeminal nerve [V], and abducen [VI] nerves, and the ophthalamic veins.

Posteriorly and towards the medial aspect of the superior orbital fissure is a large opening, the foramen rotundum, that provides passage for the maxilliary nerve. Posterior-lateral to the foramen rotundum is the foramen ovale. The mandibular nerve, accessory meningeal artery, the lesser superficial petrosal artery and the emissary veins pass through this large opening.

Finally, on the border of the spheno-occipital junction, posterior-lateral to the foramen ovale is a smaller opening, the foramen spinosum. This opening may be absent or combined with the foramen ovale. It normally allows passage of the middle meningeal artery and a branch of the mandibular nerve, the spinous nerve, which divides into an anterior and posterior branch to innervate the dura mater.

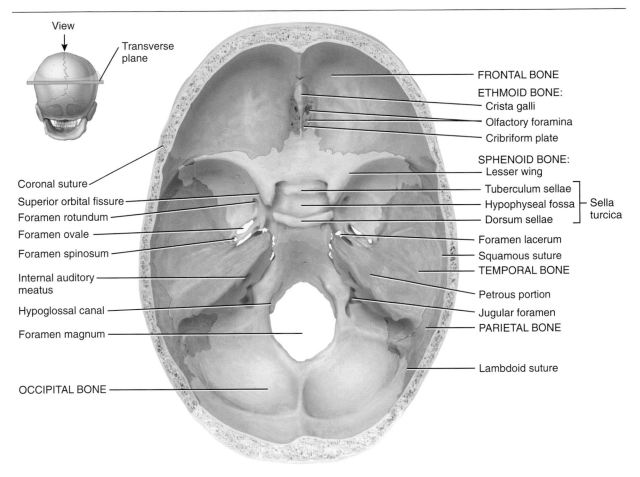

(a) Superior view of sphenoid bone in floor of cranium

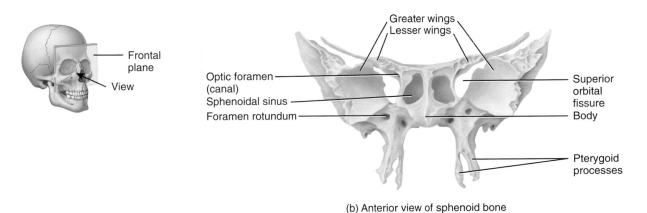

(b) Anterior view of sphenoid bone

Figure 2.2 Sphenoid bone. (a) Superior view of the sphenoid bone in floor of cranium. (b) Anterior view of sphenoid bone. Reproduced from *Principles of Anatomy and Physiology 12e* by Gerard Tortora and Bryan Derrickson. Copyright (2009, John Wiley & Sons). Reprinted with permission of John Wiley & Sons Inc.

The ethmoid bone

The ethmoid bone separates the nasal cavity from the cranial cavity. It has a complex shape. It forms most of the bony area between the nasal cavity and the orbits. It consists of the cribriform plate, that forms part of the anterior-basal floor of the cranial cavity. The perpendicular plate, which forms the bony part of the nasal septum and two lateral masses of bone the ethmoidal labyrinths.

The cranial cavity

In clinical practice reference is often made to the three cranial fossae that make up the cranial cavity. These are the:

- Anterior cranial fossa which accommodates the frontal lobes of the brain
- Middle cranial fossa which accommodates the two temporal lobes
- Posterior cranial fossa which houses the cerebellum and the brain stem

The vertebral column

The vertebral column (Figure 2.3) encompasses and protects the spinal cord. It also supports a number of muscles and provides fixation for ligaments as well as articular surfaces for bones of the lower limbs. Owing to this varied function the bones of the vertebral column, although similar in structure, vary in terms of projections and attachment surfaces.

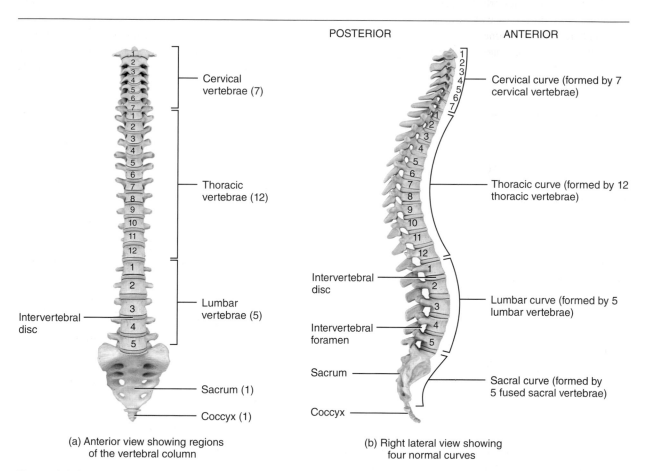

Figure 2.3 Vertebral column. The numbers in parentheses in (a) indicate the number of vertebrae in each region. (a) Anterior view showing regions of the vertebral column. (b) Right lateral view showing four normal curves. Reproduced from *Principles of Anatomy and Physiology 12e* by Gerard Tortora and Bryan Derrickson. Copyright (2009, John Wiley & Sons). Reprinted with permission of John Wiley & Sons Inc.

The vertebral column consists of 26 segments or vertebrae divided into five different regions:

- Cervical (C1–C7)
- Thoracic (T1–T12)
- Lumbar (L1– L5)
- Sacral (S1–S5, fused)
- Coccygeal (Co1–Co4, fused)

A vertebra

A typical vertebra (Figure 2.4) has two main parts. The anterior portion is centrally formed from spongy cancellous bone and surrounded by a hard external shell, the cortical rim. This part of the vertebra is known as the body or centrum and is the weight bearing region. This bone formation is clearly defined in all but the first two cervical vertebrae. Arising posteriorly from either side of the body are short bony processes called the pedicles which join with flattened plates of bone called the laminae.

Together these four bones form the vertebral (neural) arch, which provides space for the spinal cord and is known as the vertebral canal (foramen). This is the second feature shared by most vertebrae. Dorsal to the neural arch a hard spine of bone, the spinous process, is found. This structure provides attachment to different muscles and ligaments. It is poorly defined in the first cervical vertebra. Laterally on either side of the vertebra arising from the border of the body and neural arch is a further bony process known as the transverse process. These processes, like the spinous process, attach different muscles and ligaments. In addition each vertebra has 4 smaller articular processes, two superior and two inferior. These processes correspond with articular surfaces on opposing vertebrae to provide torsional strength and a degree of flexibility to the vertebral column.

Cervical vertebrae

The first cervical vertebra is known as the atlas and joins the vertebral column to the skull together with the second cervical vertebra, the axis. The atlas is devoid of a body and spinous process but has short and strong transverse processes that contain an opening, the transverse foramen,

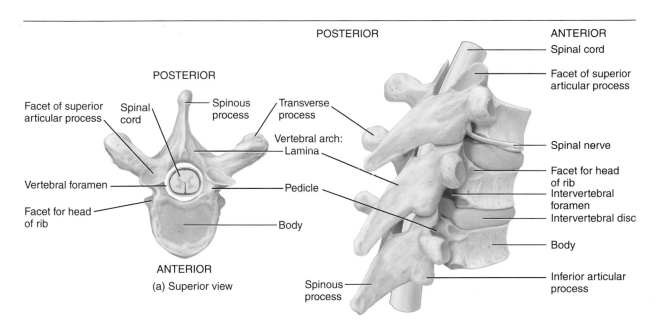

(a) Superior view

(b) Right posterolateral view of articulated vertebrae

Figure 2.4 Structure of a typical vertebra, as illustrated by a thoracic vertebra. In (b) only one spinal nerve has been included, and it has been extended beyond the intervertebral foramen for clarity. The sympathetic chain is part of the autonomic nervous system. (a) Superior view. (b) Right posterolateral view of articulated vertebrae. Reproduced from *Principles of Anatomy and Physiology 12e* by Gerard Tortora and Bryan Derrickson. Copyright (2009, John Wiley & Sons). Reprinted with permission of John Wiley & Sons Inc.

which provides passage for the vertebral artery and vein and the nerves of the sympathetic nervous system (Figure 2.5a). The second cervical vertebra, the axis, differs from the atlas in that it has a clearly defined and prominent body that projects upwards called the odontoid peg (Figure 2.5b). Together the atlas and axis allow pivotal motion of the skull. The remainder of the cervical vertebrae have a clearly defined body and spinous process with short transverse processes.

Thoracic vertebrae

The 12 thoracic vertebrae have a 'typical' vertebral shape with a well developed body, spinous and transverse processes. The thoracic vertebrae, except for the 11th and 12th, have two additional articular surfaces for each rib.

Lumbar vertebrae

The lumbar vertebrae have a well developed body with short spinous and transverse processes. The lumbar verte-

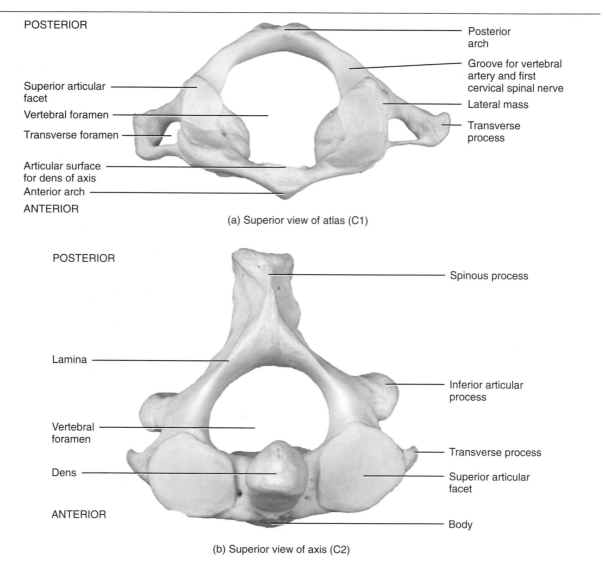

(a) Superior view of atlas (C1)

(b) Superior view of axis (C2)

Figure 2.5 Cervical vertebrae. (a) Superior view of atlas (C1). (b) Superior view of axis (C2). Reproduced from *Principles of Anatomy and Physiology 12e* by Gerard Tortora and Bryan Derrickson. Copyright (2009, John Wiley & Sons). Reprinted with permission of John Wiley & Sons Inc.

brae possess the most well developed bodies of all the vertebrae as they are the main weight bearing vertebrae. Despite this robust structure they are the vertebrae that are most commonly associated with lower back pain.

The sacrum

The sacrum is made up of five fused bones, which have strong and broad lateral processes. The bodies of the vertebrae become progressively compressed dorso-ventrally to give rise to a broad flat structure that is curved ventrally. The sacrum joins with the lumbar vertebrae superiorly, the coccyx inferiorly and to the ilium of the pelvic girdle via an articular surface and strong posterior sacroiliac ligaments. The structure of the sacrum differs between male and female. The female sacrum is broader and shorter with a more acute curvature beginning half way down the structure, whereas the male sacrum has a more evenly distributed curvature.

The coccyx

The coccyx consists of four vertebrae. Although fused, these bones show a degree of movement.

THE MENINGES AND CEREBROSPINAL FLUID (CSF)

The meninges are made up of three layers of connective tissue. From the skull inwards, they are dura mater, arachnoid mater and pia mater (Figure 2.6). The protective arrangement of these membranes is akin to the protection provided by other fibrous encasements in the body like the lung pleura and foetal amniotic sac. The inner and outer membranes (dura and pia mater) impart structural support and provide a role in reducing friction between the delicate brain tissue and the internal surface of the cranium. The arachnoid mater is bathed in cerebrospinal fluid (CSF). In addition to reducing friction, the CSF provides a buoyancy to the CNS tissue, akin to amniotic fluid providing buoy-

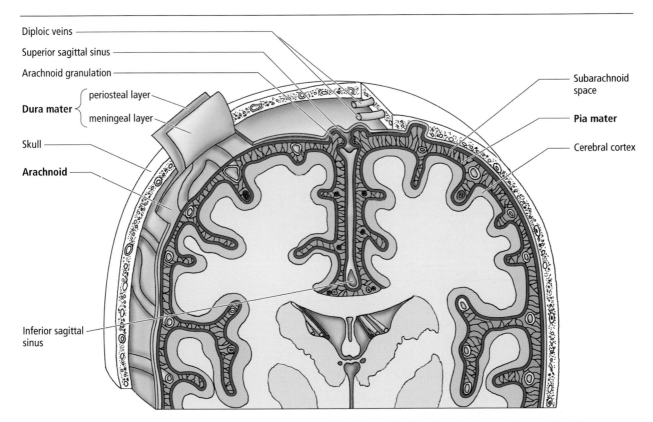

Figure 2.6 Diagram of a frontal section of the skull and brain to display the three meninges: the dura mater, arachnoid, and pia mater. Reproduced from Maria A Patestas and Leslie P Gartner, *A Textbook of Neuroanatomy*, Wiley-Blackwell, with permission.

ancy to a foetus in the womb (Kothari and Goel, 2006). Thus together the meninges provide structural support and buoyancy to the CNS protecting it from the continuous knocks and bumps it would otherwise experience in everyday life.

The choroid plexus

Cerebrospinal fluid is produced in the brain by modified ependymal cells in the choroid plexus. The choroid plexus (CP) constitutes a number of thin leafy structures found floating within but attached to some surfaces of the brain ventricles (Redzic and Segal, 2004). These surfaces include the floor and lateral aspects of the lateral ventricle and the roof of the third ventricle and fourth ventricles.

Production of CSF

The choroid plexus produces between 400 and 500 ml of CSF a day, however the distribution volume for CSF is only 150–175 ml. This leads to a pressure build-up that exceeds venous pressure in the brain and allows CSF

to be absorbed in the arachnoid villi (see Chapter 6 for further detail). CSF is a clear and odourless, normally sterile fluid. Its main constituents and characteristics are listed below:

- Specific gravity: 1.006–1.009
- Glucose: 40–80 mg/dl
- Total protein: 15–45 mg/dl
- Lactate: less than 35 mg/dl
- Leukocytes (white blood cells): 0–5/µl (adults and children); up to 30/µl (newborns)
- Differential: 60–80% lymphocytes; up to 30% monocytes and macrophages; other cells 2% or less. Monocytes and macrophages are somewhat higher in neonates
- Red blood cell count: Nil

CSF circulation

The CSF circulates from the lateral ventricles through the foramen of Monro into the third ventricle, and then through the cerebral aqueduct into the fourth ventricle (Figures 2.7, 2.8), where it exits through two lateral apertures (foramina

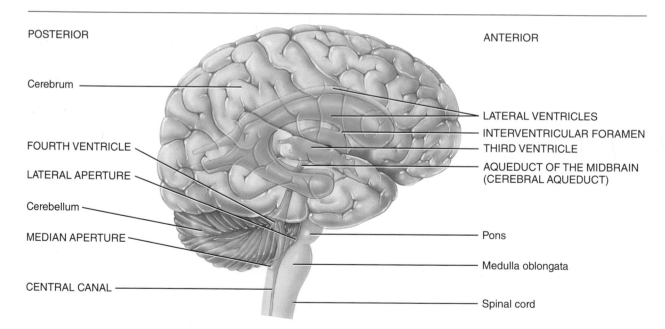

Right lateral view of brain

Figure 2.7 Locations of ventricles within a 'transparent' brain. One interventricular foramen on each side connects a lateral ventricle to the third ventricle, and the aqueduct of the midbrain connects the third ventricle to the fourth ventricle. Right lateral view of brain. Reproduced from *Principles of Anatomy and Physiology 12e* by Gerard Tortora and Bryan Derrickson. Copyright (2009, John Wiley & Sons). Reprinted with permission of John Wiley & Sons Inc.

of Luschka) and one median aperture (foramen of Magendie). It then flows through the cerebromedullary cistern down the spinal cord and over the cerebral hemispheres. From there the CSF is absorbed via the arachnoid villi.

Arachnoid villi

These structures are protrusions of the arachnoid mater into the subarachnoid space (Figure 2.8). In addition to these primary draining routes, Johnston *et al.* (2007) suggest that CSF may drain via a number of other unconventional pathways including the cavernous sinus, the adventitia of the internal carotid arteries and in lymphatic vessels emerging from the epineurium of the nerve.

Protective functions of the CSF

The unidirectional flow of CSF provides an ablutionary effect which continually removes waste and other potentially noxious substances like drugs and their metabolites from the brain (see below: CSF flow and substance clearance). The CSF provides a fluid buffer that cushions the brain against impact. Fluid buffers are particularly effective in reducing injury from impact as they decelerate the object gradually as the fluid gets compressed. The CSF

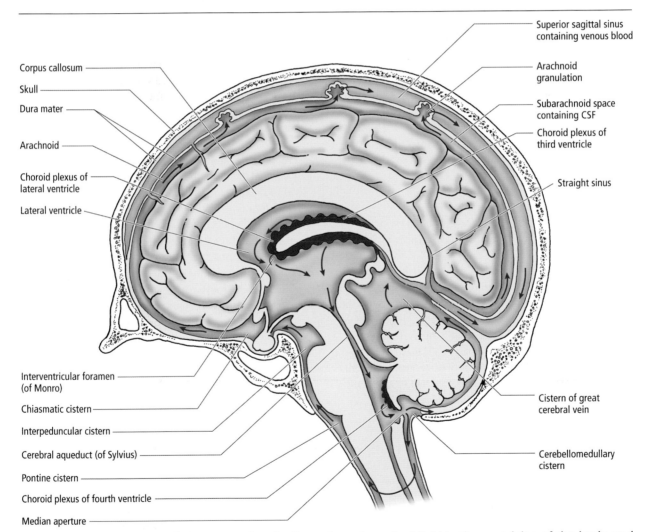

Figure 2.8 Hemisected skull demonstrating the flow of cerebrospinal fluid in the ventricles of the brain and in the subarachnoid spaces. Reproduced from Maria A Patestas and Leslie P Gartner, *A Textbook of Neuroanatomy*, Wiley-Blackwell, with permission.

lubricates the meninges to provide support and frictionless movements of the brain. Although the brain's specific gravity is higher than CSF, 1.0329 ± 0.0014 g/ml, (Lescot et al., 2005) vs 1.006–1.009 g/ml respectively, the presence of CSF provides the brain with some buoyancy reducing pressure at the base of the brain.

Circumventricular organs (CVOs)

Circumventricular organs (CVOs) include a number of structures found at and around the ventricles in the brain. In mammals, nine organs are recognised as CVOs, the most common being: pineal gland (PIN), posterior pituitary (PP), area postrema (AP) and choroid plexus (CP).

Although part of the central nervous system, they are devoid of a typical tight blood–brain barrier (BBB) and appear to function as chemical sampling areas involved in homeostasis (the area postrema acts as a chemoreceptor trigger centre for vomiting, for example). The CVO organs are associated with a well developed and permeable capillary network. Owing to this ease of communication between the blood and brain in these areas, the CVOs are called windows of the brain (Joly et al., 2007). The functions of particular CVOs differ, however the majority provide a secretory function as well as many having a sensory function.

CSF flow and substance clearance

The large fluid flow through the ventricles acts as a convection current to clear CSF-borne substances (Johanson et al., 2008). Diffusional exchange of substances between the interior of the brain and the CSF occurs via the choroid plexus, other CVOs and ependyma. Diffusional exchange of substances between the external environment of the brain and the CSF occurs via the arachnoid membranes and pia mater (Johanson et al., 2008). Apart from regulating hormonal levels in the brain and CSF, these exchanges may contribute towards removal of a number of agents from the brain and CSF. The effect of this CSF flow on drug clearance in the brain remains unclear.

BLOOD SUPPLY TO THE CNS

Cerebral blood supply

The brain is supplied with blood by four main arteries: the two internal carotid arteries and the two vertebral arteries that originate from the subclavian artery. These arteries give rise to the bilateral middle cerebral arteries, the basilar artery and the circle of Willis (Figure 2.9).

Middle cerebral arteries are essentially a continuation of the internal carotid arteries. They supply blood to the lateral surfaces of the cerebral hemispheres including the parietal and temporal lobes, also including the majority of the lateral aspects of the frontal lobe. The basilar artery is formed by the posterior inferior convergence of the two vertebral arteries. It largely supplies blood to the cerebellum and pons via the superior and inferior cerebellar arteries and the smaller bilateral pontine branches respectively.

The two internal carotid arteries interconnect via a circular arterial ring, known as the circle of Willis, the posterior margin of which also receives blood from the basilar artery. This circular ring supplies blood to the majority of the brain. Physiologically this arrangement is significant as it allows for a considerable degree of redundancy in contributing blood vessels, thus preserving cerebral blood flow when one of the main contributors become stenosed.

The bilateral anterior cerebral arteries, as their name suggests, supply blood to the anterior medial portions of the frontal and parietal lobes as well as supplying blood to the deeper anterior portions of the corpus callosum and the basal ganglia. The anterior communicating artery forms the anterior portion of the circle of Willis and when present joins the two anterior cerebral arteries.

The posterior cerebral arteries give rise to ganglionic and cortical branches. The ganglionic branches provide blood to the area around the third ventricle and thalamus, whereas the cortical branches supply blood to the posterior-most part of the occipital lobe and the inferior aspects of the parietal and temporal lobes. The posterior communicating artery forms the main part of the collateral communication between the ipsilateral anterior, middle and posterior cerebral arteries. It supplies blood to the thalamus, hypothalamus and optic chiasm.

Arterial blood supply to the spinal cord

The spinal cord is supplied with blood by three main arteries and a reticular arterial network the vasocorona. The anterior two thirds of the spinal cord is supplied with blood by the anterior spinal arteries that arise bilaterally from the two vertebral arteries. These run caudally to the origins of the basilar artery and run to the filum terminale in the sacrum. These two arteries converge within the cervical area to form a singular anterior spinal artery that runs medially on the anterior surface of the spinal cord.

The posterior spinal arteries run bilaterally on the posterior surface of the spinal cord. Similar to the anterior spinal artery the posterior spinal artery arises from the ipsilateral vertebral artery just below the medulla and runs down to the cauda equina. The two posterior arteries give rise to a reticular network of arterioles that form an arte-

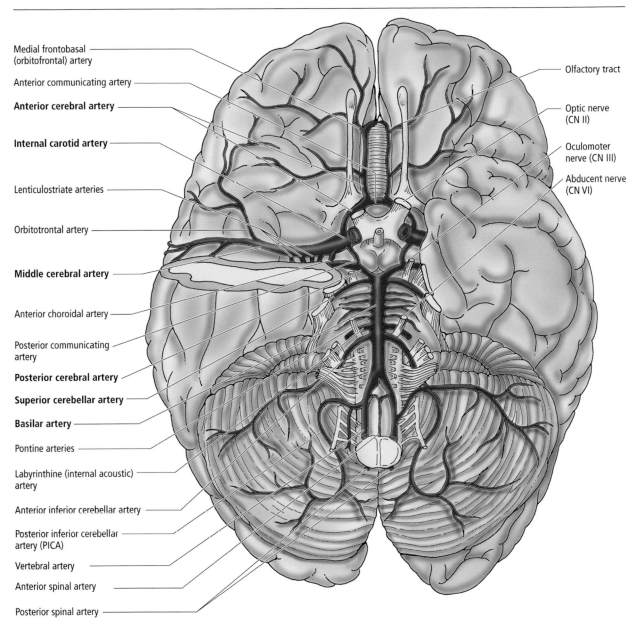

Figure 2.9 Arterial supply of the brain. Note that the frontal lobes are spread apart somewhat to show the anterior cerebral arteries and that the right temporal lobe is severed to show the path and branches of the middle cerebral artery. Reproduced from Maria A Patestas and Leslie P Gartner, *A Textbook of Neuroanatomy*, Wiley-Blackwell, with permission.

riolar plexus on the dorsal surface of the spinal cord known as the vasocorona.

The posterior spinal artery supplies blood to the posterior-most portion of the spinal cord. The vasocorona supplies blood to the superficial layer of the anterior lateral surface of the spinal cord.

Venous drainage of the CNS

The venous drainage of the brain consists of a number of sinuses formed between the two layers of the dura mater. These sinuses receive blood from superficial areas of the brain, the cranium and scalp. In turn these sinuses are interconnected to eventually drain into the two internal jugular veins. There is also a network of deeper veins that drains blood from internal structures of the brain.

Venous sinuses

The most prominent sinuses include the superior and inferior sagittal sinuses that run along on the superior and inferior borders of the falx cerebri respectively. The superior sagittal sinus drains blood largely from the superficial surface of the cerebrum via the superior cerebral veins. It also drains blood from within the diploe of the skull via the diploid veins and from the external surface of the cranial cavity via emissary veins. These veins have particular clinical significance, as they can provide passage for pathogens to enter the cranial cavity. The inferior sagittal sinus largely drains blood from the falx cerebri and a few cerebral veins.

The occipital sinus is small and is located at the base of the falx cerebri. It drains blood from the cerebellum and opens into a swollen sinus junction known as the confluence of sinuses that also drains blood from the superior sagittal sinus. The straight sinus also drains into the confluence of sinuses after receiving blood from the inferior sagittal sinus, the great cerebral vein, the posterior cerebral veins and the superficial cerebellar veins. The confluence of sinuses drains blood into the bilateral transverse sinuses. These sinuses run horizontally on the plane of the confluence of sinuses after which they inferiorly and medially form the sigmoid sinuses to eventually meet with the internal jugular veins (Figure 2.10).

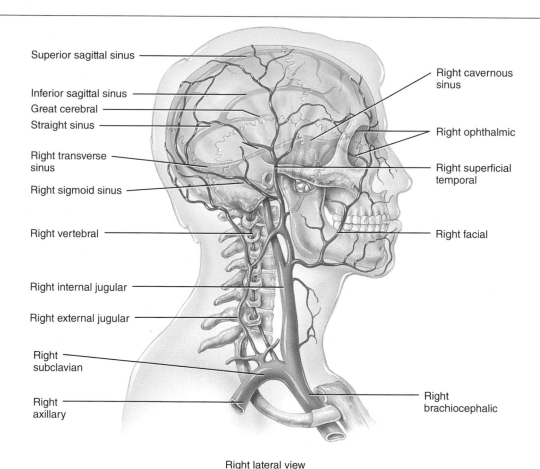

Right lateral view

Figure 2.10 Principal veins of the head and neck. Reproduced from *Principles of Anatomy and Physiology 12e* by Gerard Tortora and Bryan Derrickson. Copyright (2009, John Wiley & Sons). Reprinted with permission of John Wiley & Sons Inc.

Veins of the brain

The two groups of veins that drain the brain are the cerebral and cerebellar veins. These veins can be further divided into superficial and deep veins. Superficial cerebral veins include the superior middle and inferior cerebral veins.

THE BLOOD–BRAIN BARRIER (BBB)

The final element of protection for the brain is the so called blood–brain barrier (BBB). The BBB is a selectively exclusive barrier that dynamically restricts the entry of water and many lipid-soluble substances from the blood into the brain. Initially the BBB was thought to be made up of the microvessels or capillaries that perfuse the brain tissue. However, it is now increasingly apparent that the BBB is the product of a combination of effects derived from influences of a number of cellular components. The BBB effect may be separated into structural and chemical properties. The majority of these properties are attributed to structural and functional changes in brain capillary endothelial cells.

The structural properties of the BBB include:

- Exceedingly tight cell–cell junctions
- A reduced capillary lumen surface area
- A lack of fenestrations in the capillary endothelial cell wall

Chemical properties of the BBB include:

- A higher energy yield in brain capillary endothelial cells afforded by a greater mitochondria concentration when compared to other capillary endothelium
- The presence of a diverse number of drug efflux proteins that reduce lipid-soluble drug entry from the blood to the brain
- The presence of a significant number of enzymes that metabolise medication, enhancing their removal from brain capillary endothelium or rendering the medication ineffective on entering the brain

The combination of cells that confer these BBB properties on brain endothelial cells is known collectively as the neurovascular unit (NVU). The concept of the neurovascular unit allows an explanation of how different cells interact to produce the exclusive BBB. At present the cells known to influence the BBB include: brain capillary endothelium (brain microvessels), astrocytes, pericytes, neurons, microglia (Figure 2.11).

Therefore the BBB is a physico-chemical barrier between the blood in brain capillaries and the brain matter

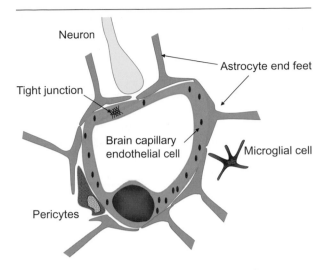

Figure 2.11 Cells of the neurovascular unit.

on the other side of the capillary. Although the physical barrier appears to be formed by the brain capillary endothelium under influence of other cells in the neurovascular unit, it may be possible that the other cells of the neurovascular unit play a direct role in barrier formation.

The structural BBB and protection of the brain

The brain is physically protected by the BBB. The brain endothelium forms a continuous cell layer between the blood and brain. The endothelium of brain capillaries has very tight cell to cell junctions that virtually eliminate movement of substances from the blood to the brain via the passage formed between two neighbouring cells, although the strength of these tight junctions changes constantly under influence of the systemic environment (Khan, 2008). The presence of tight junctions together with a limited number of fenestrations and a reduced surface area of the brain capillary, means that the only route available for entry into the brain for most medications is via the diffusion pathway. Fat soluble substances diffuse from the blood through the luminal surface of the brain capillary and then from inside the brain capillary cell through the abluminal (brain side) wall of the cell into the brain.

Active drug efflux in the BBB

As the BBB presents an exclusive barrier, water-soluble substance entry into the brain is controlled and limited by transport mechanisms in the endothelial cell membrane. These include ion channels and substrate transport proteins, as well as receptor mediated movement of larger

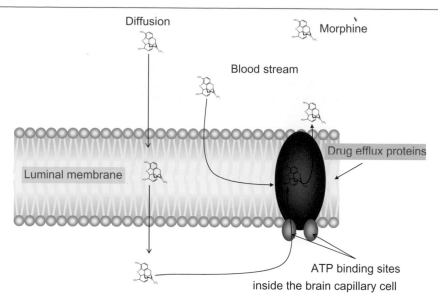

Figure 2.12 Active drug efflux in the blood–brain barrier.

molecules via transcytosis. For a more detailed review of these mechanisms at the BBB see Hawkins and Davis (2005). Entry of fat (lipid) soluble substances into the brain occurs by diffusion. As a large number of toxins, natural and synthetic, are lipid-soluble, the brain is vulnerable to their effects. To reduce the entry of noxious lipidic substances into the brain, membranes on a number of cells of the neurovascular unit possess different types of efflux proteins. These efflux proteins remove lipid soluble molecules from the membrane or cell as they pass through the BBB. These transport proteins belong to the ATP-binding cassette (ABC) superfamily of transport proteins. The common feature of these proteins is that they utilise ATP to transport their substrates against the substance's diffusion gradient, i.e. they actively transport the diffusing substances out of the cells of the BBB back into the blood stream, thus limiting the entry of these substances into the brain (Figure 2.12).

These mechanisms, although physiologically useful, present an obstacle to delivering drugs to the brain. Owing to the comprehensive protection that the drug efflux proteins collectively provide, few CNS-active medications gain access to the brain without being limited by these BBB-located defences. In addition to their constitutive presence, there is evidence to suggest that the number of these transport proteins in NVU cell membranes may increase when exposed to therapeutic levels of CNS active drugs (Tischler *et al.*, 1995; Marchi *et al.*, 2003; Kwan and Brodie, 2005; Volk and Löscher, 2005). The increased number of these proteins in the BBB may contribute towards the drug resistance observed in treatment of chronic CNS pathologies like epilepsy.

SUMMARY

The brain is protected by a number of mechanisms. Structurally it is protected primarily by the bony cranium and a balanced intracranial pressure maintained by haemodynamic and CSF regulation. Chemically the brain is protected from toxic insult by a complex inter-player of a number of cells making up the so called neurovascular unit. These interactions give rise to the blood–brain barrier a syncytium of characteristics which confers both structural and chemical protection to the brain against damage from water or lipid soluble substances.

REFERENCES

Hawkins BD, Davis TP (2005) The blood-brain barrier/ neurovascular unit in health and disease. *Pharmacological Reviews* 57(2):173–185.

Johanson CE, Duncan JA 3rd, Klinge PM *et al.* (2008) Cerebrospinal fluid functions: New challenges in health and disease. *Cerebrospinal Fluid Research* 5:10–42.

Johnston M, Armstrong D, Koh L (2007) Possible role of the cavernous sinus veins in cerebrospinal fluid absorption. *Cerebrospinal Fluid Research* 4:3–8.

Joly J-St, Os'orio J, Alunni A *et al.* (2007) Windows of the brain: Towards a developmental biology of circumventricular and other neurohemal organs. *Seminars in Cell and Developmental Biology* 18:512–524.

Khan EU (2008) Understanding the use of corticosteroids in managing cerebral oedema. *British Journal of Neuroscience Nursing* 4(4):156–162.

Kothari M, Goel A (2006) Maternalizing the meninges: A pregnant Arabic legacy. *Neurology India* 54(4):345–346.

Kwan P, Brodie MJ (2005) Potential role for drug transporters in the pathogenesis of medically intractable epilepsy. *Epilepsia* 46(2):224–235.

Lescot T, Bonnet MP, Zouaoui A *et al.* (2005) A quantitative computed tomography assessment of brain weight, volume, and specific gravity in severe head trauma. *Intensive Care Med* 31(8):1042–1050.

Marchi N, Cucullo L, Moddel G *et al.* (2003) Pharmacological and pathological significance of MDR1 expression in human epileptic brain. *Epilepsia* 44 (Suppl 9) 98.

Redzic ZB, Segal MB (2004) The structure of the choroid plexus and the physiology of the choroid plexus epithelium. *Advanced Drug Delivery Reviews* 56:1695–1716.

Tishler DM, Weinberg KT, Hinton DR *et al.* (1995) MDR1 gene expression in brain of patients with medically intractable epilepsy. *Epilepsia* 36:1–6.

Volk HA, Löscher W (2005) Multidrug resistance in epilepsy: rats with drug-resistant seizures exhibit enhanced brain expression of P-glycoprotein compared with rats with drug-responsive seizures. *Brain* 128:1358–1368.

3

The Anatomy and Physiology of the Brain

Chris Eberhardie, Sue Woodward and Ann-Marie Mestecky

INTRODUCTION

A clear knowledge of the anatomical structures of the brain and an understanding of their normal physiological function is essential in neuroscience nursing. When disease, injury or disorder affect all or part of the brain the sufferer is often bewildered by it and cannot understand why they can no longer achieve something that once was second nature to them. Detailed knowledge of the normal structure and function of the brain can often lead to helping the patient and his carers to understand what is causing their distress.

DESCRIBING ANATOMICAL STRUCTURES

The terms used to describe the anatomical structures of the brain are:

- Anterior: lying in front of
- Posterior: lying behind or at the back of
- Rostral: towards the head (top)
- Ventral: the front or anterior
- Caudal: towards the tail (bottom)
- Superior: lying above
- Inferior: lying below
- Sagittal: medial plane, divides the body into two symmetrical halves
- Parasagittal: any plane parallel to the sagittal plane
- Coronal: parallel to the long axis of the body and perpendicular to the sagittal plane, divides the body into back and front

- Transverse or axial: divides the body into head and tail portions
- Lateral: viewed from the side

FOETAL DEVELOPMENT OF THE BRAIN

The foetal nervous system develops from the third week of pregnancy. The neural plate develops from the ectodermal layer of the amniotic sac. It then forms neural folds, which fuse to become the neural tube (Figure 3.1). The neural tube changes shape and develops into a tadpole like structure with the rostral section developing into the brain and the caudal end becoming the spinal cord.

The emerging shape of the brain and spinal cord can be seen throughout the pregnancy. By the fourth week there are three distinct sections to the developing brain, the prosencephalon or forebrain, the mesencephalon or midbrain and the rhombencephalon or hindbrain (Figure 3.2) (Patestas and Gartner, 2006). The prosencephalon further divides into the telencephalon and the diencephalon. The telencephalon goes on to become the cerebral cortex and the corpus striatum in the fully developed brain. The diencephalon develops into the thalamus and hypothalamus. The mesencephalon becomes the midbrain and the rhombencephalon develops into the pons varolii, cerebellum and medulla oblongata (Fitzgerald *et al.*, 2007).

THE GROSS ANATOMY OF THE BRAIN
CEREBRUM

The cerebrum (Figure 3.3) is the largest part of the brain. The outer layer of the cerebrum is known as the cortex and has a complex pattern of folds giving rise to the brain's convoluted appearance. There are two parts to each fold:

Neuroscience Nursing: Evidence-Based Practice, 1st Edition.
Edited by Sue Woodward and Ann-Marie Mestecky
© 2011 Blackwell Publishing Ltd

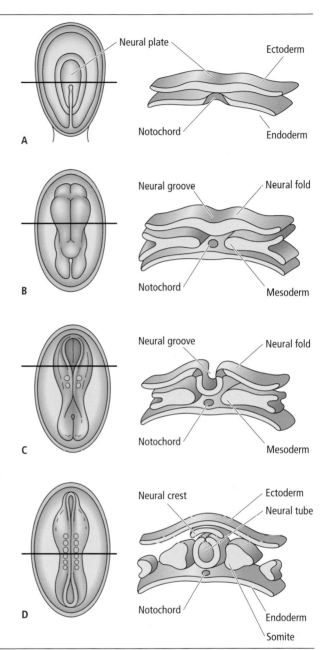

Figure 3.1 Formation of the neural tube. (a) The notochord is responsible for inducing the overlying ectodermal cells to form the neural plate. (b, c) As the embryo continues its development, it enters the stage of neurulation, the process whereby the forming nervous system is brought into the body by the formation of an intermediary neural groove, and finally a neural tube, the precursor of the brain and spinal cord. (d) Note that the neural crest, initially the lateral aspect of the neural plate, becomes separated as the neural tube is formed. Cells of the neural crest give rise to all of the ganglia of the peripheral nervous system as well as to numerous additional structures of the developing embryo. Reproduced from Maria A Patestas and Leslie P Gartner, *A Textbook of Neuroanatomy*, Wiley-Blackwell, with permission.

the area that is raised – the gyrus (pl. gyri) and that which sinks down – the sulcus (pl. sulci). Deep sulci are known as fissures. The cerebrum is almost completely divided into the left and right cerebral hemispheres by the longitudinal fissure. The cerebral hemispheres communicate with each other via three major commissures (Figure 3.4) (thick collections of nerve fibres):

- Corpus callosum – running between and connecting corresponding regions of the cerebral hemispheres (except temporal regions)
- Anterior commisure – running transversely connecting inferior and middle temporal gyri
- Hippocampal commisure – running transversely connecting the two hippocampi

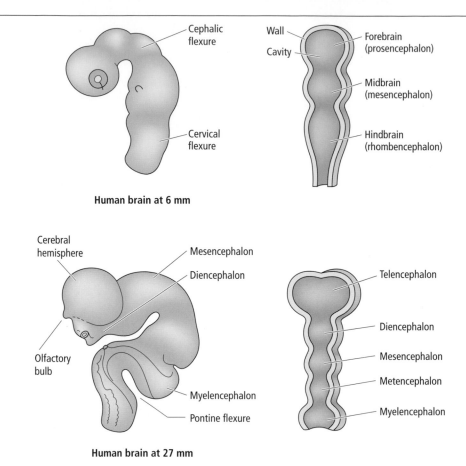

Human brain at 6 mm

Human brain at 27 mm

Figure 3.2 Development of the brain. Three-dimensional representation of the human brain (left) and its longitudinal section (right; as if the brain were stretched out) at 6 and 27 mm of development. Note that the three primary brain divisions of the 6 mm embryo give rise to the five divisions of the 27 mm embryo. Reproduced from Maria A Patestas and Leslie P Gartner, *A Textbook of Neuroanatomy*, Wiley-Blackwell, with permission.

The cerebrum is separated from the cerebellum by the tentorium cerebelli, a fold of dura, and the transverse sinus.

The outer layer of each cerebral hemisphere is known as the cerebral cortex and is made up of neuronal cell bodies and dendrites. When viewed by the naked eye a post-mortem specimen of the cerebral cortex looks grey, in contrast to the white matter lying below it which is made up of neuronal axons which appear paler (Figure 3.5). This gives rise to the terms grey matter and white matter respectively.

The lobes of the cerebrum

The lobes of the cerebrum take their names from the bones which lie above them. There are four lobes: the frontal,

parietal, temporal, and occipital lobes. Each lobe is interconnected but has specific functions. Some areas of the cerebral cortex have clearly defined functions whereas others are either unknown or less well understood.

There are two theories about cerebral function which have developed over the last hundred years. The first of those theories was that each area of cerebral cortex 'mapped' to a specific function. Brodmann (1909–1994) developed a cortical map based on visual appearance, but this is not necessarily directly related to function. Golgi developed the net theory of neural integration that challenged Brodmann's work (Clarke and O'Malley, 1996). Magnetic resonance imaging (MRI) and computerised axial tomography have contributed much to the study of neuroanatomy, but the development of positron emission

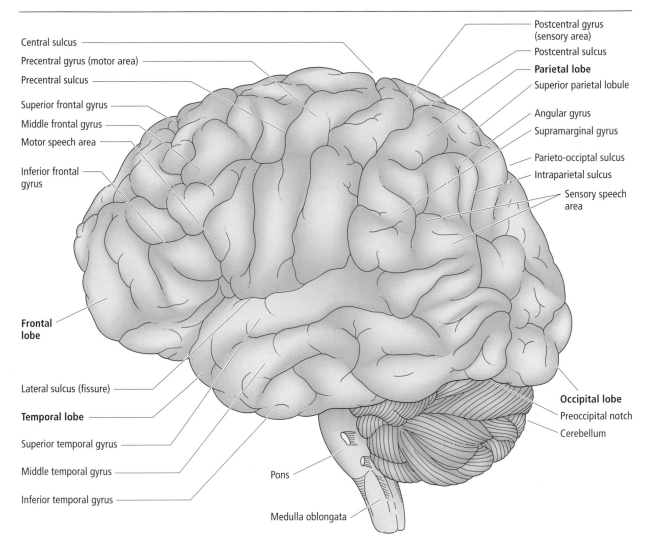

Central sulcus

Precentral gyrus (motor area)

Precentral sulcus

Superior frontal gyrus

Middle frontal gyrus

Motor speech area

Inferior frontal
gyrus

**Frontal
lobe**

Lateral sulcus (fissure)

Temporal lobe

Superior temporal gyrus

Middle temporal gyrus

Inferior temporal gyrus

Pons

Medulla oblongata

Postcentral gyrus
(sensory area)

Postcentral sulcus

Parietal lobe

Superior parietal lobule

Angular gyrus

Supramarginal gyrus

Parieto-occipital sulcus

Intraparietal sulcus

Sensory speech
area

Occipital lobe

Preoccipital notch

Cerebellum

Figure 3.3 Diagram of the brain from a lateral view. Reproduced from Maria A Patestas and Leslie P Gartner, *A Textbook of Neuroanatomy*, Wiley-Blackwell, with permission.

tomography (PET scanning) which demonstrates brain function over time, and functional MRI, continue to contribute to a greater understanding of brain physiology. In particular PET has demonstrated that there is both localisation and integration of neural activity.

FRONTAL LOBE

The frontal lobe is separated from the parietal lobe by the central sulcus, and from the temporal lobe by the lateral sulcus (Figure 3.3). The frontal lobe lies in the anterior cranial fossa. On the inferior surface of each frontal lobe lie the olfactory bulb and the olfactory tract.

One of the principal functions of the frontal lobe is the organisation of muscle movement. The primary motor cortex (motor strip) is situated in the precentral gyrus. It is in this area that muscle movement involving groups of muscles, known as muscle synergy, is initiated. For example when lifting a pen not only are the muscles of the hand involved, but the arm and the shoulder too. The axons extending from the motor cortex to the spinal cord (corticospinal tracts) pass through the internal capsule to the medulla oblongata in the brain stem where the fibres cross to the other side of the body. Therefore the motor strip in the left hemisphere activates the right side of the

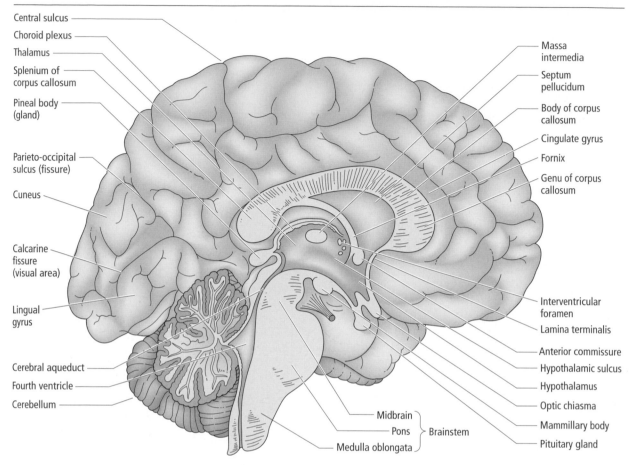

Central sulcus
Choroid plexus
Thalamus
Splenium of corpus callosum
Pineal body (gland)
Parieto-occipital sulcus (fissure)
Cuneus
Calcarine fissure (visual area)
Lingual gyrus
Cerebral aqueduct
Fourth ventricle
Cerebellum

Massa intermedia
Septum pellucidum
Body of corpus callosum
Cingulate gyrus
Fornix
Genu of corpus callosum
Interventricular foramen
Lamina terminalis
Anterior commissure
Hypothalamic sulcus
Hypothalamus
Optic chiasma
Mammillary body
Pituitary gland

Midbrain
Pons   } Brainstem
Medulla oblongata

Figure 3.4 Diagram of the medial view of a sagittal section of the brain. Reproduced from Maria A Patestas and Leslie P Gartner, *A Textbook of Neuroanatomy*, Wiley-Blackwell, with permission.

body and vice versa. Damage to the motor areas of the frontal lobe can result in spastic hemiplegia, as in a stroke or trauma.

Primary motor and pre-motor cortex

One half of the body is represented in the primary motor cortex of each cerebral hemisphere, as if the feet were hanging on to the sagittal sinus with the head near to the temporal lobe. The body's representation on the cortex is related to the amount and complexity of motor activity involved. For example, if a homunculus is drawn the face, lips, hands and fingers are huge, but the elbow and trunk are tiny in comparison (Figure 3.6). This is because more 'information processing power', and therefore a larger number of cerebral neurones, are required to control fine finger movements than gross movements of the trunk.

The pre-motor cortex lies directly in front of the primary motor strip. Stimulation of this area induces less focused movement and it is thought to co-ordinate learned movements (Crossman and Neary, 2005). It is involved in the planning and sequencing of movement. The pre-motor cortex communicates directly with the motor cortex; axons from the pre-motor cortex also extend to the striatum (corticostriate pathway) and contribute to the corticospinal pathway. Damage to this area results in impairment of skilled movement and difficulty with visuomotor skills (Barker and Barasi, 2008).

Broca's area

Broca's area is unilateral and lies anterior to the motor strip on the inferior frontal gyrus of the dominant hemisphere, (usually the left) (Crossman and Neary, 2005). This area

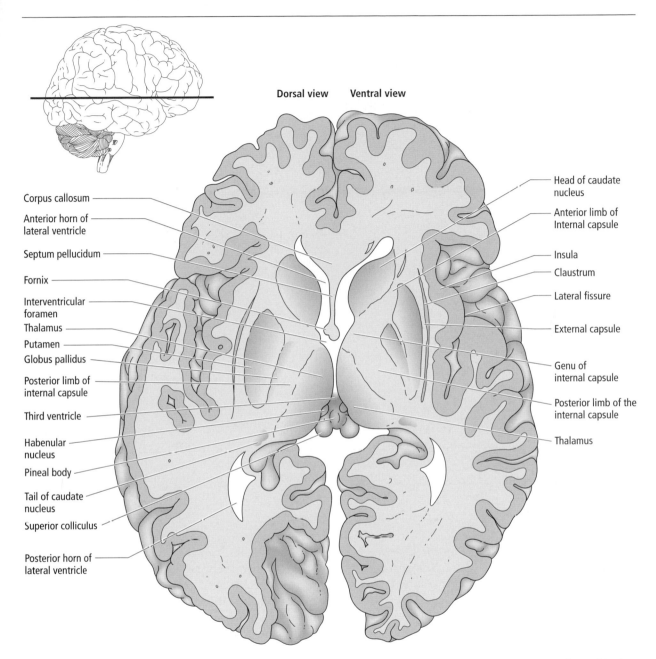

Dorsal view   Ventral view

Corpus callosum

Anterior horn of lateral ventricle

Septum pellucidum

Fornix

Interventricular foramen

Thalamus

Putamen

Globus pallidus

Posterior limb of internal capsule

Third ventricle

Habenular nucleus

Pineal body

Tail of caudate nucleus

Superior colliculus

Posterior horn of lateral ventricle

Head of caudate nucleus

Anterior limb of Internal capsule

Insula

Claustrum

Lateral fissure

External capsule

Genu of internal capsule

Posterior limb of the internal capsule

Thalamus

Figure 3.5 Diagram of a coronal section of the brain displaying the basal ganglia. Reproduced from Maria A Patestas and Leslie P Gartner, *A Textbook of Neuroanatomy*, Wiley-Blackwell, with permission.

plays an important role in the motor aspects of speech, enabling the individual to form, articulate, pronounce and express the spoken word (Edmans *et al.*, 2001). Impairment of the neuronal tissue in this area can result in aphasia and oral dyspraxia (see Chapter 12). Broca's area communicates with Wernicke's area in the temporal lobe of the same hemisphere via a pathway of fibres called the arcuate fasiculus.

Prefrontal cortex

The prefrontal cortex is a large area of the frontal lobes that has extensive neural connections with all the other

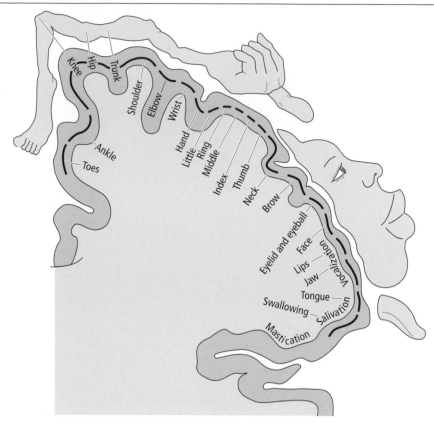

Figure 3.6 Coronal section through the primary motor cortex showing the motor homunculus. Note the somatotopic mapping. The cortical area devoted to each body part is proportional to the motor innervation received by the corresponding body part. Reproduced from Maria A Patestas and Leslie P Gartner, *A Textbook of Neuroanatomy*, Wiley-Blackwell, with permission.

cerebral lobes. This area is involved with personality and higher cognitive functions of reasoning, understanding, thinking and foresight. Damage to this area by trauma, ischaemia or disease results in behavioural changes such as disinhibition, apathy, inattentiveness and poor problem-solving.

PARIETAL LOBE

The anterior part of the parietal lobe is separated from the frontal lobe by the central sulcus, from the temporal lobe by the lateral sulcus and from the occipital lobe by the parieto-occipital sulcus (Figure 3.3). The primary somatosensory cortex is found in the postcentral gyrus. It is involved with the initial processing of sensory information, specifically related to touch, vibration and proprioception (joint position sense). Damage affecting this area will result in loss of fine touch and proprioception. The

proximity of the primary somatosensory cortex to the primary motor cortex facilitates rapid motor response to sensory stimuli.

The body is represented in the primary somatosensory cortex as if hanging by a foot from the sagittal sinus with the face, lips and pharynx adjacent to the temporal lobe. The body is not represented in the same way as in the motor cortex and if a homunculus is drawn of the sensory strip it shows a body with very large lips, face and fingers, as these are very sensitive areas (Figure 3.7). The sensory strip in the right hemisphere receives sensory information from the left side of the body and vice versa.

Posterior to the primary somatosensory cortex lies the somatosensory association area. This area enables recognition of objects just by feeling them rather than looking at them. This is known as stereognosis, e.g. the ability to tell the difference between different coinages. Loss of this

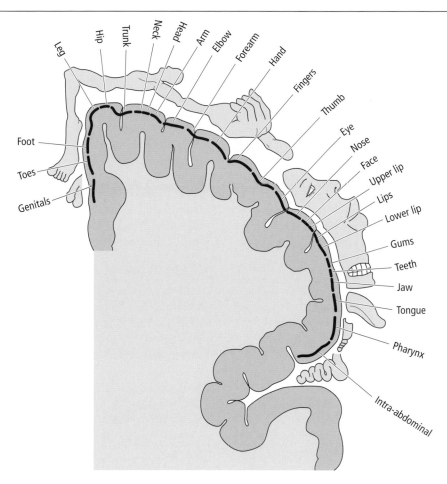

Figure 3.7 Coronal section through the primary somatosensory cortex (postcentral gyrus), showing the sensory homunculus. Note that the amount of cerebral cortex representing each body part is proportional to the extent of its motor innervation. Reproduced from Maria A Patestas and Leslie P Gartner, *A Textbook of Neuroanatomy*, Wiley-Blackwell, with permission.

ability is termed astereognosis. The parieto-occipital association areas play a key role in spatial perception. Damage to this area can cause unilateral neglect (inattention) in which the patient may deny the existence of one half of the body, constructional and dressing dyspraxia, which is particularly noticeable in patients with a right parietal lesion (Edmans *et al.*, 2001). In lesions of the left parietal lobe the patient is likely to be left with one or more of the following deficits: inability to calculate (acalculia) difficulty with writing (dysgraphia), difficulty reading (dyslexia) and difficulty naming objects (Edmans *et al.*, 2001; Crossman and Neary, 2005). Partial seizures in the parietal lobe give rise to bizarre and unique sensations.

The visual pathways pass through the parietal lobes as the optic radiations. Damage to these pathways will result in a loss of vision in the same quarter of each eye (homonymous quadrantanopia) (see Chapter 13).

TEMPORAL LOBE

The temporal lobe is separated from the frontal lobe by the lateral sulcus, which is very deep, and has 'an island' of brain tissue, called the insula cortex, within it (discussed under the limbic system). The posterior boundaries of the temporal lobe are less well defined (Figure 3.3).

This lobe plays an important role in the interpretation of specialist sensory information such as taste, smell, hearing and sensory memory. The primary auditory cortex is found near the lateral fissure and receives auditory information from the cochlea of the ear via the medial geniculate nucleus in the thalamus. It distinguishes sound quality e.g. loudness, tone. The auditory information is further processed in the auditory association areas which are linked to Wernicke's area.

The medial parts of the temporal lobes are concerned with memory, learning and emotional behaviour; however, the specific structures involved form part of the limbic system and so will be discussed later.

Lesions in the temporal lobe can also result in altered taste, auditory or olfactory hallucinations. The unique symptoms experienced in temporal lobe epilepsy (see Chapter 30) demonstrate the importance of this lobe in specialist sensory processing and emotional behaviour.

Wernicke's area

Wernicke's area is located in the superior temporal gyrus in the dominant temporal lobe. This area is crucial in understanding spoken language. Damage to Wernicke's area results in an inability to understand (receptive dysphasia) or produce language (expressive dysphasia).

OCCIPITAL LOBE

The occipital lobe is separated from the parietal lobe by the parieto-occipital sulcus. Another important sulcus on the medial surface is the calcarine sulcus. The primary visual cortex lies adjacent to the calcarine sulcus. The principal function of the occipital lobe is the recognition, interpretation and storage of visual images and memories.

Visual association cortex

Vision is not totally perceived in the primary visual cortex. Each part of the cortex only 'sees' a small part of the visual field and to perceive objects or entire scenes these small portions of visual information have to be combined in visual association areas. Visual information is transmitted from the primary visual cortex to the inferior temporal cortex, which functions in object recognition, and the posterior parietal cortex, which is associated with the location of objects.

Damage to the occipital cortex can result in homonymous hemianopia which is a defect in the same hemifield on both eyes (see Chapter 13 for further detail). Bilateral lesions of the occipital cortex may cause cortical blindness. Diffuse posterior lesions affect visual association areas within the temporal and parietal lobes. This can result in aperceptive visual agnosia, which is the inability to recognise objects in a whole or meaningful way even

though visual pathways and visual acuity are intact (Ghadiali, 2004). This is a failure in early stage visual processing and results in the inability to perceive visual information.

Associative visual agnosia is more common. Objects that are presented visually can be perceived but the person cannot understand or assign meaning to the object, face or word. It is usually the result of bilateral damage to the inferior temporo-occipital junction. Prosopagnosia is the inability to recognise faces, which is a much less severe form of visual agnosia. Patients can recognise a face as a face, but cannot recognise the person (Ghadiali, 2004). Most cases of visual agnosias occur when damage to the occipital lobes is diffuse and bilateral, but it can also occur in right hemisphere damage alone (Carlson, 2006).

LIMBIC SYSTEM

The limbic system is made up of several important structures that form a border round the brain stem. Its primary functions relate to basic instincts, motivation and emotional drives (fear, sex, hunger, sleep). Structures of the limbic system include the:

- Amygdala
- Hippocampus
- Septum pellucidum
- Cingulate gyrus
- Insula
- Parahippocampal gyrus
- Fornix
- Mamillary bodies

The structures of the limbic system have connections with the olfactory tract, the hypothalamus and the upper reticular formation within the midbrain. The hypothalamus is involved in limbic functions and in some texts some hypothalamic nuclei are considered structures of the limbic system. The functions of the limbic system are expressed through endocrine, visceral, somatic and behavioural reactions.

The link between the hippocampus and the hypothalamus via the pathways of the limbic system plays an important role in learning and memory, including the association of sights, sounds and smells with emotions e.g. a couple may have a favourite song which evokes strong emotions. It is also associated with distressing memories and fear. The limbic system links to the cerebral cortex and can modify behaviour; in some cases emotions may override rationale thought. Functions of specific structures of the limbic system are discussed below.

AMYGDALA

The amygdala is situated in the anterior temporal lobe. It is an island of nuclear grey matter, which has connections with the hypothalamus and the prefrontal cortex. Its main function is the formation and storage of memories of emotional experiences, particularly strong emotions such as fear, anger and those associated with sexual behaviour. The amygdala has a regulatory function in control of aggression (Cohen, 1999) and the physiological responses to these emotions are controlled by the hypothalamus. Damage to the amygdala results in a deficit in emotional learning.

HIPPOCAMPUS AND MEMORY

The hippocampus is a forebrain structure of the temporal lobe and lies on both sides of the cerebrum, stretching along the floor and medial wall of the inferior horn of the lateral ventricle (Patestas and Gartner, 2006). There appears to be communication in the form of a loop from the hippocampus to the fornix, mamillary body, thalamus, cingulate gyrus and then returning to the hippocampus (Lindsay and Bone, 2004). The main role of the hippocampus is in the formation of memory. There are several different forms of memory and an understanding of each of them is important in the diagnosis and care of patients with a number of neurological disorders such as traumatic brain injury, stroke and Alzheimer's disease.

Short-term or working memory is the ability to retain small amounts of information for a short period, lasting seconds to a few minutes, such as remembering a new telephone number while you search for a pen, and is limited to seven items ± two.

Long-term memory can be broken down into declarative and procedural memory:

- Declarative memory – enables a wide variety of facts or events to be recalled and is controlled by the hippocampus.
  - Episodic memory – helps the individual to recall whole episodes of their personal experience, e.g. life as a student or first love.
  - Semantic memory – focuses on remembering written or spoken words.
- Procedural memory – facilitates learned motor responses or procedures, e.g. playing an instrument after a number of years, primarily involving the pre-motor cortex, visual association areas and basal ganglia, rather than the hippocampus.

(Fitzgerald *et al.*, 2007)

Organisation of memory

The way in which the brain organises and lays down new memory is not completely understood. The hippocampus is active during the original experience and is thought to tie together a sequence of perceptions (context and events). It is also thought to be involved in converting short-term to long-term memories (Carlson, 2006).

When a memory is formed new connections are made between neurones in cortical networks involving the hippocampus (Bliss *et al.*, 2006). The synapses between these neurones are reinforced and strengthened over time (long term potentiation, LTP) resulting eventually in plastic changes to the structure of pathways within cortical networks (Whitlock *et al.*, 2006). Rather than memory being uniformly distributed throughout the hippocampus, it is now also known that synaptic change associated with new memory is located in specific spots within the hippocampus (Bliss *et al.*, 2006). Storage of episodic memory becomes a function of the neocortex over time (Sacktor, 2008).

Damage to the hippocampus can result in loss of both the ability to lay down new memory (anterograde amnesia) and the ability to retrieve old memories (retrograde amnesia). In addition to the hippocampus, the mamillary bodies and anterior thalamus are involved in formation of memory and damage to these structures, e.g. due to Korsakoff psychosis or Alzheimer's disease, will result in anterograde amnesia (Patestas and Gartner, 2006). If the function of the temporoparietal cortex is impaired, e.g. due to Alzheimer's disease, memory storage and retrieval is compromised (Barker and Barasi, 2008).

MAMILLARY BODIES

These two round masses lie inferior to the hypothalamus and relay information coming from the amydalae and hippocampi to the thalamus. They are thought to play a role in memory, wakefulness and a sense of well-being (Carlson, 2006) as well as expression of emotions (Patestas and Gartner, 2006).

SEPTUM PELLUCIDUM

The septum pellucidum separates the anterior part of the lateral ventricles. It has been reported that stimulation of this area is important in defensive rage (Cohen, 1999).

CINGULATE GYRUS, INSULA AND PARAHIPPOCAMPAL GYRUS

These structures are thought to connect the conscious behaviour of the cortex with the subconscious behaviour of the limbic system.

Cingulate gyrus

Stimulation of this cortex in animals results in an increase in calling and emotional vocalisation (Cohen, 1999), although the role in language generation in humans is unclear. This gyrus co-ordinates sensory input with emotions, such as the emotional response to pain, and regulates aggressive behaviour. It is important in complex motor control and social interaction.

Damage to the cingulate gyrus can result in reduced pain perception, aggression and vocalisation, leading to altered social behaviour. Overstimulation, e.g. during an epileptic seizure, can result in changes to autonomic function, increased vocalisation and complex movements (Barker and Barasi, 2008).

Insula

The insula is an area of cortex that is situated deep to the brain's lateral surface. The insula is the source of many human emotions (lust, disgust, pride, humiliation, guilt) and is responsible for responding to hunger and craving. Functional MRI has demonstrated that the insula is active during pain perception or anticipation, empathy with others, humour, listening to music and eating chocolate and is thought to be important in suppressing natural urges (Lerner *et al.*, 2008). Impairment of the insula may lead to obsessive compulsive disorder, tics, hyperactivity, post-traumatic stress and addiction (Lerner *et al.*, 2008).

Parahippocampal gyrus

The parahippocampal gyrus is a key structure in declarative memory processing.

CEREBELLUM

Cerebellum means 'small cerebrum' and, like the cerebrum, there are two cerebellar hemispheres that are joined at the midline by the vermis, a wormlike structure. The cerebellum is convoluted and has numerous deep fissures. The gyri of the cerebellum are known as folia (Figure 3.8).

The cerebellar cortex is divided into three lobes:

• Anterior
• Posterior
• Flocculonodular

The cerebellum is connected to the brain stem by three paired tracts, called the inferior, middle and superior cerebellar peduncles. The inferior and superior peduncles contain both afferent and efferent fibres allowing two way communication between the cerebellum and the brain stem, whereas the middle peduncles contain afferent fibres only. Each of the three pairs of peduncles conveys specific information.

Afferent and efferent pathways

Afferent fibres from the spino-cerebellar, olivo-cerebellar, vestibulo-cerebellar and ponto-cerebellar tracts arrive at the cerebellar cortex via the inferior, middle and superior peduncles.

Sensory spino-cerebellar fibres arrive in the anterior lobe via the inferior and superior cerebellar peduncles and carry proprioception information. The main function of the anterior lobe is the processing of unconscious proprioceptive information. It influences lower motor neurones via the rubrospinal tracts. Patients with lesions in this area suffer from increased muscle tone and postural instability.

Cortico-pontine fibres from the cerebral cortex synapse with ponto-cerebellar fibres in the pons where they cross over before entering the posterior lobe of the cerebellum via the middle cerebellar peduncle. These fibres form the largest input to the cerebellum and provide feedback to the cerebellum about movements as they are happening. This allows for constant monitoring and co-ordination of the movements (Patestas and Gartner, 2006) and is important for skilled voluntary movement, e.g. typing or playing a piano. Efferent fibres project to the thalamus and to the cerebral cortex, thereby co-ordinating movement. Patients with problems in this area may suffer from intention tremor and lack of co-ordination.

Olivo-cerebellar fibres arise from the inferior olivary nucleus, which receives input mainly from the primary and secondary motor and somatosensory cortex. These fibres decussate and enter the cerebellum via the inferior cerebellar peduncle (Patestas and Gartner, 2006). The inferior olivary nucleus plays an important role in learning new motor skills.

Vestibulo-cerebellar fibres pass through the inferior cerebellar peduncle to the inferior and medial vestibular nuclei of the flocculonodular lobe from the vestibular system, transmitting sensory information about head position. This lobe is responsible for postural adjustments to gravity, balance (equilibrium) and gait and is involved in controlling eye movements. The flocculonodular lobe projects efferent fibres to the vestibular nuclei and thence via the vestibulospinal tracts to synapse with the motor neurones within the spinal cord that control gait and balance (Patestas and Gartner, 2006). Patients with lesions in this area can be described as having flocculonodular syndrome in which they are unable to maintain equilibrium and develop nystagmus and an ataxic, broad based gait.

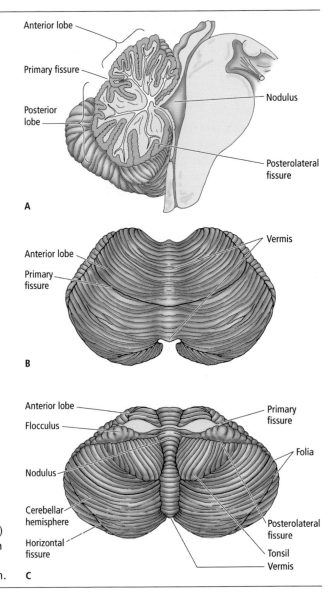

Figure 3.8 The cerebellum: (A) midsagittal view, (B) dorsal view, and (C) ventral view. Reproduced from Maria A Patestas and Leslie P Gartner, *A Textbook of Neuroanatomy*, Wiley-Blackwell, with permission.

Unlike the cerebrum the fibres exiting from one side of the cerebellum control the ipsilateral side of the body. Damage to one hemisphere of the cerebellum therefore produces lack of co-ordination, with an unsteady gait (ataxia) and tremor on the same side of the body as the lesion (Patestas and Gartner, 2006), without accompanying weakness or sensory loss. More widespread dysfunction of the cerebellar hemispheres results in a wide-based, unsteady gait (cerebellar ataxia), lack of coordination of both arms, intention tremor, nystagmus, and slowness and slurring of speech (dysarthria).

BASAL GANGLIA AND THE THALAMUS

Basal ganglia

The basal ganglia are collections of nuclei in the cerebrum, lying laterally to the thalamus, and consisting of the corpus striatum (caudate nucleus, putamen and globus pallidus), substantia nigra, and the subthalamic nucleus. The caudate nucleus and putamen form the neostriatum; the putamen and the globus pallidus form the lentiform nucleus. The basal ganglia have neural connections with the cerebral cortex and play an important role in the control of movement and thought.

Functional anatomy of the basal ganglia

Corticospinal tracts are referred to as pyramidal tracts, so named as the fibres pass through a pair of structures on the surface of the medulla, known as pyramids. All other descending tracts, including those that pass through the basal ganglia are 'extrapyramidal' tracts. The two systems are intimately related. 'Extrapyramidal' is considered an out-dated term, but is still widely used. Generally speaking the basal ganglia facilitate constant readjustment during voluntary movement and enable fine motor control due to a number of feedback mechanisms (Figure 3.9), facilitating ongoing movement and inhibiting unwanted movement.

Movement is initiated from the cortex and fibres pass from here both to corticospinal tracts and to the neostria-

tum (the main input to the basal ganglia). From the neostriatum fibres connect to the rest of the basal ganglia through both a direct pathway that promotes movement and an indirect pathway that inhibits unwanted movement (Figure 3.10).

Neostriatum (caudate + putamen)

The putamen lies laterally to the internal capsule and globus pallidus. The caudate nucleus has a large head and a tapering curved tail that descends into the temporal lobe. The neostriatum receives the main input to the basal ganglia, which primarily arises from the motor regions of the frontal lobes. Input also comes from the thalamus and the substantia nigra. The corticostriatal pathways are excitatory and use glutamate as the neurotransmitter, which stimulates the neostriatum to influence other structures within the basal ganglia through both direct and indirect pathways (Figure 3.10). This will ultimately facilitate ongoing movement and inhibit unwanted movements. Damage to the neostriatum will result in hyperkinetic movement disorders such as Huntington's disease as the motor areas of the cortex are overstimulated, resulting in excess and unwanted movements (Patestas and Gartner, 2006).

Globus pallidus

The globus pallidus lies medially to the putamen and is divided into two (internal and external segments). Together with the substantia nigra, the globus pallidus provides the main output from the basal ganglia. The globus pallidus uses the inhibitory neurotransmitter gamma amino butyric acid (GABA) and fibres from this nucleus pass to the primary motor and pre-motor cortex via the thalamus. The effect of activation of this pathway is to support or facilitate ongoing movements.

Subthalamic nuclei

The subthalamic nucleus lies against the internal capsule, below the thalamus as the name suggests, and uses the excitatory neurotransmitter glutamic acid. Fibres from this nucleus pass to the globus pallidus and subthalamic nucleus and the effect of activation of this pathway is to inhibit unwanted movements (Crossman and Neary, 2005).

Substantia nigra

Functionally the substantia nigra of the midbrain acts as part of the basal ganglia and has both inhibitory and excitatory effects. Axons extend from the substantia nigra to the striatum – the nigrostriatal pathway. The neurotransmitter used within the nigro-striatal pathway is dopamine.

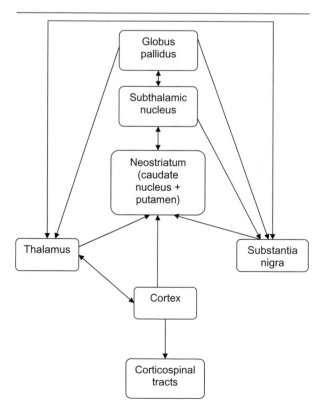

Figure 3.9 Connections of the basal ganglia (simplified).

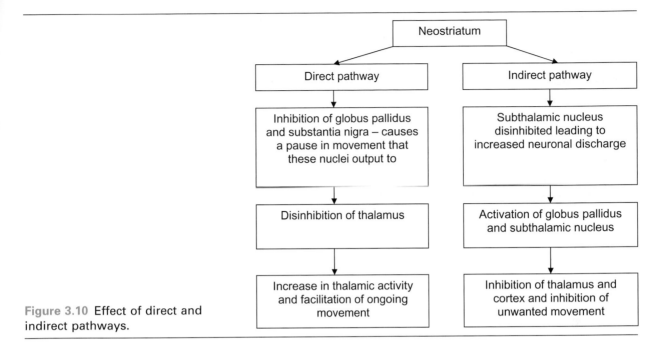

Figure 3.10 Effect of direct and indirect pathways.

This pathway plays an essential role in muscle tone and movement. When there is a degeneration of dopamine producing neurones in this pathway, there is an imbalance of neurotransmitter activity in the basal ganglia, which brings about the symptoms of Parkinson's disease.

Thalamus

The thalamus is the dorsal part of the diencephalon and is the largest mass of grey matter lying deep in the brain. It forms the superior and lateral walls of the third ventricle. The thalamus is ovoid in shape and lies on either side of the midline of the brain. Most afferent pathways to the cerebrum (including all sensory pathways except olfaction) pass through the thalamus, where information is sorted and relayed to the appropriate region of the cortex. The thalamus therefore has widespread projections to many areas of the cortex and generally causes excitation of the areas it connects to.

The thalamus is made up of several nuclei some of which have very specific roles:

- The medial geniculate nuclei form part of the auditory pathway. Information is relayed from the inferior colliculus in the midbrain to the primary auditory cortex.
- The lateral geniculate nuclei relay visual information from the retina to the visual cortex.
- The lateral dorsal nucleus is connected to the cingulate cortex and is important in laying down memory.

- The mediodorsal nucleus relays information from parts of the limbic system to the pre-frontal cortex and is associated with thought, reasoning and mood.
- The ventrolateral nucleus conveys information from the cerebellum to the primary motor cortex.

In addition to its primary function as a relay station the thalamus plays a significant role in the perception of pain and temperature, focusing attention and has links with the reticular activating system (Crossman and Neary, 2005).

Internal capsule

The internal capsule lies between the thalamus, the caudate nucleus and the putamen. This small, but critical area contains large bundles of both sensory and motor tracts (Crossman and Neary, 2005). All sensory tracts projecting to the cortex from the spinal cord pass through the internal capsule on leaving the thalamus and all corticospinal tracts pass through this area before entering the brain stem and thence the spinal cord. Patients who have had a stroke in this area suffer from sensory loss and hemiplegia on the opposite side of the body.

THE HYPOTHALAMUS

The hypothalamus lies within the diencephalon. It lies inferior to the thalamus and forms the floor and lateral walls of the third ventricle. The optic chiasma and the midbrain lie inferior to the hypothalamus. It is linked to the pituitary gland by the infundibulum, which is also referred to as the pituitary stalk (Figure 3.11).

It is made up of small nuclei, which are vital to survival and homeostatic regulation of the body. The masses of specialised nuclei grouped within each of these regions are discussed below. The whole hypothalamus weighs less than five grams, but despite its size, it controls much of the limbic, neuro-endocrine and autonomic nervous system functions of the body (Box 3.1) (see also Chapter 5).

Hypothalamic nuclei

The hypothalamus is divided into twelve areas of hypothalamic nuclei (preoptic, supraoptic, suprachiasmatic, paraventricular, dorsomedial, lateral, ventromedial, arcuate, posterior, mamillary, tuberomamillary and dorsal nuclei). Some of the functions of the hypothalamus are carried out by more than one of these nuclei, but others appear to function independently (Table 3.1).

Sensory input comes from many regions of the brain and other organs including the:

- Limbic system
- Thalamus
- Reticular formation
- Retina
- Olfactory pathways
- Sensory and nociceptive pathways
- Internal organs

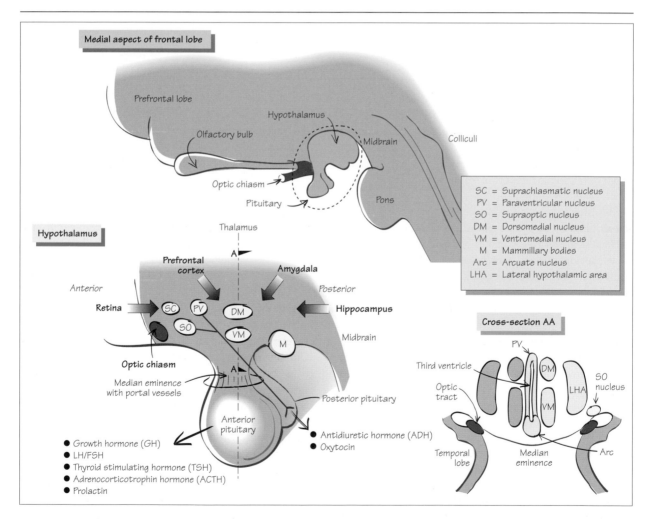

Figure 3.11 Medial aspect of frontal lobe and hypothalamus. Reproduced from Roger Barker and Stephen Barasi, *Neuroscience at a Glance 3e,* Wiley-Blackwell, with permission.

Table 3.1   Hypothalamic nuclei and their functions

Nucleus	Functions
Preoptic + medial preoptic	Sexual arousal (controls release of reproductive hormones from pituitary)
Suprachiasmatic	Circadian rhythms and the sleep/wake cycle
Paraventricular + supraoptic	Produces the hormones oxytocin (uterine contraction and milk production) and anti-diuretic hormone (ADH)
Posterior	Regulates sympathetic nervous system and body temperature through heat production and conservation (thermostat)
Lateral + ventromedial	Appetite, hunger and satiety. Lateral also regulates sympathetic nervous system
Anterior	Regulates parasympathetic activity and body temperature through heat loss regulation

The majority of the afferent input to the hypothalamus is from the limbic system and many connections to the hypothalamus are bi-directional, having a component of efferent pathways as well. The limbic system provides sensory input on hunger, thirst and sex drive and in response to this sensory input the hypothalamus regulates eating and drinking. The hypothalamus receives input from the retina, which enables it to influence the body's circadian rhythms and it also controls and regulates the two branches of the autonomic nervous system (see Chapter 6).

The hypothalamus also receives afferent nociceptive input from both the spinal cord and reticular formation. The hypothalamus responds by influencing neuroendocrine and cardiovascular responses, producing both autonomic and reflex responses to pain (Patestas and Gartner, 2006). At the same time collateral nociceptive branches from the spinal cord and trigeminal pain pathways link to the reticular formation, this results in the individual becoming more alert to the noxious stimulus and able to respond appropriately.

Hypothalamic hormones

The hypothalamus secretes two hormones: antidiuretic hormone (ADH/vasopressin) and oxytocin. The hormones are transported by the hypothalamic–hypophyseal tract to the posterior pituitary (neurohypophysis), from where they are released. The hypothalamus also produces releasing and inhibiting factors which stimulate or attenuate the synthesis and release of hormones from the anterior pituitary gland (adenohypophysis). The releasing factors are detailed in Table 3.2. Inhibiting factors produced by the hypothalamus are as follows:

- Somatostatin – inhibits growth hormone and thyroid stimulating hormone.
- Prolactin-inhibitory factor (dopamine) – inhibits prolactin.
- Melanocyte-stimulating hormone inhibitory factor – inhibits melanocyte stimulating hormone.

(Patestas and Gartner, 2006; Fitzgerald *et al.*, 2007)

PITUITARY GLAND (HYPOPHYSIS)

The pituitary gland or hypophysis is a small cherry like structure, which lies inferior to the hypothalamus and optic chiasma. It is joined to the hypothalamus by the infundibulum or pituitary stalk. The posterior part of the infundibulum contains the hypothalamo-hypophyseal tract. The pituitary gland is divided into two parts the anterior pituitary (adenohypophysis) and the posterior pituitary (neurohypophysis) (Figure 3.11).

Table 3.2 Hypothalamic releasing factors and pituitary hormones

Anterior Pituitary		
Releasing factor (from hypothalamus)	Hormone	Action
Somatotropin-releasing factor	Growth hormone (somatotropin)	Stimulates cell growth by stimulating protein synthesis, lipid mobilisation and catabolism
Corticotropin-releasing factor	Adrenocortiocotrophic hormone (ACTH)	Stimulates adrenal glands to secrete cortisol
TSH-releasing factor	Thyroid stimulating hormone (TSH)	Stimulates the thyroid gland to secrete thyroxine and triiodothyronine
Prolactin-releasing factor	Prolactin	Production of breast milk
Gonadotropin-releasing factor	Follicle-stimulating hormone (FSH)	In females stimulates immature Graafian follicles within the ovary to mature, culminating in ovulation.
Gonadotropin-releasing factor	Luteinising hormone (LH)	In males enhances spermatogenesis
Melanocyte stimulating hormone (MSH) releasing factor	Melanocyte stimulating hormone	Triggers ovulation in females and stimulates testosterone production in males
		Skin darkening
Posterior Pituitary		
Hormone	Action	
Anti-diuretic hormone (ADH)	Increases water re-absorption in the distal convoluted tubules resulting in more concentrated urine. Raises blood pressure by inducing some vasoconstriction	
Oxytocin	Stimulates uterine contractions	

Anterior pituitary

The adenohypophysis is stimulated to synthesise and secrete or inhibit hormones by releasing or inhibiting factors from the hypothalamus. The hormones which are secreted from the pituitary gland are detailed in Table 3.2.

Posterior pituitary

The posterior pituitary stores and releases the hormones ADH and oxytocin that have been secreted by the hypothalamus.

Pineal body

The pineal gland lies in the epithalamus, anterior to the superior colliculi in the midline of the brain. It becomes calcified after the onset of puberty and can easily be seen on skull x-rays, providing a useful landmark for clinicians looking for signs of a midline shift of the brain.

The pineal gland plays a role in regulating the onset of puberty and in the regulation of the body's circadian rhythms (menstrual, reproductive cycle, sleep cycles). Humans have a diurnal rhythm, which means that they have a period of wakefulness and a period of sleep in any twenty-four hour period (Waterhouse *et al.*, 1990), which is influenced by this small gland. The pineal gland, historically known as 'the third eye', is able to detect light on the retina of the eye and synthesises melatonin, a metabolite of 5-hydroxytryptamine (serotonin) in periods of darkness. The level of melatonin influences the sleep-wake cycle. People who wake up as soon as it is daylight appear to be particularly sensitive to retino-pineal stimulation (Wu and Swaab, 2005). Lack of melatonin can result in disruption of body functions that would normally be slowed down in the hours of darkness, such as bowel function and reduction in urinary output. Jet lag or shift work can affect the production of melatonin resulting in irritability, loss of appetite, and menstrual, sleep, or gastrointestinal disturbances.

BRAIN STEM

The brain stem consists of the midbrain, pons varolii (usually abbreviated to pons) and the medulla oblongata. Structures and tracts running throughout the brain stem are shown in Figure 3.12. They include:

- The reticular formation
- Afferent sensory pathways
- Efferent motor pathways

Midbrain

The midbrain develops from the mesencephalon, lies inferior to the diencephalon and superior to the pons and is divided into three parts. The midbrain provides the main connection between the cerebral hemispheres and lower parts of the brain. The dorsal part of the midbrain is known as the tectum which means 'roof' and incorporates the superior and inferior colliculi or corpora quadrigemina (four bumps on the surface) (Carlson, 2006). The superior colliculi are nuclei that process visual information from the eyes and control reflexes triggered by this information e.g. an object coming into your field of vision unexpectedly will

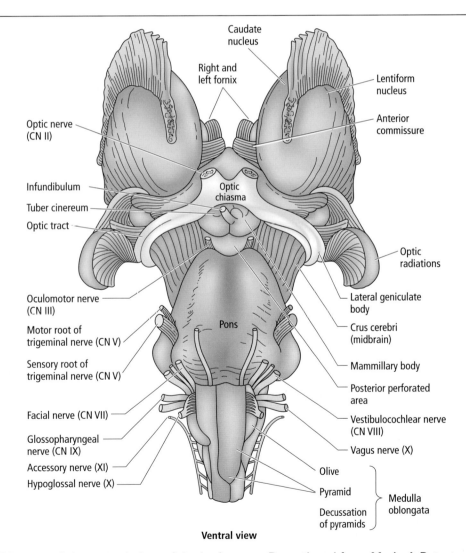

Ventral view

Figure 3.12 Diagram of the ventral view of the brain stem. Reproduced from Maria A Patestas and Leslie P Gartner, *A Textbook of Neuroanatomy*, Wiley-Blackwell, with permission.

cause a reflexive response (sudden movement of the eyes and turning of the head). The inferior colliculi process auditory information from the ears and control reflexes triggered by this information. The upper part of the midbrain contains the nuclei for the oculomotor (III) and trochlear (IV) cranial nerves (refer to Chapter 13). The cerebral aqueduct (aqueduct of Sylvius), runs through the centre of the midbrain connecting the third and fourth ventricles.

The cerebral peduncles form part of the anterior surface of the midbrain, these contain the large pyramidal (coritcospinal) motor tracts. The superior cerebellar peduncles connect the midbrain to the cerebellum (discussed under cerebellum). The substantia nigra sits within the base of the midbrain, alongside the cerebral peduncles (Crossman and Neary, 2005). The red nucleus lies within the midbrain, deep to the substantia nigra. It is a relay station for some descending motor tracts that affect upper limb position and tone. Efferent fibres descend from the red nucleus in the rubrospinal tract.

Pons varolii

The term pons means bridge and the pons links the midbrain and the medulla oblongata (Figure 3.12). Corticospinal tracts run through the pons and pontine nuclei relay information between the motor cortex and the cerebellum via the middle cerebellar peduncles. The pons contains several cranial nerve nuclei, namely, the trigeminal (V), abducens (VI), facial (VII) and acoustic (VIII) nerves, as well as containing the fourth ventricle. In addition the pons contains a portion of the reticular formation, including nuclei that are important in sleep and arousal (Carlson, 2006). The pneumotaxic and apneustic centres, which play a role in the control of breathing (refer to Chapter 15 for more detail) are also located within the pons.

Medulla oblongata

The medulla oblongata lies inferior to the pons and is the gateway to the brain for all afferent sensory fibres and efferent motor fibres exiting the brain. The medulla contains the lower portion of the fourth ventricle.

In the middle of the medulla there is an area that looks like pyramids macroscopically. It is here that decussation (crossing-over) of the cortico-spinal pathways as well as some sensory pathways occurs. As a result the right cerebral cortex regulates motor function on the left side of the body. The inferior cerebellar peduncles connect the medulla to the cerebellum (discussed under cerebellum). The inferior olivary nuclei relay motor information from the motor cortices to the cerebellum about voluntary motor commands as they are happening.

The nuclei of the glossopharyngeal nerve (IX), the vagus nerve (X) and the accessory nerve (XI) are found in the nucleus ambiguous of the medulla. The nucleus of the hypoglossal nerve (XII) lies inferior to the fourth ventricle in the posterior part of the medulla. The solitary nucleus and the solitary tract lie in the posterior part of the medulla. They receive visceral and gustatory information from the vagus, glossopharyngeal and facial nerves.

The medulla contains three vital reflex centres: the cardiac centre which regulates heart rate and force of contraction, the vasomotor centre which regulates the diameter of blood vessels, and the medullary rhythmicity centre which adjusts the basic rhythm of breathing. The former two are discussed in Chapter 14 and the latter in Chapter 15. The medulla also regulates other functions, including coughing, sneezing, vomiting and hiccoughing.

RETICULAR FORMATION AND RETICULAR ACTIVATING SYSTEM

Reticular formation

The reticular formation is a net-like structure of neurones, which is found throughout the brain stem. It is a complex structure that has neural connections with long axons that spread widely throughout the brain and connections from the spinal cord, through the brain stem, subthalamus, hypothalamus and thalamus to cerebral hemispheres. It forms the central core of grey matter within the brain stem, containing more than 100 nuclei (Patestas and Gartner, 2006) and the neurones are interlaced between ascending and descending pathways. The reticular formation receives input from sensory systems and plays a role in controlling skeletal muscle tone, attention, somatic and visceral sensation, autonomic (it forms part of the cardiovascular and respiratory centres of the pons and medulla) and endocrine functions, as well as influencing sleep, arousal and consciousness through the reticular activating system (Crossman and Neary, 2005; Patestas and Gartner, 2006).

Reticular activating system (RAS)

The reticular activating system (RAS) derives from the reticular formation, extends from the lower brain stem to the cerebral cortex and plays a key role in attention and consciousness. It can be divided into two portions: brain stem and thalamic (Crossman and Neary, 2005). The brain stem portion activates the whole brain to wakefulness, while the thalamic portion activates the cerebrum and cerebellum to achieve full consciousness and perception. The RAS may selectively activate specific areas of the cerebral cortex during mental activities, but is active and stimulates the cortex throughout the day as the cerebral cortex would be unable to maintain consciousness without this input (Patestas and Gartner, 2006).

The RAS is capable of rousing the individual independently of any external stimuli, but also receives input from auditory and other sensory pathways. It is the reticular activating system which arouses an individual to the sound of an alarm clock, fire alarm or a baby crying when they are asleep and will also wake an individual with pain.

Brain stem lesions

Lesions in the brain stem frequently result in profound coma and death, but where the lesion is unilateral and the patient survives, some or all of the following clinical signs and symptoms may present:

- Ipsilateral (same side as the lesion) cranial nerve deficits
- Contralateral (opposite side to the lesion) spastic hemi-plegia and sensory loss
- Ipsilateral loss of coordination

Consciousness, brain stem testing and brain stem death will be discussed in Chapter 8.

SUMMARY

Every nurse caring for patients with neurological conditions needs to have a working knowledge of neuroanatomy and physiology. Advances in imaging and neuroscience mean that our understanding of the inner workings of the brain continues to develop. With this knowledge nurses will be able to appreciate the pathophysiology affecting patients and the signs and symptoms that this produces.

REFERENCES

Barker RA, Barasi S (2008) *Neuroscience at a Glance* (3rd edition). Oxford: Blackwell Publishing.

Bliss TVP, Collingridge GL, Laroche S (2006) ZAP and ZIP, a story to forget. *Science* 313:1058–1059.

Carlson MR (2006) *Physiology of Behaviour* (9th edition). San Fransisco: Pearson Higher Education.

Clarke E, O'Malley CD (1996) *The Human Brain and Spinal Cord* (2nd edition). San Francisco: Norman Publishing.

Cohen H (1999) *Neuroscience for Rehabilitation* (2nd edition). Philadelphia: Lippincott.

Crossman AR, Neary D (2005) *Neuroanatomy* Edinburgh: Churchill Livingstone.

Edmans J, Champion A, Hill L *et al.* (eds) (2001) *Occupational Therapy and Stroke* London: Whurr.

Fitzgerald MJT, Gruener G, Mtui E (2007) *Clinical Neuroanatomy and Neuroscience* (5th edition). Philadelphia: Elsevier Saunders.

Ghadiali E (2004) *Agnosia: advances in clinical neuroscience and rehabilitation* Available from: http://www.acnr.co.uk/pdfs/volume4issue5/v4i5cognitive.pdf Accessed July 2010.

Lindsay KW, Bone I (2004) *Neurology and Neurosurgery Illustrated* (4th edition). Edinburgh: Churchill Livingstone.

Lerner A, Bagic A, Hanakawa T *et al.* (2008) Involvement of the insula and cingulate cortices in control and suppression of natural urges. *Cerebral Cortex* doi:10.1093/cercor/bhn074.

Patestas MA, Gartner LP (2006) *A Textbook of Neuroanatomy.* Oxford: Blackwell Publishing.

Sacktor TC (2008) *Protein kinase C ispzymes in long-term hippocampal synaptic plasticity and memory persistence.* Available from: http://www.downstate.edu/pharmacology/faculty/sacktor.html Accessed July 2010.

Waterhouse J, Minors D, Waterhouse M (1990) *Your Body Clock.* Oxford: Oxford University Press.

Whitlock JR, Heynen AJ, Shuler MG *et al.* (2006) Learning induces long-term potentiation in the hippocampus. *Science* 313:1094–1097.

Wu YH, Swaab DF (2005) The human pineal gland and melatonin in ageing and Alzheimer's disease *Journal of Pineal Research* 38(3):145–152.

4

The Spinal Cord

Maureen Coggrave

INTRODUCTION

The spinal cord is essential to the conscious and unconscious control of the body. It transmits and manages the flow of information continuously between the brain and the rest of the body, and facilitates homeostasis in response to changes within and outside the body. The significance the spinal cord is such that damage due to trauma or disease can result in catastrophic losses of function. For example, traumatic damage to the cervical spinal cord can result in the loss of voluntary movement and sensation in all limbs and the trunk; impaired respiratory function, sometimes requiring permanent mechanical ventilation; loss of normal bowel, bladder and sexual function and control; and the disruption of autonomic homeostatic mechanisms resulting in hypotension, spasticity and the risk of autonomic dysreflexia.

Knowledge of the complex anatomy and physiology of the spinal cord enables the health care professional to understand the outcomes of insults to this important part of the central nervous system, and to plan management and rehabilitation effectively.

GROSS ANATOMY

The spinal cord is a cylindrical structure forming a major part of the central nervous system. It is flattened posteriorly and anteriorly, and divided incompletely into right and left sides longitudinally by the anterior median fissure and posterior median sulcus (Figure 4.1).

Neuroscience Nursing: Evidence-Based Practice, 1st Edition.
Edited by Sue Woodward and Ann-Marie Mestecky
© 2011 Blackwell Publishing Ltd

The cord begins as a continuation of the medulla oblongata and extends through the foramen magnum of the occipital bone usually to the upper border of the second lumbar vertebra, though it may terminate between the twelfth thoracic vertebra and the third lumbar vertebra (Figure 4.2). In adults it measures approximately 2.5 cm in circumference, and 42–45 cm in length. It lies within the vertebral column and is protected by it and its associated ligaments and muscles, and by the meninges and cerebrospinal fluid.

The cord has two enlargements: the cervical enlargement which extends from the fourth cervical to first thoracic vertebra from which arise nerves supplying the arms (brachial plexus), and the lumbar enlargement extending from ninth to twelfth thoracic vertebrae (spinal segments L1–S3) from which arise nerves supplying the legs (lumbosacral plexus).

Below the lumbar enlargement the cord tapers and becomes conical; this area is called the conus medullaris. The cord is anchored to the base of the vertebral column by the filum terminale, a continuation of the pia mater composed of non-nervous tissue which extends from the conus medullaris and attaches to the coccyx.

The spinal cord does not grow to the same length as the vertebral column; it fills only the upper two thirds of the vertebral space. As a result spinal nerves from the lower parts of the cord travel downwards within the vertebral space before exiting. The nerves of the lumbar and sacral area resemble a horse's tail as they travel down through the vertebral space and are known as the cauda equina (Figure 4.2).

Nerves leave and enter the spinal cord in 31 pairs (Figure 4.2), one pair for each segment of the cord. The

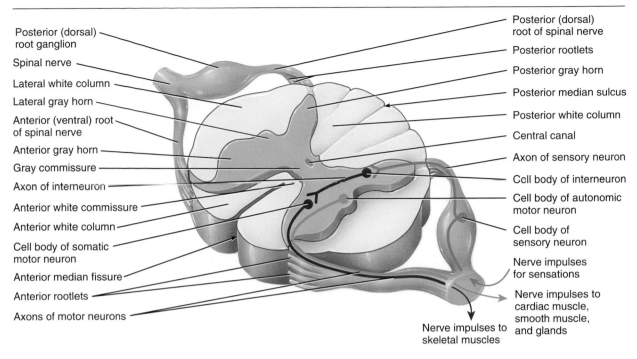

Figure 4.1 Internal anatomy of the spinal cord: the organisation of grey matter and white matter.
Reproduced from *Principles of Anatomy and Physiology 12e* by Gerard Tortora and Bryan Derrickson.
Copyright (2009, John Wiley & Sons). Reprinted with permission of John Wiley & Sons Inc.

anterior or ventral roots of each nerve carry motor fibres away from the cord. The posterior or dorsal roots carry sensory fibres into the cord. There are 8 cervical segments and nerve pairs, 12 thoracic, 5 lumbar, 5 sacral and 1 coccygeal. The term 'segment' defines the area of cord from which a pair of nerves arises. However there is no structural segmentation within the cord; it is continuous throughout its length and its structure changes only gradually. The spinal nerves are named and numbered according to where they emerge from the vertebral column. Cervical nerves 1–7 emerge above their respective vertebrae. Cervical 8 emerges between the seventh cervical and first thoracic vertebrae. The remaining nerves are named for the vertebra below which they emerge. Each muscle or group of muscles innervated from a spinal segment is called a myotome (see Figure 4.3).

Structure

The meninges which cover and protect the spinal cord, and the spinal blood supply are described in Chapter 2.

The spinal cord consists of grey and white matter (Figure 4.1). White matter is composed of sensory, motor and interneurone fibres and surrounds the grey matter. The grey matter forms a central H or butterfly shaped mass and is composed of the cell bodies of sensory neurones, lower motor neurones and interneurones, unmyelinated fibres and dendrites of interneurones and motor neurones lying at right angles to the long axis of the cord. The grey matter is rich in blood vessels and glial cells and is pierced by a central canal. This small channel extends from the fourth ventricle of the brain through the length of the cord and contains cerebrospinal fluid.

The grey matter

The grey matter is divided into regions called horns, linked together by the grey commisure. The horns of grey matter are named for their location:

- Anterior (ventral) grey horns – contain cell bodies of somatic motor nerves which carry impulses to skeletal muscles.
- Posterior (dorsal) grey horns – contain the cell bodies of somatic and autonomic sensory neurones.
- Lateral grey horns –contain cell bodies of autonomic motor neurones that regulate activity of smooth muscle, cardiac muscle and glands.

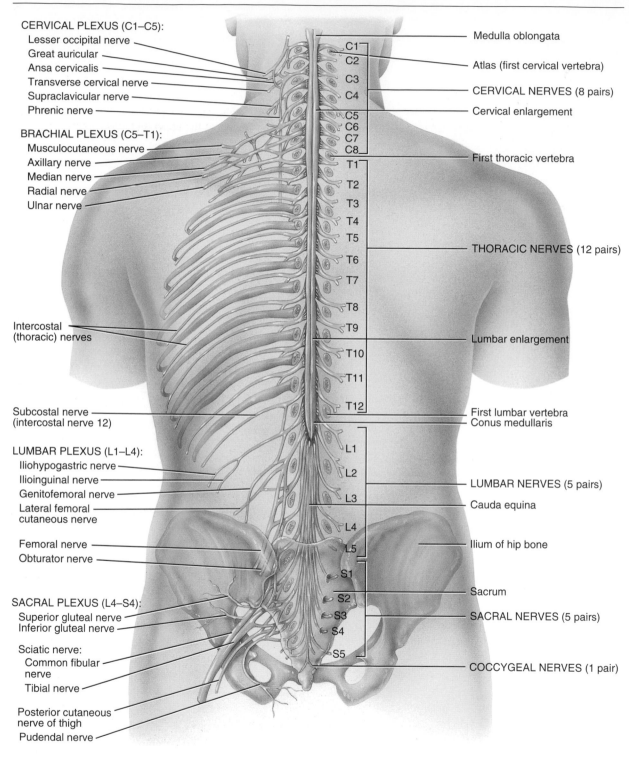

CERVICAL PLEXUS (C1–C5):
- Lesser occipital nerve
- Great auricular
- Ansa cervicalis
- Transverse cervical nerve
- Supraclavicular nerve
- Phrenic nerve

BRACHIAL PLEXUS (C5–T1):
- Musculocutaneous nerve
- Axillary nerve
- Median nerve
- Radial nerve
- Ulnar nerve

Intercostal (thoracic) nerves

Subcostal nerve (intercostal nerve 12)

LUMBAR PLEXUS (L1–L4):
- Iliohypogastric nerve
- Ilioinguinal nerve
- Genitofemoral nerve
- Lateral femoral cutaneous nerve

Femoral nerve
Obturator nerve

SACRAL PLEXUS (L4–S4):
- Superior gluteal nerve
- Inferior gluteal nerve

Sciatic nerve:
- Common fibular nerve
- Tibial nerve

Posterior cutaneous nerve of thigh
Pudendal nerve

Medulla oblongata
Atlas (first cervical vertebra)
CERVICAL NERVES (8 pairs)
Cervical enlargement
First thoracic vertebra
THORACIC NERVES (12 pairs)
Lumbar enlargement
First lumbar vertebra
Conus medullaris
LUMBAR NERVES (5 pairs)
Cauda equina
Ilium of hip bone
Sacrum
SACRAL NERVES (5 pairs)
COCCYGEAL NERVES (1 pair)

C1, C2, C3, C4, C5, C6, C7, C8
T1, T2, T3, T4, T5, T6, T7, T8, T9, T10, T11, T12
L1, L2, L3, L4, L5
S1, S2, S3, S4, S5

Posterior view of entire spinal cord and portions of spinal nerves

Figure 4.2 External anatomy of the spinal cord and the spinal nerves. Posterior view of entire spinal cord and portions of spinal nerves. Reproduced from *Principles of Anatomy and Physiology 12e* by Gerard Tortora and Bryan Derrickson. Copyright (2009, John Wiley & Sons). Reprinted with permission of John Wiley & Sons Inc.

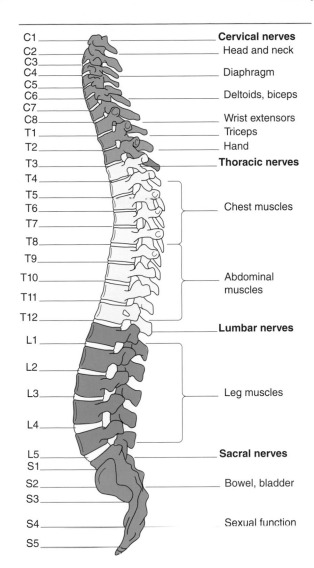

C1 ——— **Cervical nerves**
C2 ——— Head and neck
C3
C4 ——— Diaphragm
C5
C6 ——— Deltoids, biceps
C7
C8 ——— Wrist extensors
T1 ——— Triceps
T2 ——— Hand
T3 ——— **Thoracic nerves**
T4
T5
T6 ——— Chest muscles
T7
T8
T9
T10 ——— Abdominal
T11   muscles
T12
L1 ——— **Lumbar nerves**
L2
L3 ——— Leg muscles
L4
L5 ——— **Sacral nerves**
S1
S2 ——— Bowel, bladder
S3
S4 ——— Sexual function
S5

Figure 4.3 The spinal nerves and their areas of innervation. Reproduced from Peate I, Nair M, eds (2011) *Fundamentals of Anatomy and Physiology for Student Nurses.* Oxford: Blackwell Publishing Ltd., with permission.

The anterior and posterior horns run the entire length of the cord. The small lateral horns project from the cross bar portion of the H from the second thoracic segment to the first lumbar segment only. All neurones with their cell bodies lying in the grey matter are multipolar.

The anterior horns contain some interneurones but are mostly composed of the cell bodies of somatic motor neurones. The axons of these cells leave the spinal cord via the anterior roots to travel to their effector organs, the skeletal muscles. The varying size of the ventral horns at different levels of the spinal cord reflects the varying amounts of grey matter present; the cervical and lumbar enlargements are due to the greater number of motor axons needed to innervate the upper and lower limbs.

The lateral horn neurones are sympathetic autonomic motor neurones serving the visceral organs. Their axons leave the cord via the ventral roots. The ventral roots carry both somatic and autonomic motor neurones.

The dorsal horns are composed entirely of afferent interneurone fibres from peripheral visceral and somatic sensory receptors whose cell bodies are found in the dorsal root or spinal ganglion. After entering the spinal cord via the dorsal root these axons may follow a number of paths. Some immediately enter the posterior white matter of the cord and travel upwards to synapse at a higher cord level or in the brain. Others synapse with interneurones in the dorsal horn grey matter at their entry level.

Within the grey matter neurone cell bodies form functional groups called nuclei. Motor nuclei provide output to effector tissues via motor neurones. Sensory nuclei receive input from sensory receptors via sensory neurones.

White matter

The white matter is composed of myelinated and unmyelinated nerve fibres and is organised as three columns on each side of the spinal cord:

- The ventral column lies between the ventral grey horn and the anterior median fissure.
- The dorsal column lies between the dorsal grey horn and posterior median sulcus.
- The lateral column lies between the anterior and posterior columns.

The anterior white commissure lies in front of grey commissure, connecting the white matter on left and right sides of cord. Each column is divided into tracts. A tract, or funiculus, is a distinct bundles of nerve fibres with a common origin or destination carrying the same type of information (Figure 4.4). The fibres within each tract are uniform in their diameter, myelination and conduction speeds. Sensory ascending and motor descending tracts are continuous with motor and sensory tracts in the brain. Tracts are named for their location, origin and destination, and direction of transmission, e.g. the spinothalamic tract carrying impulses from the spinal cord to the thalamus, or the corticospinal tract carrying impulses from the cortex to the spinal cord.

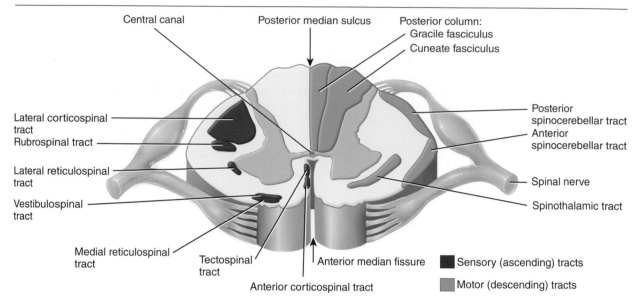

Figure 4.4 Locations of major sensory and motor tracts, shown in a transverse section of the spinal cord. Sensory tracts are indicated on one half, and motor tracts on the other half of the cord, but actually all tracts are present on both sides. Reproduced from *Principles of Anatomy and Physiology 12e* by Gerard Tortora and Bryan Derrickson. Copyright (2009, John Wiley & Sons). Reprinted with permission of John Wiley & Sons Inc.

Most tracts will cross from one side of the central nervous system to the other at some point in their journey; this may occur in the brain or the spinal cord. Most tracts include two or three neurones along their length. All tracts are paired, with one half of the pair on each side of the spinal cord or brain. The centres and tracts that link the brain and the rest of the body are called pathways.

Sensory ascending pathways carry impulses from the periphery to the brain. There are three main ascending pathways:

1. The nonspecific or anterolateral pathway carries impulses from many different sensory receptors to the brain stem. It is formed mostly of the lateral and anterior spinothalamic tracts. Decussation occurs in the spinal cord (Figure 4.5). It transmits temperature, pain and coarse touch which are not clearly localised.
2. The specific ascending pathway or the medial lemniscal system carries precise transmission of impulses from a single type of sensory receptor or a small number of related sensory receptors which can be precisely located on the body surface i.e. discriminative touch, vibration and proprioception. It is formed mostly by the dorsal column (fasciculus cuneatus and the fasciculus gracilis)

in the spinal cord and the medial lemniscus tracts which arise in the medulla and terminate in the thalamus, from where impulses are forwarded to the somatosensory cortex (Figure 4.6).

3. Anterior and posterior spinocerebellar tracts transmit impulses from muscle and tendon stretch to the cerebellum, where they are used to coordinate skeletal muscle activity. The pathways either do not decussate or do so twice so that information arises from and terminates on the same side.

Motor descending neurones carry impulses from the brain to peripheral effectors. There are two major descending pathways, the direct system and the indirect system:

• Direct. The pyramidal or corticospinal tract, arising mainly in the pyramidal neurones of the precentral gyrus, carries impulses through the brain without synapsing until they reach the spinal cord (Figure 4.7). Here they synapse with interneurones or ventral horn motor neurones. This direct pathway carries impulses for fast or skilled movement.
• Indirect. The extrapyramidal tract includes all pathways outside the pyramidal tract (see Chapter 3). The term

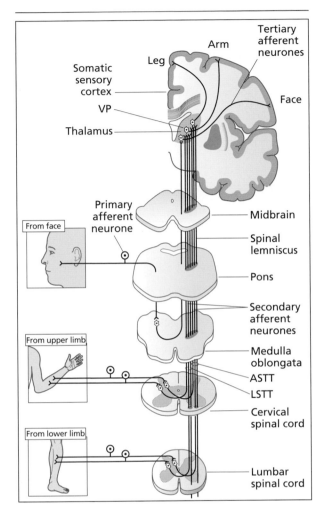

Figure 4.5 Sensation. The spinothalamic pathway. ASTT, anterior spinothalamic tract; LSTT, lateral spinothalamic tract; VP, ventral posterior nucleus of thalamus. Reproduced from C. Clarke *et al.*, *Neurology: A Queen Square Textbook*, Wiley-Blackwell, with permission.

tory stimuli. Table 4.1 provides more detail of each of the motor tracts.

PHYSIOLOGY

Unipolar sensory nerves enter the spinal cord through the posterior roots; their cell bodies form the posterior root ganglia. Sensory nerve tracts in the posterior horns carry afferent, ascending impulses generated by cutaneous receptors in the skin in response to pain, temperature, light touch and pressure, to the brain. A series of three neurones carry these impulses to the opposite cerebral hemisphere, where the sensation is perceived (Figure 4.5). Pain and temperature sensations travel to the cerebral hemispheres within the lateral spinothalamic tracts and cross over or decussate on entry to the cord. The anterior spinothalamic pathways carry information about pressure/coarse touch and itching and also decussate within a few segments of their entry to the spinal cord. The area of skin monitored for sensory information by a specific pair of spinal nerves is called a dermatome (Figure 4.8).

Sensory nerve tracts also carry vibration and light touch (discriminative, e.g. stereognosis) information from the skin, and 'conscious proprioception' from proprioceptors in tendons, joints and muscles. Proprioceptors provide information about balance and posture and the position of the body in space (see Chapter 11). It is referred to as conscious proprioception as this is information about position of which we are aware. These impulses may be carried by a three neurone pathway to the opposite cerebral hemisphere or by a two neurone pathway to the cerebral hemisphere on the same side. The impulses ascend within the dorsal or posterior columns (fasciculus cuneatus and the fasciculus gracilis) and decussate at the medulla (see Figure 4.6).

Motor nerve tracts carry efferent, descending impulses from the brain to the periphery resulting in contraction of voluntary, involuntary and cardiac muscle, and secretion by glands controlled by the autonomic system. Motor pathways use two neurones, upper motor neurones and lower motor neurones. The cell bodies of upper motor neurones supplying voluntary muscle lie in the motor cortex. The nerve fibres decussate in the medulla oblongata and, in the spinal cord, form the lateral corticospinal or pyramidal tracts (Figure 4.7).

The cell bodies of upper motor neurones supplying involuntary muscle lie in the mid-brain, brain stem, cerebellum or spinal cord. They form the extrapyramidal rubro-, reticulo-, tecto- and vestibulospinal tracts, some of which decussate while others do not. These tracts influence muscle activity that maintains posture and balance, coor-

extrapyramidal has been superceded as it is now known that pyramidal tract neurones project into and influence the activity of much of the extrapyramidal tract. The complex, multisynaptic pathway is now referred to as the indirect or multi-neuronal pathway, or by the individual tracts of which it is comprised. The reticulospinal and vestibulospinal tracts maintain balance by varying the tone of postural muscles. The rubrospinal tracts controls flexor muscles and the tectospinal tracts mediate head and eye movements in response to visual and audi-

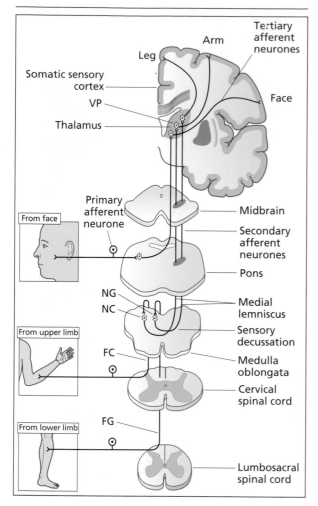

Figure 4.6 Sensation. The posterior column → medial lemniscal pathway. FC – fasciculus cuneatus; FG – fasciculus gracilis; NC – nucleus cuneatus; NG – nucleus gracilis; VP – ventral posterior lateral and ventral posterior medial nuclei of thalamus. Reproduced from C. Clarke *et al.*, *Neurology: A Queen Square Textbook*, Wiley-Blackwell, with permission.

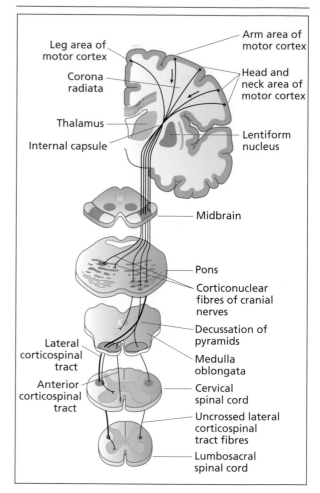

Figure 4.7 Corticospinal (pyramidal) motor pathways. Reproduced from C. Clarke *et al.*, *Neurology: A Queen Square Textbook*, Wiley-Blackwell, with permission.

dinates voluntary muscle movement and maintains muscle tone. Table 4.1 provides a summary of the main motor spinal tracts.

All upper motor fibres synapse with lower motor neurones in the anterior horns of grey matter. The lower motor nerve fibre leaves the spinal cord in the anterior root, joining with afferent sensory fibres to form a spinal nerve (Figure 4.9) which passes through an intervertebral foramen. The cell bodies of the lower motor neurones

are stimulated and inhibited by various upper motor neurones and interneurones within the spinal cord which work together to produce smooth coordinated movement. The lower motor neurone forms the final common pathway for conduction of impulses to voluntary, skeletal muscle.

Spinal nerves

The spinal nerves form part of the peripheral nervous system, carrying communication between the periphery of the body and the central nervous system. After leaving the cord, spinal nerves branch extensively to innervate the

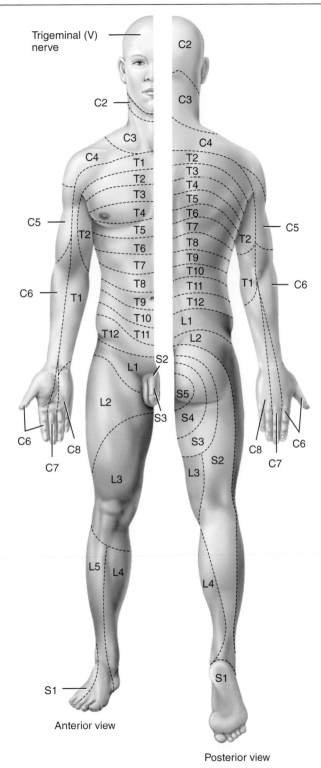

Trigeminal (V) nerve

Anterior view

Posterior view

Figure 4.8 Distribution of dermatomes. Reproduced from *Principles of Anatomy and Physiology 12e* by Gerard Tortora and Bryan Derrickson. Copyright (2009, John Wiley & Sons). Reprinted with permission of John Wiley & Sons Inc.

Table 4.1 Descending motor tracts of the spinal cord.

Tract	Column	Origin	Point of decussation	Termination	Function
Direct (pyramidal)					
Lateral corticospinal	Lateral	Pyramidal neurones of the motor cortex	Medulla Spinal cord	Synapse with lower motor neurones and interneurones in the ventral horns	Voluntary motor movement
Anterior corticospinal	Anterior	Pyramidal neurones of the motor cortex		As above	Voluntary motor movement
Indirect (extrapyramidal)					
Tectospinal	Anterior	Midbrain and pons	Spinal cord	Synapse with ventral horn interneurones influencing motor neurones	Coordinated reflex movement of the head, neck, upper limbs and eyes in response to visual stimuli
Vestibulospinal	Anterior	Brain stem	No decussation	Synapse with ventral horn lower motor neurones and interneurones influencing motor neurones	Maintenance of standing or moving posture and balance by regulation of muscle tone, innervation of ipsilateral limb and trunk extensor muscles and innervation of muscles moving the head
Rubrospinal	Lateral	Midbrain and pons	Brain stem	As above	Control of skilled muscle movement, muscle tone and posture
Reticulospinal (anterior, medial and lateral)	Anterior	Brain stem – pons and medulla, crossed and uncrossed fibres	Medullocervical junction	As above	Muscle tone, visceral motor functions, unskilled movements

trunk and limbs. As previously stated, each spinal nerve has two points of attachment to the spinal cord, a posterior or dorsal root containing sensory nerve fibres and an anterior or ventral root containing motor fibres. The two roots combine into a single mixed nerve. Immediately after exiting the intervertebral foramina the spinal nerves branch into three strands or rami (Figure 4.9):

- The ventral rami supply the anterior and lateral aspects of the body. In some areas the anterior rami unite almost immediately to form plexuses before going on to supply skin, bone, muscles and joints.
- The posterior rami pass backwards and supply the skin and muscles of a small area of the back of the head, neck and trunk.

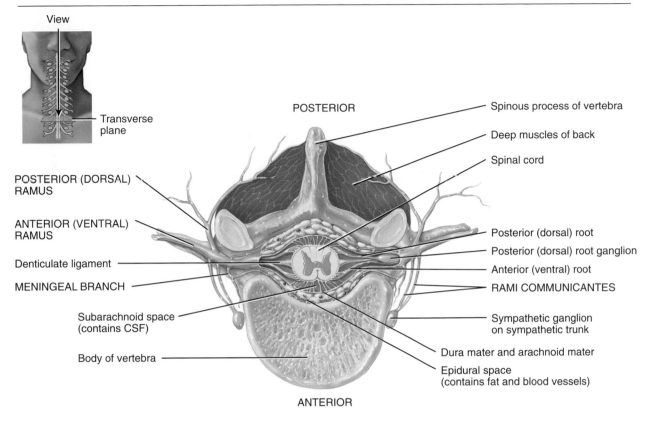

View

Transverse plane

POSTERIOR

Spinous process of vertebra

Deep muscles of back

Spinal cord

POSTERIOR (DORSAL) RAMUS

ANTERIOR (VENTRAL) RAMUS

Denticulate ligament

MENINGEAL BRANCH

Subarachnoid space (contains CSF)

Body of vertebra

Posterior (dorsal) root

Posterior (dorsal) root ganglion

Anterior (ventral) root

RAMI COMMUNICANTES

Sympathetic ganglion on sympathetic trunk

Dura mater and arachnoid mater

Epidural space (contains fat and blood vessels)

ANTERIOR

Figure 4.9 Branches of a typical spinal nerve, shown in transverse section through the thoracic portion of the spinal cord. Reproduced from *Principles of Anatomy and Physiology 12e* by Gerard Tortora and Bryan Derrickson. Copyright (2009, John Wiley & Sons). Reprinted with permission of John Wiley & Sons Inc.

- The rami communicantes arise from the base of the ventral rami in the thoracic and upper part of the lumbar spine and carry sympathetic fibres. The rami communicantes have two branches, white and grey (see Chapter 5).

A plexus is a complex interwoven network of nerves serving a particular area of the body, i.e. the cervical plexus serving the neck, the brachial plexus serving the upper limbs and the lumbosacral plexus serving the lower limbs (Figure 4.2). During the developmental process small skeletal muscles innervated by different ventral rami fuse to become larger muscles but retain their original sensory and motor nerve innervation. This results in convergence of the ventral rami of adjacent spinal nerves; their fibres blend to produce a series of compound nerve trunks which make up a plexus.

The cervical plexus is composed of the first five cervical spinal nerves. It is found at the level of the first to fourth cervical vertebrae, covered by muscle. This plexus includes the phrenic nerve which originates from C3, 4 and 5 and passes through the chest to supply the diaphragm, a key respiratory muscle. Other component nerves innervate the neck muscles and the skin of the neck and upper chest.

The brachial plexus is composed of rami from spinal nerves C5–8 and T1. This plexus supplies the skin and muscles of the arms, shoulders and some chest muscles. It lies in the neck, shoulder and axilla. It gives rise to five large nerves:

- The axillary nerve supplies the deltoid muscle, shoulder joint and overlying skin
- The radial nerve, the largest branch, supplies the triceps, wrist extensors, and the skin of the thumb, first two fingers and the lateral half of the third finger
- The musculocutaneous nerve supplies the muscles of the upper arm and the skin of the forearm.

- The median nerve supplies the muscles of the front of the forearm, and the small muscles and skin of the thumb, first two fingers and lateral half of the third finger
- The ulnar nerve supplies the muscles of the ulnar aspect of the forearm and the palm of the hand, and the skin of the little finger and medial aspect of the third finger

The lumbar plexus is comprised of the ventral rami of the first three and part of the fourth lumbar nerves. It lies in front of the transverse processes and behind the psoas muscle. The main branches are:

- The iliohypogastric, ilioinguinal and genitofemoral nerves supplies the muscles and skin of the lower abdomen, upper and medial aspects of the thigh and the inguinal region
- The lateral cutaneous nerve of the thigh supplies the skin of the lateral aspect of the thigh
- The femoral nerve divides into cutaneous and muscular branches to supply the skin and muscles of the front of the thigh. The saphenous nerve is another branch of the femoral nerve and it supplies the medial aspect of the leg, ankle and foot
- The obturator nerve supplies the adductor muscles of the thigh and skin of the medial aspect of the thigh down to the knee
- The lumbosacral trunk travels to the pelvis and combines with the sacral plexus

The sacral plexus is comprised of the ventral rami of L4 to S3. It lies in the posterior wall of the pelvic cavity. The main branches are:

- The sciatic nerve, the largest in the body, supplies the hamstring muscles and then divides into:
  - the tibial nerve, serving the muscles and skin of the posterior lower leg, sole of foot and toes, the heel, the lateral aspect of the ankle and some of the dorsum of the foot
  - and the common peroneal nerve, serving the skin and muscles of the anterior aspect of the lower leg and dorsum of the foot and toes.
- The pudendal nerve (S2–4) serves the external anal and urethral sphincters and surrounding skin

The coccygeal plexus is small, comprised of part of the fourth and fifth sacral and coccygeal nerves, and serves the skin around the coccyx and anal area.

The spinal nerves T2 to T11 do not form plexuses. They are called the intercostal nerves and pass directly to the structures they innervate. These include the intercostal muscles between the ribs, abdominal muscles and the skin of the chest and back.

Reflex activity in the spinal cord

A reflex is an immediate, rapid, involuntary, predictable sequence of motor actions that occur in response to a particular sensory stimulus. Reflexes may be inborn, such as the protective withdrawal reflexes seen in response to pain. These reflexes result from connections made between neurones during development. The reflex response of limb withdrawal may be so rapid that perception of pain in the cerebrum and withdrawal of affected part may be simultaneous. Reflexes may also be acquired, i.e. a driver responds to a danger on the road ahead by putting a foot on the break. These complex motor patterns are rapid and automatic, but learned rather than innate and are strengthened by repetition. Most reflexes, acquired or innate can be modified or suppressed.

A reflex arc is the pathway followed by the nerve impulse that produces a reflex action. The building blocks of a reflex arc are:

1. Sensory receptor – a specialised cell or the distal end of a sensory nerve
2. Sensory neurone along which the impulse is conducted into the central nervous system grey matter. In some reflex pathways branches of the neurone also relay impulses to the brain, bringing conscious awareness of the reflex action
3. Interneurone (association neurone) in the spinal cord to carry the impulse from sensory to motor neurones
4. Motor neurone to carry impulse to the effector organ that will respond
5. Effector organ – this may be a muscle or gland

If the effector is skeletal muscle, then the reflex is a somatic reflex. If the effector is smooth muscle, cardiac muscle or a gland it is a visceral (autonomic) reflex (autonomic reflexes are presented in Chapter 5).

Reflexes may be monosynaptic or polysynaptic. In monosynaptic reflex arcs, such as the stretch reflex, the response is very rapid. Polysynaptic reflexes produce more complex responses; the interneurones of the arc may synapse with nerves serving several different muscle groups.

The patellar stretch reflex is an example of a monosynaptic reflex arc (Figure 4.10). Stretch reflexes cause muscles to contract in response to stretching of the muscle (increase in muscle length) providing automatic regulation

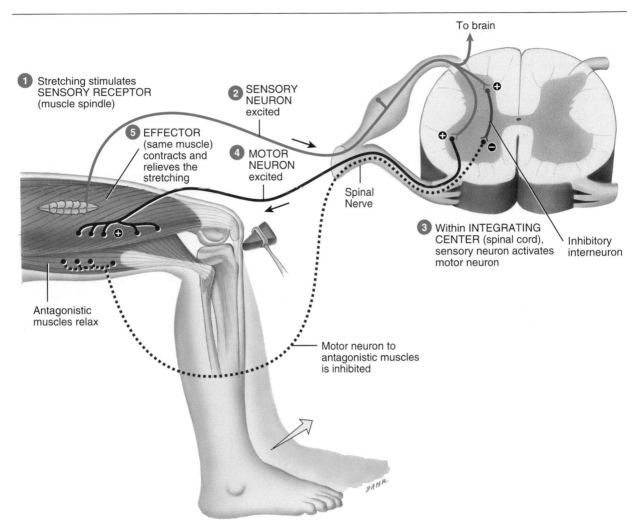

Figure 4.10 Stretch reflex. This monosynaptic reflex arc has only one synapse in the CNS – between a single sensory neurone and a single motor neurone. A polysynaptic reflex arc to antagonistic muscles that includes two synapses in the CNS and one interneurone is also illustrated. Plus signs (+) indicate excitatory synapses; the minus sign (–) indicates an inhibitory synapse. Reproduced from *Principles of Anatomy and Physiology 12e* by Gerard Tortora and Bryan Derrickson. Copyright (2009, John Wiley & Sons). Reprinted with permission of John Wiley & Sons Inc.

of muscle length. The patellar stretch reflex is triggered by the stretching of sensory nerve endings in the patellar tendon and the thigh muscle spindles by a hammer strike to the tendon. An impulse travels along the sensory nerve into the spinal cord to the cell body of the lower motor neurone in the anterior grey horn. The ensuing motor impulse results in sudden contraction of the thigh muscle and an extension of the limb with a forward kick of the foot (Figure 4.10). Loss of this reflex indicates damage somewhere in the reflex pathway and, because it is easy to provoke, this reflex is commonly used as a diagnostic tool.

Although this simple stretch reflex is monosynaptic, a polysynaptic reflex arc is triggered simultaneously to relax the antagonistic muscles in an example of reciprocal inhibition (Figure 4.10). Reciprocal inhibition serves to stop the antagonistic muscles resisting the shortening of the stretched muscle which is essential for smooth coordinated movements. While the stretch reflex occurs automatically, higher centres in the brain are informed through ascending tracts of the degree of muscle stretch (length) and can subsequently modify the muscle activity through descending fibres.

Superficial reflexes are elicited by stroking of the skin with an object. The plantar response or Babinski response is the most clinically important. Stroking the sole of the foot should produce a plantar reflex (curling of the toes), but if there is damage to the motor cortex or the corticospinal tracts an abnormal response will occur causing the big toe to extend and the other toes to spread out laterally (Babinski response or sign). This response is present in infants but disappears as inhibitory descending motor pathways develop, if the higher centres or the descending pathways are damaged, the Babinski sign re-emerges. Superficial reflexes depend both on functional reflex arcs and on corticospinal tracts. The Babinski sign indicates an upper motor lesion.

Voluntary and reflex activities are often combined in stereotyped motor patterns embedded in the spinal cord. While walking, running or jumping are voluntary movements, assistance with coordination and control of muscle tone is maintained by spinal reflexes under the control of higher centres via the rubro-, reticulo-, vestibulo-, and tectospinal tracts.

Removal of descending input from the brain, as in spinal cord injury or stroke results in increased tone or spasticity of muscles below the level of injury. Damage to the reflex pathway, as in cauda equina injury, results in loss of muscle tone or flaccidity of muscles below the level of injury.

SUMMARY

This chapter has described the complex structure of the spinal cord and shown how its functions are both integral and essential to the somatic and autonomic functions of the body. Even a rudimentary understanding of the structure and functions of this intricate part of the central nervous system will aid the understanding of conditions such as traumatic spinal cord injury, cauda equina syndrome, poliomyelitis and motor neurone disease, facilitating and promoting patient education and care.

SUGGESTED READING

Marieb EM (2004) *Human Anatomy and Physiology.* (6th edition). San Francisco, Ca: Pearson Benjamin Cummings.

Martini FH (2006) *Fundamentals of Anatomy and Physiology.* (7th edition). San Francisco, Ca: Pearson Benjamin Cummings.

Tortora GJ, Derrickson SR (2006) *Principles of Anatomy and Physiology.* (11th edition). Hoboken, NJ: John Wiley and Sons.

5

The Autonomic Nervous System

Chris Brunker

INTRODUCTION

The autonomic nervous system (ANS) controls the body's vital functions, maintaining homeostasis in ever-changing circumstances. It performs this complex and unceasing task largely unnoticed by the conscious brain (hence *autonomic*, or self-regulating). This chapter describes the contrasting anatomy of the two branches of the system before considering the neurotransmitters and receptors that are specific to the ANS. The sensory components are discussed, followed by a review of autonomic function. The final section looks at the integration of the entire system and its relationship with consciousness.

The ANS maintains the balance of the body's vital functions in response to changing demands from within the body itself and from the outside environment. The ANS has two divisions that contrast in their anatomy, physiology and effects on the body. The *sympathetic* division comprises nerve pathways originating in the thoracic and upper lumbar spinal cord; its overall effect is to increase bodily activity and it is crucial in organising responses to stress and threat. The *parasympathetic* division comprises nerve pathways originating both in the brain and in the sacral levels of the spinal cord; it functions most effectively with the body at rest, and it is vital in controlling digestion and excretion. Many of the body's organs are innervated by both branches, typically with opposing effects.

ANATOMY

As discussed in Chapter 4 the somatic nervous system is made up of nerves projecting from the central nervous system (brain or spinal cord) all the way to the target organ, i.e. skeletal muscle and skin. The autonomic nervous system is different: myelinated neurones emerging from the brain or spinal cord (pre-ganglionic neurones), terminate in ganglia (*sing.* ganglion), small clumps of neuronal junctions, where they synapse with other, non-myelinated neurones (post-ganglionic neurones) whose axons project to the target organs.

The sympathetic division

The cell bodies of pre-ganglionic neurones of the sympathetic division of the ANS originate in the lateral horns of the spinal cord at levels T1 down to L2, and it is therefore sometimes called the *thoracolumbar* division (Figure 5.1). Neurones emerge from the cord along the anterior roots of the spinal nerves, branching off to enter the paravertebral chain as the white communicating rami.

The paravertebral chain

The biggest group of ganglia in the ANS is the paravertebral chain, a major part of the sympathetic division. The paravertebral chain is also known as the sympathetic chain or sympathetic trunk ganglia. Pairs of ganglia lie either side of the spinal column, each linked above and below to form a belt running from C1 down to the coccyx. There are three pairs of cervical ganglia, twelve thoracic, five lumbar, five sacral and a single fused ganglion (the *ganglion impar*, or unpaired ganglion) at the coccyx, linking right and left sides. Post-ganglionic neurones leave the chain, either to join the spinal nerves (via the grey com-

Neuroscience Nursing: Evidence-Based Practice, 1st Edition.
Edited by Sue Woodward and Ann-Marie Mestecky
© 2011 Blackwell Publishing Ltd

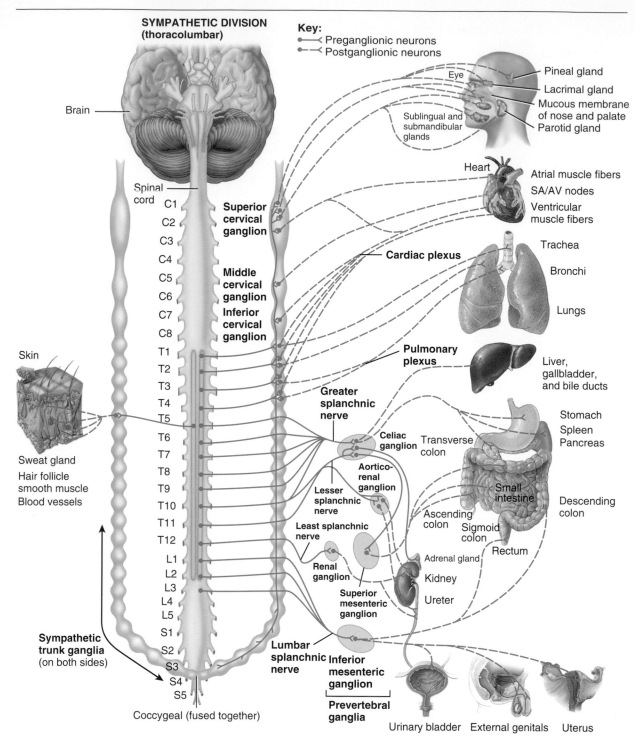

Figure 5.1 Structure of the sympathetic division of the autonomic nervous system. Solid lines represent pre-ganglionic axons; dashed lines represent post-ganglionic axons. Although the innervated structures are shown for only one side of the body for diagrammatic purposes, the sympathetic division actually innervates tissues and organs on both sides. Reproduced from *Principles of Anatomy and Physiology 12e* by Gerard Tortora and Bryan Derrickson. Copyright (2009, John Wiley & Sons). Reprinted with permission of John Wiley & Sons Inc.

municating ramus), or to project to their target organs by other routes.

Post-ganglionic fibres leave the *superior cervical ganglia* (sited at the level of C2 and C3 vertebrae) and form a network around the carotid, scalp and facial arteries to reach the dilator muscles of the irises, the sweat glands and erector pili muscles of the head and face, the salivary glands and the small vessels of the scalp, face, mouth and nose. Post-ganglionic fibres also leave the ganglia to join spinal nerves C1 to C4 while another group forms the *superior cardiac nerve*, part of the nervous supply to the heart.

The *middle cervical ganglia* lie either side of the C6 vertebra. These smaller ganglia project post-ganglionic fibres out to spinal nerves C5 to C7 as well as to the oesophagus, trachea and thyroid, along with the *middle cardiac nerve* to the heart.

Neurones from the *inferior cervical ganglia* form the *inferior cardiac nerve* as well as feeding into spinal nerves C7 to T1. Post-ganglionic neurones from ganglia below the inferior cervical ganglia down to the T5 level project to the lungs and bronchi.

Prevertebral ganglia

Pre-ganglionic neurones entering the paravertebral chain from T5 to L2 do not synapse within the chain but pass through it, synapsing in the *prevertebral ganglia* lying along the anterior surface of the aorta and its main branches (Figure 5.1). Neurones from T5 to T9 form the *greater splanchnic nerve* which itself divides. One portion synapses in the *celiac ganglion*, whose post-synaptic neurones supply the stomach, small bowel, liver, kidney and spleen.

Another portion of the greater splanchnic nerve reaches the *superior mesenteric ganglion* which is also supplied by neurones from T10 and T11 forming the *lesser splanchnic nerve*. Post-synaptic neurones from the superior mesenteric ganglion project to the small bowel and colon. A separate branch of the greater splanchnic nerve projects to the adrenal medulla. There is no synapse here; instead, stimulation of the medulla prompts it to release the neurotransmitters adrenaline and noradrenaline directly into the bloodstream.

Neurones from T12 (the *least* or *lowest splanchnic nerve*) and L1, L2 (the *lumbar splanchnic nerve*) synapse in the *inferior mesenteric ganglion*. From here post-ganglionic neurones project to the distal colon, the bladder, rectum and reproductive organs.

The parasympathetic division

The pre-ganglionic neurones of the parasympathetic division of the ANS derive from two distinct regions of the central nervous system: the brain, via cranial nerves III, VII, IX and X; and the spinal cord at segments S2, S3 and S4. The parasympathetic branch is sometimes called the *cranio-sacral* division (Figure 5.2). Parasympathetic neurones synapse in or close to their target organs, so the pre-ganglionic segments are relatively long compared with their sympathetic counterparts.

Pre-ganglionic fibres in cranial nerve III (oculomotor) synapse in the *ciliary ganglion* at the rear of the orbit of the eye. Post-ganglionic neurones project to the smooth muscles of the lens (the ciliary muscles) and the constrictor muscles of the iris.

Neurones from cranial nerve VII (facial) synapse in the *pterygo-palatine ganglion* which lies between the sphenoid and palatine bones of the base of the skull. From here, post-ganglionic neurones innervate the lacrimal glands and the nasal and oral mucosa. Other fibres from the VIIth nerve synapse in the *sub-mandibular ganglion* before projecting the short distance to the sub-mandibular and sub-lingual salivary glands.

Parasympathetic elements of cranial nerve IX (glossopharyngeal) make a brief journey to the *otic ganglion* near the foramen ovale at the base of the skull. Post-ganglionic neurones reach the parotid salivary glands.

If the parasympathetic elements of nerves III, VII and IX are limited in reach and focused in scope, the same cannot be said for cranial nerve X (vagus) which makes up about 80% of the parasympathetic branch. Pre-ganglionic neurones originate in the dorsal motor nucleus of the medulla and project down the thorax and abdomen before synapsing in ganglia in the walls of the target organs (*intramural ganglia*). Post-ganglionic axons are correspondingly short. Vagal parasympathetic ganglia lie in the walls of the bronchi, heart, stomach, pancreas, liver, gall-bladder, small bowel and the transverse and descending colon.

Pre-ganglionic neurones of the sacral component of the parasympathetic division emerge from the spinal cord at segments S2, S3 and S4 to form the *pelvic splanchnic nerves*. These spread to ganglia in the walls of the ascending and sigmoid colon, rectum, ureters, bladder and the genitalia.

Dual innervation

The sympathetic and parasympathetic branches of the ANS are anatomically distinct and in many cases neurones of each division reach the same organ by markedly different routes: note how the eye is innervated by the parasympathetic (a short route via cranial nerve III) and the sympathetic (a lengthier journey from the thoracic spine

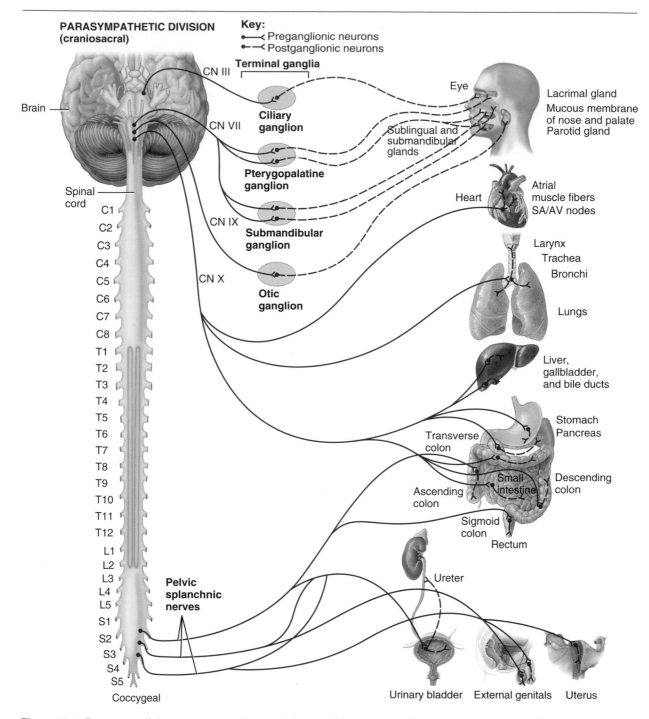

Figure 5.2 Structure of the parasympathetic division of the autonomic nervous system. Solid lines represent pre-ganglionic axons; dashed lines represent post-ganglionic axons. Although the innervated structures are shown for only one side of the body for diagrammatic purposes, the parasympathetic division actually innervates tissues and organs on both sides. Reproduced from *Principles of Anatomy and Physiology 12e* by Gerard Tortora and Bryan Derrickson. Copyright (2009, John Wiley & Sons). Reprinted with permission of John Wiley & Sons Inc.

Table 5.1 Summary of the distribution and effects of the autonomic nervous system.

Effector organ	Sympathetic innervation	Receptor	Sympathetic effect	Parasympathetic innervation (muscarinic receptors)	Parasympathetic effect
Eye Radial muscle of iris	Superior cervical ganglia	Alpha-1	Pupil dilation	None	Nil
Circular muscle of iris	None	None	Nil	Cranial III	Pupil constriction
Ciliary muscle	Superior cervical ganglia	Beta-2	Relaxation (accommodation to distance vision)	Cranial III	Contraction (accommodation to near vision)
Lacrimal glands			Nil	Cranial VII	Increased tear secretion
Skin Erector pili muscles	Superior cervical ganglia, spinal nerves	Alpha-1	Erection	None	Nil
Sweat glands	Superior cervical ganglia, spinal nerves	Muscarinic ACh	Increased secretion	None	Nil
Sweat glands (palms and soles)	Spinal nerves	Alpha-1	Increased secretion	None	Nil
Gastro-intestinal tract Salivary glands	Superior cervical ganglia	Alpha-1	Constriction of vessels: reduced salivation	Cranial VII and IX	Increased salivation
Cardiac sphincter	Celiac ganglion	Alpha-1	Constriction of sphincter	Cranial X	Relaxation of sphincter
Stomach	Celiac ganglion	Alpha-2, Beta-2	Reduced motility and secretion	Cranial X	Increased motility and secretion
Pyloric sphincter	Celiac ganglion	Alpha-1	Constriction of sphincter	Cranial X	Relaxation of sphincter
Liver	Celiac ganglion	Alpha-1, Beta-2	Conversion of glycogen to glucose. Decreased bile production.	Cranial X	Conversion of glucose to glycogen. Increased bile production

Continued

Table 5.1 *Continued*

Effector organ	Sympathetic innervation	Receptor	Sympathetic effect	Parasympathetic innervation (muscarinic receptors)	Parasympathetic effect
Gall-bladder	Celiac ganglion	Alpha-1	Relaxation – reduced bile secretion	Cranial X	Contraction – increased bile secretion
Small intestine	Celiac ganglion, superior mesenteric ganglion	Alpha-2, Beta-2	Reduced motility and secretion	Cranial X	Increased motility and secretion
Colon	Superior mesenteric ganglion, inferior mesenteric ganglion	Alpha-2, Beta-2	Reduced motility and secretion	Cranial X, Sacral 2,3,4	Increased motility and secretion
Rectum	Inferior mesenteric ganglion	Alpha-1	Constriction	Sacral 2,3,4	Relaxation
Renal system					
Kidney	Celiac ganglion	Beta-1	Increased rennin secretion – reduced urine formation	None	Nil
Anterior pituitary	Superior cervical ganglia	Beta-1	Increased anti-diuretic hormone, reduced urine formation	None	Nil
Bladder	Inferior mesenteric ganglion	Alpha-1, Beta-2	Relaxation of bladder, constriction of sphincter	Sacral 2,3,4	Contraction of bladder and relaxation of sphincter
Respiratory system					
Oral and nasal mucosa	Superior cervical ganglia	Alpha-1	Increased secretion	None	Nil
Trachea and bronchi	Paravertebral ganglia T1–4	Beta-2	Dilation of airways	Cranial X	Constriction of airways
Adrenal medullae	T5 (unganglionated)	Nicotinic ACh	Secretion of adrenaline and noradrenaline into circulation	None	Nil

Organ	Tissue	Sympathetic ganglia	Receptor	Sympathetic effect	Parasympathetic source	Parasympathetic effect
Heart	Sino-atrial/atrio-ventricular nodes	Superior cervical ganglia	Beta-1	Increased excitability: raised heart rate	Cranial X	Reduced excitability: lowered heart rate
	Cardiac muscle	Superior, middle and inferior cervical ganglia	Beta-1	Increased rate and force of contraction	Cranial X	Restricted innervation of ventricular muscle – little effect
Blood vessels (arteriolar smooth muscle)	Cardiac	Superior, middle and inferior cervical ganglia	Alpha-1, Alpha-2 Beta-2	Constriction Dilation	None	Nil
	Lung	Paravertebral ganglia T1–4	Alpha-1 Beta-2	Constriction Dilation	None	Nil
	Renal	Celiac ganglion	Alpha-1	Constriction	None	Nil
	GI tract	Ganglia as above	Alpha-1 Beta-2	Constriction Dilation	None	Nil
	Skeletal muscle	Spinal nerves	Alpha-1 Beta-2 Muscarinic ACh	Constriction Dilation Dilation	None	Nil
	Skin	Superior cervical ganglia, spinal nerves	Alpha-1 Muscarinic ACh	Constriction Dilation	None	Nil
Adipose tissue		Spinal nerves	Alpha-1, Beta-1, Beta-3	Lipolysis, release of fatty acids into circulation	None	Nil
Reproductive system	Male	Inferior mesenteric ganglion	Alpha-1	Ejaculation	S2,3,4	Erection, production of semen
	Female				S2,3,4	Erection of clitoris, increased secretion

up into the skull). A review of Table 5.1 shows that many organs are innervated by only one branch, notably blood vessels and sweat glands (sympathetic only). Even when the same organ is innervated by both branches, different structures are often involved: the pupil is dilated by sympathetic control of the radial muscle of the iris, but constricted by parasympathetic control of the circular muscle. However many organs, particularly the thoracic and abdominal viscera, receive *dual innervation* by both branches via *autonomic plexuses*, i.e. bundles of nerve fibres from different sources forming networks in the region of their target organs.

The *cardiac plexus* is formed of sympathetic fibres from the superior, middle and inferior cervical ganglia (the superior, middle and inferior cardiac nerves) bundled with fibres from cranial nerve X, all bound for the heart. Similarly the *pulmonary plexus* supplying the trachea, bronchi and lungs is a bundle of sympathetic axons from the paravertebral chain along with parasympathetic fibres, again from cranial nerve X. The *oesophageal plexus*, with fibres from a branch of the greater splanchnic nerve and cranial nerve X, supplies the oesophagus and stomach.

The abdominal viscera are innervated via a series of autonomic plexuses named for the major arteries nearby. The *celiac plexus* (also called the *solar plexus* because of its star-like appearance) consists of the sympathetic prevertebral celiac ganglia and parasympathetic fibres (again cranial nerve X) distributed to the stomach, liver, gall bladder, pancreas, kidneys, and spleen. Sympathetic fibres to the adrenal medullae also pass through the celiac plexus.

The *superior mesenteric plexus* and *inferior mesenteric plexus* innervate the small intestine and colon. The *hypogastric plexus* and *pelvic plexus* are made up of fibres from the lowest and lumbar splanchnic nerves (sympathetic) and pelvic splanchnic nerves (parasympathetic) and supply the colon, bladder and genitalia.

NEUROTRANSMITTERS AND RECEPTORS

Nerve impulse transmission in the ANS involves two synapses: the first between two neurones (pre-ganglionic and post-ganglionic) at a ganglion, and the second between the post-ganglionic neurone and the effector organ (Figure 5.3). The exception to this is transmission to the adrenal medulla, which has a single neurone and synapse.

Autonomic synapses are of two main types. All ganglionic synapses and all parasympathetic post-ganglionic synapses are *cholinergic*, using acetylcholine (Figure 5.3). Post-ganglionic sympathetic synapses are *adrenergic*, using adrenaline or noradrenaline (except for sweat glands and some blood vessels in skeletal muscle, whose post-

ganglionic supply is cholinergic). The effect of the neurotransmitters on the target organ (excitation or inhibition) depends on specific receptors in the synaptic membrane of the target organ.

Cholinergic receptors: nicotinic and muscarinic

Cholinergic receptors are of two types, both of which bind acetylcholine but each of which also binds a specific chemical not naturally present in the synapse: n*icotinic* receptors which bind nicotine and m*uscarinic* receptors which bind muscarine (a toxin found in certain mushrooms and rotting fish).

Nicotinic receptors are *excitatory* in their effect on the post-synaptic cell and are found at all ganglionic synapses. Muscarinic receptors are found at all synapses between parasympathetic post-ganglionic neurones and their effector organs; these synapses may be *inhibitory* or excitatory in effect depending on the tissue concerned: in the sino-atrial node of the heart, for example, they inhibit activity; in the wall of the bowel they excite it. Muscarinic receptors are also found at the synapse between sweat glands and their sympathetic neurones; these synapses are excitatory.

Adrenergic transmission

With the exception of innervations to sweat glands and some blood vessels in skeletal muscle, sympathetic post-ganglionic transmission is *adrenergic*, using the catecholamines noradrenaline and adrenaline. There are two mechanisms at work: specific neurone-to-organ synapses with noradrenaline as the transmitter, and the diffuse effects of the adrenaline and noradrenaline released into the bloodstream by the adrenal medulla.

Sympathetic post-ganglionic synapses: noradrenaline

Sympathetic post-ganglionic synapses are structurally very different from cholinergic synapses or the neuromuscular junctions of the somatic nervous system (presented in Chapter 4). Rather than a distinct synaptic bulb, the axon forms chains of *varicosities*, bulges along the nerve fibre that resemble beads on a string. These chains branch to form a net spread around or close to the surface of the effector organ. There are no specialised post-synaptic membranes either: rather the surface of the effector cell is dotted with receptors.

Each axonal varicosity stores noradrenaline in vesicles to prevent it being degraded by the monoamine oxidase attached to mitochondria. Depolarisation of the axon prompts the vesicles to bind with the wall of the varicosity and expel the noradrenaline which binds with specific receptor sites. Noradrenaline has a longer duration of

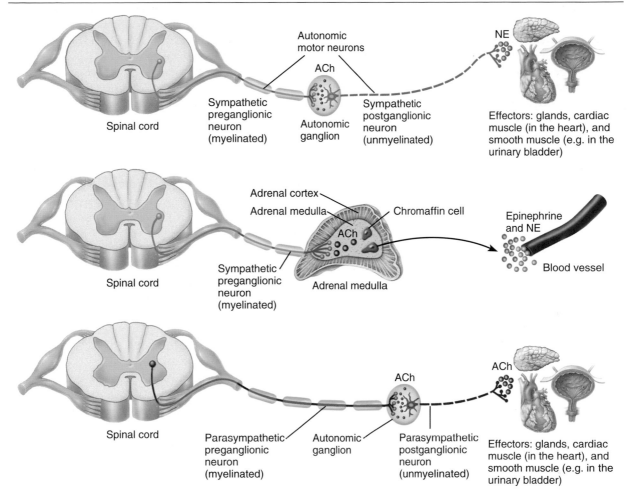

Figure 5.3 Motor neurone pathways in the autonomic nervous system (ANS). Note that autonomic motor neurones release either acetylcholine (ACh) or noradrenaline (NE): somatic motor neurones release ACh. Reproduced from *Principles of Anatomy and Physiology 12e* by Gerard Tortora and Bryan Derrickson. Copyright (2009, John Wiley & Sons). Reprinted with permission of John Wiley & Sons Inc.

effect than acetylcholine and will continue working on the effector cell until removed, either actively by the axon (which re-captures up to 80%), or by diffusing away into surrounding tissues where it is inactivated by an enzyme called catechyl-O-methyl transferase (COMT).

The adrenal medulla and sympathetic stimulation

The ardrenal medulla is directly innervated by a branch of the greater splanchnic nerve (spinal levels T5 to T9). When stimulated in response to stress it releases adrenaline and noradrenaline (in proportions of about 3 to 1 respectively) directly into the bloodstream. As these catecholamines circulate they enhance the effect of noradrenaline released by post-ganglionic sympathetic fibres but also act on tissues that have the required receptors but no direct sympathetic innervation. Levels of adrenaline and noradrenaline remain raised for some time; the adrenal aspect of the sympathetic system, therefore, has widespread, unspecific and prolonged effects on the body.

Adrenergic receptors

There are two classes of adrenergic receptor: *alpha* and *beta*. Noradrenaline affects alpha receptors more strongly than beta receptors while adrenaline (the dominant circulating catecholamine) activates both alpha and beta. Each class has distinct sub-types.

Alpha-1 receptors respond predominantly to noradrenaline with an excitatory effect. As the noradrenaline binds to the receptor, it triggers the liberation of calcium (a positive ion) bound in the effector cell's endoplasmic reticulum. This increases the electrical potential of the cell, bringing it closer to the depolarisation threshold. Alpha-1 receptors are found in the smooth muscle walls of the blood vessels of the skin, mucosal membranes, salivary glands, kidneys and abdominal digestive organs as well as in the radial muscles in the iris of the eye, sphincters of the digestive tract and the bladder and the vas deferens of the male reproductive system. Activation of alpha-1 receptors prompts the contraction of these muscles. Alpha-1 receptors activate sweat glands on the palms of the hands and soles of the feet (all other sweat glands have cholinergic transmission). Refer to Table 5.1 for the specific effect on each effector organ.

Alpha-2 receptors are found at some neuro-muscular and neuro-glandular junctions including the smooth musle walls of some blood vessels and the insulin-secreting Beta cells of the pancreas. They respond to noradrenaline by reducing levels of cyclic AMP (cAMP) inside the effector cell, and so inhibiting their function.

Beta receptors are *metabotropic receptors* (refer to Chapter 1); their activation prompts a rise in the levels of cyclic-AMP (cAMP), a second messenger, inside the cell. **Beta-1** receptors are found on the cells of the sino-atrial and atrio-ventricular nodes of the heart, and in the cardiac muscle. They respond to noradrenaline secreted locally by sympathetic fibres from the paravertebral ganglia but more strongly to circulating adrenaline released from adrenal medullae. The effect is excitatory, increasing the rate and force of cardiac contraction. Beta-1 receptors are also found in the posterior pituitary gland where they stimulate the release of anti-diuretic hormone and in the kidneys where they prompt the secretion of renin which in turn initiates the release of angiotensin II. Both ADH and angiotensin II are powerful vasoconstrictors and serve to raise the blood pressure as well as reducing urinary volume.

Beta-2 receptors are inhibitory in effect, relaxing muscle. They are found in the walls of the trachea and bronchi and in blood vessels feeding the heart, liver and skeletal muscle. They are also present in the muscles of stomach, intestines and bladder wall as well as the ciliary muscle of the eye.

Beta-3 receptors are found in adipose tissue. They promote the breakdown of triglycerides into fatty acids which are then available for use by other organs.

Sympathetic cholinergic transmission

Some sympathetic fibres use acetylcholine as a neurotransmitter. Sweat glands (except those of the palms and soles)

are innervated in this way, as are small blood vessels of the skeletal muscle. Sympathetic release of noradrenaline tends to constrict blood vessels (which have no parasympathetic innervation), so these specific sympathetic terminals release acetylcholine to maintain dilation in muscles needed for increased physical activity while the noradrenaline constricts vessels supplying less immediately relevant tissues.

Sympathetic transmission with nitric oxide

Nitric oxide is used as transmitter by some sympathetic neurones innervating blood vessels to skeletal muscles and to the brain. These synapses dilate the vessels affected, preserving blood supply to key regions in conditions of stress.

THE SENSORY COMPONENT

The autonomic nervous system requires a constant flow of information about the body's organs if it is to fulfil its goal of maintaining homeostasis under ever-changing conditions.

Autonomic reflexes

Autonomic, or *visceral*, reflexes begin with information provided by sensory receptors in the tissues. These are sensitive to specific stimuli, i.e. the degree of stretch in the muscle wall of a blood vessel, or irritation of the internal surface of the trachea and so on. Autonomic sensory neurones form elements of spinal and cranial nerves, relaying stimuli back to the central nervous system. Here, within the brain or spinal cord, sensory neurones synapse with *interneurones* which in turn synapse with the preganglionic neurones of the motor component of the system. Autonomic reflexes are invariably *polysynaptic* unlike the single-synapse arcs of simpler somatic reflexes.

Parasympathetic reflexes tend to be localised and specific, such as the triggering of the sequence of muscle contractions involved in swallowing when food or liquid is moved from the mouth into the pharynx. Sympathetic reflexes, on the other hand, tend to be more generalised in their effect, such as the generalised vasoconstriction provoked by a sudden fall in arterial blood pressure.

THE ENTERIC NERVOUS SYSTEM

Some autonomic reflex arcs do not involve the central nervous system at all. Instead, sensory neurones link to motor neurones via interneurones in autonomic ganglia within the tissues. A huge number of these *short reflex* arcs are concentrated in the gastro-intestinal system in the *myenteric* and *sub-mucous* plexuses within the gut wall.

Much of the neural control of digestion is managed by these plexuses responding to local sensory information, ensuring regular smooth peristalsis and release of digestive secretions as food passes through. Many authorities have treated this *enteric nervous system* as an independent entity, and it has been estimated that there are as many interneurones in the gut as in the spinal cord, leading some to refer to a 'gut-brain'.

VISCERAL PAIN

Autonomic pain neurones run along the same pathways as somatic pain fibres; this may explain why the brain interprets damage to visceral organs as pain in the somatic distribution involved. For example, cardiac ischaemia is signalled by autonomic neurones along spinal nerves T1 to T5 on the left side of the body. The patient experiences pain in the upper left chest wall extending down the medial aspect of the left arm – the pain is *referred* to cutaneous areas innervated by spinal nerves T1–5.

THE FUNCTION OF THE AUTONOMIC NERVOUS SYSTEM

The major concerns of the parasympathetic branch are digestion and excretion. These are relatively slow processes involving chains of inter-dependent events. The processing of food from salivation to defecation requires the co-ordination of mechanical and chemical functions in an orderly sequence along a journey of several metres and many hours. Parasympathetic activity needs to be localised and specific: at any given moment different tissues need to be stimulated or inhibited as part of an overall pattern. Not all parasympathetic-controlled functions are slow (coughing and pupil constriction are relatively rapid reactions) but they are limited in scope to the tissues concerned: sudden bright light doesn't make you want to defecate.

The principle work of the sympathetic division, by contrast, is the management of the cardiovascular system. This requires constant fine tuning across the entire body simultaneously: not just heart rate and contractility, but the dilation and constriction of vessels both at tissue level and globally to match blood supply to changing demand. In an emergency, when the body needs to move suddenly and fast, the cardiovascular system must respond at once, increasing cardiac output and directing maximum blood supply to the immediately vital organs (brain, heart and lungs, liver and skeletal muscle). Sympathetic activity, therefore, must be rapid and global in its effects when necessary. Much of the work of the sympathetic division is specific to the organs that need to be mobilised: turning

the lights off does not make you break into a sweat. The influence of the adrenal medullae in times of stress is powerful. High levels of circulating adrenal hormones stimulate tissues around the entire body and the effects endure for some time after the threat recedes; consider the time it takes for your heart to stop pounding after you have been startled.

Some functions are controlled by both systems in rough equilibrium, notably the eye's accommodation to light and distance, but dual innervation typically does not imply symmetry of control. The sympathetic division has strong input into the gastro-intestinal system from salivary glands to rectum but it only exercises control in an emergency and does so in typically sympathetic fashion: it inhibits motility, constricts sphincters and reduces blood supply all along the tract so as to direct blood flow to more immediately useful tissues. The sophisticated management needed to digest food is the work of the parasympathetic branch.

The integrated working of the ANS

Autonomic reflexes are limited in scope and central control is needed if the body is to respond to the range of challenges posed by differing circumstances. Specific autonomic functions have specialised control centres in the medulla oblongata such as heart rate and blood vessel diameter. These centres are in turn regulated by the hypothalamus (See Chapter 3).

THE HYPOTHALAMUS

Along with the range of functions discussed in Chapter 3, the hypothalamus also controls and balances the two branches of the ANS. Parasympathetic control is centred in the *anterior hypothalamic nucleus*, sympathetic control in the *posterior hypothalamic nucleus*. The constant fine tuning of impulses within each branch of the ANS and the balancing of the entire system is a constant and dynamic process referred to as autonomic tone (refer to Chapter 14 for more detail).

THE AUTONOMIC NERVOUS SYSTEM, EMOTION AND THE CONSCIOUS BRAIN

The word *autonomic* was derived from *autonomy* (self-regulation) specifically as a term for the elements of the nervous system which maintain bodily functions without the need for conscious control. As a description, however, the word is a little misleading. Some autonomic functions do go on entirely hidden from the conscious brain: we are unaware of and cannot control the dilation and constriction of blood vessels, for example. Other autonomic effects are more apparent, particularly when the responses are strong: we are all aware when our heart pounds with excitement. Some autonomic responses demand conscious attention: the release of the sphincters of the bladder and rectum, for example, ordinarily requires voluntary control. In such cases, signals between autonomic nerves and the cerebral cortex are relayed by the hypothalamus.

In the same way emotion, memory and conscious thought can affect the ANS. This is not surprising: the sympathetic branch in particular is geared to respond to stress and there is a huge evolutionary advantage in being physiologically ready before a threat becomes an attack. Such responses can involve aspects of the limbic system (fear, aggression and sexual attraction), sensory perception, memory and higher intellectual processing, which all feed into the hypothalamus and prompt responses from the ANS. Sympathetic activity, for example, can be triggered by fears that are innate (unknown dark spaces, heights and so on) or learned (an unattended bag on a train) or even by fears that the subject knows are fictional: a good writer of thrillers can make your hair stand on end even as you sit quietly reading in your perfectly safe home. Parasympathetic responses of salivation and a rumbling stomach can be reliably set off by watching cookery programmes on television, a fact cheerfully exploited by advertisers. The human nervous system is far too complex and subtle to be neatly parcelled up into its component parts.

SUMMARY

The complex network of cells and fibres of the two divisions of the ANS act to control the activities of the body's vital functions. By triggering a host of physiological responses, which are highly coordinated, the sympathetic division acts to prepare the body for activity (fight, flight or fright), whereas the parasympathetic division generally promotes restorative functions (rest and digest).

SUGGESTED READING

Kandel ER, Schwartz JH, Jessell TM (2000) *Principles of Neural Science* (4th edition). New York City, NY: McGraw Hill.

Marieb EM (2004) *Human Anatomy and Physiology* (6th edition). San Francisco, Ca: Pearson Benjamin Cummings.

Martini FH (2006) *Fundamentals of Anatomy and Physiology* (7th edition). San Francisco, Ca: Pearson Benjamin Cummings.

Tortora GJ, Derrickson SR (2006) *Principles of Anatomy and Physiology* (11th edition). Hoboken, NJ: John Wiley and Sons.

Turlough Fitzgerald MJ, Gruener G, Mtui E (2007) *Clinical Neuroanatomy and Neuroscience* (5th edition). Edinburgh: Elsevier Saunders.

6
Intracranial Physiology

Ann-Marie Mestecky

INTRODUCTION

An understanding of the concepts of intracranial pressure (ICP) and the physiology of cerebral blood flow is a prerequisite for managing patients with raised ICP. This knowledge is fundamental for practitioners to be able to make informed decisions about the nursing management of the patient and to make sense of the management strategies and interventions that are employed to treat raised ICP. This chapter reviews the concepts of ICP and describes the factors that regulate cerebral blood flow (CBF); raised ICP and its management are presented in Chapter 7.

INTRACRANIAL PRESSURE

The intracranial vault is almost filled to capacity with three components. The brain parenchyma (tissue) contributes approximately 83% of the intracranial volume, cerebral blood volume (CBV) accounts for 8% and the third component, cerebrospinal fluid (CSF), makes up the remaining 9%. All three components are largely incompressible given that they are essentially fluid, therefore there is only minimal capacity for expansion of the contents within the bony encasement of the skull. Brain parenchyma is made up of 75% water, most of which is contained within cells (intracellular) and the remainder bathes the cells of the brain (interstitial fluid).

The pressure exerted by the three components within the rigid confines of the skull is referred to as the intracranial pressure. Normal values for ICP are between 0 and 10 mmHg, with an upper limit of 15 mmHg in the supine position. ICP is not a static pressure; minor rhythmic changes occur with arterial pulsations (a rise during systole and fall during diastole) and with the respiratory cycle. The cerebral venous system is continuous with the central venous system so any increase in the pressure of the central veins, e.g. due to coughing or valsalva manoeuvre, will impede venous outflow from the intracranial vault with a subsequent transient increase in ICP. In health these elevations are transient and are easily accommodated.

Monro–Kellie hypothesis

An important concept for understanding how changes in the volume of the components of the intracranial vault are accommodated within the rigid confines of the skull is the modified Monro–Kellie hypothesis.

As the three components are contained within the rigid skull, the total volume of the intracranial contents remains fairly constant. Total volume is expressed as:

$$Vc = Vbrain + Vblood + VCSF$$

V – volume; Vc – total volume of the intracranial contents

The Monro–Kellie hypothesis states that if there is an increase in the volume of one of the intracranial components, there must be a compensatory equal decrease in one or both of the other two components to maintain homeostasis of ICP. If the components are unable to compensate for the increase in volume then ICP will increase. This is one of the fundamental principles on which treatment of raised ICP is based.

Compensatory mechanisms to maintain normal ICP

The compensatory mechanisms that maintain normal ICP when increases in the total volume of intracranial contents (Vc) occur are:

Neuroscience Nursing: Evidence-Based Practice, 1st Edition.
Edited by Sue Woodward and Ann-Marie Mestecky
© 2011 Blackwell Publishing Ltd

- Displacement of CSF from the intracranial cavity to the low pressure distensible space that surrounds the base of the spinal cord, called the lumbar theca. It is the distension of the spinal dura mater that allows for greater volumes of CSF to be accommodated in this space.
- Compression of the thinned walled veins by the increasing intracranial volume which displaces the cerebral venous blood out of the intracranial cavity more rapidly.
- An increase in the rate of CSF absorption, but only when ICP rises. This is because absorption of CSF is dependent on the pressure gradient between the CSF in the subarachnoid space and the venous blood in the venous sinuses; the higher the CSF pressure the greater the rate of CSF absorption into the venous sinuses.

In addition to these compensatory mechanisms, the brain parenchyma is capable of considerable distortion to accommodate increases in volume. This will be discussed in detail in Chapter 7. The compensatory mechanisms occur much more readily when there is a slow increase in the volume, e.g. a brain tumour. When acute increases in volume occur, as is the case with a significant acute intracranial haemorrhage, the brain is less able to compensate for the changes by the mechanisms outlined above and ICP can rapidly increase.

Pressure/volume curve

The pressure volume curve (also referred to as the elastance curve) illustrates the effect of changes in volume on ICP and the compensatory reserve (see Figure 6.1). The horizontal axis represents the volume and the vertical axis the ICP. As the volume increases the compensatory mechanisms maintain normal ICP by displacing CSF and

venous blood from the intracranial cavity. This is illustrated on the pressure/volume curve as point a. At this point the system is described as being *compliant* or as having good compensatory reserve i.e. it can accommodate changes in volume without resultant changes in ICP. As volume increases the system becomes less compliant even though normal ICP is maintained. However a continued increase in volume will eventually exhaust the compensatory mechanisms. Point b (the steepest part of the curve) depicts low compensatory reserve; therefore any further increases in volume above this point will result in an exponential increase in ICP. At this critical point the compliance is said to be low.

Elastance is another term used to describe the effects of changes in volume on ICP; it describes the stiffness of the system (or the resistance offered to the addition of volume). Compliance is the inverse of elastance i.e. when compliance is high elastance is low and vice versa. ICP monitoring can provide information about how compliant the system is (see Chapter 7). The speed at which the critical level is reached (point b) depends on the cause of the increase in volume and varies between individuals. The critical level is often reached almost immediately following acute changes in volume, e.g. following a large intracranial bleed.

CEREBRAL BLOOD FLOW (CBF)

The brain weighs approximately 2–3% of the body weight, so a person weighing 70 kg would have a brain weighing approximately 1.5 kg. This small organ requires a disproportionate cerebral blood flow (CBF) for its size; it receives blood at a rate of 50 to 60 ml/100 g/min, i.e. approximately 750 ml/min which is 15% of the cardiac output. The brain is dependent on this apparently luxurious blood flow to maintain its high requirements for oxygen and glucose.

Factors that regulate CBF are:

- Cerebral metabolism
- Cerebral perfusion pressure and autoregulation
- Chemoregulation

(Ropper *et al.*, 2004)

Cerebral metabolism and CBF

In the absence of cerebral insult, local CBF will either increase or decrease to match the regional metabolic demands of the brain. Some areas of the brain are more metabolically active than others and therefore the CBF is unequally distributed within the brain. The metabolic

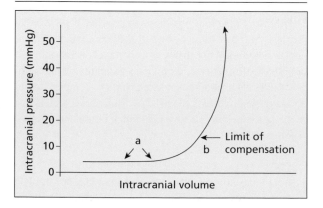

Figure 6.1 Pressure/volume curve.

activity of the cerebral cortex by far exceeds that of the underlying white matter and during normal neuronal activity regional increases in CBF occur. The changes in CBF to match activity is termed coupling of flow and metabolism (Bowler 2000). This coupling ensures that the functioning tissue receives additional oxygen and glucose to meet its metabolic requirements. The coupling is almost immediate; within seconds there is increased CBF to meet increased local metabolic demands (Barzo, 1996). Functional neuroimaging demonstrates the coupling of flow to metabolism.

The mechanism by which matching of CBF to local metabolic needs occurs is not completely understood. Increases in the concentration of hydrogen (H^+), potassium (K^+) and adenosine in the interstitial fluid of brain tissue are thought to be the main mediators of vasodilation and increased CBF (Barzo, 1996). The vasodilators neuronal nitric oxide and endothelial nitric oxide (NO) have also been found to be crucial in flow–metabolism coupling (Bowler, 2000). Following cerebral injury uncoupling may occur, i.e. the CBF may not increase to match the metabolic demands of the brain which predisposes the brain to ischaemic damage (Ropper *et al.*, 2004).

Cerebral perfusion pressure (CPP) and autoregulation

Cerebral perfusion pressure is the result of the pressure gradient driving blood through the cerebral circulation, i.e. arterial blood pressure driving blood to the brain against the opposing pressure within the cranial vault (ICP):

$$CPP = \text{mean arterial pressure (MAP)} - ICP$$

In health, MAP is in the region of 70–100 mmHg and ICP is between 5 and 10 mmHg. Therefore in a healthy person CPP would be approximately:

$$MAP\,(70 \text{ to } 100 \text{ mmHg}) - ICP\,(5 \text{ to } 10 \text{ mmHg})$$
$$= CPP \text{ between 60 and 95 mmHg.}$$

Globally, CBF remains fairly constant despite changes in CPP between the levels of 50 mmHg and 140 mmHg (Figure 6.2). This constant state is made possible by a mechanism termed autoregulation. As changes occur in systemic blood pressure the cerebral vessels respond by dilating or constricting to maintain a constant CBF. For example, if CPP was to fall from 70 to 60 mmHg due to a drop in systemic blood pressure, cerebral vessels, particularly the microcirculation, will dilate to decrease vascular resistance and thereby keep CBF unchanged. Conversely,

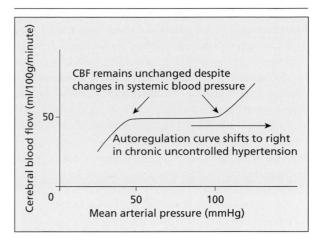

Figure 6.2 Changes in cerebral blood flow (CBF) in response to changes in cerebral perfusion pressure (CPP).

if there is an increase in systemic blood pressure, the cerebral vasculature would respond by constricting thereby maintaining a constant CBF. Under these circumstances there is a direct correlation between CBF and CBV. CBF and CBV will both increase as vessels dilate and both decrease as vessels constrict (Warlow *et al.*, 2007).

However there are limits to autoregulation. If CPP falls below 50 mmHg, due either to an increase in ICP or a fall in MAP, or if CPP rises to >140 mmHg, the cerebral vessels lose their ability to autoregulate. The CBF therefore becomes passively dependent on CPP and, hence, on MAP (Ropper *et al.*, 2004). Loss of autoregulation therefore leaves the brain unprotected against potentially harmful effects of changes in blood pressure (see Figure 6.2).

Autoregulation can become impaired due to any of the following:

- Any major cerebral insult
- Ischaemic stroke
- Cerebral vasospasm
- Acute hypertension

Autoregulation functions at higher levels than normal for people with long-term hypertension, so for example it may be that autoregulation will be intact with CPPs up to 160 mmHg. The lower level will also be higher so in such cases the values shift to the right of normal. Therefore hypertensive patients with raised ICP will require higher CPPs to perfuse cerebral tissue.

The mechanism by which autoregulation occurs is most likely to be a direct response of the smooth muscle of the blood vessels to the changes in intra-arterial pressure (myogenic theory). Decreased intraluminal pressure results in dilation of the smooth muscle to maintain a constant CBF; conversely increased intraluminal pressure brings about vasoconstriction to maintain the steady CBF. Autoregulation involves global slower control of CBF whereas coupling of flow to metabolism is important in regional rapid control and occurs almost immediately in response to increased metabolic demands (Bowler, 2000; Ropper *et al.*, 2004).

Chemoregulation

Chemoregulation refers to the response of cerebral vessels and consequently of CBF to changes in arterial carbon dioxide partial pressure ($PaCO_2$) and oxygen partial pressure (PaO_2). $PaCO_2$ is a powerful regulator of CBF. Increases in $PaCO_2$ cause the cerebral vessels to dilate with a subsequent increase in CBF. The increase in flow is a protective mechanism to remove metabolic waste more efficiently from the brain.

Figure 6.3 illustrates the relationship between $PaCO_2$ and CBF. There is a linear relationship between $PaCO_2$ and CBF between 4 kPa and 9 kPa. Within this range the CBF increases by approximately 8–16 ml per 100 g/min for every 1 kPa increase in $PaCO_2$. This equates to an increase in CBF of approximately 240 ml/min for each 1 kPa increase in the $PaCO_2$. A $PaCO_2$ of less than 4 kPa (hypocapnia) causes the cerebral vessels to vasoconstrict with a subsequent decrease in CBF.

CBF is only minimally affected by arterial oxygen levels (PaO_2), that is, until the pressure falls to hypoxic levels (8 kPa). Once arterial oxygen pressure reaches this level there is a significant increase in CBF which is proportional to the decrease in PaO_2 as is illustrated in Figure 6.3. This response is a protective mechanism to try to maintain oxygen delivery to the brain when hypoxia occurs. The impact of increased CBF and CBV resulting from hypercapnia and/or hypoxia for the patient with raised ICP is presented in Chapter 7.

OXYGEN AND GLUCOSE REQUIREMENTS

Within normal functioning the above mechanisms ensure that the brain has the rich supply of the substrates that it requires to function optimally. The rate of cerebral oxygen consumption, termed the cerebral metabolic rate of oxygen ($CMRO_2$), has a mean of 2.9 ml/100 g/min (range 1.4–4.9 ml/100 g/min), the grey matter requiring nearly three times as much as the white matter (Bowler, 2000).

The brain's oxygen consumption is 20% of the total oxygen consumption of the body at rest. Gram for gram the brain extracts more oxygen than any other organ in the body (Williams, 2000). The normal functioning brain will extract 30–40% of oxygen that is available from the arterial supply, so there is a massive reserve. When CBF is no longer coupled to metabolism (e.g. following stroke) and brain tissue is hypoperfused, the oxygen extraction fraction (OEF) can be increased up to the theoretical maximum of 100% (Warlow *et al.*, 2007).

Unlike other tissues of the body the brain is dependent on glucose as its energy source. It utilises approximately 5 mg/100 g/min of glucose. The brain does not have the capacity to use other substrates, e.g. free fatty acids to provide energy and has little capacity to store glucose. Because of this dependence on glucose, cerebral function is rapidly affected by disturbances in carbohydrate metabolism (Williams, 2000).

Up to 60% of the brain's energy requirements are used to fuel the sodium–potassium adenosine triphosphate (Na^+/K^+) pumps (Williams, 2000), which are essential to maintain the membrane potential and, consequently, the generation of impulses. If CBF cannot meet the metabolic demands of the brain, ischaemia results (see Chapter 22).

Ischaemia

When CBF falls by approximately 60% (below 20 ml/100 g/min) there is an accumulation of lactic acid with a subsequent drop in the intracellular pH owing to the switch to anaerobic metabolism (Williams, 2000). When CBF falls below 15 ml/100 g per minute, electrical activity ceases due to insufficient energy substrates being delivered to fuel the pumps. As a consequence of pump failure Na^+ moves

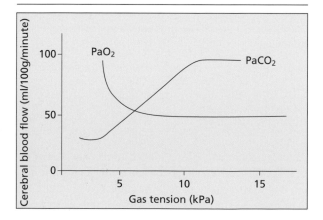

Figure 6.3 The effect of arterial oxygen partial pressure (PaO_2) on cerebral blood flow (CBF).

into the cells and water follows by osmosis leading to cytotoxic oedema. These events are reversible if CBF is rapidly restored. The exact duration of ischaemia necessary for neuronal death to occur is not exactly known, but some areas of the brain are more susceptible to ischemia than others, e.g. the hippocampus is particularly vulnerable. It is generally accepted that changes begin to occur in neurones following approximately five minutes of complete global ischaemia.

SUMMARY

Compensatory mechanisms maintain homeostasis of intracranial pressure when changes in intracranial volume occur. However, these mechanisms have a limited capacity, beyond which the contents lose compliance and deleterious increases in ICP occur. A constant cerebral blood flow is essential for normal cerebral function. A number of factors regulate the flow to maintain a constant CBF in order to provide the brain with its rich demand for the energy substrates required to maintain optimal function. When flow and metabolism become uncoupled and the limits of autoregulation are exceeded the brain becomes dependent upon the mean arterial pressure to perfuse the brain. An understanding of the physiology presented in this chapter will enable nurses to manage patients more effectively following cerebral insult.

REFERENCES

Barzo P (1996) Physiology of cerebral blood flow. In: Palmer JD (ed) *Manual of Neurosurgery*. London: Churchill Livingstone.

Bowler JV (2000) Cerebral blood flow supply. In: Crockard A, Haywad R, Hoff J (eds) *Neurosurgery: The Scientific Basis of Clinical Practice* (3rd edition). Oxford: Blackwell Science.

Ropper AH, Gress DR, Diringer MN *et al.* (2004) *Neurological and Neurosurgical Intensive Care*. (4th edition). Philadelphia: Lippincott Williams and Wilkins.

Warlow C, Van Gijin J, Dennis M *et al.* (2007) *Stroke Practical Management*. Oxford: Blackwell Publishers.

Williams S (2000) Energy supply for the maintenance of brain function. Cited in: Crockard A, Haywad R, Hoff J (eds) *Neurosurgery: The Scientific Basis of Clinical Practice* (3rd edition) Oxford: Blackwell Science.

Section II
Assessment, Interpretation and Management of Specific Problems in the Neurological Patient

7

Assessment and Management of Raised Intracranial Pressure

Ann-Marie Mestecky

INTRODUCTION

A number of intracranial conditions can cause an increase in intracranial pressure (ICP). The increase can occur either suddenly, e.g. following an intracranial haemorrhage, or gradually, e.g. with a slow growing brain tumour. Any pathological process that causes an increase in volume of one or more of the intracranial components (cerebrospinal fluid (CSF), cerebral blood, brain tissue) or a mass lesion, will result in an increase in ICP when the intracranial compensatory mechanisms have been exhausted. ICP is generally regarded as raised when ICP is greater than 20 mmHg, and interventions to reduce ICP are generally instituted when ICP reaches this level.

Nursing patients with raised ICP requires an understanding of the concepts presented in the previous chapter, as well as a knowledge of the signs and symptoms of raised ICP, the current evidence to support nursing interventions and the treatment options that are available. With this knowledge the nurse is better equipped to interpret assessment data, to plan evidence based care and to make effective decisions which ultimately could affect the outcome of the patient.

There are a number of different measures to treat raised ICP, all of which aim to reduce the volume of one or more of the three intracranial components. Most of the recommendations for the management of raised ICP have evolved from research involving patients with traumatic brain injuries (TBI). The specific management of raised ICP for this patient group is similar to that for other pathol-

ogies that give rise to raised ICP, however there are some exceptions. Where specific recommendations for other pathologies exist, e.g. spontaneous intracerebral haemorrhage, it will be clearly stated within the text. Otherwise it can be assumed that each of the measures/treatments presented in this chapter are instituted to treat raised ICP regardless of pathology.

CAUSES OF RAISED ICP

There are a number of pathological processes that can result in raised ICP which include:

- Brain oedema
- Hydrocephalus
- Vascular engorgement
- Mass lesions
- Idiopathic intracranial hypertension (IIH) also known as benign intracranial hypertension (see Chapter 25)

Brain oedema

Brain oedema is an increase in fluid in either the intracellular and/or interstitial spaces in the brain; the resulting increase in brain volume can cause an increase in ICP. Oedema can be localised or generalised. There are four types of cerebral oedema: vasogenic, cytotoxic (cellular), interstitial and hypo-osmolar (osmotic).

Vasogenic oedema

This type of oedema occurs due to disruption to the integrity of the blood–brain barrier (BBB). The loosening of the tight junctions between endothelial cells of the cerebral capillaries results in the BBB becoming more permeable. A protein rich fluid enters freely from the blood into the interstitial fluid of the brain, causing vasogenic oedema. It

Neuroscience Nursing: Evidence-Based Practice, 1st Edition.
Edited by Sue Woodward and Ann-Marie Mestecky
© 2011 Blackwell Publishing Ltd

has been hypothesised that the breakdown in the BBB is caused by mediator substances released or generated within necrotic brain tissue (Unterberg and Sarrafzadeh, 2000).

Newly formed capillaries that supply blood to brain tumours lack the tight junctions that are integral to a functioning BBB and this can also lead to vasogenic oedema. Vasogenic oedema typically surrounds cerebral tumours, particularly malignant gliomas and metastatic tumours. It is also found surrounding cerebral abscesses. Vasogenic and cytotoxic oedema often co-exist following stroke and traumatic brain injury. Vasogenic oedema primarily affects the white matter because the cells are less tightly packed than in the grey matter; the white matter therefore offers less resistance to the accumulation of fluid.

Cytotoxic (cellular) oedema

The movement of water between intracranial fluid spaces in the brain is largely determined by the movement of sodium. Water will move by osmosis in the direction where sodium is most concentrated. The sodium–potassium (Na^+- K^+) pumps within the cell membranes (refer to Chapter 1) are dependent on a continual supply of oxygen to maintain their function of moving sodium (Na^+) out of the cells and moving potassium (K^+) in against their concentration gradients. When there are insufficient energy substrates available to power the Na^+- K^+ pumps, e.g. due to ischaemia, Na^+ rapidly accumulates inside the cells and water follows by osmosis. This increase in cellular volume is called cytotoxic or cellular oedema.

Another cause for influx of Na^+ into the cells is the increase in the neurotransmitter, glutamate, in the interstitial fluid. This occurs following traumatic brain injury and ischaemia (Kimelberg, 1995). Glutamate triggers the opening of Na^+ channels, with subsequent influx of Na^+ and water. In addition, more energy is utilised by the cells to reduce the concentration of glutamate in the interstitial space; this mopping up operation of glutamate reduces the available energy to power the Na^+- K^+ pumps. Irrespective of the cause for the influx of Na^+, the subsequent accumulation of water inside the cells causes them to swell. Cytotoxic oedema is common following cerebral hypoxia, ischaemia and TBI. The grey and white matter are equally affected.

Interstitial oedema

Interstitial oedema is associated with hydrocephalus. When the pressure in the ventricles is increased, the CSF is forced out through the lining of the ventricles into the surrounding white matter.

Hypo-osmolar (osmotic) oedema

Water diffuses easily across the BBB and is largely determined by osmolar forces. Hypo-osmolar oedema occurs when the serum osmolality falls acutely below normal levels. The hypo-osmolality of the blood leads to the movement of water by osmosis across the BBB into the interstitial fluid of the brain. The most common causes are the syndrome of inappropriate secretion of anti diuretic hormone (SIADH), and the administration of excessive volumes of 5% glucose resulting in dilutional hyponatraemia and a fall in plasma osmolality. If changes in serum osmolality occur slowly the hypo-osmolar state is less likely to cause oedema due to the fact that the brain can compensate for the gradual change (see Chapter 16).

Hydrocephalus

Any abnormality affecting the production, circulation or absorption of CSF may result in hydrocephalus. The excessive volume of CSF causes an increase in ICP.

Vascular engorgement

Vascular engorgement is a less common cause for an increase in ICP. Any pathological process that obstructs venous drainage of the intracranial vault will result in an increase in cerebral blood volume (CBV) with a subsequent increase in ICP. Tumours that compress or invade the large venous sinuses, e.g. meningiomas, will obstruct venous outflow, as will a large thrombosis of a venous sinus, e.g. sagittal sinus thrombosis.

Vascular engorgement can also occur with severe hypoxia and hypercapnia because they both cause dilation of the cerebral vasculature resulting in a significant increase in cerebral blood volume.

Mass lesions

Mass lesions can be slow growing, e.g. meningiomas, or rapidly expanding, e.g. intracranial haematomas. Mass lesions include tumours, haematomas and abscesses.

Summary of the causes of ICP

Table 7.1 provides a summary of specific causes of raised ICP categorised by the component of the intracranial cavity that is primarily affected.

SIGNS AND SYMPTOMS

The signs and symptoms of raised ICP will differ according to the speed with which the ICP increases and in the case of mass lesions, their location. When acute increases in intracranial volume occur as for example with acute intracranial haematomas, the compensatory

Table 7.1 Causes of increased intracranial pressure (ICP).

Brain	CSF	Blood	Mass lesions
Oedema: vasogenic, cytotoxic, interstitial and hypo-osmolar	Hydrocephalus which can be caused by subarachnoid haemorrhage, intracranial infections, mass lesions that obstruct the CSF pathway, or congenital conditions	Obstruction to venous outflow, e.g. cerebral venous thrombosis Vascular engorgement due to severe hypoxia and severe hypercapnia	Haematomas, i.e. subdural (SDH), extradural (EDH), intracerebral (ICH) Tumours, abscesses, arteriovenous malformations

mechanisms that usually maintain homeostasis of ICP become overwhelmed and signs and symptoms that indicate the patient's condition is critical will be apparent. In patients with intracranial lesions that are slow growing, particularly those in non functional areas, the signs and symptoms will progress slowly and be more subtle.

Because of the compensatory mechanisms and the visco-elastic properties of the brain (see Chapter 6) a slow growing mass lesion will often grow to a considerable size before the symptoms become apparent. However, if the lesion is enlarging in an eloquent (functional) area of the brain then the patient will be symptomatic earlier due to direct compression and disruption of the local functional tissue and its blood supply, irrespective of whether there is an increase in ICP or not.

It is essential for the neuroscience nurse to recognise and interpret signs and symptoms of a rising ICP to enable early and appropriate measures to be taken.

Early signs and symptoms

Early signs and symptoms are commonly associated with gradual increases in intracranial volume, for example with tumours, abscesses, and hydrocephalus. Early signs include:

- Headache, which is usually worse in the morning and increases in severity with coughing, straining and bending
- Vomiting, usually in the morning often without nausea and can progress to projectile vomiting
- Papilloedema, which is swelling of the optic disc. The raised ICP is transmitted from the subarachnoid space through to the optic nerve sheath which impedes venous drainage from the retina resulting in the capillaries becoming tortuous and dilated. This congestion and dilatation of the retinal blood vessels results in a swollen optic disc often with superficial retinal haemorrhages.

Papilloedema will eventually lead to blurring of vision and in rare cases loss of vision can occur. Papilloedema will not usually be present if the ICP is of recent onset, i.e. within 24 hours
- Seizures
- Focal neurological signs can occur, but are not necessarily due to raised ICP. They can be due to the mass lesion directly compressing functional tissue and its blood supply, e.g. a lesion compressing Broca's area will result in dysphasia which can occur without an increase in ICP

Later signs and symptoms

Pathologies that result in sudden increases in ICP and slow growing lesions that are left untreated can develop the following:

- Decrease in level of consciousness, which can occur due to the distortion and compression of anatomic structures related to consciousness and/or as a result of a compromised cerebral perfusion pressure (CPP). As ICP increases it becomes more difficult for blood to flow into the brain, the CPP subsequently falls and the brain has insufficient substrates to maintain normal neuronal function.
- Seizures.
- Changes in the pupil size and the reaction of the pupils to light as a direct result of compression of the oculomotor nerve/s (cranial nerve III) (discussed below).
- Other specific signs and symptoms associated with herniation of the brain which are presented below.

Herniation syndromes

When the intracranial vault has reached maximum capacity and can no longer accommodate any further increase in volume, the brain will shift to the area of least resistance which is usually downwards. The term herniation refers to the shift of brain tissue downwards through a rigid opening.

It occurs due to pressure gradients between different intracranial compartments; the compartments are created by large folds of dura mater. The large fold of dura mater that almost separates the cerebral hemispheres longitudinally is called the falx cerebri (Figure 7.1). The fold of dura that separates the posterior portions of the cerebral hemispheres from the cerebellum is called the tentorium cerebelli or tentorium. The compartment above the tentorium is referred to as supratentorial and below as infratentorial. There is a central opening in the tentorium (tentorial hiatus) which allows for communication between the supratentorial and infratentorial compartments (Figure 7.1).

As the brain herniates it becomes damaged by mechanical forces and by alteration to cerebral blood flow as the cerebral vessels become compressed. Herniation can also obstruct CSF pathways which will contribute further to the increase in ICP.

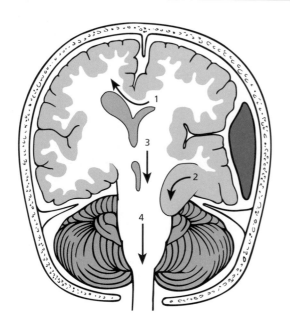

Figure 7.1 Brain herniations. A lateral supratentorial mass will cause displacement of the lateral ventricles with: (1) subfalcine herniation of the cingulate gyrus below the falx cerebri; (2) herniation of the uncus into the tentorial hiatus; (3) caudal displacement of the brain stem. Raised pressure within the posterior fossa may cause herniation of the cerebellar tonsils into the foramen magnum (4). Reproduced from Andrew Kaye, *Essential Neurosurgery*, Wiley-Blackwell, with permission.

There are four recognised herniation syndromes which can occur in isolation or can happen in rapid succession depending on the site and dynamics of the expanding lesion. For the purpose of explanation each will be described in turn.

Subfalcine herniation

Although not a herniation syndrome in the true sense of the word it is commonly described as one. A unilateral mass lesion located in either the right or left cerebral hemisphere will compress adjacent tissue and cause a shift of brain tissue from the affected hemisphere to the non affected hemisphere. A shift of part of the frontal lobe (the cingulate gyrus) under the falx cerebri to the opposite hemisphere is referred to as subfalcine herniation. It is often not associated with any specific neurological signs or symptoms, but occasionally it can cause compression of the anterior cerebral artery resulting in contralateral leg weakness. Subfalcine herniation is illustrated as number 1 in Figure 7.1. Unilateral mass lesions left untreated will eventually result in further shifts of brain tissue downwards (transtentorial herniation).

Transtentorial herniation

The downward movement of brain from the supratentorial compartment through the opening in the tentorium is called transtentorial herniation. Transtentorial hernation can be either central or unilateral (uncal).

Central transtentorial herniation

Central herniation occurs when there is a central lesion or diffuse oedema of the cerebral hemispheres. Downward movement of the cerebral hemispheres forces the central structures, i.e. the diencephalon, through the opening in the tentorium. The initial compression of the diencephalon results in a deterioration in conscious level; the pupils will be small, making it difficult to determine reactivity to light. If the herniation continues the midbrain will be compressed, the pupils become unreactive to light and are midsized (about 5 mm) (Lee and Hoff, 2000). There is loss of consciousness and Cheyne stokes breathing will become apparent. The breathing pattern can rapidly change to central neurogenic hyperventilation when the pons is compressed. There will be progressive dysfunction of the pons and medulla as the downward herniation continues. Flexor posturing will progress to extensor posturing.

The very late response to critical elevations in ICP is the Cushing's response which includes the triad of signs: bradycardia, hypertension and erratic breathing (refer to Chapter 14 for a comprehensive account of Cushing's response). This is followed by apnoea and at this stage the pupils become dilated (Lee and Hoff, 2000). If the herniation progresses rapidly not all of the signs and symptoms will be apparent. Hyperthermia and diabetes insipidus can also occur due to compression of the hypothalamus. Central herniation is illustrated as number 3 in Figure 7.1.

Uncal transtentorial herniation

The initial presentation of uncal herniation differs from central herniation because the diencephalon is not centrally compressed. A unilateral supratentorial mass lesion will result in herniation of a part of the temporal lobe called the uncus, on the same side as the lesion (ipsilateral) through the opening in the tentorium. This will result in compression of the midbrain on the same side. Early signs are confusion and restlessness which can rapidly progress to loss of consciousness depending on the dynamics of the mass lesion.

The pupil ipsilateral to the lesion becomes dilated and sluggishly reactive to light (Lee and Hoff, 2000) due to compression of the oculomotor nerve (CN III). Initially the patient will have a contralateral hemiparesis, or very occasionally ipsilateral hemiparesis can occur due to compression of the cerebral peduncle (within the midbrain) against the tentorial notch on the opposite side of the mass lesion (Lee and Hoff, 2000). If herniation is uninterrupted, the pons and medulla become displaced and compressed and the final signs and symptoms will therefore be the same as for central herniation. Uncal herniation is illustrated as number 2 in Figure 7.1.

Tonsillar herniation

Lesions situated in the infratentorial compartment can result in either a downward shift of brain tissue through the foramen magnum or an upward shift into the supratentorial space. The latter is relatively rare and will occur if the pressure in the infratentorial compartment is greater than in the supratentorial compartment. A downward shift results in the cerebellar tonsils being forced through the foramen magnum (tonsillar herniation), compressing the pons, medulla oblongata and upper cervical spinal cord. There will be loss of consciousness, erratic breathing and tetraparesis leading to respiratory and cardiac arrest. Tonsillar herniation is illustrated as number 4 in Figure 7.1.

Hypertension as a sign of raised ICP

The point is made in Chapter 14 that hypertension is caused by many factors and is not in itself a reliable sign of raised ICP. Acute intracranial haemorrhages, e.g. sub-

arachnoid haemorrhage and intracerebral haemorrhage will usually cause sudden increases in blood pressure. This is most likely to be the result of a significant sympathetic response following the insult to the brain and is often referred to as a 'reactive hypertension'. The blood pressure usually settles within hours to days. The extreme elevation in blood pressure that occurs as part of the Cushing's response is a terminal event by which stage the patient is unconscious.

INVESTIGATIONS

Computed tomography (CT Scan)

Patients presenting with signs of raised ICP will have an urgent CT scan performed. A CT scan will provide valuable information about the cause, and more specifically the size and location of the lesion (if present), and whether brain shifts have occurred. Dilated ventricles of the brain will indicate that there is obstruction to the flow of CSF, whereas a decrease in the size of the ventricles without obstruction along the pathway can indicate increased displacement of CSF to the lumbar theca (a compensatory mechanism, discussed in Chapter 6). With raised ICP the cortical sulci disappear and the basal cisterns are compressed.

Lumbar puncture (LP)

Intracranial pressure can be determined by taking a measurement of the intrathecal (lumbar cerebrospinal fluid) pressure. CSF conducts pressure from the CSF pathways in the brain to the lumbar theca, therefore readings reflect the ICP. A lumbar CSF pressure measurement may be performed in patients with hydrocephalus and idiopathic intracranial hypertension (IIH) to determine the need for further management, e.g. a shunt. Lumbar puncture is contraindicated if there is a mass lesion present because removal of CSF can create a pressure gradient which could result in downward herniation of the brain.

ASSESSMENT

Neurological assessment

The frequency of the neurological assessment will be dependent on the condition of the patient. A patient who is alert but has some early signs of raised ICP due to a cerebral tumour and is awaiting surgical excision will require less frequent observations than a patient who has just been admitted with a Glasgow Coma Score (GCS) of 10 following a traumatic brain injury (TBI). Nurses must make a decision with medical colleagues on an individual patient basis and be able to justify that decision. In patients who are unconscious and ventilated, ICP cannot be reliably estimated by observing any clinical feature; pupillary dilation and abnormal posturing can occur in the absence of raised ICP (Hlatky *et al.*, 2003). In such patients ICP monitoring provides essential information about the patient's ICP.

ICP monitoring

Monitoring is most often utilised in the critical care area to guide treatment during the acute period, for patients with the following: moderate to severe brain injury, significant intracranial haemorrhages, acute intracranial infections, large ischaemic strokes and encephalopathies. It is less frequently used for diagnostic purposes, e.g. for IIH, and only very occasionally used to determine the need for a shunt in patients with hydrocephalus. In such cases the monitoring is for a period of approximately 24 hours.

In the critical care setting ICP monitoring enables the practitioner to detect promptly increases in ICP. This allows early, appropriate management to be instituted to reduce ICP and to maintain optimal CPP, thereby potentially preventing further damage to the brain. There are however variations in the use of ICP monitoring in patients who are being actively managed for raised ICP. Many believe that it is unacceptable not to measure ICP in patients with severe brain injuries in the acute period, arguing that any delay in detecting an acute deterioration in a comatosed patient is associated with unjustifiable mortality and morbidity risk (Stover *et al.*, 2006; Brain Trauma Foundation (BTF), 2007). However, ICP monitoring was reported to be used in less than 50% of severely brain injured patients for whom it was indicated (Hesdorffer *et al.*, 2002); figures for frequency of use for other pathologies are not available.

The variations in the use of ICP monitoring to guide treatment may be due to the fact that its use has never been subject to a randomised controlled trial, so there is little evidence to demonstrate that outcomes are improved for patients who have ICP monitored (Forsyth *et al.*, 2010). Insufficient expertise in placing and cost may also be factors that contribute to ICP monitoring devices not being used in non-specialist centres. Infections and bleeding complications resulting from the use of ICP monitoring devices are rare and are not considered to be justifications for not using them (BTF, 2007).

The BTF recommend (2007) that ICP is monitored in the following groups:

- All salvageable patients with a severe traumatic brain injury (TBI) (GCS 3–8 after resuscitation) and an abnormal CT scan.

- Severe TBI with a normal CT scan if two or more of the following are noted on admission: age >40 years, unilateral or bilateral motor posturing, or systolic blood pressure <90 mmHg (BTF, 2007).

The American Heart Association and the American Stroke Association (AHA/ASA, 2007) guidelines for the management of patients following a spontaneous intracerebral haemorrhage (ICH) recommend that ICP is monitored when aggressive therapies to decrease ICP are being implemented (they include mannitol and hypertonic saline as aggressive therapy). There are no other specific guidelines for the use of ICP monitoring for other pathologies.

ICP devices

The ICP devices are in most cases inserted via a burr hole in the skull. ICP devices are most commonly placed in the brain parenchyma or within the lateral ventricle and less commonly in the extradural, subdural and subarachnoid spaces (Figure 7.2). There are a number of different devices available for monitoring ICP. The most regularly used devices to measure ICP in the UK are the fluid-filled (fluid-coupled) system, the fibreoptic system and micro strain gauge devices (Brunker, 2006).

ICP devices placed in the ventricle most accurately reflect the ICP. As discussed under herniation syndromes, pressure within the intracranial vault can be compartmentalised. For this reason devices placed in the parenchyma or on the surface of the brain in one hemisphere may not always accurately reflect the ICP in other compartments. Sahuquillo *et al.* (1999) demonstrated differences of up to 15 mmHg between right and left hemispheres with unilateral mass lesions. Therefore if the patient's neurological assessment data does not reflect the ICP reading, and if there is any doubt about possible deterioration in the patient's condition, medical staff should be informed immediately and the patient should have an urgent CT scan.

Fluid-filled systems

Intraventricular fluid-coupled devices

Intraventricular fluid-coupled devices are regarded as the gold standard for ICP monitoring in terms of accuracy, cost and reliability (BTF, 2007). The intraventricular fluid-coupled catheter is connected to an external pressure transducer which converts the pressure transmitted from the CSF in the ventricles, via the fluid-filled pressure tubing, into an electrical signal. The ICP reading and waveform are displayed on a monitor (Figure 7.3). Because the catheter is placed within the ventricle, most commonly the right lateral ventricle, it is a more accurate measure of

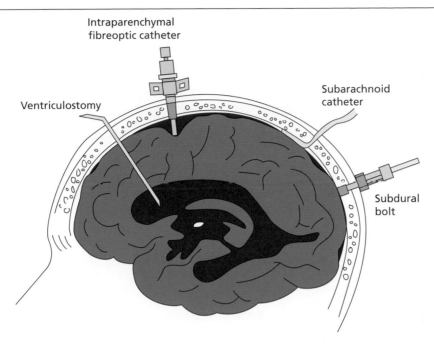

Intraparenchymal
fibreoptic catheter

Ventriculostomy

Subarachnoid
catheter

Subdural
bolt

Figure 7.2 ICP devices situated in the lateral ventricle (ventriculostomy), the brain parenchyma, subarachnoid and subdural spaces.

global ICP. This system has the added advantage of being able to drain CSF when ICP rises (see below: Drainage of CSF). However measuring ICP and draining cannot be done concurrently.

The catheter is most commonly tunneled under the skin a short distance from the burr hole which helps to immobilise the catheter and to reduce the risk of ventriculitis. There is a very small risk of haemorrhage occurring post insertion (approximately1.1%) (BTF, 2007). Holloway *et al.* (1996) reported a rising risk of infection over the first 10 days following insertion (n=584); but more importantly they found that patients in whom catheters were replaced prior to 5 days did not have lower infection rates than those whose catheters were exchanged at more than 5 days (Holloway *et al.*, 1996). They concluded that catheters should be removed as quickly as possible, but if required for longer than 5 days, there is no benefit in changing the catheter.

In patients with displaced or compressed ventricles due to mass lesions this system may be difficult to place and another option may be indicated.

Specific management of the ventricular fluid-filled system

The external transducer must be consistently level with the position of the catheter in the ventricle. If the transducer is positioned above or below this level then a pressure gradient will exist resulting in inaccurate readings. The anatomical reference points most commonly cited with which to align the transducer are the external auditory meatus or tragus of the ear (Pope 1998; Ropper *et al.*, 2004); these points correspond with the bridge of the nose when the patient is in the lateral position. Local protocols should agree the anatomical reference point to ensure that all staff are consistently using the same point. The transducer should be aligned using a laser or carpenter's level (Bisnaire and Robinson, 1997) to ensure accuracy of the reading.

Excessive and non compliant (soft) tubing, bubbles or debris in the tubing can all be causes of a dampened pressure waveform and will lead to underestimation of the ICP. The catheter can be flushed with saline solution (usually less than 1 ml) under strict asepsis by experienced competent practitioners if it should become blocked with debris.

External transducers drift from zero reference point over time which will lead to inaccurate readings if the monitoring system is not re-zeroed (Davoric, 2002). Local protocols should therefore include frequent re-zeroing of the monitoring system to eliminate the influence of changeable atmospheric pressure.

Most local protocols include the sending of daily CSF samples for microscopy, culture and sensitivity (MC&S)

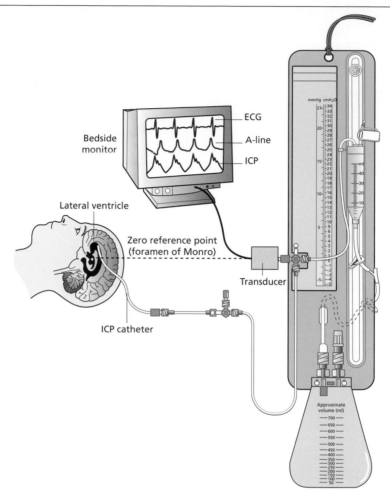

Figure 7.3 Fluid-filled system draining cerebrospinal fluid and monitoring intracranial pressure. From Mestecky AM, Brunker C, Connor J, Hanley C (2007) Understanding the monitoring of intracranial pressure: a benchmark for better practice. *British Journal of Neuroscience Nursing* 3(6):277. Reproduced with permission of MA Healthcare Limited.

to identify infection early. There is no evidence to support the prophylactic use of antibiotics whilst the intraventricular device is in-situ.

Subarachnoid bolt

A fluid-filled system can also be placed in the subarachnoid space, often referred to as the subarachnoid bolt. This device is seldom used in the UK. It is less accurate than the intraventricular catheter and it is also more likely to become blocked by brain tissue.

Fibreoptic and micro strain gauge devices

In contrast to the fluid-filled system, the transducers of these devices are placed within the intracranial vault at the tip of the catheters.

The most frequently used fibreoptic system is the Camino® ICP monitoring catheter (Integra NeuroSciences Camino®). This system is most commonly placed in the parenchyma of the frontal lobe and less often in the ventricle and subarachnoid space. There is a moveable diaphragm at the tip of the narrow fibreoptic catheter. Changes in the intracranial pressure will result in changes in the amount of light reflected off the diaphragm; the changes in light intensity are interpreted in units of pressure by the transducer at the tip of the fibreoptic catheter. An ICP pressure reading with or without a waveform can be displayed, depending on the type of monitor to which it is attached. Care must be taken with the handling the Camino catheter as kinks in the catheter and extreme bending can affect the performance of the fibreoptic transducer.

The most common micro strain gauge device is the Codman MicroSensor (Codman; Johnson & Johnson, Raynham, MA). The microchip transducer is positioned at the distal tip of a long flexible tube. This system is most commonly placed in the parenchyma of the brain but it can also be placed in the lateral ventricle. Changes in pressure will cause a silicone diaphragm to deflect a small amount, inducing strain in the embedded resistor. This resistance change is reflected in the form of a differential voltage which is then converted into units of pressure and displayed on the ICP Express Box™. Using an additional cable, the ICP Express Box™ can be connected to a patient monitor to display the ICP pressure reading and waveform.

The advantage of the fibreoptic and micro strain gauge devices is that they are virtually artefact free because the transducer is at the distal end of the catheter in the brain. Unlike the fluid-filled system these devices are calibrated prior to insertion and cannot be recalibrated following insertion, which eliminates the need for leveling. A disadvantage of both devices is that zero drift can occur with time, which means that overestimation or underestimation of ICP can occur (Martinez-Manas *et al.*, 2000, Koskinen *et al.*, 2005).

Both these devices are now available to be placed in the ventricle with an additional catheter to allow for drainage of CSF thereby providing similar benefits to the intraventricular fluid-filled system.

Nursing management of all devices

Table 7.2 shows a summary of the nursing management of an ICP device.

Interpretation of ICP waveforms

Changes seen in waveform with increasing ICP

Monitors will usually display the mean ICP but some may include the diastolic and systolic pressures. The normal ICP waveform is sawtooth in appearance with three characteristic peaks or waves: P1, P2, P3 (Figure 7.4). These peaks reflect changes in a single cardiac cycle. P1 is called the percussion wave, it is the most prominent wave and

Table 7.2 Care required for an ICP monitoring device.

Nursing management	Rationale
Maintain a sterile occlusive dressing over the site where the catheter breaches the skin	To allow for early identification of infection at the catheter site
Set realistic alarm parameters for ICP and CPP. Accurately record ICP and CPP at intervals appropriate to the patient's condition	To allow for prompt detection of significant changes in ICP and CPP
The scale of the display screen should be adjusted so that the whole waveform is visible	To ensure accurate readings of ICP and interpretation of waveforms
Monitor waveform for significant changes and report any that are clinically significant	ICP waveforms can provide additional information about compliance (refer to section on waveforms)
Identify and troubleshoot promptly possible causes of a dampened waveform and take relevant action	A dampened waveform can give an inaccurate ICP reading
Document interventions and stimuli that result in significant changes in ICP	Measures should be in place to prevent subsequent increases when the interventions are repeated

For additional specific management of the fluid-filled system refer to: Fluid-filled systems.
Adapted from A. Mestecky *et al.*, 2007.

appears as a rapid upstroke, and corresponds with the arterial systolic pressure. It is due to the arterial pulsation being transmitted to the brain tissue and CSF. P2, the tidal wave, represents the rebound (or elastance) of the brain structures, an echo of the arterial pulse (Mestecky *et al.*, 2007). P3 is known as the dicrotic notch which corresponds with the arterial dicrotic notch.

As ICP increases and the compensatory reserve diminishes, each arterial pulsation provokes a bigger pressure

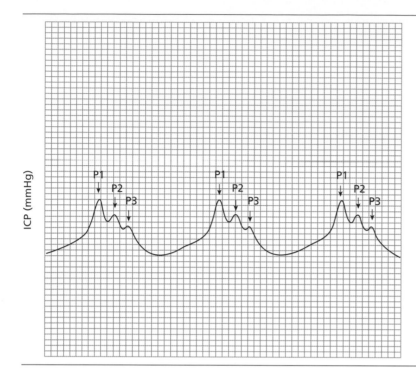

Figure 7.4 Normal ICP waveform with 3 characteristic peaks: P1, P2, P3.

response which is evident by the increase in the amplitude (height) of the whole waveform. When the contents of the intracranial vault lose the ability to absorb changes in pressure, i.e. compliance is low and elastance is high, the P2 wave increases in amplitude to a greater extent than P1 or P3 (Figure 7.5). This change in the P2 wave can occur before there is any significant change in ICP. The presence of the tall P2 wave exceeding the P1 wave can alert practitioners that any further increase in volume will potentially result in a disproportionate increase in ICP lasting longer than a few minutes (Kirkness *et al.*, 2000). Therefore utmost care and appropriate measures are taken when performing any interventions that are known to increase ICP.

Although a peak of P2 can be predictive of a disproportionate increase in ICP and loss of compensatory reserve, it is possible for patients to have a normal mean ICP with no peak of P2 and have disproportionate increases in ICP, and vice versa. The ICP responses to noxious stimuli and nursing interventions must be observed and care planned according to the response. When ICP climbs steeply and stays elevated following an intervention, e.g. suctioning, it indicates that compliance is low. If further interventions were conducted in quick succession without allowing the ICP to return to baseline, herniation of the brain may potentially ensue. If the patient's ICP rises during the intervention but rapidly returns to baseline it indicates that

compensatory mechanisms are still functioning. In such cases it is not necessary for nursing interventions to be staggered but nurses should not ever be complacent; continual monitoring of responses is still required.

TREATMENT OF RAISED ICP

Current treatment is directed at reducing ICP and achieving optimal levels for cerebral perfusion pressure (CPP). The primary aim of this ICP/CPP directed therapy is to limit further damage to brain tissue.

The management of patients with raised ICP has evolved over the last 2 decades from research primarily focused on the traumatic brain injured (TBI) population. Until the 1990s the mainstay of treatment was directed solely at reducing ICP, but some of the treatments used to reduce ICP often did so at the cost of reducing cerebral blood flow (CBF) which resulted in cerebral ischaemia (e.g. hyperventilation and restricting fluid input).

In the 1990s, CPP guided therapy was introduced, which aimed to maintain a CPP >70 mmHg to minimise ischaemia. It was found to provide better outcomes than previous studies that focused treatments solely at reducing ICP (Rosner and Daughton, 1990; Rosner *et al.*, 1995). However subsequent studies and retrospective reviews have found that aggressively treating to achieve a CPP >70 mmHg is associated with a significant increase in

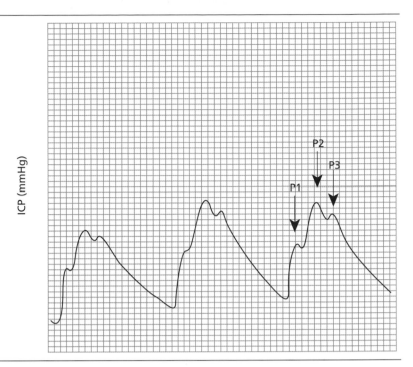

Figure 7.5 Waveform showing low compliance.

complications such as acute respiratory distress syndrome (ARDS) (Robertson *et al.*, 1999; Juul *et al.*, 2000; Clifton *et al.*, 2001). It is however well established that a CPP <50 mmHg in patients with TBI results in ischaemia and should be avoided (Nordstrom *et al.*, 2003). So although current management aims to avoid cerebral ischaemia by reducing ICP and by maintaining optimal CPP, there is uncertainty about what the optimal target level is for CPP.

The Brain Trauma Foundation (BTF) has published evidence based guidelines for the management of severe TBI patients with raised ICP, in which they recommend that the target for CPP lies between 50 and 70 mmHg, and for patients with intact autoregulation the level may be higher (BTF, 2007). The guidelines also recommend that additional monitoring such as jugular venous bulb oximetry (SjvO$_2$), brain tissue oxygen tension (PbtO$_2$) and microdialysis (MD) can facilitate CPP management by providing additional information about the adequacy of CBF. MD provides information about the degree of metabolic disturbance caused by ischaemia whereas SjvO$_2$ and PbtO$_2$ assess the adequacy of cerebral oxygenation. The additional information can assist clinicians in determining the patient's optimal CPP level. This offers a more individualised approach to managing patients with raised ICP (BTF, 2007). These monitoring techniques are discussed in Chapter 32.

Where additional monitoring is not being used, a CPP of 60–70 mmHg is generally the target level for patients with raised ICP. Exceptions are patients with raised ICP caused by spontaneous intracerebral haemorrhage. These patients generally present with hypertension and the majority would require the blood pressure to be lowered to achieve a CPP of <70 mmHg, which would increase the risk of ischaemia. The American Heart Association and the American Stroke Association (AHA/ASA, 2007) produced evidence based guidelines for the management of this patient population; it is recommended that CPP should be maintained >70 mmHg when there is evidence of raised ICP.

Target level for ICP

Correlation between elevated ICP (>20 mmHg) and poor outcomes is well documented in the severely head injured population (Saul and Ducker, 1982; Eisenberg *et al.*, 1988; Marmarou *et al.*, 1991; Miller and Dearden, 1992). The BTF (2007) guidelines recommend (based on class II evidence) that treatment should be initiated with ICP thresholds above 20 mmHg (see Chapter 32). Most authorities recommend 20 mmHg as the threshold above which treatment should be initiated (Hlatky *et al.*, 2003).

Treatments to reduce ICP

The specific management will depend on the cause of the raised ICP and the condition of the patient. If the cause can be safely treated with surgery, e.g. evacuation of a haematoma or tumour, then this is performed at the earliest possible time to prevent further deleterious effects to brain tissue. Box 7.1 outlines the surgery for each condition and any specific medical management. If the patient is conscious and being nursed in the ward setting, and has suspected raised ICP, then the general measures and nursing care discussed below will form the basis of care and treatment (see Box 7.3). If the patient is unconscious due to raised ICP, their management will include instituting more aggressive treatments (discussed below). These patients will be intubated and ventilated and managed in a critical care unit. All care and management discussed below will apply to this patient group.

Treatments instituted to reduce ICP generally reduce the volume of one or more of the intracranial components, i.e. brain, blood volume or CSF. However, none of the treatments offer the perfect solution and most are associated with adverse effects. The treatments are instituted incrementally; the safer and simpler treatments of sedation, analgesia, normothermia, head elevation and tight control of arterial blood gases are instituted early. When these measures fail to control ICP, treatment progresses to first line measures which may include ventricular drainage of CSF, mannitol, and mild hyperventilation. Second line therapies are instituted as clinically indicated when ICP fails to respond to first line treatments (refractory raised ICP). These may include, moderate hypothermia, mild to moderate hyperventilation and, as a last resort, barbiturate coma and decompressive craniectomy may be considered (Sahuquillo and Arikan, 2006).

Despite this aggressive goal-directed therapy, ICP will fail to be controlled in a minority of cases.

Treatment of raised ICP has evolved around patients with TBI, so the majority of the literature presented in the

following section is based on the TBI population. Where a specific treatment is not indicated for a specific diagnosis (e.g. tumours, stroke, etc.) then it will be clearly stated, otherwise, it can be assumed that the treatment is used to lower ICP regardless of the pathology.

GENERAL MEASURES AND NURSING CARE FOR PATIENTS WITH RAISED ICP OR SUSPECTED RAISED ICP

Respiratory management

In addition to ensuring optimal CPP, it is also essential that respiratory function is optimised to provide the brain with the best chance of receiving adequate oxygen to reduce the possibility of further neuronal damage. The relationship between hypoxia and CBF and subsequent increase in ICP has been presented in Chapter 6. The aim is for a partial pressure of oxygen (PaO_2) of 13 kPa (Maas *et al.*, 1997; NICE, 2007). Parameters for $PaCO_2$ are discussed below under 'First Line Measures' and in Box 7.3. The conscious patient should be taught and encouraged to do regular deep breathing exercises.

The utmost care must be taken to avoid hypoxia when suctioning; patients should be hyperoxygenated for 1 minute prior to suctioning (Wong, 2000). Suctioning should be limited to <15 seconds, with a maximum of two suction passes (Wainwright and Gould, 1996). Hyperventilation is discussed below under first line measures.

Positioning

There have been a number of small, well designed studies that have observed the effects of head positioning on ICP, CPP and, more recently, cerebral oxygenation. The majority conclude that 30° head elevation is associated with a small reduction in ICP (Durward *et al.*, 1983; Feldman *et al.*, 1992; Winkleman, 2000; Ng *et al.*, 2004). The physiological basis for 30° head elevation is that it increases venous return via the jugular veins, thereby decreasing the venous cerebral blood volume (CBV) with a subsequent decrease in ICP.

Although the average CPP in the above studies was not affected by the 30° head of bed elevation, some individual patient responses to the measure did result in lowering of their blood pressure with a subsequent fall in CPP, thereby potentially negating any benefit in the reduction in ICP. A fall in BP in response to head elevation is most likely to occur in patients who are hypovolaemic and where cerebral autoregulation is impaired. Individual patient responses to head elevation should therefore be monitored.

Box 7.1 Surgical management for specific diagnosis

- Tumours: dexamethasone, surgical excision or debulking (see Chapter 21)
- Abscess: Intravenous antibiotics, aspiration or excision (see Chapter 24)
- Hydrocephalus: CSF shunt or endoscopic third ventriculostomy (see Chapter 25)
- Intracranial haematomas (acute and chronic): burr hole, craniotomy or craniectomy for evacuation (see Chapter 20)

The head should always be kept in a neutral position as slight flexion can impede venous return; when the patient is lying in the lateral position a towel rolled and placed under the pillow should be sufficient to support the neck in a neutral alignment.

Positioning a patient in a head down position (Trendelenburg position) will elevate the ICP and should always be avoided. Care should be taken to avoid extreme hip flexion which can elevate intra-abdominal pressure, displacing the diaphragm upward and increasing intrathoracic pressure and central venous pressure. The increase in pressure will reduce venous return and increase ICP.

Nursing interventions

Nursing activities and noxious stimuli can increase ICP. The response will vary amongst individuals and depends on the patient's level of compensatory reserve, i.e. compliance, and whether autoregulation is impaired. If ICP is being monitored then individual responses to specific nursing interventions and to stimuli can be determined and care and management can be adjusted accordingly. However in patients not being monitored it should be borne in mind that any activity or stimulus that results in an increase in blood pressure, an increase in intrathoracic or intraabdominal pressures, or impedes venous drainage from the brain, can potentially increase ICP in patients with poor compliance. Box 7.2 lists some stimuli and interventions that are known to increase ICP.

Bowel management

It is important to monitor and accurately record bowel movements and to take appropriate measures to avoid patients becoming constipated. To prevent straining with bowel movements stool softeners should be administered regularly and laxatives may also be required. Patients who are aware and confined to bed must be assured that their privacy will be maintained during toileting and appropriate care should be taken to maintain the dignity of the patient. Patients are often reluctant to use the bedpan as they find it undignified, which can cause them to become constipated.

Auditory stimuli

Some environmental noises (monitor alarms, phones, staff communicating) can be distressing for patients, and can evoke the stress response. The sympathetic response will elevate blood pressure which, for patients with impaired autoregulation, will result in an increase in CBF and a subsequent increase in ICP. Every attempt should be made to reduce environmental noise, i.e. reducing the volume of

---

> **Box 7.2 Stimuli and interventions known to increase ICP**
>
> - Blocked catheter
> - Pain
> - Coughing
> - Straining with bowel movements
> - Cervical collars secured too tightly (see Chapter 33)
> - Endotracheal ties secured too tightly
> - Suctioning (see Chapter 15)
> - Positive end expiratory pressure (PEEP) (see Chapter 15)
> - Auditory stimuli

---

the ward phone ring tone and the alarms of the bedside monitors. Small studies have not demonstrated any adverse effects of family visits on ICP (Hendrickson 1987; Walker *et al.*, 1998), however given the small sample size of the studies it would be unwise to make recommendations based on their findings. Individual responses are likely to be influenced by a number of factors, e.g. what is being discussed and the patient's level of consciousness. Conversations about the patient that might be distressing for the patient should take place away from the bedside.

Seizure control

Seizures will result in an increase in CBF which could further increase ICP. Prophylactic anti-epileptic drugs (AEDs) may or may not be used in the short term depending on the pathology. The use of AEDs is recommended in the short term following spontaneous intracerebral haemorrhage (ICH) (AHA/ASA, 2007) and TBI (BTF, 2007). Phenytoin is generally preferred because it can be administered parenterally and is rarely sedating (Ropper *et al*, 2004). If seizure activity occurs, rapid control is required to prevent ischaemic damage which can rapidly ensue due to the increased metabolic demands of the brain.

Fluid management

The aim is to maintain normovolaemia. Hypovolaemia can result in hypotension and a fall in CPP, which can predispose the brain to ischaemia, whereas hypervolaemia can potentially exacerbate cerebral oedema. Regular assessment of the patient's hydration status is essential and a strict fluid balance should be maintained. Central venous pressure will also be monitored in the critical care patient to provide a more detailed assessment of the patient's fluid status.

Intravenous fluids containing dextrose should be avoided. Dextrose solutions will lower plasma osmolality, which will cause water to move by osmosis across the BBB and will contribute further to cerebral oedema. Serum osmolality is for this reason maintained on the higher side of normal. This is achieved by administering isotonic fluids and limiting free water (Ropper *et al.*, 2004). Refer to Chapter 16 for further detail on the management of fluids and electrolytes.

Corticosteroids

Glucocorticoids are very effective at reducing vasogenic cerebral oedema that typically surrounds brain tumours and abscesses. The reduction in oedema will reduce the local mass effect on adjacent functional tissue and lower ICP. Glucocorticoids have a tightening effect on the damaged blood–brain barrier (BBB) making it less permeable and thereby preventing the indiscriminate movement of substances from the blood into the brain (Khan, 2008). Dexamethasone 16 mg daily in divided doses is the typical starting dose for patients with tumours (see Chapter 21 for patient education/advice). The majority of patients will demonstrate marked improvement in their neurological symptoms within 48 hours of their first dose (Ropper *et al.*, 2004). When patients with brain tumours deteriorate acutely due to raised ICP, a bolus dose of up to 100 mg of dexamethasone is administered intravenously (Ropper *et al.*, 2004) in addition to implementing other measures to reduce the ICP.

Similar favourable effects have not been associated with the use of corticosteroids in patients with cerebral oedema secondary to traumatic brain injury. The CRASH trial (Corticosteroid Randomisation After Significant Head Injury) found that high dose methylprednisolone for raised ICP following TBI failed to demonstrate any beneficial effect on outcome (Alderson & Roberts, 2005; CRASH Trial Collaborators, 2005). There is also limited evidence to support the efficacy of steroids following stroke (AHA/ASA, 2007; Wiebers *et al.*, 2006). Steroids are therefore not generally administered for raised ICP in the stroke and head injured population.

Analgesia

It is imperative to keep the patient comfortable and to prevent the elevations in blood pressure and ICP that can occur as a result of pain or headache in patients whose autoregulation is impaired. The adequacy of sedatives and analgesics should be assessed regularly. In the ward setting codeine based analgesia and paracetamol (acetaminophen) are the most commonly used analgesics for patients who have headache associated with raised ICP, whereas in the critical care setting the opioids fentanyl and morphine sulphate are commonly used.

Opioid analgesics can compromise blood pressure so careful monitoring is required, particularly in patients who are haemodynamically unstable. Constipation is a common side-effect of opioid analgesics which should be managed before it becomes a problem by ensuring adequate hydration, a balanced diet and the use of prophylactic aperients. There is insufficient evidence for recommendations to be made about which analgesics are the most effective and have the least undesirable side-effects in patients with raised ICP.

Summary of nursing management

A summary of the measures taken to nurse patients with raised ICP or suspected raised ICP is shown in Box 7.3. Refer to page 542 for more detail on the immediate checks that should be made if an acute increase in ICP is observed.

FIRST LINE MEASURES TO REDUCE ICP

Tight control of arterial carbon dioxide (PaCO$_2$) and hyperventilation

Some patients with raised ICP are ventilated to protect and maintain the airway and also to control arterial carbon dioxide (PaCO$_2$) levels. The relationship between PaCO$_2$ and CBF is well established (see Chapter 6). Hypocapnia causes cerebral vasoconstriction and thereby reduces CBF and ICP. Hypocapnia occurs through hyperventilation either by increasing the respiratory rate or tidal volume or both.

Until the early 1990s aggressive hyperventilation was used as a prophylactic measure to reduce ICP. However, the benefit of lowering the ICP is offset by the reduction in CBF which can result in cerebral ischaemia. Head injured patients were found to have significantly poorer outcomes when they were prophylactically hyperventilated to induce hypocapnia compared to those who were not (Muizelaar *et al.*, 1991).

Aggressive prophylactic hyperventilation is no longer recommended as a treatment for patients with raised ICP. However because small increases in PaCO$_2$ significantly increase CBF and therefore ICP, levels are tightly controlled usually between 4.5 and 5 kPa (normocapnia) as part of the general management from the outset of treatment. If ICP has not been controlled by the measures outlined thus far, then mild hyperventilation is generally employed as a temporary measure to reduce ICP. In such cases controversy exists about the degree of hypocapnia that should be used and for how long. BTF guidelines recommend (based on class III evidence) that hyperventilation is only used as a temporary measure to reduce ICP.

Box 7.3 Summary of nursing management of patients with suspected raised ICP in the ward setting

- Frequent monitoring of neurological observations to allow for early detection of deterioration
- Maintain adequate BP to provide CPP >60 mmHg (CPP = MAP–ICP)
- Maintain normovolaemia: regular assessment of hydration status and maintain an accurate record of fluid balance
- Promote optimal respiratory function; this requires regular assessment of respiratory function. Ensure patient has an adequate depth and rate of breathing to allow for effective clearance of CO_2. Patients who are drowsy are at risk of partial airway obstruction and hypoventilation which could lead to retention of CO_2. Encourage regular deep breathing exercises. Maintain $SpO_2 > 96\%$.Hyperoxygenate prior to suctioning, limit each suction to <15 seconds and a maximum of two suction passes
- Treat pyrexia with antipyretics and cooling methods
- The head should always be kept in a neutral position. Avoid head and neck positions that impede venous return
- Maintain patient comfort by adequately treating pain and headache
- Reduce unnecessary auditory stimuli
- Avoid constipation by ensuring adequate hydration, a balanced diet and the use of prophylactic aperients
- Provide explanations for all interventions, regular reassurance and support

CPP – cerebral perfusion pressure; ICP – intracranial pressure; MAP – mean arterial pressure; SpO_2 – saturation of haemoglobin with oxygen as measured by pulse oximetry.

A review of the literature by Stocchetti *et al.* (2005) concluded that the general consensus is in favour of a short duration of hyperventilation in head injured patients, but that $PaCO_2$ levels should be maintained above a $PaCO_2$ of 4 kPa (30 mm Hg). Because there is a possibility of mild hyperventilation causing ischaemia, it is recommended that jugular venous oxygen saturations ($SjvO_2$) or brain tissue oxygen tension ($PbtO_2$) are monitored to guide treatment (BTF, 2007; Ropper *et al.*, 2004; Helmy *et al.*, 2007). Refer to Chapter 32 for further detail on $SjvO_2$ and $PbtO_2$. A fall in CBF would manifest as a fall in $SjvO_2$; a fall

below 50% is considered a sign of excessive hyperventilation (Ropper *et al.*, 2004).

Hyperventilation is generally avoided in patients who have symptomatic vasospasm following aneurysmal subarachnoid haemorrhage (ASAH) and in the first 24 hours following traumatic brain injury when CBF is known to be significantly reduced.

Sedation

Ventilated patients whose ICP is unstable are heavily sedated for the purpose of preventing increases in ICP related to: agitation, nursing and medical interventions, fighting against the ventilator, coughing, and other noxious stimuli. Propofol is usually the preferred choice of sedative (Citerio and Cormio, 2003) and is titrated to minimise increases in ICP. It allows for a more rapid recovery from sedation enabling reassessments of neurological function. Propofol also has neuroprotective properties; it decreases cerebral metabolic rate of oxygen consumption ($CMRO_2$), CBF and ICP (Martin and Smith, 2004). Propofol is also thought to have antioxidant properties. It is being compared with midazolam in a study to determine whether its anaesthetic effect is supplemented by a reduction in intracerebral oxidative stress (Aarabi and Simard, 2009).

Propofol can induce hypotension and in large doses can induce hepatic dysfunction so careful monitoring of CPP and hepatic function are required. Intravenous fluids and noradrenaline are administered to counter the hypotension. Midazolam is most commonly prescribed as an alternative to propofol if side-effects are apparent or if an additional sedative is required to treat ICP when maximum doses of propofol have not adequately reduced it. All sedatives will cause respiratory depression so careful monitoring of arterial $PaCO_2$ or end tidal CO_2 is required.

Drainage of CSF

Drainage of CSF is an effective measure to temporarily reduce the intracranial volume thereby lowering ICP and improving CPP. It is generally used as a first line measure to reduce ICP in severely head injured patients (Sahuquillo and Arikan, 2006; Corteen *et al.*, 2007) and is commonly employed in patients with subarachnoid haemorrhage (SAH) and hydrocephalus.

Despite its frequent use, there are no large randomised studies examining the efficacy of this measure in the head injured population. In a small study (n=58) of head injured patients, drainage of just 3 ml of CSF significantly lowered ICP (by an average of 10%) and increased CPP (Kerr *et al.*, 2001). Although these changes in ICP are small the study demonstrated an incremental volume related decrease in ICP, so further drainage in CSF is likely to result in further decreases in ICP. Regardless of the volume drained the response is transient. Patients with SAH and hydrocephalus have a better response to CSF drainage than TBI patients (Mehta *et al.*, 1996, Ropper *et al.*, 2004).

The guidelines for the management of spontaneous intracerebral haemorrhage recommend CSF drainage to reduce ICP (AHA/ASA, 2007). The external ventricular drain (EVD) will either be permanently open, in which case it will be set to drain when the ICP reaches a certain level e.g. >20 mmHg, or the drain may be turned on intermittently to drain a specific volume when the ICP reaches a predetermined level. For the management of an EVD refer to Chapter 25.

Hyperosmolar therapy (osmotherapy)

Mannitol

Mannitol is a 6-carbon sugar. It works by increasing plasma osmolality, i.e. by making the blood hyperosmolar. An osmotic gradient is thereby established between the intravascular and the interstitial spaces which results in fluid being drawn by osmosis from the oedematous brain. This osmotic effect will temporarily increase the intravascular volume and reduce blood viscosity which improves cerebral blood flow and oxygen delivery (Cruz *et al.*, 1990). It has been proposed that the improvement in CBF and oxygenation results in autoregulatory cerebral vasoconstriction, thereby decreasing CBV and ICP (Muizelaar *et al.*, 1984).

There are a number of possible side-effects that the nurse needs to monitor following administration. The potent diuretic effect occurs within 15–25 minutes which can lead to a reduction in blood pressure. Hypotension will reduce the CPP which could potentially negate the benefit of a reduction in ICP. It is therefore necessary to be vigilant for a fall in blood pressure and to administer additional intravenous fluids if necessary to maintain intravascular volume and blood pressure. The diuresis causes the plasma osmolality to increase, so it is necessary to monitor it regularly as values >320 mOsm/kg can cause acute renal failure. Acute elevation of plasma osmolality to more than 20 mOsm/kg above the patient's baseline could result in encephalopathy (Wiebers *et al.*, 2006).

With repeated doses mannitol affects the integrity of the blood–brain barrier (BBB). This results in mannitol crossing into the brain and causing a rebound effect, i.e. it draws fluid from the intravascular space into the brain, contributing to further oedema.

Mannitol is administered as an intravenous bolus at a dose of 0.25–1 g/kg. In patients without ICP monitoring its use is generally restricted to those showing acute progressive neurological deterioration. Its use is recommended in TBI patients (BTF, 2007) and in haemorrhagic stroke patients (AHA/ASA, 2007).

The BTF guidelines (2007) recommend (based on class II evidence) mannitol as a first line treatment for control of raised ICP following TBI, however there is a lack of evidence to support repeated and prolonged use of mannitol over several days.

Hypertonic saline (HTS)

In some hospitals HTS is being used as an alternative form of hyperosmolar therapy. By increasing serum sodium levels to the higher side of normal the osmotic gradient is altered and water is drawn from an area of lower osmolality, i.e. the brain parenchyma, into the intravascular space.

A few small clinical studies have demonstrated that HTS is effective at reducing ICP in adults with raised ICP from ischaemic stroke and TBI (Shwarz *et al.*, 2002, Qureshi *et al.*, 1998, Suarez *et al.*, 1999). However, the studies are difficult to compare owing to the differences in study design, i.e. differences in the hypertonic solution preparations, dosing regimens and patient populations. Large randomised controlled trials are required before recommendations can be made. The question of whether HTS is more efficacious than mannitol also needs to be studied further by a large randomised controlled trial.

There is the risk of central pontine myelinolysis when administering HTS to patients who have an existing hyponatraemia (see Chapter 16). It is therefore essential that serum sodium levels are established prior to administration. HTS is contraindicated for patients with existing cardiac and pulmonary problems due to the increased risk of developing pulmonary oedema.

Temperature and induced hypothermia

Fever is associated with increases in ICP (Rossi *et al.*, 2001). Increases in body temperature can be detrimental to patients with raised ICP for one of two reasons. Coupling of CBF and metabolism may be impaired in patients with raised ICP (refer to Chapter 6 for more detail) so when additional CBF is required to meet the metabolic demands that occur with a raised temperature, the brain is susceptible to ischaemia because that additional CBF is not achieved. A 1 °C increase in body temperature increases the cerebral metabolic rate for oxygen ($CMRO_2$) by approximately 6 – 9%. Secondly, if the coupling is intact, the increase in CBF will result in further increases in ICP. It is therefore general practice to treat elevated temperatures in patients with raised ICP.

Reducing the body temperature therapeutically to decrease the metabolic demands of the brain is a measure employed to reduce ICP in patients who have not responded to measures outlined thus far. Although there have been a number of studies to determine the efficacy of this treatment there is still uncertainty whether the side-effects of induced hypothermia outweigh the benefits of lowering the ICP and ultimately whether they result in improved patient outcomes. The studies that have been conducted are difficult to compare owing to the differences in study design, i.e. differences in the duration of the hypothermic treatment, the target temperatures, the methods employed to cool and to measure temperature.

A large multicentred clinical trial (n = 392) found that there was no significant difference in outcomes in TBI patients (at 6 months following injury) who had moderate hypothermia treatment (33 °C) when compared to the normothermia group (Clifton *et al.*, 2001).The hypothermic group had a higher rate of complications and longer hospital stays.

Other smaller randomised studies have found that therapeutic hypothermia does improve patient outcomes (Polderman *et al.*, 2002; Jiang *et al.*, 2006; Qiu *et al.*, 2007). The study by Jiang *et al.* (2006) on the use of mild hypothermia in TBI patients with refractory raised ICP, found that the outcomes for patients who had 5 days of (long-term) cooling were significantly better than those that received 2 days of (short-term) cooling. Incidentally, the Clifton study induced hypothermia for 48 hours only. It may be that longer periods of induced hypothermia are required to improve overall outcomes.

There is a belief that a modified protocol, with a shorter time from the accident to the start of active cooling, longer cooling and rewarming time, and better control of blood pressure and intracranial pressure would be beneficial for TBI patients. This belief has led to the instigation of new trials in adults and in children, including these types of protocol adjustments (Grande *et al.*, 2009).

There is currently insufficient evidence to demonstrate that therapeutic hypothermia improves patient outcomes. Despite a lack of evidence many neuroscience units induce mild hypothermia (35 °C) in patients with refractory ICP.

When inducing hypothermia it is important to consider which method of cooling is the most effective and the possible systemic side-effects (refer to Chapter 14 for a detailed account of the methods available).

Barbiturate coma

Thiopentone is a powerful barbiturate anaesthetic which is sometimes used when all other measures have failed to control ICP (refractory raised ICP). By heavily sedating the brain with thiopentone (barbiturate coma), the brain's metabolic rate and therefore its requirement for energy substrates and ultimately blood flow are reduced, thereby reducing ICP and the risk of ischaemia.

Thiopentone is titrated to decrease neuronal activity which can be determined by continuous EEG. The maintenance dose is 1 mg/kg/hr. Approximately 50% of the metabolic activity of the brain is electrical activity so by sedating the brain to the point of suppressing EEG activity – 'electrical burst suppression' – the $CMRO_2$ is decreased to minimal levels. In some units new technology known as bispectral index (BIS) monitoring is used as an alternative to the traditional EEG. It essentially analyses the EEG and processes the result into a single number. A BIS of 0 equals EEG silence whereas near to 100 is the expected value in someone who is awake and aware. The value for a patient in barbiturate coma would be expected to be in the range of 10–20. BIS uses a forehead sensor rather than the traditional EEG electrodes to the scalp.

Although barbiturate coma effectively reduces ICP, there is insufficient evidence to suggest that barbiturate coma improves outcome. The BTF guidelines (2007) recommend its use (based on class II evidence) as a last resort for ICP which is refractory to all other treatments. This treatment is used in patients with TBI, malignant cerebral infarction, subarchnoid haemorrhage and encephalitis when all other measures have failed (Corteen *et al.* 2007).

Barbiturates can have significant side-effects which include: hypotension, vasodilation and suppression of myocardial contractility. The hypotensive effect can significantly reduce CPP which can offset the beneficial effect of the treatment (Roberts and Sydenham, 2009). Increased doses of vasopressors are usually required to maintain adequate CPPs. Such high doses of barbiturates will result in the pupils becoming small making it often very difficult to assess reaction to light.

Withdrawal of thiopentone treatment should be gradual to avoid rebound hypertension. Thiopentone accumulates in adipose tissue which can take many days to clear from the body when the drug is stopped, which makes it difficult to establish the patient's level of consciousness.

Neuromuscular blocking drugs

Neuromuscular blocking drugs are rarely used as their use is associated with respiratory complications and longer stays in ITU (Hsiang *et al.*, 1994). Their use can also prevent detection of seizure activity in patients where continuous EEG monitoring is not being used. They may however be necessary when a patient is regularly posturing or to prevent shivering when hypothermic treatment is being used as a measure to decrease ICP.

Decompressive craniectomy (DC)

When all treatments have failed to control raised ICP, a decision may be taken to perform a decompressive craniectomy (DC). By removing a part of the cranium the swollen brain is no longer restricted within the rigid confines of the skull and can expand upwards. There are two surgical options: a unilateral fronto-temporal craniectomy for unilateral hemisphere swelling and a bilateral fronto-temporal-parietal craniectomy for diffuse brain swelling (Corteen *et al.*, 2007). DC is considered for selected patients with large hemispheric infarction (Wiebers *et al.*, 2006) and TBI patients.

Recent reports of severely head injured patients who did not respond to maximal medical management suggest that patients can have a favourable outcome following DC (Morgalla *et al.*, 2008; Aarabi *et al.*, 2006). There is currently no level I evidence to support this practice as a measure to reduce unfavourable outcomes. However the RESCUEicp study is currently being conducted. This is a large multicentred randomised study comparing the outcomes for patients who undergo DC to those that have medical intervention only (Corteen *et al.*, 2007; Hutchinson *et al.*, 2009).

Brain lobectomies are rarely performed to reduce the ICP due to the high probability of causing severe permanent disability.

Acute deterioration in the ward setting as a result of raised ICP

Wards that regularly manage patients with raised ICP should have appropriate equipment by the bedside and in designated areas to allow for rapid intervention if sudden deterioration occurs, i.e. herniation syndromes. Patients who show signs of transtentorial herniation will be immediately intubated and mannitol will be administered (except in cases where a decision is taken not to continue active management). The patient can be manually hyperventilated as an immediate measure to try to control ICP, by increasing the number of breaths delivered by the bag valve mask or by increasing the volume delivered if a portable ventilator is not readily available. Mannitol will cause a diuresis so a urinary catheter will need to be inserted at the earliest possible time, if one is not already in-situ. The patient will be scanned immediately and a decision will be taken as to whether the patient would benefit from decompressive surgery.

SUMMARY

The goals of management for raised intracranial pressure are to protect the brain from further insult by maintaining optimal cerebral perfusion pressure and reducing ICP. There are a number of therapeutic measures to treat raised ICP which are instituted incrementally. Only a few of the measures have been subject to large randomised trials and many are associated with adverse effects. The risk benefit relation of each therapeutic measure should therefore be assessed on an individual patient basis.

Research into the efficacy of a number of the treatments for raised ICP are ongoing and changes to current management will no doubt continue to evolve based on the findings of these and future studies.

Nurses can optimise outcomes for patients with raised ICP by: vigilant assessment of the patient, early recognition and interpretation of changes in the patient's condition, and by being equipped with the necessary knowledge and skills to respond to and manage changes based on the best available evidence.

REFERENCES

Aarabi B, Simard JM (2009) Traumatic brain injury. *Current Opinion in Critical Care* 15(6):548–553.

Aarabi B, Hesdorffer D, Ahn E *et al.* (2006) Outcome following decompressive craniectomy for malignant swelling due to severe head injury. *Journal of Neurosurgery* 104:469–479.

Alderson P, Roberts I (2005) Corticosteroids for acute traumatic brain injury. *Cochrane Database of Systematic Reviews* 25(1):CD000196.

American Heart Association and the American Stroke Association (AHA/ASA) (2007) Guidelines for the management of spontaneous intracerebral haemorrhage in adults. *Stroke* 38:2001–2023.

Bisnaire D, Robinson L (1997) Accuracy of leveling intraventricular collection drainage systems. *Journal of Neuroscience Nursing* 29(4):261–268.

Brain Trauma Foundation (BTF), American Association of Neurological Surgeons, Congress of Neurological Surgeons AANS/CNS (2007) Joint section on neurotrauma and critical care: Guidelines for the management of severe traumatic brain injury. *Journal of Neurotrauma* 24(Suppl):S1–S95.

Brunker C (2006) Assessment of sedated head-injured patients using the Glasgow Coma Scale: An audit. *British Journal of Neuroscience Nursing* 2(6):276–280.

Citerio G, Cormio M (2003) Sedation in neurointensive care: advances in understanding and practice. *Current Opinion in Critical Care* 9(2):120–126.

Clifton GL, Miller ER, Choi SC *et al.* (2001) Lack of effect of induction of hypothermia in acute brain injury. *New England Journal Medicine* 344:556–63.

Corteen E, Timofeev I, Kirkpatrick P *et al.* (2007) The RESCUEicp study of decompressive craniectomy: Implications for practice. *British Journal of Neuroscience Nursing* 3(9):428–33.

CRASH Trial Collaborators (2005) Final results of the Medical Research Council CRASH trial, a randomised placebo-controlled trial of intravenous corticosteroid in adults with head injury – outcomes at 6 months. *Lancet* 365:1957–9.

Cruz J, Miner M, Allen S *et al.* (1990) Continuous monitoring of cerebral oxygenation in acute brain injury: injection of mannitol during hyperventilation. *Journal of Neurosurgery* 73:725–730.

Davoric G (2002) *Haemodynamic Monitoring: Invasive and noninvasive clinical application.* (3rd edition). Philadelphia: W.B. Saunders.

Durward QJ, Amacher L, Del Maestro RF (1983) Cerebral and cardiovascular responses to changes in head elevation in patients with intracranial hypertension. *Journal of Neurosurgery* 59:938–944.

Eisenberg HM, Frankowski RF, Contant CF *et al.* (1988) High-dose barbiturate control of elevated intracranial pressure in patients with severe head injury. *Journal of Neurosurgery* 69:15–23.

Feldman Z, Kanter MJ, Robertson CJ *et al.* (1992) Effects of head elevation on intracranial pressure, cerebral perfusion pressure and cerebral blood flow in head-injured patients. *Journal of Neurosurgery* 76:207–211.

Forsyth RJ, Wolny S, Rodrigues B (2010) Routine intracranial pressure monitoring in acute coma. *Cochrane Database of Systematic Reviews 2010, Issue 2.* Art. No.: CD002043. DOI: 10.1002/14651858.CD002043.

Grande PO, Reinstrup P, Romner B (2009) Active cooling in traumatic brain-injured patients: a questionable therapy. *Acta Anaesthesiologica Scandinavica* 53(10):1233–1238.

Helmy A, Vizcaychipi M, Gupta AK (2007) Traumatic brain injury: intensive care management. *British Journal of Anaesthesiology* 99(1):32–42.

Hendrickson S (1987) Intracranial pressure changes and family presence. *Journal Neuroscience Nursing* 19: 14–17.

Hesdorffer D, Ghajar J, Iacono L (2002) Predictors of compliance with the evidence – based guidelines for traumatic brain injury care: a survey of the United States Trauma Centres. *Journal of Trauma* 52:1202–1209.

Hlatky R, Valadka AB, Robertson CS (2003) Intracranial hypertension and cerebral ischaemia after severe traumatic brain injury. *Neurosurgical Focus* 14(4):1–4.

Holloway K, Barnes T Choi S *et al.* (1996) Ventriculostomy infections: the effect of monitoring duration and catheter exchange in 584 patients. *Journal of Neurosurgery* 85:419–424.

Hsiang JK, Chestnut RM, Crip CB *et al.* (1994) Early, routine paralysis for intracranial pressure control in severe head injury: is it necessary? *Critical Care Medicine* 22:1471–1476.

Hutchinson PJ, Corteen E, Czosnyka M *et al.* (2009) Decompressive craniectomy in traumatic brain injury: the randomised multicenter RESCUEicp study (www.RESCUEicp.com). *Acta Neurochirurgica Suppl* 96:17–20.

Jiang JY, Xu W, Li WP *et al.* (2006) Effect of long-term mild hypothermia or short-term mild hypothermia on outcome of patients with severe traumatic brain injury. *Journal of Cerebral Blood Flow and Metabolism* 26(6):771–776.

Juul N, Morris GF, Marshall SB *et al* (2000) Intracranial hypertension and cerebral perfusion pressure: influence on neurological deterioration and outcome in severe head injury. The Executive Committee of the International Selfotel Trial. *Journal of Neurosurgery* 92:1–6.

Kerr ME, Weber BB, Sereika SM *et al.* (2001) Dose response to cerebrospinal fluid drainage on cerebral perfusion in traumatic brain-injured adults. *Neurosurgical Focus* 11(4):1–7.

Khan E (2008) Understanding the use of corticosteroids in managing cerebral oedema. *British Journal of Neuroscience Nursing* 4(4):156–162.

Kimelberg HK (1995) Current concepts of brain oedema. Review of laboratory investigation. *Journal of Neurosurgery* 83:1051–1059.

Kirkness CJ, Mitchell PH, Burr RL *et al.* (2000) Intracranial presure waveform analysis: Clinical and research implications. *Journal of Neuroscience Nursing* 32(5):271–276.

Koskinen LO, Olivercrona M *et al.* (2005) Clinical experience with intraparenchymal intracranial pressure monitoring Codman microsensor system. *Neurosurgery* 56:693–698.

Lee KR, Hoff JT (2000) Raised intracranial pressure and its effects on brain function. In: Crockard A, Haywad R, Hoff J (eds) *Neurosurgery: The Scientific Basis of Clinical Practice* (3rd edition). Oxford: Blackwell Science.

Maas AI, Dearden M, Teasdale GM *et al.* (1997) EBIC-guidelines for management of severe head injury in adults: European Brain Injury Consortium. *Acta Neurochirurgica (Wien)* 139:286–294.

Marmarou A, Anderson RL, Ward JD *et al.*(1991) Impact of ICP instability and hypotension on outcome in patients with severe head trauma. *Journal of Neurosurgery* 75: Suppl S59–S66.

Martin D, Smith M (2004) Medical management of severe traumatic brain injury. *Hospital Medicine* 65(11):674–680.

Martinez-Manas RM, Santamarta D, de Campos JM *et al.* (2000) Camino intracranial pressure monitor: prospective study of accuracy and complications. *Journal of Neurology, Neurosurgery and Psychiatry* 69:82–86.

Mehta V, Holness RO, Connolly K *et al.* (1996) Acute hydrocephalus following aneurysmal subarachnoid hemorrhage. *Canadian Journal of Neurological Sciences* 23:40–45.

Mestecky A, Brunker C, Connor J *et al.* (2007) Understanding the monitoring of intracranial pressure: a benchmark for better practice. *British Journal of Neuroscience Nursing* 3(6):276–282.

Miller JD, Dearden NM (1992) Measurement, analysis and the management of raised ICP. In: Teasdale GM, Miller JD (eds). *Current Neurosurgery. Edinburgh:* Churchill Livingstone,.

Morgalla MH, Will BE, Roser F *et al.* (2008) Do long-term results justify decompressive craniectomy after severe traumatic brain injury? *Journal of Neurosurgery* 109(4): 685–690.

Muizelaar J, Lutz H, Becker D (1984) Effect of mannitol on ICP and CBF and correlation with pressure autoregulation in severely head-injured patients. *Journal of Neurosurgery* 61:700–706.

Muizelaar JP, Marmarou A, Ward JD *et al.* (1991) Adverse effects of prolonged hyperventilation in patients with severe head injury: a randomised clinical trial. *Journal of Neurosurgery* 75:731–739.

National Institute of Health and Clinical Excellence (2007) *Head injury: Triage, assessment, investigation and early management of head injury in infants, children and adults.* London: National Collaborating Centre for Acute Care, Royal College of Surgeons of England.

Ng I, Lim J, Wong HB (2004) Effects of head posture on cerebral haemodynamics: Its influence on ICP, CPP and cerebral oxygenation. *Neurosurgery* 54:593–597.

Nordstrom CH, Reinstrup P, Xu W *et al.* (2003) Assessment of the lower limit for cerebral perfusion pressure in severe head injuries by bedside monitoring of regional energy metabolism. *Anesthesiology* 98:809–814.

Polderman KH, Tjong JR, Peerdeman SM *et al.* (2002) Effects of therapeutic hypothermia on intracranial pressure and outcome in patients with severe head injury. *Intensive Care Medicine* 28:1563–1573.

Pope W (1998) External ventriculostomy: A practical application for the acute care nurse. *Journal of Neuroscience Nursing* 30(3):185–190.

Qiu W, Zhang Y, Sheng H *et al.* (2007) Effects of therapeutic mild hypothermia on patients with severe traumatic brain injury after craniotomy. *Journal of Critical Care* 22(3):229–235.

Qureshi AL, Suarez JI, Bhadwaj *et al.* (1998) Use of hypertonic saline (3%) saline/acetate infusion in the treatment of cerebral oedema: effect on intracranial pressure and lateral displacement of the brain. *Critical Care Medicine* 26:440–446.

Roberts I, Sydenham E (2009) Barbiturates for acute traumatic brain injury. *Cochrane Database of Systematic Reviews* Issue 4: Art.No: CD000033.

Robertson CS, Valadka AB, Hannay HJ, *et al* (1999) Prevention of secondary ischaemic insults after severe head injury. *Critical Care Medicine* 27:2086–2095.

Ropper AH, Gress DR, Diringer MN *et al.* (2004) *Neurological and Neurosurgical Intensive Care* (4th edition) Philadelphia: Lippincott Williams and Wilkins.

Rosner MJ, Daughton S (1990) Cerebral perfusion pressure management and head injury. *Journal of Trauma* 30:933–940.

Rosner MJ, Rosner SD, Johnson AH (1995) Cerebral perfusion pressure: management protocol and clinical results. *Journal of Neurosurgery* 83:949–962.

Rossi S, Zanier ER, Mauri I *et al.* (2001) Brain temperature, body core temperature and intracranial pressure in acute cerebral damage. *Journal of Neurology, Neurosurgery and Psychiatry* 71:448–445.

Sahuquillo J, Arikan F (2006) Decompressive craniectomy for the treatment of refractory high intracranial pressure in traumatic brain injury. *Cochrane Database of Systemic Reviews 1*: CD003983.

Sahuquillo J, Poca MA, Arribus M *et al.* (1999) Interhemispheric supratentorial intracranial pressure gradients in head injured patients: are they clinically important? *Journal of Neurosurgery* 90:16–26.

Saul TG, Ducker TB (1982) Effect of intracranial pressure monitoring and aggressive treatment on mortality in severe head injury. *Journal of Neurosurgery* 56:498–503.

Schwarz S, Georgiadas D, Aschoff A (2002) Effects of hypertonic (10%) saline in patients with raised intracranial pressure *Stroke* 33:136–140.

Stocchetti N, Maas A, Chieregato A *et al.* (2005) Hyperventilation in head injury: A review. *Chest* 127(5):1812–1827.

Stover JF, Steiger P, Stocker R (2006) Need for intracranial pressure monitoring following severe traumatic brain injury. *Critical Care Medicine* 34(5):1582–1583.

Suarez JI, Qureshi AL, Bhadwaj A *et al.* (1999) Treatment of refractory intracranial hypertension with 23.4% saline. *Critical Care Medicine* 26:1118–1122.

Unterberg AW, Sarrafzadeh AS (2000) Brain oedema. In: Crockard A, Haywad R, Hoff J (eds). *Neurosurgery: The scientific basis of clinical practice* (3rd edition). Oxford: Blackwell Science.

Wainwright SP, Gould D (1996) Endotracheal suctioning in adults with severe head injury: Literature review. *Intensive Care Critical Care Nurse* 12:303–308.

Walker J, Eakes G, Siebelink E (1998) The effects of familial voice interventions on comatose head injured patients. *Journal of Trauma Nursing* 5(2):41–45.

Wiebers DO, Feigin VL, Brown RD (2006) *Handbook of Stroke.* (2nd edition). Philadelphia: Lippincott Williams & Wilkins.

Winkleman C (2000) Effect of backrest position on intracranial pressure and cerebral perfusion pressures in traumatically brain-injured adults. *American Journal Critical Care* 9:373–380.

Wong F (2000) Prevention of secondary brain injury. *Critical Care Nurse* 20(5):18–27.

8

Assessment, Interpretation and Management of Altered Consciousness

Neal Cook and Sue Woodward

INTRODUCTION

The phenomenon of consciousness has intrigued mankind for centuries, with its complexity leaving many questions unanswered as to its origins, control and exact nature. The role of consciousness is to process all information within the brain in order that the brain can then plan ahead, detect deviations from normal, make decisions and rationalise, all while regulating language (Koch and Tsuchiya, 2007). The assessment of consciousness informs us of the global functioning of the brain. However, the complexity of consciousness makes assessment challenging and, despite the many advances in neurosciences, the same methods of assessing consciousness largely continue today as they did 30 years ago.

CONSCIOUSNESS

Consciousness can be defined as a state of awareness of self and the environment, implying arousal in the brain and perceptual processing of an experience (Mashour, 2006). Consciousness has two components: arousal and cognition. Arousal is determined mainly by the functioning of the reticular activating system (RAS) (see Chapter 3), through neurones that communicate with both the thalamus and cortex. Arousal is a pre-requisite for awareness and information processing, selective attention and purposeful responses, but does not imply awareness. Cognition and awareness require simultaneous functioning of both the cerebral hemispheres and an intact RAS (Laureys *et al.*, 2004). Control of consciousness is there-

fore brought about through a complex network of activating structures (Zeman, 2001) (Table 8.1). Sensory input from multiple pathways is channelled through the reticular formation and onwards to the thalamus and cerebral cortex (Figure 8.1).

SLEEP

Sleep is a regularly occurring state of inactivity during which consciousness is lost and responses to external stimuli are reduced. Consciousness is lost during both sleep and coma, but the two states are very different. During sleep the brain remains highly active and cerebral oxygen uptake is similar to that when awake. Sleep is divided into two distinct phases: non rapid eye movement (NREM) or slow wave sleep, and rapid eye movement (REM) sleep. During NREM sleep thalamocortical cells are inhibited resulting in reduced cortical stimulation. During REM sleep the cerebral cortex is highly active, almost identically to that of an awake state, but the peri-locus ceruleus suppresses muscle tone (atonia), preventing the body from reacting to such cortical activity (Nadeau *et al.*, 2004).

The suprachiasmatic nucleus is the timekeeper of consciousness, maintaining wakefulness and sleep cycles. It is stimulated by light on the retina being transmitted to the hypothalamus. In healthy people, there is a circadian cycle over a 24 hour period between deep sleep with low arousal and very little conscious experience to increasing arousal and conscious sensation.

ASSESSMENT OF CONSCIOUSNESS

When assessing the neurological system, there are five key components which need to be considered: level of consciousness (both arousal and cognition), pupil reaction,

Neuroscience Nursing: Evidence-Based Practice, 1st Edition.
Edited by Sue Woodward and Ann-Marie Mestecky
© 2011 Blackwell Publishing Ltd

Table 8.1 Structures involved in maintaining consciousness.

Area of the brain	Function in consciousness
Reticular formation (including RAS)	Relay station for sensory information; coordinates somatic and autonomic activity; regulates arousal and awareness by controlling stimuli sent to the thalamus
Thalamus	Mediates arousal, communicating activity in the sensory systems from the brain stem and the optic nerve to the cerebral cortex and achieves cortical stimulation
Prefrontal cortex	Executive functioning, e.g. integration of perceptual functioning and formulating a response (Dietrich, 2003)

motor function, sensory function and vital signs. While this chapter will discuss level of consciousness (LOC), Chapters 13, 14 and 11 will review the assessment and interpretation of pupil reaction, vital signs, and motor and sensory function respectively.

Consciousness cannot be measured directly, but is observed through behavioural indicators and responses to certain stimuli (Zeman, 2001). Changes in LOC are felt to be the most important indicators of damage to the brain, but may be small and subtle. Rapidly changing LOC is a key indicator of neurological deterioration as it is occurring. Competence and accuracy in assessment are therefore crucial in nursing practice if subtle changes are to be detected.

The AVPU Scale

The AVPU (Alert, Voice, Pain, Unresponsive) scale (Box 8.1) has gained in popularity in recent years as a rapid assessment of LOC (Kelly *et al.*, 2004), but it is not an evidence-based tool and is inadequate for assessing LOC in a patient with a neurological condition. The full extent of the alteration to consciousness must be established,

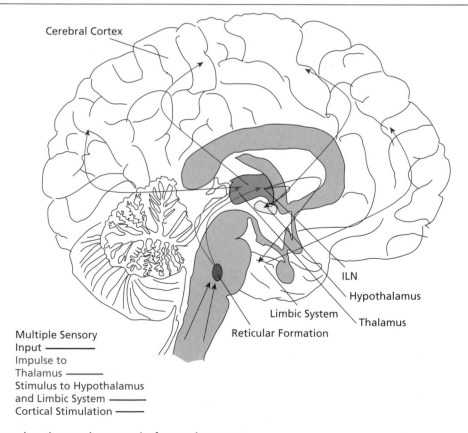

Figure 8.1 Neural pathways in control of consciousness.

requiring the nurse to perform a more in-depth assessment that cannot be achieved using the AVPU score.

The Glasgow Coma Scale (GCS)

The gold standard for assessment of consciousness throughout the world is the Glasgow Coma Scale (GCS). The GCS was first developed as a 14 point objective scale that assessed behavioural responses to a stimulus (Teasdale and Jennett, 1974), but was then adapted into a 15 point scale, with the addition of 'abnormal flexion' to the motor response category (Teasdale and Jennett, 1976). The GCS was developed to assess the impairment of consciousness and coma, primarily in those who have sustained a head injury, but it is now used more widely to assess LOC in patients with a range of neurological problems.

The scale is divided into three sections: eye opening, verbal response and motor response. Each of the above categories contain several possible behavioural responses to stimuli from which to choose. The GCS should be documented by using dots and recorded as a graph on a neurological assessment chart (Figure 8.2). Scores have been appended to each of these responses, with the lowest possible score in each category being 1. Thus the minimum possible score that can be obtained using the GCS is 3 (comatose and unresponsive) and the maximum possible score is 15 (fully conscious). However in clinical practice, summing scores is fairly meaningless, unless the total score is either 3 or 15. A GCS of 10 could be achieved in many different ways and the score for each category should be documented separately if the scores are to be used at all (e.g. E-4, V-3, M-3, rather than total GCS-10).

Validity and reliability of GCS

The GCS has been shown to have moderate (Gill *et al.*, 2004) to high inter-rater reliability (Cavanagh and Gordon, 2002). Education/training, qualifications and previous neurosurgical experience are statistically significant in

---

Box 8.1 AVPU scale

- A – Alert
- V – Responds to voice
- P – Responds to pain
- U – Unresponsive

Neurological Observation Chart

			1	2	3	4	5	6	7	8								
Glasgow Coma Scale	**Eye Opening**	Open spontaneously (4)	•														(C) = Eyes closed due to swelling
		Open to speech (3)		•	•												
		Open to pain (2)				•	•										
		Closed (1)						•	•	•							
	Verbal Response	Orientated (5)															(T) = intubated
		Confused (4)	•	•	•												
		Inappropriate words (3)				•	•										
		Incomprehensible sounds (2)						•	•								
		No verbal response (1)								•							
	Motor Response	Obeys commands (6)	•	•													Record Best Arm Response
		Localises to pain (5)			•												
		Flexion withdrawal (4)				•	•										
		Abnormal flexion (3)						•									
		Extension to pain (2)							•								
		No movement (1)								•							
		Total (out of 15)	14	13	12	9	9	6	5	3							

Figure 8.2 Documentation of the Glasgow Coma Scale (GCS).

improving accuracy in using GCS, particularly in nursing (Heron *et al.*, 2001) and video demonstration of scoring the GCS has been shown to improve accuracy (Lane *et al.*, 2002), reinforcing the need for consistency in education. It is also contended that the motor component of the GCS is more clinically important than the entire GCS itself, as it is more accurate in predicting patient outcome (Healey *et al.*, 2003). The assessment of a sedated patient using the GCS is contentious due to the need for repeated application of painful stimuli and its use should be weighed up against whether the result of such an assessment will influence treatment (Brunker, 2006).

Assessing eye opening

Eye opening is a measure of arousal, but does not imply that awareness is present. Eye opening is split into four levels of response (see Figure 8.2). If a patient has their eyes open on approach, this is recorded as spontaneous eye opening. To record an individual as 'eye opening to speech' then the patient must open their eyes to a verbal stimulus of some kind. It is often necessary to raise the volume of the verbal stimulus incrementally until you are sure that there is no response to a loud stimulus.

Only then should the assessor move on to assess whether the eyes will open in response to pain. No response to any stimulus is the lowest possible score in this section. The assessor should also consider the patient who may be deaf. Light touch on a person's shoulder may be sufficient to cause a patient to open their eyes. In this instance, it would be reasonable to assume a score of 3 (eyes open to speech) as pain was not applied to achieve the response. If a patient's eyes are closed due to swelling, 'C' should be documented on the chart and the score for this category cannot be used.

There is much debate about how to apply a painful stimulus. Some painful stimuli will cause the patient to grimace and stop the eyes from opening. Teasdale and Jennett (1974) identified that applying a painful stimulus to the finger was appropriate for assessing eye opening. Failure to use this method may lead to understimulation and application of pressure to the side of a finger-tip, using the barrel of a pen, should be used to determine an eye opening response (Edwards, 2001). This pressure should not be applied to the nail bed, due to the potential risk of damage to the underlying nerves and microcirculation, among other structures (Shah, 1999). It is recommended that the first and second fingers are not used due to their heightened sensitivity (Davidhizar and Bartlett, 1997). While this stimulus may be considered peripheral, the intensity of the application of the stimulus can result in it being central and not simply a reflex response.

Assessing verbal response

Verbal response is divided into five levels. Speech is a higher cerebral function, and assessing verbal response will measure awareness or cognition. To score someone as orientated they should be orientated to time, place and person and should know where they are and the month and year. Other questions are often used to vary the assessment, such as asking what season it is. It is essential that the questions you are asking refer to current orientation and not to information that may be laid down in long-term memory. For example, asking someone to name a relative does not indicate orientation. An orientated person will be able to answer the questions asked correctly. However, in order for someone to be orientated, they must also be orientated in conversation. If someone can just answer these questions, but their general conversation is confused in nature, then they are not orientated. It is unfair to ask a patient what day or date it is, as every day in a hospital can appear the same to a patient. In addition, care should be taken to avoid the use of closed questions requiring a yes/no response to establish the patient's awareness of their orientation (Edwards, 2001).

To record someone as confused, they must be talking in grammatically correct sentences while maintaining their attention on the nurse, but may be unable to answer the above three questions correctly or may be confused in conversation. If the patient does not understand the question, then this may also be interpreted as confusion, bearing in mind potential language barriers.

A patient who is clearly articulating words, but not constructing a sentence should be scored as using 'inappropriate words'. They may be using a single word repetitively that has no relationship to the question asked. The use of swear-words usually results in a score in this category, as long as all the other criteria are met (i.e. expletives are used outside of a complete sentence). Incomprehensible sounds are characterised by moaning and groaning to a physical stimulus. These sounds may occur spontaneously.

The lowest response in this category is no verbal response to any stimulation. If a patient is intubated, then a 'T' should be recorded on the chart and the score for this category cannot be used. However, someone with a tracheostomy may be able to verbalise, and thus we can establish their level of awareness. Although this is not strictly a verbal response, it does establish level of awareness, which is the goal of assessment in this section of the GCS.

When assessing verbal response it is important to reiterate that dysphasia does not impact on consciousness, and so it should not be assumed that someone with dysphasia is confused or has impaired awareness. Often, people with dysphasia are scored with a 'D' placed in either the confused box or inappropriate words box on the observations chart, but this is not standard practice and should not be done. It is essential for nurses to score what they see. The GCS becomes a futile tool if practitioners attempt to second guess what they are observing. Patterns and trends are important in monitoring LOC, and therefore this should be the focus – working from a baseline, i.e. if a verbal deficit occurs as a result of damage to the speech and language centres in the brain, this will not change.

Assessing motor response

Assessing motor response has been shown to be problematic for nurses, with one study identifying that 35% of nurses record motor responses incorrectly (Heron *et al.*, 2001). While this study has a small sample size, the findings are concerning considering the significance of motor response. Muscle relaxants and paralysing agents prevent accurate assessment of motor response.

Assessment of motor function begins by asking the patient to follow a specific and distinctive command that is not difficult to follow, does not elicit a reflex response, and is not something that the patient is mimicking (Edwards, 2001), e.g. 'Stick your tongue out'. Care must be taken not to 'act out' the command and only to give verbal instructions to prevent a patient from mimicking the correct response. In patients who have sustained a spinal injury, the elicitation of a motor response may be inhibited by paralysis, but tongue movement will still determine if a patient is able to obey a command. Asking a patient to squeeze your hand/fingers may trigger a primitive grasp reflex and so should not be used.

If a patient is unable to obey a command, then the motor response to pain is elicited. Motor response to pain is assessed *only* from the motor response of the arms and the best observed response is recorded. Correct application of painful stimulus is again essential and nurses need to ensure that a reflex reaction is not triggered erroneously in an attempt to assess motor response, e.g. the plantar reflex. Alternative methods of applying a painful stimulus are recommended for assessing motor response to pain and it is vital that a central stimulus rather than a peripheral stimulus is applied. Peripheral stimuli evaluate spinal responses (Edwards, 2001) and are therefore not useful for assessing consciousness. Trapezius squeeze/pinch, supra-orbital pressure and sternal rub are all forms of central stimuli, but are not all appropriate (Teasdale and Jennett, 1974).

Sternal rub

A sternal rub can cause marked bruising, despite its effectiveness in eliciting a central stimulus, and should not be used.

Supra-orbital ridge pressure

Supra-orbital ridge pressure is a common form of stimulation used to elicit a pain response. However, it must not be applied to any patient who has orbital fractures or other facial injuries. In one study 11% of patients who have sustained a blunt head trauma have facial fractures, and non-surviving patients who had low GCS scores also had mid and upper facial fractures (Plaisier *et al.*, 2000). Additionally, placing a thumb on the supra-orbital ridge can be a potential hazard to the patient with reduced awareness, who has the potential to move suddenly and sustain injury to their eye from the practitioner's thumb and nail. This makes the practice of supra-orbital ridge pressure unjustifiably risky.

Trapezius pinch

This is the most suitable method of applying a central stimulus to assess motor response, but may result in understimulation if not correctly performed and can be difficult to perform on obese patients. Trapezius pinch is performed by grasping approx 3 cm of the muscle between the thumb and forefinger and twisting. The painful stimulus should be applied for a maximum of 30 seconds and it may take up to 20 seconds to elicit the true response.

To record a patient as 'localising to pain', they should move their arm(s) across the midline of the body towards the site of the stimulus, or attempt to stop the application of the stimulus. A patient who bends their elbows and withdraws their hands, but makes no attempt to localise to the stimulus, should be scored as flexing to pain. It is important to note that the patient abducts their hand away from the midline of the body during this response, but there is no rotation of the wrist. Abnormal flexion is distinctly different from flexion/withdrawal and is characterised by flexion at the elbow, adduction of the upper arm and pronation of the wrists in response to a central stimulus. Extension to pain is very distinct with straightening of the elbows, rotation of the arms towards the body, and flexion of the wrists. A score of no response is given to a patient who shows no movement to a central stimulus.

INTERPRETATION OF GCS FINDINGS

It should be remembered that the GCS is not designed to diagnose the cause of an altered state of consciousness, but simply to measure the LOC. Therefore, nurses should not second guess an assessment score and the golden rule is always to 'score what you see', i.e. always document the patient's actual responses. Generally speaking the lower the GCS, the lower the LOC, and a patient with a GCS of 8 or below, with no eye opening is in a coma. In order to determine the cause of the change in LOC, e.g. raised ICP or reduced cerebral perfusion due to hypovolaemia, the GCS needs to be considered in conjunction with pupil responses (see Chapter 13), assessment of limb movements (see Chapter 11) and systemic observations (see Chapter 14). Clearly, the identification of patients who are deteriorating due to raised ICP using GCS is vital. The interpretation and recognition of this has been discussed in Chapter 7.

Motor function illustrates the complexity of cerebral functioning, and represents the patient's ability to process information and elicit an appropriate response. It is the most valuable component within the GCS and a reduction in motor response indicates a significant deterioration in neurological functioning (Fischer and Mathieson, 2001; Balestreri *et al.*, 2004).

Using GCS as a prognostic indicator

While admission GCS can be used to grade the severity of head injury (see Chapter 32), it is not an accurate predictor of outcome following a deterioration in LOC (Balestreri *et al.*, 2004). Duration of unconsciousness, however, is statistically significant in predicting outcome (Ratan *et al.*, 2001). Teasdale *et al.* (1998) advocated the use of a different scale, the Glasgow Outcome Scale (GOS), to predict outcome following head injury (see Chapter 32). It is has since become apparent that baseline GOS score is a reliable predictor of outcome in patients with no or mild disability, but not in patients with severe disability (Miller *et al.*, 2005).

A GCS score can inform clinical decision making through assessment of existing neurological impairment or by demonstrating deterioration in consciousness. The GCS also has a role to play in decision making at time of resuscitation. A score of 3/15 on the GCS with fixed dilated pupils indicates that the patient has no realistic chance of survival, whereas a score of 3/15 without fixed dilated pupils is an indicator for aggressive resuscitation (Lieberman *et al.*, 2003). Further research has demonstrated that the GCS is effective in allocating triage priority in emergency care situations (Norwood *et al.*, 2002)

and in monitoring those with organophosphate poisoning (Grmec *et al.*, 2004).

ALTERED STATES OF CONSCIOUSNESS

Altered states of consciousness occur when there is damage to the neural pathways and structures that are required to maintain consciousness. Aetiology of altered consciousness can be divided into intracranial and extracranial causes (Box 8.2).

Coma

Coma is an altered state of consciousness characterised by absence of arousal or conscious awareness (Whyte *et al.*, 2005). Sleep-wake cycles are absent, and this altered state of consciousness must last for more than one hour before the term coma is applied. Outcome from coma is related to the cause, and is independent of the patient's initial presentation, length of time in the coma, or 'depth' of the coma (Bates, 2001). Some clinical signs are also important prognostic indicators (Box 8.3), but in many cases, the prognosis and outcome of coma is difficult to predict with any degree of certainty.

Many investigators have tried interventions, such as music therapy and thalamic stimulators, in an attempt to promote recovery from coma, all without success (Wijdicks

---

Box 8.2 Aetiology of altered consciousness

Intracranial causes

- Intracranial haemorrhages
- Ischaemia and infarction
- Infections (meningitis, encephalitis, cerebral abscess)
- Tumours
- Cerebral oedema
- Trauma
- Epilepsy

Extracranial causes

- Hypo/hypertension
- Infection and septicaemia
- Metabolic causes (hypo/hyperglycaemia, electrolyte disorders, hypoxia, carbon monoxide poisoning, hypercarbia, hepatic encephalopathy, uraemic encephalopathy
- Drug induced (e.g. sedatives, opioids, alcohol)
- Substance misuse
- Drug and alcohol withdrawal

Box 8.3 Prognosis following coma	
	Likelihood of recovery (%)
Cause:	
• Metabolic/septic	25
• Hypoxic/ischaemic	10
• SAH/stroke	5
Clinical signs:	
• Eye opening within 6 hours	20
• Flexion response	15
• No motor response	3
• Verbal groans	30
• No verbal noise	8
Duration:	
• 1 day	10 (good recovery)
• 3 days	6
• 7 days	3
• 14 days	2

Adapted from Bates, 2001.

Box 8.4   Characteristics of persistent vegetative state (PVS)

- Preservation of circadian rhythms such as sleep wake cycles
- Preservation of autonomic responses of the hypothalamus and brain stem
- Incontinence of urine and faeces
- Possible cranial and spinal nerve reflexes present
- Inconsistent motor actions (non purposeful movement, facial grimacing, chewing, verbal sounds)
- Inconsistent sensory responses to auditory and oculomotor stimulation

Source: Howard and Miller, 1995.

and Cranford, 2005). Some medications (amphetamines, amantadine, methylphenidate and bromocriptine) have been investigated and shown to have some positive effects on improving coma after traumatic brain injury (Richer and Tell, 2003), but improvements have been limited and further large scale trials are required. Medical management of conditions that result in coma and advances in life support provision are thought to increase chances of survival from coma, but there is no concrete evidence that advances in care do improve chances of survival (Bates, 2001).

Those patients who die while in a comatose state normally do so early in the course of coma. Those who survive coma generally show a gradual improvement in consciousness within 2–4 weeks. The extent of recovery will vary, with some patients remaining in a minimally conscious state or vegetative state, while others have a good recovery (Laureys *et al.*, 2002).

Persistent/permanent vegetative state

Persistent vegetative state (PVS) is a chronic neurological syndrome that is characterised by preserved wakefulness, but voluntary interaction with the environment is absent, and there is complete loss of all cognitive functioning (Kotchoubey *et al.*, 2005). In other words, there is a preserved capacity for spontaneous or stimulated arousal, but

it is not purposeful (Giacino and Kalmar, 2005). 'Persistent' refers to the vegetative state continuing for at least one month, but this does not necessarily imply permanency or irreversibility. PVS is characterised by certain characteristics (Box 8.4). The individual may still be able to hear, but may lack the high order activities for processing what they hear.

PVS has to be distinguished from other neurological states, such as coma or locked-in syndrome. A diagnosis of PVS cannot be made if there is any degree of voluntary/purposeful movement, sustained/consistent visual tracking (pursuit and fixation), or if the individual reacts to threatening interaction (Howard and Miller, 1995; Laureys *et al.*, 2002). Currently there is no treatment available which is effective in reversing PVS. Zolpidem has shown promising effects in improving LOC (Clauss and Ncl, 2006), but the sample in this study was only three patients and further research is indicated.

The diagnosis of *permanent* vegetative state is usually applied when an individual has remained in a vegetative state for longer than six months and this is normally considered to be irreversible (Laureys *et al.*, 2002).

Minimally conscious state (MCS)

The MCS state is 10 times more common than PVS, and is associated with a better prognosis for recovery (Wijdicks and Cranford, 2005). An individual who is in a MCS has a limited, but definite, awareness of themselves or environment, distinguishing this state of consciousness from a vegetative one (Whyte *et al.*, 2005). This limited awareness must be reproducible or sustained, and must be associated with one or more of four particular behaviours (Giacino *et al.*, 2004; Laureys *et al.*, 2004) (Box 8.5).

Box 8.5   Diagnostic criteria for minimally conscious state

- Following simple commands
- Response with gestures or yes/no (accuracy is not relevant)
- Displays intelligible speech
- Purposeful behaviour that is not reflexive activity
  - Crying, smiling or laughter in response to a emotional stimulus
  - Vocalisation or gestures in response to a verbal stimulus
  - Purposefully reaching for an object
  - Accommodation of the size and shape of an object when holding or touching it
  - Tracking or fixation of the eyes in response to a stimulus

---

There is a degree of cognitive processing, and the diagnosis is reliant on some language and motor system integrity being present (Giacino and Kalmar, 2005).

While patients in this state may meet the four criteria above, they are usually doubly incontinent, require nutritional support, and are unable to make complex decisions (Wijdicks and Cranford, 2005). Therapies that involve sensory stimulation may improve prognosis, and active rehabilitation should be engaged with (Taylor *et al.*, 2007). Deep brain stimulation (DBS) of the thalamus has received increasing attention in recent years as an intervention that promotes arousal and can significantly improve LOC (Schiff *et al.*, 2007).

Locked-in syndrome

Locked-in syndrome, sometimes referred to as pseudocoma, is characterised by quadriplegia and anarthria (partial or total loss of motor speech control) and is commonly caused by ventral pontine and brain stem lesions. Awareness of the environment is present, as is sustained eye opening, aphonia or hypophonia and vertical or lateral eye movement. Blinking responses are also present, with eye movement being the only method of communication, as patients have no limb movements or facial expressions (Laureys *et al.*, 2005). Communication can be difficult as the patient can become exhausted trying to communicate by eye movements alone.

Life expectancy, once homeostatic stability has been achieved, can be several decades and quality of life can often be reported to be meaningful. Patients may be able to give valid and informed consent, having the cognitive abilities to make choices about treatment. These patients are vulnerable, however, and nurses must recognise this as well as the potential for patient's human rights to be breached. This often requires the nurse to be proactive in communicating, establishing the needs of the patient and acting as an advocate when necessary.

Cataplexy and sleep states

Cataplexy is a phenomenon that occurs when REM sleep atonia (loss of muscle tone) intrudes into a state of wakefulness (Chakravorty and Rye, 2003), thereby affecting consciousness. While in a state of cataplexy there is no loss of awareness, but the patient is unable to respond to the environment due to the loss of motor tone. Cataplexy is usually triggered by experiencing a strong emotion, e.g. anger, laughter, or intense sadness, as cataplexy is linked with the limbic system that controls emotion (see Chapter 3). Cataplexy is one of the four main features of narcolepsy, a neurological disorder associated with insufficient production of hypocretin. Hypocretin is a neurotransmitter released by the hypothalamus; it links physiological arousal, appetite and neuro-endocrine homeostasis (Selbach *et al.*, 2003).

REM sleep disorders and parasomnias, such as sleepwalking (somnambulism) and sleep paralysis (a form of cataplexy), are also considered disorders of consciousness. The affected individual experiences either a loss of awareness or they are aware, but unable to respond to the environment. This is similar in akinetic mutism, where damage to the frontal lobe causes inhibition that results in the patient being mute and akinetic (unmoving). In akinetic mutism, there is reduced voluntary movement, speech and thought, but there is no disruption to arousal (Lim *et al.*, 2007). Akinetic mutism can occur after stroke, subarachnoid haemorrhage, malignancy or carbon monoxide poisoning and usually involves damage to subcortical structures such as the thalamus, basal ganglia, and mid brain; all of which are areas vital to controlling consciousness.

BRAIN STEM DEATH

Brain stem death results from raised intracranial pressure leading to tonsillar herniation (see Chapter 7), and subsequent cerebrocirculatory arrest (Shemie *et al.*, 2007). Brain stem death can also occur with isolated injury to the brain stem, such as brain stem stroke/infarction. The haemodynamic impact of brain stem death is presented in Chapter 14. The concept of brain stem death was defined in 1976 and is accepted as death of the individual in the

UK (Inwald *et al.*, 2000). Death is defined as 'the irreversible loss of the capacity for consciousness, combined with the irreversible loss of the capacity to breathe' (DH, 1998 p 7).

The concept of 'death' is challenging to people from all backgrounds and has diverse interpretation across cultures. The advances of medical science and sophisticated life-support systems have added to this challenge, blurring the boundaries of traditional concepts and definitions of death. It is now more difficult to determine the point at which disorders are irreversible, when treatment is no longer effective, and when death is considered to have occurred (Shemie *et al.*, 2007). The practices of organ donation further add to the confusion, particularly in relation to brain stem death. The appropriate use of specific terms such as death and brain stem death are crucial in helping families to understand and accept the end of life of a loved one. When the term 'brain death' was used instead of 'death' with relatives of brain-dead patients, there was a 20% reduction in consent for organ donation, largely as a result of an inability to accept death based on the terminology used (Tessmer *et al.*, 2007).

Assessment of brain stem death

Gaining consent to testing for brain stem death is largely dependent on culture and religion (Aldawood *et al.*, 2007), the terminology used (Tessmer *et al.*, 2007) and the quality and process of information provided to families throughout the patient's care (Rocker *et al.*, 2006).

The Department of Health (1998) set out the following conditions and subsequent diagnostic criteria for brain stem death (Box 8.6).

The patient may be moderately hypothermic, flaccid, and with a depressed metabolism at the time of testing. Ventilation with 100% oxygen should take place for 10 minutes and subsequently with 5% CO_2 in oxygen for five minutes (if available) prior to testing. The ventilator should be disconnected for 10 minutes, with oxygen delivered by catheter into the trachea at 6 l/min. Those with pre-existing chronic respiratory disease require expert opinion.

Testing is normally undertaken by two different medical consultants, often 24 hours apart. However, this largely depends on the stability of the patient, and considerations of potential organ donation. When the patient's condition makes aspects of this testing difficult or impossible, the ITU consultant normally collaborates with the multidisciplinary team and colleagues in order to reach a consensus on how to proceed. While the criteria for brain stem death testing are explicit, interpretation of results can vary. Bell *et al.* (2004) demonstrated that marked variations in the

---

Box 8.6 Diagnostic criteria for brain stem death
Conditions under which the diagnosis should be considered:
• Confirmation that the patient's condition is due to irremediable brain damage of know aetiology
• The patient is deeply unconscious and that this state is not induced by drugs, hypothermia, or by potentially irreversible circulatory, metabolic or endocrine disorders
• There is inadequate or absent spontaneous respirations
Diagnostic criteria:
• Absence of brain stem reflexes
• Pupils are fixed and unresponsive to sharp changes in incidental light intensity
• Absence of corneal reflexes
• Absence of vestibulo-ocular reflexes (normal reflex is deviation of the eyes away from the side of the stimulus) in response to instilling 50 ml of ice cold water, over one minute, into each external auditory meatus, ensuring access to tympanic membrane and head is maintained at 30°
• Absence of motor response (from stimulation of somatic area within cranial nerve distribution). This includes no limb response to supraorbital pressure
• Absence of gag reflex or reflex response to bronchial stimulation
• Absence of respiratory movement on disconnection from mechanical ventilation, with the arterial carbon dioxide levels exceeding the threshold for spontaneous respiratory stimulation ($PaCO_2$ >6.65 kPa)
Source: Department of Health, 1998.

---

interpretation of the UK guidelines occur, mainly as a result of confounding variables, how the apnoea test and brain stem reflexes are performed, and the repetition of testing. They highlight that guidelines do not replace professional judgement, and thus the process and the results may not be rigidly applied.

NURSING MANAGEMENT OF A PATIENT WITH ALTERED CONSCIOUSNESS

Caring for the unconscious patient

Caring for the unconscious patient is a nursing privilege. This group of patients have lost the ability to protect their dignity, provide valid informed consent and meet their own personal care needs. Ultimately, a skilled nurse is required to identify the patient's needs and proactively manage them. Other chapters will focus on specific aspects of care, such as managing respiratory function (see Chapter 15), raised ICP (see Chapter 7) and meeting fluid and nutritional requirements (see Chapter 16). This section will discuss specific care of the unconscious patient.

Immediate priorities in the patient who becomes unconscious

In the immediate phase of loss of consciousness, vital functions central to survival become the focus of care. The maintenance of an airway, support of breathing (either through artificial ventilation or other respiratory support), cardiovascular support, evaluation of the extent of neurological compromise, and assessment as to the cause of the loss of consciousness are the immediate priorities. This is in keeping with the A (airway), B (breathing), C (circulation), D (disability), E (exposure) model of assessment and care advocated by the Resuscitation Council UK (2005). The extent of support required in each area will determine the nursing care required.

Preventing complications of bed rest

Patients with a reduced LOC often experience significantly reduced mobility, resulting in the potential for patients to develop pressure sores, deep vein thrombosis (DVT), muscular atrophy and contractures (see also Chapter 11).

Pressure area care

Patients at high risk for developing pressure sores are more likely to be male, older, unconscious and in a post-operative phase of healing (Uzun and Tan, 2007). The catabolic state that may present in the acutely ill neuroscience patient may contribute to low body mass index and low serum albumin, which increase the risk. The accurate assessment of risk, using reliable validated tools, such as the Braden Scale (Bergstrom et al., 1987), and the implementation of risk reducing strategies such as frequent turning, use of pressure relieving mattresses, management of continence and optimisation of nutrition and hydration, can reduce the incidence of pressure necrosis (Brillhart, 2005).

Patient repositioning is well established as a key intervention in the prevention and management of pressure ulcers. Anecdotal evidence often suggests that the patient's position should be changed every two hours in order to reduce/eliminate pressure while maintaining microcircula-

tion to at-risk pressure points (Reddy et al., 2006). However, the evidence base for turning regimens is weak. Defloor et al. (2005) determined that four hourly turns, combined with the use of low-pressure foam based mattresses, significantly reduced the development of pressure ulcers in comparison to two hourly turns on a standard hospital mattress. This study, however, does not evaluate the evidence on turning alone and so makes it difficult to ascertain the effectiveness of this intervention (Reddy et al., 2006). Salcido (2004) argues that while the evidence on the frequency of turning is weak, the evidence on the effect of the mechanical forces of shearing and pressure on the development of pressure ulcers is strong and that the reduction of such forces by turning is a logical basis for the intervention. On this basis, and in the absence of greater evidence to the contrary, the greater the frequency of turning, the more likely is the reduction in such forces, and thus the prevention of ulceration (Salcido, 2004).

There is a strong body of evidence that supports the use of foam-based low pressure mattresses and overlays, and pressure relieving/alternating mattresses in the prevention of pressure ulceration development (Cullum et al., 2004). This is supported by various studies comparing these devices with standard hospital mattresses (Russell et al., 2003; Gray and Campbell, 1994). Vanderwee et al. (2005) determined that alternating pressure air mattresses reduced the incidence of pressure ulcer development, particularly at the heels. However, the evidence that exists relates to specific types of mattresses and often in relation to the care of specific groups of patients. It is therefore necessary to evaluate each mattress type on the basis of its use for neuroscience patients alongside professional judgement. NICE (2005) provides a flow chart to apply the evidence alongside such professional judgement, which stems from guidelines developed by the Collaborating Centre for Nursing and Supportive Care (2004).

Deep vein thrombosis (DVT) prophylaxis

Deep vein thrombosis (DVT) is a further complication of bed-rest. The aetiology of venous thrombosis is explained by Virchow's Triad:

- Hypercoagulability (systemic or local)
- Venous stasis from poor venous return and
- Injury to the venous intima (specifically the endothelium)

(Malone and Agutter, 2006)

All unconscious patients will be at risk of developing DVT and appropriate interventions should be followed. NICE

(2007) provides guidelines to prevent DVT formation (Box 8.7). In addition, passive limb movements can help venous return to the heart, while also helping to prevent contractures and muscular atrophy (Geraghty, 2005).

The use of low molecular weight heparin is controversial for some neuroscience patients, particularly when there is a risk of further haemorrhage. A risk assessment strategy should be adopted to determine potential benefits/ risks of administering low molecular weight heparin on an individual basis. NICE (2007) provides guidance for specific clinical conditions.

Bladder and bowel care

Many patients with an altered LOC will develop urinary incontinence that often necessitates the insertion of an indwelling urethral catheter in the early stages when an accurate fluid balance is required. Long-term management many require the consideration of urinary sheaths in males or incontinence pads (Geraghty, 2005). Additionally, unconscious patients are at a greater risk of constipation, requiring proactive prevention through a high fibre enteral feed, use of laxatives as appropriate and accurate assessment and documentation of bowel function (Geraghty, 2005). Adequate hydration is also important in reducing constipation (see Chapter 18 for further details).

Box 8.7   Deep vein thrombosis (DVT) prophylaxis

- Mechanical prophylaxis except where contraindicated – graduated compression or antiembolism stockings, intermittent pneumatic compression (IPC), or foot impulse devices. Compression stockings should meet the following criteria – compression should be about 18 mmHg at the ankle, 14 mmHg at the mid-calf, and 8 mmHg at the upper thigh when using thigh length stockings. Correctly sized and applied stockings will normally achieve these requirements
- The administration of low molecular weight heparin, unless contraindicated
- Ensure optimal hydration
- Consideration of the risks and benefits of discontinuing anticoagulation or antiplatelet therapy that may have been in place on admission

Source: National Institute of Health and Clinical Excellence, 2007.

Oral, aural and nasal hygiene

Debris can build up around the oral cavity in the unconscious patient, which can be exacerbated by unhumidified oxygen therapy. In critically ill patients increased levels of oral flora have been reported and these bacteria adhere to the surface of teeth, creating a biofilm and eventually leading to the build up of dental plaque (Berry & Davidson, 2006). Poor oral hygiene has also been associated with ventilator acquired pneumonia (VAP) due to build up of bacteria within plaque. The introduction of oral care protocols has been shown to reduce the incidence of VAP (Ross and Crumpler, 2007; Powers and Brower, 2007; Sona *et al.*, 2009).

Pearson and Hutton (2002) demonstrated that a soft-bristled toothbrush is most effective for removing the bacterial biofilm and dental plaque. For unconscious patients, oral hygiene with a toothbrush and toothpaste or water twice daily should suffice, but for ventilated patients additional recommendations exist. While there is limited evidence, oral hygiene using antiseptics such as chlorhexidine is recommended for this patient group (NICE, 2008) and anaphylaxis and serious respiratory complications associated with chlorhexidine are rare. Nasal mucosa and external aural canals may also require cleansing to remove debris.

Eye care

Unconscious patients will not have a protective blink reflex, and the tears required to cleanse and hydrate the eyes will not be spread over the surface of the cornea. Eyelid closure is also often incomplete. Critically ill and unconscious patients are at risk of corneal dehydration, keratitis, abrasions and in extreme cases ulceration, perforation, scarring and possibly permanent visual impairment due to the loss of these fundamental protective mechanisms (So *et al.*, 2008). It is essential that regular eye care is provided, although regimes often vary between units and evidence in favour of one regime over another is lacking (Marshall *et al.*, 2008).

Gentle cleansing of closed eyes with normal saline and gauze is advocated (Geraghty, 2005). Maintaining hydration through prescribed lubricating drops, ointments, or polyethylene covers is required (Dawson, 2005) and the nurse should check that the eye lids remain closed to prevent keratitis and epithelial erosion. In one recent study, So *et al.* (2008) identified that there was no difference between the effectiveness of polyethylene covers and lanolin eye ointment in preventing corneal abrasions.

Management of pain and comfort

Assessment and management of pain and comfort in the unconscious patient can be a complex task. Uncertainty exists as to whether patients with altered states of consciousness experience pain and to what degree. Neural pathways in those in a vegetative state are incomplete, resulting in pain being processed at only a primary (reflex) level (Schnakers and Zasler, 2007). However, in the minimally conscious state these neural pathways are largely intact, meaning secondary processing takes place. When it is difficult to isolate which of these two states the patient is in, it is important to recognise that pain may be experienced, and should be assumed when physiological and non-verbal cues indicate. Further detail of pain assessment and management is presented in Chapter 17.

Communication needs of patients and family

Verbal communication and interaction received by the unconscious patient is less than that received by patients who are verbally responsive (Alasad and Ahmad, 2005).

Alasad and Ahmad (2005) highlight how nurses often find communicating with patients who are unresponsive to be challenging, largely due to the lack of feedback from the patient and the uncertainty of its benefit. While it is not always possible to determine how much verbal and non-verbal communication is processed by patients with lower levels of consciousness, communication underpins practice and keeps the patient central to care (see Chapter 12).

Communication needs to extend to the family members who will often be experiencing a traumatic situation. Azoulay and Pochard (2003) highlight the need for family centred care that emphasises better communication and involvement of family in the process of care throughout.

Psychological support for the patient's family

Regardless of the environment, family support is crucial as the crisis event they have encountered may be prolonged and family members may find themselves taking on the role of carer. Family carers experience many challenges, with male family members known to experience higher levels of emotional distress and neuroticism than female members (Chiambretto et al., 2001). As time progresses and the patient's condition remains unchanged, caregivers use fewer coping strategies, report increasingly unsatisfactory family relationships, and experience advancing emotional distress (Chiambretto et al., 2001). Care givers report symptoms of depression and anxiety linked with thoughts of the possible death of the patient.

The impact upon the caregiver's life is significant as social interaction is reduced, their independence is curtailed and they often feel alone in coping.

Nurses are ideally placed to offer support to families, listen to their concerns and explain everything that is happening. Relatives may feel helpless and can appreciate opportunities to become involved in patient care, but equally may be reluctant to get involved and so should not be put under pressure to participate.

NURSING MANAGEMENT OF A PATIENT WITH BRAIN STEM DEATH

Care of the family

The experience of the relatives of those diagnosed as brain stem dead is undoubtedly traumatic. Some describe the process of testing as 'macabre' and 'harrowing' (Pugh et al., 2000). The experience is confrontational, with relatives having to process the experience of their relative presenting as 'living-dead' (Frid et al., 2007). There is debate as to whether relatives should be present during testing, and whether this would help or hinder acceptance. Pugh et al. (2000) determined that 42% of nurses had experienced relatives being present during brain stem death testing, with 69% of these nurses reporting this process as helpful in facilitating acceptance. Fundamental to the success of this process was the explanation of the procedure and the patient responses that may occur.

Evidence suggests that nurses currently underestimate the levels of anxiety surrounding end of life issues (Rocker et al., 2006), and the key factor that determines decision-making around end of life is the nature of the interaction between health care professional and family members. Honesty, compassion and completeness of information are key issues, requiring the nurse to dedicate time and attention to ensuring that the family are sufficiently cared for.

A patient who has been diagnosed with brain stem death may still exhibit spinal reflex responses that may be misinterpreted as purposive actions by relatives. 85% of nurses report that spinal reflexes are a significant issue requiring advanced warning and explanation by nurses to minimise their effect on relatives (Pugh et al., 2000). Although often considered rare, approximately 19% of patients who are brain stem dead exhibit reflex movements such as periodic leg movements (Han et al., 2006).

It is crucial for nurses to be proactive in assisting relatives to understand the concept of brain stem death (Tessmer et al., 2007). This has the potential to increase consent for organ donation, but more importantly may help the family in grieving for their loved one. This can be particularly challenging outside of critical care areas, but nurses should remember that non-heart-beating donors are also eligible for organ donation.

Organ donation

A high percentage of neuroscience patients diagnosed with brain stem death meet the criteria for organ donation. Those with a GCS of 7 or less are identified as having potential to be eventual organ donors (Bustos *et al.*, 2006). For parents and next-of-kin consent to donation is influenced by personal factors, the conditions under which the request to consider donation is made, prior knowledge and experience with organ donation or serious illness, and interpersonal factors (Bellali and Papadatou, 2006). Religion and culture may also influence the decision to consent and it is essential to recognise the multicultural nature of society and discuss issues sensitively.

In the UK, US, Germany and Australia, informed consent is required before cadaveric organ procurement occurs, usually determined by an organ donor registration card. Other countries in Europe perform cadaveric organ procurement based on the principle of presumed consent, whereby a potential donor is identified by the absence of explicit opposition to donation before death (Abadie and Gay, 2006). However, contemporary practice is to make such decisions in conjunction with the family.

Currently in the UK the Human Tissues Act (DH, 2004) (covering England, Wales and Northern Ireland, with Human Tissues Act (2006) covering Scotland) specifies that organ retrieval from the deceased (cadaveric donation) must adhere to the fundamental principle of consent. The removal, use or storage of human organs or tissues is unlawful for scheduled purposes (e.g. transplantation) without appropriate consent.

Consent has to be established in one of two ways. Either the decision of a deceased person to consent or not to consent must have been in force immediately prior to his/her death or, if no such consent is in place, then consent is required from either a nominated representative or a person in a qualifying relationship, usually next of kin. However, the UK chief medical officer's report for 2006 (DH, 2007), makes the following recommendations in terms of organ donation, which may alter this position in the near future:

- an opt-out system for organ donation should be created within UK legislation
- an increase in donation in hospital should be facilitated by the creation of opportunities to maximise organ transplantation and

- ethnic minority groups should be targeted with campaigns aimed at increasing organ donation

(DH, 2007)

SUMMARY

The complexity of consciousness brings with it significant challenges. The nature of altered consciousness depends on the extent of disruption within the central nervous system. It requires nurses to have the knowledge and understanding of the principles behind assessment of consciousness and its various states, the presentation of these, and the evidence-based nursing practice for both the patient and family.

REFERENCES

Abadie A, Gay S (2006) The impact of presumed consent legislation on cadaveric organ donation: a cross-country study. *Journal of Health Economics* 25(4):599–620.

Alasad J, Ahmad M (2005) Communication with critically ill patients. *Journal of Advanced Nursing* 50(4): 356–362.

Aldawood A, Al Qahtani S, Dabbagh O, *et al.* (2007) Organ donation after brain death: experience over five-years in a tertiary hospital. *Nasrat Amrad Wa Ziraat Alkulat* 18(1):60–64.

Azoulay E, Pochard F (2003) Communication with family members of patients dying in the intensive care unit. *Current Opinion in Critical Care* 9(6): 545–550.

Balestreri M, Czosnyka M, Chatfield DA *et al.* (2004) Predictive value of Glasgow Coma Scale after brain trauma: change in trend over the past ten years. *Journal of Neurology, Neurosurgery and Psychiatry* 75(1):161–162.

Bates D (2001) The prognosis of medical coma. *Journal of Neurology, Neurosurgery and Psychiatry* 71(Suppl 1): i20–i23.

Bell MDD, Moss E, Murphy PG (2004) Brainstem death testing in the UK – time for reappraisal? *British Journal of Anaesthesia* 92(5):633–640.

Bellali T, Papadatou D (2006) The decision-making process of parents regarding organ donation of their brain dead child: A Greek study. *Social Science and Medicine* 64(2):439–450.

Bergstrom N, Braden BJ, Laguzza A *et al.* (1987) The Braden scale for predicting pressure sore risk. *Nursing Research* 36(4):205–210.

Berry AM, Davidson PM (2006) Beyond comfort: oral hygiene as a critical nursing activity in the intensive care unit. *Intensive and Critical Care Nursing* 22:318–328.

Brillhart B (2005) Pressure sore and skin tear prevention and treatment during a 10-month program. *Rehabilitation Nursing* 30(3):85–91.

Brunker C (2006) Assessment of sedated head-injured patients using the Glasgow Coma Scale: An Audit. *British Journal of Neuroscience Nursing* 2(6):276–280.

Bustos JL, Surt K, Soratti C (2006) Glasgow Coma Scale 7 or less surveillance program for brain death identification in Argentina: Epidemiology and outcome. *Transplantation Proceedings*. 38(10):3697–3699.

Cavanagh SJ, Gordon VL (2002) Grading scales used in the management of aneurysmal subarachnoid hemorrhage: a critical review. *Journal of Neuroscience Nursing* 34(6): 288–295.

Chakravorty SS, Rye DB (2003) Narcolepsy in the older adult: epidemiology, diagnosis and management. *Drugs and Aging* 20(5):361–376.

Chiambretto P, Rossi Ferrario S, Zotti AM (2001) Patients in a persistent vegetative state: caregiver attitudes and reactions. *Acta Neurologica Scandinavica.* 104(6):364–368.

Clauss R, Nel W (2006) Drug induced arousal from the permanent vegetative state. *Neurorehabilitation* 21(1):23–28.

Collaborating Centre for Nursing and Supportive Care (2004) *Clinical Practice Guidelines: The use of pressure-relieving devices (beds, mattresses and overlays) for the prevention of pressure ulcers in primary and secondary care.* London: Royal College of Nursing.

Cullum N, McInnes E, Bell-Syer SE *et al.* (2004) Beds, mattresses and cushions for pressure sore prevention and treatment. *Cochrane Database Systematic Reviews.* 2000;(2):CD001735.

Davidhizar R, Bartlett D (1997) Management of the patient with minor traumatic brain injury. *British Journal of Nursing* 6(9):498–503.

Dawson D (2005) Development of a new eye care guideline for critically ill patients. *Intensive and Critical Care Nursing* 21(2):119–122.

Defloor T, De Bacquer D, Grypdonck MH (2005) The effect of various combinations of turning and pressure reducing devices on the incidence of pressure ulcers. *International Journal of Nursing Studies.* 42:37–46.

Department of Health (1998) *A Code of Practice for the Diagnosis of Brain Stem Death.* London: DH.

Department of Health (2004) *The Human Tissue Act.* London: DH.

Department of Health (2007) *On the State of Public Health: Annual report of the chief medical officer 2006.* London: DH.

Dietrich A (2003) Functional neuroanatomy of altered states of consciousness: the transient hypofrontality hypothesis. *Consciousness and Cognition* 12(2):231–256.

Edwards SL (2001) Adult/elderly care nursing. Using the Glasgow Coma Scale: analysis and limitations. *British Journal of Nursing* 10(2):92–101.

Fischer J, Mathieson C (2001) The history of the Glasgow Coma Scale: implications for practice. *Critical Care Nursing Quarterly* 23(4):52–58.

Frid I, Haljamae H, Ohlen J *et al.* (2007) Brain death: close relative's use of imagery as a descriptor of experience. *Journal of Advanced Nursing* 58(1):63–71.

Geraghty M (2005) Nursing the unconscious patient. *Nursing Standard* 20(1):54– 65.

Giacino JT, Kalmar K (2005) Diagnostic and prognostic guidelines for the vegetative and minimally conscious states. *Neuropsychological Rehabilitation* 15(3–4): 166–174.

Giacino JT, Kalmar K, Whyte J (2004) The JFK Coma Recovery Scale-Revised: measurement characteristics and diagnostic utility. *Archives of Physical Medicine and Rehabilitation* 85(12):2020–2029.

Gill MR, Reiley DG, Green SM (2004) Interrater reliability of Glasgow Coma Scale scores in the emergency department. *Annals of Emergency Medicine* 43(2):215–223.

Gray DG, Campbell M (1994) A randomised clinical trial of two types of foam mattresses. *Journal of Tissue Viability* 4:128–132.

Grmec S, Mally S, Klemen P (2004) Glasgow Coma Scale score and QTc interval in the prognosis of organophosphate poisoning. *Academic Emergency Medicine* 11(9): 925–930.

Han SG, Kim GM, Lee KH *et al.* (2006) Reflex movements in patients with brain death: a prospective study in a tertiary medical center. *Journal of Korean Medical Science* 21(3):588–590.

Healey C, Osler TM, Rogers FB, *et al.* (2003) Improving the Glasgow Coma Scale score: motor score alone is a better predictor. *Journal of Trauma* 54(4):671–680.

Heron R, Davie A, Gillies R *et al.* (2001) Inter-rater reliability of the Glasgow Coma Scale scoring among nurses in sub-specialties of critical care. *Australian Critical Care* 14(3):100–105.

Howard RS, Miller DH (1995) The persistent vegetative state. *British Medical Journal* 310:341–342.

Inwald D, Jakobovits I, Petros A (2000) Brain stem death: managing care when accepted medical guidelines and religious beliefs are in conflict. *British Medical Journal* 320:1266–1268.

Kelly CA, Upex A, Bateman DN (2004) Comparison of consciousness level assessment in the poisoned patient using the Alert/Verbal/Painful/Unresponsive Scale and the Glasgow Coma Scale. *Annals of Emergency Medicine* 44(2):108–113.

Koch C, Tsuchiya N (2007) Attention and consciousness: two distinct brain processes. *Trends in Cognitive Sciences* 11(1):16–22.

Kotchoubey B, Lang S, Mezger G *et al.* (2005) Information processing in severe disorders of consciousness: vegetative state and minimally conscious state. *Clinical Neurophysiology* 116(10):2441–2453.

Lane PL, Baez AA, Brabson T *et al.* (2002) Effectiveness of a Glasgow Coma Scale instructional video for EMS providers. *Prehospital and Disaster Medicine* 17(3):142–146.

Laureys S, Faymonville ME, Peigneux P *et al.* (2002) Cortical processing of noxious somatosensory stimuli in the persistent vegetative state. *NeuroImage* 17(2):732–741.

Laureys S, Owen AM, Schiff ND (2004) Brain function in coma, vegetative state, and related disorders. *The Lancet* 3(9):537–546.

Laureys A, Pellas F, Van Eeckhout P *et al.* (2005) The locked-in syndrome: what is it like to be conscious but paralyzed and voiceless? *Progress in Brain Research* 150:495–511.

Lieberman JD, Pasquale MD, Garcia R *et al.* (2003) Use of admission Glasgow Coma Score, pupil size, and pupil reactivity to determine outcome for trauma patients. *Journal of Trauma* 55(3):437–443.

Lim YC, Ding CSL, Kong KH (2007) Akinetic mutism after right internal watershed infarct. *Singapore Medical Journal* 48(5):466–468.

Malone PC, Agutter PS (2006) The aetiology of deep venous thrombosis. *Quarterly Journal of Medicine* 99(9):581–593.

Marshall AP, Elliott R, Rolls K *et al.* (2008) Eyecare in the critically ill: clinical practice guideline. *Australian Critical Care* 21:97–109.

Mashour GA (2006) Integrating the science of consciousness and anesthesia. *Anesthesia and Analgesia* 103(4):975–982.

Miller KJ, Schwab KA, Warden DL (2005) Predictive value of an early Glasgow Outcome Scale score: 15-month score changes. *Journal of Neurosurgery* 103(2):239–245.

Nadeau SE, Ferguson TS, Valenstein E *et al.* (2004) *Medical Neuroscience* Philadelphia: WB Saunders.

National Institute for Health and Clinical Excellence (2005) *The Prevention and Treatment of Pressure Ulcers.* London: NICE.

National Institute for Health and Clinical Excellence (2007) *Reducing the Risk of Venous Thromboembolism (deep vein thrombosis and pulmonary embolism) in Inpatients Undergoing Surgery.* London: NICE.

National Institute for Health and Clinical Excellence (2008) *Technical Patient Safety Solutions for VAP in Adults.* London: NICE.

Norwood SH, McAuley CE, Berne JD *et al.* (2002) A prehospital Glasgow Coma Scale score less than or equal to 14 accurately predicts the need for full trauma team activation and patient hospitalization after motor vehicle collisions. *Journal of Trauma* 53(3):503–507.

Pearson LS, Hutton J (2002) A controlled trial to compare the ability of foam swabs and toothbrushes to remove dental plaque. *Journal of Advanced Nursing* 39:480–489.

Plaisier BR, Punjabi AP, Super DM *et al.* (2000) The relationship between facial fractures and death from neurologic injury. *Journal of Oral and Maxillofacial Surgery* 58(7):708–712.

Powers J, Brower A (2007) Impact of oral hygiene on prevention of ventilator-associated pneumonia in neuroscience patients. *Journal of Nursing Care Quality* 22(4):316–321.

Pugh J, Clarke L, Gray J *et al.* (2000) Presence of relatives during testing for brain stem death: questionnaire study. *British Medical Journal* 321:1505–1506.

Ratan SK, Pandey RM, Ratan J (2001) Association among duration of unconsciousness, Glasgow Coma Scale, and cranial computed tomography abnormalities in head-injured children. *Clinical Pediatrics* 40(7):375–378.

Reddy M, Gill SS, Rochon PA (2006) Preventing pressure ulcers: A systematic review. *Journal of the American Medical Association* 296(8):974–984.

Resuscitation Council (2005) *Resusciation Guidelines 2005.* London: Resuscitation Council.

Richer E, Tell L (2003) Indications, efficacy and tolerance of drug therapy in view of improving recovery of consciousness following a traumatic brain injury. *Annales de Readaptation et de Medecine Physique* 46(4):177–183.

Rocker GM, Cook DJ, Shemie SD (2006) Brief review: Practice variation in end of life care in the ICU: implications for patients with severe brain injury. *Canadian Journal of Anesthesia* 53:814–819.

Ross A, Crumpler J (2007) The impact of an evidence-based practice education program on the role of oral care in the prevention of ventilator-associated pneumonia. *Intensive and Critical Care Nursing* 23:132–136.

Russell LJ, Reynolds TM, Park C *et al.* (2003) Randomised clinical trial comparing 2 support surfaces: Results of the Prevention of Pressure Ulcers Study. *Advances in Skin and Wound Care* 16(6):317–327.

Salcido R (2004) Patient turning schedules: why and how often? *Advances in Skin and Wound Care.* 17(4 Pt 1):156.

Schiff ND, Giacino JT, Kalmar K *et al.* (2007) Behavioural improvements with thalamic stimulation after severe traumatic brain injury. *Nature* 448(7153):600–603.

Schnakers C, Zasler ND (2007) Pain assessment and management in disorders of consciousness. *Current Opinion in Neurology* 20(6):620–626.

Selbach O, Eriksson KS, Haas HL (2003) Drugs to interfere with orexins (hypocretins). *Drug News and Perspectives* 16(10):669–681.

Shah S (1999) Neurological assessment. *Nursing Standard* 13(22):49–55.

Shemie SD, Pollack MM, Morioka M *et al.* (2007) Diagnosis of brain death in children. *The Lancet Neurology* 6(1):87–92.

So HM, Lee CCH, Leung AKH *et al.* (2008) Comparing the effectiveness of polyethylene covers (Gladwrap™) with lanolin (Duratears®) eye ointment to prevent corneal abrasions in critically ill patients: A randomized controlled study. *International Journal of Nursing Studies* 45:1565–1571.

Sona CS, Zack JE, Schallom ME *et al.* (2009) The impact of a simple, low-cost oral care protocol on ventilator-associated pneumonia rates in a surgical intensive care unit. *Journal of Intensive Care Medicine* 24(1):54–62.

Taylor CM, Aird VH, Tate RL *et al.* (2007) Sequence of recovery during the course of emergence from the minimally conscious state. *Archives of Physical Medicine and Rehabilitation* 88(4):521–525.

Teasdale G, Jennett B (1974) Assessment of coma and impaired consciousness. *Lancet* ii:81–84.

Teasdale G, Jennett B (1976) Assessment and prognosis of coma after head injury. *Acta Neurochir (Wien)* 34:45–55.

Teasdale GM, Pettigrew LE, Wilson JT *et al.* (1998) Analyzing outcome of treatment of severe head injury: a review and update on advancing the use of the Glasgow Outcome Scale. *Journal of Neurotrauma* 15(8):587–597.

Tessmer CS, da Silva AR, Barcellos FC *et al.* (2007) Do people accept brain death as death? A study in Brazil. *Progress in Transplantation* 17(1):63–67.

Uzun O, Tan M (2007) A prospective, descriptive pressure ulcer risk factor and prevalence study at a university hospital in Turkey. *Ostomy/Wound Management* 53(2): 44–46.

Vanderwee K, Grypdonck MH, Defloor T (2005) Effectiveness of an alternating pressure air mattress for the prevention of pressure ulcers. *Age and Ageing.* 34(3):261–267.

Whyte J, Katz D, Long D *et al.* (2005) Predictors of outcome in prolonged posttraumatic disorders of consciousness and assessment of medication effects: a multicenter study. *Archives Physical Medicine and Rehabilitation* 86:453–462.

Wijdicks EFM, Cranford RE (2005) Clinical diagnosis of prolonged states of impaired consciousness in adults. *Mayo Clinic Proceedings* 80(8):1037–1046.

Zeman A (2001) Consciousness. *Brain* 124(Pt 7):1263–1289.

9
Assessment, Interpretation and Management of Impaired Cognition

Thom Aird

INTRODUCTION

Cognitive problems, such as lapses in memory and attention, difficulties in organisation, planning and problem solving, apathy, disinhibition and lack of insight can impact significantly on daily living for individuals with neurological disease. Cognitive problems following brain injuries or dementia, for example, are known to impact not only on the individual, but also on their families, and are often cited as the reason for relationship breakdown.

Many neurological diagnoses (including stroke, traumatic brain injury, multiple sclerosis, Parkinson's disease, dementia, encephalitis) will be accompanied by cognitive deficits, which can present a significant challenge for health care professionals and families in the care of patients. The nature of the phenomenon can often result in those affected becoming virtual strangers to those around them. The prevalence of head injury survivors living with chronic impaired cognitive functioning is thought to be 100–150 per 100,000 (Select Committee on Health, 2001), although this may be an underestimate.

Neurosurgical patients may also develop cognitive impairment that contributes to determining their outcome and depends on surgical techniques, as well as on the primary disease and the surgeon's operative skills (Agner *et al.*, 2002). It has been reported, for example, that those patients who underwent a surgical procedure for anterior communicating artery aneurysms had significantly decreased scores in logical memory, language and frontal lobe executive functions when compared to endovascular and non invasive groups (Fontanella *et al.*, 2003).

Delirium is characterised by a rapidly occurring acute impairment in cognitive function. It is also a common manifestation of acute brain dysfunction in critically ill patients, occurring in up to 80% of critically ill patients in intensive care units (Girard *et al.*, 2008) and 21% of elderly patients undergoing neurosurgery (Oh *et al.*, 2008).

The identification of cognitive impairments is paramount to the effective management of patient problems and it is vital that nurses are aware of those who may be at risk of developing delirium and cognitive impairment (NICE, 2010) and be able to respond and manage the impairments effectively.

PHYSIOLOGY OF COGNITION

The complex nature of cognitive functioning necessitates consideration of the neurophysiological basis of brain structures contributing to cognitive processes and the subsequent impact that deviations from normal may have on these processes. In order to respond to the environment in which we find ourselves, human brains work on the principle of stimulus-response. We are confronted with a vast amount of information from which we must choose the relevant information, convert it into a meaningful format and then elicit a response. Schmitt *et al.* (2005) refer to cognition as a complex system of inter-related parts which generally include the following six domains:

- Memory
- Planning and abstract reasoning (executive functions)
- Language
- Attention
- Perception and
- Psychomotor skills

Neuroscience Nursing: Evidence-Based Practice, 1st Edition.
Edited by Sue Woodward and Ann-Marie Mestecky
© 2011 Blackwell Publishing Ltd

Further details of these six domains, associated problems and suggested management strategies can be found in Table 9.1.

Memory

Memory systems in the nervous system are necessary if the incoming sensory information is to be understood. Memory does not represent a single system, brain structure or cellular mechanism, but is rather a complex combination of memory subsystems (Bear *et al.*, 2001). Learning is the acquisition of new information or knowledge, and alterations in behaviour as a result of experience. Memory is the retention of this learned information (see Chapter 3).

Executive functions

The frontal lobes, particularly the pre-frontal areas, are important in maintaining the integrity of higher-order cognitive and executive functions (reasoning, planning, concept formation, evaluation and strategic thinking) (Box 9.1).

Language

Language is the complex signal system used by individuals to communicate with one another and is fundamental to cognitive processing. The key area for the recognition of sounds as language and where the meaning of words is understood is Wernicke's area. This concept area is connected to Broca's area, which is responsible for the generation of speech (see Chapter 12). Similar simple models can be used for explaining the reading and writing aspects of language.

Attention

Attention is the ability to focus on a topic long enough to be able to understand it or make an appropriate response to it. Bear *et al.* (2001:659) refer to attention as the preferential processing of sensory information and define selective attention as 'the act of differentially processing simultaneous sources of information'. Certain behaviours can be performed with little, if any, focused attention, whereas others are highly sensitive to the allocation of attention. Concentration is sustained attention by which the individual is able to remain fixed on a topic over a period of time.

The particular areas of the brain that govern attention will depend on the nature of the behavioural task being performed. For example, there is increased activity in specific areas of the visual cortex when attention is focused on performance of a visual task. How attention is controlled remains unknown, but an area of the thalamus called the pulvinar nucleus is thought to play a role in guiding attention (Bear *et al.*, 2001).

Perception

Perception is the ability to interpret and give meaning to sensory information and is a subjective experience. Our sensory impressions are affected by the contexts in which they take place, by our emotional states, and by our past experiences (Kolb and Whishaw, 2003). This includes somatic peripheral, visual, auditory, and olfactory information. Many older adults experience sensory and perceptual impairments which can influence cognitive processing and may in turn influence the individual's ability to fully attend to sensory information (Glogoski *et al.*, 2001).

Psychomotor skills

Psychomotor skills include initiation or the ability to begin and/or complete a task as well as the ability to figure out the sequence of steps necessary to complete the task.

Cognitive processing

The efficient functioning of one cognitive process is often dependent on the integrity of various other cognitive processes. For example storage of new information in long term memory systems cannot occur without proper attention (Schmitt *et al.*, 2005). Cognitive functioning can be modulated by a number of other factors including arousal, mood, motivation and physical well being.

PATHOPHYSIOLOGY AND ALTERED COGNITION

Confusion

The terminology used to describe the effects of impaired cognitive function is an area for potential misunderstanding of a patient's problem. The word 'confused' is ill-defined, ambiguous because of discrepancies in its use between different groups of health professionals (Simpson, 1984) and should be avoided. It has been used to mean muddled thinking, disorientation, clouding of consciousness or delirium (Jacques and Jackson, 2000). Neelon *et al.* (1996) also use the term 'acute confusion' defining it as 'an acute organic brain syndrome encompassing a broad spectrum of psychophysiological manifestations, from mild disorientation to agitated delirium, altered consciousness, and physiological deterioration.'

Patients are often described as 'confused', but their cognitive deficit may be caused by two main underlying pathologies: delirium or dementia. In an attempt to avoid the creation of a definition quagmire it is recommended that a common language is established. Given the

Table 9.1 Cognitive problems and suggested management strategies.

Function	Area of brain	Problem	Management
Executive functions	• Frontal lobes, particularly the prefrontal cortex	Often subtle and difficult to assess: • Poor at self motivated learning • Failure to plan, lack of organisation • Chaotic lifestyle, unrealistic goal setting • Increased demand on limited cognitive ability • Repeated failure, loss of confidence and frustration • Avoidance, withdrawal, anxiety, suspiciousness. • Increased dependency, isolation	• Establish routines and structure to daily living (ensure the routines are within a framework of a concrete and predictable environment) • Use calendars and/or diaries to plan activities in advance • Make checklists to help the individual to work through complex tasks on their own • Encourage them to think about the views of others, and take time to listen to them • Over learning of routines and skills within different environments
Memory	• Limbic system • Hippocampus	Variable depending on the aetiology – refer to Table 9.2 for differentiation between delirium and dementia: • Forgetfulness • Language impairment • Decline in motor skills • Disorientation • Loss of recognition skills	• Use external memory aids (for example computers or personal organisers) • Use cueing devices (devices with alarms, electronic diaries, • Adapt the environment • Use routines • Repetitive practice • Allow extra time to take in and retrieve information • Encourage the development and use of internal strategies; these include artificial mnemonics, repetitive practice
Attention (this includes vigilance, concentration and persistence)	• Reticular activating system • Thalamus • Multiple cortical association areas in the pre frontal, parietal and temporal lobes	• Easily distracted if interrupted • Difficulty concentrating for long periods • Difficulty in inhibiting immediate, but inappropriate, responses • Impulsivity • Slowness in information processing • Disorientation in time and place owing to impaired attention	• Keep number of distractions to a minimum • Work on one task at a time • Activities should be planned so that the tasks that demand more should be undertaken at the best time • Pace activities • Schedule rest periods

Continued

Table 9.1 *Continued*

Function	Area of brain	Problem	Management
Language	• Left posterior-superior temporal area (Wernicke's area) for sensory elements of language and the • Left inferior frontal cortex (Broca's area) for motor elements of language. • Both areas communicate via a bundle of association fibres called the arcuate fasciculus	• Sensory or receptive dysphasia: poor comprehension, fluent but often meaningless speech, no repetition • Motor or expressive dysphasia: preserved comprehension, non-fluent speech, no repetition • Aphasia: loss of language function • Dysarthria	• For receptive problems stand close to the patient so they can observe lip movements, speak slowly and clearly, use simple gestures as an added cue, repeat or rephrase any instructions if they are not understood • For expressive problems stimulate conversation and ask open-ended questions, allow patient time to express themselves, be supportive and accepting of the patients behaviour as they deal with the frustration of finding the right words of expression, use pictures of common objects so that the patient can point to the picture when unable to say the word
Perception	• Parietal lobe (especially right side for two and three dimensional shapes	• Apraxia: the inability to perform certain skilled, purposeful movements despite normal motor power, sensation and coordination • Body scheme disorder: a decreased awareness of the relationship of the body and its parts, often leading to neglect of the affected side • Spatial relations disorder: the inability to recognise form, depth, and position of objects and to understand their relationship to oneself and the environment • Agnosia: the inability to recognise familiar objects using a given sense, although the corresponding sensory organ is undamaged • If a perceptual deficit is present in conjunction with a sensory impairment, the risk of injury to the individual will be greater	• Compensatory techniques specific to the deficit encountered • Often requires assessment using specific perceptual assessment tools • For apraxia encourage the patient to participate in normal activities, correct any misuse of equipment or incorrect actions, re-teach any forgotten skills • For body scheme disorders, approach the patient from the affected side, place food, call bells, etc. toward the unaffected side, and use verbal cues to guide the patient to the affected side • For spatial disorders as for body scheme, plus provide verbal cues and do not allow the patient to wander alone • For agnosia use other intact senses to identify environmental stimuli

Table 9.1 *Continued*

Function	Area of brain	Problem	Management
Psychomotor	• Primary motor cortex • Pre motor cortex • Basal ganglia • Brain stem • Cerebellum	• Hyperalert: restless, excitable, vigilant, shouting, laughing, crying • Increased physical activity and repetitive purposeless behaviour such as picking • Autonomic signs such as tachycardia, sweating, and pupillary dilatation • Hypoalert: quiet and motionless, drifts of to sleep if not stimulated. • Reduced psychomotor activity. • Speech is typically sparse and slow and answers are stereotypical and often incoherent	• May be related to any combination of the above listed problems and appropriate management of them may improve motor signs • May be due to a secondary cause (see section on delirium), which needs to be identified and managed

The above management strategies are general principles and are by no means exhaustive. Sources: Hodges, 1994; Cermak and Lin, 1997; Haase, 1997; Morgans and Gething, 2002.

Box 9.1   Cognitive functions attributed to the frontal lobe.

• Adaptive behaviour
• Abstract conceptual ability
• Set-shifting/mental flexibility
• Problem solving
• Planning
• Initiation
• Sequencing of behaviours
• Temporal-order judgements
• Personality, especially drive, motivation and inhibition
• Social behaviour

Source: Hodges, 1994.

---

characteristic defining features of delirium and dementia, these are the preferred terms to use, rather than 'confusion' and will be referred to throughout the chapter. The use of terms such as 'appears confused' implies that some form of behaviour has been observed leading to such a conclusion and should be avoided in favour of a more descriptive account.

It is important to differentiate between acute and chronic impairment of cognitive function, i.e. between delirium and dementia. The two syndromes vary widely in their presentation, course and outcome. The onset of dementia is normally slow and progressive, in comparison to the acute, rapid onset observed in delirium. The main differences between delirium and dementia are listed in Table 9.2. It is important to remember that individuals with dementia are at risk of developing delirium superimposed on their pre-existing dementia and for that reason it is crucial to be aware of the differing presentations and risk factors for developing delirium. The time course of dementia, chronic brain damage and delirium are illustrated in Figure 9.1.

Delirium

Delirium is characterised by a rapidly occurring acute impairment in cognitive function. It may present with increased or decreased psychomotor activity and is prevalent in patients with acute medical and surgical disorders. The British Geriatric Society (2006) reports that up to 30% of all elderly medical patients may be affected by delirium. Delirium is also a common manifestation of acute brain dysfunction in critically ill patients, occurring in up to 80% of critically ill patients in intensive care units (Girard *et*

Table 9.2 Comparison of delirium and dementia.

Feature	Delirium	Dementia
Onset	Acute/sub acute depending on cause but relatively sudden – over a period of hours or days	Chronic and generally insidious, depending on cause
Course	Short. Fluctuates throughout the day, worse at night and on awakening	Progressive but stable over time
Progression	Abrupt	Slow but even
Duration	Hours to less than one month, seldom longer	Months or years
Awareness	Reduced	Clear
Alertness	Abnormally low or high	Usually normal
Attention	Impaired, causing distractibility; fluctuation over the course of the day	Relatively unaffected
Orientation	Usually impaired for time; tendency to mistake unfamiliar places and persons	Impaired in the later stages
Short-term (working) memory	Always impaired	Normal in the early stages
Episodic memory	Impaired	Impaired
Thinking	Disorganised, delusional	Impoverished
Perception	Illusions, delusions and hallucinations, usually visual. Difficulty in distinguishing between reality and misperceptions	Absent in earlier stages, common later
Speech	Incoherent, hesitant, slow or rapid	Difficulty in finding words
Sleep-wake cycle	Always disrupted	Usually normal or fragmented
Psychomotor behaviour	Variable, hypokinetic, hyperkinetic and mixed	Normal, may have apraxia
Associated features	Variable affective changes, symptoms of autonomic hyperarousal, exaggeration of personality type, associated with acute physical illness	Affect tends to be superficial, inappropriate, and labile; attempts to conceal deficits in intellect; personality changes, aphasia, agnosia may be present; lacks insight
Mental status testing	Distracted from task, numerous errors	Failings highlighted by family, frequent 'near miss' answers, struggles with test, great effort to find an appropriate reply, frequent requests for feedback on performance

Adapted from Hodges 1994; Foreman and Zane 1996.

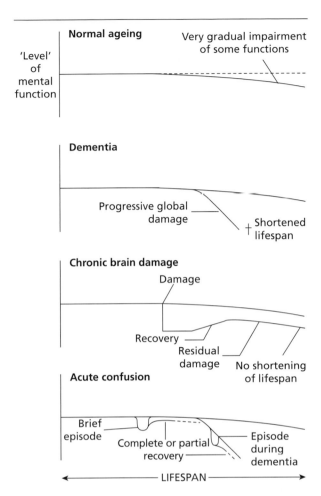

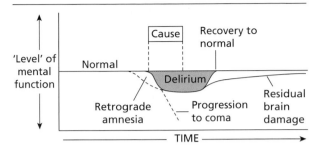

Figure 9.2 The course of delirium. This article was published in *Understanding Dementia* (3rd edition). A Jacques and GA Jackson, Figure 2.2 Copyright Elsevier (2000).

Figure 9.1 The time course of dementia, chronic brain damage and delirium, compared to normal ageing. This article was published in *Understanding Dementia* (3rd edition). A Jacques and GA Jackson, Figure 2.1 Copyright Elsevier (2000).

'a disturbance of consciousness with inattention, accompanied by a change in cognition or perceptual disturbance that develops during a short period (hours to days) and fluctuates over time, with evidence from history, physical examination or laboratory findings that the disturbance is:

1. *Physiological consequence of general condition*
2. *Caused by intoxication*
3. *Caused by medication*
4. *Caused by more than one aetiology'*

The course of delirium is illustrated in Figure 9.2.

The pathophysiological basis for delirium remains unclear. Truman and Ely (2003) suggest an imbalance in neurotransmitters, including dopamine and acetylcholine that modulate the control of cognitive function, behaviour and mood. A disturbance in oxidative metabolism causing a change in cholinergic transmission is suggested by Schuurmans *et al.* (2001).

Dementia

Dementia is defined and discussed further in Chapter 29

AETIOLOGY AND PRESENTATION OF DELIRIUM

Underlying conditions associated with delirium are often divided into cerebral and extra-cerebral disorders (Table 9.3). Risk factors for delirium are divided into predisposing and precipitating factors. Predisposing factors are present at the time of hospital admission. Precipitating factors are noxious insults or hospital-related factors that may contribute to the development of delirium (Schuurmans *et al.*, 2001).

There are three subtypes of delirium:

al., 2008) and 21% of elderly patients undergoing neurosurgery (Oh *et al.*, 2008). Bhat and Rockwood (2002) estimated hospital mortality rates for patients with delirium to range from 6 to 18% and delirium has been associated with death and on-going cognitive decline following discharge. The cause for cognitive deterioration in medically ill patients remains unclear, but severity of the illness may be a contributing factor, with the delirium potentiated by features of their illness (Jackson *et al.*, 2004).

The American Psychiatric Association Diagnostic and Statistical Manual of Mental Disorders (DSM) (1994) define delirium as:

Table 9.3 Causes of delirium

Cerebral	Extra-cerebral
• Post-epileptic states • Trauma • Transient ischemic attacks • Encephalitis • Primary or secondary tumours	• Drugs – all psychotropic drugs, anti-Parkinson's drugs, anti-convulsants, and analgesics. Drugs are associated with delirium in the elderly • Drug and alcohol withdrawal • Metabolic abnormalities – anoxia, hypoglycaemia, hypothyroidism, vitamin deficiencies (thiamine and B), electrolyte disturbances, hepatic failure and anaemia • Infections. This has been found to be a major causative factor in elderly patients (O'Keeffe and Lavan, 1997) • Constipation and urinary retention

Box 9.2   Risk factors for delirium

- Infection
- Dehydration
- Hypokalaemia
- Hyponatraemia
- Hyperglycaemia and hypoglycaemia
- Hyperthermia and hypothermia
- Decreased cardiac function
- Congestive heart failure
- Decreased respiratory function
- Hypoxia
- Trauma

1. Hyperactive – characterised by an agitated state, constant motion, usually displaying non-purposeful, repetitive movement, and most often involving verbal behaviours.
2. Hypoactive – characterised by an inactive, withdrawn and sluggish state, with limited, slow, and wavering verbalizations.
3. Mixed – characterised by the patient fluctuating unpredictably between hypo- and hyperactivity.

Behavioural manifestations of delirium may become problematic. Patients may wander in an attempt to escape the environment (often resulting in falls), remove medical equipment (e.g. intravenous lines, catheters), vocalise (e.g. screaming, calling out, complaining, cursing, muttering) and may develop a predilection to attack others (Rapp *et al.*, 2001).

ASSESSING PATIENTS WITH IMPAIRED COGNITION

Cognitive changes may be subtle and nurses often rely on family members to alert them to the change in the patient's cognitve, behavioural and emotional functioning.

Relatives however may dismiss what they perceive as small changes in these functions, often believing/expecting that these changes will resolve with time. It is essential that cognitive impairments are identified early to enable appropriate post acute care and support for the patient and their family.

Observation forms a key element to the assessment of cognitive function and any observed behaviour, physical or verbal, considered to deviate from the norm for that patient should be accurately described. This would allow for comparison of the same observed behaviour within a variety of settings and at differing times during a 24 hour period. Delirium is commonly undetected and therefore untreated (Neelon *et al.*, 1996). This may be because the manifestations fluctuate in severity and nature, even in the same patient, and patients are not consistently or systematically assessed.

Physical parameters

Since a number of physical disorders can directly affect cerebral functioning it is important to monitor vital signs and laboratory results. Alterations in systemic metabolic processes may impact on the neuronal cell environment and ultimately higher cerebral functions. Potential risk factors (Box 9.2) should be systematically excluded as a potential cause of delirium.

Assessing cognition

The establishment of a baseline of normal higher cerebral functioning for the individual is essential in order to determine the extent of the problem. The British Geriatric Society (BGS) (2006) recommend that cognitive testing should be carried out on all elderly patients admitted to hospital. Regardless of age, serial cognitive measurements in neurological patients at risk may detect the development of delirium. A history from a relative or carer of the onset and course of the 'confusion' is helpful in distinguishing between delirium and dementia, and diagnosis of delirium can be facilitated using an appropriate screening instrument.

Cognition assessment tools

Mini Mental Status Examination

The Mini Mental Status Examination (MMSE) (Table 9.4) (Folstein *et al.*, 1975) is the most widely used bedside assessment chart for the identification of cognitive problems. It is an eleven item open ended questionnaire. It is not intended to diagnose cognitive problems, rather it is used as a quick screen to rule out or confirm cognitive impairment. The MMSE is therefore useful in determining if a more in-depth cognitive assessment is required.

The MMSE is essentially divided into two sections. The first section requires vocal responses to the questions posed by the examiner. This tests orientation, memory, and attention. In the second section of the test, the patient is asked to follow verbal and written instructions, testing the patient's auditory and visual language processing. The maximum score possible is 30. A score of 24 or more is considered within normal limits.

On average the test takes about 10 minutes to complete and, although the MMSE has been found to provide a

Table 9.4 Mini Mental Status Examination (MMSE).

Function assessed	Test	Score
Orientation	Ask patient to state the year, month, day, date and season (prompts are allowed for omitted items)	1 point for each item (max 5)
	Ask patient to identify the country, county/district, town, hospital and ward/room	1 point for each item (max 5)
Registration	Name three objects (e.g. tree, flag, ball) and ask patient to repeat them	1 point for each item (max 3)
Attention	Ask the patient to count backwards in serial sevens, i.e. to subtract 7 from 100 and so on five times (100, 93, 86, 79, 72). Do not correct errors	1 point for each item (max 5)
	Alternatively ask the patient to spell the word WORLD backwards	
Recall	Ask the patient to repeat the three objects learned earlier (e.g. tree, flag, ball)	1 point for each item (max 3)
Language	Point to a watch and a pencil – ask the patient to name them	1 point for each item (max 2)
	Ask the patient to repeat 'No ifs, ands or buts'	Score 1 if correct
	Ask the patient to follow a three-step verbal command e.g. 'take this piece of paper in your right hand, fold it in half and put it on the floor/chair'	1 point for each action (max 3)
	Write 'Close your eyes' on a piece of paper and ask the patient to read and follow the instruction	Score 1 if correct
	Ask the patient to write a sentence, which makes sense and contains a subject and a verb	Score 1 if correct
	Ask the patient to copy the diagram of two intersecting pentagons	Score 1 if correct (i.e. 10 corners and 2 intersecting lines

Adapted from Folstein *et al.*, 1975.

sensitive and specific measurement of mental status, it has its limitations. In order to complete the test, patients must be able to see well enough, read and converse in English, copy a figure, and have sufficient musculoskeletal function to use a pencil. Folstein *et al.* (1975) recommended that the patient's educational level and cultural background should be taken into consideration when administering the test, and that longer times may be necessary for patients with known low IQ and physical impairments to complete the test. The MMSE is biased heavily towards assessment of orientation and language and fails to include more robust indices that assess early dementia, e.g. frontal lobe dysfunction. It does not assess features of acute confusional states (Neelon *et al.*, 1996).

The MMSE is favoured because it is brief and easy to administer and can be further enhanced by the addition of a clock drawing task during the screening process. When screening for cognitive impairment in dementia the clock drawing task is also considered to be a brief but effective and useful tool (Heruti *et al.*, 2002). During this task the patient is presented with a circle and asked to draw the numbers on a clock face. The next command requires the patient to draw the hands of the clock at 3 o'clock. This simple test assesses the patient's ability to plan and visiospatial skills. Patients with dementia will fill in the clock face from the figure 12 or 1, with uneven or inaccurate spacing between the figures (Figure 9.3). Unimpaired indi-

viduals normally start the task by writing in the figures 12, 3, 6 and 9 at the four quadrants.

When screening patients with dementia, the MMSE is helpful only in the early stages and is not sensitive enough to accurately rate patients with severe dementia (Brown and Hillam, 2004). It is also recommended that all patients are assessed using the MMSE after a stroke (Royal College of Physicians, 2008).

The NEECHAM Confusion Scale

The NEECHAM Confusion Scale (Table 9.5) (Neelon *et al.*, 1996) was developed for rapid and unobtrusive assessment and monitoring of acute confusion/delirium. Screening tests that require patients to respond to specific questions or commands may not be feasible with acutely ill older patients and most are not designed for frequent testing. Consequently they are not helpful when monitoring rapid changes in cognitive functioning and behaviour with delirium (Neelon *et al.*, 1996). The NEECHAM scale consists of nine scaled items, divided into three subscales: cognitive processing, behaviour and vital functions.

The NEECHAM scale is easy to use for screening of elderly hospitalised patients and takes only one shift to observe (Schuurmans *et al.*, 2003). This is in comparison to other scales which require completion over a number of consecutive shifts.

The Confusion Assessment Method (CAM)

The Confusion Assessment Method (CAM) (Inouye *et al.*, 1990) provides a structured format which considers three of the four cardinal features of delirium: acute onset, fluctuating symptoms, and changes in cognition. It is reported to be valid and reliable in identifying delirium. The assessment can be incorporated into routine activities and is estimated to take 5–10 minutes to complete. The assessment is dependent on observations, so some of the information may need to be obtained from family members or other staff. The CAM instrument assesses the areas outlined in Box 9.3.

A modified version of the CAM for use in critical care areas (CAM-ICU) has also been developed. Disorganised thinking is the most subjective of the four areas and the hardest to assess (Truman and Ely, 2003). Mechanical ventilation and loss of fine motor movement can limit the expressive ability of patients. The CAM-ICU is designed to be used in conjunction with other assessment tools such as the Glasgow Coma Scale and/or a sedation scale and is recommended for the assessment of delirium in hospitalised adults (NICE, 2010).

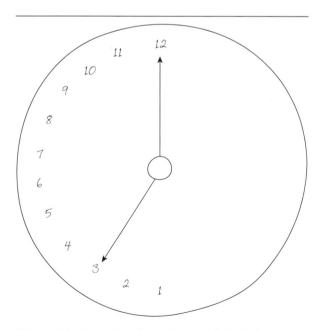

Figure 9.3 Example of an abnormal clock face.

Table 9.5 NEECHAM scale

Subscale	Observations
Subscale 1: Cognitive processing (max 14 points)	**Attention** • Full attentiveness/alertness (responds appropriately) (4 points) • Short or hyper attention/alertness (3 points) • Attention/alertness inconsistent or inappropriate (2 points) • Attention/alertness disturbed (1 point) • Arousal/responsiveness depressed (0 points) **Command** • Able to follow a complex command (5 points) • Slowed complex command response (4 points) • Able to follow a simple command (3 points) • Unable to follow a direct command (2 points) • Unable to follow visually guided command (1 point) • Hypoactive/lethargic (0 points) **Orientation** • Orientated to time, place and person (5 points) • Orientated to person and place (4 points) • Orientation inconsistent (3 points) • Disorientated and memory/recall disturbed (2 points) • Disorientated, disturbed recognition (1 point) • Processing of stimuli depressed (0 points)
Subscale 2: Behaviour (max 10 points)	**Appearance** • Controls posture, maintains appearance, hygiene (2 points) • Either posture or appearance disturbed (1 point) • Both posture and appearance disturbed (0 points) **Motor** • Normal motor behaviour (4 points) • Motor behaviour slowed or hyperactive (3 points) • Motor movement disturbed (2 points) • Inappropriate, disruptive movements (1 point) • Motor movement depressed (0 points) **Verbal** • Initiates speech appropriately (4 points) • Limited speech initiation (3 points) • Inappropriate speech (2 points) • Speech sound disturbed (1 point) • Abnormal sounds (0 points)
Subscale3: Vital functions (max 6 points)	**Vital signs** • Blood pressure, heart rate, temperature, respiration within normal range (2 points) • Any two of the above in abnormal range (1 point) • Two or more in abnormal range (0 points)

Continued

Table 9.5 *Continued*

Subscale	Observations
	Oxygen saturation • Normal range (2 points) • 90–92 or is receiving oxygen (1 point) • Below (0 points) Urinary incontinence • Maintains bladder control (2 points) • Incontinent of urine in last 24 hr or has condom catheter (1 point) • Incontinent now or has indwelling or intermittent catheter or is anuric (0 points)

Total score 30

Helpful hints for scoring the NEECHAM Confusion Scale

- Score the NEECHAM at the completion of the interaction. Read all scoring options for each item before selecting item score.
- In scoring a patient, it is not uncommon for a 1 or 2 point difference to occur between ratings – a change of more than 2 points is considered clinically significant and warrants a more complete assessment.
- Be creative, develop an approach that is comfortable and gets the necessary information. The key is to be consistent in assessment and scoring.
- Cognitive ability may fluctuate even in a short 15 minute period. Should this occur, score the lowest level observed during the entire interaction.
- Pay attention to the patient's awareness or reaction to surroundings as well as what occurs in your interaction.
- Avoid asking yes and no questions as the basis for scoring.
- Record only what you observe during the present interaction, not what was seen previously.
- Score patient as observed regardless of possible cause (recent sedation or narcotic medication, etc.). Make a note of circumstances that might affect scoring.

Source: Neelon, 1997.

Box 9.3   Areas assessed by the Confusion Assessment Method (CAM)

1   Acute onset
2A Inattention (e.g. easily distracted)
2B If inattention present, did this fluctuate
3   Disorganized thinking (e.g. rambling or illogical flow of ideas)
4   Level of consciousness

Disorientation
Memory impairment

7   Perceptual disturbances (e.g. hallucinations)
8A Psychomotor agitation (e.g. restlessness, picking at bedclothes, tapping fingers)
8B Psychomotor retardation (e.g. sluggishness, staring into space or moving very slowly)
9   Altered sleep-wake cycle (e.g. excessive daytime sleepiness with insomnia at night)

Both the NEECHAM and the CAM are primarily observation based and therefore place few demands on the patient during assessment (Wakefield, 2002). In addition, the relative ease of use for both tools enables screening to take place in a relatively short period of time.

INTERPRETATION OF ASSESSMENT FINDINGS

When reporting clinical observations of behaviours, Ross (2002) suggests that the following ABC sequence is helpful:

(1) Analyse the events before the behaviour occurred (antecedents) (A)
(2) Analyse the behaviour itself (what exactly happened) (B) and
(3) Analyse the actions that followed the behaviour (consequences) (C)

The context and environment in which the assessment is taking place, e.g. in response to a problem, time of day, when other people are around, following change in routine, must be considered. This is discussed further in Chapter 10.

Interpreting the Mini Mental Status Examination

A score of 17 or below indicates severe cognitive impairment (dementia) and consists of marked memory impairments that, in combination with impairments of other cognitive functions, lead to complete disadaptation of the patient to daily life. A MMSE score below 24, in the absence of the features of delirium, is a fairly good marker of dementia (Hodges, 1994). Mild cognitive impairments on the other hand are subtle and can only be detected with detailed and in-depth neuropsychological testing.

Cognitive changes associated with normal ageing include subjective memory complaints, frequent problems with name retrieval, and minor difficulties in recalling detailed events, all of which are annoying but not disabling problems (Franken, 2000). Moderate cognitive impairment MMSE between 24 and 17 is a clinically characteristic syndrome of memory and/or other cognitive impairments clearly beyond age norms, but not reaching the severity of dementia and not resulting in disadaptation to daily life. The MMSE is vulnerable to the effects of age, education and socio-economic status (Hodges, 1994) and the usefulness of mental status questionnaires has been questioned (Milisen *et al.*, 2005).

Interpreting the NEECHAM Confusion Scale

NEECHAM scores range from zero (minimal function) to 30 (normal function). The following cut-off points have been recommended for clinical practice:

- 0–19 indicates acute and moderate confusion, to severe confusion and/or delirium to non responsiveness
- 20–24 indicates mild disturbance in information processing, to mild or early development of confusion and/or delirium
- 25–26 indicates risk for confusion and/or delirium
- scores equal to or greater than 27 indicate normal cognitive functioning.

(Milisen *et al.*, 2005)

The CAM Diagnostic Algorithm

The diagnosis of delirium using the Confusion Assessment Method (see Figure 9.4) requires the patient to display the following features: presence of acute onset and fluctuating course; *and* inattention; *and either* disorganised thinking (disorganised or incoherent speech); *or* altered level of consciousness (usually lethargy or stuporose).

---

1. Acute onset and fluctuating course
Is there evidence of an acute change in mental status from the patient's baseline? Did this behaviour fluctuate during the past day, that is, tend to come and go or increase and decrease in severity?

and

2. Inattention
Does the patient have difficulty focusing attention, for example, being easily distractible, or having difficulty keeping track of what was being said?

and

3. Disorganised thinking	*or*	**4. Altered level of consciousness**
Is the patient's speech disorganised or incoherent, such as rambling or irrelevant conversation, unclear or illogical flow of ideas, or unpredictable switching from subject to subject?		Overall, how would you rate this patient's level of consciousness? – Alert (normal) – Vigilant (hyperalert) – Lethargic (drowsy, easily aroused) – Stupor (difficult to arouse) – Coma (unarousable)

Figure 9.4 The CAM Diagnostic Algorithm. Reproduced from Inouye SK, vanDyck CH, Alessi CA, Balkin, S, Siegal, AP, Horwitz, RI. Clarifying confusion. The Confusion Assessment Method: a new method for detection of delirium. *Ann Intern Med* (1990) 113:941–948 with permission. *Confusion Assessment Method: Training Manual and Coding Guide* Copyright 2003 Sharon K. Inouye, M.D., MPH.

Inouye (2003) suggests rating the severity of delirium by adding each score for the four designated symptoms listed above. Each symptom of delirium, except acute onset/fluctuation, can be rated as: absent (0 points), mild (1 point) or marked (2 points). Acute onset and fluctuation is rated as absent (0 points) or present (1 point). The sum of these ratings yielded a delirium-severity score, ranging from 0 to 7, with higher scores indicating increased severity. While these scores were shown to correlate with persistence and duration of delirium, they have not been independently validated.

NURSING MANAGEMENT OF DELIRIUM

The management of delirium is primarily directed to identifying and treating the underlying physical cause. Strategies recommended for the management of specific cognitive problems can be found in Table 9.1

The 'slowing of cognitive functioning that often accompanies ageing' may result in elderly patients being easily distracted, especially when combined with illness, fatigue, and anxiety (Foreman and Zane, 1996). Patients with pre-existing cognitive or functional impairment are at greater risk of experiencing delirium. Declining sensation (peripheral, visual, auditory), cognition, nutrition, and general health further predispose to the development of acute confusion.

The following principles should guide the effective prevention and treatment of delirium. Prevent, eliminate, or minimise aetiological factors. Strategies include the judicious administration of medications (especially antidepressants, antipsychotic drugs and sedatives), preventing infection, maintaining fluid volume, and promoting electrolyte balance. A therapeutic environment and general supportive nursing care should always be provided (Foreman *et al.*, 1999).

The onset of delirium is sudden and the symptoms normally persist as long as the causative factors are present. Once the causative factors have been eliminated, the symptoms of delirium will usually recede over a period of between three to seven days.

Preventative measures

A number of simple preventative measures may decrease the incidence of delirium (Henry, 2002). Compensate for sensory deficits by providing the patient with glasses and hearing aids. If the patient has any visual field defect (e.g. bitemporal or homonymous hemianopia) it is important to ensure that any objects or food are placed within the patient's intact visual field. When communicating with the patient, ensure that they are able to see you. Encourage

ambulation or range-of-motion activities three times a day and minimise the use of immobilising devices such as indwelling catheters and physical restraints. Encourage fluid intake in order to maintain hydration and avoid multiple new medications.

Supportive measures

Physical

The impact of physical disorders on the patient's level of cognitive functioning will depend on a number of factors. These include effects, side-effects and drug interactions of prescribed medications, the patients underlying health problems and their current health status. It is therefore imperative to identify and correct underlying problems which contribute to the development of acute delirium. Age related changes may alter the effect that drugs will have on an individual (Foreman and Zane, 1996). These include slowed hepatic detoxification and renal clearance of drugs, resulting in a potential prolonged half-life of administered drugs. Protein malnourishment may also result in drugs that normally bind to serum proteins circulating freely and producing increased effects. Drugs particularly worthy of attention are detailed in Box 9.4.

It is vital that any alterations from normal physical parameters, such as fluid and electrolyte or endocrine disturbances and hypoxia are identified and corrected. Patients attempting to get out of bed are often trying to get to the bathroom, and a bedside commode or frequent toileting may be a useful solution (Rogers and Boccino, 1999).

Sensory

Sensory impairment of visual and auditory stimuli may result in misperceptions such as hallucinations, illusions, misidentification of people and objects. Nursing interventions should minimise the effects of sensory impairment as described above. In addition, reduce unnecessary visual and auditory stimuli which may distract the patient, especially when communicating. Speak clearly, slowly and precisely; do not shout, and repeat phrases as necessary.

Box 9.4   Drugs to be considered

- Those producing anticholinergic activity: amitriptyline, neuroleptics, tricyclic antidepressants
- Histamine blocking agents: cimetidine, ranitidine
- Analgesics: non-steroidal anti-inflammatory drugs
- Sedative-hypnotics: benzodiazepines
- Cardiovascular drugs: nifedipine, beta blockers

If the patient is hard of hearing, speak into their best ear. Face the patient directly when speaking to them, they may find lip reading helpful in enhancing their understanding of the conversation. Statements should be direct, concise and unambiguous.

The multiple stimuli encountered in a hospital environment and the distraction of acute illness may result in complex messages overwhelming the patient (Foreman and Zane, 1996). Touch may also be an effective method of communicating with patients with visual or hearing loss as well as providing reassurance. It is important to respect social and cultural norms with regards to whom one should touch, where and when (Ross, 2002). If using written materials to communicate, use large print with lighter coloured objects on darker backgrounds. Place them directly in front of the patient, and use indirect lighting to reduce or eliminate glare.

Environmental

Environmental factors such as noise, light, or isolation from cues which help in orientation may result in sensory overload or sensory deprivation. This can result in visual or auditory hallucinations and ultimately may lead to psychosis and challenging behaviour, as is often seen in neuroscience and critical care environments. Nursing interventions can minimise the effects of these environmental factors. Avoid the relocation of the patient to different ward areas. If relocation is necessary ensure that a thorough explanation of the move and orientation to the new ward area is given. Provide stimuli which help to orientate the patient (NICE, 2010), e.g. a clock, radio, television, newspapers or personal items such as photographs from home; but excessive and unnecessary stimuli, e.g. continuous background noise from TV or radio, may be counterproductive and use should be carefully monitored. Switch off the television or radio when not required and remove unused and unnecessary equipment from the bed area or room.

Whenever possible limit the number of staff involved in the care of the patient
and maintain continuity by allocating the same staff to look after the patient.

Ensure that a routine for balancing rest with activity is established and maintained, and encourage social interaction with family and friends. Excessive activity, however, may lead to fatigue, which can present as acute confusion as the individual lacks energy for attending to and processing of information. Conversely inadequate activity and stimulation may lead to apathy and little desire to attend to information (Foreman and Zane, 1996).

Restraint

The increased psychomotor activity associated with delirium often makes patient's behaviour challenging and management difficult. Restraint may then be used to prevent harm to the patient or others. Restraint is defined as 'restricting someone's liberty or preventing them from doing something they want to do' (RCN, 2004). Within neurosciences nurses may employ restraint to stop a patient injuring themselves by removing tracheostomy tubes, ventricular catheters or central lines, for example (Waterhouse, 2007), but it should be used with caution as it has been associated with a number of adverse outcomes (Box 9.5). Restraint and management of challenging behaviour is discussed further in Chapter 10.

In addition to the physical impacts that restraint may have, Mott *et al.* (2005) suggest that restraint may exert significant psychological and emotional effects, and may contribute to regressive, disorganised and unsocial behaviour, as well as to loss of self-image, disorientation, withdrawal, feelings of discomfort, dependency, resistance, fear and anger.

Restraint should only ever be used as a last resort in managing challenging behaviour and only after an appropriate risk assessment has been undertaken (Evans *et al.*, 2003; Waterhouse, 2007). Nurses should seek to prevent and reduce the use of restraint, but should maintain patient safety by following a simple stepwise approach to managing the behaviour, initially identifying possible causes for altered behaviour (Box 9.6).

MULTIDISCIPLINARY TEAMWORKING

The National Service Framework (NSF) (DH, 2005) stresses the need to work across traditional service boundaries and models of care, as well as the need for

---

Box 9.5   Adverse outcomes associated with restraint

- Increased mortality
- Increased hospitalisation and failure to discharge
- Nosocomial infections
- Pressure sores
- Increased confusion
- Damage from the restraining device e.g. lacerations, bruising or strangulation
- Falls and falls related injury

Source: Evans *et al.*, 2003; Braine, 2005; Waterhouse 2007).

Box 9.6 Causes of altered behaviour

Easily treatable causes:
* Pain
* Full bladder/bowel
* Pyrexia
* Hypoxia
* Metabolic/electrolyte disturbance
* Anxiety/frustration
* Communication difficulties
* Sleep deprivation
* Environmental factors (e.g. lighting, noise)

Other causes (may take longer to resolve):
* Brain injury
* Memory impairment
* Ictal or post-ictal state
* Drug or alcohol dependency/withdrawal
* Neurodegenerative disorder (e.g. dementia, Parkinon's disease)
* Other mental health disorders

Adapted from Waterhouse, 2007.

---

collaborative, multi agency approaches to the delivery of services. Nurses should ensure that appropriate and timely referrals to other team members are made.

Although all members of the multidisciplinary team involved in the patient's care have a role in assessing and managing patient problems, it is often the occupational therapist or speech therapist that will normally perform cognitive assessments. It is important, however, that all members of the multidisciplinary team are involved in any discussions concerning patients' cognitive functioning. This will help to determine the need for further neuropsychological testing. The identification of cognitive problems is important for the planning, implantation and evaluation of treatment plans.

The occupational therapist's approach to cognitive skills tends to emphasise the processing of visual, tactile and spatial information; functions largely mediated by the right cerebral hemisphere. Information regarding visual-perceptual functions can be provided by the physiotherapist during gross motor and ambulation tasks.

Neuropsychologists may also become involved in cognitive assessment and are able to administer a range of standard cognitive tests that assess all major skill areas, which may take several hours to complete. Testing is indicated to identify specific cognitive deficits, differentiate depression from dementia, determine the course of an illness, assess neurotoxic effects (such as memory loss and substance abuse), evaluate the effects of treatment, and evaluate learning disorders (Sadock and Sadock, 2009). The occupational therapist, however, is able to observe the patient in functional occupations, which may be an advantage (Haase, 1997). Any formal testing and reporting needs to considered alongside self and family reports, observations of both nursing and other staff, and parallel assessments completed by other professionals (Carpenter and Tyerman, 2006).

POST-DELIRIUM COUNSELLING

The British Geriatrics Society (2006) recommends the provision of support and counselling for patients who have experienced delirium. Delirium is an unpleasant experience and patients are often left with unpleasant half-recollections of the events and of the delusions held during the delirious period.

SUMMARY

The identification of acute changes in cognitive functions is a key role in the management of patients, in both hospital and community settings. A number of factors place vulnerable patients at risk of developing delirium. A number of assessment tools are available for bedside testing of higher cerebral functions. These tools can be used in conjunction with other assessment strategies and will help in the implementation of appropriate care strategies. It is important that risk factors are identified and acted upon in an attempt to reduce the occurrence of delirium and its associated problems. Observation during routine nursing interventions is a valid method of identifying changes in behaviour and thought processes which may be suggestive of cognitive impairment.

REFERENCES

Agner C, Dujovny M, Gaviria M (2002) Neurocognitive assessment before and after cranioplasty. *Acta Neurochir.* 10:1033–1040.

American Psychiatric Association (1994) *Diagnostic and Statistical Manual of Mental Disorders.* (4th edition) Washington DC: American Psychiatric Association.

Bear MF, Connors BW, Paradiso MA (2001) *Neuroscience: Exploring the brain.* (2nd edition) Baltimore: Lippincott Williams and Wilkins.

Bhat RS, Rockwood K (2002) The prognosis of delirium. *Psychogeriatrics* 2(3):165–179.

Braine ME (2005) The minimal and appropriate use of physical restraint in neuroscience nursing. *British Journal of Neuroscience Nursing* 1(4):177–184.

British Geriatric Society (2006) Guidelines for the prevention, diagnosis and management of delirium in older people in hospital. Available from: http://www.bgs.org.uk

Brown J, Hillam J (2004) *Your Questions Answered: Dementia*. Edinburgh: Churchill Livingston.

Carpenter K, Tyerman A (2006) Working in clinical neuropsycholgy. In: Hall J, Llewelyn S (eds.) *What is Clinical Psychology* (4th edition) Oxford: Oxford University Press.

Cermak SA, Lin KC (1997) Assessment of perceptual dysfunction in the adult. In: Van Deusen J, Brunt D (eds.) *Assessment in Occupational Therapy and Physical Therapy*. London: WB Saunders.

Department of Health (2005) *The National Service Framework for Long-term Conditions*. London: Department of Health.

Evans D, Wood J, Lambert L (2003) Patient injury and physical restraint devices: a systematic review. *Journal of Advanced Nursing* 41(3):274–282.

Fick DM, Hodo BA, Lawrence F *et al.* (2007) Recognising delirium superimposed on dementia. *Journal of Gerontological Nursing* 33(2):40–47.

Folstein M, Folstein S, McHugh P (1975) Mini-Mental State: A practical method for grading the cognitive state of patients for the clinician. *Journal of Psychiatric Research* 12:189–198.

Fontanella M, Perozzo P, Ursone R *et al.* (2003) Neuropsychological assessment after microsurgical clipping or endovascular treatment for anterior communicating artery aneurysm. *Acta Neurochir* 18:867–872.

Foreman M, Mion LC, Tryostad L *et al.* (1999) Standard of practice protocol: Acute confusion/delirium. *Geriatric Nursing* 20(3):147–152.

Foreman MD, Zane DBA (1996) Nursing strategies for acute confusion in elders. *American Journal of Nursing* 96(4):44–51.

Franken J (2000) Dementia. In: Atchison BJ, Direite DK (eds) *Conditions in Occupational Therapy: Effect on Occupational Performance*. London: Lippincott Williams & Wilkins.

Girard TD, Pandharipande PP, Ely EW (2008) Delirium in the intensive care unit. *Critical Care* 12 (Suppl3):s3.

Glogoski C, Milligan NV, Wheatly CJ (2001) Evaluation and treatment of cognitive dysfunction. In: McHugh Pendleton HM, Schultz-Krohn W (eds) *Occupational Therapy, Practice Skills for Physical Dysfunction* (6th edition). St Louis: Mosby.

Haase B (1997) Cognition In: Van Deusen J, Brunt D (eds) *Assessment in Occupational Therapy and Physical Therapy*. London: WB Saunders.

Henry M (2002) Descending into delirium. *American Journal of Nursing* 102(3):49–56.

Heruti RJ, Lusky A, Danker R *et al.* (2002) Rehabilitation outcome of elderly patients after a first stroke: Effect of cognitive status at admission on the functional outcome. *Archives of Physical Medicine and Rehabilitation* 83:742–749.

Hodges JR (1994) *Cognitive Assessment for Clinicians*. Oxford: Oxford University Press.

Inouye SK (2003) *The Confusion Assessment Method (CAM): Training manual and coding guide*. Connecticut: Yale University School of Medicine.

Inouye SK, vanDyck CH, Alessi CA *et al.* (1990) Clarifying confusion. The Confusion Assessment Method: a new method for detection of delirium. *Annals of Internal Medicine* 113:941–948.

Jackson JC, Gordon SM, Hart RP *et al.* (2004) The association between delirium and cognitive decline: A review of the empirical literature. *Neuropsychology Review* 14(2):87–98.

Jacques A, Jackson GA (2000) *Understanding Dementia*. (3rd edition) Edinburgh: Churchill Livingstone.

Kolb B, Whishaw IQ (2003) *Fundamentals of Human Neuropsychology*. (5th edition) New York: Worth Publishers.

Milisen K, Foreman MD, Hendrickx A *et al.* (2005) Psychometric properties of the Flemish Translation of the NEECHAM Confusion Scale. *BMC Psychiatry* 5(16) doi:10.1186/1471-244X-5-16.

Morgans L, Gething S (2002) Cerebrovascular accident In: Turner A, Foster M, Johnson SE (eds.) *Occupational Therapy and Physical Dysfunction*. Edinburgh: Churchill Livingstone.

Mott S, Poole J, Kenrick M (2005) Physical and chemical restraints in acute care: Their potential impact on the rehabilitation of older people. *International Journal of Nursing Practice* 11:95–101.

National Institute for Health and Clinical Excellence (2010) *Delirium: Diagnosis, prevention and management*. London: National Guideline Development Group, NICE.

Neelon VJ (1997) The NEECHAM Confusion Scale. University of North Carolina at Chapel Hill.

Neelon VJ, Champagne MT, Carlson JR, Funk SG (1996) The NEECHAM Confusion Scale: Construction, validation and clinical testing. *Nursing Research* 45(6):324–330.

Oh YS, Kim DW, Chun HJ *et al.* (2008) Incidence and risk factors of acute postoperative delirium in geriatric neurosurgical patients. *Journal of Korean Neurosurgical Society* 43(3):143–148.

O'Keeffe ST, Lavan L (1997) The prognostic significance of delirium in older hospital patients. *Journal of the American Geriatric Society* 45:174–178.

Rapp CG, Mentes J, Titler MG (2001) Acute confusion/delirium protocols. *Journal of Gerontological Nursing* 27(4):21–33.

Ritchie K (2004) Mild cognitive impairment: An epidemiological perspective. *Dialogues in Clinical Neuroscience* 6(4):401–407.

Rogers PD, Boccino N (1999) Restraint-free care: Is it possible? *American Journal of Nursing* 99(10):26–34.

Ross C (2002) Managing cognitive impairment in older people. *Nursing and Residential Care* 5(11):529–532.

Royal College of Nursing (2004) *Restraint Revisited: Rights, risks and responsibilities – guidance for nursing staff.* London: RCN.

Royal College of Physicians (2008) *National Clinical Guidelines for Stroke.* (3rd edition) London: RCP.

Sadock BJ, Sadock VA (2009) *Synopsis of Psychiatry: Behavioural sciences/clinical psychiatry,* (9th edition) London: Lippincott Williams & Wilkins.

Schmitt AJ, Benton D, Kallus KW (2005) General methodological considerations for the assessment of nutritional influences on human cognitive functions. *European Journal of Nutrition* 44(8):459–464.

Schuurmans MJ, Deschamps PI, Markham SW *et al.* (2003) The measurement of delirium: Review of scales. *Research and Theory for Nursing Practice: An International Journal* 17(3):207–224.

Schuurmans MJ, Duursma SA, Shortridge-Baggett LM (2001) Early recognition of delirium: review of the literature. *Journal of Clinical Nursing* 10:721–729.

Select Committee on Health Third Report (2001) *Head Injury Rehabilitation.* London: House of Commons Publications and Records.

Simpson CJ (1984) Doctors' and nurses' use of the word confusion. *British Journal of Psychiatry* 145(10):441–443.

Truman B, Ely EW (2003) Monitoring delirium in critically ill patients: Using the Confusion Assessment Method for the intensive care unit. *Critical Care Nurse* 23(2):25–37.

Wakefield BJ (2002) Risk for acute confusion on hospital admission. *Clinical Nursing Research* 11(2):153–172.

Waterhouse C (2007) Development of a tool for risk assessment to facilitate safety and appropriate restraint. *British Journal of Neuroscience Nursing* 3(9):421–426.

World Health Organisation (1992) *ICD-10. Classification of Mental and Behavioural Disorders. Clinical descriptions and diagnostic guidelines.* Geneva: World Health Organisation.

Yakhno NN, Zakharov VV, Lokshina AB (2007) Impairment of memory and attention in the elderly. *Neuroscience and Behaviour Physiology* 37(3):203– 208.

10
Assessment and Management of Challenging Behaviour

Mary Braine

INTRODUCTION

The nature and magnitude of challenging behaviour presents one of many challenges to neuroscience nurses, mainly because of the threat posed to the safety of the patient, staff and others.

Brain injury, traumatic (TBI) or acquired (ABI), can result in a constellation of cognitive deficits, mood disturbances, personality changes and behavioural problems. These may either be temporary or permanent and may result in partial or total disability. Brain injury strikes at those fundamental structures that determine a person's humanity and self-identity (Groswasser and Stern, 1998). This presents the victim with the challenge of reconstructing and reorganising their identity. The nature and severity of neurobehavioural outcomes depends on a number of factors including: the nature, location and severity of the injury, diffuse effects, secondary mechanisms of injury, and the presence of seizures. In addition, the age, medical health, history of previous brain injury, pre-morbid level of function, history of any substance abuse (drugs/alcohol), psychiatric history and psychosocial factors, e.g. poor socio-economic background, and culture or experience of violence, also interact with the injury itself to affect outcome.

In the acute setting, behavioural changes are common following brain injuries and may present as acute confusional states. This is most common in the acute recovery phase of the severe TBI patient, who may experience a period of post-traumatic amnesia (PTA), manifested by disorders of orientation, attention, memory, and a

decreased capacity to respond to environmental cues, that may last weeks or months (Weir *et al.*, 2006). During this period, and often for some time afterwards, the patient may experience what Groswasser and Stern describe as:

> *'... having lost control over everything. They are physically, emotionally and cognitively dislocated.'*
> (Groswasser and Stern, 1998)

The term 'challenging behaviour' was introduced in North America in the 1980s to describe the problematic behaviours of people with learning difficulties. It is a term that is now widely used across the spectrum of health disciplines. Whilst the literature offers many definitions of challenging behaviour, the most widely used definition is offered by Emerson:

> *'... culturally abnormal behaviour of such an intensity, frequency or duration, that the physical safety of the person or others is likely to be placed in jeopardy, or behaviour that is likely to seriously limit use of, or result in the person being denied access to ordinary community facilities.'*
> (Emerson, 1995 pp. 4–5)

The term does not carry any diagnostic significance; rather it describes the behaviour of an individual. Challenging behaviour may also be described as 'anti-social' behaviour, which carers and services may find difficult to manage and may take several forms (see Box 10.1).

Survival rates following severe brain injury have improved dramatically in recent years due to technological advances in acute care. This has, however, surpassed our ability to treat the long-term sequelae, placing increasing demands on specialist neurorehabilitation services. Chronic

Neuroscience Nursing: Evidence-Based Practice, 1st Edition.
Edited by Sue Woodward and Ann-Marie Mestecky
© 2011 Blackwell Publishing Ltd

Box 10.1   Examples of challenging behaviour

Behavioural changes may include:
- Confusion, disorientation
- Presence of impulsive behaviour (impulsivity)
- Excitement
- Perseveration – tendency for a memory or idea to persist or recur without any apparent stimulus for it, or the act of continual repetition of a particular behaviour
- Belligerence (anger and impulsivity)
- Acts of aggression and destruction
- Akathisia – a constant sense of inner restlessness, which may or may not be manifested in motor activity, ranging from bouncing legs and fidgeting hands to pacing behaviour (inability to keep still, restlessness)
- Disinhibition – loss of inhibition, unrestrained behaviour, e.g. swearing

Emotional disturbances may include:
- Agitation – generally regarded as a disturbed behavioural pattern often accompanied by over-activity. Patients may be uncooperative, incoherent, abusive and irritable
- Anxiety
- Depression, suicidal thoughts
- Apathy – disinterest, inertia, lack of motivation
- Anger, paranoia, emotional lability (feeling up and down emotionally)
- Confabulation (creation of false memories, perceptions, or beliefs)
- Frustration and lack of tolerance
- Lack of empathy
- Alexithymia – cannot interpret the emotional communication of others correctly

Source: Sandel and Mysiw, 1996; Ducharme, 1999; Rao and Lyketsos, 2000.

Box 10.2   Specific behavioural sequelae of traumatic brain injury (TBI)

- Anger and impulsivity (Hanks *et al.*, 1999)
- Childish behaviour (Brooks *et al.*, 1986)
- Agitation (Lombard and Zafonte, 2005)
- Aggression (Baguley *et al.*, 2006)
- Alexithymia (Henry *et al.*, 2006)
- Lack of self-awareness

---

bances. Although the aetiology of emotional and behavioural deficits remains unclear, it is clear that the pre-injury demographic and personality characteristics of the patient may contribute to their adjustment difficulties after brain injury. Although the list of dysfunctional behavioural problems as a result of brain injury is long (see Box 10.1), specific behavioural difficulties associated with TBI have been identified (see Box 10.2). These often interact causing frustration, intolerance and reduced capacity to control mood, giving rise to the so called *frontal lobe syndrome*.

Frontal lobe syndrome vs executive dysfunction syndrome

One of the first accounts of frontal lobe syndrome was recorded by Bigelow (1850), who described the case of American railway labourer, Phineas Gage, who suffered marked personality changes after an accidental prefrontal leucotomy. Since then the literature has provided many accounts of frontal lobe dysfunction, but with little consensus as to what constitutes frontal lobe syndrome. The term implies that the frontal lobe is the only part of the brain that is damaged, whereas in fact several areas of the brain are affected and cause the clinical presentation.

It is argued that the disturbance should be referred to as *executive dysfunction syndrome* (Lyketsos *et al.*, 2004), reflecting the impact on the executive system rather than an anatomical dysfunction. Executive dysfunction encompasses a wide range of deficits: problem solving, poor organising and planning skills, perseveration, and inability to inhibit actions. Typically these patients exhibit attention problems, their language lacks coherence, is socially inappropriate and disinhibited. They may also confabulate, perseverate or stereotype. They may be unable to switch from one line of thinking to another and their activities are reduced, showing apathy, lack of drive and lack of concern.

EPIDEMIOLOGY

The prevalence of challenging behaviour has been most extensively studied in learning disability populations,

deficiencies in specialist service provision for these patients means that they are often managed within services that are not specifically designed for them. These behaviours have also been increasingly reported to cause significant stress and be a burden on their families and carers.

PATHOPHYSIOLOGY

Damage to the frontal and temporal lobes, along with disruption to the nearby limbic system, are frequently cited as causative factors in emotional and behavioural distur-

reflecting the longer established use of the term in this field. Prevalence of challenging behaviour in neuroscience populations is less well understood, although it is acknowledged as being a significant problem. Thornhill and colleagues (2000) found that specific problems of cognition and mood were consistently reported in all survivors of mild, moderate and severe TBI (47%, 48% and 76% respectively). Johnson and Balleny (1996) reported that behavioural problems were identified in about 30% of severely brain injured patients while they were in hospital, but that this figure increased to approximately 80% once these patients had returned home to their families.

Although the prevalence of emotional and behavioural problems after mild traumatic brain injury (MTBI) is unknown, the proliferation of published literature on the subject over the last five years has highlighted that the sequelae are distinct and commonly referred to as the post-concussion syndrome. Post-concussion syndrome occurring after head injury (with loss of consciousness) may be accompanied by a reduction in cognitive function, and specific neurobehavioural symptoms, i.e. feelings of depression or anxiety, emotional lability and irritability (Powell, 2005). According to Mittenberg and Strauman (2000) the emotional and behavioural sequelae of MTBI are distinct and should be considered separately.

By definition, MTBI is characterised by a GCS of 13–15 at the time of hospital admission, which means that the majority of these patients will only receive treatment in the accident and emergency department, or may not seek treatment at all (Shah *et al.*, 2004). Despite most of these patients never reaching a neuroscience centre they present a significant health care problem as they account for up to 75% of all TBI (Bazarian *et al.*, 2005) and can develop adverse, long-term neuropsychological outcomes (Vanderploeg *et al.*, 2005).

ASSESSMENT

Before a management plan is agreed and implemented, it is essential that a comprehensive clinical assessment is undertaken and a diagnosis made. Often this process is hindered by the challenging nature of the patient's behaviours and ideally the clinical assessment should be multidisciplinary. Exclusion of possible medical, surgical and metabolic causes of the behaviour (see Chapter 9) is important as many treatable factors can contribute to challenging behaviour. It is equally important to establish whether the patient has an underlying mental health problem that may necessitate detention under either section 2 or 3 of the Mental Health Act (Department of Health, 2007).

Many behavioural disturbances are functional for patients, i.e. they serve a particular purpose and may be communicating a need. Functional assessment of behaviour seeks to identify the function(s) that a specific behaviour serves for the individual, based on the premise that all behaviour serves some purpose. The function or purpose of the patient's behaviour is not always obvious, especially in the acute setting, and assessment helps to determine what purpose the behaviour serves and what factors are maintaining the behaviour. The purpose of the behaviour(s) may be to communicate a need, gain attention, escape from or avoid an unpleasant situation/activity, e.g. exhibiting an aggressive episode in response to a painful procedure or treatment, or to gain access to a need, e.g. wanting to leave, or to release built up tension/frustration.

Identifying and describing the behaviours in observable terms, including where and when they occurred, what usually happens before the behaviour and what happens after the behaviour, i.e. how did people react, form the basis of functional behavioural analysis. One simple analysis tool is the 'ABC' chart (Wesolowski and Zencius, 1994). The tool analyses the behaviour of the patient according to possible triggers (**A**ntecedents) of the **B**ehaviour, and possible maintainers (**C**onsequences) of the behaviour. These ABC charts (see Figure 10.1) enable all members of the multidisciplinary team to participate in data collection and encourage a systematic observational assessment to determine the conditions associated with problem behaviours. Careful analysis of these charts can lead to the planning and implementation of appropriate behavioural plans, normally determined by the neuropsychologist.

The assessment and analysis of the behaviour may indicate that the observed behaviours occur at specific times or in specific environments, e.g. constant background noise or demands made during therapy. Equally, the analysis may provide information regarding stimuli that are associated with a desirable behaviour. Thus by creating an atmosphere and environment in which the patient's needs and wishes are anticipated in advance, many incidents of behavioural disturbance can be prevented.

Agitated Behavioural Scale (ABS)

Despite the difficulties in assessing challenging behaviour, a number of scales have been developed for rating agitation and aggression. The Agitated Behavioural Scale (ABS) (Corrigan, 1989), offers a valid and reliable measure of agitation specifically in the TBI population (Sandel and Mysiw, 1996). Its quantitative and qualitative measures,

| Name: | | | | |
| Hospital number: | | | | |
Date & time	Antecedent (What happened before the behaviour?)	Behaviour (Describe the behaviour including location & other aspects of the environment)	Consequence (What happened thereafter? What did you do or not do? How did others react?)	Final outcome (What did the observed person do after the incident was over?)

Figure 10.1 Antecedent, behaviour and consequence data collection form (ABC).

based on rating 14 different behaviours, are easy to use and usually completed within 10 minutes. At the end of each observation period, nurses can assign a number ranging from 1 (absent) to 4 (present to an extreme degree) for each item, representing the frequency of the agitated behaviour and/or the severity of a given incident. Total scores range from 14 (no agitation) to 56 (extremely severe agitation).

Overt Aggression Scale (OAS)

Another frequently used scale is the Overt Aggression Scale (OAS) (Yudofsky *et al.*, 1986), a 16-point scale designed for rating aggressive behaviour, which originated in the psychiatric setting. It has subsequently been modified for neurorehabilitation (OAS-MNR) (Alderman *et al.*, 1997). The OAS measures global aggression as well as four subscales: verbal, physical towards objects, physical towards self and physical towards others.

Assessing emotional disturbances

Whilst there may be no consensus as to the most appropriate scale for measuring emotional disturbances following brain injury, the Katz Adjustment Scale (KAS) (Katz and Lyerly, 1963) is frequently reported in the literature. Designed for the non-professional, it is a short and relatively easy scale to use, covering a wide range of emotional behaviours observed in the TBI population.

Assessment of post-traumatic amnesia (PTA)

Post-traumatic amnesia (PTA) should also be assessed (Weir *et al.*, 2006) (see also Chapter 32). It is a valid measure for predicting outcome after TBI (Tate *et al.*, 2001), but also provides guidance for commencing further

functional assessment and active therapy. Carrying out active treatment whilst the patient is suffering PTA is not advisable as this may increase confusion, agitation and aggression, due to an inability to process new information.

There are a number of prospective measurement scales available: for example, the Westmead PTA Scale (Shores *et al.*, 1986), the Oxford PTA Scale (Artiola *et al.*, 1980), the Galveston Orientation and Amnesia Test (GOAT) Levin *et al.*, 1979) and the Julia Farr Centre PTA Scale (Geffen *et al.*, 1991). All of these measurements provide nurses and other health care professionals with detailed, objective information to plan and determine the effectiveness of the treatment for these patients. They also provide valuable information for nursing teams in determining actual and potential risk to staff and others, supporting the case for additional staffing or the relocation of the patient to a more appropriate setting.

Other forms of assessment

In order to conduct a more holistic and comprehensive assessment of challenging behaviour, nurses can also provide useful accounts of observations in practice. Nurses are well placed to observe the nuances that occur in non-verbal and verbal cues that may indicate an escalation in unwanted behaviours, such as agitation and aggression. Picking up changes in the patient's facial expression, deeper firmer tone, increased volume and speed of the patient's speech, as well as what the patient says are all important predictors of aggression (Pryor, 2005). Although prediction of changes in behaviour is not always possible, with careful monitoring and observation nurses may be able to moderate some of these challenging behaviours.

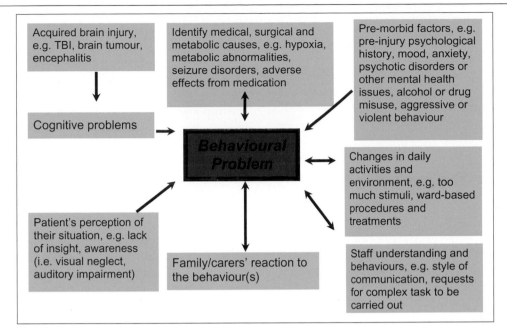

Figure 10.2 Illustration of contributory factors that can lead to behavioural problems. Adapted from Braine (2005).

MANAGEMENT

General principles

Assessment and management may not always be distinguishable, as continuous reassessment and treatment often merge together. It is important to recognise that intervention strategies may not work the first time or every time and that every patient is different. The management of these patients must always start with the least restrictive interventions, such as changes to the environment and general approaches of staff (see Chapter 9) in redirecting and de-escalating behaviour. This may require progression to pharmacological intervention. Figure 10.2 illustrates the complexity of the different factors that may influence the behaviour of the patient.

The principal aim is to reduce the frequency of the behaviours and the risks associated with the behaviours for both patients and staff. Any intervention must take into account the physical, emotional, and medical needs of the patient and whether it is in the patient's best interests. Assessment of best interest must consider the patient's physical health, psychological health, beliefs and values when competent, quality of life, spiritual and religious welfare as well as the views of others involved in the care of the patient.

Human rights' issues must always be taken into consideration (see Chapter 36) as these patients are at risk of deprivation of liberty. Maximising the patient's participation in medical and other treatments, including rehabilitation, is an important consideration in order to minimise long-term difficulties which may develop as a result of acquired impairments and learned inappropriate behaviour patterns. Any intervention should be applied consistently by all staff members and reviewed on a regular basis. A summary of the guiding principles of the management of these patients is provided in Box 10.3.

ENVIRONMENTAL AND BEHAVIOURAL MANAGEMENT STRATEGIES

The environment plays an important part in contributing to the patient's rehabilitation and can contribute to an exacerbation of unwanted behaviour. The key to effective management is the identification of any underlying cause and environmental triggers, defined as anything outside the patient's immediate control that causes distress and/or confusion for the patient. These environmental triggers can come from a variety of sources and have already been discussed in detail in Chapter 9.

Box 10.3   Guiding principles for the management of challenging behaviour

- Maintain the safety of patients at all times
- Maximise potential and enhance recovery
- Prevent escalation/minimisation of inappropriate and aggressive behaviour
- Perform a comprehensive clinical assessment and reassessment
- Consider the patient's best interests, human rights and the capacity to consent
- Any interventions must take account of the physical, emotional, and medical needs of the individual patient
- Provide appropriate interventions
- Commence with the least restrictive intervention
- Management of these patients must be multidisciplinary
- Care must be provided by appropriately trained and educated health care practitioners

Over-stimulation and under-stimulation

The busy ward environment can provide many known stressors such as excessive sensory stimulation and loud noises. These may not always be controllable, but strategies to reduce over-stimulation are advocated. Pryor (2004), sought to identify key environmental factors that irritated patients with acquired brain injury (ABI) and concluded that too much stimulation, too many restrictions and staff interaction, especially the staff style, were key. Placing the patient in a quieter area of the ward or a side-room, if the clinical condition of the patient permits, may help. However, patients should not change beds within the ward unless it is likely to reduce distress and behavioural problems, as this in itself has the potential to increase disorientation and distress further. Rest periods should be scheduled into the patient's timetable and any tasks should be presented one at a time so as to prevent overload of information.

Patients may also be under-stimulated, especially in hospital settings where staffing levels and routines do not permit or sustain intensive patient involvement. Under-stimulation has been reported to be a more common source of agitation than over-stimulation (Ducharme, 1999). Nurses need to balance the need for a safe environment with one that provides activities that these patients can engage with in a meaningful way. Further interventions are discussed in Chapter 9.

Wandering

Perhaps one of the most frequent, difficult and dangerous forms of behaviour following brain injury is wandering or 'excessive walking'. Although there is no consensus as to what constitutes wandering or how to measure it, patients may exhibit pacing and straying, often off the ward/unit. Patients more likely to exhibit this behaviour are typically male, often with sleep problems and often with a pre-morbid active lifestyle (Arthur and Lai, 2003). Wandering can be problematic for both the patient and their carers, as patients can put themselves at risk of harm and cause distress to others. Understanding the reason for the wandering may help in providing some solutions. It may be that the patient is searching for somebody, or is disorientated in place. Excessive walking may be a continuance of a lifetime habit, e.g. delivering mail or dog walking, but may also be an attempt to orientate themselves, searching for landmarks that make sense to them, or an attempt to relieve boredom.

Several different intervention strategies are identified in Table 10.1. The research to support these interactions is sparse, and largely carried out in the dementia population (Price *et al.*, 2002). Due consideration needs to be given to alternative care packages and details of the systematic reviews should be clearly documented, so that compliance with the law can be more easily demonstrated.

Sleep-wake disturbances

These patients often have disturbances of their sleep-wake cycle, ranging from mild insomnia or daytime sleepiness to a complete reversal of their sleep-wake cycle. Several researchers have identified the link between the role of the hypothalamus in the sleep-wake cycle and TBI resulting in sleep disturbances post injury (Fichtenberg *et al.*, 2002; Parcell *et al.*, 2006; Baumann *et al.*, 2007). It may even be the first symptom of an evolving problem. Strategies to manage the 'timelessness' of being in hospital may include turning lights off and on at appropriate times, opening and closing curtains, keeping wall clocks accurate and repeated reorientation by staff and carers in a non-confrontational manner. Pharmacological interventions, such as the administration of night sedation, to reverse the sleep-wake cycle may also be helpful.

STAFF INTERACTIONS AND BEHAVIOURS

Patients often experience difficulties in perceiving and processing information accurately. This can lead to misperceptions where patients misinterpret helpful intentions of nursing and therapy staff. This can lead to irritability and even hostile reactions by the patient, as he/she feels threatened by their environment. Many patients may per-

Table 10.1 Possible strategies to manage wandering (excessive walking).

Strategy	Rationale
One-to-one monitoring	
Staff to carry mobile telephone whilst escorting the patient	To support and maintain the patient's individual agreed treatment plan whilst at the same time maintaining their safety and the safety of others. For those who are at risk of falling, escorting the patient may reduce the associated risks
Specific environments – wandering areas, i.e. enclosed court yards or creating a home environment in the ward/unit. Digital lock and keypads to gain access and exit to the ward /unit	Facilitates the patient's need for walking within the confines of the ward/unit reducing the risk of absconding and reduces the restriction of freedom
Use of subjective barriers such as camouflaging doors or door handles, mirrors placed in front of the door, patterns on the floor	Depending on the patient's level of cognition this may be helpful in confining them within the ward/unit environment without the need for digital locks
Structured activities – exercise classes, music therapy, occupational therapy	Physical activity diverts energy that may be otherwise focused on agitation or aggression. May help to relieve the patient's boredom
Installation of a security system that alarms speech/buzzer/lights when the patient attempts to enter an area	Alerts the staff to attempts to abscond and may reduce the number of attempts by the patient
Electronic tagging and tracking devices, e.g. bracelets	Unobtrusive means of restraint which has the potential to improve patient safety and alerts staff to attempts to abscond (Miskelly, 2004). Allows the patient to wander within a designated area

ceive certain tones of voice as being punitive or patronising and this may serve to increase their irritation (Gervasio and Matthies, 1995). Nurses also need to be aware that other interaction, such as physical contact (e.g. family members playing with the patient's hair), may be a source of irritation.

To help with reorientation, incorrect information should be corrected. However, this must be done sensitively to avoid a patient feeling humiliated, e.g., saying '*you are 28*' rather than '*no you are not 20*' and then move the conversation onto another topic. Distraction techniques may also be used to prevent challenging behaviour from escalating. Staff should make themselves aware of topics of conversations or alternative activities that may appeal to the patient and serve to distract him/her from the inappropriate behaviour pattern. In addition, behavioural programs may also be considered, such as structured activities during the day.

Other interactions

Multisensory stimulation (Snoezelen therapy) is an alternative therapy that is gaining attention world wide. It involves controlled sensory stimulation, involving all

sensory systems, in a non-threatening secure environment (Hulsegge and Verheul, 1987). This multi-sensory stimulation is thought to reduce tension and pressure, thus improving general behaviour, but very few studies have addressed the efficacy of the therapy in the brain injured population. Decreased agitation and an overall benefit have been reported in children recovering from severe brain injury (Hotz *et al.*, 2006). Research in other populations, i.e. learning disabilities and dementia, is much more prolific and cites many positive behavioural changes as a result of the therapy (Shapiro *et al.*, 1997; Hogg *et al.*, 2001), but the evidence does not support its general application. Further research is clearly required to explore the benefits, both in the short and long-term, especially in the ABI population.

Other alternative interactions that might be employed in the management of challenging behaviour are illustrated in Box 10.4. This is not an exhaustive list and each patient needs to be assessed and managed individually.

PHARMACOLOGICAL MANAGEMENT

Whilst there are a number of measures that neuroscience nurses can use to modify the patient's environment and

---

> **Box 10.4　Example of alternative interventions**
>
> Physical interventions
> - Covering over lines with pyjamas, long sleeve clothing, and abdominal bandaging placed over padded gastrostomy tube, using bandages or stockinet to keep tubing, such as IV lines, out of the patient's field of vision
> - Providing physical activities to diffuse and distract behaviours e.g. giving the patient soft squeeze balls or small soft hand-held objects to divert their attention away from medical devices
> - One-to-one monitoring – providing constant observation
> - Reducing the use of medical devices, e.g. lines or tubes as soon as possible
> - Pressure sensors – bed or chair to act as an alert to the movement of patients who are at risk, i.e. falls
> - Strategies to assess and manage pain, nicotine withdrawal, alcohol withdrawal and other drug withdrawal (e.g. recreational)
>
> Psychological interventions
> - Involve the family in the care which may help to identify the cause of the behaviour
> - Families play a key role in helping a person recover from injury or illness

behaviour and to protect them from harm, these may not always be successful. Pharmacological management may then be used, but not as a substitute for environmental and behavioural interventions. Medication may help to moderate the individual's response to difficult environmental conditions and provide rehabilitation staff with the opportunity to teach more adaptive strategies for self-management (Ducharme, 1999).

Chemical restraint is:

'... the deliberate and incidental use of pharmaceutical products to control behaviour and/or restrict freedom of movement ...'

(Mott *et al.*, 2005)

This, however, has the potential for abuse. The over-prescription of medication for the purpose of sedation and restraint have been commonly reported in older patients (House of Commons Health Committee, 2004), but no evidence is available as to the extent of this within neuro-science practice. The over-prescription and inappropriate use of medication or the failure to review prescriptions regularly can constitute abuse. There does not appear to be agreement as to the best pharmacological treatment for these patients, which is further complicated by the diversity of the behaviours as previously identified. A systematic review of drug treatment for agitation and aggression following ABI revealed a lack of substantial evidence as to which drugs were effective and identified that the best evidence of effectiveness was for the use of beta-blockers i.e. propranolol (Fleminger *et al.*, 2006). Without firm evidence of efficacy it is important to choose drugs with few side-effects and to monitor their effect.

Key considerations

Once the decision has been made to use pharmacological interventions, each drug needs to be the considered for its positive and negative effects in the management of the neurobehavioural sequelae. Nurses need to be aware that no one single therapeutic intervention is a panacea for all symptoms, but rather that each drug needs to be considered separately. Several factors need to be considered when choosing the drug; these include drug metabolism, excretion and interaction with other prescribed medication. Anti-epileptic and anti-spasmodic medications, for example, often interact with neuroleptic agents to alter pharmacokinetics or pharmacodynamics. If sedating agents are used, nurses need to monitor sedation levels carefully to avoid over sedation.

Whilst there may be no agreement as to the best treatment for neurobehavioural symptoms, some drugs (e.g. neuroleptics) have been shown to have a negative effect on the patient. Over 20 years ago the use of haloperidol in head injured patients was found to hinder patient recovery, and the drug's side-effects included restlessness (akithisia) and increased confusion (Feeney *et al.*, 1982). Similar findings have since been reported (Mysiw *et al.*, 2006; Elovic *et al.*, 2008). Antipsychotic drugs, e.g. haloperidol and chlorpromazine, should be avoided as they may adversely affect neuronal recovery, reduce seizure threshold, increase sensitivity of patients with ABI to extrapyramidal effects, increase the risk of neuroleptic malignant syndrome and impair motor and cognitive function.

More recent evidence provides support for the use of benzodiazepines and anti-epileptic drugs (AEDs) in the management of behavioural problems, but further trials are required to clarify the role of these medications. A summary of pharmacological interventions and their rationale is presented in Table 10.2.

Table 10.2 Pharmacological management of challenging behaviours

Drug	Rationale
Benzodiazepines	
If an immediate response is necessary lorazepam is the drug of choice (orally, via PEG or intra-muscularly)	Benzodiazepines, e.g. lorazepam, oxazepam and alprazolam, have fewer adverse side-effects than neuroleptics (antipsychotic drugs)
If a more prolonged period of sedation is required, diazepam can be administered (orally, enterally (via NG or PEG), or PR)	Lorazepam has a shorter duration of action and less potential for accumulation than diazepam
Intranasal midazolam of the parenteral preparation is also an alternative	
Anti-epileptic drugs (AEDs)	
AEDs can be beneficial in reducing agitation and aggression, e.g. carbamazepine and valproic acid	Both these anti-convulsants are effective mood stabilisers and it is likely that this is the mode of action following ABI (Fleminger *et al.*, 2006; Francisco *et al.*, 2007). May be useful in agitation, irritability and aggression, although there is no firm evidence of their effectiveness
Carbamazepine	Carbamazepine is advocated for its low sedative effects, its perceived efficacy and lack of cognitive side-effects (Fugate *et al.*, 1997)
Valproic acid can be used if benzodiazepines are ineffective or contra-indicated. It may be beneficial when carbamazepine is not.	Valproic acid reduces destructive and aggressive behaviour in ABI patients (Wroblewski *et al.*, 1997; Lonergan *et al.*, 2004)
Valproate semisodium is an alternative	May be useful in patients who are alert, labile, impulsive and disinhibited (Chatham-Showalter and Kimmel, 2000)
Beta blockers	
Propranolol can also be used either alone or in combination with an antiepileptic	May reduce the physiological reaction to anxiety which can perpetuate agitation. Beta-blockers offer the best quality evidence, although it is still limited (Fleminger *et al.*, 2006)

PHYSICAL RESTRAINT

In cases where there is no obvious antecedent to the behaviour and all other methods to control and manage the behaviour(s) have failed, then physical restraint may be required as a last resort to protect the patient and others. Physical restraint is defined as:

'... any device, material or equipment attached to or near a person's body and which cannot be controlled or easily removed by the person and which deliberately prevents or is deliberately intended to prevent a person's free body movement to a position of choice and/or a person's normal access to their body.'

(Retsas, 1998)

Put simply, it is any limitation on an individual's freedom of movement. Physical restraint can be viewed in three broad categories as follows:

- The direct use of physical contact between the patient and the nurse
- The use of barriers such as locked doors to limit freedom of movement
- The use of materials or equipment to restrict or prevent movement

The National Institute for Health and Clinical Excellence (NICE, 2005) guidelines on the short-term management of disturbed/violent behaviour in psychiatric in-patient settings, and accident and emergency departments, clearly states that:

'The level of force applied must be justifiable, appropriate, reasonable and proportionate to a specific situation and should be applied for the minimum possible amount of time.'

(NICE, 2005)

Both the Royal College of Nursing (2004) and the Mental Health Act (DH, 2007) provide additional guidance on the use of physical restraint. Whilst this guidance is aimed at the psychiatric setting, the guiding principles undoubtedly have relevance for the neuroscience nurse. Based upon the available literature from both government and professional bodies, some general guiding principles on the use of physical restraint are offered (Box 10.5).

Neuroscience nurses are often faced with ethical tensions of risk versus duty of care, or when the nurse's duty to 'do good' places the nurse at risk, as in the case of managing the violent and aggressive patient. Fowler (1989) asserts that it is here that some ethical principles, such as the principles of beneficence and non-maleficence apply. Restraint may be considered ethical if:

- the patient is at significant risk of harm, danger, or loss
- the nurse's interventions will probably prevent that harm to the patient
- the good outweighs the harm that the nurse could sustain
- the risk is no more than would be expected.

Box 10.5   Principles of using physical restraint

- Restraint should be used as a last resort when all other strategies in a hierarchy of interventions have been explored including behavioural, environmental and pharmacological interventions
- The decision to use physical restraint must be multi-disciplinary and involve the family/carers whenever possible
- The patient's self respect, dignity, privacy and cultural values should be taken into consideration at all times
- The minimum and correct restraint device/measure should be used
- Consent should be obtained whenever possible
- The patient should be closely monitored/observed
- The need for restraint should be continually assessed and documented
- Nurses should record the decision and the reasons for physical restraint and document and review every episode of physical restraint
- Restraint should be carried out by nurses who have received the relevant training

---

The use of physical restraint is a frequent intervention performed by neuroscience nurses across the UK, but is an issue that raises many ethical and practical concerns. The adverse effects incurred as a result of restraining patients are well documented (see Table 10.3). The law, however, is quite clear that, with limited exceptions such as reasonable defence, reasonable chastisement or reasonable everyday contact, to touch someone or cause someone to be touched against their will is unlawful (Human Rights Act) (HMSO 1998; DH, 2005).

In reality, the assessment of 'best interests' is often a balancing exercise, i.e. weighing up the various interests of the patient in order to reach a reasoned decision. For example, it may be appropriate to lock doors where the purpose is to keep the patient safe from harm. However, this may breach the patient's right to liberty under Article 5 of the European Convention of Human Rights if the purpose is to prevent the patient from leaving the hospital. Each patient needs to be considered carefully and regularly reviewed on a case-by-case basis in light of the particular circumstances pertaining to that patient.

Physical restraint should only be used when all other strategies have been tried and found to be unsuccessful, or in an emergency, when the risks of not employing physical restraint are outweighed by the risks of using force. Under Common Law, any individual is entitled to apprehend and restrain a person who is mentally disordered and presents an imminent danger to themselves or others. However, the degree of medical or physical restraint should be sufficient and proportionate to the individual circumstances, that is the minimum to achieve the needs of the individual, but no greater. Nurses also have an ongoing duty of care to the patient, themselves and other members of staff.

The importance of completing a risk assessment (see Chapter 36) to identify those who are at risk as well as the benefits and risks associated with the restraint intervention strategy is therefore critical in guarding against unnecessary harm (Waterhouse, 2007). An inadequate assessment and failure to deploy appropriate measures to manage risks can have serious or even fatal consequences, e.g. the patient's airway being compromised due to self-extubation. If it is decided that restraint is in the patient's best interests then all the legal and ethical implications need to have been considered. There may be several situations in neuroscience practice when physical restraint may be deployed when all other strategies have failed (see Box 10.6). The use of physical restraint devices, however, is not without

Table 10.3 Examples of physical intervention/restraint

Mechanism of restraint	Intervention
Bodily contact	• Holding a patient's hands to prevent them from hitting out/pulling at medical devices • Control and restraint
Mechanical	**Whilst in bed** • Bed rails • The use of bedclothes (sheets) • 'Posey' mitts • Arm-cuffs/limb holders • Vest **Whilst in a chair** • Chairs with reclining actions, e.g. Buxton chair • Securing table tops onto chairs • Placing tables in front of chairs • Wheel chair belts /straps • Body restraints – vests, jacket **Whilst mobile** • Limb restraints – arm-cuffs, arm splints, mitts/boxed hands –'Posey mitts' • Body restraints – vests, jackets • Removing walking sticks/frame and other walking aids • Removing visual aids, i.e. glasses
Environmental changes	• Forced seclusion within the ward with key-padded doors • Covers over door handles • Electronic tagging and tracking, e.g. electronic wrist tags

---

Box 10.6   Situations when physical restraint may be considered

• To maintain the safety of the patient, preventing them from harming themselves, e.g. by pulling out central lines or tracheostomy tubes, or falling
• When staff are put in immediate danger and thus need to take control of the situation
• To manage dangerous, threatening or destructive behaviour
• To provide postural support and sitting balance
• To facilitate treatment and/or to prevent therapy disruption

---

hazards, and carries a risk of serious adverse incidents (Box 10.7).

SUMMARY

The management of challenging behaviours is complicated and should involve a multidisciplinary, individualist approach. Nurses have a critical role to play in the assessment of these patients, which must include the patient's best interests, human rights and the capacity to consent. There are a number of assessment tools available to support nurses and the multidisciplinary teams in the assessment process. Nursing care should be focused upon a holistic approach with the employment of the least restrictive intervention from a hierarchy, commencing with behavioural and environmental interventions.

Box 10.7   Adverse outcomes associated with restraint

Indirect injury
- Increased hospitalisation and failure to discharge
- Reduced physiological potential and functional capacity
- Increased risk of hospital acquired infections (HAI), e.g. urinary tract, chest infection
- Pressure ulcers
- Contractures
- Increased confusion
- Psychological damage, e.g. loss of self image, withdrawal, increased confusion and agitation

Direct injury
- Damage from the restraining device, e.g. lacerations, bruising or strangulation and death
- Nerve injuries from wrist devices
- Ischaemic injuries from tight restraint devices
- Falls and falls-related injury

Source: Paterson *et al.*, 2003; Evans *et al.*, 2003; Mott *et al.*, 2005; Waterhouse, 2007.

REFERENCES

Alderman N, Knight C, Morgan C (1997) Use of a modified version of the Overt Aggression Scale in the measurement and assessment of aggressive behaviour following brain injury. *Brain Injury* 11 (7):503–523.

Arthur DG, Lai CKY (2003) Wandering patients with dementia. *Journal of Advanced Nursing* 44(2):173–182.

Artiola I, Fortuny L, Briggs M *et al.* (1980) Measuring the duration of post traumatic amnesia. *Journal of Neurology, Neurosurgery and Psychiatry* 43:377–379.

Baguley IJ, Cooper J, Felmingham K (2006) Aggressive behaviour following traumatic brain injury: how common is common? *Journal of Head Trauma Rehabilitation* 21(1):45–56.

Baumann CR, Werth E, Stocker R *et al.* (2007) Sleep wake disturbances 6 months after traumatic brain injury: a prospective study. *Brain* 130(7):1872–1883.

Bazarian J, McClung J, Shah M *et al.* (2005) Mild traumatic brain injury in the United States. *Brain Injury* 19(2):85–91.

Bigelow HJ (1850) Dr Harlow's case of recovery from the passage of an iron bar through the head. *American Journal of the Medical Sciences* 19:13–22.

Braine ME (2005) The management of challenging behaviour and cognitive impairment. *British Journal of Neuroscience Nursing* 1(2):67–74.

Brooks N, Campsie L, Symington C, Beattie A, McKinlay W (1986) The five year outcome of severe blunt head injury. A relative's view. *Journal of Neurology, Neurosurgery and Psychiatry* 49:764–770.

Chatham-Showalter PE, Kimmel DN (2000) Agitated symptom response to divalproex following acute brain injury. *Journal of Neuropsychiatry Clinical Neuroscience* 12(3):395–397.

Corrigan JD. (1989) Development of a scale for assessment of agitation following traumatic brain injury. *Journal of Clinical and Experimental Neuropsychology* 73: 320–323.

Department of Health (2005) *Mental Capacity Act.* London: The Stationery Office.

Department of Health, Home Office (2007) *Mental Health Act.* London: Stationery Office.

Ducharme JM (1999) Subject review: A conceptual model for treatment of externalising behaviours in acquired brain injury. *Brain Injury* 13(9):645–668.

Elovic EP, Jasey NN, Eisenberg ME (2008) The use of atypical antipsychotics after traumatic brain injury. *The Journal of Head Trauma Rehabilitation* 23(2):132–135.

Emerson E (1995) *Challenging Behaviour. Analysis and intervention in people with learning difficulties.* Cambridge: Cambridge University Press.

Evans D, Wood J, Lambert L (2003) Patient injury and physical restraint devices: a systematic review. *Journal of Advanced Nursing* 41(3):274–282.

Feeney DM, Gonzalez A, Law WA (1982) Amphetamine, haloperidol, and experience interact to affect the rate of recovery after motor cortex surgery. *Science* 217:855–857.

Fichtenberg NL, Zafonte RD, Putnam S *et al.* (2002) Insomnia in a post-acute brain injury sample. *Brain Injury* 16(3):197–206.

Fleminger S, Greenwood RJ, Oliver DL. (2006) Pharmacological management for agitation and aggression in people with acquired brain injury. *Cochrane Database of Systematic Reviews* (4) CD003299. DOI: 10.1002/14651858.pub2.

Fowler MDM (1989) Ethical decision making in clinical practice. Ethics, Part II Application to clinical practice. *Nursing Clinics of North America* 24(4):955–965.

Francisco GE, Walker WC, Zasler ND *et al.* (2007) Pharmacological management of neurobehavioral sequelae of traumatic brain injury: A survey of current psychiatric practice. *Brain Injury* 21(10):1007–1014.

Fugate l P, Spacek LA, Kresty LA *et al.* (1997) Measurement and treatment of agitation following traumatic brain Injury: II A survey of the Brain Injury Special Interest Group of the American Academy of Physical Medicine and Rehabilitation. *Archives of Physical Medicine and Rehabilitation* 78:924–928.

Geffen GM, Encel JS, Forrester GM (1991) Stages of recovery during post-traumatic amnesia and subsequent everyday memory deficits. *Neuroreport* 2(2):105–108.

Gervasio AH, Matthies BK (1995) Behavioural management of agitation in the traumatically brain injured person. *Neurorehabilitation* 5:309–316.

Groswasser Z, Stern MJ (1998) A psychodynamic model of behaviour after acute central nervous damage. *Journal of Head Trauma and Rehabilitation* 13(1):69–79.

Hanks R A, Temkin NR, Machamer J *et al.* (1999) Emotional and behavioural adjustment following traumatic brain injury. *Archives of Physical Medicine and Rehabilitation* 80:991–997.

Henry JD, Philips LH, Crawford JR *et al.* (2006) Cognitive and psychological correlates of alexithymia following traumatic brain injury. *Neuropsychologia* 44:62–72.

Her Majesty's Stationery Office (1998) *Human Rights Act* London: HMSO.

Hogg J, Cavet J, Lambe L *et al.* (2001) The use of 'Snoezelen' as multisensory stimulation with people with intellectual disabilities: A review of the research. *Research in Developmental Disabilities* 22:353–372.

Hotz G, Castelblanco A, Lara I *et al.* (2006) Snoezelen: A controlled multi-sensory stimulation therapy for children recovering from severe brain injury. *Brain Injury* 20(8):879–887.

House of Commons Health Committee (2004) *Elder Abuse Health – Second Report of Session 2003–04*, Health Committee Publications. HC111–1.

Hulsegge J, Verheul A (1987) *Snoezelen: Another World*. Chesterfield: ROMPA International Ltd.

Johnson R, Balleny H (1996) Behavioural problems after head injury: incidence and need for treatment. *Clinical Rehabilitation* 10:173–181.

Katz MM, Lyerly PR (1963) Methods for measuring adjustment and social behaviour in the community: I. Rationale, description, discriminative validity and scale development. *Psychological Reports* 13:503–535.

Levin HS, O'Donnell VM, Grossman RG (1979) The Galveston Orientation and Amnesia Test: a practical scale to assess cognition after head injury. *Journal of Nervous and Mental Disease* 167:675–841.

Lombard LA, Zafonte RD (2005) Agitation after traumatic brain injury: Considerations and treatment options. *American Journal of Physical Medicine and Rehabilitation* 84 (10):797–812.

Lonergan ET, Cameron M, Luxenberg J (2004) Valproic acid for agitation in dementia. *Cochrane Database Systematic Review* (2):CD003945.

Lyketsos CG, Rosenblatt A, Rabins P (2004) Forgotten frontal lobe syndrome or 'executive dysfunction syndrome' *Psychosomatics* 45(3):247–255.

Miskelly F (2004) A novel system of electronic tagging in patients with dementia and wandering. *Age and Ageing* 33(3):304–307.

Mittenberg W, Strauman S (2000) Diagnosis of mild head injury and the post concussion syndrome. *Journal of Head Trauma Rehabilitation* 15(2):783–791.

Mott S, Poole J, Kenrick M. (2005) Physical and chemical restraints in acute care: Their potential impact on the rehabilitation of older people. *International Journal of Nursing Practice* 11(3):95–101.

Mysiw WJ, Bogner JA, Corrigan JD *et al.* (2006) The impact of acute care medications on rehabilitation outcome after traumatic brain injury. *Brain Injury* 20(9):905–911.

National Institute for Health and Clinical Excellence (2005) *Violence. The short-term management of disturbed/violent behaviour in in-patient psychiatric settings and emergency departments*. National Collaborating Centre for Nursing and Supportive. London: NICE.

Parcell DL, Ponsford JL, Rajaratnam SM *et al.* (2006) Self-reported changes to night-time sleep after traumatic brain injury. *Archives Physical Medicine Rehabilitation* 87(2):278–285.

Paterson B, Bradley P, Stark C *et al.* (2003) Deaths associated with physical restraints in the health and social care setting in the UK – The results of a preliminarily survey. *Journal of Psychiatric and Mental Health Nursing* 10:3–15.

Powell J. (2005) Improving follow-up for head injury patients in a nurse-led post-concussion clinic. *British Journal of Neuroscience Nursing* 1(4):185–190.

Price JD, Hermans DG, Grimley-Evans J (2002) Subjective barriers to prevent wandering of cognitively impaired people. (Cochrane Review) In: *The Cochrane Library*, Issue 2 2002 Oxford: Update Software.

Pryor J (2004) What environmental factors irritate people with acquired brain injury? *Disability and Rehabilitation* 26(16):974–980.

Pryor J (2005) What cues do nurses use to predict aggression in people with acquired brain injury? *Journal of Neuroscience Nursing* 37(2):117–121.

Rao V, Lyketsos C. (2000) Neuropsychiatric sequelae of traumatic brain injury. *Psychosomatics* 41(2):95–103.

Retsas AP (1998) Survey findings describing the use of physical restraints in nursing homes in Victoria, Australia. *International Journal of Nursing Studies* 35(3):184–191.

Royal College of Nursing (2004) *Restraint Revisited: rights, risks and responsibilities. Guidance for nursing staff.* London: Royal College of Nursing.

Sandel E, Mysiw J (1996) The agitated brain injured patient. Part 1: Definition, differential diagnosis and assessment. *Archives of Physical Medicine and Rehabilitation.* 77:617–623.

Shah M, Brazarian J, Mattingly A *et al.* (2004) Patients with head injuries refusing emergency medical services transport. *Brain Injury* 18(8)765–773.

Shapiro M, Parush S, Green M *et al.* (1997) The efficacy of the 'Snoezelen' in the management of children with mental retardation who exhibit maladaptive behaviours. *British Journal of Developmental Disabilities* 43:140–155.

Shores EA, Marosszeky JE, Sandanam J *et al.* (1986) Preliminary validation of a clinical scale for measuring the duration of post-traumatic amnesia. *The Medical Journal of Australia* 144:569–572.

Tate RL, Perdices M, Pfaff A *et al.* (2001) Predicting duration of post traumatic amnesia (PTA) from early PTA measurements. *Journal of Head Trauma Rehabilitation* 16(6):525–542.

Thornhill S, Teasdale GM, Murray G D *et al.* (2000) Disability in young people and adults one year after head injury: prospective cohort study. *British Medical Journal* 320(7250):1631–1635.

Vanderploeg RD, Curtiss G, Belanger HG (2005) Long-term neuropsychological outcomes following mild traumatic brain injury. *Journal of the International Neuropsychological Society* 11(3):228–237.

Waterhouse C (2007) Development of a tool for risk assessment to facilitate safety and appropriate restraint. *British Journal of Neuroscience Nursing* 3(9):421–426.

Weir N, Doig EJ, Fleming JM *et al.* (2006) Objective and behavioural assessment of the emergence from post-traumatic amnesia (PTA) *Brain Injury* 20(9):927–935.

Wesolowski MD, Zencius AH (1994) *A Practical Guide to Head Injury Rehabilitation: A focus on post-acute residential treatment.* New York and London: Plenum Press.

Wroblewski BA, Joseph AB, Kupfer J *et al.* (1997) Effectiveness of valproic acid on destructive and aggressive behaviours in patient with acquired brain injury. *Brain Injury* 11(1):37–48.

Yudofsky SC, Silver JM, Jackson W *et al.* (1986) The Overt Aggression Scale for the objective rating of verbal and physical aggression *The American Journal of Psychiatry* 143(1):35–39.

11

Assessment, Interpretation and Management of Altered Perceptual, Motor and Sensory Function

Iain Bowie and Sue Woodward

INTRODUCTION

The somatic nervous system controls voluntary movement and sensation that is consciously perceived (see Chapter 4) and can be assessed to provide information about the functioning of the nervous system. Because areas of the central nervous system control specific functions, and nerve impulses travel in identified pathways, it is possible to locate neurological malfunction by careful analysis of the findings of clinical examination. In this chapter some of the fundamental assessment techniques will be discussed as well as information on the specific care of people with sensory and motor impairments. Sensory impairment of vision and hearing is discussed in Chapter 13.

SENSATION

Sensation refers to the function by which the central nervous system (CNS) gains information about the status of the world around us. Perception is the interpretation of that information, obtained by the sensory nerves distributed throughout the body. The brain is insensitive to the environment and so requires the sensory organs to detect stimuli from the environment, and the sensory pathways to transmit the information in the form of action potentials to the brain.

The sensory nervous system consists of receptor organs or receptor cells and the pathways via the spinal cord (see Chapter 4) or cranial nerves (see Chapter 13) to the brain

and the cortical and subcortical areas that process the incoming information. As discussed in Chapter 4, it is possible to map the sensory dermatomes, which may be useful in interpreting sensory function.

The vital function of sensation in the body may be overlooked compared to the apparent importance of the motor system. However, the motor system *cannot* operate effectively without sensory input. All movements are subject to sensory feedback from proprioceptors, which enable fluid and effective motion. Vision is important in locomotion, and sensory information from the vestibular system together with proprioception from joints is essential for maintaining balance, which in turn is essential for movement. People with defective sensory input will have impaired motor function.

Sensory receptors and axons

Receptors are considered to be transducers because they convert one form of energy: light, heat, movement or chemical stimulus, into an action potential. Action potentials are the 'currency' of the nervous system and the only way that information can be passed on and interpreted within the nervous system. Receptors adapt to the stimulus, that is, they become less responsive to a repeated or constant stimulus. Receptors adapt at different rates therefore different aspects of the stimulus can be discriminated. Some adapt quickly and these generally transmit information about the duration or variation within the stimulus. Receptors that show slow adaptation transmit information about location and intensity of the stimulus.

Neuroscience Nursing: Evidence-Based Practice, 1st Edition.
Edited by Sue Woodward and Ann-Marie Mestecky
© 2011 Blackwell Publishing Ltd

The axons from the receptors to the spinal cord vary in diameter and whether they are myelinated or not. These structural differences affect conduction velocity along the axons:

- Myelinated fibres conduct impulses faster than unmyelinated fibres
- Large diameter fibres conduct more rapidly than narrow diameter fibres

The conduction of pain and noxious stimuli may be modified by utilising this difference in conduction velocity between large and narrow diameter fibres (see Chapter 17).

Each sensation that the nervous system can interpret is transmitted via a specifically adapted receptor (Table 11.1). The receptors involved in the somatic nervous system will now be discussed in further detail.

Mechanoreceptors and thermoreceptors

Mechanoreceptors detect physical forces such as movement and pressure. Mechanoreceptors are found throughout the skin where they detect light touch, pressure and stretch (Figure 11.1). Mechanoreceptors sensitive to light touch are found in the dermal papillae, which are close to the surface, and are rapidly adapting. Some types of receptor are found deeper in the dermis and are slowly adapting receptors. They are also found in the ear where the hair cells of the scala media in the cochlea detect pressure changes in the endolymph and this is interpreted as sound. Mechanoreceptors are also found in the vestibular system where movement is detected and sent to the brain to help maintain equilibrium. Receptors for pressure are found in the dermis and subcutaneous tissue. Vibration is detected

by the rapid and repeated stimulation of dermal mechanoreceptors (Tortora and Derrickson, 2006).

Thermoreceptors detect heat and are found widely throughout the body although the distribution may vary according to physiological need which, of course, is similar to the distribution of most receptor cells. Thermoreceptors detect heat in the range of 10 to 40° Celsius. Temperatures greater or less than this stimulate nociceptors (Tortora and Derrickson, 2006).

Proprioceptors

Proprioceptors provide a specific sense which relates to body position. It is mediated by stretch receptors in tendons and muscles and these are essential for locomotion. There are two types of proprioception which are carried in different spinal pathways. The proprioceptive information ascending in the dorsal columns is sometimes referred to as 'conscious proprioception' as this is the information about position of which we are aware (see Chapter 4). These pathways crossover (decussation) to the opposite hemisphere of the brain in the medulla. Axons carrying proprioceptive information to the cerebellum do not cross, as the cerebellar hemispheres serve the same side of the body, unlike the cerebral hemispheres. This proprioceptive information which is below the level of consciousness ascends in the spinocerebellar tracts on the lateral side of the cord.

Nociceptors

Nociceptors are free nerve endings distributed throughout the body except in the brain itself, although cerebral blood vessels and the meninges do contain nociceptors (see Chapter 17). Thermal, mechanical and damage from chemicals can produce pain if the intensity of the stimulus is sufficient.

SENSORY ASSESSMENT

A standard neurological testing set may contain items such as: a test tube to hold cold and warm water to assess temperature sensation, a clinical tuning fork (with a base plate) to assess vibration, disposable neurotips™ which have a sharp and a blunt point on them, and cotton wool balls to assess light touch. Neurotips™ should always be used to assess pinprick sensation rather than hypodermic needles, which will pierce the skin. Monofilament nylon is available to provide a test for discrimination. The amount the filament bends when applied to the patient's skin corresponds to the pressure exerted, enabling the examiner to discover the threshold for touch. This is useful in peripheral neuropathy as it enables a comparison to be made with earlier readings.

Table 11.1 Receptor types and sensations.

Receptor	Sensation transmitted
Photoreceptor (rods and cones)	Electromagnetic radiation in visible spectrum (light)
Chemoreceptor	Chemicals within both internal and external environment
Mechanoreceptor	Movement, pressure and stretch
Proprioceptor	Joint position
Thermoreceptor	Temperature
Nociceptor	Painful or unpleasant (noxious) stimuli

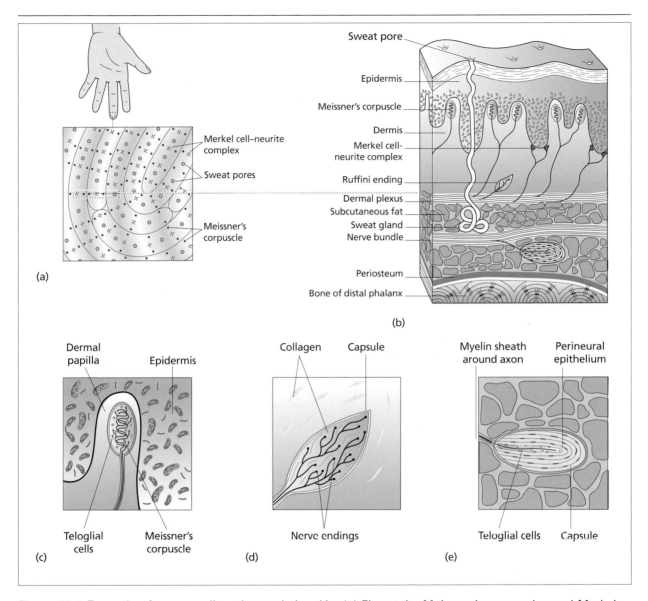

Figure 11.1 Example of nerve endings in non-hairy skin. (a) Finger tip: Meissner's corpuscles and Merkel cell–neurite complexes. (b) Section through skin of finger tip. (c) Meissner's corpuscle. (d) Ruffini ending. (e) Pacinian corpuscle. Reproduced from C. Clarke *et al.*, *Neurology: A Queen Square Textbook*, Wiley-Blackwell, with permission.

The two point discrimination test shows the effectiveness and distribution of touch receptors over the surface of the body. To perform this test monofilament is used to detect the point at which the patient can no longer distinguish between one and two points with their eyes closed (Fuller, 2004). It is important to compare the right side with the left and to compare findings with normal values. For example, on the finger tips the minimum discrimina-tion distance is about 2 mm, but on the back the two points can be applied to the skin as far as 70 mm apart before the patient can identify two distinct sensations, due to the different number of sensory receptors within these two areas. This test is useful in cortical lesions as it may help to localise the lesion. It is also useful in peripheral nerve lesions and carpal tunnel syndrome as it will help to identify which peripheral nerves are not working optimally.

Assessing light touch, pressure, vibration and temperature

Sensory testing should be systematic and, depending on the condition, must include data from the fingers, hands, forearms, upper arms, toes, legs and thighs, abdomen, chest, and top and bottom of the back. Long axons are often affected first in peripheral neuropathy so hands and feet will require special attention. Both sides of the midline need to be tested on the trunk as each side has separate innervation.

Where necessary the patient should be tested with closed eyes so that visual clues do not affect the response. Sensory testing is carried out as follows:

- Ask the patient if you have warm or cold water in a test tube applied to the skin to test for heat sensation.
- Ask the patient if the sensation of pressure from a neurotip is sharp or blunt. Ask if the patient can feel the vibrations of a vibrating tuning fork (most sensitive over bony prominences).
- Test for light touch using a wisp of cotton wool or a monofilament. Accurate interpretation of the data will need to take account of a sensory dermatome map (see Chapter 4) e.g. absence of sensation in the thumb and index finger may indicate a lesion at the level of C6.

Because pain and temperature sensation are carried in the same pathway it is not necessary to test both sensations unless peripheral neuropathy is suspected, when the examiner is testing the receptors rather than the pathways.

Assessing proprioception

Proprioception is tested by asking the patient, with closed eyes, to state where their limbs are when positioned by the examiner. Alternatively ask the patient to touch the end of their nose with the index finger or to touch the ends of each finger with the thumb rapidly in turn. Proprioception may also be tested by asking a recumbent patient to run the heel of one foot along the shin of the other leg. These movements should be smooth and coordinated. Romberg's test (see Chapter 13) can also be used to test proprioception. Romberg's test assesses proprioception by testing the ability to balance the whole body when standing. The sensory input for this is from the proprioceptors in the trunk and limbs, and the vestibular system for head position (Khasnis and Gokula, 2003).

Stereognosis

Stereognosis (see Chapter 3) is a perceptual rather than sensory process and relates to the ability to recognise objects by touching them and feeling the texture and shape. Stereognosis can be tested by placing everyday objects in the patient's hand with their eyes closed. Suitable objects might be a comb, pen, coins (denomination should be easy to assess due to size, shape and texture, e.g. milling on the edge of higher denomination coins) or keys.

SENSORY IMPAIRMENT

Numbness and paraesthesia

Paraesthesia means altered sensation and refers to any unusual sensation experienced such as burning, tingling or pricking in the absence of a physical stimulus. It commonly refers to the 'pins and needles' sensation. Numbness is sometimes known as anaesthesia but note that this is the physiological term and it does not entirely overlap with the medical term, so to avoid confusion numbness is sometimes included in the definition of paraesthesia.

There are several causes of paraesthesia. The ones most recognised include reduced circulation to a body part often caused by awkward positioning which is transient and the sensation disappears when the position is relieved. There are many other causes, including hyperventilation, not all of which are neurological. Paraesthesia is also associated with certain medications such as acetazolamide, carbamazepine and topiramate and some other anticonvulsants. It is a relatively common drug side-effect so the British National Formulary or similar text should be consulted. In neurological terms, chronic paraesthesia occurs with many conditions such as: multiple sclerosis, Guillain–Barré syndrome and peripheral neuropathies such as diabetic neuropathy (Perkins *et al.*, 2000). Where numbness is a long-term problem care should be taken that the patient does not suffer injury without awareness. For this reason chiropody may be required in patients with, for example, diabetic neuropathy.

Perceptual deficits

Cerebral lesions or injury in areas which process tactile sensations, i.e. the somatosensory association area in the parietal lobes, may produce perceptual problems that appear as sensory deficits. It is important to differentiate between sensory and perceptual problems as these will be treated differently. Loss of the ability to recognise objects by touching them and feeling the texture and shape, stereognosis, is termed astereognosis. There are other specific agnosias where the patient is unable to recognise various classes of objects or materials (Table 11.2). The visual agnosias are discussed in Chapter 3.

Table 11.2 Common agnosias.

Name of agnosia type	Inability to recognise
Anosognosia	Disease processes. This is fairly common after stroke where the patient does not acknowledge any deficit
Associative agnosia	What is seen. The patient can describe what they are looking at but cannot say what the scene is. For example, they can describe a tree, a ladder, a sack, apples and picking but they cannot say that apples are being harvested
Phonagnosia	Voices. The patient can repeat words but cannot identify the voice of the speaker
Prosopagnosia	Faces
Visual agnosia	Objects. The patient can see and describe parts of an object but cannot identify it

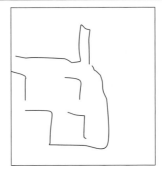

Figure 11.2 A house drawn by a patient with neglect.

Hemi-inattention/neglect

Unilateral neglect or hemi-inattention occurs after damage to the brain, i.e. following head injury, stroke or any other disorders that affect the hemispheres. Although either hemisphere may be involved it is most likely to occur when the right parietal lobe is affected (Ringman *et al.*, 2004) more specifically the parieto-occipital association area. Neglect may also occur after damage to the temporal and frontal lobes and/or deeper structures such as the thalamus.

The patient may not be able to perceive objects or events occurring in the affected side (i.e. the left of the patient when the right hemisphere is damaged). Neglect can cause the patient to lose awareness of the space and its contents on the affected side even to the extent of world knowledge. For example, a routine test is asking a patient to draw a simple house or clock face. They may only complete details on the right side (Figure 11.2).

The patient may have an accompanying agnosia that prevents their recognition of the deficit (anosognosia), or an accompanying motor deficit. Observable signs include failure to wash or dress one side of the body, arms or legs on the affected side hanging out of bed, head turned to unaffected side, or ignoring stimuli on the affected side. Patients may start to read from the centre of a page. Food and drink left on the neglected side will be ignored. The patient may only eat from one half of a plate.

There are several bedside tests which will strengthen the diagnosis of neglect, such as the line bisection test. In this test the patient is asked to draw a vertical line to divide a horizontal pre-drawn line in half. Normal individuals will have no problem in estimating the centre but patients with neglect may draw their line considerably to one side of the true centre. Patients with neglect will have difficulty in using a pain scale that requires them to show their pain level on a horizontal line, leading to poor pain management. In these circumstances use a vertical scale. Another test uses a grid of equally spaced letters and asks the patient to cross out all instances of a given letter, e.g. all the Cs. The patient with neglect may only cancel from one half of the grid. Formal testing is usually performed by an occupational therapist or a clinical psychologist.

Management is aimed at helping the patient by using all sensory modalities to attend to the neglected space. This may involve touch, auditory stimuli such as speech or music, visual stimuli such as lighting, television, etc. These should be presented from the neglected side, but it may be necessary to start at the midline and gradually move the stimuli over to the unattended side. There is little point in placing a patient's locker on the unattended side if this results in the locker being 'ignored'.

Some equipment may help such as spectacles with prisms to change the visual axis towards the neglected side (Frassinetti *et al.*, 2002). Cueing or prompting the patient to attend to the neglected area may be useful. For instance one technique to ensure that meals are eaten is to cue the patient to turn their plate a one quarter turn after each mouthful so that the whole plate receives attention. Clothes should be laid out upside down (e.g. presenting a shirt buttons down rather than the more usual up) so that it removes the need for the patient to make the reversal (which may be difficult in cases of neglect) before donning their clothing. Safety is, at all times, the main consideration. Rehabilitative efforts maybe difficult if the patient has accompanying anosognosia. Treatment and management are usually initiated by an occupational therapist or a clinical psychologist.

Care of the patient with sensory impairment

The patient who has impaired sensation is at risk, e.g. damage may occur to the feet of patients with peripheral neuropathy. Safety and protection from harm is the aim of care and must take account of the sensory modalities affected. Table 11.3 is a danger checklist to help identify actions in care to promote safety.

PHYSIOLOGY OF MOVEMENT

The complexity of the motor system is apparent in the number of areas, i.e. the premotor and motor cortices, the basal ganglia and the cerebellum, that are involved in movement (see Chapter 3). For each movement there may be a conscious intention to act and some unconscious moderating activity. When someone initiates the action of walking it is normally unnecessary to think how to move each leg in turn and to maintain balance, etc. This unconscious moderating component of movement can be affected in some diseases, notably Parkinson's disease and ataxic syndromes. People with Parkinson's disease may have problems initiating movement. People with dyspraxia may also have problems with initiation of an action.

Agonist and antagonist muscle groups

A further level of complexity occurs in the spinal cord and lower motor neurones (see Chapter 4), which cause the contraction of one muscle or group and inhibit the contraction of antagonist muscles. An agonist muscle produces a movement and an antagonist muscle produces the opposite muscle action: for example, the biceps produces elbow flexion (agonist) and the triceps produces elbow extension, which is antagonist to flexion. Sometimes both agonist and antagonist muscle groups contract to produce a rigid limb for stability, for example, the legs in standing upright.

Skeletal muscle

At the effector end of the pathway, the neuromuscular junction, there are both intrafusal and extrafusal muscle fibres. Each has its own input from the lower motor neurone and a complex feedback system via the sensory nerves (Figure 11.3), as much movement is governed at the level of spinal reflex. Sensory feedback from the proprioceptors in the muscle and tendons, the vestibular system and the eyes, is required to monitor effective movement. The extrafusal fibres are supplied by the alpha (α) motor nerve and the intrafusal fibres are supplied by the gamma (γ) motor nerve. The gamma motor neurones stimulate the intrafusal fibres to contract so that they remain equal to the contraction of the surrounding extrafusal fibres. If this did not happen the intrafusal fibres would slacken off during contraction of the extrafusal fibres and the stretch reflex (see Chapter 4) would diminish with increasing stretch.

Table 11.3 Danger checklist.

Sensation and affected pathway	Danger or effects of loss	Possible action
Temperature pathways	Burns and scalds	• Check bath temperature • Monitor smoking to prevent burns • Care when placing near electric fires and radiators • Help with cooking and using kettles
Pressure, vibration and proprioceptive pathways	Pressure sores Trips and falls Problems with gait Problems handling and using utensils and machines	• Conduct falls assessment • Change position • Remove hazards and obstructions • Correct fitting shoes • Chiropody referral as required • Observe pressure areas and provide relief • Referral to occupational therapy

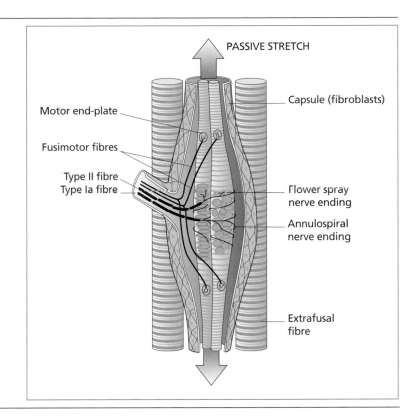

PASSIVE STRETCH

Motor end-plate

Fusimotor fibres

Type II fibre
Type Ia fibre

Capsule (fibroblasts)

Flower spray
nerve ending

Annulospiral
nerve ending

Extrafusal
fibre

Figure 11.3 The muscle spindle. Reproduced from C. Clarke *et al.*, *Neurology: A Queen Square Textbook*, Wiley-Blackwell, with permission

Myotomes

The relationship of a pair of lower motor neurones and their distribution is known as a myotome. Myotomes are discussed further in Chapter 4.

Normal tone

Normal muscle tone (or postural tone) is the slight state of contraction of muscles. Muscle tone is important in maintaining normal posture and is usually stronger in those muscle groups which maintain posture against gravity. Normal tone allows for normal movement and upright posture as well as being a basis for skilled movements. For example, when standing upright in a relaxed manner, the arms are slightly flexed at the elbows because of muscle tone, which is greater in the flexor muscles than the extensors. Normal tone is also required to keep the jaw closed at rest. Without this the lower jaw would gape due to the effects of gravity.

Tone is highest when the posture is upright because the base of support, the soles of the feet, covers a small surface area. Tone is lowest when lying because the base of support is much greater and therefore lying is a more stable position. Muscles need to increase the strength of contrac-

tion against the work they perform – the load. The stretch receptors in the muscle spindle and Golgi tendon organs send feedback via the stretch reflexes in order to increase the contraction to perform the action. This phenomenon is called recruitment. When reflexes are increased (hyperreflexia), due to upper motor neurone damage, recruitment may increase contraction of a stretched muscle beyond its functional requirement. This contraction is not useful functionally and is called a muscle spasm, or spasticity.

ASSESSMENT OF MOVEMENT

The motor nervous system is assessed by examining the function, quality and performance of motor activity including:

- Muscle power/strength
- Muscle tone
- Reflexes
- Gait
- Tremor

Muscle strength gives information about the neuromuscular junction and the lower motor neurone. Gait describes the quality and performance of walking, a motor activity. Abnormal movements can pinpoint the location of a lesion as in *cerebellar* ataxia. Assessment of movement can also enable nurses to gain an appreciation of how the person is managing in their daily activities.

Muscle strength/power

Muscle strength is tested using the Medical Research Council (MRC) scale (James, 2007). It is quite a simple test but does need practice to produce reproducible and consistent results. Muscle groups are tested separately and on both sides of the body. A reduced version is included on many standard neurological observation charts. A score of 0 to 5 is allocated according to set criteria (Table 11.4).

The muscles tested depend on the reason for the investigation, but a simple test consists of asking the patient to push the examiner away using the arms. Legs can be tested by asking the patient to lie down, flex the hip and knee and then straighten the leg against resistance. In more in depth testing fingers, hand, wrist, elbow and shoulder movements are tested for the upper limbs. Ankle, knee and hip movement may be assessed in the lower limbs (Fuller, 2004). It is not necessary to test each level of the scale, but to select the level by intuition.

Table 11.4 Medical Research Council (MRC) muscle strength grading system.

Score	Assessment criteria
0	There is no visible or palpable movement
1	There is minimal movement when patient moves muscle on request
2	There is movement in the muscle being tested but the patient cannot overcome the force of gravity (e.g. can move arm but cannot raise it off bed surface)
3	There is movement against gravity but not against resistance from the examiner (e.g. can raise arm from bed but not if the examiner restrains gently)
4	There is movement against gravity and against resistance (e.g. can raise arm with moderate restraint applied by the examiner)
5	Full strength (e.g. can raise arm even against firm resistance from examiner)

Source: James, 2007.

Power should be graded according to the maximum power the patient is able to achieve, no matter for how briefly this is achieved (Fuller, 2004). If any weakness is apparent decrease the resistance applied to a limb in a stepwise sequence, moving down the scale, until the assessment is completed and the power graded. Muscles may be weak because of intrinsic muscular disease as well as neurological impairment. Consider that even when the patient has 'full strength' pain, joint disease, fractures and soft tissue injury etc., may interfere with the results of this test.

Muscle tone

A simple bedside measure of tone is the Ashworth scale (Ashworth, 1964). The Ashworth scale is widely used and has been found to be valid in some studies, but inter-rater reliability has been questioned (Burridge *et al.*, 2005; Platz *et al.*, 2005). It needs careful practice to assess the criteria of the score levels and does not distinguish rigidity from spasticity. Table 11.5 shows the modified Ashworth scale where the 1+ level has been added to the original scale to give a six point scale. Spasticity is felt by the examiner as a resistance to passive movement. A limb with no tone is flaccid.

Spasticity may lead to other phenomena, such as reduced range of movement at a joint. This can be measured objectively using a goniometer, which measures the angle at a joint. While a variety of assessment measures are used in research and clinical practice, some more subjective than others, in practice many of these fail to assess the functional problems caused to the patient by a change in muscle tone (Burridge *et al.*, 2005). It is recommended that a range of methods be undertaken in producing a clinically useful assessment of spasticity.

Reflexes

Reflexes are tested by applying a stimulus and eliciting and observing a reflex response. It is necessary to use separate assessment scales for stretch reflexes and superficial reflexes. The notation for superficial reflexes is different because they cannot be brisk nor have clonus. Stretch reflexes are assessed by stretching a tendon, which produces a reflex contraction of the muscle as the stretch receptors in the muscle are stretched passively. Usually the stimulus is applied by a light tap to the tendon with a patellar hammer or by using the fingers, which then stretch the tendon producing the reflex response (Figure 11.4). Superficial reflexes are usually elicited by stroking the skin with a finger, the pointed end of a patellar hammer or using a cotton bud. Sometimes it is possible to reinforce a reflex

Table 11.5 Modified Ashworth scale.

Score	Assessment criteria
0	No increase in tone
1	There is a slight increase in muscle tone. There may be a catch and release (clasp knife phenomenon) when moving the limb passively or there may be slight resistance at the end of the normal range of motion for the joint when it is flexed or extended
1+	There is a slight increase in muscle tone and a catch in the movement after which there is minimal resistance in the remainder of the range of motion but in less than half of the range
2	There is a more noticeable increase in muscle tone during the whole range of motion. Passive movement is still easy
3	Muscle tone is very strong and therefore passive movement is difficult to perform
4	The joint is rigid and it cannot be moved passively

Adapted from Bohannon and Smith, 1987.

if it is difficult to obtain a response: for upper limb reflexes ask the patient to clench their teeth while testing the reflex; for lower limb reflexes ask the patient to grasp their fingers with each hand and try to pull apart. In the reflex table (Table 11.6) the abdominal reflex is a superficial reflex.

Table 11.6 shows the most common stretch reflexes, the notation used and interpretative information.

It will not be possible to elicit a reflex if the sensory nerve is impaired. Other problems can affect reflex responses such as injury, pain, swelling or muscle weakness and should be taken into account during the assessment. A brisk response to a reflex suggests that there is no cerebral inhibition of the reflex and so an upper motor neurone lesion may be present. Absent reflexes suggest that either there is a sensory loss or lower motor neurone lesion. If sensation is intact, that is the patient can feel the stimulus, lower motor neurone lesions may be suspected. Superficial reflexes are not associated with muscle tendons so a brisk response is not possible and a different scale is utilised (see Table 11.6).

Gait

Normal gait is determined by the neurological control of movement, the physical status of the person, the texture and slope of the surface being walked on and by the suitability of footwear and clothing. An experienced adult will know that walking on ice or other slippery surface requires a different gait from walking on a surface with good traction. The slope determines step length and effort in the gait. Poor footwear or restrictive clothing may impede normal gait. Musculo-skeletal problems may affect gait. A patient with unequal limb length will limp and, if there is a painful joint, antalgic gait is typical, that is walking in such a manner to avoid pain. It must be remembered that people with a neurological condition may have a coexisting orthopaedic or psychological problem and these non-neurological causes need to be excluded during examination.

Neurological control of gait depends on motor input to move the limbs, sensory feedback for information about limb position (and pain), and cerebellar pathways to coordinate all the muscle groups involved in the limbs, trunk and balance. Balance is essential in human bipedal gait and therefore an intact vestibular system is required. Neurological dysfunction and trauma to any of these pathways may produce abnormal gait.

To assess gait, ask the patient to walk and observe all four limbs as they do this. Assess if the gait is symmetrical or not and consider:

- Size of paces
- Posture
- Arm swing
- Lateral distance between feet
- Knee lift
- Rotation of pelvis and shoulders

(Fuller, 2004).

The patient may also be asked to walk 'heel to toe', on their heels or on tiptoes. Gait assessment is subjective and requires specialist training and equipment, however it is important to recognise the patterns and significance of gait disorders.

Other assessments

Of course it is one thing knowing how strong the muscles are, whether they are coordinated or not, or whether there is high or low tone, but often these tests can be misleading in terms of the patient's functional ability. People with motor and sensory deficits may appear to cope with everyday activities. For this reason some form of functional

Table 11.6 Basic reflexes.

Reflex	Method	Normal response	Spinal level	Assessment Scale
Biceps	Tap the biceps tendon at the elbow	Forearm flexes	C5	*Stretch Reflexes* Absent = 0
Brachioradialis (called supinator reflex in some texts)	Tap the radial tuberosity	Forearm flexes	C6	Normal = + Reinforced = ± Brisk = ++ Very brisk (maybe with clonus) =+++
Triceps	Tap the triceps tendon at the elbow	Elbow extends	C7	*Superficial Reflexes* Absent = 0
Finger flexor	Tap the palm gently	Fingers flex	C8	Present = +
Abdominal	Gently stroke the skin on one side of the abdomen with cotton bud towards the midline	Abdominal wall muscle contract on the stimulated side	T8 and T9 above navel T10 and T11 below navel (see comment on notation)	Equivocal = ±
Patellar	Tap the patellar ligament below the patella	Knee extends	L3 and L4	
Ankle	Hold the ball of the foot and tap gently	Foot plantar flexes at the ankle	S1 and S2	

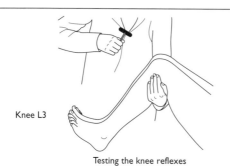

Knee L3

Testing the knee reflexes

Figure 11.4 Testing the knee reflexes. Reproduced from Robert Turner and Roger Blackwood, *Lecture Notes on Clinical Skills 3e.*, Wiley-Blackwell, with permission.

assessment may be useful to identify whether the patient requires help with activities.

There are several functional assessment measures available, but a commonly used one, which is easy to apply and has good reliability is the Barthel index (Table 11.7)

(Mahoney and Barthel, 1965). There are some modifications to the Barthel index with different scoring schemes available. The Barthel index compares favourably to other more elaborate functional assessment measures such as FIM (Functional Independence Measure) (Sangha *et al.*, 2005). The total for the Barthel index gives a level of functional ability score that is related to movement.

Another simple but effective test is the timed 'up and go' test. In this test an unimpaired person should be able to rise from a chair, walk a straight 3 metre line, turn and return to sitting in the chair in about ten seconds. Times longer than this, and especially when over twenty seconds, require further investigation (Bischoff *et al.*, 2003). The test is found to be valid and reliable in a number of clinical settings such as elderly, orthopaedic and neurological patients. The results of this test also depend on joint flexibility, pain, respiratory function and other factors such as in-growing toenails, corns and bunions. For this reason it provides useful information about the patient's functional ability which may be due to factors other than neurological deficits.

Table 11.7 Modified Barthel index.

Activity	Score
Continence of bowels	0 = Incontinent (or requires enemas) 1 = Occasional accident 2 = Continent
Bladder control	0 = Incontinent (or unable to manage catheter) 1 = Occasional accident 2 = Continent (or manages catheter unaided)
Personal care and hygiene	0 = Needs help 1 = Independent
Toilet use	0 = Dependent 1 = Needs some help but can do some tasks alone 2 = Independent (on and off toilet, dressing, wiping)
Eating	0 = Unable to eat unassisted 1 = Needs help 2 = Independent
Transferring	0 = Unable 1 = Major help 2 = Minor help 3 = Independent
Mobility	0 = Immobile or less than 50 meters 1 = Wheel chair independent 2 – Walks with help 3 = Independent
Dressing and undressing	0 = Dependent 1 = Needs help but can do about half unaided 2 = Independent
Managing stairs	0 = Unable 1 = Needs help 2 = Independent
Bathing	0 = Dependent 1 = Independent

Adapted from Mahoney and Barthel, 1965.

ABNORMAL MOVEMENTS AND MOVEMENT DISORDERS

There are a number of abnormal movements that indicate motor dysfunction; most are involuntary, but some occur in association with voluntary movement. Abnormal movement is known as dyskinesia and there are a number of recognised abnormal movements (Table 11.8).

Upper motor neurone lesions

When the upper motor neurone is damaged there is no control over the effector muscles, which then operate without cortical inhibition. This results in 'spastic paralysis' because the lower motor neurone produces reflex muscle contraction in the absence of useful movement. Upper motor neurone lesions result in increased tone, increased reflexes and extensor plantar responses (Fuller, 2004). In spastic paralysis the first order sensory nerve and the lower motor neurone remain intact. When there is an intact lower motor neurone, muscles keep a dysfunctional nerve supply therefore muscle wasting is in theory preventable with good management, but rarely achievable in practice regardless of the location of the lesion. In spastic paralysis reflexes are strong and maybe exaggerated as there is no control over the extent of the reflex response from the higher centres. Diseases which affect the upper motor neurone include stroke, brain injury, multiple sclerosis and some forms of motor neurone disease.

Lower motor neurone lesions

When the lower motor neurone is damaged there is no input at all to the muscles from the spinal cord and the result is called 'flaccid paralysis' because muscles remain uncontracted or with reduced tone. In lower motor neurone lesions and flaccid paralysis, reflexes are absent and the muscle will waste, producing characteristic loss of shape to the limbs and fasciculation (fine, subcutaneous movement – contraction of a motor unit) may occur (Fuller, 2004). Diseases which affect the lower motor neurone include spinal injury, some spinal disease processes, Guillain–Barré syndrome and motor neurone disease.

Dyspraxia

Dyspraxia is a condition where the patient lacks the ability to perform a skilled action in the absence of any other neurological deficit, e.g. paralysis, movement disorder, an intellectual or a language disorder.

Dyspraxia occurs when in there is damage to areas of the cortex where movement is planned, that is the areas where the 'programming' for complex, skilled movement is located, such as the premotor cortex in the frontal lobes.

Table 11.8 Abnormal movements.

Name	Description	Causes/conditions
Akinesia	Inability to initiate voluntary movement	Parkinson's disease
Ataxia	Uncoordinated movement/unsteadiness of gait	Disorders of the cerebellum (cerebellar ataxia) or vestibular system, excess alcohol intake
Athetosis	Slow, writhing movement when awake. Not associated with voluntary movement	Cerebral palsy, Huntington's disease
Bradykinesia	Slow voluntary movements	Parkinson's disease (see Chapter 26)
Chorea	Rapid, jerky movements without purpose. May be associated with athetosis (choreo-athetosis)	Huntington's disease, post-streptococcal rheumatic fever and obsessive compulsive disorder (Sydenham's chorea)
Clonus	Rapid contraction and relaxation of a muscle or muscle group following a stretch reflex in that muscle. May be marked leading to the person requiring repositioning	Common in upper motor neurone disorders, e.g. MS, stroke, head injury
Dystonia (See Chapter 26)	Movements associated with muscle contraction with increased tone in both agonist and antagonist muscles	Writer's cramp, torticollis, cerebral palsy, brain injury, drug induced
Spasm and spasticity	Involuntary contraction of voluntary muscles or muscle groups. It can also affect involuntary muscle, e.g. bronchospasm and sphincters. Spasticity results in increased tone	Muscle spasm can occur below the level of the injury following spinal damage. It can occur in MS and other CNS lesions, e.g. stroke and head injury. It may have non-neurological causes such as dehydration and electrolyte imbalances. Cramp is a common example
Tics	Rapid, localised contractions. Often associated with the facial muscles leading to grimacing. Tics can also occur in the vocal tract leading to phonic tics which are audible. May be suppressed voluntarily	Tourette's syndrome
Tremor	Rapid, rhythmic contractions of a muscle group, producing characteristic shaking movements	Disorders of the basal ganglia and cerebellum, peripheral neuropathy, psychiatric disorders, metabolic changes e.g. hypoglycaemia, thyroid disease, drug induced or idiopathic (essential tremor)

The 'programming' for some learned movements is in the left parietal lobe and lesions here, too, can lead to dyspraxia. Dyspraxia may be congenital but it may also occur following stroke, tumours or dementia. One characteristic of dyspraxia is that the patient is frequently unaware of the loss of the skill.

Testing for dyspraxia involves asking the patient to demonstrate the use of a particular object such as a comb, an item of cutlery, scissors, etc. The objects do not necessarily have to be present as the patient can mime their use. Observation of the patient performing activities of daily living will also provide diagnostic data.

There are several types of dyspraxia, based on the functional ability which is affected by the condition, such as:

- Ideomotor dyspraxia, where the patient cannot imitate a skilled action such as combing the hair
- Buccofacial dyspraxia, where there is poor control of actions of the mouth muscles (the patient may not be able to mime a kiss or blow out a match) and
- Constructional dyspraxia, where the patient cannot copy drawings or build models

Abnormal gait

Common gait disorders are seen in hemiplegia where the usual pattern is a flexed and adducted arm and an extended, abducted leg. In bilateral upper motor neurone damage (e.g. multiple sclerosis) the legs are usually abducted resulting in a lurching gait where the track of each leg might cross the path of the other. In lower motor neurone damage foot drop may occur causing the affected leg to be raised high to keep the trailing foot clear of the floor.

Parkinsonian gait typically involves a slow start to movement, poor stopping ability and small and increasingly rapid steps known as festinating gait (from Latin *festinare* meaning to hurry or hasten). Parkinsonian gait is stooping and shuffling but has no arm swing. Ataxic gait is associated with cerebellar disorders and the movement is often swaying and unbalanced. When the dorsal columns in the spinal cord are damaged following injury or syphilis, proprioception is lost so that the patient walks with an ataxic broad based gait. *Marche à petits pas* (walking on small steps) is a gait pattern with small shuffling steps, but unlike Parkinsonian gait the torso is upright and there is normal arm swing. *Marche à petits pas* is found in cortical dysfunction and lacunar stroke. It is sometimes called gait dyspraxia.

Tremor

Tremor is a rhythmical, alternating movement. Tremor should be observed and the examiner should note whether the tremor occurs at rest, with movement, with the contraction of muscles against gravity (as in holding the arms out) or with the intention to move. Tremor that occurs at rest is indicative of Parkinsonism. Tremor that occurs with movement or muscle contraction against gravity (postural or action tremor) may be due to benign essential tremor, physiological tremor (due to hyperthyroidism) or more rarely liver or renal failure and withdrawal from alcohol (Fuller, 2004). Intention tremor is indicative of cerebellar disease.

SPASTICITY, RIGIDITY AND CONTRACTURE

High muscle tone (hypertonia)

There are two main types of abnormal high muscle tone that occur in neurological disorders: spasticity and rigidity. They may not be easy to distinguish in practice, but there are some key features that define them (Table 11.9).

Spasticity

Spasticity is a manifestation of a hyperactive, abnormal stretch reflex. There are many stimuli that occur which can trigger spasms and spasticity in affected individuals (Box 11.1).

A defining characteristic of spasticity is the increased tone in muscle groups, usually in flexor groups although extensor spastic patterns do occur. Spasticity does not occur in flexor and extensors of the same joint although an abnormal response called co-contraction can occur in spasticity when an antagonist muscle contracts simultaneously with the agonist. Spasms are sudden, involuntary movements that may be painful. These are transient, but may be superimposed on spasticity and are often considered part of the same phenomenon (Thompson *et al.*, 2005).

In severe cases clonus may be present (see Table 11.8). Spasticity can cause major problems for the patient including pain, incontinence, loss of function (e.g. walking, transferring, washing, dressing, speech, sexual activity), contractures, sleep disturbance, weight loss, pressure sores and limb or trunk deformity. Other problems associated with spasticity are altered body image, emotional disturbance and depression (Jarrett, 2004). Patients may also experience negative behaviour from other people who may assume intellectual impairment (Nicholson and Anderson, 2001). On the other hand spasticity may be useful in mobilising a patient, allowing them to stand or walk when otherwise they may not be able to due to weakness (Thompson *et al.*, 2005), for example following stroke or head injury.

Table 11.9 Hypertonia.

Sign	Spasticity	Rigidity
Velocity dependent	Yes – increase in tone is dependent on the velocity of the stretch stimulus	No – velocity of the stimulus has no effect on the increased tone
Resistance to passive movement	Clasp knife – initial resistance to passive movement which is followed by catch and release. In severe spasticity the resistance may be throughout the whole range of movement	Cogwheel – a constant resistance to passive movement which releases suddenly and for short duration and movement range. This is the result of superimposed tremor on high tone Lead pipe – there is constant resistance to passive movement throughout the normal range
Symmetry at joints	Asymmetrical – there is resistance in one muscle group at the joint (e.g. flexors but not corresponding extensors)	Symmetrical – there is equal high tone in both flexors and extensors (or other agonist – antagonist muscle group)
Reflexes	Exaggerated and hyperactive due to loss of cortical inhibition via the upper motor neurone	Normal response or difficult to observe due to high tone. Postural reflexes in advanced Parkinson's disease may be slow or diminished
Clonus	May be present	Not present although tremor maybe present in Parkinson's disease with a similar appearance.
Pathophysiology	Defective upper motor neurone	Basal ganglia defect

Adapted from Lance, 1980.

Box 11.1   Stimuli that trigger spasticity/spasm

- Constipation or diarrhoea (the sensory stimulus is the trigger)
- Urinary retention or infection
- Bladder calculus
- Tight clothing including orthotics and leg bags.
- Pressure sores
- Draughts
- Sudden movements
- In-growing toenails
- Wounds
- Burns (including sunburn)
- Any other noxious stimuli

Rigidity

Rigidity is commonly associated with Parkinson's disease when there is damage to the basal ganglia. Rigidity, unlike spasticity, occurs in agonist and antagonist muscle groups simultaneously causing characteristic 'lead pipe' rigidity: that is the rigidity remains constant when passive stretching is applied. If tremor is present the rigidity may be described as 'cog-wheel', where there is a characteristic catch and release response to passive movement; the effect is rather as if the joint is operated on a ratchet. The presence of rigidity usually places the pathology in the extrapyramidal pathways. Care needs to be used with the term rigidity which refers both to a specific neurological sign as well as to the more general stiffness from muscular or orthopaedic causes.

Contractures

In contractures the soft tissues (muscles and tendons) have atrophied and shortened. They are the result of immobility. However, contractures frequently coexist with spasticity and rigidity and, if the increased tone is not relieved contractures, are likely to occur. In contractures, the stiffness is also often referred to as 'lead pipe' rigidity as there is no release at all when passive stretching is applied. It is not always easy to distinguish between spasticity, rigidity and contractures. Contractures must be actively prevented wherever possible by active and passive exercise, careful positioning, and the use of splints and orthotics.

Contractures are difficult to release once formed and surgery may be necessary to improve function or posture.

NURSING CARE OF THE PATIENT WITH MOTOR IMPAIRMENT

Multidisciplinary care of the patient aims to maximise functional ability by providing time, space for activities, aids and equipment, preventing injury and promoting safety. Preventing injury must be one of the highest priorities in caring for a patient with motor impairment. There is an increased risk of falling if the balance, gait and muscle strength are affected. People with motor impairment will have difficulty in maintaining activities of daily living, including personal hygiene, dressing, toileting/continence, nutrition and leisure activities. Every effort should be put into allowing the patient to achieve maximum independence within the limits of the impairment. In long term illness this is an essential priority, so early assessment and intervention from an occupational therapist and physiotherapist is important if the problems are likely to persist for more than a few days.

Immobility and disuse syndrome

Immobility is, of course, a major issue when people have motor deficits. Pressure sores are a serious risk in immobile patients and the risk is increased if the patient has sensory loss as well and cannot perceive the discomfort caused by pressure or shearing forces. Pressure area care is discussed in Chapter 8. Immobility can also cause deep vein thrombosis, which is also discussed in Chapter 8. The well known adage 'use it or lose it' is fundamental in neurological disease or trauma: even after a few days of bed rest legs feel wobbly and weak on mobilising. After many months or a lifetime of immobility the body undergoes many changes. The resulting immobility increases the problem, and so on: a vicious circle. The aim of care in all these potential problems is to preserve the patient's functional ability as much as possible and to prevent the sequelae of immobility. The management of common problems are discussed below.

Impact on musculo-skeletal system

Calcium is lost from bones when the patient is no longer weight bearing (Bischoff *et al.*, 1999). This is not only an issue in illness as astronauts lose calcium from bones during weightlessness in space and astronauts are very fit and healthy. Muscle mass is lost and the loss happens quite quickly with recordable changes in only a few days (Nissen, 1997). In some cases of neurological impairment, such as following spinal injury, new bone can be laid down in tendon tissues, especially at the shoulder joint (Hudson and Brett, 2006). This is called heterotopic ossification which can be painful and lead to further immobility.

Tendons and ligaments that are not in use will shorten leading to contractures. Contractures are very difficult to treat once they have occurred. Many of these problems are self sustaining because immobility increases when muscle weakness and contractures occur. Active or passive movements and application of splints to promote alignment where possible are vital and a key part of the nurse's role as well as educating others about their potential to form. Serial splinting may be used to 'stretch out' contacted tissues and increase range of movement at a joint. The limb is straightened to a comfortable maximum and a straighter splint is applied every 7 to 10 days (Barnes and Ward, 2005).

The aim of care should be to prevent the complications occurring. Moving and handling risk assessment should be undertaken, according to local policy, for all patients. Weight bearing is vital to prevent calcium loss (Porth, 2005; Bloomfield, 1997). Early mobilisation and the use of a standing frame or tilt table, usually in the physiotherapy department, will help. Careful positioning (see below) will help prevent spasticity and the development of contractures. Passive exercises can help to maintain range of joint movement, prevent contractures avoid joint stiffness and pain and prevent loss of muscle bulk (Dawe and Curran-Smith, 1994). Koch *et al.* (1996) found that passive exercise may be safe in patients with raised intracranial pressure. The use of standing frames, tilt tables and standing transfer hoists allow passive weight bearing by patients who cannot move or maintain posture and should be encouraged in neuroscience nursing practice.

Bladder and bowel care

The calcium lost from bone is removed from the blood by the kidneys and as calcium is poorly soluble in water there is an increased risk of renal or bladder calculi (Pieltrow and Karellas, 2006). If there is decreased muscle power it may not be possible to completely empty the bladder during micturation as bearing down with the muscles of the abdominal wall is important in emptying the bladder. Where this is not possible there is increased risk of high residual volume, which can further increase calculus formation and risk of urinary tract infection. If there is an indwelling catheter the risk of urinary tract infection is greater. An adequate fluid intake will help to reduce calculus formation and the risk of urinary tract infection.

Long term use of an indwelling catheter is best avoided (see Chapter 18).

The digestive tract works best when people are mobile and active and immobility can lead to constipation and possible impaction. For the same reasons as described above with emptying the bladder, defecation is more effective when the abdominal wall can be tensed to increase intra-abdominal pressure. Bowel function should be assessed and measures taken to prevent constipation (see Chapter 18).

Respiratory care

Respiration may be impaired if there is weakness of the respiratory muscles or the patient is lying down and full lung expansion is prevented. This can lead to chest infection, pneumonia or even atelectasis (Moore and Duffy, 2007). All these complications contribute to poor oxygenation. Breathing and coughing exercises and assisted coughing may help keep the respiratory system clear (see Chapter 15). The use of a standing frame may give better expansion and oxygenation.

Cardiovascular care

Perfusion of all organs, including the skin, may be affected by immobility. The heart rate usually drops in long term immobility. The control of the blood pressure by the baroreceptors in the aortic arch and carotid sinuses may be lost due to deconditioning (Dampney *et al.*, 2002). Like all physiological processes, the baroreceptors need to have positional change to keep them working and with lack of movement they become deconditioned.

When mobilising patients it is important to raise patients to an upright position slowly to avoid orthostatic hypotension (Hollister, 1992). The use of the standing frame or early mobilisation will help maintain good circulation. The use of compression stockings, anticoagulants and sometimes intermittent pneumatic compression devices will assist in the prevention of thrombi (Cayley, 2007) (see Chapter 8).

Nutritional management

Bed rest and supine positioning increase the risk of oesophageal reflux. Many neurological conditions are hypermetabolic leading to increased calorie expenditure (Hill, 1998), but immobility often results in decreased appetite. This can lead to malnutrition and weight loss. A dietician should be consulted in each case to ensure optimum nutrition related to needs. Nursing care should involve monitoring of the diet and the use of food charts or food diaries to identify nutritional needs (see Chapter 16).

SPECIFIC NURSING MANAGEMENT OF SPASTICITY

Management of spasticity includes:

*   Preventing stimuli that trigger spasms (see Box 11.1)
*   Physiotherapy and maintaining passive/active movement
*   Occupational therapy and use of assistive devices and orthotics
*   Drug therapy

There is no agreed evidence-based model (Thompson *et al.*, 2005), but it is widely accepted that education of the patient and their family/carers, multidisciplinary approaches and continuity of care between the acute and primary care sectors are vital. Spasticity is a common feature of many long-term neurological conditions and a key nursing role involves educating and empowering the patient to self-manage their condition, as most of their time will be spent at home (Jarrett, 2004). Key elements of the nursing role in management of spasticity are detailed in Box 11.2.

Positioning

Handling and positioning play a part in maintaining neutral alignments and minimising postural reflexes. Some 'primitive' reflexes become suppressed during infancy, including the grasp reflex, the sucking reflex, the rooting reflex and a group of reflexes known as the tonic neck reflexes. The symmetrical tonic neck reflex occurs when the neck is flexed forwards and in response the arms flex and the legs extend. When the head is extended backwards the response is for the arms to extend and the legs to flex. When the head is turned to one side, a reflex called the asymmetric tonic neck reflex occurs. When an infant's

---

> **Box 11.2   Key nursing roles in managing spasticity**
>
> *   Prevent noxious stimuli
> *   Posture and positioning
> *   Moving and handling
> *   Drug education
> *   Pain management
> *   Sexual dysfunction
> *   Emotion/depression
> *   Impact on employment/socialising
>
> Adapted from Jarrett, 2004.

head is turned to the left, for example, the left arm and leg extend and the right arm and leg flex. This is sometimes known as the fencing posture because it resembles the posture adopted by fencers when *en garde*. The converse happens when the head is turned to the right. These primitive reflexes may be 'released' (i.e. no longer suppressed) if there is significant neurological damage as in some head injuries or strokes, especially where the frontal lobe is damaged (Schott and Rossor, 2003). Patient positioning is important so that these primitive reflexes, especially the grasp reflex and the tonic neck reflexes, do not stimulate spasm and possible contractures in the longer term.

Patients need to be positioned in a neutral alignment at all times so that these primitive reflexes are not triggered, but it is particularly important in the early stages of a motor impairment such as stroke or head injury to prevent complications such as spasticity becoming established. In order to achieve this, the patient should be positioned so that the midline is not crossed by limbs and the head and neck are not tilted. Side lying is important so that pressure sores are avoided but the limbs should be placed so that they do not cross the midline and for this pillows will be needed for support. The side lying position (Figure 11.5) is similar to the recovery position but well supported. When the patient lies supine, the arms and legs need to be in a neutral alignment and supported by pillows to prevent external rotation of the limbs (Figure 11.6). The affected arm and shoulder should be supported so that the paralysed shoulder does not drop down to the mattress. A pillow placed under the arm and shoulder will facilitate this position. Good support for the arms and legs is needed when the patient is sitting in a chair (Figure 11.7). Pillows may be necessary on a table to support the arms and shoulders, and a footrest may be needed to keep the knees level with or slightly higher than the hips.

Sitting in bed is not recommended as sitting with extended legs and flexed hips is uncomfortable and unnatural. However, sitting in bed may be needed for short periods during meal times or a visit. If a patient is required to sit up in bed a profiling bed should be used and an element of knee flexion introduced to prevent pain at the knee joint. Most profiling beds will introduce this small amount of knee flexion automatically on raising the head of the bed. A wedge or foam roll may also be used under the knees to flex them when there is no profiling bed (Jarrett, 2004).

To prevent stimulation of the grasp reflex nothing should be placed in the patient's hand. If this does occur the fingers may flex and contract making functional recovery difficult.

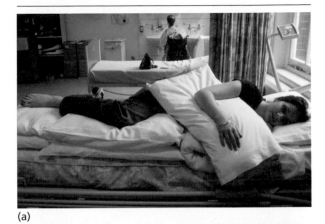

(a)

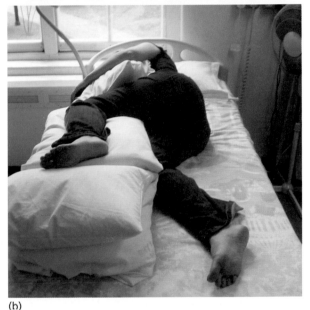

(b)

Figure 11.5 Side-lying on unaffected side.

Preventing triggers

Nurses need to help patients and carers learn to identify and prevent specific trigger stimuli (Jarrett, 2004). For instance, urinary tract infections might be noted and treated or care taken to avoid over tight leg bag straps. Not every trigger stimulus will produce spasm in every patient. Carers or the patients themselves will apply splints and orthotics and therefore careful training in their use is required.

Moving and dressing patients

Nurses may be familiar with the phenomenon that pulling the arm to straighten it may cause an increase in spasm

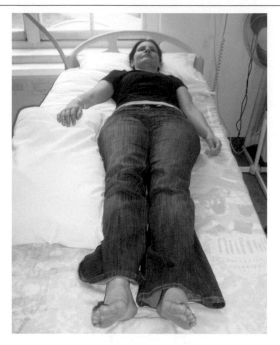

Figure 11.6 Lying supine with pillows on affected side.

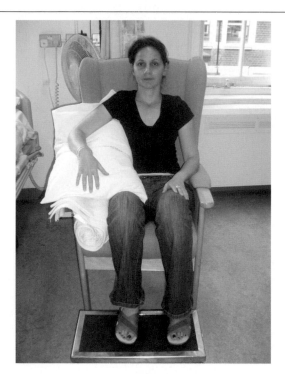

Figure 11.7 Sitting out with pillows supporting affected side.

when dressing a patient with spasticity. The harder you pull to straighten the arm to get it into a sleeve the harder it is to straighten. Spasticity is velocity dependent, i.e. if you pull quickly on the forearm to passively extend the elbow in a spastic arm the tone will increase and the arm will stiffen. Gentle, slow pressure will help the straightening more effectively. Occupational therapists and physiotherapists should assess the patient to provide the optimum management plan for moving and dressing individual patients.

Patients may experience sudden spasms during movement, which can risk the safety of both themselves and their carers. Getting a patient up in the morning can be the most troublesome, but using a profiling bed to assist the patient into a sitting position and break up the extensor spasm may help (Jarrett, 2004). When transferring patients using a sliding board, they should be encouraged to keep their feet on the floor and pass weight through them, which may also help (Jarrett, 2004). Patients and their carers can also be taught how to perform stretching and exercise programmes in their daily routine, an example of which is detailed in Stephenson and Jarrett (2006).

Drug therapy

A number of drugs are effective in controlling spasticity although each one of them has some contraindications. Nurses need to be aware of the problems associated with any medication they administer so that side-effects are recognised and therapeutic outcome is achieved. Nurses will also need to advise the patients and carers on the correct administration of drugs.

Systemic drugs

Baclofen is commonly used and may be given orally or intrathecally. Oral baclofen can produce flaccidity, causing further problems, if the dose is not carefully titrated. It acts by binding to GABA receptors on the lower motor neurone and thus prevents overstimulation associated with spasticity.

Dantrolene sodium works at the muscle and moderates calcium ion transfer necessary for contraction thereby reducing spasticity. It has several side-effects, including liver toxicity.

Diazepam, like baclofen, blocks GABA receptors and so damps down muscle activity. Diazepam also has anxiolytic properties and may be useful in managing some of the emotional issues in spasticity. The dependence on diazepam and other benzodiazepine drugs make it less useful for long term management.

Gabapentin is another GABA analogue drug and has been used in managing spasticity increasingly since its development in 1994. It has fewer side-effects than some other drugs.

Tizanidine is an alpha-2 adrenergic agonist (chemically similar to adrenaline), which works in the CNS to reduce tone.

Intrathecal drugs

Baclofen administered intrathecally can be given in lower doses and is therefore less likely to cause flaccidity or systemic side-effects, but this does require the surgical insertion of a pump (Stephenson and Jarrett, 2006). Patients and carers will need education on the use and maintenance of a pump. It is useful in cases where the spasticity of the lower limbs is a management issue and poor control is achieved with oral medication.

Phenol is a potent drug that causes damage to both motor and sensory nerves at the level of injection. The effect is long lasting, but bowel, bladder and sexual function may be affected. Before phenol is given a trial with a long acting local anaesthetic is given so that the effects can be monitored and the functional range established.

Topical drugs

Botulinum toxin has been injected locally into spastic muscles with good effect although repeat injections are required (see Chapter 26).

Functional electrical stimulation for spasticity of the foot

Drop foot is the inability to lift the foot and toes when walking and can occur as a result of either lower motor neurone lesions or upper motor neurone lesions such as stroke, multiple sclerosis and head injury for example (NICE, 2008). The spastic pattern of knee and ankle straightening results in the foot dragging while walking, producing an abnormal, slow and unsafe gait. First line management is normally physiotherapy and an ankle–foot orthosis, but there is evidence that functional electrical stimulation (FES) is also effective (Robbins *et al.*, 2006).

FES aims to stimulate muscle contractions that mimic normal movement by applying electrical stimuli to the common peroneal nerve via either surface or implanted electrodes (NICE, 2008). The effects of FES are to improve gait, reduce effort and pain while walking, reduce falls and improve quality of life. Patients receiving FES via surface electrodes need to be trained to apply the electrodes and must follow the regime prescribed, often long-term, to

obtain any benefit. FES via implanted electrodes does not require the patient to site the electrodes, but there have been some reports of skin erythema (Daly *et al.*, 2006) and wound infection (Burridge *et al.*, 2007) using this approach.

SPECIFIC NURSING MANAGEMENT OF FLACCIDITY

Patients with lower motor neurone or muscular disorders (e.g. Guillain–Barré syndrome, peripheral neuropathies, motor neurone disease) may have low muscle tone or flaccidity. Flaccidity and reduced tone affects all levels of activity and interferes with normal function. If the flaccidity is generalised the patient may not be able to hold their head up and thus make eye contact with carers and visitors, increasing social isolation.

Management of flaccidity is aimed at maintaining function and preventing injury. Affected limbs need to be supported in a good 'functional' position, e.g. feet at 90° to the ankle to enable walking. Muscles provide much of the stability at a joint and patients may experience painful joints if these are unsupported, allowing hyper-extension injuries to develop. Profiling beds can help to support a patient with flaccidity in a functional position. Patients with flaccidity are also particularly at risk of DVT as the deep veins have reduced support within the muscles. DVT prophylaxis is essential (see Chapter 8).

Early involvement of a physiotherapist and occupational therapist is essential. Orthotics and splints may be used to provide stability for a flaccid limb and ankle–foot orthoses will support a drop foot during mobilisation. If such splints are used it is essential to remove them at least once per day to provide for hygiene needs and inspect pressure areas. While FES is effective in treating drop foot of central neurological origin, it has no benefit for lower motor neurone lesions. Passive movements of the affected joint are also essential to maintain range of movement. Wheelchair-bound patients may require supports such as belts, knee braces and head supports to maintain a suitable position. Special seating is available which positions the patient avoiding belts and straps.

SUMMARY

Most, if not all, neurological disorders will have some manifestation affecting the sensory, motor (or autonomic) nervous systems. Although some disorders affect only the brain itself the damaged integrative and perceptual functions may appear as sensory or motor impairment. For this reason most of the issues discussed in this chapter will have implications for the testing, treatment and nursing care of most neurological patients.

REFERENCES

Ashworth B (1964) Preliminary trial of carisoprodal in multiple sclerosis. *Practitioner* 192:540–542.

Barnes MP and Ward AR (2005) *Oxford Handbook of Rehabilitation Medicine*. Oxford: Oxford University Press.

Bischoff HA, Stähelin HB, Monsch AU *et al.* (2003) Identifying a cut-off point for normal mobility: a comparison of the timed 'up and go' test in community-dwelling and institutionalised elderly women. *Age and Ageing* 32(3):315–320.

Bischoff HA, Stähelin HB, Vogt P *et al.* (1999) Immobility as a major cause of bone remodelling in residents of a long-stay geriatric ward. *Calcified Tissue International* 64(6):485–489.

Bloomfield SA (1997) Changes in musculoskeletal structure and function with prolonged bed rest. *Medicine and Science in Sports and Exercise* 29(2):197–206.

Bohannon RW, Smith MB (1987) Inter-rater reliability of a Modified Ashworth Scale of muscle spasticity. *Physical Therapy* 67(2):206–206.

Burridge JH, Haugland M, Larsen B *et al.* (2007) Phase II trial to evaluate the ActiGait implanted drop-foot stimulator in established hemiplegia. *Journal of Rehabilitation Medicine* 39:212–218.

Burridge JH, Wood DE, Hermens HJ *et al.* (2005) Theoretical and methodological considerations in the measurement of spasticity. *Disability and Rehabilitation* 27:69–80.

Cayley W E (2007) Clinical review – Preventing deep vein thrombosis in hospital patients. *British Medical Journal* 335:147–151.

Daly JJ, Roenigk K, Holcomb J *et al.* (2006) A randomised controlled trial of functional neuromuscular stimulation in chronic stroke subjects. *Stroke* 37:172–178.

Dampney RAL, Coleman MJ, Fontes MAP *et al.* (2002) Central mechanisms underlying short- and long-term regulation of the cardiovascular system. *Clinical and Experimental Pharmacology and Physiology* 29(4):261–268.

Dawe D, Curran-Smith J (1994) Going through the motions. *Canadian Nurse* 90(1):31–33.

Frassinetti F, Angeli V, Meneghello F, Avanzi S, Ladavas E (2002) Long-lasting amelioration of visuospatial neglect by prism adaptation. *Brain* 125(3):608–623.

Fuller G (2004) *Neurological Examination Made Easy*. (3rd edition). Edinburgh: Churchill Livingstone.

Hill G (1998) Implications of critical illness, injury and sepsis on lean body mass and nutritional needs. *Nutrition* 14(6):557–558.

Hollister AS (1992) Orthostatic hypotension – Causes, evaluation and management. *Western Journal of Medicine* 157:652–657.

Hudson SJ, Brett SJ (2006) Heterotopic ossification – a long-term consequence of prolonged immobility. *Critical Care* 10(6):174.

James MA (2007) Use of the Medical Research Council muscle strength grading system in the upper extremity. *The Journal of Hand Surgery* 32(2):154–156.

Jarrett L (2004) The role of the nurse in the management of spasticity. *Nursing and Residential Care* 6(3):116–119.

Khasnis A, Gokula R (2003) Romberg's test. *Journal of Postgraduate Medicine* 49(2):169–172.

Koch S, Fogarty S, Signorino C *et al.* (1996) Effects of passive range of motion exercises on intracranial pressure in neurosurgical patients. *Journal of Critical Care* 11(4):176–179.

Lance JW (1980). Symposium synopsis. In: Feldman RG, Yound RR, Koella WP, eds. *Spasticity: Disordered motor control*. Chicago: Year Book Medical 485–494.

Mahoney F, Barthel DW (1965) Functional evaluation: the Barthel Index. *Maryland State Medical Journal* 14(2):56–61

Moore S, Duffy E (2007) Maintaining vigilance to promote best outcomes for hospitalized elders. *Critical Care Nursing Clinics of North America* 19(3): 313—319.

National Institute for Health and Clinical Excellence (2008) *Interventional Procedure Overview of Functional Electrical Stimulation for Drop Foot of Central Neurological Origin*. London: NICE. Available from: http://www.nice.org.uk/nicemedia/pdf/657_FES_overview_post%20IPAC%20II%20190109.pdf Accessed June 2010.

Nicholson P, Anderson P (2001) The psychosocial impact of spasticity-related problems for people with multiple sclerosis: a focus group study. *Journal of Health Psychology* 6(5):551–567.

Nissen S (1997) Measurement of muscle proteolysis and the impact on muscle wasting. *Proceedings of the Nutrition Society* 56:793–799.

Perkins BA, Olaleye D, Zinman B, Bril V (2000). Simple screening tests for peripheral neuropathy in the diabetes clinic. *Diabetes Research and Clinical Practice* 50(Suppl 1):270–271.

Pieltrow PK, Karellas ME (2006) Medical management of common urinary calculi. *American Family Physician* 74(1):86—94.

Platz T, Eickhof C, Nuyens G *et al.* (2005) Clinical scales for the assessment of spasticity, associated phenomena and function: a systematic review of the literature. *Disability and Rehabilitation* 27:7–18.

Porth CM (2005) Activity, tolerance and fatigue. In: *Pathophysiology: Concepts of altered health*. Philadelphia: Lippincott Williams Wilkins.

Ringman JM, Saver JL, Woolson RF, Clarke WR, Adams HP (2004) Frequency, risk factors, anatomy, and course of unilateral neglect in an acute stroke cohort. *Neurology* 63(3):468–474

Robbins SM, Houghton PE, Woodbury MG *et al.* (2006) The therapeutic effect of functional and transcutaneous electrical stimulation on improving gait speed in stroke patients: a meta-analysis. *Archives of Physical Medicine and Rehabilitation* 87:853–859.

Sangha H, Lipson D, Foley N *et al.* (2005) A comparison of the Barthel Index and the Functional Independence Measure as outcome measures in stroke rehabilitation: patterns of disability scale usage in clinical trials. *International Journal of Rehabilitation Research* 28(2):135–139.

Schott JM, Rossor MN (2003) The grasp and other primitive reflexes. *Journal of Neurology Neurosurgery and Psychiatry* 74:558–560.

Stephenson VL, Jarrett L (2006) *Spasticity Management.* Oxford: Informa Healthcare.

Thompson AJ, Jarrett L, Lockley L (2005) Clinical management of spasticity. *Journal of Neurology, Neurosurgery and Psychiatry* 76:459–463.

Tortora G, Derrickson B (2006) *Principles of Anatomy and Physiology.* (11th edition). London: Wiley.

12

Assessment, Interpretation and Management of Altered Speech and Swallowing

Jane Dundas and Kathryn Chappell

INTRODUCTION

A large number of people suffer from altered speech and swallowing as a result of a neurological condition (Box 12.1) and each individual suffering from a particular disorder may be affected in different ways (British Brain and Spine Foundation, 1998). In many cases the lives of both the patient and their families are drastically changed. It may also transform the way in which they are perceived by others in their daily lives, impacting on their self-esteem and quality of life. It is therefore vital for neuroscience nurses to be well informed of the nature and consequences of speech and swallowing difficulties and to implement evidence based practice. There are many ways in which nursing care can influence outcome.

OVERVIEW OF ALTERED SPEECH

The ability to communicate is central to our daily lives and is something that can easily be taken for granted. We use communication to express our individuality, to form and sustain relationships and it is necessary for both work and leisure. People who have communication difficulties may become ignored, isolated and unable to participate (Liechty and Buchholz, 2006); they may become angry, frustrated and depressed. Therefore speed is of the essence to treat the affected person using individualised strategies to optimise recovery. If full recovery is not expected it is important to establish a reliable method of communication by any means possible.

The umbrella term 'speech' incorporates two separate components, i.e. speech and language. It is important to differentiate between these for the purpose of assessment and diagnosis of specific communication impairments, however, when considering the physiology of speech it is impossible to separate the two.

The physiology of speech

Normal speech production requires the integration of cognitive, neuromuscular and musculoskeletal activities. The cerebral functions involved in the production of speech act as components in a process, each as indispensable as the next (Table 12.1).

Structures involved in the cortical activation and programming of speech and language are shown in Figure 12.1.

Neuroanatomy of language

The principal regions of the brain which are activated during speech were originally identified in the nineteenth century and are named after the physicians who first discovered them. Broca's area lies in the left frontal lobe just in front of the motor face area and Wernicke's area sits in the posterior part of the left superior temporal gyrus (Brodal, 2004) in the dominant hemisphere (see Chapter 3). More recently functional positron emission tomography (PET) and functional magnetic resonance imaging (fMRI) has shown that there are some other areas of cortical involvement (Demonet *et al.*, 2005).

Neuroscience Nursing: Evidence-Based Practice, 1st Edition.
Edited by Sue Woodward and Ann-Marie Mestecky

Box 12.1   Neurological causes of altered speech or swallowing

- Vascular: stroke, sub-arachnoid haemorrhage
- Neoplastic: primary or secondary tumours
- Trauma: head injury
- Infective: abcess, HIV encephalopathy, encephalitis, tuberculosis, prion disease, e.g. Creutzfeldt–Jacob disease (CJD)
- Structural: hydrocephalus, demyelination
- Degenerative: Parkinson's disease (PD), multiple sclerosis (MS), Alzheimer's disease, Huntingdon's disease, motor neurone disease (MND)

The right cerebral hemisphere (more commonly non-dominant) is important for many cognitive functions which underpin language:

- Visuo-spatial processing and perception
- Integration of incoming stimuli
- Understanding and producing facial expression and intonation
- Attention and selective attention to a task

(Love and Webb, 2001)

Language is believed to rely on a complex interplay of many different brain areas rather than isolated, defined

Table 12.1 Components of speech.

Component	Description
Conceptualisation	• Formulating ideas • Desire/intention to communicate Relies on sensory and motor integration. Requires alertness and attention, cannot be attributed to a localised area, but to the brain as a whole.
Linguistic planning (language processing mechanism)	• Higher function combining linguistic and cognitive skills • Expression of thoughts, feelings and emotions Cerebral cortex organises and activates the language system to form a verbal message. The process requires knowledge of word meaning (semantics), development of phonological representation, e.g. forming the word 'bath' by the ordering of speech sounds: 'b', 'ah', 'th', and ability to place words together in a sequence according to grammatical rules of language (syntax).
Motor planning or programming	• Programmes speech articulation movements • Production of fluent, intelligible speech Pre-motor area of the inferior frontal gyrus (Broca's area) and sensory cortex.
Performance	The four components of performance require the integration and coordination of respiratory and voice systems: • Respiration: air passes through the vocal cords of the larynx, causing them to vibrate • Phonation: production of sound on exhalation • Articulation: muscles involved in articulation are stimulated by both the direct and indirect activation pathways and lower motor neurones. An interruption to any of these pathways will cause an alteration in speech processes • Resonance: the sound is changed as it passes through the oral and/or nasal cavities
Feedback	• Sounds must be heard, understood and interpreted by the listener in order to generate a response; communication is a two way process, involving both the speaker and the listener Speech production is modified according to sounds relayed back via the acoustic nerve. This concept is important in language rehabilitation since the conversation partner can play an active treatment role in therapy.

Adapted from Duffy, 1995.

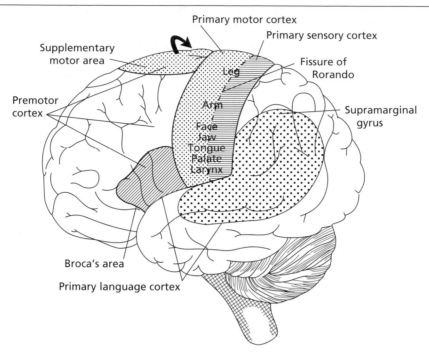

Figure 12.1 The major cortical components of the direct and indirect activation pathways and the motor speech programmer. This figure was published in *Motor Speech Disorders* by Joseph R. Duffy, p42, Copyright Elsevier (1995). Reprinted with permission.

areas. Our knowledge and understanding of aphasia is continuing to evolve as imaging techniques improve (Basso, 2003).

THE ASSESSMENT AND INTERPRETATION OF COMMUNICATION

One of the principal roles and responsibilities of the speech and language therapist (SLT) is to assess and diagnose the following impairments of communication:

- Language – APHASIA
- Motor speech programming – DYSPRAXIA
- Motor production – DYSARTHRIA
- Cognitive communication disorder
- Altered voice quality – DYSPHONIA

Following diagnosis the SLT will prescribe an individually tailored treatment plan consisting of a combination of strategies and exercises.

Aphasia

Aphasia is a communication disorder most commonly caused by a lesion in the dominant hemisphere, i.e. the left

in the majority of cases. The location and extent of neurological damage will determine both the type and the severity of the aphasia. Assessment models of language processing have changed in recent years in response to evidence gained from research. The classic nineteenth century localisationist models of aphasia, e.g. Broca's aphasia and Wernicke's aphasia, were based on limited research studies and purported to have discovered that specific areas of the brain were responsible for particular language functions. Damage to these areas could therefore produce selective communication disorders (Basso, 2003). Although these models may still be encountered there is some controversy as to their validity. Today the most commonly used approach employs a combination of cognitive neuropsychological and functional assessment to establish levels of language processing, and to identify acquired speech and language problems through closely monitoring the contextual use of language and social interaction (Laine and Martin, 2006).

The term *aphasia* is commonly used to describe a complete inability to use language, and the term *dysphasia* refers to less severe language impairment. Language is far too complex to categorise in this way and, in practice, these terms are used interchangeably. Even minimal language impairment can cause major disruption to the life of an individual, destroying the pleasure of reading or conversation; it may also cause an increase in feelings of social isolation. It is easy to falsely perceive that a person with aphasia understands more than they actually do, for example when a non-verbal social response such as smiling or nodding appears appropriate.

A broad definition of aphasia is that there is difficulty across all communication modalities, e.g. speech output, auditory comprehension, reading comprehension and writing, and that this has arisen as a consequence of an acquired brain injury or disease process.

We all experience occasional word-finding difficulties, but these are nothing in comparison to the profound deficit experienced by the person with aphasia. The ways in which words are retrieved or understood even in normal conversation, results from a complex interaction of *semantics* (the meaning of words or expressions), *syntax* (grammatical rules) and *pragmatics* (the way in which language is used in practice, e.g. implied or intended meaning). There are limitless combinations of these interactions where it is possible for a breakdown to occur, leading to different degrees of disability (Ward, 2006).

Word-finding problems might be demonstrated by the use of the following word choices:

- Paraphasia (a word which has a similar meaning sound)
- Neologism (a word that does not resemble a known word)

In *jargon aphasia* the patient's use of numerous paraphasias renders their speech incomprehensible although it may be fluent (Basso, 2003).

Dyspraxia

Dyspraxia is the term used to describe an inability to perform purposeful, voluntary movements even though the neuromuscular systems are intact (Darley *et al.*, 1975). The speaker knows what they want to say, but is unable to co-ordinate the right sequence of muscle movements to produce the right sounds. The person with verbal dyspraxia may be able to produce automatic speech or gesture, such as to say hello and smile, but would be unable to repeat this sequence when asked. Dyspraxia often occurs concurrently with dysarthria and dysphasia, but is managed quite differently.

Dysarthria

Dysarthria is a collective name for motor speech disorders affecting the neuromuscular execution of speech (Duffy,

1995). It refers to oral communication difficulties, particularly slurred speech, due to paralysis, weakness or incoordination of speech musculature (Darley *et al.*, 1975).

Damage to the nerve supply to any of the following muscle groups and structures may cause dysarthria:

- Abdominal muscles and diaphragm
- Intercostal muscles
- Laryngeal structures
- Tongue and pharyngeal muscles
- Facial muscles
- Muscles involved in jaw movement

A person with dysarthria alone is able to understand what is said to them, and to read and write without difficulty; language and cognition are not affected.

Dysphonia

Dysphonia is a disorder of voice production resulting in hoarseness or a breathy voice or other voice qualities, e.g. creak, aphonia. This disorder may be difficult to classify, with a mixed picture of symptoms, either physical, psychological or functional (vocal strain) (Syder, 1992). Physical symptoms may be due to unilateral or bilateral vocal cord paralysis, e.g. following a medullary infarct, nerve palsy or neoplastic disease (Lindsay and Bone, 2004).

It should be noted that people affected by neurogenic disorders of speech and language may also suffer from acute dysfunctions of numeracy (*dyscalculia),* reading *(dyslexia)* or writing (*dysgraphia*).

ASSESSMENT OF COMMUNICATION

Nursing assessment of communication

Communication needs are an important component of nursing assessment. Assessment should be carried out in a quiet and non-distracting environment. The nurse should position themselves with sensitivity to the person's disability, e.g. sitting to the unaffected side of someone with a hemiplegia or hemianopia, and at the same eye level. Visual material should also be presented to the unaffected side, ensuring that, if a person needs glasses or a hearing aid, these are in place. It may be necessary to obtain a history from relatives or friends if the patient has a severe communication difficulty, although the patient should be included in exchanges. Eye contact, tone of voice and touch are important measures to ensure that communication links are maintained with the patient. Relevant background information is also required (Box 12.2).

Patients with altered speech should be referred as quickly as possible to a SLT for assessment and provision

Box 12.2   Examples of assessment criteria

- Diagnosis and past medical history
- Handedness
- Medications which may have an indirect effect on speech quality
- Case history:
  a. Presenting communication difficulties and symptoms identified
  b. Patient's first language and pre-morbid language skills, literacy, education, culture
  c. How does the problem affect daily life?
  d. Employment: language skills required – letter writing, numeracy, answering the telephone
  e. With whom does the person interact on a daily basis?
  f. Communication history: work, hobbies, friends, type of personality
- Information from carers: any difficulties or changes encountered, levels of family support, living arrangements
- Informal observation: interaction with family and friends/staff, strategies used

of communication strategies and aids if necessary. The provision of accurate background information will ensure that appropriate patients are seen as quickly as possible.

Nursing assessment of understanding and expressive ability

Comprehension may be assessed by asking the patient simple questions such as their name and address. A conversational tone is more natural and provokes less anxiety than direct questioning. In this way it is also possible to assess levels of attention, concentration and memory which are important foundations for language reception (see Chapter 9). Expressive ability may be assessed using both speech and writing, e.g. naming an object or reading aloud. The ability to form a sentence can be ascertained by asking an open question or by asking the person to describe a picture. It is important to establish if there is a history of memory loss which may cause word–finding difficulties. Refer the patient to occupational therapy for cognitive assessment and treatment if any deficit is known or suspected.

SLT assessment of communication

Formal assessment of communication by a highly skilled SLT is essential to determine the ongoing management and

therapy for each individual patient. Treatment strategies are prescribed and adapted to take into account the patient's level of insight, motivation and their desire or ability to change and co-operate in therapy. For example, fatigue may compromise tolerance and necessitate shorter treatment sessions. The complex and diverse nature of communication deficits means that performing a formal assessment which isolates language ability from cues or from a cognitive communication disorder is often necessary. Standardised assessment and diagnostic tools may also be used by SLTs to determine an objective baseline which can then be repeated after therapy to identify and measure improvement.

NURSING MANAGEMENT OF ALTERED COMMUNICATION

Communication skills are a fundamental nursing requirement, but in patients with altered speech and language good communication may actively assist recovery (Hemsley *et al.*, 2001). The ability and readiness to listen, interpret and understand as well as to explain and inform in a way which is comprehensible, is central to quality of care (Sundin and Jansson, 2003). Nurses play an important role in the lives of patients with communication disorders since they are usually the first point of contact and have responsibility for the following:

- Rapid identification of altered speech and immediate referral to a SLT
- Informing the SLT of changes in the patient's communication
- Exercising empathy to establish communication by the best available method, seeking advice from the SLT
- Protection of the patient's interests and dignity
- Recognition of potential psychological problems and informing clinicians
- Ensuring that the patient and their carers receive all the information they need in a format that they can understand, in partnership with the SLT (Brennan *et al.*, 2005)

Barriers faced by patients with aphasia/dysarthria/dysphonia/dyspraxia or cognitive communication disorder are much less tangible than those obstructing the person who is wheelchair dependent, but they may be equally disabling. An important aspect of the nursing management is to recognise these barriers and to realise that nurses can go a long way to ensure that barriers are removed by raising awareness of dysphasia and communication diagnoses at all levels.

Strategies to help in communicating with people with comprehension difficulties

Each patient should be assessed and treated as an individual and the following strategies are given only as a guide. Distractions should be limited to assist and improve concentration, for example: remove background noise such as television or music, draw curtains around the bedspace to prevent sudden interruptions and visual distractions. Use simple language, but do not talk down to the patient. Speak slowly and clearly and do not shout. Families and friends may be anxious to fill a silence, but they must be encouraged to slow down and give the dysphasic person time to think and reply.

The patient will be able to communicate with greater ease if they are relaxed; slowing the rate of your speech whilst maintaining intonation and rhythm will allow time for the content to be processed. Be prepared to repeat and rephrase if you are not understood. Ambiguity, humour or sarcasm may also lead to a lack of understanding and consequent distress (Syder, 1992). The person with aphasia will have good days and bad days and fatigue should be acknowledged. The use of pauses between phrases is also helpful in allowing time to absorb meaning or to have a rest. Skilled questioning is important and closed questions with one word answers should be used. Alternative communication methods, such as pen and paper for writing or drawing, props such as photos or maps may help and appropriately designed and illustrated material can be used to highlight important points.

Strategies to help in communicating with people with expressive difficulties

Aphasia alone does not diminish a person's intellect although there may be accompanying cognitive impairment (Liechty and Garber, 2004). The 'does he take sugar?' syndrome persists and health professionals should ensure that individuals are not ignored or talked over. Patients may become anxious and excluded if they are unable to draw attention, so you need to ensure that they have a means of doing so at all times. All attempts at speech should be encouraged, but patients should not be pushed too hard. Positive feedback should be given by acknowledging when you understand and encouraging the person to continue. Coping strategies should be developed, for example allowing rest breaks and protected mealtimes, maintaining visiting restrictions when the patient is fatigued.

Before any attempt at communication the nurse should ensure that the patient is wearing spectacles and/or hearing aids if required. Take time to listen. Try not to interrupt or finish sentences and encourage family members to do the same. People who seem socially appropriate, who nod and smile in the right places, may lead the nurse to believe that what they are saying is appropriate and that they can understand and carry out anything you ask them to. But this may not be the case. Try different ways to communicate and encourage relatives and friends to do the same: use diagrams, drawings and photographs; use a communication board if prescribed by a SLT. Always confirm and check understanding and don't make assumptions; confirm by using 'yes' or 'no'. Eye contact should be maintained and the nurse should watch for non-verbal cues and body language; add animation or gestures to get the message across. Prompts should be offered; assess what the person is trying to say and help them by giving them the first sound of the word or by putting the word into a sentence, e.g. 'It's a c...' 'You drink from a c ...'

Above all the nurse should recognise that every attempt at communication is a huge leap of faith on the part of the patient. It is important to provide encouragement and to celebrate success no matter how small. Do not pretend to understand if the meaning of what the patient is saying is unclear. When the pretence is inevitably discovered it will leave the dysphasic person feeling more vulnerable than ever since trust has been destroyed. If things are proving too difficult, take a break and make an agreement to return in a few minutes. No-one is perfect and sometimes enrolling another person with fresh ideas can make a difference.

Nursing contribution to therapy

Language/speech exercises should be continued on the ward and family members encouraged to complete exercises with the patient. Ensure that others are aware of the best strategies for communication and inform the SLT of any deterioration or alteration in ability which may require reassessment.

Communication difficulties can be tiring and stressful for everyone involved since it is both difficult to understand and to be understood. Even experienced nurses may have difficulty communicating with patients with severe speech disorders (Hemsley *et al.*, 2001). A current government strategy (DH, 2004a) emphasises training in communication skills, but until this becomes widely available nurses should develop a close working relationship with SLTs whose expertise is a valuable resource for the development of nurses' skills and knowledge. Some charitable organisations (Connect (www.ukconnect.org) and Speakability (www.speakability.org.uk)) provide training and resources for both health care professionals, and individuals with aphasia and their carers.

MEDICAL MANAGEMENT RELATED TO ALTERED COMMUNICATION

Recognition and treatment of depression

Patients with aphasia may be at risk of developing depression, but the data are incomplete due to the difficulty in screening patients with communication impairment (Dennis *et al.*, 2000). Standard methods of assessment for depression require written and verbal communication skills; it is also difficult to carry out psychiatric assessment since patients may have difficulty in expressing emotions and feelings (Sutcliffe and Lincoln, 1998). If signs of depression or altered mood are suspected it is important to take this into account so that the patient may be treated rapidly. A depression screening tool has been developed and validated – the Stroke Aphasic Depression Questionnaire (SADQ), (Bennett *et al.*, 2006) to facilitate the identification of depression in stroke patients with aphasia. Other visual analogue scales (Visual Analogue Self-Esteem Scale- Brumfitt and Sheeran, 1999, and the Visual Analogue Mood Scales- Stern, 1997) may be useful in identifying patients at risk of emotional dysfunction, but their use in severe communication impairment is cautioned (Vickery, 2006).

OVERVIEW OF ALTERED SWALLOWING (DYSPHAGIA)

Eating and drinking are at the core of human existence. Not only do they support life through the intake of nutrients, they offer pleasure, structure cultures and provide opportunities for social relationships. Imagine then that the ability to eat and drink is taken away. The consequences of dysphagia can be devastating both psychologically and physically, with sensory deprivation, social embarrassment, aspiration pneumonia, choking and even death possible. People with dysphagia can become frightened at mealtimes and avoid eating with others leading to feelings of isolation, loss of self esteem and relationship breakdown (Ekberg *et al.*, 2002).

Dysphagia is usually defined as an abnormal transfer of a bolus from mouth to stomach (Groher, 1997). An alternative definition expands its meaning to incorporate all the sensory, motor and behavioural acts in preliminary swallow preparation (Box 12.3). Prevalence in the general population over 50 years of age has been estimated at 22% (Lindgren and Janzon, 1991).

Unmanaged, dysphagia may lead to the development of complications such as malnutrition, dehydration, aspiration pneumonia, disability and death, (Ekberg *et al.*, 2002; Marik and Kaplan, 2003). It may also lead to an increased length of stay in hospital (Low *et al.*, 2001) and to patients

---

Box 12.3 Sensory and cognitive functions affecting preliminary swallow preparation

- Vision
- Smell
- Appetite
- Mood: depression may lead to a reduction in a desire to eat
- Cognition: reduced awareness and recognition or memory of food
- Coordination: Dyspraxia (breakdown in planning and executing voluntary movement), e.g. transferring food from plate to mouth during eating. Motor sequence may be further compromised by presence of weakness or paralysis
- Spatial awareness: visual field and perceptual deficits may mean that a person does not see food on one half of the plate or lacks the spatial awareness to accurately move it from the plate to their mouth.

Adapted from Leopold and Kagel, 1996.

---

being newly institutionalised at discharge (Groher, 1997). Patients with dysphagia are also at risk of skin breakdown, fatigue and muscle weakness (Elmstahl *et al.*, 1999), poor nutrition and weight loss (Wright *et al.*, 2005).

Physiology of normal swallowing

The swallowing centre is believed to be located in the reticular formation of the medulla oblongata and involves several of the brain stem cranial nerve nuclei: olfactory, trigeminal, facial, glossopharyngeal, vagus, accessory and hypoglossal. The sensory recognition centre is contained within the lower brain stem, in the nucleus solitarius. Incoming sensory information is decoded and sent to the nucleus ambiguous in the medulla, which then initiates the pharyngeal motor movement via the IX cranial nerve (Figure 12.2) (Ertekin and Aydogdu, 2003). It is known that there is bilateral cortical involvement in the swallowing process (Hamdy and Rothwell, 1998). The cerebral cortex is important for recognition of food and liquid and placing the bolus in the mouth prior to initiation of the oral phase.

Swallowing is a highly complex function requiring the sensory and motor integration of at least 26 sets of muscles. It consists of voluntary and involuntary movements and is carried out approximately a thousand times a day to swallow saliva. Figure 12.3 shows the main anatomical structures involved in swallowing. Once food is placed in

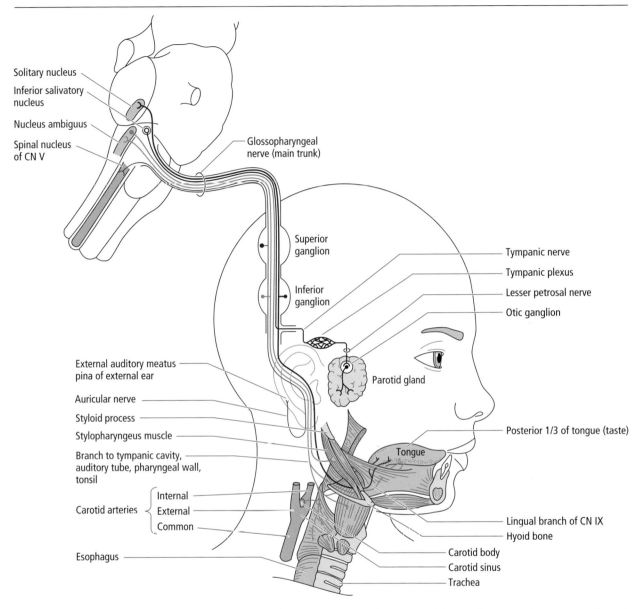

Figure 12.2 The origin and distribution of the glossopharyngeal nerve and its major branches. Reproduced from Maria A Patestas and Leslie P Gartner, *A Textbook of Neuroanatomy*, Wiley-Blackwell, with permission.

the mouth, the initiation of swallowing begins. Swallowing is classically described in four phases:

- Oral preparatory phase
- Oral phase
- Pharyngeal phase
- Oesophageal phase

(Logemann, 1998, see Table 12.2).

AETIOLOGY OF NEUROGENIC DYSPHAGIA

The most common causes of neurogenic dysphagia are shown in Box 12.4. These may broadly be divided into two sub-groups:

- Acute, from which it is hoped the patient will recover, at least partially

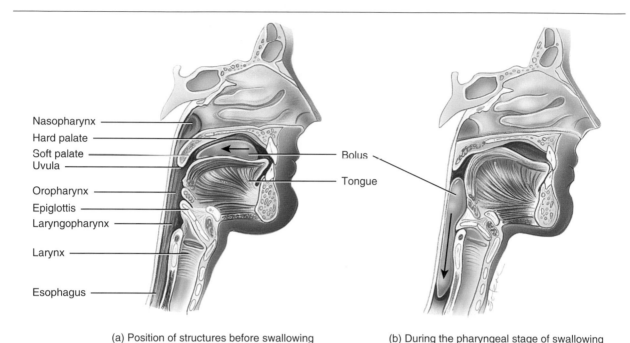

(a) Position of structures before swallowing (b) During the pharyngeal stage of swallowing

Figure 12.3 Deglutition (swallowing). During the pharyngeal stage of deglutition (b) the tongue rises against the palate, the nasopharynx is closed off, the larynx rises, the epiglottis seals off the larynx, and the bolus is passed into the oesophagus. Reproduced from *Principles of Anatomy and Physiology 12e* by Gerard Tortora and Bryan Derrickson. Copyright (2009, John Wiley & Sons). Reprinted with permission of John Wiley & Sons Inc.

• Degenerative, in which swallowing will gradually deteriorate

ASSESSMENT OF DYSPHAGIA

Nurses have a responsibility to ensure that patients' nutritional needs are met (Perry, 2001a) and to protect patients from harm. It is critical that neuroscience nurses are aware of the signs and symptoms of dysphagia (Box 12.5) so that patients at risk may be identified. A detailed history and assessment should be undertaken to detect these signs and symptoms. Swallow should be assessed as early as possible if dysphagia is likely, using a simple, validated bedside screening protocol, and certainly within 24 hours of stroke (Royal College of Physicians, 2008). Between 20 and 40% of healthy, normal swallowing adults do *not* have a gag reflex (Davies *et al.*, 1995). The gag reflex has been shown to be an unreliable indicator of swallowing

function (Leder, 1996) and should not be used to assess swallowing.

Nurse dysphagia screening

The primary consideration is the assessment of aspiration risk and the suitability of the patient for oral feeding. Swallow screening should only be carried out by nurses who have been trained and deemed competent in a dysphagia screening protocol, following structured education in their local health care areas in close partnership with SLTs (Davison and Giles, 1996; Herbert, 1996; Perry, 2001b). An example of a nurse dysphagia screening protocol is shown in Figure 12.4.

Within the United Kingdom no one specific screening protocol is used although the expansion of nurses' knowledge and skills dovetails with the requirements of the Knowledge and Skills Framework (DH, 2004b). Ten

Table 12.2 Phases of swallowing

Phase	Innervation	Activity
Oral preparatory phase (voluntary control) Airway is open as the larynx and pharynx are relaxed, nasal breathing takes place as the mouth is closed to prevent spillage	VII	Bolus containment – labial (lip) seal and cheek tension
	XII	Food is softened by the action of the tongue combined with saliva
	V, VII, XII	Chewing (mastication) breaks down solid food to form a cohesive ball (bolus). Duration depends on size and consistency of the bolus, dentition, oral motor efficiency and enjoyment of savouring the taste (Love and Webb, 2001)
Oral phase (voluntary control)	V, VII, XII	The tongue begins the posterior transition of the bolus. Thicker foods require more pressure to propel them efficiently through the oral cavity. The oral phase should take 1 to 1.5 seconds
Pharyngeal phase (involuntary control)		Backward movement of bolus stimulates sensory receptors in oropharynx transmitting sensory information to the cortex and brain stem (Jean, 2001) triggering the swallow. A number of movements (below) occur simultaneously. If not triggered at this point, the trigger is described as delayed which is an important indicator of aspiration risk (Smith *et al.*, 1999).
	X	1. Elevation of velum (soft palate) to prevent material entering nasal cavity
	V	2. Tense anterior velum and open auditory tube
	XII	3. Elevation and anterior movement of hyoid and larynx
	X	4. Respiration ceases and airway is protected through closure of larynx at three sphincters: true and false vocal cords and epiglottis
	X	5. Relaxation of the cricopharyngeal (or upper oesophageal) sphincter allows passage of material into oesophagus
	XII	6. Base of tongue becomes ramped in shape, enabling food to be directed into pharynx
	IX, X, XII	7. Tongue and contraction of pharyngeal walls propel bolus downwards
		Duration: approximately 1 second
Oesophageal phase (involuntary)	X	Bolus is propelled by peristalsis through the oesophagus into the stomach
		Normal transit time is 8 to 20 seconds

Adapted from Logemann, 1998.

years ago the Collaborative Dysphagia Audit Study (CODA, 1997) recognised that nurse screening for dysphagia had many advantages:

- A reduction in the numbers of patients who were kept nil-by-mouth unnecessarily
- A reduction in the number of patients who had either inappropriate or no feeding restrictions when they were at risk of aspiration

- A noticeable improvement in the quality of referral to a SLT

Sensitivity and reliability of bedside tests have been found to be variable (Ramsey *et al.*, 2003) and dependent on the experience of the assessor.

The screening process

Before proceeding with the screening process it is essential to ascertain that the patient is able to maintain a sufficient

---

Box 12.4   Causes of neurogenic dysphagia

- Disorders of the cerebral hemispheres and brain stem, e.g. stroke, traumatic brain injury, neoplasm, congenital defects
- Demyelinating diseases, e.g. multiple sclerosis (MS)
- Cerebellar and extrapyramidal disorders: disorders of movement, e.g. Parkinson's disease, Huntingdon's disease
- Dementia, e.g. Alzheimer's disease
- Motor abnormalities, e.g. amyotrophic lateral sclerosis (ALS), motor neurone disease (MND), Guillain–Barré syndrome
- Muscular dystrophies and other myopathies, e.g. inflammatory myopathies (polymyositis, dermatomyositis)
- Connective tissue disease, e.g. scleroderma, Sjögren's syndrome

---

Box 12.5   Signs and symptoms of dysphagia

- Inability to recognise food, difficulty in placing food in mouth
- Incomplete mouth emptying, pocketing of food between teeth and gums
- Taking inappropriately sized bites
- Delayed swallowing trigger, difficulty in chewing
- Avoiding certain consistencies of food
- Chest or throat discomfort, food feels as if it is 'stuck'
- Prolonged mealtimes
- Regurgitation, either nasal or oral
- Coughing or choking, throat clearing during eating or drinking
- Weight loss for no other reason
- History of chronic chest infection, spiking pyrexia
- Unexplained sudden change in diet or avoidance of mealtimes
- Drooling, loss of lip seal
- Difficulty managing secretions, wet or gurgly voice

---

level of alertness and an upright position; they must also be able to co-operate.

Following an explanation of the procedure and obtaining verbal consent the patient should be positioned comfortably at 90°, supported with pillows if necessary. The patient is asked to open their mouth; the oral cavity is inspected taking particular note of oral hygiene, dentition and secretion management. Basic oro-motor function is assessed by looking for adequate lip seal and movement of the tongue. The patient is asked to cough to ensure their ability to protect the airway. If the cough is weak or if there is any existing respiratory compromise, or suspicion of respiratory distress, the screen should be stopped at this stage and the patient kept nil-by-mouth since they are at risk of aspiration. Urgent assessment by a SLT is then indicated.

Patients deemed as safe for assessment are first tested with sips of water and monitored for signs of respiratory distress or coughing, gurgly or wet voice and laryngeal movement. Patients with no obvious difficulties are then offered larger quantities of water and continuously monitored; the screen may then proceed to trials with yoghurt and then soft or normal texture food if there are no signs of dysphagia. Patients without problems may be given a normal diet but their intake and vital signs should be monitored for the first 48 hours for signs of silent aspiration. (Box 12.6).

Assessment of respiratory function is also required. The patient should be monitored for shortness of breath and difficulty co-ordinating breathing and swallowing.

Although pulse oximetry is a useful adjunct to swallowing assessment (Smith *et al.*, 2000; Westergren, 2006) it cannot be relied upon to detect silent aspiration, therefore the utmost caution should be exercised and the assessment terminated if silent aspiration is suspected. Patients considered to be at risk of dysphagia should immediately be referred to a SLT for urgent detailed assessment and management.

Dysphagia assessment by the SLT

Formal clinical assessment of swallowing takes place by the SLT (Box 12.7).

Physical examination

Assessment by the SLT begins with an examination of the oral structures (lips, hard and soft palate, tongue, uvula, faucal arches, sulci) and inspection of the oral cavity for scarring, lesions, asymmetry and fasciculations (fine, involuntary muscle contractions). Dentition and ability to manage oral secretions is assessed. Oro-motor examination is then conducted to identify any deficit in cranial nerve function by evaluating the strength, range, rate and accuracy of movement of the lips, tongue, jaw, palate and the efficiency of airway closure. Sensory oral awareness can be ascertained by testing taste, texture and temperature (sweet, sour, bitter, hot, cold) to identify optimum sensation and the patient's reaction.

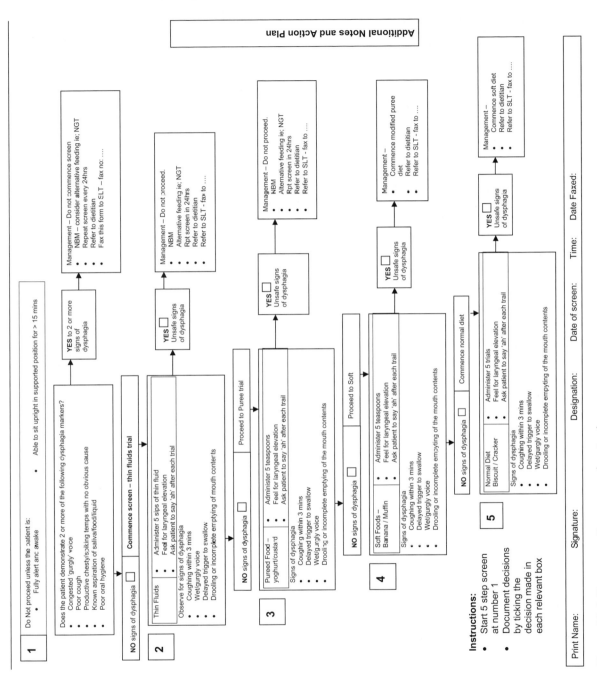

Figure 12.4 Nurse swallow screening tool.

Box 12.6   Signs of silent aspiration

- Pyrexia
- Tachycardia
- Altered breathing: increase in respiratory rate, audible breath sounds, reduced air entry
- Abnormal chest x-ray
- Raised white cell count

Box 12.7   Speech and language therapist (SLT) dysphagia assessment considerations

- Presenting condition
- Pre-morbid oral intake
- Vital signs (blood pressure, pulse, respirations, oxygen saturation level, temperature)
- Consciousness level
- Nutritional status – are nil by mouth restrictions in place?
- Current chest status
- Current and past medical history
- Medication – some medications affect saliva production or alter alertness
- Insight and vigilance
- Cognition
- Posture
- Positioning

Abnormal oral reflexes may be seen in patients with neurological impairments, e.g. tongue thrusting or a tonic bite reflex, which hinders the normal swallow (Logemann, 1998). It is important to identify the location in the mouth where these are triggered and the nature of the stimulus which triggers them so that techniques may be employed either to avoid eliciting or to desensitise the reflex (Logemann, (1998). To avoid injury (to both the patient and the clinician) where an abnormal bite reflex is present food should be placed in the mouth using a spoon which will not break easily.

Further assessment – food/fluid challenge

A SLT assesses the patient's swallow function using different textures of liquid and food depending on information gathered during initial oro-motor assessment. During this time, the oral and pharyngeal phases of the swallow are observed (Table 12.3).

Dysphagia investigations

In 40% of cases clinical bedside assessment alone does not detect aspiration (Logemann, 1998). Therefore objective assessments are often required (see Table 12.4).

NURSING MANAGEMENT OF DYSPHAGIA

Nurses play an important part in ensuring that all dysphagic patients are identified rapidly and receive the best possible care. Prime areas of responsibility are detailed in Box 12.8. The management of dysphagia is crucially important particularly because of the potential for life-threatening airway obstruction and aspiration pneumonia (Perry and Love, 2001). Following assessment and discussion with the patient and/or carer, the SLT will recommend safe swallowing strategies if oral feeding is appropriate, and alternative methods of providing nutritional intake if not. Cognitive or behavioural problems make concordance with strategies or advice difficult; this will be taken into account when recommendations are made.

Written guidelines are placed at the patient's bedside and discussed with the nurse responsible for coordinating the patient's care. Documentation should be clear and available to all staff, the patient and their family. Nurses are ideally placed to monitor the patient throughout the day, supplying information, education and assistance to patients and their families in the use of compensatory techniques (Travers, 1999). They also have an important role in the rehabilitation process by encouraging and reinforcing exercise regimes (Perry, 2001a).

The two main components for the effective management of dysphagia are:

- The prevention of aspiration
- The maintenance of sufficient nutritional intake

Prior to oral feeding, it must be determined whether the person is sufficiently alert and well enough to attempt to swallow. If these criteria are not met, any attempts to eat or drink may put the individual at risk of aspiration (Ramsey and Smithard, 2005). Nurses are often the first to observe dysphagia since they supervise patients when they are eating (Travers, 1999). Nurses must therefore be aware of the signs and symptoms of dysphagia and aspiration in order to initiate prompt interventions and avert critical complications (see Boxes 12.5 and 12.6).

Aspiration

Aspiration occurs when there is a malfunction in the mechanisms of airway protection during swallowing (Ramsey and Smithard, 2005). As the patient inhales after swallow-

Table 12.3 Speech and language therapist (SLT) observations during swallowing

Phase	Observations
Oral	Adequacy of lip seal, nasal breathing, spillage and drooling of material, speed and efficiency of chewing, whether any food residue is left in the mouth
Pharyngeal	Palpation of the larynx: the extent of laryngeal elevation is assessed using light touch (no pressure). The index finger is placed under the chin to feel movement of the tongue base, the middle finger on the hyoid bone, third finger at the top and the fourth at the bottom of the thyroid cartilage. • Timing of swallow trigger is judged from when chewing ceases and hyoid and laryngeal movement begins. The number of swallows taken for each bolus is noted; depending on consistency multiple swallows may be an indication of weak pharyngeal contraction • Laryngeal penetration is indicated by coughing during the swallow or up to three minutes afterwards, or a wet or gurgly voice

Table 12.4 Dysphagia investigations

Investigation	Description of procedure
Videofluoroscopy	The patient sits at 45–90° and is asked to swallow a variety of food/fluid consistencies containing a contrast agent. Imaging of the swallowing process is observed and video recorded in real time. Used to detect silent aspiration, diagnose the nature of the problem and assess different compensatory techniques. Not suitable for repeated use due to radiation exposure.
Fibreoptic endoscopic evaluation of swallowing (FEES)	A flexible endoscope is inserted into the nose to observe the process of swallowing from the soft palate. Food and/or drink contains a dye to distinguish it from oral secretions. Assesses secretion management and airway closure, and evaluates the use of swallowing strategies such as the supra-glottic swallow. No radiation exposure and portable. Good for physically immobile or very frail patients, but may not be well tolerated.

ing, material retained in the laryngeal vestibule, valleculae or piriform spaces is sucked into the trachea. Normally when this occurs, a protective cough prevents aspiration, but in dysphagia this protective reflex can be weak or absent. Liquid or food entering the airway may result in infection (Galvan, 2001). Aspiration may also occur before swallowing due to a delayed trigger, or during swallowing due to incomplete airway closure.

Silent aspiration

Silent aspiration cannot be detected at bedside assessment since it is by definition without cough or other indication of distress (Ramsey *et al.*, 2005). Detection depends on other objective methods of assessment such as videofluoroscopy (see Table 12.4). There is an increased incidence of silent aspiration following brain stem stroke (Teasell *et al.*, 2001) and in Parkinson's disease (Leopold and Kagel, 1997).

Swallowing strategies

Following assessment the SLT decides whether to provide therapy by working *directly* on swallowing, by introducing food into the mouth, or *indirectly* using exercises to improve neuro-motor control, or to practice swallowing saliva only. Specific techniques (Table 12.5) designed to change pharyngeal dimensions and redirect food flow by altering the patient's head or body posture can be an effective way of reducing aspiration risk (Logemann, 1998). These should always be prescribed by a SLT as incorrect use can result in increased risk to the patient.

Werner (2005) suggests simple nursing interventions which may also help to prevent complications (Box 12.9).

Oral care

Special attention should be given to the maintenance of oral hygiene since swallowing saliva from a neglected and

---

Box 12.8   Prime nursing responsibilities

- Prompt identification of patients with dysphagia and referral to a speech and language therapist (SLT)
- Ensuring that those thought to be at risk of aspiration are kept nil-by-mouth and referred urgently to a SLT
- Taking steps to ensure that patients are properly hydrated and receive nutrition within 24 hours, (particularly if it is necessary to keep the patient nil-by-mouth until a formal SLT assessment)
- Maintaining an accurate record of fluid and nutritional intake
- Maintaining oral hygiene and comfort
- Provision of information, education and emotional support
- Informing physicians and SLT if any deterioration is noted
- Supporting patients and their families in complying with SLT recommendations

---

bacteria laden mouth is a common cause of chest infections in the person suffering from dysphagia. Good oral health can also prevent aspiration pneumonia in the elderly (Marik and Kaplan, 2003). Dependence on others for oral care has been shown to predict pneumonia (Langmore *et al.*, 1998), therefore patients should be encouraged to brush their own teeth after meals if they are able. If the patient is dependent for activities of daily living, national guidelines for correct oral care procedures should be followed (BSDH, 2000).

Nutrition and feeding

Food must be of the correct consistency to minimise aspiration risk, but at the same time to meet nutritional requirements (Perry, 2001a). Food should be presented in such a way as to stimulate appetite. The dysphagic patient may be put off by the sight of a large portion of food; a smaller amount may appear more enticing. Patients should be offered food when hungry and enteral feeding should be stopped at least an hour prior to mealtimes if oral intake is commencing. If the patient is hungry and food is attractively presented and smells good, salivation will increase and improve bolus formation (Galvan, 2001).

Table 12.5 Posture and compensatory techniques

Technique	Description of technique
Chin tuck	The airway entrance is narrowed and the valleculae space is widened. Helpful for patients with a delayed swallow, provides greater airway protection
Head turn	To the damaged side to close the weaker side of the pharynx. More food flows down the normal side
Head tilt	Uses gravity to drain food down the non-affected side providing better control
Supra-glottic swallow	Hold breath while swallowing and cough after swallow to clear any residue. Closes vocal cords before and during swallow
Mendelsohn manoeuvre	Prolongs laryngeal elevation during swallow and improves swallowing coordination. The patient is told to hold the swallow for several seconds as their 'Adam's apple' rises
Effortful swallow	As the patient swallows they are told to squeeze hard with muscles of tongue and throat, this improves clearance of the bolus from the valleculae
Increased sensory stimulation	For patients with reduced food recognition during the oral stage or slowed oral transit, e.g. increased downward pressure of the spoon against the tongue, different food textures or cold temperature, strong flavours, use of thermal stimulation to trigger swallowing
Exercises designed to strengthen swallowing musculature	e.g. Masako and Shaker techniques

> **Box 12.9   Simple nursing interventions to prevent complications of dysphagia**
>
> - Avoid using straws
> - Proper positioning
> - Avoid using drinks to wash food down (unless recommended by the speech and language therapist)
> - Ensure that the environment is free of distractions; talking and laughing while eating increases risk of aspiration (Galvan, 2001)
> - Protect mealtimes
> - Ensure that staff are trained in correct feeding techniques
> - Encourage self-feeding
> - Reinforce prescribed feeding strategies
>
> Adapted from Werner (2005).

Feeding a dysphagic patient is a skilled process requiring awareness of the potential dangers for the patient and knowledge of correct feeding methods. It must not be rushed; patients should be allowed sufficient time to allow them to eat in an unhurried manner, and food should be offered in a manageable form and consistency. The management strategy of dysphagia will usually consist of a combination of dietary texture modification in conjunction with compensatory postures or manoeuvres (see Table 12.5).

For further information refer to the national guidelines on texture modification and fluid thickness which have been agreed between dietitians and SLTs (BDA and RCSLT, 2002). The person feeding should monitor for signs of fatigue and deteriorating swallowing, ensuring good mouth clearance by checking cheeks for pocketing of food residue. Patients' weight and nutritional status should be monitored and the SLT and dietician informed of any deterioration or concerns, it may be necessary to instigate an alternative feeding strategy.

Artificial nutritional support

Enteral feeding may be required to minimise malnutrition and discomfort for the patient. The decision to begin artificial feeding should be based on several factors. Informed consent should be obtained, where possible. Prognosis should also be considered in weighing up the benefits versus risks, i.e. is the patient likely to recover swallowing function and if so how quickly.

The dietician will advise on the choice of feed and devise an appropriate feeding regimen tailored to individual need. Partial oral feeding may be continued alongside enteral feeding. A decision must then be made as to the choice of feeding tube to be used. Fine-bore nasogastric tubes are better tolerated and more comfortable, allowing for potential recovery of swallowing since a more flexible tube is less obstructive when the patient makes attempts to swallow (Negus, 1994).

Patients who cannot tolerate a naso-gastric tube or who suffer from prolonged, severe dysphagia may be considered for insertion of a percutaneous endoscopic gastrostomy tube (PEG). A PEG may achieve superior feed delivery and be preferred by patients and staff, but the procedure is invasive and is associated with an increase in morbidity and mortality (Perry, 2001b). Patients with permanent dysphagia may require a long term PEG. This may be a considerable psychological burden both for the patient and family, and has a profound impact on quality of life (Rickman, 1998) including:

- Loss of enjoyment of food and drink
- Problems encountered with administration and storage of feed
- Changes in lifestyle, relationships and body image
- Impact on sexuality

It is vital for the patient and their family to receive education and information about the administration of feeding and long term care of a gastrostomy prior to discharge to the community. They should also be linked in to the appropriate agencies for long term follow-up and support. Further detail of enteral feeding and nursing management is presented in Chapter 16.

Impact of dysphagia on drug administration

When dysphagic patients are unable to swallow tablets whole it is necessary to liaise with the pharmacist to seek liquid rather than solid preparations. Chewing or sucking tablets may lead to alterations in the pharmokinetics of the drug, or lead to additional side-effects (Morris, 2005). Medication may be given through either a naso-gastric or gastrostomy tube, but it is imperative to seek the correct drug formulation; crushing oral tablets or opening capsules can alter the way in which medication is absorbed and may cause tube erosion and occlusion (Morris, 2006). Crushing and mixing tablets with food or drink without the patient's consent may be construed as covert administration of medication and is to be avoided.

SUMMARY

Communication and swallowing disorders may result from many diverse neurological conditions, either acute or chronic and may cause life threatening complications or devastating psychological effects. Neuroscience nurses have a pivotal role in ensuring the best outcomes for patients and families affected by these problems, which may range from the prompt identification of the risk of aspiration to the sympathetic understanding of the frustrations felt by the person who cannot speak, and finding ways to establish a reliable method of communication. Nurses should be aware that this cannot be achieved in isolation and an important factor in achieving positive outcomes is the development of a close working partnership with the SLT.

REFERENCES

Basso A (2003) *Aphasia and Its Therapy*. Oxford: Oxford University Press.

Bennett HE, Thomas SA, Austen R *et al.* (2006) Validation of screening measures for assessing mood in stroke patients. *British Journal of Clinical Psychology* 45:367–376.

Brennan A, Worrall L, McKenna K (2005) The relationship between specific features of aphasia-friendly written material and comprehension of written material for people with aphasia: An exploratory study. *Aphasiology* 19(8):693–711.

British Brain and Spine Foundation (1998) *Speech, Language and Communication Difficulties: A guide for patients and carers*. London: BBSF.

British Dietetic Association and the Royal College of Speech and Language Therapists joint document. (2002) *National descriptors for texture modification in adults*. Available from: http://www.slodrinks.com/images/National%20 Descriptors.pdf. Accessed June 2010.

British Society for Disability and Oral Health (2000) *Guidelines for the development of local standards of oral health care for dependent, dysphagic, critically and terminally ill patients*. Available from: www.bsdh.org.uk/ guidelines/depend.pdf. Accessed June 2010.

Brodal P (2004) *The Central Nervous System: Structure and function*. (3rd edition). Oxford: Oxford University Press.

Brumfitt S, Sheeran P (1999) *Visual Analogue Self-esteem Scale (VASES)*. UK, Winslow Press Ltd.

CODA Collaborators (1997) Guidelines for screening and management of stroke patients with dysphagia. Collaborative Dysphagia Audit Study. Cited by Davies S. (2002) An interdisciplinary approach to the management of dysphagia. *Professional Nurse* 18(1):22–25.

Darley FL, Aronson AE, Brown JR (1975) *Motor Speech Disorders*. Philadelphia: WB Saunders.

Davies AE, Kidd D, Stone SP *et al.* (1995) Pharyngeal sensation and gag reflex in healthy subjects. *Lancet* 345(8948):487–488.

Davison A, Giles J (1996) SLT and nursing: partners in dysphagia. *Royal College of Speech and Language Therapist's Bulletin* December: 10–11.

Demonet JF, Thierry G, Cardebat D (2005) Renewal of the neurophysiology of language: Functional neuroimaging. *Physiology Reviews* 85:49–95.

Dennis M, O'Rourke S, Lewis S *et al.* (2000) Emotional outcomes after stroke: factors associated with poor outcome. *Journal of Neurology, Neurosurgery Psychiatry* 68:47–52

Department of Health (2004a) *Better Information, Better Choices, Better Health*. London: The Stationery Office.

Department of Health (2004b) *The NHS Knowledge and Skills Framework and the Development Review Process*. London: The Stationery Office.

Duffy JR (1995) *Motor Speech Disorders: substrates, differential diagnosis, and management*. USA: Mosby.

Ekberg O, Hamdy S, Woisard V *et al.* (2002) Social and psychological burden of dysphagia: its impact on diagnosis and treatment. *Dysphagia* 17:139–146.

Elmstahl S, Bulow M, Ekberg O *et al.* (1999) Treatment of dysphagia improves nutritional conditions in stroke patients. *Dysphagia* 14:61–66.

Ertekin C, Aydogdu I (2003) Neurophysiology of swallowing. *Clinical Neurophysiology* 114:2226–2244.

Galvan TJ (2001) Dysphagia: Going down and staying down. *American Journal of Nursing* 101(1):37–42.

Groher ME (1997) *Dysphagia: Diagnosis and management*. (3rd edition). Newton, USA, Butterworth-Heinemann.

Hamdy S, Rothwell JC (1998) Gut feelings about recovery after stroke: the organisation and reorganisation of human swallowing motor cortex. *Trends in Neuroscience* 21(7):278–282.

Hemsley B, Sigafoos J, Forbes R *et al.* (2001) Nursing the patient with severe communication impairment. *Journal of Advanced Nursing* 35(6):827–835.

Herbert S (1996) A team approach to the treatment of dysphagia. *Nursing Times* 92(50):26–29.

Jean A (2001) Brain stem control of swallowing: neuronal network and cellular mechanisms. *Physiological Reviews* 81(2) 929–969.

Laine M, Martin N (2006) *Anomia: theoretical and clinical aspects*. Hove: Psychology Press.

Langmore SE, Terpenning MS, Schork A *et al.* (1998) Predictors of aspiration pneumonia: How important is dysphagia? *Dysphagia* 13:69–81.

Leder SB (1996) Gag reflex and dysphagia. *Head and Neck* 18:138–141.

Leopold NA, Kagel MA (1996) Prepharyngeal dysphagia in Parkinson's disease. *Dysphagia* 11:14–22.

Leopold, NA, Kagel MA (1997) Pharyngo-oesophageal dysphagia in Parkinson's disease. *Dysphagia* 12(1):11–18.

Liechty JA, Buchholz J (2006) The sounds of silence – relating to people with aphasia. *Journal of Psychosocial Nursing* 44(8):53–55.

Liechty JA, Garber DW (2004) Dealing with aphasia: Three simple rules. *Rehabilitation Nursing* 29(1):3–4.

Lindgren S, Janzon L (1991) Prevalence of swallowing complaints and clinical findings among 50–70 year old men and women in an urban population. *Dysphagia* 6:187–192.

Lindsay KW, Bone I (2004) *Neurology and Neurosurgery* (4th edition). Edinburgh: Churchill Livingstone.

Logemann J (1998) *Evaluation and Treatment of Swallowing Disorders.* (2nd edition). Austin, Texas: Pro-Ed.

Love RJ, Webb WG (2001) *Neurology for the Speech Language Pathologist.* (4th edition). Boston: Butterworth-Heinemann.

Low J, Wyles C, Wilkinson T *et al.* (2001) The effect of compliance on clinical outcomes for patients with dysphagia on videofluoroscopy. *Dysphagia* 16:123–127.

Marik PE, Kaplan D (2003) Aspiration pneumonia and dysphagia in the elderly. *Chest* 124:328–336.

Morris H (2005) Audit highlights prevalence of dysphagia. *Professional Nurse* 16(12):590–593.

Morris H (2006) Dysphagia in the elderly – a management challenge for nurses. *British Journal of Nursing* 15(10):558–562.

Negus E (1994) Stroke-induced dysphagia in hospital: the nutritional perspective. *British Journal of Nursing* 3(6):263–269.

Perry L (2001a) Dysphagia: the management and detection of a disabling problem. *British Journal of Nursing* 10(13):837–844.

Perry L (2001b) Screening swallowing function of patients with acute stroke. Part one: identification, implementation and initial evaluation of a screening tool for use by nurses. *Journal of Clinical Nursing* 10:463–473.

Perry L, Love C (2001) Screening for dysphagia and aspiration in acute stroke: A systematic review. *Dysphagia* 16:7–18.

Ramsey DJ, Smithard DG (2005) Assessment and management of dysphagia. In *Stroke: Therapy and Rehabilitation.* Ed: White R. pp113–123 London: Quay books.

Ramsey DJ, Smithard DG, Kalra L (2003) Early assessments of dysphagia and aspiration risk in acute stroke patients. *Stroke* 34:1252–1257.

Ramsey DJ, Smithard DG, Kalra L (2005) Silent aspiration: What do we know? *Dysphagia* 20:218–225.

Rickman J (1998) Percutaneous endoscopic gastrostomy: psychological effects. *British Journal of Nursing* 7(12):723–729.

Royal College of Physicians (2008) *National Clinical Guidelines for Stroke.* (3rd edition). London: RCP.

Smith C, Logemann J, Colangelo L *et al.* (1999) Incidence and patient characteristics associated with silent aspiration in the acute care setting. *Dysphagia* 14(1):7.

Smith HA, Lee SH, O'Neill PA *et al.* (2000) The combination of bedside swallowing assessment and oxygen saturation monitoring of swallowing in acute stroke: a safe and humane screening tool. *Age and Ageing* 29:495–499.

Stern RA (1997) *Visual Analogue Mood Scales.* Odessa, FL: Psychological Assessment Resources.

Sundin K, Jansson L (2003) 'Understanding and being understood' as a creative caring phenemenon – in care of patients with stroke and aphasia. *Journal of Clinical Nursing* 12:107–116.

Sutcliffe L, Lincoln N (1998) The assessment of depression in aphasic stroke patients: the development of the Stroke Aphasic Depression Questionnaire. *Clinical Rehabilitation* 12:506–513.

Syder D (1992) *An Introduction to Communication Disorders.* USA: Singular publishing.

Teasell R, Foley N, McRae M *et al.* (2001) Utilization of percutaneous gastrojejunostomy feeding tubes in stroke rehabilitation patients. *Archives of Physical Medical Rehabilitation* 82:1412–1415.

Travers PL (1999) Poststroke dysphagia: implications for nurses. *Rehabilitation Nursing* 24(2):69–73.

Vickery C (2006) Assessment and correlates of self-esteem following stroke using a pictorial measure. *Clinical Rehabilitation* 20(12):1075–1084.

Ward J (2006) *The Student's Guide to Cognitive Neuroscience.* Hove: Psychology Press.

Werner H (2005) The benefits of the dysphagia clinical nurse specialist role. *Journal of Neuroscience Nursing* 37(4):212–215.

Westergren A (2006) Detection of eating difficulties after stroke: a systematic review. *International Nursing Review* 53:143–149.

Wright L, Cotter D, Hickson M *et al.* (2005) Comparison of energy and protein intakes of older people consuming a texture modified diet with a normal hospital diet. *Journal of Human Nutrition and Dietetics* 18:213–219.

13

Assessment, Interpretation and Management of Cranial Nerve Dysfunction

Iain Bowie and Sue Woodward

INTRODUCTION

The cranial nerves arise mainly from the brain stem and pass through the foramina of the cranium. There are twelve pairs of cranial nerves which are traditionally numbered using Roman numerals. The numbering reflects the order in which they arise from the CNS, with the first cranial nerve most anterior and the twelfth cranial nerve most inferior. The first spinal nerve (C1) is immediately behind the twelfth cranial nerve. Traditionally the cranial nerves were divided into sensory nerves, motor nerves or mixed nerves (i.e. both sensory and motor). However, only two cranial nerve pairs (the olfactory nerves and the optic nerves) are purely sensory and all other nerves are mixed to some extent. These two nerves differ from the others in that they are specialised extensions of the brain (Wilkinson and Lennox, 2005).

Cranial nerves mainly serve the neurological functioning of the head and neck structures, except the vagus, glossopharyngeal and spinal accessory nerves. The vagus nerve forms the parasympathetic nerve supply to the viscera, with some branches extending as far as the sigmoid colon. There is some spinal nerve supply to the head as the first thoracic nerve supplies the sympathetic input to the radial fibres of the iris muscle and the salivary and lacrimal glands. This explains the constricted pupil in Horner's syndrome which is sometimes associated with neck or thoracic lesions.

Neuroscience Nursing: Evidence-Based Practice, 1st Edition.
Edited by Sue Woodward and Ann-Marie Mestecky
© 2011 Blackwell Publishing Ltd

In this chapter each cranial nerve will be treated separately (except the third, fourth and sixth nerves, which are considered together). Function and testing is described, followed by a discussion of the common disorders affecting the cranial nerves. Most cranial nerve disorders do not require admission, but patients with underlying neurological conditions, such as stroke or multiple sclerosis, may have cranial nerve involvement and may require inpatient care.

FUNCTIONS OF THE CRANIAL NERVES

The olfactory nerve (I)

The olfactory nerve is the first cranial nerve. It is a sensory nerve, taking information about chemicals in the air to the brain for interpretation. The sense of smell is socially important to humans and occasionally physically important, e.g. alerting an individual to the smell of smoke. Receptor cells in the nasal mucosa detect chemicals that bind with receptor proteins. Receptors are specific to odorous chemicals and the nose is capable of discriminating thousands of different molecules. The sensory endings are in the top of the nasal cavity and nerve fibres pass through a series of perforations, called the cribriform plate of the ethmoid bone, into the cranium where they form the olfactory bulbs. The olfactory nerve sends signals to the olfactory cortex in the temporal lobe, but there are also connections to other areas of the brain, such as the limbic system, accounting for the emotional aspect of olfactory perception. Smell can also be extremely evocative of memories, known as the Proust phenomenon.

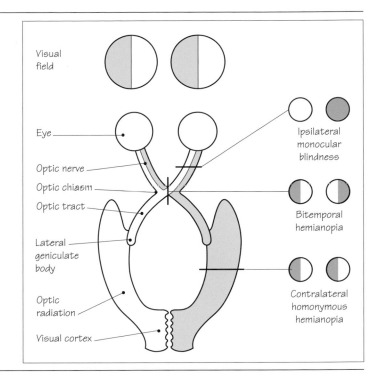

Figure 13.1 The anatomy of the visual pathways, and the three common types of lesion occurring therein. Reproduced from Iain Wilkinson and Graham Lennox, *Essential Neurology*, Wiley-Blackwell, with permission.

The optic nerve (II)

The optic nerve supports the sensory function of the retina, which is comprised of two types of peripheral receptors: rods (for night/twilight vision) and cones (for day/colour vision). The macula contains the greatest concentration of cones and is the most important area of the retina for visual acuity. The ganglion of the optic nerve forms a layer within the retina, with axons converging at the optic disc. As the optic disc has no sensory cells it is often known as 'the blind spot'. The ganglion cells are connected to the sensory rod and cone cells of the retina by bipolar neurons and receive their blood supply from tributaries of the central retinal artery. Defects of this circulation are analogous to stroke and often precede or co-occur with stroke involving the anterior circulation.

The axons of the optic nerve are bundled together and protected by the dura, which is continuous with and histologically similar to the sclera of the eye. The optic nerves enter the cranium via the optic foramen at the back of the orbital cavity from where they converge at the optic chiasma, located superior to the pituitary gland. The fibres from the nasal side of each retina then cross over to the opposite side and proceed to the contralateral hemisphere. This forms an arrangement where each optic nerve beyond the chiasma carries information from the nasal field of the contralateral eye and the temporal field of the ipsilateral

eye (Figure 13.1). The optic nerves end at the lateral geniculate bodies in the thalamus and connect to the optic radiations that form the pathway to the visual cortex in the occipital lobes where visual information is interpreted.

The oculomotor (III), trochlear (IV) and abducens (VI) nerves

The third, fourth and sixth cranial nerves are concerned with eye movements. The lateral rectus muscle is supplied by the abducens nerve, the superior oblique muscle is served by the trochlear nerve and all the other eye muscles (inferior, medial and superior rectus and inferior oblique) are served by the oculomotor nerve (Figure 13.2) (Ginsberg, 2005). While these three nerves are predominantly motor nerves, they also contain some sensory fibres gathering proprioceptive data. This information tells us in which direction we are looking even with our eyes closed.

The root of the oculomotor nerve is immediately above the tentorium and then the nerve passes through the tentorium alongside the brain stem. The efferent, parasympathetic fibres of the oculomotor nerve control constriction of the pupil, but the dilator muscles of the iris are also served by sympathetic fibres from the first thoracic nerve (Ginsberg, 2005). The relative dilation or constriction of the pupil is in a dynamic state as both sympathetic and parasympathetic systems 'compete' to exert their effects

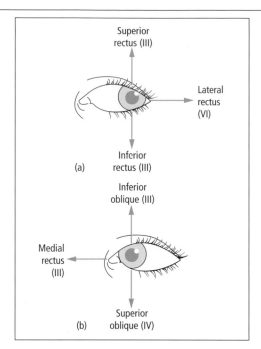

Figure 13.2 Actions and innervation of the extraocular muscles (left eye). When the eye is abducted (a), the superior and inferior rectus muscles are responsible for elevating and depressing the eyeball, respectively. In adduction (b), these actions are taken by the inferior and superior oblique muscles, respectively. Reproduced from Lionel Ginsberg, *Lecture Notes: Neurology*, Wiley-Blackwell, with permission.

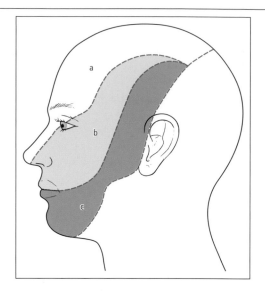

Figure 13.3 Sensory divisions of the trigeminal nerve: (a) ophthalmic, (b) maxillary, (c) mandibular. Note the trigeminal nerve is also responsible for innervation of noncutaneous structures – the eye, particularly the cornea, the frontal and maxillary air sinuses, the nasal and oral cavities, including jaws, teeth and anterior two-thirds of tongue, and the temporomandibular joint and anterior wall of the external auditory meatus. Reproduced from Lionel Ginsberg, *Lecture Notes: Neurology*, Wiley-Blackwell, with permission.

on the pupil. The oculomotor nerve also controls the levator palpebrae superioris muscle that raises the eyelid. A lesion affecting the oculomotor nerve may therefore cause ptosis.

The trigeminal nerve (V)

The three branches of the trigeminal nerve (ophthalmic, maxillary and mandibular) support functions with a fairly wide distribution in the face, mouth and jaw. The ophthalmic branch provides sensation to the forehead, upper eyelid, cornea and front part of the scalp. The maxillary branch serves the cheeks, lower eyelid, and upper lip and the mandibular branch serves the lower jaw and touch sensation to the anterior part of the tongue (Figure 13.3). Motor fibres serve the muscles of biting, chewing and some aspects of swallowing. Because the jaw muscles are important in speech production, people with trigeminal nerve defects may have communication problems.

The facial nerve (VII)

The facial nerve contains motor fibres that supply the muscles of the face and autonomic fibres to the lacrimal and salivary glands. It also contains sensory fibres from the anterior two thirds of the tongue carrying information about taste. The facial nerve is important in speech production as complex lip movements are necessary for clear speech.

The vestibulocochlear nerve (auditory or acoustic nerve) (VIII)

The vestibulocochlear nerve is a mainly sensory nerve serving the cochlea for hearing and the vestibular system for balance information. The nerve also contains some motor fibres that can moderate the tension of the hair cells within the ear and so moderate the perception of sounds. The vestibular apparatus of the inner ear (labyrinth) transmits information to the brain stem nuclei and cerebellum (Ginsberg, 2005). Vestibular nuclei also connect to the III, IV and VI cranial nerve nuclei, cerebellum and cerebral hemispheres.

Glossopharyngeal nerve (IX)

The glossopharyngeal nerve does not have a nucleus of its own within the CNS, but fibres connect to several nuclei shared with other cranial nerves. The glossopharyngeal nerve shares some of its distribution with the vagus nerve and the carotid body that monitors blood pressure is served by glossopharyngeal fibres. The glossopharyngeal nerve provides motor input to the muscles of the pharynx and parasympathetic input to the parotid (salivary) glands as well as sensory fibres to the posterior third of the tongue, pharynx and middle ear. This nerve is very important in the coordination of swallowing.

Vagus nerve (X)

The branches of this nerve are widely distributed from the ear to the rectum, providing most of the parasympathetic output to the abdominal and thoracic viscera. The main distribution of the vagus nerve is given in Table 13.1. See Chapter 5 for its role in the parasympathetic nervous system.

Table 13.1 Distribution of the vagus nerve.

	Motor	Sensory
Head	Palatoglossal muscle	Skin behind ear Outer surface of ear drum (inside surface supplied by glossopharyngeal nerve) External auditory meatus
Neck	Muscles on the pharynx	Taste from pharynx
Thorax	Parasympathetic supply to the smooth muscle in the thorax Exocrine glands in the thorax	Larynx, oesophagus, trachea, thoracic viscera, baroreceptors in the aortic arch, chemoreceptors in the aortic body.
Abdomen	Smooth muscle of the abdominal viscera	Abdominal viscera

Spinal accessory nerve (XI)

Some fibres of the spinal accessory nerve arise from the cervical spinal cord, but then pass back alongside the cord into the cranium via the foramen magnum. Other fibres arise from a nucleus in the brain stem. Fibres from the brain stem join the spinal fibres to exit from the jugular foramen in the base of the skull. It is also unusual in that some of its fibres join the peripheral distribution of the vagus nerve in the neck. It is a motor nerve and innervates the shoulder muscles, the sternocleidomastoid muscle and muscles of the palate and pharynx. Some sensory fibres serving proprioceptors in the muscles are also carried in the spinal root of the spinal accessory nerve.

Hypoglossal nerve (XII)

The hypoglossal nerve is mainly a motor nerve innervating the intrinsic muscles and all but one of the extrinsic muscles of the tongue. It also contains some sensory fibres serving proprioceptors in the tongue. This nerve is essential in swallowing as tongue movement is necessary in the preparation of the bolus. The motor fibres are also essential for speech production as the tongue is used to shape the vocal tract and the shape of the vocal tract determines both nouns and consonant sounds. The proprioceptive function of the sensory fibres is especially important in speech because spatial feedback enables exact control of tongue movement in order to render speech sounds intelligible.

TESTING CRANIAL NERVES AND INTERPRETING FINDINGS

Olfactory nerve (I)

Sense of smell is normally only tested when the patient complains of a specific problem with this. Odours can be readily improvised at the bedside using items at hand, such as lemon or lavender oils, soap, chocolate, coffee or anything with a distinctive smell. Less pleasant odours can be used, but ammonia is detected by the trigeminal nerve endings in the nasal mucosa, rather than via olfaction (Ginsberg, 2005) and should not be used. It is important that each nerve is tested individually by blocking off one nostril at a time and that the patient's mouth remains closed. The patient does not need to identify specific smells, but should be able to discern a difference.

Anosmia is the total loss of the sense of smell and can be congenital. Sense of smell may be lost temporarily with an upper respiratory tract infection or damage to the nasal mucosa, so an ENT cause for anosmia must be excluded. Temporary or permanent loss may be due to head injury (usually recovers), drugs, endocrine disorders (e.g. Addison's disease and thyrotoxicosis), tumours, and aneurysm of the Circle of Willis (Lindsay and Bone, 2004). Olfactory hallucinations may occur during complex partial seizures and migraine. The sense of smell is intimately related to the sense of taste, which may also impact on appetite. Care for people with anosmia includes advising the fitting of smoke detectors at home to protect the patient in the event of a fire.

Optic nerve (II)

Visual fields

Testing the visual fields can demonstrate damage to the ganglion cells in the retina or the pathway from the retina. Special apparatus is used to assess the visual fields, but a simple non-specialist screening test, the confrontation field test, can be performed at the bedside (Figure 13.4). This test requires the examiner to sit (or stand) facing the patient at a distance of about one metre. Both the examiner and the patient cover one eye at a time, with the examiner covering their right eye while the patient covers their left, and vice versa. The examiner moves a target such as a pencil, at arms length, from outside the visual field slowly towards the centre. The patient is instructed to say immediately when the stimulus enters the field of vision. The test relies on the examiner having a normal field of vision and therefore if the target appears in the examiner's field before the patient reports seeing it this is recorded as a potential field loss requiring further investigation. When performing a confrontation field test it is important that the patient looks directly into the examiner's eye and does not move the line of gaze. The examiner must monitor this by looking directly into the patient's eye and reminding the patient if attention is lost.

The arrangement of visual pathways produces specific patterns of visual field loss when one or both optic nerves are damaged by CNS lesions. The pattern of visual field

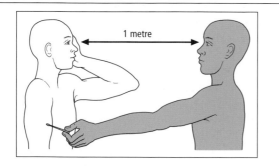

Figure 13.4 Visual field testing by confrontation. Reproduced from Lionel Ginsberg, *Lecture Notes: Neurology*, Wiley-Blackwell, with permission.

loss can be diagnostic of the site of an intracerebral lesion (Figure 13.1). Visual field loss is the end result of inflammatory, vascular or compressive optic nerve lesions (Lindsay and Bone, 2004). Defective visual fields may occur in stroke, tumours and trauma as well as other more localised neurological lesions. However there are some ophthalmic conditions that also produce field loss, such as glaucoma or retinal detachment. Therefore defects are not necessarily indicative of neurological disorders and a careful history is needed to determine pre-existing conditions.

Visual acuity

Visual acuity can test optic nerve function, but also tests the optical function of the eye. This test is done using Snellen's test type (the familiar eye test chart of letters in rows of decreasing size). Sometimes a rough guide to visual acuity is necessary, which can be achieved simply by asking the patient to read from a newspaper. One eye needs to be assessed at a time and the patient is asked to read from various examples of print size. The patient may use reading glasses if they normally wear them, as the aim is not to asses the optical resolution of the eye. A pinhole may be used to improve optical resolution if glasses are not available (Ginsberg, 2005). If the patient cannot read the print at all, the patient is asked to count the number of fingers or see a moving hand at a distance of about 30 cm. This is recorded as 'counts fingers' (c/f) or 'hand movements' (h/m). If the patient fails this test then the examiner should shine a pen light into the patient's eye and ask if the light can be seen; a positive response is recorded as 'perception of light' (p/l). These tests are sometimes difficult to perform, especially following trauma when there is periorbital swelling.

If visual acuity is normal with refractive errors corrected, then the lesion lies within the retina, visual pathway or cortex (Lindsay and Bone, 2004).

Colour vision

Colour vision is commonly tested using the book of Ishihara test plates, which consists of a number of numerals or patterns composed of coloured dots embedded in a circular matrix of dots of other colours. People with normal colour vision will see the figure designated in the answer key. People with defective colour vision will see no figure or a different figure (designated in the answer key). Detailed interpretation of the findings is complex and beyond the scope of this chapter.

Another important test of vision, but again beyond the scope of this chapter is contrast sensitivity where the ability to distinguish items from their background is tested. The most sensitive vision can distinguish shapes printed in a shade very close to the surrounding white background, but this ability may be decreased in papilloedema (Friedman and Jacobson, 2004).

Oculomotor (III), trochlear (IV) and abducens (VI) nerves

Eye movements

Testing eye movements is complex because the right eye and the left eye are capable of moving together to converge the visual axes (going cross eyed) or moving with each other so that a moving object can be tracked from left to right and vice versa. This means that the lateral rectus muscle of one eye contracts simultaneously with the medial rectus of the other eye, or both medial rectus muscles contract simultaneously to effect convergence. Vertical and torsional movement are also possible.

To test the extraocular muscle function, ask the patient to follow a target such as a pen/finger. The directions of gaze can be broken down into nine positions (upper left, centre and right, mid left centre and right, and lower left centre and right). The patient should be able to follow the target in each direction. Note any deficiencies of movement. It is necessary to test each eye separately and both eyes together to note any deficits in coordination. Testing should also take in convergence (follow the target towards the nose) and rotation by asking the patient to follow a target in both a clockwise and anticlockwise direction.

Pupil constriction

The size (in mm) of the pupil should first be estimated in normal lighting conditions (Ginsberg, 2005). Pupil constriction is then tested by shining a beam of light from a pen torch into each eye in turn. The effect of the light falling on each eye should be noted as both pupils normally constrict when either retina is stimulated by a light. Some fibres of the optic nerves branch off before the lateral geniculate bodies and pass to the nucleus of both left and right oculomotor nerves. Therefore the pupillary reflex is also a test of optic nerve function.

To conduct the pupillary reflex test, shine a pen torch across from the temple onto the eye; this avoids stimulating both eyes at once and invalidating the test. Note the speed of reaction of the pupil on the side being tested (ipsilateral) to assess the direct light response. Bring the pen-torch across the same pupil in the same way again, but watch the opposite pupil to assess the indirect (consensual) light response. Repeat the test on the other pupil. In some cases it may be difficult to see a patient's pupils, especially if they

have dark-coloured irises. Under these circumstances the nurse should darken the environment, causing a normal pupil to dilate and making it easier to see. Any abnormalities must be reported immediately and documented accurately on the neurological observations chart.

Pupils should be circular and equal in size (Turner and Blackwood, 1997). Pupil size is normally 2–6 mm and depends on the balance between sympathetic and parasympathetic stimulation. Pupil inequality (anisocoria) affects 20% of the population and is distinguished from other pathological causes by a normal response to light (Lindsay and Bone, 2004). Pupil size may be affected by drugs, e.g. topical anticholinergics will cause dilatation, while opiates may cause pinpoint pupils (Ginsberg, 2005). Other causes of pupil dilatation include III nerve palsies and migraine, while constriction may occur with Horner's syndrome.

Both pupils should normally react briskly, simultaneously and equally to light. If a patient has raised intracranial pressure the pupils may react sluggishly or not at all due to compression of the oculomotor nerve. This is a sign of trans-tentorial herniation (see Chapter 7). If you have to keep looking – then the pupil is not reacting! Pupils may also change shape under these circumstances and appear oval or irregular rather than circular, but shape changes may also be the result of eye trauma (Ginsberg, 2005).

If the optic nerve (or retina) is not functioning the pupil will not constrict. This is called an afferent pupillary defect and is usually an ophthalmological sign. It is often caused by eye disease preventing light reaching the retinal cells (Figure 13.5), but may also occur in optic neuritis. When the pupil in the opposite eye constricts but not in the stimulated eye this indicates that the oculomotor nerve on that side is affected. This is known as an efferent pupillary defect. Efferent pupillary defects can be a very serious neurological sign, hence the fundamental importance of checking the pupil reactions accurately. Pupillary defects are often early signs of supratentorial brain shifts.

Trigeminal nerve (V)

Testing of the trigeminal nerve involves assessing touch, taste, and motor function of jaw and cheek movements and lip closure. To assess motor function, palpate the bulk of the masseter and temporal muscles with the jaw closed, then ask the patient to open their jaw. If one side is weak, the jaw will deviate towards the affected side (Ginsberg, 2005).

Sensation in the areas served by the three branches of the trigeminal nerve (Figure 13.3) is assessed by touching

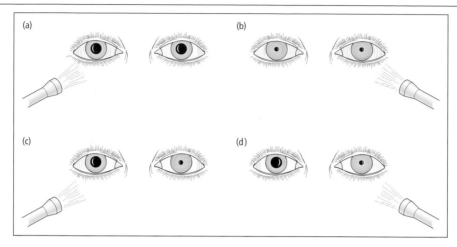

Figure 13.5 Afferent and efferent pupillary defects. (a, b) Afferent defect – when the torch shines in the affected eye (a), light is not perceived and neither pupil constricts. When the normal eye is tested (b), its pupil constricts, as does the other pupil consensually. (c, d) Efferent defect – light is perceived by the affected eye but the pupil cannot respond (c). The other pupil constricts consensually. When the torch shines in the unaffected eye (d), there is direct pupillary constriction but no consensual response from the affected eye. Reproduced from Lionel Ginsberg, *Lecture Notes: Neurology*, Wiley-Blackwell, with permission.

the skin lightly with cotton wool to establish threshold levels of touch; a neurotip™ can be used to check sharp sensation. Testing should be performed with the patient's eyes closed so that visual clues do not interfere with the patient's answers. Peripheral lesions affect sensation in the corresponding anatomical divisions (Ginsberg, 2005).

The corneal reflex is tested by touching the cornea of each eye lightly with a wisp of cotton wool and should elicit a blink bilaterally. The blink efferent pathway is from the facial nerve.

Unilateral facial sensory loss in combination with unilateral hearing loss may indicate a cerebello-pontine angle lesion, e.g. acoustic neuroma (Ginsberg, 2005).

Facial nerve (VII)

The motor function of the facial nerve can be assessed by asking the patient to smile, frown and to blow out the cheeks with the lips closed. The assessor should note and obvious facial asymmetry at rest and if there is any difference in the movement of either side of the face. The patient should be asked to raise their eyebrows, close their eyes tight, purse their lips, inflate their cheeks and whistle. Gentle tapping on the inflated cheeks should not cause air loss if there is good lip seal. Poor eye closure may result from loss of facial nerve innervation to the orbicularis oculi muscle. If the eye cannot be closed properly care

must be taken to avoid drying and subsequent damage to the cornea (see: Medical and nursing management of common cranial nerve disorders/ Bell's palsy). Patients may also report reduced lacrimation or salivation on one side (Lindsay and Bone, 2004).

Taste can be tested by dropping solutions of salt, sugar, lemon juice or strong coffee onto the patient's tongue, to provide the basic flavours of salt, sweet, sour and bitter. The taste test should be done on each side of the tongue to check each nerve; each taste used can be placed anywhere on the anterior two thirds of the tongue.

Vestibulocochlear nerve (VIII)

Simple hearing tests involve whispering to the patient and asking them to repeat what was said. The other external auditory meatus should be blocked by the assessor. If a whisper cannot be heard, the volume of speech should be gradually increased until a threshold level is reached. Tests using a tuning fork can also provide valuable information and can help to distinguish between conductive hearing loss (a problem conducting sound waves through the outer or middle ear) and sensory hearing loss. Two common and simple tests are Rinne's test and Weber's test (see Figure 13.6). More complex tests such as audiometry, which tests perception and thresholds of loudness and frequency of sound, are beyond the scope of this chapter and are

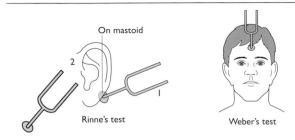

Figure 13.6 Rinne's test: Place a high pitched vibrating tuning fork on the mastoid (1 in figure). When the patient says the sound stops, hold the fork at the meatus (2 in figure).
- If still heard: air conduction > bone conduction (normal or nerve deafness)
- If not heard: air conduction < bone conduction (middle ear conduction defect)

Weber's test: Hold a vibrating tuning fork in the middle of the patient's forehead. If the sound is heard on one side, middle ear deafness exists on that side or the opposing ear has nerve deafness. Reproduced from Robert Turner and Roger Blackwood, *Lecture Notes on Clinical Skills 3e.*, Wiley-Blackwell, with permission.

normally conducted in an ENT department. Auditory evoked potentials are discussed in Chapter 19.

Rinne's test

Rinne's test assesses conductive and sensorineural (cochlear and VIII nerve) hearing loss and is carried out by placing a tuning fork with the prongs vibrating near the external auditory meatus and then placing the base of the fork on the skin overlying the mastoid process. The patient is asked to state which is louder: the air conduction tested at the meatus, or the bone conduction tested on the mastoid.

Air conduction is normally louder. If bone conduction is reported as louder the patient may have a conductive hearing loss. If sensorineural hearing is impaired, air conduction will be louder than bone conduction, but will be reduced compared to the unaffected side (Ginsberg, 2005).

Weber's test

Weber's test is carried out by placing the base of the vibrating tuning fork on the vertex of the forehead. The patient is asked to say whether the vibration is heard in one or both ears, and whether either is louder. In conductive hearing loss the vibrations will be louder in the affected ear, while with sensorineural hearing loss sound

is perceived to be louder in the unaffected ear (Ginsberg, 2005).

Assessing balance

Balance and the vestibular system can be assessed by asking the patient to walk along a narrow line. The vestibular system can also be tested simply by using Romberg's test, although this is also a test of proprioception. The patient is asked to stand with their feet and legs together looking forward for thirty seconds, after which the patient is asked to close both eyes. People with normal balance will sway a little after a few seconds, but Romberg's sign is positive if the patient sways so much that it is necessary to move a leg to steady the sway. If this happens it will be the leg on the same side as the damaged vestibular system that moves.

Caloric test

This test is used to identify severe damage to the superior brain stem in an unconscious patient. During this test 50 ml of iced water is irrigated into the external auditory meatus, which will have a cooling effect on the fluid in the adjacent semicircular canals (Figure 13.7). Normally there is conjugate deviation of both eyes towards the side of the stimulus. This sign is absent when there is severe damage superior to the brain stem and can be one sign used for determining brain death. There is a close relationship between eye movements and the vestibular system. People who spin round until they feel dizzy will have nystagmus which is subjectively reported as the 'room spinning' although it is their eyes that are moving and not the room. Note the similarity with motion sickness where the room might indeed be moving.

Glossopharyngeal nerve (IX)

Testing of the glossopharyngeal nerve involves testing taste on the posterior third of the tongue (discussed above), the gag reflex and swallowing movements. A gag reflex (contraction of the pharynx, retraction of the tongue and palatal elevation) is elicited by touching the posterior pharyngeal wall with an orange stick. The efferent fibres of the gag reflex pass through the vagus nerve (Ginsberg, 2005). Swallowing assessment begins by asking the patient to swallow clear water in small amounts (approximately 5 ml) and observing for difficulty. Clear water must be used first because, when impairment is present, swallowing anything else could irritate the respiratory tract in the event of aspiration. Swallowing assessment should always be carried out by specially trained personnel and is explained further in Chapter 12.

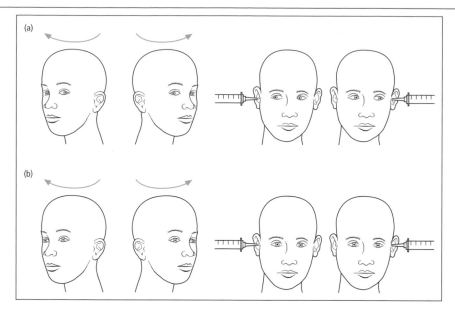

Figure 13.7 Testing the vestibulo-ocular reflex. (a) Intact brain stem – head rotation produces transient eye movement in the opposite direction – oculocephalic or doll's head reflex. Note this reflex also applies to vertical eye movements in response to neck flexion/extension. Caloric testing – instillation of 50 ml iced water into the external auditory meatus produces conjugate deviation of the eyes towards the stimulus. (b) Brain stem death – absent oculocephalic and caloric responses. Reproduced from Lionel Ginsberg, *Lecture Notes: Neurology*, Wiley-Blackwell, with permission.

Vagus nerve (X)

Because the vagus nerve has such wide ranging effects in the body, testing the function needs to be broken down by the different branches. The palatoglossal muscle moves the soft palate and is tested by asking the patient to say 'Ahh' with the tongue depressed. If the muscle works the soft palate can be seen rising and lowering. If a weakness is present the uvula will deviate towards the unaffected side.

Sensation can be tested on the skin behind the ear or carefully in the external auditory meatus. Swallowing must be assessed (see Chapter 12) to evaluate the innervation of the muscles of the pharynx. The visceral sensory and motor nerves cannot be tested simply, but blood pressure, especially lying and standing contrast, heart rate and blood gases may give practical information on function (see Chapters 14 and 15).

Spinal accessory nerve (XI)

The spinal accessory nerve can be tested by asking the patient to shrug their shoulders or turn their head. Muscle power can be tested by applying pressure to the shoulders and asking the patient to shrug against the resistance.

Lesions of this nerve are very rare, but may be caused by surgical trauma. Damage causes loss of function in the shoulder and an inability to raise the arm (Wilkinson and Lennox, 2005).

Hypoglossal nerve (XII)

The hypoglossal nerve can be tested by asking the patient to stick out the tongue. If the hypoglossal nerve on one side is not functioning, the tongue will be thrust forward by the muscles on the unaffected side, deviating towards the affected side because the weak side does not provide a counterbalance to the forward movement of the tongue.

CRANIAL NERVE DISORDERS

There are a number of relatively common conditions that affect the cranial nerves, although some are not managed within neurology practice. Impairment of vision is usually treated in an ophthalmology department, and vestibulocochlear nerve problems are often treated in an ENT department. Cranial nerves may also be affected by general central nervous system pathology such as stroke or multiple sclerosis.

Disorders of olfaction

Olfactory nerve function declines with age (Wilkinson and Lennox, 2005). Loss of olfaction or changes to the sense of smell may be due to: certain drugs, head trauma especially when there is ethmoid bone damage, frontal lobe tumours (Ginsberg, 2005), tumours (e.g. meningiomas) arising from the floor of the anterior fossa, and other lesions such as Parkinson's disease and dementia with Lewy bodies (Bromley, 2000).

Disorders of vision

Visual field loss

The most common visual defects are monocular blindness, bitemporal hemianopia and homonomous hemianopias (Figure 13.1).

Monocular blindness

This can occur transiently with migraine or be due to embolism in the ophthalmic artery. If infarction of the optic nerve or retina occurs, then this blindness will be permanent. Monocular blindness can also occur with giant cell arteritis and in multiple sclerosis (Wilkinson and Lennox, 2005).

Bitemporal hemianopia

This occurs when the optic chiasma is compressed, for example due to pituitary adenoma (see Chapter 21), craniopharyngioma, meningioma, third ventricle tumours or large internal carotid artery aneurysms (Wilkinson and Lennox, 2005).

Homonomous hemianopia

Central vision may be spared and the patient only becomes aware of the field loss by bumping into things on their affected side. If central vision is lost the patient complains of only being able to see half of the object they are looking at (Wilkinson and Lennox, 2005). Homonomous hemianopias are caused by posterior cerebral artery occlusion, occipital lobe infarcts or infarcts affecting the internal capsule, and abscesses and tumours in the posterior half of the cerebral hemisphere which affect the fibres of the optic radiation.

Impaired acuity

Optical anomalies due to the physical shape of the eye such as myopia and astigmatism will affect visual acuity. Loss of visual acuity can also be related to ophthalmic conditions such as cataract, uveitis and corneal ulceration, but may point to neurological damage within the visual pathway.

Impaired colour vision

Colour vision is a cone function, but may be impaired by drug side-effects, especially with antiepileptic drugs (Lopez *et al.*, 1999) and digoxin (Lawrenson *et al.*, 2002). Cataracts, which are a yellowish brown, filter certain wavelengths from visible light causing colour defective vision. Congenital colour vision defects are almost exclusively found in men, but acquired defects, such as those caused by optic neuropathy, are found in both sexes.

Disorders of eye movement and pupillary defects

Ptosis

Ptosis is drooping of the upper eyelid caused by palsy of the oculomotor nerve; the margin of the upper eyelid should not normally cover the pupil in wakefulness. Ptosis is a feature of several neurological conditions, such as III nerve palsies (see Box 13.1), Horner's syndrome and myasthenia gravis (see Chapter 31).

Diplopia (double vision)

If the patient has problems with coordination of eye movements this may be reported subjectively as double vision (diplopia). Impairments in the movement of one eye will result in an image being focused on the macula of the unaffected eye and just to the side of the macula in the affected eye – a false image (Lindsay and Bone, 2004). Binocular diplopia disappears if the patient closes one eye and is a symptom of neurological disease (Ginsberg, 2005). If diplopia is significant an eye pad can be placed over one eye and alternated from one eye to the other on a daily basis (Philips, 2007). Patients should be advised to avoid driving or operating machinery until they are used to wearing the patch.

Horner's syndrome

Horner's syndrome is uncommon and is caused by a lesion that impairs the sympathetic nerve supply from the hypothalamus to the eyelid (Ginsberg, 2005). This sympathetic

---

Box 13.1   Causes of III nerve palsies

- Brain stem tumours
- Aneurysm (basilar, cavernous sinus, posterior communicating arteries)
- Trans-tentorial herniation
- Brain stem stroke
- Inflammation of basal meninges
- Medical causes (e.g. diabetes, hypertension, giant cell arteritis, systemic lupus erythematosus (SLE)

innervation is derived from the hypothalamus and descends ipsilaterally via the brain stem and spinal cord to the sympathetic chain (see Chapter 5) via the motor root of T1. The fibres run alongside the outer sheath of the common carotid artery and the ophthalmic branch of the internal carotid artery (Wilkinson and Lennox, 2005). Horner's syndrome presents with partial ptosis and pupil constriction due to the resultant unopposed parasympathetic activity. Management of this symptom depends on the underlying cause (see Box 13.2).

Other eye movement disorders

Squint

Squint can occur in adults and should always be investigated as there may be an underlying neurological problem, such as a nerve palsy or a vascular condition such as giant cell arteritis. Paralytic squint is invariably due to a nerve or muscle lesion. The patient presents with little movement in the affected eye, diplopia and may tilt the head to minimise this diplopia (Lindsay and Bone, 2004).

Nystagmus

Irregular eye movements, such as nystagmus, can be related to eye muscle function, but can also be a sign of vestibular disorders. Nystagmus is an involuntary, rhythmic oscillation of the eyes in either a horizontal or vertical plane (Ginsberg, 2005). It may be congenital or acquired. Central nystagmus occurs in vascular disease, multiple sclerosis, neoplasms, Wernicke's encephalopathy, alcohol intoxication and drug toxicity, e.g. phenytoin (Lindsay and Bone, 2004).

Trigeminal nerve disorders

Herpes zoster ophthalmicus (HZO)

Herpes zoster ophthalmicus is caused by an infection of the ganglion of the nerve with herpes zoster virus (shingles), and commonly affects the ophthalmic branch. Vesicular lesions appear on the scalp and may affect the tip of the nose and the cornea of the eye (nasociliary branch), causing severe pain. The incidence of HZO is approximately 2 per 1000 and increases with age (Liesegang, 2008). If there is involvement of the cornea an urgent ophthalmic referral is required (Wilkinson and Lennox, 2005). Treatment with either oral or intravenous antiviral drugs (e.g. aciclovir) has been shown to limit the duration of the disease, reduce complications (Colin *et al.*, 2000) and is essential if the cornea is involved. Pain following infection can last for several months after the lesions have healed and adequate analgesia is essential throughout the course of the disease.

Trigeminal neuralgia

Trigeminal neuralgia (tic douloureux) is a painful condition that is usually unilateral. The severe facial pain is often accompanied by eye watering and is the most common condition affecting the trigeminal nerve. It is a rare condition, with an incidence of 4.3 per 100,000 per annum (Katusic *et al.*, 1990), predominantly affecting older women. The cause of trigeminal neuralgia is unknown, but it is thought to be caused by irritation of the nerve as it enters the brain stem (e.g. by an adjacent blood vessel or a cerebello-pontine angle tumour) or within the brain stem (e.g. due to multiple sclerosis) (Bennetto *et al.*, 2007). Attacks of paroxysmal, sharp, stabbing, shooting pain last days or even weeks and may be precipitated by chewing, speaking, washing the face, brushing teeth or cold winds. MRI may be used to screen for structural causes, which may be identified in 15% of cases (Gronseth *et al.*, 2008).

Disorders of the facial nerve

Facial nerve weakness

Lower motor neurone lesions arise from damage to the facial nerve or its nucleus within the brain stem (see Box 13.3). Upper motor neurone lesions arise between the cortex and the pons (e.g. tumours/stroke).

Hemifacial spasm

A hemifacial spasm produces unilateral, shock-like contractions of the face and predominantly affects older women. The aetiology is unknown (Lindsay and Bone, 2004), but may result from irritation of the nerve from blood vessels, tumours, multiple sclerosis or it may follow Bell's palsy. Hemifacial spasm can be successfully treated with botulinum toxin injections (Costa *et al.*, 2005).

Box 13.2   Common causes of Horner's syndrome

- Stroke
- Multiple sclerosis
- Tumours (pituitary, skull base, spinal cord, lung)
- Trauma (neck)
- Syringomyelia
- Chiari malformation
- Cluster headaches and migraine
- Herpes zoster infection
- Thoracic aortic aneurysm

> **Box 13.3   Causes of facial nerve palsies**
>
> - Brain stem
>   - Tumour
>   - MS
>   - Stroke
>   - Trauma
> - Acoustic neuroma
> - Middle ear infections
> - Bell's palsy
> - Parotid tumour/surgery/trauma
> - Guillain–Barré syndrome
> - Lyme disease
> - Sarcoidosis

Bell's palsy

Bell's palsy is an idiopathic, unilateral facial paralysis. It is thought to be of viral or post-viral origin, with some evidence supporting a herpes simplex infection or reactivation within the ganglion (Linder *et al.*, 2005). Herpes zoster and Lyme disease have also been implicated. It has a rapid onset (hours–days), but usually within 24 hours. Lacrimation is unaffected, but drainage of tears may be affected and the eyelid fails to close, leading to the eye watering on the affected side. The cornea is vulnerable to damage due to failure of eye closure, and speaking, eating and drinking become difficult. Loss of taste sensation (ageusia) can also occur. The prognosis is poor if the paralysis is complete, taste is lost, or in pregnant or elderly individuals.

Disorders of the vestibulocochlear nerve

Damage to the vestibulocochlear nerve can result in hearing loss, tinnitus and ataxia because of the role of the vestibular system in balance. CNS conditions, such as stroke or multiple sclerosis, may affect hearing or balance and some drugs, such as aminoglycoside antibiotics, may be ototoxic and result in sensorineural hearing loss (Forge and Schacht, 2000).

Deafness

There are two main types of deafness: conductive deafness, where the outer or middle ear fails to conduct vibrations to the cochlea (e.g. wax, ear infections); or sensorineural deafness where the eighth nerve fails to send impulses to the auditory cortex in the temporal lobe (e.g. acoustic neuroma, trauma).

Tinnitus

Tinnitus is either a continuous or intermittent sensation of noise, often buzzing or ringing. It may be unilateral or bilateral and either high or low pitched. Any lesion causing deafness can also cause tinnitus.

Acoustic neuroma

This is a benign tumour affecting the sheath of the acoustic nerve (a branch of the vestibulocochlear nerve). Although it is benign it is nevertheless a space occupying lesion that requires surgical intervention. The affected nerve will produce a sensorineural hearing loss that may be identified using Rinne's and Weber's tests (see Figure 13.6). Acoustic neuroma is discussed further in Chapter 21.

Vertigo

Vertigo is a false perception of movement and orientation of the body in space due to an imbalance of the vestibular apparatus (Ginsberg, 2005). It may be associated with nausea, vomiting, loss of balance and/or nystagmus. Common causes include acute labyrinthitis (viral or post-viral), Ménière's disease, vertebrobasilar ischaemia or multiple sclerosis within the brain stem. Vertigo is also a common drug side-effect associated with some antibiotics (streptomycin and gentamicin) if toxic levels are reached, and with anticonvulsants, barbiturates and alcohol.

The mainstay of treatment for vertigo is with vestibular suppressants (centrally acting anticholinergics and antihistamines or benzodiazepines) and centrally acting antiemetics such as metoclopramide, prochlorperazine and ondansetron (Hain and Uddin, 2003).

Disorders of the glossopharyngeal nerve

Damage to the glossopharyngeal nerve may cause loss of the gag and swallowing reflexes. Speech production may also become impaired as the glossopharyngeal nerve supplies the muscles used in shaping the vocal tract to produce speech sounds. Speech may be hypernasal as the velum (soft palate) cannot be raised to shut off the nasal passages during speech and air escapes through the nose. Raising the velum is also essential during swallowing to prevent nasal regurgitation and dysphagia. Hypernasal speech is distinctive and easily recognised once heard. Hypernasal speech is not the same as hyponasal speech, where the nasal resonators are shut off. Hyponasal speech results from inflammation, tumour or trauma to the nasal passages so that air cannot escape from the nose during the production of nasal sounds ('m', 'n', and 'ng' sounds in the English language).

Glossopharyngeal neuralgia is a condition in which pain along the distribution of the nerve is suddenly triggered by eating or speaking, similar to trigeminal neuralgia, lasting for a few seconds or minutes. The pain often radiates towards the ear and is triggered by swallowing. It is often of unknown origin but may be related in some cases to multiple sclerosis or nerve compression. It responds to carbamazepine in some cases, but may require surgical decompression.

Disorders of the hypoglossal nerve

The hypoglossal nerve is affected in neurological diseases such as multiple sclerosis, stroke and trauma. As it is a motor nerve it can also be affected in pseudobulbar palsy and motor neurone disease (see Chapter 27). When the hypoglossal nerve is affected the tongue may also show fasciculation (a tremor like movement). More rarely the hypoglossal nerve can be affected in meningitis and intracranial tumours.

Bulbar palsy

Bilateral impairment of the IX, X and XII cranial nerves results in bulbar palsy. This is commonly caused by motor neurone disease, stroke, skull-base tumours, Guillain–Barré syndrome and myasthenia. It results in speech and swallowing problems (see Chapter 12).

MEDICAL AND NURSING MANAGEMENT OF COMMON CRANIAL NERVE DISORDERS

Trigeminal neuralgia

Carbamazepine in doses up to 1200 mg per day can be effective and is recommended (Gronseth *et al.*, 2008), although the evidence supporting this is limited (Wiffen *et al.*, 2005). If carbamazepine is ineffective, baclofen, lamotrigine or other anti-convulsants have been reported to be effective in some patients, but evidence from controlled clinical trials is lacking (Chole *et al.*, 2007; He *et al.*, 2006).

Both ablative and non-ablative neurosurgical options are considered if the pain is unrelieved and there is now some evidence from cohort studies that earlier intervention may improve long-term outcomes and patient satisfaction (Zakrzewska *et al.*, 2005). Microvascular decompression is the only non-ablative procedure (does not result in destruction of the nerve) and is recommended for younger patients (Liu and Apfelbaum, 2004). During this procedure any vessels that are compressing the nerve are lifted and separated from the nerve by absorbable sponge to relieve the pressure. Pain is relieved in 70% of cases for up to 10 years (Zakrzewska *et al.*, 2005). Microvascular

decompression carries a mortality of 0.3% (Kalkanis *et al.*, 2003). Care of patients undergoing this procedure via a posterior fossa craniectomy is discussed in Chapter 20.

Ablative procedures, such as neurectomy, alcohol injection, radiofrequency thermocoagulation, balloon compression and stereotactic radiosurgery (gamma knife – see Chapter 20), use physical or chemical methods to destroy the nerve (Zakrzewska and Linskey, 2008).

Bell's palsy

Patients with idiopathic Bell's palsy often make a full recovery without treatment, but steroids may shorten the disease process (Salinas *et al.*, 2004). Anti-viral drugs may be prescribed, but there is no evidence of benefit (Lockhart *et al.*, 2009). Acupuncture is advocated by some, but the evidence supporting this treatment is inadequate and further research is required (He *et al.*, 2007). Facial exercises in front of a mirror are often recommended in the acute stages, but this has not been shown to influence recovery (Teixeira *et al.*, 2008). Botulinum toxin may be used for persistent facial asymmetry following Bell's palsy (Tiemstra and Khatkhate, 2007). Hypoglossal–facial anastomosis may also be considered if facial paralysis is permanent. It is an effective treatment, but can cause permanent ipsilateral tongue paralysis and atrophy (Yetiser and Karapinar, 2007).

In patients who do not recover, or those in the acute phase, drying of the cornea is a serious threat. Regular use of lubricant eye drops to prevent drying during the day and eye ointment at night is recommended (Holland and Weiner, 2004; Tiemstra and Khatkhate, 2007). Hypromellose is most commonly used and may be required as frequently as hourly to reduce soreness. Long acting ointment is used to lubricate the eye at night to prevent frequent wakening of the patient. A clear bubble shield is advocated for night wear to protect the cornea from abrasions. It must not be worn all the time as the warm moist environment that develops underneath can precipitate infections (BAO-HNS 2002). The patient should receive education on eye care prior to discharge. Protective eye wear without prescription lenses will protect the eye from dust when outdoors. Tarsorrhaphy (sewing the lid margins together) is an effective intervention (Tiemstra and Khatkhate, 2007) and can be reversed if the condition improves.

SUMMARY

Many functions of the cranial nerves are associated with the special senses. Each nerve can have specific pathology or be affected by the general pathology of the nervous system. Patients with cranial nerve problems are often seen by specific specialist departments such as ophthalmology (CN II, III, IV, VI), otolaryngology (CN VIII) and orthoptics (CN III, IV, VI). Because of the systemic and visceral effects of the vagus and glossopharyngeal nerves, many of these problems are dealt with in general medicine. Some conditions are very common and others are rare.

REFERENCES

Bennetto L, Patel NK, Fuller G (2007) Trigeminal neuralgia and its management. *British Medical Journal* 334(7586):201–205.

British Association of Otorhinolaryngologists – Head & Neck Surgeons Clinical Practice Advisory Group. (2002) *Clinical Effectiveness Guidelines: Acoustic neuroma (vestibular schwannoma)*. London: BAO-HNS Document 5.

Bromley SM (2000) Smell and taste disorders: a primary care approach. *American Family Physician* 61(2):427–438.

Chole R, Patil R, Degwekar SS *et al.* (2007) Drug treatment of trigeminal neuralgia: a systematic review of the literature. *Journal of Oral and Maxillofacial Surgery* 65(1):40–45.

Colin J, Prisant O, Cochener B *et al.* (2000) Comparison of the efficacy and safety of valaciclovir and acyclovir for the treatment of herpes zoster ophthalmicus. *Ophthalmology* 107(8):1507–1511.

Costa J, Espírito-Santo CC, Borges AA *et al.* (2005) Botulinum toxin type A therapy for hemifacial spasm. *Cochrane Database of Systematic Reviews* Issue 1. Art. No.: CD004899. DOI: 10.1002/14651858.CD004899. pub2.

Forge A, Schacht J (2000) Aminoglycoside antibiotics. *Audiology and Neuro-otology* 5:3–22.

Friedman DI, Jacobson DM (2004) Idiopathic intracranial hypertension. *Journal of Neuro-ophthalmology* 24(2): 138–145.

Ginsberg L (2005) *Lecture Notes: Neurology*. Oxford: Blackwell Publishing.

Gronseth G, Cruccu G, Alksne J *et al.* (2008) Practice parameter: the diagnostic evaluation and treatment of trigeminal neuralgia (an evidence-based review). Report of the Quality Standards Subcommittee of the American Academy of Neurology and the European Federation of Neurological Societies. *Neurology* 71(15):1183–1190.

Hain TC, Uddin M (2003) Pharmacological treatment of vertigo. *CNS Drugs* 17(2):85–100.

He L,Wu B, ZhouM (2006) Non-antiepileptic drugs for trigeminal neuralgia. *Cochrane Database of Systematic Reviews* Issue 3. Art. No.: CD004029. DOI: 10.1002/14651858.CD004029.pub2.

He L, Zhou M, Zhou D *et al.* (2007) Acupuncture for Bell's palsy. *Cochrane Database of Systematic Reviews* Issue 4. Art. No.: CD002914. DOI: 10.1002/14651858.CD002914. pub3.

Holland NJ, Weiner GM (2004) Recent developments in Bell's palsy. *British Medical Journal* 329(7465):553–557.

Kalkanis SN, Eskandar EN, Carter BS *et al.* (2003) Microvascular decompression surgery in the United States, 1996 to 2000: mortality rates, morbidity rates, and the effects of hospital and surgeon volumes. *Neurosurgery* 52(6):1251–1261.

Katusic S, Beard CM, Bergstralh E *et al.* (1990) Incidence and clinical features of trigeminal neuralgia, Rochester, Minnesota, 1945–1984. *Annals of Neurology* 27(1):89–95.

Lawrenson G, Kelly C, Lawrenson AL *et al.* (2002) Acquired colour vision deficiency in patients receiving digoxin maintenance therapy. *British Journal of Ophthalmology* 86(11):1259–1261.

Liesegang TJ (2008) Herpes zoster ophthalmicus natural history, risk factors, clinical presentation, and morbidity. *Ophthalmology* 115(2 Suppl):S3–12.

Linder T, Bossart W, Bodmer D (2005) Bell's palsy and herpes simplex virus: fact or mystery? *Otology and Neurotology* 26:109–113.

Lindsay KW, Bone I (2004) *Neurology and Neurosurgery Illustrated*. Edinburgh: Churchill Livingstone.

Liu JK, Apfelbaum RI (2004) Treatment of trigeminal neuralgia. *Neurosurgical Clinics of North America* 15(3):319–334.

Lockhart P, Daly F, Pitkethly M *et al.* (2009) Antiviral treatment for Bell's palsy (idiopathic facial paralysis). *Cochrane Database of Systematic Reviews* Issue 4. Art. No.: CD001869. DOI: 10.1002/14651858.CD001869.pub4.

Lopez L, Thomson A, Rabinowitz AL (1999) Assessment of colour vision in epileptic patients exposed to single drug therapy. *European Neurology* 41(4):201–205.

Phillips PH (2007) Treatment of diplopia. *Seminars in Neurology* 27(3):288–298.

Salinas RA, Alvarez G, Ferreira J (2004) Corticosteroids for Bell's palsy (idiopathic facial paralysis). *Cochrane Database of Systematic Reviews* Issue 3: CD001942.

Teixeira LJ, Soares BG, Vieira VP *et al.* (2008) Physical therapy for Bell's palsy (idiopathic facial paralysis). *Cochrane Database of Systematic Reviews* Issue 3. Art. No.: CD006283. DOI: 10.1002/14651858.CD006283. pub2.

Tiemstra JD, Khatkhate N (2007) Bell's palsy: Diagnosis and management. *American Family Physician* 76:997–1002.

Turner R, Blackwood R (1997) *Lecture Notes on Clinical Skills* (3rd edition). Oxford: Blackwell Science Publishing.

Wiffen PJ, McQuay HJ, Moore RA (2005) Carbamazepine for acute and chronic pain in adults. *Cochrane Database of Systematic Reviews* Issue 3. Art. No.: CD005451. DOI: 10.1002/14651858.CD005451.

Wilkinson I, Lennox G (2005) *Essential Neurology* (4th edition). Oxford: Blackwell Publishing.

Yetiser S, Karapinar U (2007) Hypoglossal–facial nerve anastomosis: a meta-analytic study. *Annals of Otology, Rhinology and Laryngology* 116(7):542–549.

Zakrzewska JJM, Linskey ME (2008) Neurosurgical interventions for the treatment of classical trigeminal neuralgia. *Cochrane Database of Systematic Reviews* Issue 3. Art. No.: CD007312. DOI: 10.1002/14651858. CD007312.

Zakrzewska JM, Lopez BC, Kim SE *et al.* (2005) Patient reports of satisfaction after microvascular decompression and partial sensory rhizotomy for trigeminal neuralgia. *Neurosurgery* 56(6):1304–1311.

14

Assessment, Interpretation and Management of Altered Cardiovascular Status in the Neurological Patient

Chris Brunker

INTRODUCTION

The human cardiovascular system is remarkably flexible and responsive, constantly adjusting to the huge range of demands placed on it. This adaptability is the result of precise control of the heart and blood vessels by the autonomic nervous system. It is not surprising, then, that damage to the nervous system can have serious effects on haemodynamic stability. As different elements of the autonomic system break down in different conditions, so the effects on the heart, blood pressure and temperature of patients vary dramatically, revealing (far more clearly than in the healthy individual) the powerful effect that the nervous system has on the body that exists to support it.

HAEMODYNAMICS

Blood pressure is the key measure of haemodynamic status. It is the force needed to perfuse oxygen and nutrients to tissues. Blood pressure is the product of the volume of blood pumped by the heart (*cardiac output*, CO) and the resistance created by the blood vessels (*systemic vascular resistance*, SVR) (see Figure 14.1).

Cardiac output depends in turn on the *heart rate* (HR) and the volume of blood pumped by the heart with each beat (*stroke volume*, SV) (see Figure 14.2)

Stroke volume depends on a combination of factors, but essentially on the amount of blood returning to the heart (*venous return*) and the strength with which the heart muscle pumps (*contractility*) (see Figure 14.3).

The autonomic nervous system (ANS) directly affects every one of the components that go together to generate a blood pressure. For a fuller explanation of the effect of the ANS on the cardiovascular system see Chapter 5.

Venous return

Venous return depends on the intravascular blood volume (how much fluid there is in the system) and the degree of constriction or dilation in the venous bed. At rest, the body's veins hold about 60–65% of the total blood volume. Under sympathetic stimulation veins constrict, pushing more blood back to the heart. There is no corresponding parasympathetic effect.

Contractility

Sympathetic stimulation increases the strength of contraction by making the cardiac muscle cells more permeable to Ca^{2+} (see Chapter 5). Again, there is no corresponding parasympathetic action. Sympathetic stimulation will also selectively dilate coronary arteries thereby increasing the blood flow to the heart muscle when it is required to work harder.

Heart rate

Heart rate is directly affected by both branches of the autonomic nervous system. Although cardiac muscle can

Neuroscience Nursing: Evidence-Based Practice, 1st Edition.
Edited by Sue Woodward and Ann-Marie Mestecky
© 2011 Blackwell Publishing Ltd

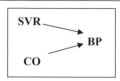

Figure 14.1 Components of blood pressure.
BP – blood pressure; CO – cardiac output; SVR – systemic vascular resistance.

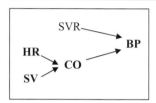

Figure 14.2 Components of cardiac output.
BP – blood pressure; CO – cardiac output; HR – heart rate; SV – stroke volume; SVR – systemic vascular resistance.

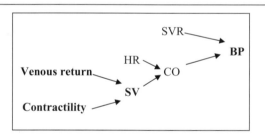

Figure 14.3 Components of stroke volume.
BP – blood pressure; CO – cardiac output; HR – heart rate; SV – stroke volume; SVR – systemic vascular resistance.

excite itself and will contract without outside stimulation, the rate at which the sinoatrial (SA) node emits waves of depolarisation and the atrioventricular (AV) node conducts them can be increased by sympathetic stimulation (excitation, see Chapter 5) and decreased by parasympathetic stimulation (inhibition).

Systemic vascular resistance

Sympathetic nerve fibres innervate the smooth muscle of blood vessel walls, causing them to constrict. Sympathetic stimulation of vascular smooth muscle is continuous, varying only in intensity: the more intense the stimulation, the more constricted the vessel. Vasoconstriction is selec-

tive, affecting vessels in the skin, abdominal viscera, kidneys, mucosal membranes and salivary glands more than those in the brain, heart and skeletal muscle. The overall effect is to raise SVR. Parasympathetic nerves innervate blood vessels only in the skin of the head. Stimulation causes vasodilation, most apparent in blushing, but this has no significance for the haemodynamic state overall.

AUTONOMIC CONTROL OF HAEMODYNAMICS

If the autonomic nervous system is to maintain blood pressure at an appropriate level it needs to receive information about the existing haemodynamic state. Bundles of baroreceptor cells are located in the walls of the aortic arch and the carotid sinuses. These are stretch receptors, responsive to changing muscle tension as the vessels stretch and relax during the pulse cycle. Baroreceptor impulses reach the cardiovascular centres of the upper medulla oblongata from the aorta via the depressor nerve (a branch of the vagus), and from the carotid sinuses via the sinus nerve (a branch of the glossopharyngeal). The impulse patterns are complex, supplying a detailed picture of mean arterial pressure, pulse pressure, heart rate and the speed of rise in pressure during systole. They also signal the rate of any change – crucial information if the system is to respond proportionately.

The cardiovascular centres in the medulla respond to change by adjusting the balance between sympathetic and parasympathetic activity. A rise in blood pressure will cause the brain to inhibit the intensity of sympathetic impulses transmitted via the spinal cord, while intensifying parasympathetic impulses relayed through the vagus nerve. A fall in blood pressure has the opposite effect. The cardiovascular centres are in turn regulated by the hypothalamus (see Chapter 5).

HAEMODYNAMIC ASSESSMENT

Given the close relationship between neurological function and haemodynamic stability, it follows that nurses caring for patients with neurological disorders need to pay careful attention to cardiovascular assessment. Advanced monitoring is only available in critical care units, but nurses in any environment, using only basic equipment, can make a very detailed assessment of their patients' cardiovascular status.

Blood pressure

Blood pressure may be regarded as a summary measure of cardiovascular status, but it must never be considered in isolation. As we have seen, blood pressure is the result of a combination of factors and the autonomic nervous system is designed to maintain a normal blood pressure by compensating for any changes in one factor by selectively altering others. This ability to compensate is limited. While it lasts, it can mask serious deterioration; once exhausted, haemodynamic collapse can be rapid and remorseless. Thorough cardiovascular assessment can detect changes before blood pressure is compromised. Moreover, once blood pressure is affected, such assessment gives vital information as to the cause and allows nurses to monitor the success of any treatment.

Heart rate

Heart rate is the easiest element of haemodynamic function to assess and often the most revealing, as the autonomic nervous system uses changes in heart rate as its first response to threatened changes in blood pressure; tachycardia will typically precede hypotension. Heart rate is best assessed manually, by taking a pulse. This gives a lot more information than the heart rate alone. The *regularity* of the pulse is important, as irregular beats indicate certain common cardiac arrhythmias (for example, atrial fibrillation or ventricular ectopic beats). This is especially helpful where continuous cardiac monitoring is not available, or where staff are not trained to interpret monitor traces. The amplitude of the pulse is also significant: a weak, thready pulse which can be easily obliterated by pressing indicates hypovolaemia (low SV), while a bounding pulse which cannot be obliterated by pressing can suggest that the patient is over-filled.

Examination of the skin

Examination of the skin, both visually and by touch, provides a good deal of information. Hot, flushed skin indicates vasodilation and the low SVR and diminished venous return typical of sepsis. Cold, pale skin demonstrates vasoconstriction and a high SVR, the autonomic nervous system's response to poor CO. Dry skin and mucous membranes suggest hypovolaemia, while oedema can be the result of cardiac failure (reduced contractility) or of the widespread inflammation encountered in sepsis.

Fluid balance

When it can be accurately established, fluid balance is very important in assessing intravascular volume and thus venous return, SV and CO. Urine output on its own is not always a reliable indicator of fluid status. Abnormal urine volume can be a complication of neurological disease, with either unusually high (cerebral salt wasting or diabetes insipidus) or low (syndrome of inappropriate antidiuretic hormone secretion) outputs. Refer to Chapter 16 for a more detailed discussion on fluid balance.

Central venous pressure (CVP)

CVP is the pressure of blood as it enters the right atrium and is a direct measure of venous return. However, measurement of CVP is not straightforward: the patient's position and changes in intrathoracic pressure during the respiratory cycle affect the readings and there can be confusion as to which anatomical reference point should be used. Moreover, raising the CVP by giving fluid will not necessarily increase the CO if the heart muscle is already at full stretch, or is damaged. The trend in CVP readings and their relationship with other observations is more useful than a single measurement.

Cardiac monitoring

Cardiac monitoring shows a continuous reading of the heart rate, but on its own this may be misleading, as electrical activity does not always translate into muscular contraction. A monitor will show arrhythmias, some types of which are common in certain neurological diseases, but monitoring is of doubtful value where nurses are not competent and confident in interpreting the traces.

Multi-parameter monitoring

Multi-parameter monitoring is generally only available in critical care areas. It allows continuous monitoring of cardiac rhythm and heart rate, arterial blood pressure and central venous pressure, as well as peripheral oxygen saturation and respiratory rate (Figure 14.4).

Advanced haemodynamic monitoring

Advanced haemodynamic monitoring is only found in critical care areas. There is a variety of devices all provid-

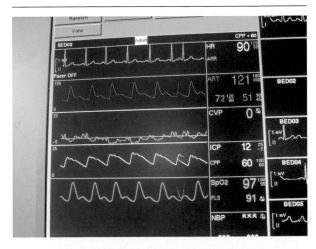

Figure 14.4 Multi-parameter patient monitoring.

ing measurements of CO, SVR and SV, as well as more accurate measurements of venous return (pulmonary artery wedge pressure, stroke volume variance or global end-diastolic volume) than can be gauged from a CVP line. This detailed monitoring can be especially useful in managing patients with neurological disease whose autonomic function may be deranged.

TEMPERATURE

The body's temperature is controlled by the hypothalamus. It receives information from two sources: hot and cold sensors in the skin (via the peripheral nerves) and the temperature of the blood as it passes though the brain itself. The temperature centre, in the pre-optic area of the anterior hypothalamus, distributes impulses to distinct heat promoting and heat reducing centres. The hypothalamus acts like a thermostat, normally set at 37°C; any deviation in temperature sets in motion both autonomic and behavioural responses.

The hypothalamus responds to the perception that the body is too cold by provoking a largely sympathetic response, but one focused on specific areas of the system. Blood vessels in the skin are constricted and hairs stand on end to minimise heat loss from the skin (although in humans piloerection has little value) while stimulation of the adrenal medullae releases adrenaline and noradrenaline, both of which accelerate the body's basal metabolic rate, generating more heat from within the body. At the same time the subject, feeling cold, adapts by putting on more clothing, moving about more (rubbing the hands and so on) and seeking the warmth of others (huddling) or of artificial heat sources. If temperature drops too far the hypothalamus stimulates motor centres in the brain stem to induce shivering and teeth-chattering; this involuntary activity generates at least some heat.

The perception that the body is too hot leads the hypothalamus to initiate responses that largely inhibit the sympathetic activity outlined above. Blood vessels in the skin dilate and hairs flatten, promoting heat loss. The basal metabolic rate reduces, generating less warmth from within. The subject, feeling hot, is inclined (where socially acceptable) to remove excess clothing, seek shade and a breeze and move around rather less. If the body is still too hot, the heat-reducing areas in the hypothalamus stimulate the cholinergic sympathetic response of sweating, increasing heat loss by evaporation. This is highly effective until air humidity reaches 100%, at which point sweat no longer evaporates.

Infection has an all too familiar effect on body temperature. Bacterial toxins induce white blood cells to release *pyrogenic* ('heat-generating') chemicals (such as interleukin-1) which prompt the hypothalamus to synthesise and release prostaglandins, adjusting the hypothalamic thermostat to a higher set-point. In some cases pyrogens may be produced by cells in the liver, initiating a neural signal to the hypothalamus via the vagus nerve. Now the hypothalamus perceives the body to be too cold and sets off the standard response: vasoconstriction, piloerection, seeking warmth and shivering. As the fever abates the thermostatic set-point falls, the body seems to be too hot and the corresponding responses ensue: flushing, sweating and the discarding of excess clothing.

Assessment of temperature

Taking a temperature may seem to be simplicity itself but is, in fact, the source of considerable ambiguity and controversy. To begin with, not all parts of the body are at the same temperature all the time. Core temperature (the temperature of blood in the central circulation) is typically higher than the temperature at peripheral sites (in the axillae, for example), but the difference is not consistent between individuals (Thomas *et al.*, 2004). Moreover, 37.0°C is not everyone's normal temperature (Smith, 2003).

To measure core temperature requires invasive monitoring: pulmonary artery catheters are regarded as the gold standard technique (Farnell *et al.*, 2005) but are only available in some ICUs. Moreover, in the acute stages of severe cerebral insult brain temperature is higher than central blood temperature, as measured at the jugular vein or rectum, and the difference varies (Rumana *et al.*, 1998; Rossi *et al.*, 2001). Rectal and oesophageal probes are impractical in most settings. Oral thermometry presents a hazard for patients who have poor levels of consciousness or who cannot control the movement of their jaws. Skin sites (axilla and groin) are usually regarded as the least reliable (Smith, 2003) and most subject to interference from ambient temperature (Farnell *et al.*, 2005).

The best type of thermometer is also the subject of disagreement; tympanic membrane thermometers have been widely criticised (Hoffman *et al.*, 1999; Giuliano *et al.*, 2000; Farnell *et al.*, 2005). Fallis *et al.* (2006) found chemical dot thermometers to be unreliable but van den Bruel *et al.* (2005) disagreed, and Farnell *et al.* (2005) found them to be better than tympanic membrane thermometers. Rajee and Sultana (2006) found chemical dot, tympanic and mercury thermometers to be interchangeable. There are also other considerations, including cost and cross-infection risks (Farnell, 2005).

It is not surprising, in the light of all this, that a survey by Childs *et al.* (2004) found no consistency in methods and equipment across the United Kingdom's 32 neurosurgical referral centres. Until an evidence-based consensus is achieved, it is important that clinicians understand the potential limitations of whatever equipment they are using.

HAEMODYNAMIC EFFECTS OF NERVOUS SYSTEM DISEASE

The way in which the nervous system controls and influences the haemodynamics of the human body can be dramatically illustrated when the system goes wrong. Nervous system disease illustrates the key fact that sympathetic and parasympathetic systems do not mirror each other anatomically or functionally, and disorder in one is not compensated for by the other, a fact that can produce some very dramatic and dangerous complications.

Neurogenic pulmonary oedema

Pulmonary oedema is usually associated with myocardial failure exacerbated by fluid overload. Some neurological patients who do not have this sort of myocardial damage can suffer a sudden-onset pulmonary oedema with dyspnoea and frothy pink sputum. The condition – neurogenic pulmonary oedema – is associated with high-energy penetrating head wounds (gun-shots or blast injuries) and, more commonly, with sub-arachnoid haemorrhage. The more severe the initial damage, the more likely the patient is to develop the condition. Reported incidence varies from 2% (Friedman *et al.*, 2003) to 23% (Solenski *et al.*, 1995) of patients with sub-arachnoid haemorrhage. Onset is anywhere from day 0 to day 7 with a peak at day 3 (Solenski *et al.*, 1995).

The precise causal mechanism for the condition is not clear, but it is likely that the hypothalamus reacts to the injury or bleed by over-stimulating the sympathetic nervous system (a so-called 'sympathetic surge'), causing a widespread and inappropriate vasoconstriction, and raising the SVR to the point where the heart cannot fully overcome the resistance. The left ventricle fails to clear with each stroke (resulting in low SV and CO) and a back pressure develops in the left atrium and pulmonary vein. High pressure in the pulmonary circulation causes fluid to leak through the arteriole-alveolar gap into the air spaces of the alveoli, creating the characteristic frothy pink sputum (Theodore and Robin, 1976; Smith and Matthay, 1997). An alternative explanation is that the sympathetic surge directly damages the endothelium of pulmonary capillaries, making them more permeable (McClellan *et al.*,

1989). It is possible that both mechanisms are at work at different stages.

Management

Neurogenic pulmonary oedema is a medical emergency requiring management in a critical care area. Diuretic therapy (the first-line treatment for *cardiogenic* pulmonary oedema) is inappropriate: neurogenic pulmonary oedema is not a problem of overload but rather of mal-distribution, i.e. too much fluid is stuck in the pulmonary circulation. Diuretics will not help: reducing circulating volume will drop the blood pressure. However, most of these patients have brains at risk of ischaemic damage from poor cerebral perfusion, and it is vital to maintain a *higher* than normal blood pressure (Friedman *et al.*, 2003). Instead, the condition is managed with a combination of dobutamine and positive end-expiratory pressure (PEEP) (Deehan and Grant, 1996).

Dobutamine has a vasodilating effect, reducing SVR, but it is also an *inotropic* agent, increasing contractility and maintaining blood pressure. PEEP raises the pressure in the alveoli at the end of expiration, thereby resisting the push of fluid through the alveolar wall by the disordered circulation. PEEP should only be reduced with caution: it is common for symptoms to recur some time after they have apparently been effectively treated..

Paroxysmal sympathetic storms

Paroxysmal sympathetic storms are bursts of uncontrolled sympathetic nervous system activity, typically accompanied by extreme hypertonic posturing. The phenomenon is most associated with severe head injury but has been linked to other types of acquired neurological damage (Diamond *et al.*, 2005). The exact cause is unclear, but it is apparent that hypothalamic control has been badly damaged, with no inhibitory mechanisms to control sympathetic activity. There is a rough consensus in the literature on the main features of sympathetic storms. These are:

- Tachycardia
- Hypertension
- Tachypnoea
- Hyperthermia
- Sweating
- Hypertonic posturing, typically extensor
- Agitation

The storms occur suddenly and repeatedly, lasting minutes to hours. They can be spontaneous or provoked by stimuli such as turning or endo-tracheal suctioning (Lemke, 2007).

Storms are upsetting to witness, as the patient appears to be agitated and distressed, sweating and straining in unnatural postures. To the unfamiliar eye, storms are easily mistaken for epileptic seizures. In fact, these episodes are not related to any epileptic brain activity (Do *et al.*, 2000). Storms seem to begin several days post-injury and Thorley and colleagues (2001) associated storms with the neuro-recovery phase. However, it may be that before this point sedatives and narcotics are masking the signs of the sympathetic storm (Lemke, 2007). Storms can persist for months (Boeve *et al.*, 1998) or wear off after as little as three weeks (Bullard, 1987). The literature to date gives little idea of the incidence: Kishner *et al.* (2006) give a figure of 15–33% of patients following brain injury, but they do not provide a basis for this figure, which seems rather high.

Management

Various treatments have been proposed. Opiates and sedatives dampen the symptoms but will delay respiratory weaning (Lemke, 2007). Bromocriptine is a dopamine receptor agonist that reduces blood pressure, temperature and sweating (Lemke, 2007). Low doses of chlorpromazine (a dopamine receptor *antagonist*) reduce temperature, but are also somewhat sedative and may spark off neuroleptic malignant syndrome (Blackman *et al.*, 2004). Propanolol (a non-selective beta-blocker) and labetalol (non-selective beta plus alpha-1 blockade) control hypertension, tachycardia and hyperpyrexia as well as reducing dystonia, but beta-1 specific antagonists such as atenolol appear to have less effect (Do *et al.*, 2000). Clonidine reduces blood pressure but is somewhat sedative (Blackman *et al.*, 2004).

Lack of a clear consensus on the best treatment reflects a paucity of thorough research. In the review by Blackman *et al.* (2004), 16 papers are cited: only two involved more than ten patients and six were based on a single patient each. Moreover, if storming is part of the recovery phase, as suggested by Thorley and colleagues (2001), it is possible that treatment of the symptoms may affect longer-term outcome, perhaps positively, perhaps negatively. There has as yet been no systematic investigation.

Neurogenic cardiac arrhythmias and ischaemia

ECG changes in patients with sub-arachnoid haemorrhage (SAH) were first described as long ago as 1954 (Burch *et al.*, 1954). Changes in ECG appearance such as T-wave inversion (see Figure 14.5), ST segment changes, and prolonged Q-T interval occur in almost all patients after SAH (Davis *et al.*, 1993) and are not in themselves associated with poor outcomes (Zaroff *et al.*, 1999). Ordinarily, such ECG changes indicate myocardial ischaemia, but only around 10% of SAH patients show left ventricular wall damage (Sato *et al.*, 1999; Banki *et al.*, 2005).

The more severe the SAH the more likely it is that the myocardium will be damaged (Banki *et al.*, 2005) and poor left ventricular function will hamper efforts to maintain the blood pressure needed to prevent cerebral ischaemia (Mayer *et al.*, 1999). More dangerous arrhythmias, including atrial fibrillation and supraventricular tachycardia occur in between 4% (Solenski *et al.*, 1995) and 8% (Wartenberg and Mayer, 2006) of patients.

The close association between SAH, arrhythmias and cardiac injury suggests neurogenic reasons for these abnormalities. In laboratory experiments, hypothalamic stimulation produces ECG changes without myocardial injury (Weinberg and Fuster, 1960) and the heart damage suffered by some SAH patients is unrelated to coronary artery disease (Zaroff *et al.*, 1999). It is likely that sympathetic nerves innervating the heart, massively overstimulated by the hypothalamus in response to the SAH, flood the tissue with noradrenaline, directly damaging muscle cells as well as receptor sites (Banki *et al.*, 2005).

Management

Cardiac arrhythmias can be managed as they occur, but left ventricular damage is more problematic. Patients with severe myocardial damage will need higher doses of inotropic drugs to maintain the blood pressure necessary to avoid cerebral ischaemia and such damage is predictive of

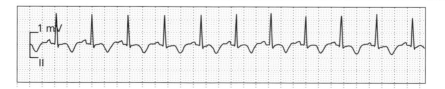

Figure 14.5 Cardiac monitor trace from a patient with sub-arachnoid haemorrhage showing the characteristic T-wave inversion.

increased risk of disability and death (Naidech *et al.*, 2005).

Spinal neurogenic shock

Sympathetic nervous supply to the heart and blood vessels is routed through the spinal cord at levels T1 to T5, while direct parasympathetic innervation is via the cranial nerves (see Chapter 5). Damage to the spinal cord in the upper thoracic or cervical spine has a dramatic effect on haemodynamic stability as the sympathetic branch is suddenly cut off from the brain. In the acute phase of cervical spinal cord injury (SCI) sympathetic stimulation is lost while parasympathetic activity continues unopposed; this is spinal neurogenic shock. The more complete the injury to the cord, the more severe the results are likely to be (Anonymous A, 2002). Symptoms occur in virtually all patients with a complete cervical spinal cord injury (Stier *et al.*, 2001).

The symptoms are exactly as one would predict from an autonomic nervous system with no sympathetic side. There is systemic vasodilation as blood vessels lose the sympathetic tone that usually maintains constriction, so SVR and venous return to the heart are both reduced (Gondim *et al.*, 2004). The heart's contractility is reduced as the muscle loses its direct sympathetic stimulation (Bilello *et al.*, 2003) and this, together with poor venous return, means a reduced stroke volume. Heart rate also falls: the heart loses the sympathetic stimulation that increases rate while the parasympathetic activity of the vagus nerve, unaffected by the injury and now working unopposed, actively slows the heart (Bilello *et al.*, 2003; Wuemser *et al.*, 2007). Low HR together with reduced SV equals poor cardiac output. Low CO together with reduced SVR equals profound hypotension. Hypotension compounds the ischaemia developing in the damaged spinal cord (Anonymous B, 2002; Wuermser *et al.*, 2007).

Temperature control is also compromised in patients with complete cervical SCI, again because of lost sympathetic activity (Stier *et al.*, 2001). This is termed 'poikilothermia' whereby the paralysed body loses the ability to actively regulate body temperature and instead takes on the temperature of the surrounding environment. In cold conditions there is no vasoconstrictor response in the peripheral vessels. Nor is there any stimulation of the adrenal medullae to increase basal metabolic rate, and the patient is unable to generate heat by movement. In a hot environment the patient's body does not sweat (Hickey, 2003). Moreover, lost sensation means that the patient may be unaware that he is becoming too hot or too cold.

Management

Spinal neurogenic shock must be managed with a view to the underlying problem of a badly unbalanced autonomic nervous system. Advanced haemodynamic monitoring in an ICU setting is essential (Bilello *et al.*, 2003).

Profound bradycardia may in extreme cases become asystole (Franga *et al.*, 2006), and some patients will need to have a pacemaker fitted (Ruiz-Arango *et al.*, 2006). In all cases, anything that stimulates the vagus nerve may evoke a worryingly low heart rate, so manoeuvres like deep tracheal suctioning must be treated warily, with preoxygenation as standard (Stier *et al.*, 2001) and atropine available as treatment or prophylaxis (Wuemeser *et al.*, 2007).

Hypotension may be complicated by hypovolaemia, but fluid replacement alone is unlikely to maintain blood pressure (Anonymous B, 2002). Inotropes should be used with care (Stier *et al.*, 2001) ideally on the basis of advanced haemodynamic monitoring (Anonymous A, 2002): the ideal combination of drugs balances HR, CO and SVR. The link between hypotension and worsened spinal cord ischaemia has been established in animal studies, and it is reasonable to assume that the same is true for humans. This has been clearly demonstrated in head injury (Anonymous A, 2002) but there is as yet no clear evidence base for setting a target blood pressure. The consensus is that a mean arterial pressure (MAP) of 85–90 mmHg is ideal in the first week after injury (Stier *et al.*, 2001; Anonymous A, 2002).

The symptoms of spinal neurogenic shock are typically at their most severe in the first week (Anonymous B, 2002) and usually resolve within three to five weeks after injury (Stier *et al.*, 2001).

Autonomic dysreflexia

Spinal neurogenic shock represents a stunning of the sympathetic nervous system when suddenly severed from cerebral control. Over time the sympathetic system reasserts itself and the symptoms of shock resolve. However, the sympathetic system is now functioning on the basis of reflex arcs via the spinal cord and lacks direct cerebral control, while the parasympathetic system is still directly controlled by the brain (Stier *et al.*, 2001). This poorly co-ordinated arrangement functions tolerably well most of the time but can easily become badly unbalanced, creating the phenomenon of autonomic dysreflexia (AD). AD is a common chronic complication in patients with SCI above T6; the more complete the cord injury, the more likely AD is to occur (Helkowski *et al.*, 2003). Symptoms typically appear from about one month post-injury, although AD can occur earlier (Krassioukov *et al.*, 2003).

An episode of AD is triggered by a noxious stimulus at a sensory level below the injury (Weaver *et al.*, 2006). Impulses from (for example) a distended bladder reach the spinal cord and, lacking inhibitory control from the hypothalamus, trigger a generalised and violent sympathetic over-reaction. The blood pressure suddenly rises and blood vessels below the injury level are constricted (Bravo *et al.*, 2004; Gondim *et al.*, 2004), producing cold, pale skin with goose bumps. However, the aortic and carotid baroreceptors are unaffected, triggering a parasympathetic response to an unwanted rise in blood pressure: the vagus nerve slows the heart rate and blood vessels in the skin above the injury level dilate, causing the skin to flush dramatically. The patient experiences a sudden pounding headache, shortness of breath, nasal congestion and blurred vision (Paralyzed Veterans of America, 2001). Some patients become confused (Khastgir *et al.*, 2007) and autonomic signs may be accompanied by painful muscle spasms (Stier *et al.*, 2001).

Management

Potential triggers for an attack of AD are: a distended bladder or bowel, ejaculation, childbirth, injections and acupuncture, ingrown toenails and so on. Management of the condition centres on avoiding and reducing exposure: careful bowel and bladder management, and care of the skin and nails are essential first steps. If an attack of AD occurs the stimulus must be identified and removed and steps taken to reduce the blood pressure. Sitting the individual up with legs lowered over the side of the bed or chair can be very effective, thanks to the orthostatic hypotension suffered by many SCI patients (Paralyzed Veterans of America, 2001). Anti-hypertensive medication may be needed.

In some ways AD resembles the signs of paroxysmal sympathetic storms after head injury: transient bursts of sympathetic over-stimulation producing dramatic hypertension. But the way in which the conditions differ illustrates the complex structure and function of the autonomic nervous system. Sympathetic storms originate in a damaged brain and parasympathetic activity is effectively dormant. In AD, both sides of the ANS are working – as if competing – but, because sympathetic and parasympathetic are not mirrors of each other, the effect of one is not cancelled out by the other. The imbalance and lack of communication make for haemodynamic chaos.

AD is extremely unpleasant for the patient and distressing for carers; it is also dangerous. Systolic blood pressure easily exceeds 200 mmHg and there is a risk of intracranial

haemorrhage (Pan *et al.*, 2005; Valles *et al.*, 2005). Vagal stimulation of the heart can produce bradyarrhythmias and heart block (Stier *et al.*, 2001). Attacks are usually limited in duration once the trigger is removed, but in rare cases of malignant AD the symptoms persist and worsen over several days (Elliott and Krassioukov, 2006).

Cushing's response

Of all situations in which neurological disease produces cardiovascular signs perhaps the best known is Cushing's response. This is a 'triad' of signs associated with a dangerously raised intracranial pressure (ICP): raised blood pressure, an erratic breathing pattern and pronounced bradycardia. It was first systematically explored by the neurosurgeon Harvey Cushing (1869–1939).

Cushing used laboratory experiments (Cushing, 1902) and clinical observation (Cushing, 1903) to uncover the link between rising ICP and the vital signs of pulse, blood pressure and respiration. Localised compression of the brain by, say, an extradural haematoma, initially produces no change in vital signs unless the medulla oblongata (the site of the cardiovascular and respiratory centres) is directly affected. But if the medulla is compressed directly, or by a global rise in ICP, marked changes occur. The high ICP (nearing the same level as the mean arterial pressure) compresses the capillaries that supply the medulla which begins to become ischaemic. The vasomotor centres are stimulated and a powerful sympathetic surge causes systemic vascular constriction and a surge in blood pressure to the point where arterial pressure is high enough to overcome the intracranial pressure, and blood supply to the medulla is restored. If the ICP rises further, the reaction occurs again, lifting the blood pressure still higher and this process may repeat unless the ICP is reduced (say, by surgery or by medical intervention). In experiments Cushing reproduced this step-wise link between ICP and BP as ICP went either up or down (Cushing, 1902).

In clinical situations, however, the intracranial compression may be remorseless as the cerebral hemispheres swell uncontrollably, lifting ICP beyond the ability of the blood pressure to match it. At this point, as the grossly oedematous cerebrum herniates through the tentorium, crushing the brain stem ('coning'), the medulla becomes terminally ischaemic. The vasomotor centres fail, respiration ceases and the blood pressure collapses. Systolic blood pressure can easily reach 300 mmHg or more in the last desperate moments.

At the same time that medullary ischaemia is producing this dramatic escalation of the blood pressure, respiration is also affected, producing the irregular Cheyne–Stokes pattern of breathing. Cushing found that as the medulla became ischaemic the breathing becomes shallow or stops altogether. When the sympathetic reaction brings up the blood pressure and restores circulation to the medulla, the breathing becomes deep but stertorous. As the ICP rises again, the breathing once again becomes shallow or stops, only to re-start again when the blood pressure rises above the ICP. But once the medulla loses circulation for good, breathing stops altogether.

The third element of the triad is pronounced bradycardia, with heart rates dropping to 40 or fewer beats per minute. This parasympathetic slowing of the heart is counter-productive: it reduces cardiac output and compromises the body's attempt to re-perfuse the medulla. Moreover, Cushing found (1902) that in subjects with spinal cords severed above the level of sympathetic outflow, very high ICP did not initiate a rising BP but *did* provoke bradycardia. He surmised that the vagal response was directly due to compression of the medulla, and not a response – however inappropriate – to the sympathetic surge in blood pressure.

In today's clinical practice, the relevance of Cushing's findings is unchanged: the triad of extreme hypertension, bradycardia and irregular respiration remains a sign of dangerously high ICP, often heralding death (Schmidt *et al.*, 2005). Less dramatic rises in blood pressure accompany more moderate rises in ICP but, given the multiplicity of factors influencing BP, it would surely be unwise to rely on it as an indicator of ICP.

BRAIN STEM DEATH

Nothing demonstrates more starkly the crucial role of the central nervous system in maintaining haemodynamic stability than the complete destruction of central nervous function: brain stem death. The death of the brain stem causes the irretrievable loss of all cerebral control of cardiovascular function, sympathetic and parasympathetic alike. Because respiratory effort is entirely the product of brain stem function, brain stem death leads almost immediately to myocardial hypoxia and cardiac arrest. But if ventilation is continued artificially, the heart may continue to beat, at least temporarily. Cushing (1902) described a case in which a patient's heart continued for twenty-three hours under artificial ventilation, and the advent of intensive care units in the later twentieth century has meant that the phenomenon of the brain stem dead patient is now almost commonplace.

The key to this situation lies in the ability of the heart to beat independently of any neural control for long periods, provided the heart muscle itself remains oxygenated. Nonetheless, the haemodynamic impact of brain stem death is profound: the sudden lack of central nervous

system control demonstrates in dramatic fashion the extent to which the cardiovascular system depends on it to function with any coherence.

The parasympathetic system's key role lies in determining the heart rate through the action of the vagal nerve on the sino-atrial node; this has a major effect on the control of blood pressure. Brain stem death stops all vagal stimulation of the heart and tachycardia results in up to 50% of brain stem dead patients (Powner and Allison, 2006).

Loss of sympathetic support produces predictable results. Complete loss of vasomotor tone means a collapse in SVR (Szabo, 2004). Venous return also falls as blood pools in dilated peripheral vessels, a situation made worse by the fluid loss caused by diabetes insipidus (Szabo, 2004). The heart muscle's contractility is seriously impaired by a combination of direct myocardial damage during the sympathetic surge of the Cushing's response and poor coronary perfusion secondary to hypotension in the period afterwards (Szabo, 2004). Any increased heart rate is thus offset by falling stroke volume and so the cardiac output cannot compensate for the loss of systemic vascular resistance (Cipolla *et al.*, 2006). Inevitably, blood pressure drops dramatically.

The situation is further complicated by the effect of brain stem death on organ function. We have seen the potentially devastating effects of a huge sympathetic surge on the lung and heart, and it is not surprising that the Cushing's response is also commonly followed by myocardial ischaemia (Dujardin *et al.*, 2001) and neurogenic pulmonary oedema (Smith, 2004). Cardiac arrhythmias occur in up to 30% of brain stem dead patients (Powner and Allison, 2006). Hypothermia is common: loss of the brain's temperature regulation means that the body's temperature tends to fall towards that of its surroundings (Pallis and Harley, 1996).

Management

Treating the chaos caused by brain stem death may seem fruitless, but it is important to maintain physiological stability until it is certain that the patient is definitely brain stem dead. Moreover, brain stem dead patients are the major source of organs donated for transplant and it is essential that a potential donor's body be kept as close as possible to normal until organ retrieval can take place or until donation has been ruled out. Failing to do so risks frustrating the wishes of the deceased patient and his or her loved ones. Management should be on the basis of protocols issued by donor transplant coordinators with the aim of anticipating problems rather than trying to correct them later. It is worth bearing in mind that an organ that is performing badly in the donor's body may do much better in a recipient who, of course, has a functioning central nervous system (Goel *et al.*, 2005). Care of patients undergoing brain stem testing is discussed further in Chapter 8.

Leaving a brain stem dead patient on a ventilator until asystole finally occurs is not a credible option. Unsupported, the blood pressure may fall to what seems to be an unsustainable level (Cushing, 1903 cites 20–30 mmHg), but the heart is tenacious and this situation can go on for hours to days (Intensive Care Society, 2004). If the patient is monitored and supported with fluids, inotropic drugs and the treatment of diabetes insipidus, the heart can survive for days to weeks (Al-Shammri *et al.*, 2003).

AUTONOMIC EFFECTS OF PERIPHERAL NERVE DISEASE

Guillain–Barré syndrome

Guillain–Barré syndrome (GBS) involves the acute inflammatory de-myelination of peripheral nerves: spinal, cranial or both. The effect is to slow or halt transmission of nerve impulses along the affected nerve axons. Up to two thirds of patients with GBS display autonomic symptoms (Seneviratne, 2000). Sympathetic and parasympathetic nervous function can be affected and symptoms vary between patients. Both tachycardia and bradycardia are reported, as are hypotension, orthostatic hypotension, cardiac arrhythmias and heart failure (Flachenecker *et al.*, 2000; Asahina *et al.*, 2002; Finkelstein and Melek, 2006; Palazzuoli *et al.*, 2006). Vagal hyper-reactivity has been found in up to 30% of patients (Flachenecker *et al.*, 1996). This can provoke serious bradycardia and even cardiac arrest (Minahan *et al.*, 1996; Zollei *et al.*, 2000).

Management of autonomic instability in patients with GBS is symptomatic and depends on careful, thorough and ongoing assessment (Hughes *et al.*, 2005).

TEMPERATURE ABNORMALITIES AND NERVOUS SYSTEM DISEASE

The nervous system sets the body's temperature and it is hardly surprising that damage to the system can produce abnormalities. Conversely, temperature disturbance can exacerbate damage to the nervous system in some common neurological diseases.

Raised temperature and acquired brain damage

There is experimental evidence that damage to brain tissue is exacerbated by even mildly raised temperatures. Several processes may be at work: pyrexia increases glutamate release (Takagi *et al.*, 1994) and the production of oxygen free radicals (Globus *et al.*, 1995); it accelerates the break-

down of the blood–brain barrier, thus aggravating cerebral oedema (Dietrich *et al.*, 1990); it also serves to break down cytoskeletal proteins (Morimoto *et al.*, 1997) and impair energy metabolism (Busto *et al.*, 1994). As will be seen, clinical evidence for a cause-and-effect relationship is less clear-cut.

Causes of pyrexia: infection and 'central' fever

Patients with acute acquired brain injury are susceptible to a variety of infections, including the upper respiratory and urinary tracts and infections of the brain, meninges and ventricles. Patients share the general infective risks of hospitalisation, restricted movement and invasive procedures, but patients with poor levels of consciousness and impaired airway control face a particularly high risk of aspiration and pneumonia (Grau *et al.*, 1999; Commichau *et al.*, 2003; Fernandez *et al.*, 2007). Some patients, however, become pyrexial without any infection being identified. While it is important to remember that no infectious screening method is 100% sensitive, the rate of unexplained fever in patients with acute cerebral disease suggests that something else may be going on.

The mechanism for what is often called a 'central' pyrexia remains unproven, and it may be that different processes operate in different circumstances. Deogaonkar *et al.* (2005) suggest that direct compression of the hypothalamus may be responsible for pyrexia in patients with ICH, citing animal experiments in support of their theory. Conversely, Schwarz and colleagues (2000) found that haemorrhage in the thalamus (which would compress the hypothalamus) did not lead to higher rates of fever than bleeds at other sites. There is a consensus that haemorrhage is more of a risk for pyrexia than ischaemic damage, especially bleeding in the sub-arachnoid space and most of all into the ventricles (Schwarz *et al.*, 2000; Fernandez *et al.*, 2007). Laboratory experiments show that blood in the CSF induces fever (Frosini *et al.*, 1999). Blood in the CSF may affect the hypothalamus directly, re-setting the body's thermostatic set-point to a higher temperature (Oliveira-Filho *et al.*, 2001; Commichau *et al.*, 2003).

Pyrexia: incidence and outcome

Pyrexia is often present during the acute phase of several common forms of acquired brain injury, with incidences reported at 48% in ischaemic stroke (Sulter *et al.*, 2004), 73% in severe head injury (Stocchetti *et al.*, 2002) and 72% in sub-arachnoid haemorrhage (Fernandez *et al.*, 2007). The more severe the initial insult to the brain, the more likely it is that fever will develop (Commichau *et al.*, 2003).

Pyrexia on admission is associated with worsened outcome in ischaemic stroke. Wang and colleagues (2000) found that for every 1°C increase in admission temperature, the risk of in-hospital mortality increased nearly four times and the risk of mortality at one year by over two times. They suggested that a higher temperature increases the metabolic demand of tissue in the penumbral area around the initial infarct; this tissue is poorly perfused and easily becomes ischaemic. Patients who are mildly hypothermic on admission are less likely to die and more likely to have an improved outcome, and this effect is independent of the severity of the stroke (Reith *et al.*, 1996). Hajat and colleagues (2000) found a less clear but still positive relationship between pyrexia after admission and poor outcome.

Intracerebral haemorrhage (ICH) presents a slightly different picture. Pyrexia is more common after ICH than after ischaemic stroke and again, pyrexia after ICH is associated with a worsened outcome (Schwarz *et al.*, 2000) although there is no association with admission temperature as such (Wang *et al.*, 2000). Schwarz and colleagues (2000) found no link between the site of the bleed and pyrexia: in particular, a bleed in the thalamus (which might be expected to disrupt hypothalamic temperature centres) was not associated with fever, but blood in the ventricles was. Conversely, Deogaonkar and colleagues (2005) found a correlation between the incidence of pyrexia and the size of the haemorrhage and, particularly, with shift of the third ventricle compressing the hypothalamus.

About 70% of patients with sub-arachnoid haemorrhage (SAH) develop pyrexia; risk factors include age and severity of the haemorrhage, but there is also a clear link with intraventricular haemorrhage and hydrocephalus (Oliveira-Filho *et al.*, 2001). Fernandez and colleagues (2007) found that for every 1°C rise in mean maximum temperature there was an eightfold increase in the odds of death, and a two-and-a-half times increase in the risk of cognitive impairment and functional disability at 90 days in survivors. Patients with symptomatic cerebral vasospasm are more likely to have a pyrexia than those who do not show symptoms (Fernandez *et al.*, 2007), but whether one causes the other is unclear and it may be that pyrexia and vasospasm are both the product of substances released into the CSF as clots break down (Oliveira-Filho *et al.*, 2001). This would imply that, rather than a cause-and-effect relationship between temperature and outcome, raised temperature and poor outcome are together the result of the severity of the original haemorrhage.

The incidence and duration of pyrexia in patients with acute head injury is associated with the initial severity of the injury. Stocchetti and colleagues (2002) found that 68 of 87 patients (78%) with a Glasgow Coma Scale (GCS) 8 or less developed pyrexia, but only 11 out of 23 patients (48%) with a GCS higher than 8 did so. However, they were unable to conclude that pyrexia actually made head injury worse. The level of intracranial pressure (ICP) was not associated with pyrexia as such, but a *change* in the brain temperature *was* related to changes in ICP: a rise in temperature was followed by a rise in ICP and a fall in temperature was associated with a fall in ICP (see also Rossi *et al.*, 2001). Most importantly there was no independent relationship between pyrexia and outcome at six months.

Efforts to demonstrate more clearly a relationship between pyrexia and outcome in, for example, head injury and SAH, are hampered by the ethical limits of clinical trials. Given the laboratory evidence that pyrexia worsens neurological damage, and the clinical evidence from ischaemic stroke and ICH that pyrexia is independently associated with poor outcome, it would be difficult to justify a trial in which some patients were not treated for pyrexia. On this basis, it is considered best practice to treat pyrexia (Kilpatrick *et al.*, 2000; Commichau *et al.*, 2003; Cormio *et al.*, 2003).

Acquired brain injury and hypothermia

If a raised temperature can worsen acute neurological damage, it may also be the case that a lowered temperature might protect the damaged brain. There is evidence from laboratory experiments that inducing hypothermia inhibits the progress of ischaemia in acutely damaged brains (Busto *et al.*, 1989a; Busto *et al.*, 1989b). Hypothermia induced after cardiac arrest improves neurological outcome (Hypothermia after Cardiac Arrest Study Group, 2002; Bernard *et al.*, 2002), but to date there is no clear clinical evidence for the benefits of induced hypothermia as a treatment for acute brain injury. Numerous studies have been undertaken but differences in inclusion criteria, time, duration and level of hypothermia make it difficult to establish a firm conclusion from all the evidence available (Alderson *et al.*, 2004). Moreover, inducing hypothermia has damaging side-effects for critically ill patients including hypotension, hypovolaemia, electrolyte disturbance and increased infection risk (Clifton *et al.*, 2001; Polderman *et al.*, 2002).

Managing raised temperature

In most situations fever is a normal physiological response to infection. Using drugs (other than antibiotics) or physical cooling to reduce moderately raised temperatures is of doubtful value in many cases (Gozzoli *et al.*, 2001) and may be positively harmful for some critically ill patients (Schulman *et al.*, 2005). However, given the evidence that raised temperatures worsen acute neurological damage, there is a consensus that pyrexia should be avoided in patients with acute brain injury (Kilpatrick *et al.*, 2000; Commichau *et al.*, 2003; Cormio *et al.*, 2003) and a good deal of research effort has been directed to this end.

Probably the most widely used antipyretic drug is paracetamol (acetaminophen). Paracetamol inhibits prostaglandin synthesis in the brain (prostaglandins trigger the upward adjustment of the hypothalamic thermostat) but has little effect at the peripheries: this explains its weak anti-inflammatory properties as well as its antipyretic effect. A study of stroke patients with pyrexias, (Sulter *et al.*, 2004), found that both paracetamol and aspirin had no effect in 35–37% of cases. Paracetamol is likewise ineffective for many patients with sub-arachnoid haemorrhage (Fernandez *et al.*, 2007; Mayer *et al.*, 2004), severe head injury and intracerebral haemorrhage (Commichau *et al.*, 2003; Badjatia *et al.*, 2006). As yet there is no way of predicting which patients will be unresponsive.

Because standard anti-pyretic medication is of variable effectiveness in acute brain injury, a lot of attention is given to physical methods of cooling patients. Techniques such as tepid or cold sponging, ice packs and air fanning have little or no evidential base. This is not altogether surprising: there are too many uncontrollable variations in technique to achieve any sort of measurable standard.

More structured methods of cooling are also available. Air-flow blankets do not appear to be effective (Mayer *et al.*, 2001; Hinz *et al.*, 2007). Water-circulating blankets are more successful but still fail to control fever in up to 60% of cases (O'Donnell *et al.*, 1997). They may also cause unpredictable fluctuations in temperature (Hinz *et al.*, 2007). This may be because water-cooled devices rely on conduction to transfer heat away from the patient's skin and there is often a poor contact between the blanket and the patient. One solution has been to circulate cold water around gel pads stuck to the skin, a device called Arctic Sun™ (Medivance, Louisville CO) (Carhuapoma *et al.*, 2003; Mayer *et al.*, 2004). Surface-cooling devices, particularly the gel pads, are prone to induce shivering, which needs to be prevented or managed with warming devices for the hands and feet, or with sedative drugs (Carhuapoma *et al.*, 2003; Mayer *et al.*, 2004).

An alternative to surface cooling is to use an intravascular cooling device (Cool Gard™, manufactured by ALSIUS Corporation of Irvine, Ca). A specially designed central venous catheter is placed in a central vein. Cold saline at a controlled temperature is circulated through two small balloons on the distal end of the catheter, cooling the patient's blood as it passes. The system has had good results in controlling temperatures prophylactically (Schmutzhard *et al.*, 2002) and in reducing fever (Diringer, 2004; Badjatia *et al.*, 2004; Hinz *et al.*, 2007) and shivering appears to be much less of a problem than with surface cooling. Although the system is obviously invasive, it also serves as a central venous catheter which many patients require.

All cooling strategies have drawbacks. Maintaining an artificially low temperature can mask newly acquired infections. Patients who are conscious are likely to find being cooled uncomfortable: 12% of neurological ICU patients in one study refused or could not tolerate a cold air blanket (Mayer *et al.*, 2001). It is hard to imagine a disorientated patient on a ward tolerating surface cooling for long. The low-tech methods like tepid sponging take up a good deal of nursing time and the more sophisticated approaches have cost implications.

None of the research to date provides any evidence as to the effect of different cooling strategies on the temperature of the brain itself. In acute cerebral damage brain temperature differs from core temperature (being typically higher) and that difference is not constant (Mellergard and Nordstrom, 1991; Rumana *et al.*, 1998; Rossi *et al.*, 2001). It is not unreasonable to ask whether artificially cooling a patient's core temperature has a predictable effect on a damaged and disordered brain. But perhaps the biggest problem is that none of the research compares the available methods for their effect on patient outcome.

SUMMARY

Given the close relationship between neurological function and haemodynamic stability, it follows that nurses caring for patients with neurological disorders need to pay careful attention to cardiovascular assessment. This chapter has illustrated how disease or injury to the nervous system can produce some very dramatic and dangerous complications. A knowledge of such complications and their management is essential for the safe and effective management of the patient.

REFERENCES

Alderson P, Gadkary C, Signorini DF (2004) Therapeutic hypothermia for head injury. *Cochrane Database of Systematic Reviews* Issue 4. Art. No.: CD001048. DOI: 10.1002/14651858.CD001048.pub2.

Al-Shammri S, Nelson RF, Madavan R *et al.* (2003) Survival of cardiac function in patients in Kuwait. *European Neurology* 49(2):90–93.

Anonymous (2002a) Blood pressure management after acute spinal cord injury. The Congress of Neurological Surgeons: Guidelines for the management of acute cervical spine and spinal cord injuries. *Neurosurgery* 50(3 Suppl):S58–62.

Anonymous (2002b) Management of acute spinal cord injuries in an intensive care unit or other monitored setting. The Congress of Neurological Surgeons: Guidelines for the management of acute cervical spine and spinal cord injuries. *Neurosurgery* 50(3 Suppl.):S51–57.

Asahina M, Kuwabara S, Suzuki A *et al.* (2002) Autonomic function in demyelinating and axonal subtypes of Guillain Barré syndrome. *Acta Neurologica Scandinavica* 105(1):44–50.

Badjatia N, Bodocck M, Guanci M *et al.* (2006) Rapid infusion of cold saline (4°C) as adjunctive treatment of fever in patients with brain injury. *Neurology* 66:1739–1741.

Badjatia N, O'Donnell J, Baker JR *et al.* (2004) Achieving normothermia in patients with febrile subarachnoid hemorrhage: feasibility and safety of a novel intravascular cooling catheter. *Neurocritical Care* 1(2):145–156.

Banki NM, Kopelnik A, Dae MW *et al.* (2005) Acute neuro-cardiogenic injury after subarachnoid hemorrhage. *Circulation* 112(21):3314–3319.

Bernard SA, Gray TW, Buist MD *et al.* (2002) Treatment of comatose survivors of out-of-hospital cardiac arrest with induced hypothermia. *New England Journal of Medicine* 346(8):557–563.

Bilello JF, Davis JW, Cunningham MA *et al.* (2003) Cervical spinal cord injury and the need for cardiovascular intervention. *Archives of Surgery* 138:1127–1129.

Blackman JA, Patrick PD, Buck ML (2004) Paroxysmal autonomic instability with dystonia after brain injury. *Archives of Neurology* 61(3):321–328.

Boeve BF, Wijdicks EF, Benarroch EE (1998) Paroxysmal sympathetic storms ('diencephalic seizures') after severe diffuse axonal head injury. *Mayo Clinic Proceedings* 73(2):148–152.

Bravo G, Guizar-Sahagun G, Ibarra A *et al.* (2004) Cardiovascular alterations after spinal cord injury: an overview. *Current Medicinal Chemistry Cardiovascular and Hematological Agents* 2(2):133–148.

Bullard DE (1987) Diencephalic seizures: responsiveness to bromocriptine and morphine. *Annals of Neurology* 21:609–611.

Burch GE, Meyers R, Abildskov JA (1954) A new electrocardiographic pattern observed in cerebrovascular accidents. *Circulation* 9:719–723.

Busto R, Dietrich WD, Globus MY (1989a) Postischemic moderate hypothermia inhibits CA1 hippocampal ischemic neuronal injury. *Neuroscience Letters* 101(3):299–304.

Busto R, Globus MY, Dietrich WD *et al.* (1989b) Effect of mild hypothermia on ischemia-induced release of neurotransmitters and free fatty acids in rat brain. *Stroke* 20(7):904–910.

Busto R, Globus MY, Neary JT, Ginsberg MD 1994 Regional alterations of protein kinase C activity following transient cerebral ischemia: effects of intraischemic brain temperature modulation. *Journal of Neurochemistry* 63(3): 1095–103.

Carhuapoma JR, Gupta K, Coplin WM *et al.* (2003) Treatment of refractory fever in the neurosciences critical care unit using a novel, water-circulating cooling device. A single-center pilot experience. *Journal of Neurosurgical Anesthesiology* 15(4):313–318.

Childs C, Hadcock J, Ray A *et al.* (2004) Temperature measurement after severe head injury. *Anaesthesia* 59(2):192–193.

Cipolla J, Stawicki S, Spatz D (2006) Hemodynamic monitoring of organ donors: a novel use of the esophageal Echo-Doppler probe. *The American Surgeon* 72 (6):500–504.

Clifton GL, Miller ER, Choi SC *et al.* (2001) Lack of effect of induction of hypothermia after acute brain injury. *New England Journal of Medicine* 344(8):556–563.

Commichau C, Scarmeas N, Mayer SA (2003) Risk factors for fever in the neurologic intensive care unit. *Neurology* 60(5):837–841.

Cormio M, Citerio G, Patruno A (2003) Treatment of fever in neurosurgical patients. *Minerva Anestesiologica* 69(4):214–222.

Cushing H (1902) Some experimental and clinical observations concerning states of increased intracranial tension. *The American Journal of the Medical Sciences* 124(3):375–400.

Cushing H (1903) The blood pressure reaction of acute cerebral compression, illustrated by cases of intracranial haemorrhage. *The American Journal of the Medical Sciences* 125:1017–1045.

Davis TP, Alexander J, Lesch M (1993) Electrocardiographic changes associated with acute cerebrovascular disease: a clinical review. *Progress in Cardiovascular Diseases* 36(3):245–260.

Deehan SC, Grant IS (1996) Haemodynamic changes in neurogenic pulmonary oedema: effect of dobutamine. *Intensive Care Medicine* 22(7):672–676.

Deogaonkar A, Georgia MD, Bae C *et al.* (2005) Fever is associated with third ventricular shift after intracerebral haemorrhage. *Neurology India* 53(2):202–207.

Diamond AL, Callison RC, Shokri J (2005) Paroxysmal sympathetic storm. *Neurocritical Care* 2(3):288–291.

Dietrich WD, Busto R, Halley M *et al.* (1990) The importance of brain temperature in alterations of the blood–brain barrier following cerebral ischemia. *Journal of Neuropathology and Experimental Neurology* 49(5): 486–497.

Diringer MN. Neurocritical Care Fever Reduction Trial Group (2004) Treatment of fever in the neurologic intensive care unit with a catheter-based heat exchange system. *Critical Care Medicine* 32(2):559–564.

Do D, Sheen VL, Bromfield E (2000)Treatment of paroxysmal sympathetic storm with labetalol. *Journal of Neurology, Neurosurgery and Psychiatry* 69:832–838.

Dujardin KS, McCully RB, Wijdicks EF *et al.* (2001) Myocardial dysfunction associated with brain death: clinical, echocardiographic and pathologic features. *Journal of Heart and Lung Transplantation* 20(3):350–357.

Elliott S, Krassioukov A (2006) Malignant autonomic dysreflexia in spinal cord injure men. *Spinal Cord* 44(6):386–392.

Fallis WM, Hamelin K, Wang X, *et al.* (2006) A multimethod approach to evaluate chemical dot thermometers for oral temperature measurement. *Journal of Nursing Measurement* 14(3):151–162.

Farnell S (2005) Are tympanic thermometers a source of cross-infection? *Nursing Times* 101(19):62–63.

Farnell S, Maxwell L, Tan S, Rhodes A *et al.* (2005) Temperature measurement: comparison of non-invasive methods used in adult critical care. *Journal of Clinical Nursing* 14(5):632–639.

Fernandez A, Schmidt JM, Claassen J *et al.* (2007) Fever after subarachnoid hemorrhage: risk factors and impact on outcome. *Neurology* 68(13):1013–1019.

Finkelstein JS, Melek BH 2006 Guillain Barré syndrome as a cause of reversible cardiomyopathy. *Texas Heart Institute Journal* 33(1):57–59

Flachenecker P, Lem K, Müllges W *et al.* (2000) Detection of serious bradyarrhythmias in Guillain Barré syndrome: sensitivity and specificity of the 24-hour heart rate power spectrum. *Clinical Autonomic Research* 10(4):185–191.

Flachenecker P, Müllges W, Wermuth P *et al.* (1996) Pressure testing in evaluation of serious bradyarrhythmias in Guillain Barré syndrome. *Neurology* 47(1):102–108.

Franga DL, Hawkins ML, Medeiros RS *et al.* (2006) Recurrent asystole resulting from high spinal cord injuries. *American Surgeon* 72(6):525–529.

Friedman JA, Pichelmann MA, Piepgras DG *et al.* (2003) Pulmonary complications of aneurysmal subarachnoid hemorrhage. *Neurosurgery* 52(5):1025–1032.

Frosini M, Sesti C, Valoti M *et al.* (1999) Rectal temperature and prostaglandin E2 increase in cerebrospinal fluid of conscious rabbits after intracerebroventricular injection of hemoglobin. *Experimental Brain Research* 126(2): 252–258.

Giuliano KK, Giuliano AJ, Scott SS *et al.* (2000) Temperature measurement in critically ill adults: a comparison of tympanic and oral methods. *American Journal of Critical Care* 9(4):254–261.

Globus MY, Busto R, Lin B, Schnippering H *et al.* (1995) Detection of free radical activity during transient global ischemia and recirculation: effects of intraischemic brain temperature modulation. *Journal of Neurochemistry* 65(3):1250–256.

Goel R, Johnson F, Mehra MR (2005) Brain injury and ventricular dysfunction: insights into reversible heart failure. *Congestive Heart Failure* 11(2):99–101.

Gondim FA, Lopes AC, Oliveira GR *et al.* (2004) Cardiovascular control after spinal cord injury. *Current Vascular Pharmacology* 2(1):71–79.

Gozzoli V, Schottker P, Suter PM *et al.* (2001) Is it worth treating fever in intensive care unit patients? Preliminary results from a randomized trial of the effect of external cooling. *Archives of Internal Medicine* 161(1):121–123

Grau AJ, Buggle F, Schnitzler P *et al.* (1999) Fever and infection early after ischemic stroke. *Journal of the Neurological Sciences* 171(2):115–120

Hajat C, Hajat S, Sharma P (2000) Effects of post-stroke pyrexia on stroke outcome: a meta-analysis of studies of patients. *Stroke* 31(2):410–414.

Helkowski WM, Ditunno JF Jr, Boninger M (2003) Autonomic dysreflexia: incidence in persons with neurologically complete and incomplete tetraplegia. *Journal of Spinal Cord Medicine* 26(3):244–247.

Hickey JV (2003) Vertebral and spinal cord injuries. In Hickey JV (ed): *The Clinical Practice of Neurological and Neurosurgical Nursing* (5th edition). Philadelphia, PA. Lippincott Williams and Williams.

Hinz J, Rosmus M, Popov A *et al.* (2007) Effectiveness of an intravascular cooling method compared with a conventional cooling technique in neurologic patients. *Journal of Neurosurgical Anesthesiology* 19(2):130–135.

Hoffman C, Boyd M, Briere B *et al.* (1999) Evaluation of three brands of tympanic thermometer. *Canadian Journal of Nursing Research* 31(1):117–130.

Hughes RA, Wijdicks EF, Benson E *et al.* (2005) Multidisciplinary Consensus Group. Supportive care for patients with Guillain Barré syndrome. *Archives of Neurology* 62(8):1194–198.

Hypothermia after Cardiac Arrest Study Group (2002) Mild therapeutic hypothermia to improve the neurologic outcome after cardiac arrest. *New England Journal of Medicine* 346:549–556.

Intensive Care Society (2004) *Guidelines for adult organ and tissue donation.* Available from: http://www.uktransplant. org.uk/ukt/about_transplants/donor_care/policy_documents/ ICS_guidelines_for_adult_organ_and_tissue_donation_ chapter_5(nov2004).pdf Accessed July 2010.

Khastgir J, Drake MJ, Abrams P (2007) Recognition and effective management of autonomic dysreflexia in spinal cord injuries. *Expert Opinion on Pharmacotherapy* 8(7):945–956.

Kilpatrick MM, Lowry DW, Firlik AD *et al.* (2000) Hyperthermia in the neurosurgical intensive care unit. *Neurosurgery* 47(4):850–856.

Kishner S, Augustin J, Strum S (2006) *Post head injury autonomic complications.* Available from: www.emedicine.com/ pmr/topic108.htm Accessed July 2010.

Krassioukov AV, Furlan JC, Fehlings MG (2003) Autonomic dysreflexia in acute spinal cord injury: an under-recognized clinical entity. *Journal of Neurotrauma* 20(8):707–716.

Lemke DM (2007) Sympathetic storming after severe traumatic brain injury. *Critical Care Nurse* 27(1):30–37.

Mayer S, Commichau C, Scarmeas N *et al.* (2001) Clinical trial of an air-circulating cooling blanket for fever control in critically ill neurologic patients. *Neurology* 56(3):292–298.

Mayer SA, Kowalski RG, Presciutti M *et al.* (2004) Clinical trial of a novel surface cooling system for fever control in neurocritical care patients. *Critical Care Medicine.* 32(12):2508–2515.

Mayer SA, Lin J, Homma S *et al.* (1999) Myocardial injury and left ventricular performance after subarachnoid hemorrhage. *Stroke* 30(4):780–786.

McClellan MD, Dauber IM, Weil JV (1989) Elevated intracranial pressure increases pulmonary vascular permeability to protein. *Journal of Applied Physiology* 67:1185–1191.

Mellergard P, Nordstrom CH (1991) Intracerebral temperature in neurosurgical patients. *Neurosurgery.* 28(5):709–713.

Minahan RE, Bhardwaj A, Traill TA *et al.* (1996) Stimulus-evoked sinus arrest in severe Guillain Barré syndrome: a case report. *Neurology* 47(5):1239–1242.

Morimoto T, Ginsberg MD, Dietrich WD *et al.* (1997) Hyperthermia enhances spectrin breakdown in transient focal cerebral ischemia. *Brain Research* 746(12):43–51.

Naidech AM, Kreiter KT, Janjua N *et al.* (2005) Cardiac troponin elevation, cardiovascular morbidity, and outcome after subarachnoid hemorrhage. *Circulation* 112(18):2851–2856.

O'Donnell J, Axelrod P, Fisher C *et al.* (1997) Use and effectiveness of hypothermia blankets for febrile patients in the intensive care unit. *Clinical Infectious Diseases* 24(6):1208–1213.

Oliveira-Filho J, Ezzeddine MA, Segal AZ *et al.* (2001) Fever in subarachnoid hemorrhage: relationship to vasospasm and outcome. *Neurology* 56(10):1299–1304.

Palazzuoli A, Lenzi C, Iovine F (2006). A case of acute heart failure associated with Guillain Barré syndrome. *Neurological Science* 26:447–450.

Pallis C, Harley DH (1996) *ABC of Brainstem Death* (2nd edition). London, BMJ Publishing Group.

Pan SL, Wang YH, Lin HL *et al.* (2005) Intracerebral hemorrhage secondary to autonomic dysreflexia in a young person with incomplete C8 tetraplegia: A case report. *Archives of Physical Medicine & Rehabilitation* 86(3):591–593.

Paralyzed Veterans of America / Consortium for Spinal Cord Medicine (2001) *Acute Management of Autonomic Dysreflexia: Individuals with spinal cord injury presenting to healthcare facilities.* Washington DC: Paralyzed Veterans of America (PVA).

Polderman KH, Tjong Tjin, Joe R *et al.* (2002) Effects of therapeutic hypothermia on intracranial pressure and outcome in patients with severe head injury. *Intensive Care Medicine* 28(11):1563–1573.

Powner DJ, Allison TA (2006) Cardiac dysrhythmias during donor care. *Progress in Transplantation* 16(1):74–80.

Rajee M, Sultana RV (2006) NexTemp thermometer can be used interchangeably with tympanic or mercury thermometers for emergency department use. *Emergency Medicine Australasia* 18(3):245–251.

Reith J, Jorgensen HS, Pedersen PM *et al.* (1996) Body temperature in acute stroke: relation to stroke severity, infarct size, mortality, and outcome. *Lancet* 347(8999):422–425.

Rossi S, Roncati Zanier E, Mauri I *et al.* (2001) Brain temperature, body core temperature and intracranial pressure in acuter cerebral damage. *Journal of Neurology, Neurosurgery and Psychiatry* 71:448–454.

Ruiz-Arango AF, Robinson VJ, Sharma GK *et al.* (2006) Characteristics of patients with cervical spinal injury requiring permanent pacemaker implantation. *Cardiology in Review* 14(4):e8–e11.

Rumana CS, Gopinath SP, Uzura M *et al.* (1998) Brain temperature exceeds systemic temperature in head-injured patients. *Critical Care Medicine* 26(3):562–567.

Sato K, Masuda T, Izumi T (1999) Subarachnoid hemorrhage and myocardial damage clinical and experimental studies. *Japanese Heart Journal* 40(6):683–701.

Schmidt EA, Czosnyka Z, Momjian S *et al.* (2005) Intracranial baroreflex yielding an early cushing response in human. *Acta Neurochirurgica – Supplement* 95:253–256.

Schmutzhard E, Engelhardt K, Beer R *et al.* (2002) Safety and efficacy of a novel intravascular cooling device to control body temperature in neurologic intensive care patients: a prospective pilot study. *Critical Care Medicine* 30(11):2481–2488.

Schulman CI, Namias N, Doherty J *et al.* (2005) The effect of antipyretic therapy upon outcomes in critically ill patients: a randomized, prospective study. *Surgical Infections* 6(4):369–375.

Schwarz S, Hafner K, Aschoff A *et al.* (2000) Incidence and prognostic significance of fever following intracerebral hemorrhage. *Neurology* 54(2):354–361.

Seneviratne U (2000) Guillain Barre Syndrome. *Postgraduate Medical Journal* 76:774–782.

Smith LS (2003) *Re-examining age, race, site and thermometer type as variableas affecting temperature measurement in adults.* BioMed Central Nursing Available from www.biomedcentral.com/1472-6955/2/1. Accessed July 2010.

Smith M (2004) Physiologic changes during brain stem death – lessons for management of the organ donor. *The Journal of Heart and Lung Transplantation* 23(9 Suppl):S217–222.

Smith WS, Matthay MA (1997)Evidence for a hydrostatic mechanism in human neurogenic pulmonary edema. *Chest* 111(5):1326–1333.

Solenski NJ, Haley EC Jr, Kassell NF *et al.* (1995) Medical complications of aneurysmal subarachnoid hemorrhage: a report of the multicenter, cooperative aneurysm study. Participants of the Multicenter Cooperative Aneurysm Study. *Critical Care Medicine* 23(6):1007–1017.

Stier GR, Schell RM, Cole DJ (2001) Spinal cord injury. In: Cottrell JE. Smith DS. (eds). *Anaesthesia and Neurosurgery* St Louis, MO: Mosby.

Stocchetti N, Rossi S, Zanier ER *et al.* (2002) Pyrexia in head-injured patients admitted to intensive care. *Intensive Care Medicine* 28(11):1555–1562.

Sulter G, Elting JW, Maurits N *et al* (2004) Acetylsalicylic acid and acetaminophen to combat elevated body temperature in acute ischemic stroke. *Cerebrovascular Diseases* 17(2–3):118–122.

Szabo G (2004) Physiologic changes after brain death. *Journal of Heart and Lung Transplantation* 23(9 Suppl):S223–226.

Takagi K, Ginsberg MD, Globus MY *et al.* (1994) Effect of hyperthermia on glutamate release in ischemic penumbra after middle cerebral artery occlusion in rats. *American Journal of Physiology* 267(5 Pt 2):H1770–1776.

Theodore J, Robin ED (1976) Speculations on neurogenic pulmonary edema. *American Review of Respiratory Disease* 113:405–411.

Thomas KA, Burr R, Wang SY *et al.* (2004) Axillary and thoracic skin temperatures poorly comparable to core body temperature circadian rhythm: results from 2 adult populations. *Biological Research for Nursing* 5:187–194.

Thorley RR, Wertsch JJ, Klingbeil GE (2001) Acute hypothalamic instability in traumatic brain injury: a case report.

Archives of Physical Medicine and Rehabilitation 82(2):246–249.

Valles M, Benito J, Portell E, Vidal J (2005) Cerebral hemorrhage due to autonomic dysreflexia in a spinal cord injury patient. *Spinal Cord* 43(12):738–740.

van den Bruel A, Aertgeerts B, De Boeck *et al.* (2005) Measuring the body temperature: how accurate is the Tempa Dot? *Technology and Health Care* 13(2):97–106.

Wang Y, Lim LLY, Levi C *et al.* (2000) Influence of admission body temperature on stroke mortality. *Stroke* 31(2):404–409.

Wartenberg KE, Mayer SA (2006) Medical complications after subarachnoid hemorrhage: new strategies for prevention and management. *Current Opinion in Critical Care* 12:78–84.

Weaver LC, Marsh DR, Gris D *et al.* (2006) Autonomic dysreflexia after spinal cord injury: central mechanisms and strategies for prevention. *Progress in Brain Research* 152:245–263.

Weinberg S, Fuster JM (1960) Electrocardiographic changes produced by localized hypothalamic stimulations. *Annals of Internal Medicine* 53:332–341.

Wuermser LA, Ho CH, Chiodo AE *et al.* (2007) Acute care management of traumatic and non-traumatic injury. *Archives of Physical Medicine and Rehabilitation* 88(Supp.1): S55–61.

Zaroff JG, Rordorf GA, Newell JB *et al.* (1999) Cardiac outcome in patients with subarachnoid hemorrhage and electrocardiographic abnormalities. *Neurosurgery* 44(1):34–40.

Zollei E, Avramov K, Gingl Z *et al.* (2000) Severe cardiovascular autonomic dysfunction in a patient with Guillain Barré syndrome: a case report. *Autonomic Neuroscience* 86(1–2):94–98.

15

Assessment, Interpretation and Management of Impaired Respiratory Function in the Neurological Patient

Anne Mcleod and Ann-Marie Mestecky

INTRODUCTION

The nervous system regulates and controls respiration and so it is not uncommon that impairment in neurological function can affect the functioning of the respiratory system. Conversely, because the central nervous system (CNS) relies on a rich supply of oxygen, respiratory compromise can rapidly lead to CNS dysfunction. Either of these situations could be life threatening, so it is important that neuroscience nurses have the necessary knowledge and skill to assess accurately and act upon changes in respiratory function. This chapter presents an overview of respiratory physiology. The elements of a systematic respiratory assessment, the interpretation of findings, and the most common respiratory interventions that are employed to optimise and support respiratory function in the neurological patient will be discussed.

A sound understanding of the physiology of the respiratory system enables the nurse to interpret assessment findings and to understand the physiological basis of respiratory interventions and support systems.

PHYSIOLOGY

The primary function of the respiratory system is to supply tissues with the oxygen required for function, and to excrete the carbon dioxide produced from cell metabolism. The respiratory centre is located in the brain stem and is the main control of respiratory function.

Neuroscience Nursing: Evidence-Based Practice, 1st Edition.
Edited by Sue Woodward and Ann-Marie Mestecky
© 2011 Blackwell Publishing Ltd

Control of respiration

The *medullary rhythmicity area* is situated within the medulla oblongata and controls the basic rhythm of respiration. Normal inspiration lasts for two seconds; expiration lasts for three. Therefore, there is a basic inspiratory: expiratory cycle approximately every five seconds. Within the medullary rhythmicity area are two regions controlling the basic respiratory cycle: the inspiratory and expiratory areas.

Nerves originating in the *inspiratory area* determine the basic rhythm of respiration. At the beginning of expiration, the inspiratory area is inactive, but after three seconds it automatically becomes active due to the intrinsic excitability of the inspiratory nerves. The nerve impulses last for approximately two seconds and innervate the diaphragm and intercostal muscles via the phrenic and external intercostal nerves respectively. At the end of two seconds, the impulses stop and the cycle starts again.

Normally expiration is a passive process and therefore the *expiratory area* is inactive until a greater volume of carbon dioxide (CO_2) removal is required, for example, during exercise or when air movement is impeded due to bronchospasm. At this time, impulses from the inspiratory area activate the expiratory area, which causes contraction of the internal intercostals and abdominal muscles. This action actively assists in reducing the size of the thoracic cavity which will result in greater volumes of CO_2 being removed.

There are two additional centres situated within the pons that can modulate the output from the medullary rhythmicity area (Figure 15.1).

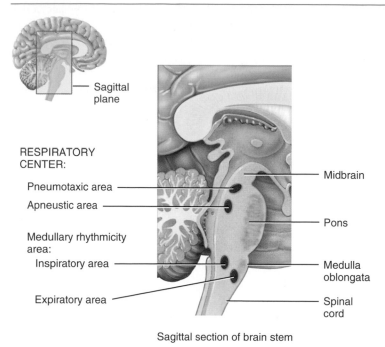

Sagittal plane

RESPIRATORY
CENTER:

Pneumotaxic area
Apneustic area

Medullary rhythmicity
area:
Inspiratory area

Expiratory area

Midbrain

Pons

Medulla
oblongata

Spinal
cord

Sagittal section of brain stem

Figure 15.1 Locations of areas of the respiratory centre. Sagittal section of brain stem. Reproduced from *Principles of Anatomy and Physiology 12e* by Gerard Tortora and Bryan Derrickson. Copyright (2009, John Wiley & Sons). Reprinted with permission of John Wiley & Sons Inc.

The pneumotaxic area

The pneumotaxic area is situated in the upper pons. Its primary function is to limit inspiration. It transmits impulses to the inspiratory area, turning it 'off' before the lungs get too full. When impulses from this area increase, inspiratory time may be as short as 0.5 seconds, thus the volume of air entering the lungs is significantly reduced. When there is a decrease in the impulses leaving the pneumotaxic area, inspiration may last for as long as five seconds, filling the lungs with greater volumes. A strong pneumotaxic signal may increase the respiratory rate to 30–40 times/minute whereas a weak signal will significantly reduce respiratory rate.

The apneustic area

The apneustic area sends impulses to the inspiratory area to prolong inspiration, particularly during quiet breathing. The apneustic area can only influence inhalation when the pneumotaxic area is inactive. When the pneumotaxic area is active it overrides the apneustic area.

Regulation of the activity of the respiratory centre

There are several influences on the respiratory centre that can modulate and alter the basic pattern of breathing:

Cortical impulses

Cortical connections allow for voluntary control of respiration, such as holding your breath. However, the duration of voluntary control is limited by the rise in arterial partial pressure of carbon dioxide ($PaCO_2$), which will stimulate the inspiratory area leading to involuntary inspiration (see chemical stimuli below).

Inflation reflex

Stretch receptors are in the walls of the bronchi and bronchioles. If they are 'overstretched', impulses are sent, via the vagus nerve, to the inspiratory and apneustic areas. This results in the inspiratory area becoming inhibited; the apneustic area is stopped from activating the inspiratory area and passive expiration occurs. This basic reflex is referred to as the Hering–Breuer reflex.

Chemical stimuli

Central chemoreceptors situated in the medulla are sensitive to changes in hydrogen ion concentration (pH) of the cerebrospinal fluid (CSF). Hydrogen is a product of CO_2 carriage, thus if there is an increase in $PaCO_2$, there will be a decrease in the pH. The increase in acidity stimulates the chemoreceptors which cause the inspiratory centre to become more active resulting in an increase in the rate and depth of respiration and an increased rate of CO_2 removal.

In addition, peripheral chemoreceptors, also known as the carotid and aortic bodies, are sensitive to changes in $PaCO_2$, pH and PaO_2 (partial pressure of oxygen) of arterial blood.

Unlike the central chemoreceptors these are also sensitive to significant decreases in oxygen concentration. If the PaO_2 drops by 40% (8 kPa), the peripheral chemoreceptors become stimulated and impulses are sent to the inspiratory area. However, as the PaO_2 continues to drop to below 6–7 kPa, the cells of the inspiratory area will eventually become hypoxic, decreasing their response. This results in fewer impulses to the inspiratory muscles and leads to a reduction in the respiratory rate.

The respiratory centre is also affected by changes in blood pressure; an increase in blood pressure reduces respiratory rate and a decrease in blood pressure will increase the rate. The changes are detected by baroreceptors and conveyed to the inspiratory centre via the vagus and glosspharyngeal nerves.

Gas exchange

There are three main processes involved in gas exchange:

- Pulmonary ventilation
- External respiration
- Internal respiration

Pulmonary ventilation ('breathing')

During this process, respiratory gases are exchanged between the atmosphere and the lungs. This occurs when a pressure gradient exists between the lungs and the atmosphere.

Inspiration

Inspiration occurs when the pressure in the lungs is lower than atmospheric pressure. The pressure reduction happens when the volume of the lungs increases through contraction of the respiratory muscles. Boyles Law explains this phenomenon: if the volume of a closed container increases, the pressure inside the container reduces and vice versa. When the volume of the container becomes decreased the pressure in the container increases.

The diaphragm is the main respiratory muscle and is innervated by the phrenic nerve. Contraction of the diaphragm, from its resting dome shape to a more flattened one, increases the vertical diameter of the thoracic cavity (Figure 15.2). This action accounts for the movement of more than two thirds of the air that enters the lungs during inspiration.

In conjunction with the diaphragm, the external intercostals muscles contract, lifting the ribs up and out, thereby increasing the anterior–posterior diameter of the thorax.

With contraction of the respiratory muscles, the pressure inside the lungs declines. The intra-alveolar pressure drops from 760 mmHg to 758 mmHg. As atmospheric pressure is 760 mmHg, a pressure gradient results, which allows air to enter the lungs and inspiration to occur. The entry of air continues until the pressures equalise.

During normal breathing, the intrapleural pressures are slightly sub-atmospheric, with a pressure of 756 mmHg prior to inspiration. During inspiration, this pressure drops to 754 mmHg, creating a vacuum effect, with the walls of the lungs being sucked outwards. This movement of the pleural membranes further aids expansion of the lungs.

Expiration

Expiration is also achieved through the creation of pressure gradients, but in this case the pressure inside the lungs becomes greater than atmospheric pressure. This results when respiratory muscles relax, the diaphragm resumes its dome shape and the intercostals relax, causing the rib cage to drop down and inwards. These actions are passive and lead to a reduction in the volume of the lungs, thus increasing the pressure inside them. Air moves out of the lungs and expiration occurs.

The alveoli have very elastic walls, and there is a risk of collapse as they recoil during expiration. The presence of surfactant within the alveoli reduces the surface tension of intra-alveolar water, thus reducing the inward pull of the surface tension and minimising the risk of collapse.

External respiration

This refers to the diffusion of respiratory gases between the alveoli and the blood. During this process, deoxygenated blood within the pulmonary capillaries is reoxygenated. Blood, as it returns back to the heart from the systemic circulation has a PaO_2 of 40 mmHg and a $PaCO_2$ of 45 mmHg. However, in the alveoli, there is a PaO_2 of 105 mmHg and a $PaCO_2$ of 40 mmHg. Therefore, a concentration gradient exists between the alveoli and the blood. Oxygen diffuses into the blood and carbon dioxide diffuses into the alveoli until the concentration becomes the same in the alveoli and blood (Figure 15.3).

There are several features of the lungs that enhance external respiration. First, the alveoli-capillary membrane is only 0.5 μm thick. Secondly, there is a huge surface area across which diffusion can occur. The lungs contain around 300 million alveoli, which creates a $70 m^2$ surface area. Each alveolus is surrounded by a capillary network so, not

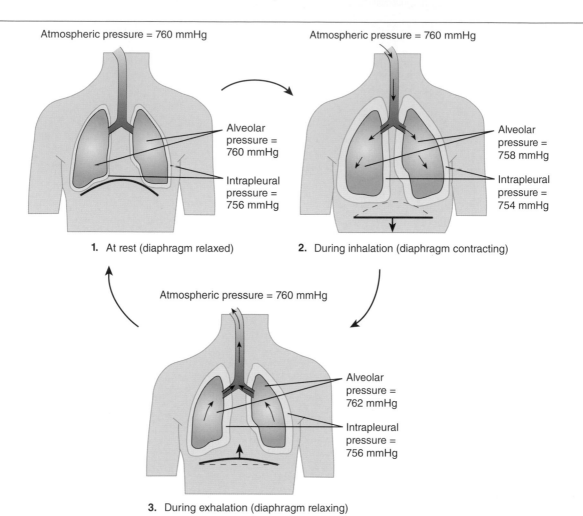

Figure 15.2 Pressure changes in pulmonary ventilation. During inhalation the diaphragm contracts, the chest expands, the lungs are pulled outward, and alveolar pressure decreases. During exhalation, the diaphragm relaxes, the lungs recoil inwards, and alveolar pressure increases, forcing air out of the lungs. Reproduced from *Principles of Anatomy and Physiology 12e* by Gerard Tortora and Bryan Derrickson. Copyright (2009, John Wiley & Sons). Reprinted with permission of John Wiley & Sons Inc.

only is there is a large surface area, but there is also a large blood supply to allow for effective gas exchange. Approximately 900 ml of blood participate in gas exchange at any one time. Furthermore, the pulmonary capillaries are so narrow that the red blood cells flow through them in single file. This allows for maximum perfusion to occur as each red blood cell can participate in gas exchange.

Internal respiration

This process refers to the exchange of gases between the blood and the cells. The left ventricle of the heart pumps blood through the arterial circulation and therefore into arterioles and capillaries. Oxygenated blood within the capillaries has a PaO_2 of 100 mmHg and a $PaCO_2$ of 40 mmHg, while cells have a PaO_2 of 40 mmHg and a $PaCO_2$ of 45 mmHg. Therefore these gases diffuse between the blood and the tissues, as a concentration gradient exists: oxygen diffuses into the tissues and carbon dioxide diffuses into the blood. The deoxygenated blood returning back to the heart has a PaO_2 of 40 mmHg and a $PaCO_2$ of 45 mmHg, where the cycle of external and internal respiration restarts (Figure 15.3).

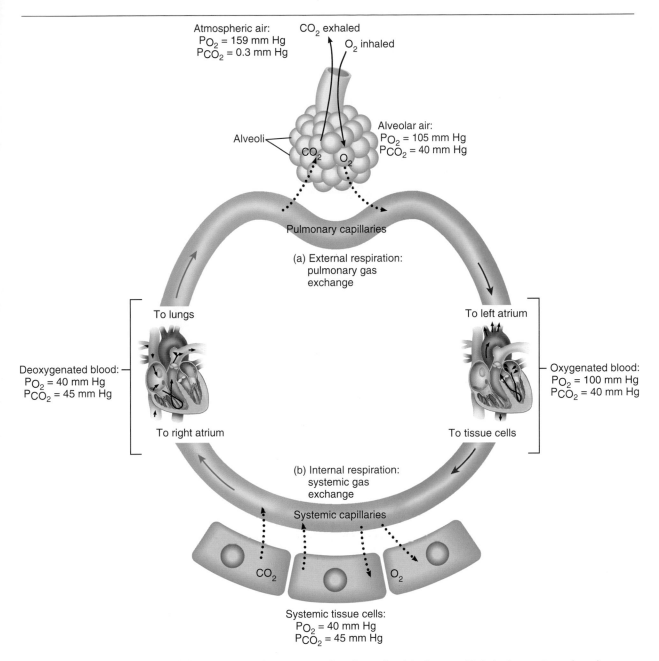

Figure 15.3 Changes in partial pressures of oxygen and carbon dioxide (in mm Hg) during external and internal respiration. Reproduced from *Principles of Anatomy and Physiology 12e* by Gerard Tortora and Bryan Derrickson. Copyright (2009, John Wiley & Sons). Reprinted with permission of John Wiley & Sons Inc.

Transport of gases

The lungs enable the oxygenation of blood and excretion of carbon dioxide; contraction of the heart and the properties of blood itself allow for the delivery and removal of the gases.

Oxygen

Oxygen does not dissolve easily in water and therefore the majority of oxygen (97%) is transported around the body in combination with the haem portion of haemoglobin. The remaining 3% of oxygen is dissolved in plasma. In

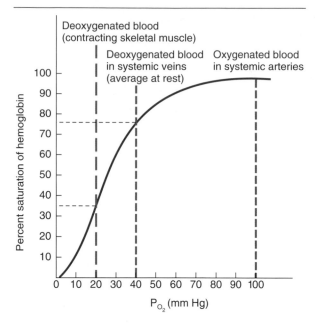

Figure 15.4 Oxygen–haemoglobin dissociation curve showing the relationship between haemoglobin saturation and PaO₂ at normal body temperature. Reproduced from *Principles of Anatomy and Physiology 11e* by Gerard Tortora and Bryan Derrickson. Copyright (2008, John Wiley & Sons). Reprinted with permission of John Wiley & Sons Inc.

resting conditions, 100 ml of blood contains about 20 ml of oxygen. Haemoglobin consists of a pigment portion called haem and a protein portion called globin. The haem portion contains four atoms of iron, each of which can combine with oxygen forming oxyhaemoglobin. This is an easily reversible reaction.

The PaO₂ is the most important factor in determining how much oxygen combines with haemoglobin. If all the haemoglobin is converted to oxyhaemoglobin, then full saturation exists. If the haemoglobin consists of both haemoglobin and oxyhaemoglobin, then partial saturation is present. The oxygen dissociation curve illustrates the degree of saturation of haemoglobin as PaO₂ changes (see Figure 15.4). From this, it is evident that when the PaO₂ is high, the haemoglobin binds with lots of oxygen and is almost totally saturated. However, when the PaO₂ is low, the haemoglobin is only partially saturated and oxygen is released for tissue use. Therefore in the pulmonary capillaries where the PaO₂ is high, lots of oxygen binds with haemoglobin, whereas in the tissues where the

PaO₂ is lower, oxygen is released for diffusion into the tissues.

The ability of oxygen to bind with haemoglobin and to be released for use by the tissues is influenced by pH, temperature and 2,3-diphosphoglycerate (DPG).

pH. Tissues releasing lactic acid and/or having a high PaCO₂ can cause a low pH (acidosis); haemoglobin gives up its oxygen readily in such an environment. This is known as the Bohr effect.

Temperature. An increase in temperature will lead to more oxygen splitting from haemoglobin. In times of increased cellular activity, cells require more oxygen. The heat that is produced due to the increase in metabolic rate will increase the amount of oxygen released from haemoglobin.

2,3-diphosphoglycerate. DPG is produced during glycolysis and can bind reversibly with haemoglobin altering its structure to release oxygen. The amount of DPG produced is greatest during times of decreased oxygen delivery to cells. Therefore, it enhances tissue oxygenation by helping to maintain the release of oxygen from haemoglobin.

Carbon dioxide

Carbon dioxide is transported around the body in several ways. About 7% is dissolved in plasma, around 23% combines with the globin portion of haemoglobin to form carbaminohaemoglobin whereas the remaining 70% is carried within plasma as bicarbonate. The formation of carbaminohaemoglobin is greatly influenced by the PaCO₂. In tissues where PaCO₂ is high, the formation of carbaminohaemoglobin is promoted whereas in the lungs where the PaCO₂ is low, CO₂ readily splits from haemoglobin and diffuses into the alveoli for excretion.

The majority of carbon dioxide is transported in the blood as bicarbonate. This comes about by CO₂ diffusing into the red blood cells where it reacts with water. This requires the enzyme carbonic anydrase, and produces carbonic acid which dissociates into hydrogen and bicarbonate. The hydrogen combines with haemoglobin and the bicarbonate leaves the red blood cell and enters the plasma. To maintain the ionic balance of the red blood cell, chloride leaves the plasma and diffuses into the red blood cell, where it combines with potassium to form potassium chloride. This is known as the chloride shift. The bicarbonate that has diffused into the plasma then combines with sodium to form sodium bicarbonate in the blood (see Figure 15.5).

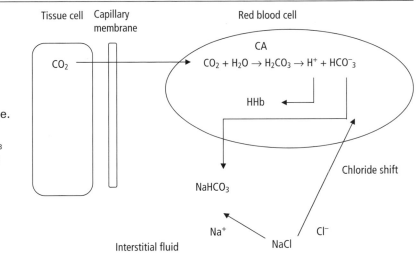

Figure 15.5 Carbon dioxide carriage. CA – carbonic anhydrase; CO_2 – carbon dioxide; H_2O – water; H_2CO_3 – carbonic acid; H^+ – hydrogen ion; HCO^-_3 – bicarbonate ion; HHb – hydrogen buffered with haemoglobin; NaCl – sodium chloride; Na^+ – sodium ion; Cl^- – chloride ion; $NaHCO_3$ – sodium bicarbonate.

Table 15.1 Examples of causes of respiratory failure.

Type 1 respiratory failure	Type 2 respiratory failure	Central nervous system causes of respiratory failure	Peripheral nervous system causes of respiratory failure
• Chest infections • Pulmonary embolism • Pneumothorax • Asthma • Pulmonary oedema • Aspiration • Acute respiratory distress syndrome	• Cerebral injury • Guillain–Barré Syndrome • Myasthenia gravis • Muscular dystrophy • Spinal cord injury • Chest wall injury/ deformity • Drug overdose • Chronic obstructive pulmonary disease	• Head injuries • Intracranial bleeds • Meningitis • Encephalitis • Status epilepticus • Spinal cord injuries • Central sleep apnoea	• Guillain–Barré syndrome (including Miller Fisher variant) • Myasthenia gravis • Motor neurone disease • Botulism

Deoxygenated blood therefore contains carbon dioxide that is transported in a variety of forms. When this blood enters the pulmonary capillaries, the above reactions and events are reversed which allows carbon dioxide to then diffuse into the alveoli.

The effect of respiratory gases on cerebral blood flow

Both CO_2 and O_2 can influence cerebral blood flow (CBF) and need to be controlled if the patient is demonstrating signs of raised intracranial pressure (ICP). Refer to Chapter 6 for a detailed description of how they affect CBF and to Chapter 7 for how CO_2 is manipulated in the management of raised ICP.

Respiratory failure

Respiratory failure is a condition in which the lungs do not properly oxygenate the blood and/or fail to adequately clear carbon dioxide. Respiratory failure is not a specific disease but is rather a result of a number of conditions that impair ventilation, compromise gas exchange or disrupt blood flow through the lungs (Porth, 2004).

There are two types of respiratory failure:

Type 1

Type 1 respiratory failure is defined as hypoxaemia without retention of CO_2 (i.e. $PaO_2 \leq 8\,kPa$ or 60 mmHg).

It is typically caused by a ventilation/perfusion (V/Q) mismatch, i.e. there are areas of low ventilation relative to perfusion (low V/Q units). This is most commonly associated with any acute disease of the lungs (see Table 15.1) which involves fluid filling or collapse of the alveoli. Regardless of the cause, haemoglobin does not become fully saturated with oxygen prior to entering the systemic circulation. This leads to a reduction in the oxygen available to the tissues and organ dysfunction can ensue.

Type 2

Type 2 respiratory failure is defined as hypoxaemia *with* retention of carbon dioxide (i.e. $PaCO_2 > 6.5\,kPa$ or 50 mmHg). This is due to ventilation failure which can occur as a result of:

* Depression of the respiratory centre
* Impairment of the muscles involved in respiration
* Degenerative lung disease
* Airway obstruction

Table 15.1 lists the specific causes of this type of respiratory failure.

With neurological illnesses, respiratory dysfunction could also be categorised in relation to whether it is due to a condition or disease of the central nervous system, or to peripheral nervous system dysfunction (see Table 15.1).

ASSESSMENT OF RESPIRATORY FUNCTION

Physical assessment skills, lung function tests and blood gas analysis are used to determine the patient's respiratory function.

Airway

Assessment of the respiratory system commences with ascertaining whether the patient is able to maintain a patent airway or whether they require an airway adjunct. Neuroscience patients may have a decreased level of consciousness affecting their ability to maintain a patent airway. Patients with a Glasgow Coma Scale (GCS) below 8 will require intubation, however partial obstruction can occur with a much higher GCS.

A fast and easy way to ascertain airway patency is to talk to the patient. If the patient verbally responds their airway is clear. Patients with a reduced level of consciousness are at risk of partial airway obstruction because the tongue becomes flaccid and falls against the posterior pharyngeal wall. Noisy breathing or snoring are signs of partial airway obstruction.

Breathing

Colour

A central cyanosis occurs when large amounts of unsaturated haemoglobin are present and can be detected when the oxygen saturation of arterial blood drops to 85–90% (Lumb, 2000). Central cyanosis is detected by the presence of a bluish greyish colour of the mucus membranes and mouth. Peripheral cyanosis indicates poor circulation.

Respiratory rate

A normal resting respiratory rate in an adult is about 10–18 breaths per minute. Bradypnoea (less than 10 breaths per minute) could indicate: depression of the respiratory centre, hypothermia, opioid overdose or a late sign of raised ICP. Tachypnoea (>20 breaths per minute) may be a sign of pain, anxiety or hypotension.

Depth of breathing

The thorax should rise and fall gently, and there should be equal expansion of the lungs. Unequal expansion could indicate lung collapse, pneumothorax or chronic fibrotic respiratory disease. Shallow breaths (hypopnea) can lead to basal collapse of the lungs and is a potential problem for patients with a reduced conscious level. Deep and rapid breaths (hyperventilation) can be a sign of a metabolic acidosis, e.g. diabetic ketoacidosis or damage to the pons (see below: Rhythms of breathing).

Effort of breathing

Increased work of breathing is evident by the use of additional respiratory muscles. Recruitment of the accessory muscles, i.e. the scalene, the sternomastoids and the external intercostals, can assist the diaphragm in increasing inspiratory effort. Expiration becomes active when the abdominal muscles and internal intercostal muscles are recruited. When the abdominal muscles contract they drive intra-abdominal pressure up, pushing up the diaphragm in the process, which raises pleural pressure, and subsequently alveolar pressure, which results in more air being expelled from the lungs.

Patients with a neuromuscular disorder or a spinal injury may not be able to increase their work of breathing and therefore these signs may be absent.

Rhythm of breathing

The following abnormal breathing patterns maybe observed in neurological patients in a coma:

Cheyne–Stokes breathing: is an irregular breathing pattern that alternates between hyperventilation and hypoventilation sometimes to the point of apnoea. It usually results from bilateral dysfunction of the deep cerebral or diencephalic structures.

Central neurogenic hyperventilation: is regular rapid deep breathing. Patients can breathe 40 to 70 times per minute. It usually results from central lesions of the pons, anterior to the cerebral aqueduct or the fourth ventricle, which result in the loss of the inhibitory influence of the apneustic and pneumotaxic areas on the medullary rhythmicity centre. Possible metabolic and pulmonary causes need to be excluded.

Apneustic breathing: is characterised by prolonged inspiration followed by a pause prior to expiration. This pattern of breathing is caused by lesions of the dorsolateral lower half of the pons, leading to loss of modulation of respiration by the pneumotaxic area.

Cluster breathing: is observed as periodic breathing with irregular frequency and amplitude, with variable pauses between the clusters of breaths. It results from high medullary damage.

Ataxic breathing, or Biot's breathing, is irregular in relation to rate, depth and rhythm. This pattern is caused by medullary lesions, and usually is a preterminal respiratory pattern (Malik and Hess, 2002).

Pain

The location, type, severity and degree of pain present on inspiration/expiration should also be assessed. Pleuritic pain is usually described as severe sharp stretching pain which is worse on inspiration. It is caused by inflammation of the parietal pleura. Musculoskeletal pain originates from the muscles or nerves of the thoracic cage. Tracheitis is described as a constant burning pain in the centre of the chest. It is most commonly caused by a staphylococcus aureus infection.

Auscultation

Auscultation involves listening to the sounds generated by breathing. A lung area on one side of the thorax should be compared to the same area of the opposite lung, i.e. apex of the right compared to apex of the left lung, right base compared to left base.

Breath sounds need to be interpreted in relation to their location, intensity, pitch and duration during inspiration and expiration.

Normal breath sounds

Normal breath sounds are:

Vesicular

These are soft and low pitched. They are heard through inspiration, continue into expiration and gently fade about a third of the way through expiration. They are heard throughout the lung fields.

Broncho-vesicular

These are louder and with a higher pitch than vesicular breath sounds. The inspiratory and expiratory sounds are about equal. These are heard centrally around the 1st and 2nd intercostal spaces.

Bronchial

These sounds are loud and have a high pitch. Expiratory sounds may last slightly longer than the inspiratory sounds. Bronchial sounds are usually heard over the trachea.

If broncho-vesicular or bronchial breath sounds are heard in locations distant from where they should be heard (usually referred to as bronchial breathing), then it is likely that the sound has been transmitted through consolidated or fluid filled lung tissue.

Adventitious sounds

Adventitious sounds are breath sounds that are heard in addition to normal breath sounds. The common adventitious sounds are:

Crackles

Crackles are intermittent, non-musical and brief sounds heard during inspiration. They can either be fine (soft, high pitched and brief) or coarse (louder, lower in pitch and heard for longer). Fine crackles are heard in diseases affecting the lower airways as the alveoli reopen, or when there is fluid in the alveoli and lower airways, e.g. pulmonary oedema. Coarse crackles occur when bronchioles open and are usually caused by copious secretions in the large airways.

Wheeze

Wheeze is a musical sound that is more commonly heard on expiration. Wheezes are high pitched and have a hissing or shrill quality. They are produced by airflow vibrating through narrowed and compressed airways as in asthma or bronchospasm.

Pleural rub

This is a rubbing sound which occurs when the pleural surfaces are roughened by inflammation, neoplasms or infection. They can be heard during inspiration and expiration, and sound like walking on snow.

Stridor

Stridor is an inspiratory musical wheeze which is loudest over the trachea. It is indicative of an obstructed trachea or larynx and requires immediate medical attention.

Breath sounds can also be absent or decreased, e.g. in atelectasis, pneumothorax, pleural effusion.

Transmitted voice sounds

If abnormally located broncho-vesicular or bronchial breath sounds are heard, it is useful to assess transmitted voice sounds. This can be performed by listening with a stethoscope over the chest wall as:

- the patient says 'ninety-nine'. Normally sounds are muffled and indistinct but if there is an area of consolidation, the sound will be louder and clearer. This test is known as bronchophony.
- the patient says 'ee'. Normally this will sound like a muffled long E sound, however over an area of consolidation it will be heard as 'ay'. This is known as egophony.
- the patient whispers 'ninety-nine'. Over an area of consolidation, this will sound louder and clearer. This is known as whispered pectoriloquy.

MONITORING AND INVESTIGATION OF RESPIRATORY FUNCTION

Sputum

Sputum should be examined for colour, consistency and quantity. A sample should be sent for microscopy, culture and sensitivity (MC&S) if infection is suspected.

Pulse oximetry

The non-invasive assessment of the arterial oxygen saturation of haemoglobin is an adjunct to the physical respiratory assessment outlined above. There are however some limitations to its use which include:

Poor peripheral circulation/hypotension

Pulse oximetry relies on a pulsatile pressure therefore the sensor may not detect a sufficiently strong signal to give an accurate reading in patients with poor peripheral circulation.

Anaemia

Haemoglobin that is fully saturated, i.e. SaO_2 98%, will not always imply adequate oxygenation. A low haemoglobin, although fully saturated, may in fact have insufficient oxygen content for adequate tissue oxygenation.

Dysheamoglobinaemias

Pulse oximetry cannot distinguish between carboxyhaemoglin (COHb) and HbO_2. Therefore in situations where COHb may be elevated, e.g. a patient suffering from smoke inhalation or carbon monoxide (CO) poisoning, the readings will be falsely high.

Pigments

Dark fingernail polish can give false readings of up to 3–5%. Dark skin pigmentation can also give inaccurate readings.

Hypercarbia

Although pulse oximetry can detect episodes of hypoxaemia it does not provide any information about levels of carbon dioxide in arterial blood.

Lung function tests

Lung function tests assist in the diagnosis of respiratory disease, but are also essential for the assessment of deterioration of ventilatory function in conditions such as Guillain–Barré syndrome and myasthenia gravis, and following acute spinal cord injury.

The lung function test that is most commonly used in the neurological setting is forced vital capacity (FVC) and forced expiratory volume in one second (FEV1) for which a spirometer is used (spirometry).

Vital capacity (VC) is the maximum volume of air that can be exhaled after a maximal inspiration; it is equivalent to the inspiratory reserve volume plus the tidal volume plus the expiratory reserve volume (Figure 15.6). To measure VC the patient is required to breathe out as hard and fast as possible after maximal inspiration (forced vital capacity, FVC). Most hand held spirometers measure FVC and FEV1. FEV1 measures the volume of air expired in the first second of the FVC. To undertake the test the patient is required to purse their lips tightly around the tube after maximal intake of breath and then to exhale until no more air can be forced out. Patients with facial weakness will find it difficult to create a seal around the mouthpiece, in such cases a face mask can be attached to the spirometer. The patient is asked to repeat the test three times, and the best of the three results is recorded.

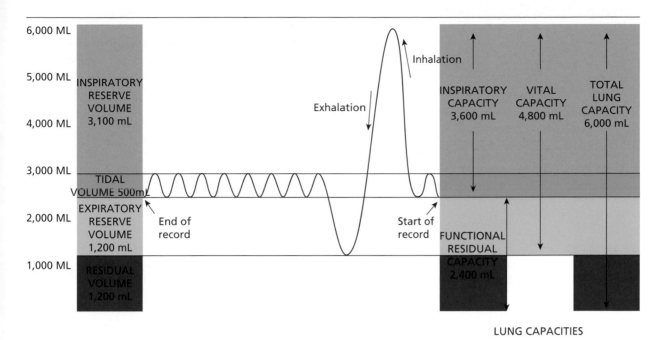

Figure 15.6 Spirogram of lung volumes and capacities.

Table 15.2 Normal blood gas values.

Measurement	Normal blood gas range
pH	7.35–7.45
PaO$_2$	10.0–13.3 kPa
PaCO$_2$	4.6–6.0 kPa
HCO$_3$	22–26 mmol/l
Base excess	−2 to +2
O$_2$ saturation	>95%

Adapted from Adam and Osbourne, 2005.

Forced vital capacity is normally approximately 65 ml/kg, and FEV1 is usually 85% of the FVC. A reduction in FVC to 30 ml/kg is associated with a poor forced cough and the patient may need supplementary oxygen. Elective intubation and mechanical ventilation is indicated if the FVC is less than 20 ml/kg (Ropper *et al.*, 2003). Other

respiratory data must be used in conjunction with the readings to make informed clinical judgements.

Arterial blood gases

In addition to these assessments, arterial blood gases provide useful information about the adequacy of pulmonary gas exchange and the acid base balance. Normal blood gas ranges are given in Table 15.2.

ACID–BASE BALANCE

Hydrogen ions and pH

The body's cells can only function effectively within a narrow range of pH. Each day the body produces hydrogen ions (H$^+$) (acidic) in abundance; these ions must be effectively eliminated from the body to maintain pH within normal range. The more hydrogen ions that are present, the lower the pH becomes. A lower pH indicates an increased relative acidity. If the blood pH falls below 7.35 it is referred to as acidaemia; the physiological change that occurs as a result of the acidaemia is called acidosis. A reduction in hydrogen ion concentration means that the blood becomes more alkaline and the pH will increase; a blood pH >7.45 is referred to as an alkalaemia, and the physiological state is called alkalosis.

As cells only function optimally within a narrow range of pH, the body requires systems to regulate and maintain pH within this range.

Body systems to regulate pH

Buffer

Buffering mechanisms allow for the binding or release of hydrogen ions thereby reducing or increasing the number of free hydrogen ions in solution. When the H^+ is buffered it becomes a much weaker acid and therefore has less effect on the pH than it would if it were unbuffered.

The degree to which the buffers are working to maintain the pH of the blood is reflected within the base excess recording of the blood gas. So in a situation where there is excess H^+, e.g. type II respiratory failure, the buffers respond by buffering the excess H^+ and the number of available buffers will subsequently be reduced. This will be reflected in the base excess reading as a negative reading (otherwise referred to as a base deficit). Conversely in a situation where H^+ concentration is decreasing, e.g. excessive vomiting, buffers will release hydrogen ions in an effort to return the pH to normal. The base excess reading, in this situation, is positive indicating that there are buffers available for hydrogen should the need arise.

Buffers include proteins, phosphates and the carbonic acid–bicarbonate system. The carbonic acid–bicarbonate system only will be briefly explained as this is essential to enable a better understanding of blood gas results. A buffer consists of a buffer pair: a weak acid, i.e. carbonic acid (H_2CO_3), and weak base, i.e. bicarbonate (HCO_3^-). Hydrogen ions produced by cells will react with the HCO_3^- (base) to produce H_2CO_3 (weak acid) which can subsequently be removed from the body by the lungs as CO_2. The H_2CO_3 is a weak acid and has much less effect on the pH than if the H^+ ions remained unbuffered. Thus when the blood becomes more acidic, the HCO_3^- level will decrease as it is used up in the buffering of the excess acids. When there is a reduction in the concentration of hydrogen ions then H_2CO_3 can release H^+ to maintain pH, and the HCO_3^- will subsequently increase.

$$H^+ \; + \; HCO_3^- \leftrightarrow H_2CO_3 \leftrightarrow H_2O + \; CO_2$$
$$\text{hydrogen ion} \; + \; \text{bicarbonate ion} \leftrightarrow \text{carbonic acid} \leftrightarrow \text{water} \; + \; \text{carbon dioxide}$$

Respiratory regulation of pH

If cells produce too much H^+ (metabolic acids) the excess can be converted into carbon dioxide (as outlined above) and eliminated from the body by the respiratory system.

The fall in pH stimulates the respiratory centre to increase the rate and depth of breathing (see: Physiology/Chemical stimuli) which results in more CO_2 being removed by the lungs, returning the pH towards normal. When pH increases the reverse will occur, i.e. a reduced rate and depth of breathing.

Renal regulation of pH (2–3 days)

The kidneys play an essential role in maintaining the pH by excreting large amounts of hydrogen ions in the urine each day. When disturbances in pH occur the kidneys can respond by changing the rates of hydrogen and bicarbonate ion excretion. Therefore if the blood becomes more acidic (fall in pH) the kidneys respond by excreting more hydrogen and reabsorbing more bicarbonate ions. When alkalaemia develops (increase in pH) the rate of hydrogen ion excretion declines and the rate of bicarbonate ion reabsorption also declines.

There are four common disturbances of acid base balance. Disturbances can be due to a respiratory or a metabolic cause and will result in either an acidosis or alkalosis.

DISTURBANCES OF ACID–BASE BALANCE

Respiratory disturbances

If the pH disturbance is due to a respiratory cause the *primary* change will be in the carbon dioxide level. Carbon dioxide is an acid when it combines with water. Therefore, an increase in carbon dioxide will result in a fall in pH ($PaCO_2$ will be high and pH will be low); this disturbance is called a *respiratory acidosis*. The reverse will happen if there is a decrease in the carbon dioxide ($PaCO_2$ will be low and pH will be high); this is called respiratory alkalosis.

The primary cause of a respiratory acidosis is type II respiratory failure (see: Respiratory failure). *Respiratory alkalosis* is much less common and it is caused by hyperventilation. In neurological patients this can be caused by lesions in the region of the pons (see: Central neurogenic hyperventilation).

Metabolic disturbances

When there is a metabolic cause for changes in pH, the *primary* change will be the bicarbonate level. A *metabolic acidosis* can result from the body producing too many acids, e.g. poor perfusion of tissues resulting in a build up of lactic acid; renal failure resulting in a failure to eliminate excess hydrogen ion and, less commonly, due to excess loss of alkaline from the body, e.g. profuse diarrhoea. Regardless of the cause, the metabolic acidosis will result in an excess of hydrogen ions which will be buffered by the bicarbonate ions. There will therefore be a reduction in the bicarbonate level (HCO_3^- will be low, pH will be low and the base excess reading will be negative).

A decrease in the concentration levels of hydrogen ions or an increase in bicarbonate levels results in a *metabolic alkalosis*, but this is relatively uncommon. It can occur due to excessive losses of acid either through the renal or gastrointestinal system, i.e. diuretics or profuse vomiting. The bicarbonate will be raised, the pH will be raised and the base excess will be positive.

Compensatory mechanisms

In certain situations, when there has been long-term derangement of either metabolic or respiratory function, compensation of the pH disturbance occurs. Blood gas analysis would reveal a normal pH, despite either the HCO_3^- or $PaCO_2$ being outside 'normal' limits. In compensation, the primary (or chronic) alteration will be compensated for by the 'opposite' system. For example, with chronic carbon dioxide retention, the high levels of carbon dioxide are compensated for by bicarbonate retention by the kidneys. Therefore, there is metabolic compensation for the respiratory problem. In metabolic acidosis, the compensation seen will be an increase in respiratory rate with a subsequent reduction in carbon dioxide. Therefore there is removal of carbon dioxide to compensate for the metabolic acidosis and thus the pH is helped to return to within a normal range.

NURSING CARE/MANAGEMENT

Airway management

Emergency airway equipment should be easily accessible by the bedside of all neurological patients. Suction equipment should be checked at least once per shift to ensure that it is in working order and that the necessary sized suction catheters are available (see below: Suctioning), in addition to a yankuer sucker to clear the mouth and orophaynx of blood, vomitus and excessive secretions. Flow meters for piped oxygen should have the appropriate nipple nozzle to enable quick attachment of oxygen tubing or bag-valve mask if required. Airway adjuncts of various sizes should also be available.

A compromised airway is managed in the first instance by head tilt and chin lift. The severity of airway compromise will determine subsequent management. Patients with a reduced level of consciousness may not be able to maintain a patent airway, therefore, an airway adjunct may be required to maintain an open, patent airway. Partial airway obstruction can lead to hypoxia and hyper-

capnia which can further compromise neuronal function, so early identification and appropriate management is essential.

Positioning the patient in the recovery position may suffice for patients who are drowsy, but continuous assessment is required to ensure that the patient is able to maintain optimal oxygenation and ventilation. Oropharyngeal airways should not be used in patients who are conscious as they will trigger the gag reflex. A nasopharyngeal airway will not trigger the gag reflex and is better tolerated in the conscious patient. Chest secretions can be suctioned via a nasopharyngeal airway. Their use is however contraindicated in patients with suspected basal skull fracture, so they should not be used following head injury until skull integrity has been confirmed on x-ray. Other contraindications include patients with nasal polyps, and, because of the high risk of causing haemorrhage during insertion, they should be used cautiously in patients who are receiving anticoagulants or who have coagulopathies.

An oropharyngeal airway can be used as a short term measure for airway maintenance if a patient is unconscious; however, this does not protect against aspiration of oral secretions such as saliva or gastric contents should the patient vomit/regurgitate. They should only be inserted by practitioners who are competent to do so, as incorrect insertion can displace the tongue into the pharynx, causing airway obstruction. If a patient has a GCS < 8, they should be assessed by an anaesthetist for intubation. An endotracheal tube maintains a patent airway and protects against aspiration of oral/gastric secretions. If a patient is intubated they will require admission to an intensive care unit for ongoing care and support.

If a patient has a longer term reduction in the level of consciousness or bulbar dysfunction resulting in an inability to maintain a patent airway for the foreseeable future, a tracheostomy may be required. A tracheostomy may also be performed if a patient is likely to require mechanical ventilation for more than seven days.

Tracheostomy management

Tracheostomy formation can either be a surgical procedure which requires a horizontal incision between the second and third tracheal ring, or a percutaneous approach may be used during which a dilator system is used to insert the tracheostomy tube; the latter is more common. There is evidence to suggest that there is less perioperative bleeding and post-operative complications associated with the percutaneous approach (Freeman *et al.*, 2000), but the decision as to which approach is used will be influenced by available resources as well as the patient's anatomy and

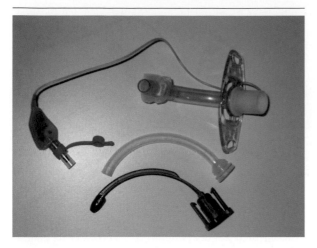

Figure 15.7 A double lumen cuffed tracheostomy tube.

medical requirements. Following insertion, the tube should remain in place for five to seven days to allow for the skin to trachea tract to form (Marino, 1998). Following this, the tube can be changed as required.

Tracheostomy tubes

There are a variety of different tubes available. The type of tube used will depend on a number of factors, e.g. the length of the time it is anticipated that the patient will require the tracheostomy, and the purpose of the tube, e.g. for clearance of secretions only or for ongoing ventilation.

Single and double lumen tubes

Single lumen tubes are typically placed when a tracheostomy is newly formed, although it is becoming more common to use double lumen tubes from the outset (Figure 15.7). After five to seven days, a single lumen tube is usually changed to a double lumen tube. The inner tube acts as a removable liner for the more permanent, outer tube. The advantage of the inner tube or cannula is that it can be withdrawn for brief periods to be cleaned, which helps to prevent blockage. If the tube did become blocked the inner cannula can be temporarily removed to leave a patent airway.

Cuffed and uncuffed tubes

A cuff is a soft balloon around the distal end of the tube that can be inflated to create a complete seal with the walls of the trachea (see Figure 15.7). The cuff provides protection of the airway and reduces the risk of aspirate reaching the lungs or, in ventilated patients, ensures that gases reach the lungs. When the cuff is inflated, the patient is unable

to phonate as air is prevented from passing over the vocal cords. An uncuffed tube is often used if a patient has a weak cough, and therefore cannot clear their secretions effectively, but has a safe swallow and is breathing spontaneously.

Fenestrated or unfenestrated

Some double lumen tubes have a fenestration (window or hole) within the outer tube. Fenestrated tubes are very useful for weaning patients off a tracheostomy. The fenestration enables air to pass through the patient's oral/nasal pharynx as well as the tracheal stoma, which helps patients to return to normal breathing. The fenestration also permits speech when the cuff is deflated, and a speaking valve is placed on the opening of the tracheostomy because exhaled air can then pass over the vocal cords.

Cuff-related complications of a tracheostomy

The cuff prevents leakage of respiratory gases through the mouth and helps to reduce the risk of aspiration of oral secretions. The cuff is designed to allow the trachea to be sealed with minimum risk of pressure-induced injury to the tracheal mucosa. The cuff pressure should be routinely checked, e.g. once a shift, and should be less than capillary closure pressure of 24–30 cm H_2O (St John, 1999). It is recommended that cuff pressures should be <25 cmH_2O. The main cuff related problems are:

Aspiration

Despite the presence of an inflated cuff, aspiration of mouth secretions and enteral nutrition can still occur. This risk can be reduced if 30° to 45° semi-recumbent positioning is used, oral secretions are regularly suctioned and cuff pressures are regularly checked.

Cuff leaks

If a leak is present respiratory gases can pass around the cuff and move out of the lungs, and oral secretions can pass down into the lungs. When this occurs in a mechanically ventilated patient, ventilation may become compromised. Cuff leaks are usually detected by sounds generated as the air passes over the vocal cords. However, cuff leaks are rarely caused by disruption of the cuff itself. It is more likely that a cuff leak results from non-uniform contact between the cuff and the trachea wall. A leak can also be caused by faulty function of the one way valve at the air injection inlet that normally keeps the cuff inflated (see Figure 15.7). If these valves leak, air can escape from the cuff. Although this is not a common problem, if the valve fails, the tracheostomy tube will need to be replaced.

Following the formation of a tracheostomy, the trachea may be inflamed and oedematous. As healing occurs, the inflammation will subside increasing the lumen of the trachea. This could lead to a cuff leak and is especially likely if the patient is receiving active treatment for inflammation, for example with steroids (Moore and Woodrow, 2004).

If a cuff leak is present, the cuff should be inflated until the sounds of a leak (e.g. gurgling, audible words or the sound of air through the patient's mouth) disappear and then the cuff pressure should be rechecked. If it is more than $25\,cmH_2O$, then the tracheal tube should be replaced as tracheal ulceration may develop (Marino, 1998).

Ulceration

Inflated cuffs place continuous pressure on the tracheal epithelium and therefore ulceration of the trachea can develop. Maintaining the cuff pressures at the lowest possible pressure to prevent a cuff leak will help to reduce the risk of ulcer development while maintaining a seal.

Loss of normal airway function

Normally, inspired air passes through the upper airways which warm, humidify and filter it. A tracheostomy by-passes the upper airway and therefore the air needs to be warmed and humidified through artificial means. Ideally a heated humidifier system should be used as this delivers $44\,mg\,H_2O/l$ at $37°C$ with a relative humidity of 100%. This is essentially the same humidification that occurs during normal breathing. A cold water humidifier only has a relative humidity of 50%. A heat moisture exchanger (HME) filter generally delivers about $25\,mg\,H_2O/l$, so there is considerably less humidification of the air when using this device.

Tracheal stenosis

Stenosis of the trachea is a late complication that can appear days to weeks following tracheal decannulation. The clinical features include dyspnoea, wheezing and in severe cases stridor. It is the result of cuff pressure and infection causing ischaemic death of tracheal cartilage and scarring. Low-pressure cuffs markedly reduce the occurrence of cuff injury.

Specific nursing care of the patient with a tracheostomy

Safety priorities

All patients who have a tracheostomy must have tracheal dilators and two spare tracheostomy tubes at their bedside at all times, for situations of accidental extubation. The replacement tubes should be the same size and one size smaller than the tube in place. A smaller tube is often required if the tracheostomy is newly formed and will be easier to insert in an emergency. Suction, oxygen, airway adjuncts, and a bag valve mask (BVM) should be available and ready to use by the patient's bedside.

Care of the stoma/prevention of site infection

The newly formed stoma is a surgical wound and therefore needs to be routinely aseptically cleaned and dressed to prevent infection. Dressings should be renewed daily (more often if indicated) and the site inspected for signs of inflammation, infection or bleeding. Normal saline (NaCl 0.9%) is sufficient to clean the site and a dry dressing such as lyofoam® is used to protect the site.

Changing the dressing always requires two people in order to prevent accidental extubation. One person undertakes the dressing whilst the second person holds the tube firmly in place, but taking care not to move the tube inwards, which will cause the patient to have explosive coughing. Following the dressing change, the ties/tube holder can be changed. This should be tight enough to allow for two fingers to slide beneath the ties so that they are not uncomfortably tight for the patient.

Inner tube management

If a double lumen tube is used, the inner tube should be used at all times and, when it is removed for cleaning, a spare inner tube should be inserted. There is no consensus on how frequently the inner tube should be cleaned. The need should be assessed on an individual patient basis as it largely depends on the amount and consistency of secretions. Inner tubes can be fenestrated or unfenestrated, but it is important to ensure that an unfenestrated inner tube is inserted prior to suctioning as the suction catheter can pass through the fenestration and damage the lining of the trachea.

Communication

A tracheostomy tube is inserted below the vocal cords so it is usual for patients who have a cuffed tube *in situ* not to be able to make sounds. Loss of speech is isolating and creates difficulties in expressing needs or concerns. The nurse should explain to the patient that this is a temporary loss and once the tracheostomy is removed, normal speech should be regained. However, information such as this must be appropriate to the individual patient; a patient who has expressive dysphasia or has dysarthria and also requires a tracheostomy may not ever regain normal speech due to the neurological dysfunction. Communication aides in the form of letter boards, pen and paper, keyboards or signs will reduce isolation and their use should be encouraged. The patient should also be encouraged to mouth words and family and friends supported to lip read.

Speaking valves can also be used. Speaking valves are one way valves which are placed on the tracheostomy opening: air enters through the tube on inspiration but closes during expiration. This allows air to pass over the vocal cords and therefore speech can be facilitated. To be able to use a speaking valve, the cuff must be deflated and therefore the patient must be able to swallow safely and have a cough reflex. This will require formal assessment by the speech and language therapist (SLT) (see Chapter 12).

Weaning and removal of the tracheostomy tube (decannulation)

Most patients with a tracheostomy will recover sufficiently to have the tracheostomy removed. Removing the tube increases work of breathing by a third (Chadda *et al.*, 2002), so the patient does need to be carefully assessed to ensure that they will be able to cope with the additional effort required and will be able to cough effectively enough to clear secretions. Assessment of the patient prior to decannulation ensures that:

* There is no ongoing requirement for mechanical ventilation that cannot be met through non-invasive methods
* There is an adequate cough (peak expiratory cough flows > 200 l/min)
* There is no physiologically significant upper airway lesion (such as overgranulation or tracheal stenosis) or swelling

(Bourjeily *et al.*, 2002)

The weaning process should be systematic and involve the multidisciplinary team (Hunt and McGowan 2005). Tracheostomy management is often undertaken by a specific tracheostomy team consisting of a SLT, physiotherapist, nurses and medical staff who will review patients with tracheostomies across the hospital. If this is not available, then the team should include at least one member of staff who is confident and competent in tracheostomy management.

The weaning process should be stepped with a flexible approach that is reflective of the patient's ability and individual needs. Braine and Sweby (2006) advocate a six stepped approach, which allows the patient to progress to decannulation safely. This may require changing the tube to a fenestrated tube or perhaps using a tube that is a smaller size.

It is advocated that prior to decannulation, the patient should have had the following procedures:

* Swallow assessed by a SLT
* Cuff deflated for at least 24 hours without an indication of aspiration or increase in chest infection
* Tracheostomy capped off for 24 hours

(Serra, 2000)

Following removal of the tube, the stoma should be covered with an occlusive dressing forming a complete seal. The stoma should close up within a few days.

RESPIRATORY SUPPORT

Depending on the underlying condition of the patient, their presentation and assessment findings, respiratory support may be required. In type 1 respiratory failure when hypoxaemia is the primary respiratory problem, efforts must be made to improve tissue oxygenation. This may be achieved through the administration of higher concentrations of oxygen and/or the use of positive end expiratory pressure (PEEP) (see below: Continuous positive airway pressure (CPAP)). In type 2 respiratory failure, there is retention of carbon dioxide so the mechanics of ventilation need to be improved. To reduce the carbon dioxide, the patient's minute volume needs to be increased; this can be achieved by either increasing the tidal volumes of the patient, or increasing the respiratory rate or, indeed, doing both. Therefore ventilatory support is needed which can be either invasive or non-invasive.

Oxygen therapy and delivery devices

Neurological patients often require oxygen therapy to optimise respiratory and neurological function. There are a number of oxygen delivery devices which generally can be categorized into those that can deliver a specific oxygen concentration (fixed performance delivery systems) and those that do not (variable performance delivery systems). The condition of the patient will determine which device is used.

Variable performance devices

Variable performance devices include nasal cannulae and simple face masks and deliver a variable concentration of oxygen. Because they deliver oxygen at flow rates below the normal patient inspiratory flow rate, the oxygen concentration that is delivered will depend on the patient's rate and depth of breathing. For example a patient breathing rapidly and deeply will entrain large volumes of room air which will dilute the supplemental oxygen being delivered. As the exact percentage being delivered cannot be determined, the prescription for oxygen should be written in litres/min and not as a percentage. The variable performance delivery systems should not be used in patients where hypoxia is a concern.

Fixed performance devices

A fixed performance device, such as the Venturi system, delivers a prescribed concentration of oxygen as stated on the valve, irrespective of the patient's breathing pattern. It delivers oxygen at rates above the normal patient inspiratory flow rate, which is made possible by the Venturi valve which accelerates the oxygen flow and mixes it with air in a precise ratio. Table 15.3 provides a summary of oxygen delivery devices, their indications for use and specific management.

Table 15.3 Oxygen delivery devices.

Oxygen delivery device	Indications for use and specific management
Nasal cannula (NC) (Variable flow)	• Delivers low concentrations of oxygen • Maximum flow rate is 5–6 l/min • Variable performance, the oxygen concentration delivered will be dependent on the patient's rate and depth of breathing • Suitable for patients requiring low flow oxygen • Can dry nasal membranes • Humidifiers are now available for NC, which should be used if administering >4 l/min • Less claustophobic than a facemask
Simple face mask, e.g. Hudson (Variable flow)	• Need to ensure adequate flow to prevent rebreathing of CO_2 (>5 l/min) • Variable performance, the oxygen concentration delivered will be dependent on the patient's rate and depth of breathing
Humidified oxygen, e.g. Aquapak	• Administers specific oxygen concentration providing flow rates are set as per flow instructions on port (determined by air entrainment port on Aquapak valve) • Provides humidification and greater patient comfort • Can be noisy at higher flow rates • Water in the tubing will cause backpressure resistance which leads to inaccurate concentrations being delivered
Venturi mask (Fixed flow)	• Delivers a specific oxygen concentration so long as the flow rate is set to the required level (as indicated on the Venturi valve) • Valves available in 24%, 28%, 35%, 40% and 60% • The large volume of entrained room air will provide adequate humidification for short term use • Most useful for patients requiring fixed low concentrations of oxygen
Nonrebreathe mask (Variable flow)	• Delivers high concentration of oxygen (up to 90%) • Used in emergency situations – where the patient is breathing spontaneously but where there is evidence of hypoxia • One way valve prevents CO_2 from entering the reservoir bag • Fill the reservoir bag before placing on the patient and ensure it remains inflated during delivery • Set the flow rate at 15 l/min • A tight fit is necessary • Short term use only

NON-INVASIVE RESPIRATORY SUPPORT

Non-invasive respiratory support avoids the use of invasive strategies. The two forms of non-invasive strategies which are used are continuous positive airway pressure (CPAP) and non-invasive ventilation (NIV).

Continuous positive airway pressure (CPAP)

CPAP is primarily used in situations of type 1 respiratory failure when higher concentrations of supplementary oxygen via a fixed delivery system (such as the Venturi system) or humidified circuit are not resolving the patient's hypoxaemia. It is also used as a way of weaning from mechanical support. Positive pressure is applied throughout the respiratory breath cycle which increases the functional residual capacity, thereby increasing the opportunity for gas exchange to take place (Keen, 2000). In addition, work of breathing is reduced as lung compliance is improved (Kannan, 1999).

The CPAP system consists of a high flow generator that is capable of delivering the required pressure throughout the breath cycle, a tightly fitting mask or T piece for use with a tracheostomy tube, and a flow resistor on the distal portion to the circuit (CPAP valve) through which the patient exhales (see Figure 15.8). The pressure from the flow generator needs to be sufficient to keep the valve within the flow resistor open throughout the breath cycle. It is usual to have an oxygen analyser within the circuit so that the prescribed oxygen concentration can be delivered.

It is essential to have a second CPAP valve within the circuit (a pressure relief valve) which requires a pressure of at least 5 cm H_2O above the prescribed CPAP level to open it: this acts as a safety valve should the CPAP valve through which the patient is exhaling become occluded or stuck (MHRA, 2000).

The CPAP mask needs to be tightly fitting to prevent air leaks and loss of pressure which patients may find difficult to tolerate. Pressure damage particularly on bony prominences may develop and the patient may experience claustrophobia. Air leaks could cause corneal dryness and abrasions. Therefore, CPAP via a face mask is seen to be a temporary measure to avoid or postpone intubation (Marino, 1998).

More recently CPAP helmets are being used in the critical care setting. These avoid some of the complications of using a CPAP mask and are generally less claustrophobic and well tolerated (Antonelli *et al.*, 2005). Patroniti *et al.* (2003) found that there was little difference between mask and helmet in the delivery of CPAP, but to avoid re-breathing of CO_2, the helmet required higher flow rates. The transparent helmet allows for better patient communication and interaction with their surroundings. Patient compliance with the mask and CPAP is enhanced when the patients is well educated, prior to the application of the CPAP, about its purpose, and by continued support from the nurse caring for the patient.

CPAP via a mask is contraindicated in patients who have a reduced level of consciousness, as there is a risk of aspira-

Table 15.4 CPAP/NIV nursing considerations.

Patient problem	Nursing actions
Mask related problems	
Tolerance	Consider use of CPAP helmet. Offer psychological support to assist patient tolerance
Claustrophobia	Ensure mask correctly sized and fitted
Eye irritation– corneal drying and abrasion	Avoid air leaks
Tissue damage	Consider use of foam backed dressings (e.g. Granuflex®) on bridge of nose/ears
Difficulties of receiving CPAP/NIV	
Communication	Use of communication aides
Eating and drinking difficult	If possible, ensure patient has breaks from using CPAP/NIV for nutrition and hydration. NB: Closely observe SpO_2 throughout and recommence CPAP/NIV as clinically indicated
Gastric distension	Consider use of nasogastric tube to decompress stomach

CPAP – continuous positive airway pressure; NIV – non-invasive ventilation.

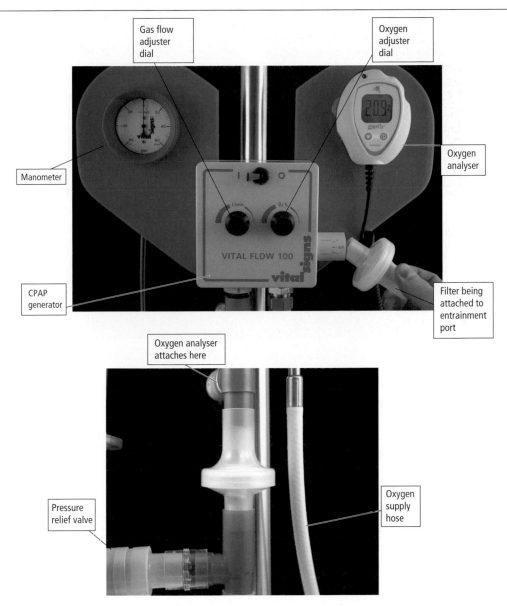

Figure 15.8 Continuous positive airway pressure (CPAP) circuit. Reproduced with permission from Vital Signs Limited.

tion if they vomit, and in patients with facial trauma. The tight mask and straps could reduce cerebral venous return and therefore could increase ICP, so the potential risk/benefit for patients with suspected raised ICP should be assessed on an individual basis. Refer to Table 15.4 for how to troubleshoot common problems of CPAP and the section below on the adverse effects of positive airway pressure support.

Non-invasive ventilation (NIV)

The British Thoracic Society (2002) recommends that NIV is indicated for:

- Chronic obstructive pulmonary disease (COPD) with a respiratory acidosis
- Hypercapnic respiratory failure secondary to neuromuscular disease, e.g. Guillain–Barré syndrome, myasthenia

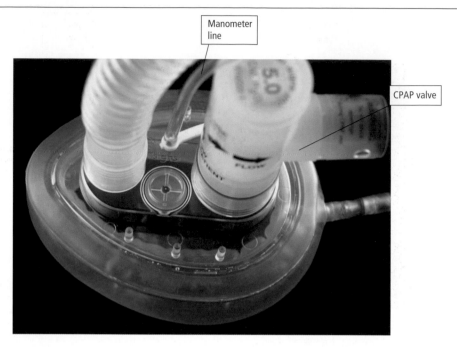

Figure 15.8 *(Continued)*

gravis, or spinal injuries, or chest wall deformity, e.g. scoliosis

NIV can also be used to improve quality of life for patients with motor neurone disease (Bourke *et al.*, 2006) (see Chapter 27), and to treat central sleep apnoea (Garner and Amin, 2006).

NIV is also referred to as Bilevel NIV and often the brand name of whatever system is used (such as NIPPY®, BiPAP®). As these machines were initially developed for domiciliary ventilation, they are often easy to use but offer relatively few options compared to the positive pressure ventilators used for invasive ventilation within the intensive care setting.

The principle of NIV is to reduce carbon dioxide by increasing the patient's spontaneous minute volume. There is alternation between two pressure levels during the breath cycle: a higher level on inspiration and a lower one on expiration. The inspiratory positive airway pressure (IPAP) provides support on inspiration so that a larger inspiratory volume is taken, which reduces the work of breathing and increases alveolar ventilation (Tully, 2002). The higher the IPAP the more air is exchanged and the more CO_2 is removed. The expiratory positive airway pressure (EPAP) creates less resistance and discomfort on expiration, prevents alveolar collapse and increases functional residual capacity (Figure 15.9). Increasing the difference between the IPAP and the EPAP increases the volume of each breath. This augmentation of the tidal volume will enhance carbon dioxide clearance.

As with CPAP, NIV is usually delivered via a tight fitting mask therefore the same complications of the mask apply. If used for domiciliary ventilation, a nasal mask can be used rather than a facemask (see Table 15.4 and Chapter 27 for nursing care considerations).

Adverse effects of positive end expiratory pressure (PEEP)

In normal breathing, i.e. without respiratory support the total volume of inhaled air with each breath (tidal volume) is exhaled completely. The normal airway pressure at the end of expiration and before inspiration is therefore equivalent to atmospheric pressure. With CPAP and NIV there is a pressure greater than that of atmospheric pressure remaining within the alveoli at the end of expiration (PEEP) therefore the distal airways are less likely to collapse, preventing atelectasis and improving oxygenation. Additionally, PEEP can reopen collapsed alveoli, improving gas exchange through alveolar recruitment.

However, there are adverse effects of PEEP that need to be considered, particularly in patients with raised ICP. The application of PEEP will increase central venous pressure

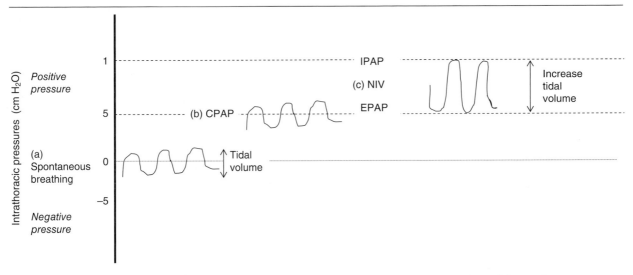

Figure 15.9 Effect of CPAP and NIV on spontaneous breathing. (a) Spontaneous breathing – the intrathoracic pressures alternate between positive and negative. (b) Once CPAP is applied – the same pattern of breathing occurs as is seen in spontaneous breathing but the intrathoracic pressures remain positive throughout. (c) If NIV is applied, the tidal volumes of spontaneous breathing are increased due to the IPAP that is applied to inspiration. The pressures are positive throughout the breath cycle. CPAP – Continuous positive airway pressure; EPAP – expiratory positive airway pressure; IPAP – inspiratory positive airway pressure; NIV – non-invasive ventilation.

which may in turn induce an increase in intracranial pressure through impeding cerebral venous return. The increase in central venous pressure (CVP) can also result in reduced cardiac filling pressures with a subsequent reduction of cardiac output and blood pressure, which could produce reductions in cerebral perfusion pressure (CPP) and may lead to cerebral ischaemia. However, this is more likely in patients who are haemodynamically unstable and who have impaired cerebral autoregulation (Muench *et al.*, 2005). Low levels of PEEP ($\leq$5 cm H_2O) are usually well tolerated without haemodynamic effects (Myburgh, 2003). Higher levels of PEEP in patients with raised ICP should be used with caution and with close monitoring of the patient's haemodynamic status and ICP. The risk/benefit of the application of higher PEEP is assessed on an individual patient basis. The benefits of adequate oxygenation may be assessed as being more important than the possible risk of increasing ICP in some patients.

Intermittent positive pressure breathing (IPPB)

Intermittent positive pressure breathing is the delivery of positive airway pressure throughout inspiration in the spontaneously breathing patient. It is most commonly used as an adjunct to physiotherapy. The most commonly used machine is called the Bird 7 ventilator (more commonly referred to as the BIRD). IPPB augments tidal volume which helps in the clearance of bronchial secretions and in improving gas exchange. It is typically used for short sessions to optimise respiratory function. In the neurological setting it is commonly used in patients with neuromuscular disease affecting the respiratory muscles, e.g. Guillain–Barré syndrome and myasthenia gravis, and following acute spinal cord injury when the respiratory muscles are affected.

If the Bird is being used by the physiotherapist to treat a patient it should form part of the patient's regular respiratory management and nurses should therefore be competent in using the equipment. By working collaboratively with the physiotherapist optimal respiratory care can be given. The Bird is fairly straightforward to use. There are three controls that are usually set by the physiotherapist. The pressure control is usually set between 12 and 15 cmH_2O. When the patient takes a breath either through a mouthpiece or mask the airflow will continue until the set pressure is reached. The ease with which a breath is triggered and the rate at which the gas flows are determined by the sensitivity and flow rate controls respectively. Patients are encouraged to take slow breaths through the mouth until the pressure is reached. A nebuliser can be incorporated into the circuit during treatment. When patients have difficulty using the mouth piece due to neuromuscular facial weakness a facemask can be used.

The Bird is often used by several patients within the same clinical area. In such cases it is imperative to prevent cross infection. Each patient's disposable breathing circuit (which attaches directly to the Bird) should be kept by the patient's bedside in an appropriate container and dated. The Bird should be cleaned as per local protocol between patients.

The management of patients requiring invasive respiratory support is beyond the scope of this book. Readers should consult a comprehensive critical care nursing text such as Adam and Osbourne (2005).

SUCTIONING

Clearing chest secretions by suctioning through either an endotracheal tube, tracheostomy tube or nasopharyngeal airway is an essential part of nursing care. There are clear indications when suctioning is required and 'routine' suctioning, for example, every 4 hours, should be avoided. The indications include:

- Coarse breath sounds on auscultation
- Spontaneous coughing
- Audible/visible secretions in tracheostomy tube
- Increased work of breathing
- Deteriorating blood gases/SpO_2 (saturation of haemoglobin with oxygen as measured by pulse oximetry)

There are inherent risks to suctioning which could be detrimental to the neurological patient. These include hypoxia and cardiac instability such as bradycardia, arrhythmias or hypotension. In patients with a spinal cord injury, there is an increased risk of these cardiovascular complications due to possible unopposed vagal stimulation (see: Neurogenic shock in Chapter 14).

Prior to suctioning, the patient should be informed of the procedure. Suctioning can be uncomfortable and adequate preparation of the patient can avoid undue anxiety and distress. Suctioning can increase ICP, so it is important to ensure that those patients who are at risk of deleterious rises in ICP are adequately sedated prior to suction. In ventilated patients Kerr and colleagues (1997) found that short duration, controlled hyperventilation with 30 breaths

per minute reduced $PaCO_2$ which resulted in a short lived reduction in cerebral blood flow. This subsequently led to fewer rises in ICP during suctioning and cerebral perfusion was maintained.

Suctioning can reduce SaO_2 so preoxygenation is recommended to avoid hypoxaemia and cardiovascular compromise (Thompson *et al.*, 2000; Wong, 2000). If atelectasis is present, several hyperinflation breaths may be useful, however its use is not without risk and should only be performed by suitably trained staff. Barotrauma, ventilator induced lung injury and patient discomfort may result (Robson, 1998). There is also an increased risk of cardiovascular instability, so suctioning should be avoided in patients with serious cardiac pathology.

A suction pressure of 100–150 mmHg or 15–20 kPa should be used during suctioning. Mucosal trauma, hypoxia and negative pressure atelectasis can occur if too high a suction pressure is used (Wood, 1998). If secretions are thick, the suction pressure should not be increased: the secretions should be made looser through humidification and saline nebulisers.

The instillation of saline does not have any proven benefit (O'Neal *et al.*, 2001). In fact, it has been shown that:

- The instillation of saline increases risk of infection (Glass and Grap, 1995)
- As saline and secretions do not mix, the secretions are not thinned (Ackerman, 1993)
- Instilled saline does not disperse beyond the main bronchi, therefore it does not affect lung periphery secretions (Hanley *et al.*, 1978)
- To elicit a cough, suction catheter stimulation is as effective as saline (Gray *et al.*, 1990)

During the suction procedure, suction should not be applied on insertion to avoid trauma, atelectasis and hypoxaemia. On withdrawing the catheter, continuous suction should be applied as this technique prevents mucus plug loss and reduces direct suction on the tracheal wall. The application of suction should be limited to a maximum of 15 seconds duration to avoid suctioning complications (McKelvie, 1998) and to a maximum of two suction passes per procedure in patients with raised ICP (Wainwright and Gould, 1996). The likelihood of these complications occurring also increases with multiple suctioning attempts.

The suction catheter should be the correct size in relation to the inner lumen of the endotrachel tube (ETT) or tracheostomy:

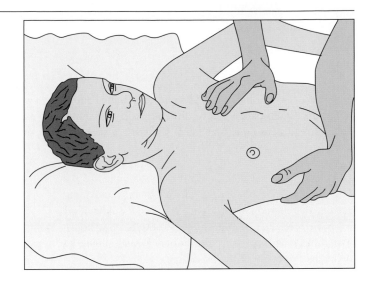

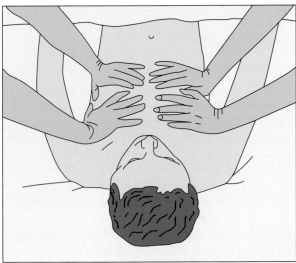

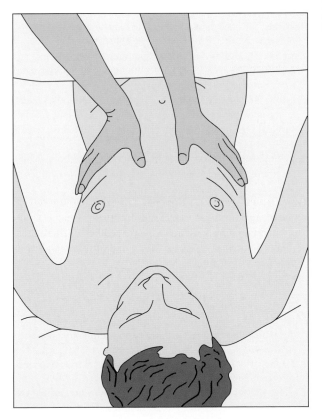

Figure 15.10 Different hand positions to give an assisted cough.

- ETT/tracheostomy size 7.5   size 10 catheter
- ETT/tracheostomy size 8   size 12 catheter
- ETT/tracheostomy size 8.5   size 12 catheter
- ETT/tracheostomy size 9   size 14 catheter

If the catheter selected is too big for the lumen of the ETT, the catheter blocks the airway during suctioning causing alveolar collapse (Dean, 1997) and the flow of air down the tube also becomes impeded (McKelvie, 1998). Suctioning is an invasive procedure so asepsis should be maintained throughout the procedure.

Closed suction units should be used when high concentrations of oxygen and PEEP are required to maintain oxygenation as they reduce the risk of arterial desaturation during suctioning (Carlton *et al.*, 1987). They also reduce the risk of environmental contamination when active chest infections are present.

ASSISTED COUGH

Patients with weakness or paralysis of the abdominal muscles will be unable to cough effectively, putting them at risk of atelectasis and chest infection. An assisted cough replaces the function of the affected muscles by manually creating increased pressure under the diaphragm. The technique should only be performed by practitioners who have been deemed competent to do so. Assisted cough is necessary for patients with neuromuscular disease affecting the respiratory muscles, e.g. Guillain–Barré syndrome and myasthenia gravis, and following acute spinal cord injury when the respiratory muscles are affected. There are three methods to give an assisted cough which require either one or two persons (Figure 15.10).

SUMMARY

Frequent, thorough respiratory assessments are essential for early detection of respiratory compromise. The nurse has a key role in monitoring the patient's respiratory status and acting promptly on the assessment findings. Nurses should be working collaboratively with physiotherapists to plan and implement individualised respiratory treatment so as to optimise the respiratory care being delivered. Neurological patients often require non-invasive and invasive respiratory support and frequent respiratory interventions which require neurological nurses to have additional knowledge, skills and competency to manage the patient safely and competently.

REFERENCES

Ackerman MH (1993) The effects of saline lavage prior to suctioning. *American Journal of Critical Care* 2 (4) 236–230.

Adam S, Osbourne S (2005) *Critical Care Nursing: Science and practice.* (2nd edition). Oxford: Oxford University Press.

Antonelli M, Pennisi MA, Montini L (2005) Clinical review: Noninvasive ventilation in the clinical setting – experience from the past 10 years. *Critical Care* 9:98–103.

Bourjeily G, Habr F, Supinski G (2002) Review of tracheostomy usage: complications and decannulation procedures Part II. *Clinical Pulmonary Medicine* 9(5):273–278.

Bourke SC, Tomlinson M, Williams *et al.* (2006) Effects of non invasive ventilation on survival and quality of life in patients with amyotrophic lateral sclerosis: a randomised controlled trial. *Lancet Neurology* 5(2):140–147.

Braine ME, Sweby S (2006) A systematic approach to weaning and decannulation of tracheostomy tubes. *British Journal of Neuroscience Nursing* 2(3):124–132.

British Thoracic Society (2002) Non-invasive ventilation in acute respiratory failure. *Thorax* 57(3)192–211.

Carlton GC, Fox SJ, Akerman RN (1987) Evaluation of a closed-tracheal suction system. *Critical Care Medicine* 15(5):522–555.

Chadda K, Louis B, Benaissa L *et al.* (2002) Physiological effects of decannulation in tracheostomized patients. *Intensive Care Medicine* 18(12):1761–1767.

Dean B (1997) Evidence- based suction management in accident and emergency: a vital component of airway care. *Accident and Emergency Nursing* 5(2):92–98.

Freeman BD, Isabella K, Lin N, Buchman TG (2000) A meta-analysis of prospective trials comparing percutaneous and surgical tracheostomy in critically ill patients. *Chest* 118(5):1412–1418.

Garner A, Amin Y (2006) The management of neuromuscular respiratory failure: A review. *British Journal of Neuroscience Nursing* 2(8):394–398.

Glass CA, Grap MJ (1995) Ten tips for safer suctioning. *American Journal of Nursing* 95(5):51–53.

Gray JE, MacIntyre NR, Kronenberger MA (1990) The effects of bolus normal saline installation in conjunction with endotracheal suctioning. *Respiratory Care* 35(8):785–790.

Hanley MV, Rudd T, Butler J (1978) What happens to intra-tracheal instillations? *American Review of Respiratory Disease* 117(Supp): 124.

Hunt K, McGowan S (2005) Tracheostomy management in the neurosciences: A systematic multidisciplinary approach. *British Journal of Neuroscience Nursing* 1(3):122–125.

Kannan S (1999) Practical issues in non-invasive positive pressure ventilation. *Care of the Critically Ill* 15(3):76-79.

Keen A (2000) Continuous positive airway pressure (CPAP) in the intensive care unit – uses and implications for nursing management. *Nursing in Critical Care* 5(3):137–141.

Kerr M, Rudy E, Weber B *et al.* (1997) Effects of short duration hyperventilation during endotracheal suctioning on intracranial pressure in severe head injured adults. *Nursing Research* 46(4):195–201.

Lumb A (2000) *Nunn's Applied Respiratory Physiology* (5th edition). Oxford: Butterworth-Heinemann.

Malik K, Hess DC (2002) Evaluating the comatose patient: rapid neurological assessment is key to appropriate management. *Postgraduate Medicine* 111(2): 38–40. Available from: http://www.ncbi.nlm.nih.gov/pubmed/11868313 Accessed July 2010.

Marino PL (1998) *The ICU Book* (2nd edition) London: Lippincott, Wiilliams and Wilkins.

McKelvie S (1998) Endotracheal suctioning *Nursing in Critical Care* 3(5):244–248.

Medicines and Healthcare products Regulatory Agency (2000) *Continuous positive airway pressure circuits: risk of misassembly*. Available from: http://www.mhra.gov.uk/Publications/Safetywarnings/MedicalDeviceAlerts/Safetynotices/CON008853 Accessed July 2010.

Moore T, Woodrow P (2004) *High Dependency Nursing Care: Observation, intervention and support*. London: Routledge.

Muench E, Bauhuf C, Roth H *et al.* (2005) Effects of positive end-expiratory pressure on regional cerebral blood flow, intracranial pressure, and brain tissue oxygenation. *Critical Care Medicine* 33(10):2367–2372.

Myburgh JA (2003) Severe head injury. In: Bernsten, A and Soni, N (eds) *Oh's Intensive Care Manual* (5th edition). Oxford: Butterworth Heinemann.

O'Neal P, Grap M, Thompson C *et al.* (2001) Level of dyspnoea experienced in mechanically ventilated adults with or without saline instillation. *Intensive and Critical Care* 17:356–363.

Patroniti N, Foti G, Mangio A *et al.* (2003) Head helmet versus face mask for non-invasive continuous positive airway pressure: physiological study. *Intensive Care Medicine* 29:1680–1687.

Porth C (2004) *Pathophysiology: Concepts of altered health states* (7th edition). London: Lippincott, Williams and Wilkins.

Robson WP (1998) To bag or not to bag? Manual hyperinflation in intensive care. *Intensive and Critical Care Nursing* 14(5):239–243.

Ropper A, Gress DR, Diringer MN *et al.* (2003) *Neurological and Neurosurgical Intensive Care*. (4th edition). Philadelphia: Lippincott, Williams and Wilkins.

Serra A (2000) Tracheostomy Care. *Nursing Standard* 14(42):45–55.

St John RE (1999) Protocols for practice: applying research at the bedside. *Critical Care Nurse* 19(4):79–83.

Thompson L, Morton R, Cuthbertson S *et al.* (2000) Tracheal suctioning of adults with an artificial airway. *Best Practice* 4(4):1–6.

Tully V (2002) Non-invasive ventilation: a guide for nursing staff. *Nursing in Critical Care* 7(6):296–299.

Wainwright SP, Gould D (1996) Endotracheal suctioning in adults with severe head injury. Literature review. *Intensive Critical Care Nurse* 12:303–308.

Wong F (2000) Prevention of secondary brain injury. *Critical Care Nurse* 20(5):18–27.

Wood CJ (1998) Endotracheal suctioning: a literature review. *Intensive and Critical Care Nursing* 14(3):124–136.

16

Assessment and Management of Fluid, Electrolytes and Nutrition in the Neurological Patient

Neal Cook

INTRODUCTION

Regulation of the body's water is dependent largely on the brain, specifically the hypothalamus and the pituitary gland. It is not surprising therefore that imbalances in fluid and electrolytes (particularly sodium) are not uncommon in the patient with acute neurological disorders. Fluid and electrolyte imbalances can further compromise neuronal function, so it is essential that such imbalances are detected early to minimise the potential adverse effects on the body and the brain. This chapter presents essential knowledge to enable effective assessment and management of disturbances in fluid and electrolytes in the neurological patient. It also gives an overview of how fluid and electrolytes are regulated in the body, how to assess a patient's fluid status and interpret the findings, and the current management of specific fluid and electrolyte disturbances that are common in neurological patients.

The second half of the chapter focuses on the assessment and management of the nutritional needs of the neurological patient. Nutrition plays a vital role in the recovery from acute neurological conditions and in the promotion of wellbeing in those with chronic neurological disorders. Meeting nutritional requirements places a structure and routine in our day, has social implications, and can be part of spiritual practices. Neurological disease or disorder often presents many challenges to this component of life. The challenges range from complete dependence on others to ensure that nutritional requirements are met, to specific neurological deficits that hinder eating and drinking. The nurse has a pivotal role in the identification, assessment, and management of such challenges, and is required to work in a multi-professional context in order to identify and implement appropriate strategies (DH, 2005).

PHYSIOLOGY OF FLUID AND ELECTROLYTE BALANCE

To understand how fluid and electrolyte imbalances can occur in neurological patients we must first appreciate the normal distribution of fluid and electrolytes in the body and how they are regulated.

Water comprises approximately 60% of the total body weight (TBW). The water is distributed in two main fluid compartments: intracellular and extracellular (see Table 16.1 for summary of approximate fluid volumes in each compartment).

The intracellular fluid (ICF) compartment

The intracellular fluid compartment refers to the fluid contained within cells. Approximately two thirds of the body's fluid volume is within this compartment (approximately 26 litres in an average 70kg adult). The main ions in the ICF are potassium (K^+) and phosphate (HPO_4^{2-}) in addition to soluble proteins (see Figure 16.1).

The extracellular fluid (ECF) compartment

Almost all of the fluid in the extracellular fluid compartment is contained in two main fluid spaces:

Neuroscience Nursing: Evidence-Based Practice, 1st Edition.
Edited by Sue Woodward and Ann-Marie Mestecky
© 2011 Blackwell Publishing Ltd

- The interstitial space (or intercellular space). This refers to the fluid that cells are bathed in, i.e. the fluid between cells (approximately 9 litres in an adult).
- The intravascular space. This refers to fluid contained within blood, i.e. plasma (approximately 3 litres in an adult).

Table 16.1 Approximate fluid volumes (70 kg person).

	% Body weight	Volume (L)	% Body water
ICF	40	26	67
ECF	20	13	33
• Plasma		3	
• Interstitial fluid		9	
• Transcellular		1	
Total	60%	39 liters	100%

ECF – extracellular fluid; ICF – intracellular fluid.

The most abundant ions in the ECF are sodium (Na^+), chloride (Cl^-), and bicarbonate (HCO_3^-). Approximately 1 litre of ECF is contained within other areas such as cerebrospinal fluid, vitreous and aqueous humours in the eyes, other serous fluids and synovial fluid. This fluid is collectively referred to as transcellular fluid.

Although water can move freely between compartments along osmotic gradients (discussed below) the movement of solutes between compartments is restricted by semipermeable membranes which allow selective movement across them. The selectivity of the semi-permeable membranes is what makes the environment inside the cells (intracellular fluid) so different from the ECF.

Movement of fluid between the interstitial space and the intracellular compartment is largely governed by osmotic forces, whereas the movement of fluid from the intravascular space to the interstitial space is also influenced by hydrostatic pressure and colloid osmotic pressure, which will be discussed later.

Osmosis is the movement of water through a selectively permeable membrane, e.g. the cell membrane, from a

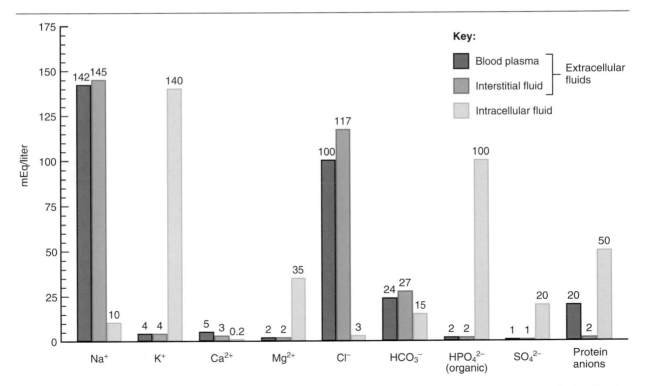

Figure 16.1 Electrolyte and protein anion concentrations in plasma, interstitial fluid and intracellular fluid. The height of each column represents the milliequivalents per litre (mEq/litre).
Reproduced from *Principles of Anatomy and Physiology 12e* by Gerard Tortora and Bryan Derrickson. Copyright (2009, John Wiley & Sons). Reprinted with permission of John Wiley & Sons Inc.

compartment that has low solute concentration to a compartment that has a high solute concentration. Therefore water moves from a dilute solution (hypotonic or one of lesser osmolality) to a more concentrated solution (hypertonic or one of higher osmolality) to achieve an osmotic equilibrium. Osmotic pressure develops when two solutions of different concentrations are separated by a selectively permeable membrane.

The osmotic pressure is the pulling power for water; the higher the solute concentration of a solution the higher the osmotic pressure and therefore its pulling power for water. Osmotic pressure controls the movement of water between the interstitial fluid space and the intracellular fluid. However, significant shifts in fluid between theses spaces are largely minimal in healthy individuals. This is because these two spaces have similar osmotic pressures, i.e. they have the same solute concentration. However, as previously discussed, the ions that make up the solute concentrations differ considerably (see Figure 16.1).

Sodium is the primary ion in the ECF; it is approximately ten times more abundant in ECF than ICF. It therefore contributes significantly to the osmotic pressure of the extracellular fluid, preventing the movement of large volumes of water to the intracellular compartment. Any change to the normal sodium concentration of the ECF will affect the movement of water between the two compartments. A rise in extracellular sodium increases the osmotic pressure of the ECF relative to the ICF, causing water to move by osmosis from inside the cell into the extracellular space. Conversely if the extracellular sodium concentration falls, the osmotic pressure of the ECF will also fall, causing the cell to swell as a result of water movement from the ECF into the cell. Changes in serum sodium levels can be a major cause of fluid shifts in the body.

Osmolality is the concentration of solutes within a solution. More specifically, in the body osmolality is: the osmolar concentration of ions, molecules and free particles dissolved in one kilogram of plasma or urine. The osmolality of the ECF is largely determined by the concentration of sodium. In health, serum osmolality is maintained between 280 and 295 mOsm/kg (milliosmoles) by mechanisms that control water balance, i.e. thirst and antidiuretic hormone (ADH).

Neurohormonal control of water and sodium balance

To maintain homeostasis water gains have to be balanced with water losses and the principal ion that has an effect on fluid balance, sodium, has to be strictly regulated to prevent adverse changes in the osmotic pressure of the ECF. Water balance is regulated by thirst and antidiuretic hormone (ADH). Sodium is largely regulated by the renin–angiotensin–aldosterone system amongst other factors.

Antidiuretic hormone (ADH)

ADH is produced in the hypothalamus and stored in the posterior pituitary (neurohypophysis). Osmoreceptors in the anterior hypothalamus respond to changes in the osmolality of blood. When an increase in osmolality is detected the supraoptic and paraventricular nuclei of the hypothalamus stimulate the posterior pituitary gland to release ADH into the circulation. Receptors for ADH are found on the cells of the distal convoluted tubules in the kidneys. The effect of the ADH on these cells is to increase water absorption, thereby returning the plasma osmolality to normal levels. The converse occurs when plasma osmolality levels are low, i.e. ADH is inhibited and urine output increases. Urine osmolality subsequently falls.

ADH is also released in response to:

* A fall in blood volume (hypovolaemia) detected by baroreceptors (see Chapter 14)
* Stress and pain
* Medications such as opioids and barbiturates
* Certain anaesthetics
* Positive pressure ventilation (McDonnell-Keenan, 1999; Terpstra and Terpstra, 2000)

Aldosterone

Aldosterone is a mineralocorticoid produced by the cortex of the adrenal glands. It is released when intravascular sodium concentration is low and that of potassium is high. It acts on the renal tubules and collecting ducts of the kidneys to cause an increase in sodium reabsorption from the filtrate; water follows by osmosis. The reabsorption is accompanied by a loss of potassium. Aldosterone is also released in response to angiotensin II as a result of activation of the rennin–angiotensin mechanism.

Thirst

Fluid intake is generally stimulated by thirst. The sensation of thirst is triggered by very small increases in the plasma osmolality. Although it is known that the hypothalamus is essential for thirst to be experienced, the specific area and neuronal pathways that stimulate the sensation of thirst in response to a rising osmolality have yet to be elucidated. Thirst is also stimulated in response to a loss of intravascular volume (haemorrhage).

Movement of water between the intravascular space and interstitial space

As presented above, the ECF is distributed between two main spaces: the intravascular fluid space and the interstitial fluid. Colloid osmotic pressure and hydrostatic pressure influence the movement of fluid between these spaces. The movement of fluid occurs at the capillaries; the veins and arteries have thick walls preventing the movement of fluid through them.

Hydrostatic pressure

Blood hydrostatic pressure is the pressure exerted by blood against the walls of the blood vessels. If this pressure was unopposed then most of the fluid in the intravascular space would be forced out of the capillaries into the interstitial fluid space. However there is an opposing pressure that counters the effect of hydrostatic pressure called colloid osmotic pressure.

Colloid osmotic pressure (COP)

Capillary membranes are freely permeable to water and electrolytes, but not to large molecules such as plasma proteins (e.g. albumin) which remain in the intravascular space. These proteins give rise to a blood colloid osmotic pressure (BCOP) that opposes the outward force of the hydrostatic pressure at the arterial end of the capillary. The hydrostatic pressure at the arterial end of the capillary is approximately 41 mmHg; the COP is approximately 28 mmHg. Therefore the resultant net pressure (13 mmHg) forces fluid out of the capillary. At the venous end of the capillary the hydrostatic pressure has dropped to 21 mmHg, but the colloid osmotic pressure has remained unchanged. Therefore the inward force is greater than the pressure forcing fluids outwards, and fluid is drawn back into the capillary at the venous end. During a 24 hour period approximately 20 litres of fluid are forced out of the arterial end of the capillaries and 17 litres are reabsorbed. The small amount of remaining fluid in the interstitial space is drained by the lymphatic system.

Through understanding what determines the movement of fluids between these two spaces, it is possible to identify factors that will result in abnormal shifts in fluids. Some of the most common are:

- Low plasma proteins (from malnutrition or chronic sepsis), causing COP to fall, thus increasing interstitial fluid volume
- Right sided heart failure, causing venous congestion, increasing the hydrostatic pressure at the venous end of the capillary, thus increasing interstitial fluid volume.

- Increased capillary permeability, as occurs in sepsis, allowing movement of proteins into the interstitial space, thereby reducing BCOP and increasing interstitial fluid
- Reduced lymphatic drainage resulting in excess fluid accumulating in the interstitial space

FLUID ASSESSMENT IN THE NEUROSCIENCE PATIENT

Nurses need to have a logical approach to fluid and electrolyte assessment, which generally includes an assessment of fluid intake and output, physical assessment of hydration status, and biochemistry results. The collective data enables a more accurate assessment to be made and decisions about the volume and type of fluid required by the patient to be determined.

Assessment of fluid intake and output

Whenever possible, nurses should assess the cumulative balance (allowing for insensible losses) over the previous few days, as a balance over a few hours may be misleading. When assessing and recording fluid intake and output, there are several sources of possible losses that need to be considered.

- Urine: Normal urine output is between 0.5 and 1 ml/kg/hr. Urine output on its own is not always a reliable indicator of fluid status; abnormal urine volume can be a complication of neurological disease and may be unusually high (cerebral salt wasting or diabetes insipidus) or low (syndrome of inappropriate anti-diuretic hormone secretion) (see: Fluid management).
- Faecal fluid losses are, on average, 200 ml/24 hr. The accuracy of measuring this is difficult and the nurse will need to rely on estimation in many cases.
- Vomiting and fluid losses from nasogastric drainage.
- Fluid from drains such as chest drains, external ventricular drainage, wound drains.
- Haemorrhagic losses should be estimated, as this will influence not only the volume of fluid replacement required but also the type of fluid.

Losses not included on the fluid balance chart (insensible loss):

- Normal loss of fluid with expiration amounts to 400 ml/24 hr approximately. There will be additional pulmonary losses when gases are poorly humidified and in patients who are tachypnoeic, which need to be taken into consideration.

- Excretory losses from sweat glands from the skin are a source of insensible loss that is also difficult to approximate. In health it is estimated that we lose 600 ml/24 hr. Additional losses associated with pyrexia need to be accounted for.
- Losses associated with burns and open surgical wounds.

Water content of ingested food is approximately 500 ml in 24 hours, with a further 500 ml generated from metabolism. In health this source of water gain generally balances the 400 ml respiratory loss and 600 ml excretory loss from the skin. The balancing effect of this is such that insensible losses are not taken into consideration unless significantly large losses are apparent.

Physical assessment of hydration status

Box 16.1 presents a summary of the physical assessment of hydration status. When water loss exceeds water intake e.g. due to excessive diarrhoea or vomiting, excessive perspiration, excessive urine production as in diabetes insipidus, or inadequate fluid intake, the body becomes dehydrated.

Signs of mild dehydration become apparent with a loss of 2–5% of total body water (TBW). The signs are: thirst, dry skin and mucus membranes, concentrated urine and fatigue. With moderate dehydration (approximately 5–8% TBW), in addition to the aforementioned signs there may be poor skin turgor, nausea, headache, muscle cramps and the intravascular volume will fall (hypovolaemia), so signs of a reduced circulatory volume will be evident (see Chapter 14). With severe dehydration (approximately 8–15% TBW) there will be significant hypovolaemia, acute renal failure, metabolic acidosis, fever which occurs due to a reduction in evaporative heat loss, and consciousness can be severely impaired.

Overhydration is much less common in clinical practice and is usually iatrogenic in origin. The other cause in the neurological setting is SIADH (syndrome of inappropriate ADH) which is discussed below. Signs of overhydration include headache, nausea, confusion and in severe cases seizures and coma.

Biochemistry results

Blood urea (BUN) and sodium will be elevated in the dehydrated patient. The causes of other common electrolyte imbalances are summarised in Table 16.2. In patients with more complex fluid and electrolyte imbalances, serum and urine osmolality can be helpful in determining the cause and degree of imbalance (see: Fluid management). The

---

Box 16.1   Physical assessment of hydration

- Thorough assessment of fluid intake and output (see under fluid assessment)
- Is the patient experiencing thirst? – thirst indicates that the body has registered a need for water
- Assessment of skin turgor (which may be unreliable in the elderly) – when the skin on the back of the hand is pinched it should quickly return to its original shape, poor skin turgor is when the skin remains pinched and indicates moderate dehydration
- Is the urine concentrated? Concentrated urine is generally a sign of being under hydrated
- Assessment of the mucous membranes (mouth and tongue) – membranes should be moist, dried membranes indicate dehydration
- Is the patient experiencing headache and/or are they irritable – may be experienced with mild–moderate dehydration
- Has the patient's weight increased/decreased? Water accounts for sixty percent of body weight; losses and gains can indicate dehydration and retention respectively
- Is the patient constipated – can be a sign of dehydration

Patients with moderate to severe dehydration will also have signs of hypovolaemia:

- Is peripheral capillary refill greater than 2.5 seconds? – indicates reduced perfusion and possible hypovolaemia (moderate – severe dehydration)
- Assess temperature of peripheries: – cold, pale peripheries may indicate vasoconstriction in response to hypovolaemia
- Assess pulse rate and volume – tachycardia will occur in moderate to severe dehydration and pulse volume will be thready. A bounding pulse and jugular venous distention are signs of volume overload.
- Assess if the pulse is regular – an irregular pulse is a sign of electrolyte imbalance (potassium, calcium or magnesium)
- Evaluate blood pressure –hypertension may be initial compensatory mechanism in hypovolaemia, low blood pressure may be due to low circulatory volume. Volume overload may present as hypertension
- A central venous pressure reading will help to evaluate fluid volume status (normal is CVP 3–9 mmHg)
- What is the patient's respiratory rate? Increased respiratory rate and depth occur with hypovolaemia (see Chapter 14 for more detail)

Table 16.2 Electrolytes: Causes and indicators of imbalances.

Serum blood test	Potential cause	Indicators
Potassium (3.5–4.5 mmol/l)	Reduced: • GI loss • Cell shift with insulin therapy • Diuretic use • Magnesium depletion Raised: • Cell membrane disorders • Decreased renal excretion • Tubular nephritis	Reduced: • ECG changes • Cardiac arrhythmias • Prolonged QT intervals • Flat T waves Raised: • Tall peaked T waves • Cardiac arrhythmias • Bradycardia • Hypotension
Sodium 135–145 mmol/l	Reduced • Net gain of water or loss of sodium rich fluid • GI, renal and skin (burns) Raised: • Pure water loss or sodium gain • Restricted access to water and ADH abnormalities	Reduced: • Irritability • Dizziness/headache • Postural hypotension • Seizures and coma Raised: • Intense thirst • Fatigue/irritability • Postural hypotension • Tachycardia • Coma
Calcium 2.2–2.6 mmol/l	Reduced: • Small bowel resection • Ulcerative bowel conditions • Liver and renal disorders • Vitamin D deficiency • Hypoparathyroidism Raised • Increased GI absorption • Vitamin D excess • Hyperparathyroidism • Thiazides, lithium	Reduced: • Tingling of fingertips • Abdominal cramps • Muscle cramps • Seizures • Prolonged QT interval Raised: • Anorexia • Constipation • Abdominal pain • Weakness/lethargy • Reduced level of consciousness • Muscular hypotonicity
Magnesium 0.7–0.9 mmol/l	Reduced • GI malabsorption • Renal wasting • Diuretics Raised: • Renal failure • Use of antacids • Laxative use	Reduced: • Cardiac arrhythmias Raised: • Hypotension • Heart block • Nausea and vomiting

normal range for urine osmolality is 50–1400 mOsm/kg and serum osmolality of 280–295 mOsm/kg.

FLUID MANAGEMENT

Poor hydration is a common problem for patients with progressive neurological conditions and can predispose the patient to additional medical problems, e.g. pressure sores (decubitus ulcers), constipation, urinary tract infections and deep vein thrombosis. It is important to identify with the patient and carers the factors that are preventing adequate fluid intake so that appropriate measures can be taken to remedy the problem. For some patients encouragement and assistance with fluids may be sufficient to restore or maintain fluid balance, whereas for others it may require short term intravenous administration. For those with dysphagia, enteral feeding will be required (see: Enteral and parenteral nutrition).

Many acute neurological patients will require intravenous fluids and assistance with taking oral fluids for which the nurse will be responsible. The patient's fluid requirements and the route of replacement will depend on a number of factors, e.g. the patient's size, hydrational status and medical condition, and will require the nurse to work collaboratively with medical colleagues to determine the patient's requirements. The specific fluid management for conditions such as subarachnoid haemorrhage, raised intracranial pressure, neurogenic shock, (following spinal injury), are addressed in the relevant chapters. The specific fluid management for hyponatraemia and hypernatraemia in neuroscience patients is presented in detail later in this chapter (see: Hyponatraemia/Hypernatraemia). The current section will focus on general principles of fluid management of the neurological patient.

Fluid therapy

Patients who are hospitalised usually require 35 ml/kg of fluid per day (Knighton and Smith, 2003). Fluid intake above this estimate is generally well tolerated without producing hyponatraemia or fluid overload. Fluid therapies for neurological patients without electrolyte imbalances aim to maintain normal osmolality. This requires the practitioner to avoid the administration of hypotonic fluids, and to opt for isotonic solutions (Bruder and Gouvitsos, 2000). Isotonic saline (0.9%) is largely the fluid of choice in acute situations where the full biochemical status of the patient remains to be determined.

Knowledge of whether a fluid is hypotonic, isotonic or hypertonic is essential for the nurse to know which fluid spaces the fluid will distribute to once in the body, (see Table 16.3). Nurses have a responsibility to ensure that the fluid prescription is appropriate for the patient.

Table 16.3 Approximate distribution of commonly used intravenous fluids.

Solution	Na$^+$ (mmol/l)	Cl$^-$ (mmol/l)	Glucose (mmol/l)	Change in ECF		Change in ICF
				Total ECF	Intravascular volume	
5% dextrose (1000 ml) (hypotonic)	0	0	278	333 ml	80 ml	667 ml
0.9% NaCl (1000 ml) (isotonic)	154	154	0	1000 ml	250 ml	0 ml
Ringer's lactate (1000 ml) (isotonic)	130	109	0	900 ml	225 ml	100 ml
Hetastarch 6% (500 ml) (colloid)	154	154	0		500 ml	0 ml
Albumin (5%) (500 ml) (colloid)	150	120–136	0	500 ml	500 ml	0 ml
Gelofusine (500 ml) (colloid)	154	120	0	500 ml	500 ml	0 ml

An isotonic fluid has the same solute concentration as plasma, therefore if a litre of isotonic fluid was administered intravenously, it would all remain in the ECF compartment. Three quarters of the litre (750 ml) would distribute to the interstitial space (as this makes up approximately three quarters of the ECF compartment) and the remaining quarter (250 ml) would remain in the intravascular space.

A hypotonic fluid has a lower solute concentration than body fluids and will distribute to all fluid spaces proportionate to the volume they occupy. For example if a litre of 5% dextrose or 0.45% sodium chloride (hypotonic) was prescribed, approximately two thirds of the litre would distribute to the intracellular space (as two thirds of the body's fluid is contained in this space). Only approximately 80 ml of the remaining third of the litre (333 ml) would remain in the intravascular space as this makes up approximately a quarter of the total ECF space (see Table 16.1). Hypotonic fluids are used to restore intracellular volume and would be inappropriate fluids to administer to a hypovolaemic patient.

Hypertonic fluids have a higher solute concentration and will remain in the intravascular space, increasing the plasma osmolality and changing the osmotic gradient. Fluid will move by osmosis from the interstitial and intracellular spaces into the intravascular space. The use of hypertonic fluids in the management of raised ICP is presented in Chapter 7.

Colloids (e.g. starches, dextrans, gelatins) remain in the intravascular space. They contain large molecules that do not readily leave the intravascular space and are therefore beneficial in volume replacement.

The use of intravenous fluids containing glucose should be strictly avoided, unless there is evident hypoglycaemia (Bruder and Gouvitsos, 2000). Even then, glucose administration must be used cautiously. Glucose administration is thought to contribute to secondary brain injury, although the mechanism of this is not yet fully understood. As discussed in Chapter 7, dextrose solutions (those containing 5% or <5%) are hypotonic and will lower plasma osmolality, which will cause water to move by osmosis across the blood brain barrier (BBB) and will contribute further to cerebral oedema.

MANAGEMENT OF COMMON CAUSES OF HYPONATRAEMIA IN THE NEUROLOGICAL PATIENT

Hyponatraemia is the most common electrolyte disturbance in the neuroscience patient. Mild hyponatraemia is classi-fied as a serum sodium less than 135 mmol/l but greater than 125 mmol/l; severe hyponatraemia is defined as a serum sodium less than 125 mmol/l. Patients with mild hyponatraemia may not be symptomatic. The consequence of hyponatraemia is a loss of osmotic pressure of the intravascular fluid which will cause fluid to move by osmosis to the interstitial and intracellular spaces. When severe this can cause osmotic brain oedema.

Sodium has a vital role to play in the nervous system, particularly in the propagation of action potentials (see Chapter 1). Hyponatraemia can result in confusion, weakness, tremors, and hyper/hypovolaemia depending on the cause. Seizure activity and coma are most likely to occur when serum sodium levels fall below 120 mmol/l, however the rate of depletion is significant, with a rapid fall more likely to result in these phenomena (Coenraad *et al.*, 2001)

Mild hyponatraemia can result from profuse diaphoresis, excessive administration of hypotonic intravenous fluids, diarrhoea and vomiting, and the use of diuretics. The primary causes of hyponatraemia in patients with intracranial disorders are the syndrome of inappropriate ADH secretion (SIADH) and cerebral salt wasting syndrome (CSWS).

Syndrome of inappropriate ADH secretion (SIADH)

SIADH is a disorder characterised by a persistently high level of ADH being released by the hypothalamus despite the existence of hypoosmolality, i.e. ADH levels do not fall as they should in response to a falling plasma osmolality. The inappropriate high level of ADH results in water retention and dilution of sodium (dilutional hyponatraemia). Head injury, encephalitis, space occupying lesions and aneurysmal rupture can all lead to SIADH (Zafonte and Mann, 1997); it can also be seen in Guillain–Barré syndrome. Non-neurological causes include medications, such as carbamazepine and haloperidol, and pulmonary tumours (Terpstra and Terpstra, 2000).

The patient may report fatigue, weakness, and dizziness which may progress to behavioural changes and drowsiness. The presence of the following confirm the diagnosis:

- Decreased plasma osmolality <280 mOsmol/l
- Hyponatraemia (serum sodium <130 mmol/l)
- Raised urine osmolality >500 mOsmol/l
- Natriuresis in the presence of hyponatraemia (>20 mmol/l) (Coenraad *et al.*, 2001)

The renal system continues to eliminate some sodium in the urine in the late stages of SIADH in an attempt to reduce blood volume (Berkenbosch *et al.*, 2002). Patients are rarely oedematous when they have SIADH, despite the likelihood of being hypervolaemic. This is because SIADH often occurs gradually, giving cells time to move osmoles out of the intracellular space, in an attempt to maintain water homeostasis. In acute SIADH, oedema can occur as there is no time for this compensatory mechanism to take place (see: Acute or chronic hyponatraemia).

Treatment

SIADH causes water retention and hypervolaemia so it is treated by fluid restricting the patient, usually to within 1000 ml in 24 hours. This promotes a negative fluid balance and sodium and plasma osmolality levels gradually move towards normal parameters. However, fluid restriction can have a negative effect on cerebral perfusion, and so meticulous hourly assessment of fluid balance and physiological responses to the restriction must be closely monitored. Hypertonic saline is sometimes administered when hyponatraemia is verging towards fatal concentrations (Coenraad *et al.*, 2001) (see: Acute or chronic hyponatraemia, for medical management to correct hyponatraemia).

Cerebral salt wasting syndrome (CSWS)

The other common cause of hyponatraemia in neuroscience patients is cerebral salt wasting syndrome (CSWS), particularly when there is insult to the hypothalamus and its connections. Unlike SIADH, CSWS results in renal loss of sodium resulting in true hyponatraemia. The aetiology of CSWS remains poorly defined (Berkenbosch *et al.*, 2002). The hormone that has been implicated in causing CSWS, is atrial natriuretic peptide (ANP) (Zafonte and Mann, 1997). ANP is produced in the atria of the heart and brain natriuretic peptide (BNP) in the ventricles of the heart (Pedersen *et al.*, 2006). These peptides are released in response to increased stretch on cardiac muscle (e.g. increased intravascular volume). The peptides increase the excretion of sodium in the urine and water follows by osmosis thus resulting in a fall in intravascular volume. The peptides exert this physiological effect by inhibiting the renin–angiotensin–aldosterone mechanism. The result of CSWS is a primary natriuresis which results in a low serum sodium and loss of intravascular volume (Coenraad *et al.*, 2001).

Assessment

In CSWS the patient experiences true hyponatraemia, elevated sodium concentration in the urine, hypovolaemia and polyuria (Berkenbosch *et al.*, 2002). The key factor here is recognising that hypovolaemia, rather then hypervolaemia (as in SIADH), is present, this distinction becomes vital in ensuring positive patient outcomes are achieved. The following will be present in CSWS:

- Hyponatraemia (serum sodium <130 mmol/l)
- High urine sodium (>25 mmol/l)
- Hypovolaemia
- Polyuria
- High blood urea (BUN)

It is recognised that in CSWS there is continual loss of sodium in the urine, while blood volume and serum sodium levels continue to fall. This is not normally seen in SIADH, except at the late stages when some natriuresis can occur (Berkenbosch *et al.*, 2002).

Treatment

In contrast to SIADH, the treatment of CSWS requires the early replacement of both water and salt requirements to the body. Accurate assessment of the patient is crucial in determining the treatment plan; making the wrong diagnosis and treating CSWS as SIADH will result in exacerbating the volume depletion with the potential risk of cerebral ischaemia, haemoconcentration and microthrombosis (Bussmann *et al.*, 2001; Berkenbosch *et al.*, 2002). Sodium should be replaced at 1 mmol/l/hr in those with acute hyponatraemia and (not exceeding) 0.5 mmol/l/hr in those with chronic hyponatraemia (Coenraad *et al.*, 2001).

Distinguishing between the two disorders requires the practitioner to have a thorough understanding of fluid and electrolyte balance and proficiency in the skills of assessment of hydration status.

Acute or chronic hyponatraemia?

In addition to considering the cause of hyponatraemia, it is also important to consider whether the hyponatraemia is acute or chronic. This will affect how the disorder is treated. Chronic hyponatraemia gives the central nervous system more time to adapt, which results in compensatory mechanisms that export osmoles out of cells in order to reduce the cellular oedema caused by the hyponatraemia (Coenraad *et al.*, 2001; Biswas and Davies, 2007). Moving osmoles into the ECF raises the osmotic pressure, and water will follow by osmosis. This can result in the cells themselves becoming dehydrated. The likelihood of cerebral oedema is therefore reduced significantly. However, this adaptation by the cells means that in chronic hyponatraemia sodium replacement has to be gradual (no more than 0.5 mmol/l/hr), as a rapid rise in sodium concentration can cause additional movement of water, and other molecules from brain cells. This sudden shift is known to lead to the destruction of myelin surrounding neurones in the area of the pons, inhibiting effective neurotransmission along the affected cells. This condition is called central pontine myelinolysis.

Acute hyponatraemia (occurs within 48 hours) does not allow time for the brain to deploy compensatory mechanisms, and so the result is cellular oedema with a subsequent increase in ICP. Sodium replacement can be quicker in acute hyponatraemia, with replacement at 1 mmol/l/hr being the replacement goal (Coenraad *et al.*, 2001). However, the patient will still require close monitoring for potential adverse effects on the CNS.

When correcting sodium deficiencies it is vital to correct any serum potassium and phosphorus deficits first to enable the cells to adapt to osmotic changes (Sedlacek *et al.*, 2006).

MANAGEMENT OF COMMON CAUSES OF HYPERNATRAEMIA IN THE NEUROLOGICAL PATIENT

While hyponatraemia is the most common sodium disturbance in the neuroscience patient, hypernatraemia (serum sodium >145 mmol/l) often presents itself as a component of the treatment of cerebral oedema (Aiyagari *et al.*, 2006) or due to diabetes insipidus. It occurs as a result of increased free water elimination when this free water is not replaced, i.e. dehydration (see Box 16.2 for other possible causes). It is less commonly caused by the over administration of hypertonic saline.

Hypernatramia is associated with raised serum urea and increases in serum osmolality and the clinical presentation will be one of dehydration. When hypernatraemia occurs

it increases the osmotic pressure of the ECF which results in water being drawn from the cells, giving rise to cellular dehydration. Treating hypernatraemia can be relatively straightforward in those without cerebral oedema or raised ICP, as it is a matter of calculating the degree of free water lost and replacing it slowly by intravenous infusion. Prior to treating hypernatraemia, replacement therapy must always evaluate the extent and length of time that the hypernatraemia has existed. When hypernatraemia is insidious in onset, compensatory mechanisms increase intracellular osmoles so as to retain water (Castilla-Guerra *et al.*, 2006). Replacement of free water in chronic hypernatraemia can therefore cause cerebral oedema. Acute hypernatraemia that is severe denies the brain the opportunity to compensate in this way, causing hypernatraemic encephalopathy.

Aiyagari *et al.* (2006) recommend reducing sodium by 12 mmol/l in a 24 hour period as the advisable rate; any faster can cause or exacerbate cerebral oedema by osmotic forces. For those with pre existing cerebral oedema and/or raised intracranial pressure, treating hypernatraemia becomes more complex, especially considering that sodium may have been raised initially by the use of osmotic diuretics to treat their intracranial disorder. In many cases, depending on the severity of the condition, the existence of the hypernatraemia may be beneficial in the management of cerebral oedema and raised ICP, and so may not require treatment. However, peak serum sodium levels >160 mmol/l are an independent predictor of mortality (Aiyagari *et al.*, 2006), and thus hypernatraemia to this extent needs to be managed proactively in consideration of the patient's overall condition. How this is best achieved is still up for considerable debate, but largely relies on dilutional intravenous fluid therapy.

Diabetes insipidus (DI)

Diabetes insipidus (DI) is a condition that is characterised by a failure to concentrate urine and an excessive urinary output. The excretion of dilute urine in large amounts can result in severe dehydration and hypernatraemia. DI can be caused by either a disturbance in synthesis and/or secretion of ADH, which is called central DI, or by failure of the kidneys to respond to the ADH, called nephrogenic DI. Polydipsia is usually reported by those experiencing DI. Central DI is the most common cause for the neuroscience patient and will be the focus of this section.

Central DI is largely associated with trauma and surgery which causes damage to the hypothalamic pituitary axis (HPA). A transient form of DI is often seen following

---

> **Box 16.2 Possible causes of hypernatraemia**
>
> - Fever
> - Nasogastric feeding (high protein)
> - Loss of thirst sensation
> - Vomiting
> - Diarrhoea
> - Hypertonic sodium bicarbonate administration
> - Use of osmotic diuretics
>
> Source: Aiyagari *et al.*, 2006; Sedlacek *et al.*, 2006; Stuart *et al.*, 2007.

pituitary surgery because the neurohypophysis may have been traumatised. The condition is more permanent when the pituitary stalk itself is damaged above the median eminence. Other causes include tumours of the hypothalamic posterior pituitary and idiopathic causes.

Assessment

There is a characteristic high dilute urine output which can be 3–20 l/day (polyuria) (Simmons-Holcomb, 2002a), however those with classic DI are more likely to have a urinary output greater than 5litres within a 24 hour period. The urine will be dilute with a specific gravity of <1.005. This can be supported by checking urine osmolality, which is less than 300 mOsm/kg in those with DI. As a result of water loss, serum osmolality is high usually >300 mOsm/kg (Simmons-Holcomb, 2002a). Patients who are conscious will have extreme thirst (polydipsia). An accurate fluid balance, supported by these biochemical markers, coupled with the patient's symptoms are the keys to arriving at a diagnosis. The role of the nurse in observing for such a pattern is crucial for such a diagnosis to be made in an accurate and timely way.

Differentials

Polyuria and polydipsia can also be signs of diabetes mellitus, therefore an assessment of urinary glucose and serum blood glucose is essential to rule out this differential diagnosis. Nephrogenic DI is more likely to occur in patients with chronic renal disease, hypokalaemia and hypercalcaemia.

Treatment

Central DI can be treated successfully with the administration of desmopressin acetate, given by injection 1–4 μg (subcutaneous, intramuscular or intravenous) in the acute period, and by the intranasal (10–40 μg) or oral route for maintenance therapy. The responsibility of the nurse is to monitor the effect of the medication and to ensure that the patient does not develop volume overload and hyponatraemia (Simmons-Holcomb, 2002b). Care should then include measuring an accurate fluid balance, monitoring of both serum and urine electrolytes and osmolality, auscultation of lung fields for crackles, and close observation of vital signs. The selection of fluids for administration should be based solely on the patient's biochemistry and haematocrit value (Simmons-Holcomb, 2002a).

The treatment often depends on the physician's preference and the degree of damage to the hypothalamic pituitary axis. If the physician believes it to be a transitory condition, they may elect not to treat with synthetic ADH but rather to replace the lost volume either by encouraging the patient to drink to thirst or if unable to do so to replace free water by a nasogastric tube with careful monitoring. This approach is taken by some because it is believed that treating with ADH can often delay recovery of the normal secretion of the ADH. If the damage is expected to be more long term the patient is often carefully monitored by the endocrinologist and synthetic ADH is prescribed.

NUTRITION IN THE NEUROSCIENCE PATIENT

There are a number of circumstances that can contribute to poor nutritional intake in neuroscience patients. The patient's functional ability to feed themselves may be impaired due to reasons such as motor/sensory impairments, reduced dexterity of the hands and cognitive impairments. Impairment of swallowing can occur in many neurological conditions, as can the loss of the ability to chew sufficiently and to produce sufficient saliva to facilitate mastication. Patients with altered conscious states will ultimately require total support to meet their nutritional needs. Emotional effects of illness, and the stress of being hospitalised can affect appetite. Patients following moderate or severe head injury have significant hypermetabolic and catabolic responses which can rapidly result in malnutrition. Malnutrition can also occur in hospital due to underfeeding. Many neuroscience patients are dependent on nurses for assistance with feeding, and without adequate planning and time allocated to assisting patients, their nutritional intake can be greatly reduced.

Patients that are undernourished are at risk of further medical complications, e.g. poor wound healing, weakened immunity and anaemia. They may have longer hospital stays and have been found to have poorer outcomes and higher mortality rates. It is essential that patients are regularly assessed and those at risk are identified early so that appropriate measures and nutritional support are instituted to optimise nutrition.

BIOCHEMICAL AND PHYSICAL ASSESSMENT

While screening tools are helpful in identifying those at risk, indeed all patients should be screened, screening tools should not replace a more holistic and in-depth patient assessment. Boxes 16.3 and 16.4 identify physical assessments and signs that will assist in determining the patient's nutritional status. It is essential to involve a dietician when a patient is identified as being at risk of malnutrition so that a more thorough assessment can be undertaken such as anthropometry, biochemical testing and indirect calorimetry. Nurses play a key role in observing patients' nutritional intake at mealtimes and identifying possible factors that could be contributing to a reduced intake. The

<table>
<tr><td>

Box 16.3   Indicators of poor nutrition

Skin and hair
- Dry, dull, thin hair, falls out easily
- Dull, rough, dry skin, acne
- Loss of subcutaneous fat
- Brittle fingernails, transverse ridging of the fingernails
- Impaired wound healing
- Oedema of the lower extremities

Oral cavity
- Ulcerated mucous membranes
- Coated or inflamed tongue
- Tooth decay

Gastrointestinal
- Nausea
- Constipation, diarrhoea
- Presence of ascites – due to low albumin levels

Musculoskeletal
- Weight loss
- Muscular atrophy
- Muscle cramps
- Joint pains
- Reduced muscle strength

Others
Fatigue, anxiety, irritability, depression, confusion, headaches, dizziness, fertility problems

Blood tests
- Albumin and prealbumin – levels will be low. Albumin has a half-life of 18 days so if the level is low it indicates the nutritional problem is longstanding. Albumin is a non-specific test as levels may also be low in liver disease and acute illness. Prealbumin is more specific of acute undernourishment as its half-life is two days
- Total lymphocyte count – low
- Vitamin and minerals such as B12, vitamin D and K and calcium and magnesium
- Iron

</td><td>

Box 16.4   Factors to consider that can affect nutritional intake

Oral assessment
- Poorly fitting dentures and tooth decay can affect the ability to bite and chew
- Painful gums and mucous membranes can affect the enjoyment of eating
- Dry and shrivelled tongue will affect swallowing
- Decreased saliva production

Gastrointestinal
- Constipation or diarrhoea – check date of last bowel movement and consistency of stool
- Nausea
- Reduced peristalsis – assess bowel sounds to determine peristaltic movement (reduced, normal or increased sounds)

Neurological
- Cognitive impairments, e.g. poor memory – forgetting to eat
- Functional loss, e.g. motor or sensory impairments
- Pain

Respiratory
- Shortness of breath – impairs appetite and intake

Hospital setting
- Poor consideration given to likes and dislikes
- Unappetising food
- Loss of appetite
- Hospital environment may not be conducive to eating
- Depression
- Medications

</td></tr>
</table>

malnutrition universal screening (MUST) tool has been widely adopted across all care settings.

Nutritional screening

The appropriateness of a screening tool for the clinical environment must be evaluated before adopting it, and nurses should determine the integrity of the tool before accepting its accuracy and specificity (Kyle *et al.*, 2006). Research has shown that many screening tools misclassify a high percentage of patients (Kyle *et al.*, 2006). Inaccuracies in weight measurement can often occur due to poorly maintained equipment and not being consistent with the time of day the weight is measured. Table 16.4 presents the strengths and limitations of each of the screening tools.

MECHANISMS OF NUTRITIONAL SUPPORT

Once a nutritional need is identified, it is essential that a proactive approach is taken to ensure that the most appropriate form of intervention is put into place. The intervention must not only meet the patient's nutritional need, but

Table 16.4 Nutritional risk screening tools.

Tool	Benefits	Weaknesses
MUST (Malnutrition Universal Screening Tool)	• Developed for screening within the community setting, assessing body mass index (BMI), weight loss over time, and acute disease parameters • Ease of use • Sensitivity and specificity compare well to other tools (Mourao *et al.*, 2004; Capra, 2007)	• Debate about the accuracy in classification of normal ranges of BMI • Does not look at functional ability, therefore limited use in those with neurological disorders and older adults (Sieber, 2006)
SGA (Subjective Global Assessment)	• Developed for those with gastrointestinal disease • Takes into account more aspects of nutrition than the MUST tool (Sieber, 2006) • Accurate predictor of complications such as wound healing problems and infection (Kyle *et al.*, 2006) • When used consistently, it is valid (Capra, 2007) • Economical as biochemical markers are not required	• Subjective, and therefore can have a degree of variation from assessor to assessor • Lack of specificity
MNA (Mini Nutritional Assessment) and MNA-SF (short form)	• Reliable and quick • Developed for the older adult population – takes into account functional ability, depression and dementia (Sieber, 2006) • Short form of the MNS is the MNA-SF, less time consuming to complete and has a high specificity (100%), sensitivity (98%), and diagnostic reliability (98%) (Rubenstein *et al.*, 2001)	• Of limited use in those with cognitive impairment • Not appropriate for use with those with enteral or parenteral nutrition • Complex to complete and many clinical environments cannot complete all the fields required (Capra, 2007)
NRS-2002 (Nutritional Risk Screening 2002)	• Created for acute setting • Positively evaluated due to its ability to be deployed without the need for in-depth physical assessment or anthropometry (Sieber, 2006) • Accounts for the age of the patient (Kyle *et al.*, 2006)	• Does not consider physical impairment in sufficient depth

must also take into account dignity, choice, and where possible promote independence. NICE (2006) emphasises the need for person-centred approaches to nutritional support, taking account of personal decisions and preferences. The nutritional plan should be evaluated regularly to ensure that it is meeting the needs of the individual patient. The neuroscience patient's condition, e.g. their cognitive function or level of consciousness, may change requiring prompt re-evaluation of the patient's nutritional care and the need to adapt the support accordingly. Failing to do so prevents the patient from receiving the dietary requirements they need and puts their health at further risk.

Oral nutritional support

Patients who continue to be able to swallow effectively, or are able to swallow through changing the consistency of food and fluids with dietary thickeners, should be provided with meals that meet their nutritional requirements, and their dietary preferences should be taken into consideration. Basic interventions such as checking the consistency of food and fluids, temperature and evaluation of the patient's ability to manage with or without assistance are essential (Gould and Lewis, 2006). Dignity should be promoted as much as possible, and the delegation of feeding assistance should not replace supervision and evaluation by the nurse. It is essential to remember that being assisted with feeding can have an impact on self-esteem, particularly when a carer appears rushed, may use protective shields for clothing, and may wipe the person's mouth from time to time (Squires, 2006). Many of these activities resemble experiences of childhood and may feel humiliating to a patient. Therefore time, patience, being fed by a family member and feeling free to make a mess (by the patient) are important considerations for the nurse. Self-esteem and body image can be altered with the realisation of the loss of independence in this activity of living.

Patients that have a poor appetite may require additional oral supplements in the form of fortified drinks or 'sip feeds', which usually provide more energy dense food in smaller volumes (Jones, 2003). While the evidence to support the benefit of sip feeds for those with neurological disorders is weak, a Cochrane review (Milne *et al.*, 2005) examined their use in the elderly, concluding that they produce a small but consistent weight gain in older people, with a possible beneficial effect on mortality. They also concluded that no evidence of improvement in clinical outcome, functional benefit or reduction in length of hospital stay exists with their use. It has been found that the reason for nutritional supplementation in the form of sip feeds, is often without rationale or supporting documentation and assessment (Brosnan *et al.*, 2001). It is important that the type of sip feed used should be based on a dietician's recommendations to avoid inappropriate prescribing, and should be provided between meals rather than as a substitute for meals.

Thickened fluids may be helpful for those with dysphagia (Squires, 2006), but often adding the thickener can make the fluids unappealing. In some cases it may be necessary to administer additional fluids via an alternative route if the patient is unable to manage sufficient volume orally.

Enteral and parenteral nutrition

Enteral nutritional is preferable to parenteral because it decreases the incidence of infection and is more cost effective (Gramlich *et al.*, 2004). Enteral nutrition also maintains

the functioning of the gastrointestinal tract and helps to maintain normal levels of intestinal flora, which is important in the prevention of translocation of micro-organisms and sepsis in vulnerable patients. Enteral nutrition also accelerates the normalisation of nutritional status when compared to parenteral nutrition (Suchner *et al.*, 1996).

The goal of enteral nutrition is to improve or maintain the patient's nutritional status until they can attain an adequate oral intake (NICE, 2006). It is advised to begin enteral feeding within the first 24 hours of admission to hospital (Wøien and Torunn Bjørk, 2006), so long as gastrointestinal activity is present (bowel sounds). Enteral nutrition can be administered via a nasogastric/jejunal, orogastric, or percutaneous endoscopic gastrostomy tube. The decision to adopt one of these measures requires the input of the multidisciplinary team, family and the patient where possible.

The use of nutritional support protocols and algorithms can result in meaningful improvements in practice, providing a structure and guidelines to practitioners in the support of their care (Wøien and Torunn Bjørk, 2006). Evidence suggests that when local protocols are in place, patients receive significantly greater volumes of their prescribed nutrition (Wøien and Torunn Bjørk, 2006). Feeds are stopped intermittently for many reasons, e.g. tube extubation, large aspirates, for investigations, which can cumulatively result in significant underfeeding. It is essential that accurate volumes are recorded and issues that prevent full volumes being administered are addressed promptly.

Table 16.5 identifies how nutritional requirements should be calculated. Patients following severe head injury often require significantly more calories and protein due to the hypermetabolic and catabolic response that follows injury. In patients who are already malnourished there is a risk of refeeding syndrome which is caused by reinstitution of nutrition too quickly. It is characterised by a rapid fall in phosphate, potassium and magnesium and an increase in ECF. It is therefore essential to recognise patients at risk (NICE, 2006) (see Table 16.6) and to commence gradual nutrition support with regular monitoring of biochemistry.

Nasogastric tubes are often used as a short-term measure until the patient can return to oral feeding that sufficiently meets their nutritional requirements. They are also used when the life expectancy of the patient may be short (Squires, 2006). Nasogastric tubes are not without complication, with the larger bore tubes being linked with pressure necrosis and the smaller bore tubes more likely to become occluded. The insertion of such tubes can also result in misplacement into the lungs, and insertion of

Table 16.5 Calculating nutritional requirements.

Non-acute/severely ill patients not at risk of refeeding syndrome	Patients at risk of refeeding syndrome
• 25–35 kcal/kg/day total energy • 0.8–1.5 g protein (0.13–0.24 g nitrogen)/kg/day • 30–35 ml fluid/kg (calculate requirements for additional losses – insensible, other forms of fluid output) • Supplement with sufficient electrolyte, mineral and micronutrients	• Commence feeding at maximum rate of 10 kcal/kg/day, increasing incrementally over 4–7 days to full requirements • Commence feeding at maximum rate of 5 kcal/kg/day in very high risk patients, with simultaneous three lead cardiac monitoring • Rehydrate and maintain circulatory volume • Administer prescribed oral thiamin 200–300 mg daily, vitamin B complex strong one or two tablets TID (or IV equivalent) and balanced multivitamin/trace element supplement daily for ten days • Where necessary, provide oral, enteral or intravenous supplements of potassium (2–4 mmol/kg/day), phosphate (0.3–0.6 mmol/kg/day) and magnesium (0.2 mmol/kg/day intravenous, 0.4 mmol/kg/day oral)

Adapted from NICE, 2006.

Table 16.6 Patients at Risk of Refeeding Syndrome.

Meet any one of these criteria:	Meet any two of these criteria:
• BMI < 16 kg/m^2 • Unintentional weight loss > 15% within previous 3–6 months • Insufficient or no nutritional intake for > 10 days • Low serum potassium, phosphate or magnesium prior to commencement of nutritional support	• BMI < 18.5 kg/m^2 • Unintentional weight loss > 10% within the last 3–6 months • Insufficient or no nutritional intake for > 5 days • History of alcohol dependency or drug use (including insulin, chemotherapy, antacids or diuretics)

Adapted from National Institute for Health and Clinical Excellence, 2006.

nasogastric tubes into patients with basal skull fractures is an absolute contra-indication due to the risk of penetration into brain tissue; orogastric tubes are usually used instead. Confirming the location of a nasogastric tube has come under considerable review in recent years, and local policy should guide the practitioner in light of the emerging evidence base behind this practice. The National Patient Safety Agency (NPSA, 2005) and NICE (2006) recommend that the pH of the aspirate should be checked using pH paper (pH <5.5 is safe to feed) and, where inconclusive, an x-ray may be required.

Before commencing enteral nutrition the nurse should assess for the presence of bowel sounds and identify if they are normal, hypoactive (very infrequent), hyperactive (loud, high-pitched) or absent. When commencing enteral nutrition, residual volumes should be checked every 2–4 hours, and the patient should be kept at a 30° angle to prevent aspiration (Mestecky, 2006). Large residual volumes usually require temporary halting of the feed administration or a slower rate of feed being commenced and the residual volume being checked again in 2–4 hours (Wøien and Torunn Bjørk, 2006). Maximising tolerance of enteral feeding can usually be achieved by administering prokinetics (metoclopramide or erythromycin). A review of the literature in relation to their effectiveness has shown that they may improve tolerance to enteral nutrition, reduce gastroesophageal reflux and pulmonary aspiration (Tischerman *et al.*, 2002).

If feed intolerance continues to be a problem for more than 72 hours, a nasojejunal tube may be required for those with a high risk of malnutrition (Mestecky, 2006). In such cases a nasogatric tube should remain *in situ* to allow for aspiration of gastric contents; in most cases the nasojejunal tube will have a gastric port.

The long term use of a nasogastric tube is not recommended due to complications associated with it (pressure necrosis, tube displacement, gastric ulceration) and often patients who require long term enteral support (i.e. >4 weeks) will usually require the insertion of a percutaneous endoscopic gastrostomy (PEG) tube (Squires, 2006).

This can have an impact on patient's self esteem and sense of dependency, often signalling to patients that there is a degree of progression of their disease. Moving to interventional forms of enteral nutrition also brings with it the loss of dignity and a heightened state of loss of ability for the patient (Shintani and Shiigai, 2004) which needs to be recognised and managed by the nurse. Patients can begin to review their body image, sexuality, the concept of ever eating again, and may experience a loss at loosing the pleasure of eating and the social role that accompanies it (Rio *et al.*, 2005). These issues and others related to PEG insertion in motor neurone disease patients are addressed in detail in Chapter 27.

Tube extubation

Enteral feeding tube extubation is a common problem for nurses working in neurosciences. Patients who are cognitively impaired, agitated or confused are high risk for such extubation. Tubes should be marked externally to allow for early identification of tube migration outwards. Whelan *et al.* (2006) highlight the necessity to replace the tube at the earliest opportunity in order that patients receive their required calculated nutritional requirements. Nasal loop (bridle) systems, used in a variety of acute settings can be effective in securing nasogastric tubes; their use is also currently being evaluated in stroke patients (Beaven *et al.*, 2007). The use of restraining devices such as padded mittens is often controversial and requires risk assessment and agreement from the multidisciplinary team (MDT) and relatives. In some patients their use may increase agitation (see Chapter 10 for further discussion of restraint).

Nurses need to consider if extubation is as a result of agitation and confusion or an expression of disapproval of the treatment itself. Determining this is difficult and often hindered by communication difficulties and the wishes of family and carers (Whelan *et al.*, 2006). The placement of PEG tubes may be a solution if the problem is persistent.

Continuous versus bolus

There is debate as to whether tube feeding should be administered on a continuous basis, by bolus feeding, or continuous with a rest period. The advantage of a rest period is that it allows gastric pH to become more acidic,

which plays a role in combating micro-organisms that enter the body through the gastrointestinal tract. NICE (2006) recommends that patients being fed into the stomach should have bolus or continuous feeding methods adopted, with consideration (where possible) for patient preference, convenience and drug administration. It may be safer to administer bolus feeds in patients who are agitated and frequently removing their tube. For those patients in intensive care, nasogastric tube feeding is recommended to be delivered continuously over 16–24 hours daily (NICE, 2006). Some patients may be hyperglycaemic and require insulin administration and in these cases NICE (2006) highlights that it is safer and often more practical to administer feeding continuously over 24 hours.

Enteral feeding and diarrhoea

Enteral feeding is not without complications. The most common and serious of these is diarhhoea (Whelan, 2007). The aetiology of diarrhoea is largely attributed to antibiotic administration, hypoalbuminaemia, and pathogenic colonisation of the colon (Whelan *et al.*, 2006; Wiesen *et al.*, 2006; Whelan, 2007). The consequences of diarrhoea are serious. Severe and life-threatening water loss can occur, as can a loss of homeostasis of sodium, potassium, magnesium and trace elements (Metcalf, 2007).

Bacterial diarrhoea is largely only treated in those who have severe infection with signs of systemic involvement, pyrexia and exhaustion (Metcalf, 2007). Diarrhoea attributed to antibiotic administration is more easily managed, most often ceasing after the attributed antibiotic has been discontinued. Fluid and electrolyte restoration, however, are still required (Metcalf, 2007). Therefore, the management of diarrhoea should include hydration and compensation for the loss of electrolytes, which may be supplemented with the use of antidiarrheal medications (Wiesen *et al.*, 2006).

The use of probiotics and prebiotics have received significant attention in recent years. Wiesen *et al.* (2006) highlight how the use of probiotics and prebiotics is not yet fully defined. However, their use has been associated with suppression of pathogenic colonisation, stimulation of immune function, and regulation of metabolism in the gastrointestinal tract (Whelan, 2007). In particular, Whelan (2007) identifies that *Saccharomyces boulardii* reduces the incidence of diarrhoea in patients receiving enteral nutrition in intensive care.

Whelan *et al.* (2006) highlight that there is a lack of evidence on whether enteral nutrition should be discontinued or the rate of the infusion slowed in the presence of diarrhoea. In the absence of such evidence, enteral feeding should be continued in order to maximise nutritional support (Whelan *et al.*, 2006; Wiesen *et al.*, 2006).

Parenteral nutrition

Parenteral nutrition becomes an option only after enteral nutritional methods have been considered as not being viable. The decision to move to parenteral nutrition is usually made on the basis that the patient is receiving inadequate or unsafe oral and/or enteral nutritional intake, or when the patient has a non-functional, inaccessible or perforated gastrointestinal tract (NICE, 2006).

The decision to commence parenteral nutrition requires the benefits to be weighed against the risks. Parenteral nutrition requires the placement of a central venous catheter in long term use and it is therefore associated with an increased risk of infection and impairment of gut-associated immunity (as a result of bypassing the GI tract) (Mestecky, 2006). Peripherally inserted central catheters (PICC) are associated with less risk of infection but can only be used for short term administration of parenteral nutrition and when the supplement feed is deemed suitable (NICE, 2006). Parenteral nutrition is costly as it has to be prepared on an individual basis under strict sterile conditions. The nurse must ensure that the solution is protected from light, as it may affect some of the micronutrients. Strict aseptic technique must be maintained when attaching and disconnecting the feed from the central line. Nutritional requirements need to be calculated specifically.

SUMMARY

Managing fluid, electrolytes and nutrition are core responsibilities for the neuroscience nurse. The complexity of these responsibilities require the nurse to be knowledgeable and intuitive in his/her practice and to work collaboratively with the multidisciplinary team. Those with neurological disorders are predisposed to nutritional and hydrational problems, which can have serious consequences for their recovery, quality of life and independence. Regular thorough assessments and an evidence-based approach has the potential to optimise the patient's nutritional and fluid status.

REFERENCES

Aiyagari V, Deibert E, Diringer MN (2006) Hypernatraemia in the neurologic intensive care unit: how high is too high? *Journal of Critical Care* 21:163–172.

Beaven J, Conroy S, Leonardi-Bee J *et al.* (2007) *Is looped nasogastric tube feeding more effective than conventional nasogastric tube feeding for dysphagia in acute stroke?*

Available from: www.trialsjournal.com/content/8/1/19 Accessed July 2010

Berkenbosch JW, Lentz CW, Jimenez DF *et al.* (2002) Cerebral salt wasting syndrome following brain injury in three pediatric patients: suggestions for rapid diagnosis and therapy. *Pediatric Neurosurgery* 36(2):75–79.

Biswas M, Davies JS (2007) Hyponatraemia in clinical practice. *Postgraduate Medical Journal* 83(980):373–378.

Brosnan S, Margetts B, Munro J *et al.* (Wessex Dietetic Managers Group) (2001) The reported use of dietary supplements (sip feeds) in hospitals in Wessex, UK. *Clinical Nutrition* 20(5):445–449.

Bruder N, Gouvitsos F (2000) Vascular loading in the first 24 hours following severe head injuries. *Annales Francaises D'Anesthesie et de Reanimation* 19(4):316–325.

Bussmann C, Bast T, Rating D (2001) Hyponatraemia in children with acute CNS disease: SIADH or cerebral salt wasting? *Child's Nervous System* 17:58–63.

Capra S (2007) Editorial: Nutrition assessment or nutrition screening – How much information is enough to make a diagnosis of malnutrition in acute care. *Nutrition* 23:356–357.

Castilla-Guerra L, Fernandez-Moreno MC, Lopex Chozas JM *et al.* (2006) Critical Review: Electrolyte Disturbances and Seizures. *Epilepsia* 47(12):1990–1998.

Coenraad MJ, Meinders AE, Taal JC *et al.* (2001) Hyponatraemia in intracranial disorders. *The Netherlands Journal of Medicine* 58:123–127.

Department of Health (2005) *The National Service Framework for Long-Term Conditions*. London: The Stationery Office.

Gould L, Lewis S (2006) Care of head and neck cancer patients with swallowing difficulties. *British Journal of Nursing* 15(20):1091–1096.

Gramlich L, Kichian K, Pinilla J *et al.* (2004) Does enteral nutrition compared to parenteral nutrition result in better outcomes in critically ill adult patients? A systematic review of the literature. *Nutrition* 20(10):843–848.

Jones J (2003) Tackling undernutrition through appropriate supplement prescribing. *British Journal of Community Nursing* 8(8):243–252.

Knighton J, Smith GB (2003) Perioperative fluid therapy. *Anaesthesia and Intensive Care Medicine* 4(10):324–326.

Kyle UG, Kossovsky MP, Larsegard VL *et al.* (2006) Comparison of tools for nutritional assessment and screening at hospital admission: a population study. *Clinical Nutrition* 25:409–417.

McDonnell-Keenan A (1999) Syndrome of inappropriate secretion of antidiuretic hormone in malignancy. *Seminars in Oncology Nursing* 15(3):160–167.

Mestecky A (2006) Metabolic responses after severe head injury and how to optimise nutrition: a literature review. *British Journal of Neuroscience Nursing* 2(2):73–79.

Metcalf C (2007) Chronic diarrhoea: investigation, treatment and nursing care. *Nursing Standard* 21(21):48–56.

Milne AC, Potter J, Avenell A (2005) Protein and energy supplementation in elderly people at risk from malnutrition. *Cochrane Database of Systematic Reviews* Issue 1. Art. No.: CD003288. DOI: 10.1002/14651858.CD003288. pub2.

Mourao F, Amado D, Ravasco P *et al.* (2004) Nutritional risk and status assessment in surgical patients: a challenge amidst plenty. *Nutrition in Hospital* 19:83–88.

National Institute for Health and Clinical Excellence (2006) *Nutrition Support in Adults: oral nutrition support, enteral tube feeding and parenteral nutrition.* London: NICE. Available from: http://www.nice.org.uk

National Patient Safety Agency (2005) *Patient Safety Alert: Reducing the harm caused By misplaced nasogastric tubes.* London: National Patient Safety Agency.

Pedersen EB, Bacevicius E, Bech JN *et al.* (2006) Abnormal rhythmic oscillations of atrial natriuretic peptide and brain natriuretic peptide in chronic renal failire. *Clinical Science* 110:491–501.

Rio A, Ampong MA, Johnson J *et al.* (2005) Nutritional care of patients with motor neurone disease. *British Journal of Neuroscience Nursing* 1(1):38–43.

Rubenstein LZ, Harker JO, Salva A *et al.* (2001) Screening for undernutrition in geriatric practice: Developing the short-form Mini-Nutritional Assessment (MNA-SF). *The Journals of Gerontology Series A: Biological Sciences and Medical Sciences* 56:M366–M372

Sedlacek M, Schoolwerth AC, Remillard BD (2006) Electrolyte disturbances in the intensive care unit. *Seminars in Dialysis* 19(6):496–501.

Shintani A, Shiigai T (2004) Survival-determining factors in patients with neurologic impairments who received home health care in Japan. *Journal of Neurological Sciences* 225:117–123.

Sieber CC (2006) Nutritional screening tools – how does the MNS® compare? Proceedings of the session held in Chicago May 2–3, 2006 (15 years of Mini Nutritional Assessment). *Journal of Nutrition, Health and Ageing* 10(6):488–494.

Simmons-Holcomb S (2002a) Diabetes insipidus. *Dimensions of Critical Care* 21(3):94–97.

Simmons-Holcomb S (2002b) Stopping the cascade of diabetes insipidus. *Nursing* 32(3):32cc1–32cc6.

Spiekermann BF, Thompson SA (1996) Fluid management. In: Stone D and Sperry RJ *et al.* (eds). *The Handbook of Neuroanaesthesia* St Louis: Mosby.

Squires N (2006) Dysphasia management for progressive neurological conditions. *Nursing Standard* 20(29):53–57.

Stuart W, Smellie A, Heald A (2007) Hyponatraemia and hypernatraemia: pitfalls in testing. *British Medical Journal* 334:473–476.

Suchner U, Senftleben U, Eckart T *et al.* (1996) Enteral versus parenteral nutrition: Effects on gastrointestinal function and metabolism. *Nutrition* 12(1):13–22.

Terpstra TL, Terpstra TL (2000) Syndrome of inappropriate antidiuretic hormone secretion: recognition and management. *Medsurg Nursing* 9(2):61–68.

Whelan K (2007) Enteral-tube-feeding diarrhoea: manipulating the colonic microbiota with probiotics and prebiotics. *Proceedings of the Nutrition Society* 66(3):299–306.

Whelan K, Hill L, Preedy VR *et al.* (2006) Formula delivery in patients receiving enteral tube feeding on general hospital wards: the impact of nasogastric extubation and diarrhea. *Nutrition* 22(10):1025–1031.

Wiesen P, Van Gossum A, Preiser JC (2006) Diarrhoea in the critically ill. *Current Opinion in Critical Care* 12(2):149–154.

Wøien H, Torunn Bjørk I (2006) Nutrition of the critically ill patient and effects of implementing a nutritional support algorithm in ICU. *Journal of Clinical Nursing* 15:168–177.

Zafonte RD, Mann R (1997) Cerebral salt wasting syndrome in brain injury patients: a potential cause of hyponatraemia. *Archives of Physical Medicine and Rehabilitation* 78:540–542.

17
Assessment and Management of Pain

Sue Woodward

INTRODUCTION

Neuroscience nurses are regularly required to care for patients in pain, which may or may not be related to their neurological condition. Headache is the most common neurological condition: 3% of the adult population in the UK present to their general practitioner with headache every year (Kernick and Goadsby, 2009). However, pain can be associated with spasticity and other neurological conditions such as multiple sclerosis, dystonia and Parkinson's disease (Schestatsky *et al.*, 2007). Neuropathic (persistent) pain can also present a significant problem within neuroscience practice, and pain, regardless of the origin, can have a significant impact on the quality of life of the individual. Pain may be acute or chronic in nature and nurses are pivotal in caring for patients in pain. They are often the 'gatekeepers' of pain relief, and careful nursing assessment is essential in effective management. Care of patients who experience pain following cranial and spinal neurosurgical procedures is addressed in Chapters 20 and 34 respectively.

DEFINING PAIN

Pain is a subjective experience, the definition of which has been the subject of much debate. There are two widely accepted definitions of pain. The International Association for the Study of Pain (IASP) have defined pain as 'an unpleasant sensory and emotional experience associated with actual or potential tissue damage, or described in terms of such damage' (Merskey and Bogduk, 1994), which is very much based on a biomedical model of under-

standing pain. This definition suggests that if a patient does not have actual or potential tissue damage, they cannot experience pain, and yet emotional or psychological distress may sometimes be perceived as a physical sensation, and a measureable cause for nociceptive pain cannot always be found. The IASP does acknowledge this and states that any sensation reported as pain by a patient should be treated as such (IASP, 2010). It also reminds us that patients who are unconscious or unable to verbalise pain may still experience it. Probably the most readily recognised definition within nursing is that 'pain is whatever the experiencing person says it is, existing whenever he says it does' (Passero and McCaffery, 1999), which stresses the subjective nature of the experience and the importance of believing patient reports of pain.

PHYSIOLOGY OF PAIN

Pain often acts as a protective mechanism to alert the individual to potential tissue damage and to cause reflex withdrawal from a painful stimulus. It can also cause behavioural responses that will limit further tissue damage and promote healing, e.g. an individual will reduce mobility following an injury or surgery. Yet pain can sometimes persist and become debilitating (Godfrey, 2005) or may occur in the absence of tissue damage.

SOMATIC AND VISCERAL PAIN

The sensation of pain is transmitted in the same way as other stimuli, the spinal pathways for which have been described in detail in Chapter 4. Specialised pain receptors (nociceptors) are located within the somatic and visceral tissues (skin, muscles, joints, visceral organs and arterial walls). There are two types of receptor channels, the first detect the noxious stimuli and the second set the stimulus

Neuroscience Nursing: Evidence-Based Practice, 1st Edition.
Edited by Sue Woodward and Ann-Marie Mestecky
© 2011 Blackwell Publishing Ltd

threshold required in order to generate an action potential (Stephan, 2005).

Noxious (painful) sensations may be caused by mechanical, thermal or chemical stimuli, which include bradykinin, prostaglandins, substance-P, serotonin and adenosine triphosphate (ATP) (Godfrey, 2005). It is thought that histamine is released from mast cells in response to painful stimuli, which results in substance P and other neurochemical release, causing a chain reaction in which ion channels open and an action potential is generated. The greater the stimulus, the greater the number of impulses produced (Godfrey, 2005) so more intense pain is felt with a more intense stimulus.

Pain is transmitted via small diameter, myelinated A-delta and unmyelinated C fibres to the dorsal horn of the spinal cord (Morinan, 2000). The A-delta fibres are able to transmit pain sensations faster than the C fibres due to their myelin sheath facilitating salutatory conduction. Pain is often initially felt as a sharp or stabbing pain and is followed by a second dull aching pain that is poorly localised. The first pain is transmitted by the A-delta fibres and the second pain by the C fibres (Craig, 2003).

Somatic/visceral pain pathways

The first-order neurones that enter the dorsal horn synapse with second-order nociceptive neurones that cross over and transmit the sensation of pain to the thalamus and reticular formation, mainly via the spinothalamic and spinoreticular tracts (Godfrey, 2005). The grey matter within the spinal cord is organised into layers, or laminae (Figure 17.1). A-delta fibres enter laminae I, V and X, while C fibres enter laminae I–V. No sensation is perceived until the impulse reaches the brain, and pain is no exception. The somatosensory cortex was thought to be responsible for differentiating pain from other sensory stimuli and for appreciation of the site, quality and intensity of pain (Craig, 2003). More recently it has been suggested that there are also specific pain centres within the brain, such as the parieto-insular cortex and anterior cingulate within the medial frontal cortex (Craig, 2010). Fibres project to all these cortical areas from the thalamus and reticular formation.

The passage of pain fibres through the reticular formation contributes to the autonomic responses exhibited by an individual in response to acute pain, e.g. sweating, tachycardia, elevated blood pressure and respiratory rate. From the thalamus pain fibres project to the hypothalamus which is also thought to contribute to the autonomic response, and to the limbic system which triggers the emotional response to pain (Godfrey, 2005).

Pain pathways within the head

The only nociceptors within the cranium lie within the dura and large intracranial arteries; there are no nociceptors within brain tissue, so the brain itself does not feel pain (Messlinger and Ellrich, 2001). A network of neurones from the trigeminal nerve surrounds the large cerebral and dural arteries and these fibres transmit pain sensation within the cranium and are responsible for headaches (Ebersberger, 2001). The fibres have been shown to have similar conduction properties to A-delta and C fibres that transmit pain from other somatic and visceral nociceptors (Ebersberger, 2001). These fibres are polymodal, i.e. they are responsive to mechanical, thermal and chemical noxious stimuli and the only sensation they transmit is pain, regardless of the stimulus (Strassman *et al.*, 2004).

These fibres then enter the pons via the trigeminal nerve and descend, transmitting the pain impulses to the spinal trigeminal nucleus, a nucleus within the medulla, which acts as the main relay station for pain from structures within the head (Messlinger and Ellrich, 2001), and to the dorsal horn of the first cervical segment (Mørch *et al.*, 2007). These trigeminal fibres also connect to other brain stem nuclei that relay impulses to the areas within the cerebral cortex where pain is perceived (Williamson and Hargreaves, 2001). Fibres from the facial, glossopharyngeal and vagus nerves also converge on the spinal trigeminal nucleus and C1 dorsal horn (Messlinger and Ellrich, 2001; Mørch *et al.*, 2007) and this convergence of nerve fibres is thought to explain referred pain (Fricke, 2001).

Chemical triggers of headache

Irritation affecting the dura, e.g. due to meningitis or subarachnoid haemorrhage, causes sensitisation and activation of the dural nociceptors through a process known as neurogenic inflammation (which involves plasma protein extravasation and vasodilatation). The chemical stimuli released during this inflammatory process (e.g. substance-P or calcitonin-gene related peptide (CGRP)) may directly influence opening of ion channels and cause an action potential to be generated, or may lead to ion channel opening via a sequence of secondary messengers (Ebersberger, 2001). CGRP is known to be released during migraine and cluster headache attacks. It causes arterial dilatation and may also have a direct effect on brain stem trigeminal neurones (Ebersberger, 2001) causing pain.

Substance-P has also been shown to be released with migraine, cluster headaches and subarachnoid haemorrhage, and substance-P can cause release of histamine from dural mast cells (Ebersberger, 2001). Inflammatory mediators, such as bradykinin, histamine, serotonin and

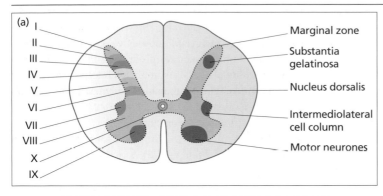

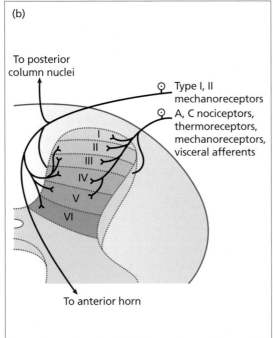

Figure 17.1 Sensation. (a) Laminae (I–X) and named cell groups at mid thoracic level. (b) Targets of primary afferent neurones in the posterior grey horn. Reproduced from Clarke, C. *et al.*, *Neurology: A Queen Square Textbook*, Wiley-Blackwell, with permission.

prostaglandins have been shown to activate cerebral nociceptors and neurones in the same way as they do in other pain pathways. Serotonin has been shown to be released following subarachnoid haemorrhage and is thought to be a key molecule in sensitising dural nociceptors and neurones (Ebersberger, 2001). There is also some evidence that nitric oxide may play a role in the vasoregulation of dural and cerebral blood vessels (Fricke, 2001) and is thought to be implicated in the onset of headache.

Gate control theory

In 1965 Melzack and Wall proposed a mechanism for neuromodulation of pain on entering the spinal cord, the *Gate Control Theory*, which has endured to this day

(Melzack and Wall, 1965; Dickenson, 2002). The theory proposes that modulation of pain sensation relies upon the stimulation of inhibitory interneurones between the first-order nociceptive neurones from the periphery and second-order nociceptive neurones within the spinal tracts. When stimulated by A-delta fibres the 'gate' is opened and these interneurones permit the transmission of painful sensations towards the brain. These interneurones are also stimulated by the neurotransmitter glutamate from large diameter A-beta sensory fibres that transmit sensations such as touch or pressure. When stimulated by A-beta fibres the transmission of pain sensations through the interneurones is inhibited and the 'gate' is said to be closed.

This theory explains why rubbing the skin over an injury reduces the sensation of pain, i.e. rubbing causes impulses to be transmitted via the A-beta fibres, which stimulates the inhibitory interneurones and closes the gate to transmission of nociceptive impulses to the second-order nociceptive neurones. The gate control theory also suggests that the inhibitory interneurones are influenced by descending inhibitory pathways from the brain, which also close the gate. These descending neurones secrete neurotransmitters, such as serotonin and noradrenaline, which excite the inhibitory interneurones and suppress the transmission of pain to the second-order neurones (Godfrey, 2005). The inhibitory interneurones secrete peptides, such as endorphins and encephalins, which act as natural opioids and inhibit the transmission of pain via the second-order neurones. These natural opioids are also thought to prevent secretion of substance-P and thereby reduce the noxious stimulation which is causing the pain.

NEUROPATHIC PAIN

Neuropathic pain follows injury to or dysfunction of the nervous system (Dworkin, 2002) and continues beyond the normal period of healing (Mann, 2008). Neuropathic pain is commonly experienced by people with peripheral neuropathies (see Chapter 35) or cranial nerve disorders (e.g. trigeminal neuralgia) (see Chapter 13), but it also occurs with many neurological and other conditions. Neuropathic pain is now also thought to be a feature of persistent pain syndromes that are resistant to standard analgesics (Mann, 2008). The mechanism and aetiology of neuropathic pain is not fully understood, but there are a number of theories, which are discussed below.

Both somatic (inflammatory) and neuropathic pain from nerve damage can produce changes in the spinal cord and brain (plasticity), which then results in persistent and altered pain sensation. Neurones that usually transmit pain can become 'sensitised' (Godfrey, 2005) and then need a lower level of stimulation to transmit a painful sensation (hyperalgesia). In neuropathic pain there is evidence that this sensitisation persists beyond the normal time for tissue healing, and minimal levels of stimulation are required to perceive pain (Mann, 2008).

Chemicals released peripherally when tissue is damaged can also sensitise other surrounding receptors. Inflammatory processes are thought to cause nociceptive fibres in neighbouring regions to become affected, and previously non-painful areas to be perceived as painful (White *et al.*, 2007; Mann, 2008). There is some recent evidence that proinflammatory cytokines (chemokines) are released from the cells of the nervous system and act on the receptors of the nervous system, causing excitation and release of substance-P (White *et al.*, 2007). Eventually this leads to abnormalities in the central processing of sensation and pain, with normal sensory stimuli, such as pressure, being abnormally recognised as pain (allodynia) (White *et al.*, 2007). There is also some evidence that the modulating effect from the descending neurones from the brain that normally close the gate to pain perception, is also lost in neuropathic pain (Mann, 2008) due to destruction of the inhibitory neurones.

Abnormal neuronal regeneration can result in neuroma formation, which can lead to spontaneous and prolonged neuronal transmission and pain (Mann, 2008). Neuronal damage may also result in proliferation in sodium channels around the site of the damage and within the dorsal horn of the spinal cord, thus increasing hyper-excitability within pain pathways (Novakovic *et al.*, 1998).

Neuropathic pain affects approximately 8% of the UK population or 7.8 million people (Donaldson, 2008), but is more common among those with diabetes (24%) and following shingles (20%) (Bennett, 2006). Neuropathic pain severely impacts on quality of life, as do all chronic pain syndromes, and the symptoms of neuropathic pain include paraesthesias (painless abnormal sensations, e.g. pins and needles), dysaesthesias (unpleasant abnormal sensations, e.g. burning/numbness), allodynia and hyperalgesia.

ASSESSMENT OF PAIN

Assessment of pain requires the nurse to consider three elements: the quality or description of the pain, the quantity or severity, and the site/distribution of the pain. Often, however, a detailed assessment of pain is not feasible and a quick assessment of the quantity of pain is all that is undertaken. Assessing intensity alone is too limited and the minimum requirements for pain assessment in any acute/emergency situation should be to evaluate the pain location, intensity and quality. As pain is a subjective experience the only way to be able to gain an understanding of a patient's pain is to ask them. Pain is underestimated on many occasions and nurses may fail to assess pain routinely and therefore to treat pain adequately (Schafheutle *et al.*, 2004).

Pain rating scales

There are a large number of valid and reliable pain rating scales available for use by nurses, many of which are freely available in different languages via the British Pain Society website (http://www.britishpainsociety.org/pub_

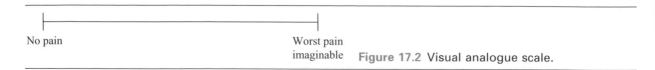

Figure 17.2 Visual analogue scale.

pain_scales.htm). Most patients are at the very least able to give a score to their pain severity. Some of the most commonly used tools will now be discussed.

Visual analogue scales (VAS)

The VAS consists of a 100 mm line marked with anchors at each end that read 'no pain' and 'worst pain imaginable' (Figure 17.2). The patient is asked to put a mark on the line that corresponds to their level of pain and the nurse then measures the distance from the 'no pain' anchor to the mark made by the patient, thereby obtaining a score in mm. The VAS has been shown to be valid and reliable as well as sensitive to change, so it can be used to assess the effectiveness of analgesia (Price *et al.*, 1983). Practical difficulties may be encountered using this tool in practice (Williamson and Hoggart, 2005) due to either poor patient dexterity or difficulty in grasping the abstract concept.

Verbal rating scales

Verbal rating scales attempt to rate severity of pain using adjectives (e.g. mild, moderate, severe) rather than numerical descriptors. Patients often prefer to use a verbal rating scale, but these can have poor sensitivity (Williamson and Hoggart, 2005).

Numerical rating scales/ pain ruler

Using a numerical rating scale, the patient is asked to rate their pain on a scale from 0–5 or 0–10, where zero equates to no pain and the largest digit relates to the worst pain imaginable. This information can be presented to patients as a numerical scale on either a horizontal or vertical line (a pain ruler) (Bourbonnais, 1981) and has been shown to be valid and reliable and to have good sensitivity (Williamson and Hoggart, 2005).

McGill pain questionnaire (MPQ)

The MPQ encompasses all aspects of pain assessment, i.e. intensity, quality and location. It has proven validity and reliability, can be used for the assessment of neuropathic pain and is often considered to be comprehensive, sensitive and accurate (Melzack, 1987). It is rarely used in clinical practice however as it can be quite time consuming to complete and is difficult to use with patients with change in level of consciousness or cognitive functioning.

Assessing pain in unconscious patients

The assessment of pain in the unconscious patient is complex as a result of the impaired ability of the patient to communicate. Nurses must often rely on physical indicators of pain and intuitive judgement, but tools have been designed to facilitate such assessment. Gelinas and Johnston (2007) report on the validity of the Critical Care Pain Observation Tool (CPOT), which was found to be reliable and valid. The CPOT has also been shown to have moderate to high inter-rater reliability, regardless of the level of consciousness (Gelinas *et al.*, 2006). The researchers also report that, while behavioural indicators provide more valid information in pain assessment than physiologic indicators, these are likely to be suppressed in the unconscious patient and nurses need to be vigilant in observing for signs of distress and proactive in pain management (Fullarton, 2002). Fluctuations in haemodynamic parameters are not always accurate indicators of pain, and Young and co-workers (2006) present another tool, the Behavioural Pain Scale (BPS), that is reliable and valid in assessing pain in those with altered states of consciousness, including patients who are sedated and ventilated.

Assessing pain in cognitively impaired patients

Patients with cognitive impairment may have difficulty in using standard pain assessment tools and nurses have had to rely on subjective behavioural indicators of pain (Box 17.1), which are notoriously unreliable. Pain can easily be overlooked in such patients as they are unable to communicate this effectively and they are less likely to receive adequate analgesics. The most common reason that patients' pain goes undetected is that no-one asks about it (McClean, 2003), often because it is incorrectly thought that patients cannot adequately report their symptoms. For patients with mild to moderate impairment a number of tools can be used, but a verbal rating scale is probably best, written down and focusing on the current pain experience. At the very least nurses should be able to elicit a yes/no response to a simple question about whether a patient has any pain, ache or discomfort.

<table>
<tr><td>

Box 17.1   Non-verbal/behavioural signs of pain

- Facial expressions
- Vocalisation (e.g. calling out, moaning)
- Posture/movement (e.g. rigidity, fidgeting, increased/restricted movement)
- Aggression
- Agitation
- Withdrawal
- Change in appetite
- Change in sleep pattern
- Crying
- Increased confusion
- Irritability
- Obvious distress
- Physiological changes (stress response in acute pain only, i.e. within initial 24 hours)

</td><td>

Box 17.2   Factors that influence nurses' assessments of patient pain

- Assessor's background
  - Ethnic origin (Leiderman-Davitz and Davitz, 1978; Davitz *et al.*, 1976)
  - Length of clinical experience (Lenberg *et al.*, 1970)
- Patient factors
  - Age (Short *et al.*, 1990; McCaffrey and Ferrell 1991a)
  - Presence/absence of physical pathology (Halfens *et al.*, 1990)
  - Non-verbal expression of pain (Baer *et al.*, 1970; McCaffrey and Ferrell, 1991b)
  - Physiological changes in systemic observations (McCaffrey and Ferrell, 1992a)
  - Lifestyle (McCaffrey and Ferrell, 1992b)
  - Gender (McCaffrey and Ferrell, 1992c)

</td></tr>
</table>

Pain assessment scales for use with cognitively impaired individuals need to be simple and easy to apply in clinical practice (van Iersel *et al.*, 2006) and while a number of tools are available, some are more complex than others. Most scales, such as the Abbey Pain Scale (Abbey *et al.*, 2004) and the Pain Assessment in Advanced Dementia (PAINAD) Scale (Warden *et al.*, 2003) rely on observations of non-verbal signs of pain by nurses. It is thought that facial expression, vocalisation and body language are the most reliable indicators of physical pain in those with cognitive impairment and these appear in all the non-verbal pain scores (van Iersel *et al.*, 2006). Physiological changes are considered to be less reliable indicators, unless the patient is in acute pain, which is less common than chronic pain among people with cognitive impairment

Assessing neuropathic pain

Neuropathic pain often results in unique sensations, so using verbal descriptors can be useful (Bennett, 2006). Several pain scales have been developed specifically for the assessment of neuropathic pain. The Neuropathic Pain Scale (Galer and Jensen, 1997) was the first to be developed and is available free to clinicians for use in clinical practice: http://www.mapi-trust.org/services/questionnairelicensing/cataloguequestionnaires/74-nps.

The Leeds Assessment of Neuropathic Symptoms and Signs Pain Scale (LANSS) (Bennett, 2001) was developed subsequently and has proven validity and sensitivity. The LANSS assessed five symptoms and examined allodynia and pinprick testing, so had to be administered by a clinician. This has since been adapted into a self-report instrument for completion by patients (Bennett *et al.*, 2005). Other tools include: the Neuropathic Pain Symptom Inventory (NPSI) (Bouhassira *et al.*, 2004), the Douleur Neuropathique 4 (DN4) (Bouhassira *et al.*, 2005) and the Neuropathic Pain Questionnaire (NPQ) (Krause and Backonja, 2003), but these have not all been prospectively validated.

Factors influencing nursing assessment of patients' pain

Seminal work undertaken in the 1970s and 80s identified that nurses do not always rely on patient reports of pain and that decision making may be influenced by a number of factors (Box 17.2). Nurses were shown to rate older patients' reports of pain more highly, but were less likely to administer analgesics over fears of respiratory depression and other side-effects. Nurses were also seen to be influenced by non-verbal signs of pain, such as facial expression, behaviour and changes in vital signs and may seek confirmation of patient self-reports of pain from such factors. Yet physiological changes will usually normalise within 24 hours of the onset of acute pain and therefore cannot be reliably used to confirm patients' verbal ratings. Patients may also 'put a brave face' on their pain, particularly if they do not wish to show that they are in pain in front of visitors, or might use distraction (e.g. watching TV or talking to others) as a form of pain relief. Not all patients in pain will lie still in bed and grimace.

A number of further studies have since identified a discrepancy between patient reports of pain and nurses' documented assessments (McCaffery *et al.*, 2000, Solomon 2001). Nurses continue to underestimate patients' pain (Sloman *et al.*, 2005) and, although education programmes have improved assessment practice, nurses still fail to administer adequate analgesia (Ene *et al.*, 2008). It is essential that patients' reports of pain are believed and acted upon if adequate pain relief is to be achieved.

HEADACHE

A headache can result from a specific process (e.g. migraine) or be symptomatic of lesions affecting cranial structures (e.g. inflammation, bleeding or raised ICP). The global prevalence of headache is 47% (Stovner *et al.*, 2007) and it is one of the ten most disabling conditions in the world. Central sensitisation (see: Neuropathic pain) is thought to be the mechanism by which headaches become chronic (Fernandez-de-las-Penas, 2008).

Classification of headaches

The International Headache Society has classified headache disorders into: (1) primary headaches, (2) secondary headaches and (3) cranial neuralgias, central and primary facial pain and other headaches (IHS, 2010). The main primary headaches include migraine, tension-type headaches (TTH), cluster headaches and other trigeminal autonomic cephalalgias. Secondary headaches are those caused by other neurological conditions, such as vascular, traumatic or infectious disorders. If the patient's history is suspicious of a secondary headache, brain imaging will be undertaken to inform differential diagnosis (Kernick and Goadsby, 2009). Cranial neuralgias and facial pain are discussed in Chapter 13.

Migraine

Epidemiology

The estimated global prevalence of migraine is approximately 10% of the population, but is most common in Europe where it affects 15% of the adult population (Stovner *et al.*, 2007) and causes significant disease burden. Migraine costs 27 billion Euros per annum throughout Europe (Goadsby, 2007) and is the most costly neurological disorder. The World Health Organisation ranks migraine as the 19th leading cause of disability in the world and rates a day spent with migraine the same as a day spent quadriplegic (Menken *et al.*, 2000). Migraine is also associated with depression, anxiety disorders, e.g. panic and phobias, substance misuse and some mood disorders (Radat and Swendsen, 2004), with increased psychiatric co-morbidity with migraine with aura. Some studies have shown a higher prevalence of migraine among females (Mett and Tfelt-Hansen, 2008), but this has not been demonstrated universally (Kelman, 2006).

Aetiology

Stimulation of the large cerebral, meningeal and temporal arteries produces throbbing pain and, in particular, stimulation of the middle meningeal artery causes pain localised behind the eye and associated with nausea (Williamson and Hargreaves, 2001). Migraine was therefore previously thought to be of vascular origin, triggered by vasodilatation. Elevated levels of CGRP have also been demonstrated in migraine, activating the trigeminal nerve (Williamson and Hargreaves, 2001), suggesting that neurogenic inflammation contributes to the onset of migraine. CGRP can be released by perivascular trigeminal nerve fibres following stimulation of the trigeminal ganglion and causes vasodilatation (Williamson and Hargreaves, 2001). Migraine is therefore now thought to be an inherited brain stem disorder of the pathways that regulate sensory information (Kernick and Goadsby, 2009), which results in a disturbance of the perception of normal sensory input.

Migraine attacks may be precipitated by a number of factors and neurophysiological studies of sufferers have shown that the brain has heightened sensitivity to internal and external triggers, such as sound, light, movement, smell and other sensory stimuli (Kelman, 2007). Many triggers have been identified (Box 17.3), but not all sufferers can identify any specific triggers for their attacks.

Box 17.3 Known triggers for migraine

- Stress
- Hormonal changes (e.g. menstrual cycle) in women
- Sexual activity
- Not eating
- Climatic conditions
- Sleep disruption/sleeping late
- Perfume or odours
- Neck pain
- Alcohol intake
- Smoking
- Heat
- Some foods
- Exercise

Source: Kelman, 2007.

Signs and symptoms

Migraine episodically causes a moderate to severe headache, which may be described as throbbing, aching, stabbing or pressure and is sometimes aggravated by activity. The pain is usually unilateral, but may be bilateral and patients describe sensitivity to light, sound and smell (Goadsby, 2003). Almost half of migraines are at their worst within an hour of onset and can last between 4 and 72 hours (IHS, 2010). 34.6% of patients report either waking with or being woken by migraine (Kelman, 2006) and these migraines often last longer and are associated with vomiting. Migraine may recur after a period of headache relief in up to 40% of patients (Kelman, 2006), on average within 10 hours. A migraine lasting for more than three days is defined as status migrainosis (Kernick and Goadsby, 2009).

Migraine is sub-divided into migraine with aura (formerly classical migraine) and migraine without aura (formerly common migraine) (Kernick and Goadsby, 2009). Migraine is accompanied by aura (visual disturbances) in approximately 10–20% of patients (Mett and Tfelt-Hansen, 2008). While visual symptoms are the most common presentation of aura, paraesthesia (30%), motor symptoms (e.g. hemiplegic migraine) (18%) and delusions, déjà vu and hallucinations may also occur (Kernick and Goadsby, 2009). An aura usually precedes the headache, but can occur at the same time, or even without the headache developing.

Tension-type headache (TTH)

Epidemiology

Tension-type headaches are the most common type of primary headaches. The global prevalence of TTH is around 40% and they may be described as chronic if they occur for 15 days per month or for 3 months or longer (Stovner *et al.*, 2007). TTH has been shown to cause as much of an economic burden as migraine, with the number of working days lost due to TTH being three times higher than due to migraine because of the higher prevalence (Stovner *et al.*, 2007). TTH is more common among women than men and is sub-divided into episodic and chronic TTH.

Aetiology

Muscular, vascular and psychological factors have been considered as possible causes of TTH. It is thought that TTH is triggered by myofascial trigger points (tender spot under a taut band of muscle), which have been identified in the shoulder, neck and head muscles, from where the pain is referred to the head (Fernandez-de-las-Penas, 2008). TTH was previously thought to be caused by prolonged muscular contraction due to stress or emotional distress, but this is now considered unlikely (Kernick and Goadsby, 2009). It is now thought more likely that central sensitisation to pain is involved in the condition becoming chronic.

Signs and symptoms

TTH is less intense and debilitating than migraine, but may occur on an almost daily basis in some individuals. It is generally described as a 'featureless' bilateral headache that does not impact on physical activity (Kernick and Goadsby, 2009). The pain is usually described as dull and aching, rather than throbbing and can affect any part of the head, lasting for a few hours to days.

Cluster headache (CH)

Epidemiology

Cluster headaches are quite rare, affecting approximately 0.2% of the population and more males than females (Kernick and Goadsby, 2009). Once it develops (usually during the third or fourth decade, CH is thought to be a lifelong condition. Cluster headaches can severely impact on quality of life and can result in anxiety and depression.

Aetiology

The aetiology of CH is unknown, but it is now thought to be of neurovascular origin and may have a similar trigeminal aetiology to that of migraine (Goadsby and Edvinsson, 1994). The posterior hypothalamus, which is involved in control of circadian rhythms and sleep-wake cycles, has also been implicated in the onset of cluster headaches and differences in the grey matter density between sufferers and healthy controls has been found (May, 2008). There is also an increased incidence of CH in some families, suggestive of a genetic component to development (Bjorn Russell, 2004).

There is also evidence of both sympathetic dysfunction (e.g. unilateral ptosis and facial sweating) and parasympathetic dysfunction (e.g. rhinorrhoea, lacrimation and nasal congestion) and it has been suggested that the condition may be caused by an inflammatory or vasculitic lesion within the cavernous sinus (Dodick and Capobianco, 2001). Many bouts of CH occur during summer months and may be triggered in some by an allergic rhinitis (hay fever). Other triggers include stress, extreme temperatures, relaxation and afternoon naps, certain foods, alcohol, smoking and sexual activity.

Signs and symptoms

Cluster headaches are excruciating, unilateral headaches that present with a remitting-relapsing pattern and normally occur seasonally and at regular times of day, often at night during the early hours of the morning (Dodick and Capobianco, 2001). Each individual headache may last from 15 minutes to three hours and these occur in bouts lasting two to three months, during which several attacks of the headaches occur (Kernick and Goadsby, 2009). In cluster headaches the facial nerve also becomes activated, causing periorbital redness, tears and nasal congestion that is characteristic of the disorder (Williamson and Hargreaves, 2001). The pain is described as stabbing or boring and will often be located around the orbit or temple.

Other causes of headache and facial pain

Post lumbar puncture (LP) headache

Following a lumbar puncture an amount of CSF has been lost and may continue to leak out of the subarachnoid space via a dural tear. It is hypothesised that this loss of CSF results in a reduction in buoyancy and a corresponding increase in relative brain weight. This additional weight puts tension onto the pial connective tissue, stimulating mechanoreceptors and causing headache (Fricke *et al.*, 2001). Care of patients with headache following LP is discussed in Chapter 19, although there is no evidence of benefit from routine bedrest and the role of fluid administration is uncertain (Sudlow and Warlow, 2001).

Medication-overuse headache (MOH)

MOH is the most common secondary cause of chronic daily headache (Dodick, 2009). The prevalence of MOH is approximately 1%. Many of these patients have suffered from chronic migraine or TTH and resort to taking various over-the-counter medications on a regular basis. MOH is treated by withdrawing and/or limiting the frequency of medication use.

Mobile phone headache

Headache has often been attributed to mobile phone use and some experimental studies on healthy individuals have shown changes in cerebral blood flow, EEG and excitability to transcranial magnetic stimulation from the electromagnetic fields of mobile phones (Oftedal *et al.*, 2008). However more recently double-blind sham-controlled studies have shown that radiofrequency emission from mobile phones does not produce headache, even in allegedly susceptible individuals (Oftedal *et al.*, 2008).

MEDICAL AND NURSING MANAGEMENT OF PAIN

Pain management should always be patient-centred and should take account of the views and preferences of patients regarding pain management. Good communication is an essential component of pain relief, supported by evidence-based interventions. The following sections discuss pain management interventions for patients with headaches and other pain syndromes that may be encountered in neuroscience nursing practice.

MANAGEMENT OF HEADACHE

Migraine

Many patients with migraine will know that, if an attack occurs, the pain may be exacerbated by light and/or movement, and they will seek to lie down in a darkened room. In addition pharmacological and other interventions are utilised to both treat an acute attack and to prevent future migraine occurrence.

Pharmacological interventions for acute migraine

Treatment of a migraine attack often begins with simple non-disease specific analgesics such as aspirin, paracetamol or other NSAIDs, which can be effective. Paracetamol 1 g, ibuprofen 400–600 mg and domperidone 10 mg is recommended when a headache is beginning (Kernick and Goadsby, 2009). Gut motility and stomach emptying is reduced in migraine and gastric stasis can contribute to nausea and vomiting, so addition of anti-emetics such as domperidone or metoclopramide can help (Goadsby, 2003). When these simple measures are ineffective, disease-specific treatments, such as triptans, are recommended. When early vomiting is a problem both domperidone and diclofenac can be administered per rectum.

Anti-migraine drugs are thought to work by inhibiting neurogenic inflammation (Williamson and Hargreaves, 2001), but the exact mechanism of action of many is unclear. Valproate is also thought to inhibit neurotransmission within the trigeminal nucleus, NSAIDs have been shown to have additional inhibitory effects within the brain stem, and aspirin and ketorolac are also thought to have antimigraine effects by reducing brain stem trigeminal neuronal activity (Williamson and Hargreaves, 2001).

Serotonin receptor agonists (triptans) interact with presynaptic serotonin receptors on the trigeminal nerve fibres, causing vasoconstriction and inhibiting the release of CGRP, thereby reducing neurogenic inflammation (Williamson and Hargreaves, 2001). They are also thought to have a central effect on the spinal trigeminal nucleus, preventing sensitisation, and have been shown to be effective in treating acute migraine (McCrory and Gray, 2003). One of the main difficulties with triptans is the vascular side-effects produced. Triptans such as sumatriptan and almotriptan, all have similar efficacy, but newer triptans (e.g. almotriptan) are better tolerated due to a lower side-effect profile than others (Mett and Tfelt-Hansen, 2008). Current research is focusing on the development of CGRP receptor antagonists (Goadsby, 2007).

Opioids, such as morphine, may be used in acute migraine attack which is intractable to other drugs. Morphine has also been shown to reduce the extravasation associated with neurogenic inflammation (Williamson and Hargreaves, 2001). More recently studies of treatment of acute attacks with corticosteroids (IV dexamethasone) have been undertaken, although some recommend that this is used only for status migrainosis (Friedman *et al.*, 2007) and it has not been shown to reduce recurrence after discharge (Rowe *et al.*, 2007).

Physical therapy/exercise

Some studies have suggested that manipulative therapy may be effective for migraine (Fernandez-de-las-Penas, 2008) and exercise has increased endorphin levels (Köseoglu *et al.*, 2003). A recent review has suggested that regular exercise may have a part to play in migraine treatment programmes, but that most studies are of poor methodological quality and have not shown significant reduction of headache frequency or duration (Busch and Gaul, 2008). There is also some evidence that spinal manipulation may also be effective for migraine prophylaxis (Brønfort *et al.*, 2004), but evidence for transcutaneous electrical nerve stimulation (TENS) is less substantive.

Lifestyle changes

Nurses and neurologists need to assist patients to identify potential triggers and to modify lifestyle. Keeping regular habits such as sleep, exercise, meals and work/relaxation, may help to reduce headache frequency (Goadsby, 2003). Trigger avoidance needs to be individualised and severe dietary restrictions are not helpful, but some patients may find that certain foods trigger their attacks and so may avoid them. It has been shown that nurse-led education for people with migraine increases confidence and that patients were more satisfied with their ability to manage migraine (Cady *et al.*, 2007).

Pharmacological migraine prophylaxis

Most patients will not require preventative management, but if the attacks are more frequent than three times per month this may be necessary (Goadsby, 2003). The most useful proven treatments for migraine prophylaxis include tricyclic anti-depressants (e.g. amitryptilline) and anticonvulsants (Chronicle and Mulleners, 2004), although there is little evidence of one over another. However, many treatments have significant side-effects such as cognitive dysfunction, weight gain, tiredness and erectile dysfunction (Goadsby, 2007). Selective serotonin-reuptake inhibitors (SSRIs) have also been tried, but have not been shown to be effective for migraine prophylaxis (Moja *et al.*, 2005). Occipital nerve stimulation has also been tried with some effect. It is based on the premis that second order neurones from these spinal afferents converge on the trigeminal spinal nucleus (Kernick and Goadsby, 2009).

Acupuncture

There is some evidence that acupuncture is as effective as pharmacological migraine prophylaxis, has fewer side-effects (Linde *et al.*, 2009a) and should therefore be considered for those who might be willing to try this intervention.

Tension-type headaches (TTH)
Pharmacological interventions for acute TTH

Simple analgesics, such as paracetamol and NSAIDs will usually be effective for TTH (Kernick and Goadsby, 2009). If the headaches become frequent, the patient should be assessed for medication overuse headaches. When TTH becomes a chronic problem the focus shifts from treatment of acute attacks to prophylaxis.

Physical therapy/exercise

There is insufficient evidence of the efficacy of physical therapy and exercise for TTH (Fernandez-de-las-Penas *et al.*, 2006), although it has been proposed that physical therapies (e.g. manipulative therapies) may help by reducing peripheral sensitisation from muscle trigger points and thereby reduce central sensitisation. Regular exercise has also been shown to have general hypoanalgesic effects (Fernandez-de-las-Penas, 2008). A Cochrane review has identified that there may be some benefit from spinal manipulation in the treatment of TTH (Brønfort *et al.*, 2004), but that the evidence for other non-invasive physical therapies, such as therapeutic touch, TENS and cranial electrotherapy is weaker.

Pharmacological prophylaxis

Many different interventions have been used to prevent chronic TTH, including non-steroidal anti-inflammatory drugs (NSAIDs), tricyclic antidepressants, relaxation therapies, and muscle relaxants (Aponte and Deantonio, 2006). SSRIs have not been shown to be as effective as tricyclic antidepressants for chronic TTH (Moja *et al.*, 2005). It is thought that centrally acting muscle relaxants (e.g. baclofen, dantrolene and diazepam) may be useful in TTH prophylaxis, due to the possible muscular origin of the headaches (Aponte and Deantonio, 2006). This is the subject of an ongoing Cochrane review, although these drugs are not currently recommended due to their adverse effects (Kernick and Goadsby, 2009).

Acupuncture and other non-invasive therapies

Acupuncture has been shown to be a potentially valuable treatment for frequent episodic or chronic TTH (Linde *et al.*, 2009b) although the evidence is limited. There is also some evidence that cognitive behavioural therapy (CBT) may be useful in individuals who are suffering from stress (Kernick and Goadsby, 2009).

Cluster headaches (CH)

Pharmacological interventions for acute attack

Sumatriptan administered subcutaneously is effective in treating an acute attack, but not in preventing an attack occurring (Dodick and Capobianco, 2001). Sumatriptan can also be administered via a nasal spray, but this is less effective (Kernick and Goadsby, 2009).

Surgical and other interventions

Surgical interventions are normally a last resort, but may become necessary in treating intractable CH. Deep brain stimulation of the posterior hypothalamus has been shown to be effective in up to 60% of patients with otherwise intractable cluster headaches (May, 2008). Occiptial nerve stimulation is also demonstrating promising results (Kernick and Goadsby, 2009).

Normobaric and hyperbaric oxygen therapy has been utilised in the treatment of cluster headaches (Bennett *et al.*, 2008). Hyperbaric oxygen therapy (HBOT) involves the administration of 100% oxygen at greater than one atmosphere, while normobaric oxygen therapy (NBOT) delivers oxygen at atmospheric pressure. NBOT is much cheaper and easy to administer in a clinical setting, while HBOT is costly and can only be delivered within a hyperbaric chamber. There is weak evidence of the effectiveness of NBOT for cluster headaches and a suggestion of the effectiveness of HBOT from one small scale, underpowered study (Bennett *et al.*, 2008). Nurses will be required to administer 100% oxygen at 7–12 l/min to in-patients for approximately 15–30 minutes to abort an acute attack (Kernick and Goadsby, 2009) via a non-rebreathing face mask.

Pharmacological prophylaxis

Corticosteroids are the most effective prophylactic treatment, but cannot be continued long-term due to the side-effects. Prevention therefore begins with oral prednisolone, up to 60 mg per day for five days, which is then tailed off (Kernick and Goadsby, 2009). As the dose of steroid is reduced another prophylactic agent is introduced, such as methysergide, verapamil, lithium or an anti-convulsant. Methysergide, verapamil and lithium are all proven to be effective in preventing CH, but the evidence supporting use of anti-convulsants is as yet unproven (Kernick and Goadsby, 2009).

MANAGEMENT OF NEUROPATHIC, SOMATIC AND VISCERAL PAIN

Pharmacological interventions for somatic and visceral pain

Pain has a significant impact on health and daily living and is often inadequately managed in hospital (Godfrey, 2005). The World Health Organisation has suggested that a 'pain ladder' is used to guide the management of cancer pain (WHO, 2010) and these general principles can also be applied to the management of other pain. The best option for the patient is to achieve adequate pain relief with the lowest side-effects possible. The pain ladder states that analgesics should be administered promptly when a patient reports pain, beginning with nonopioids for mild pain (e.g. aspirin and paracetamol), followed by mild opioids (e.g. codeine) for unrelieved mild or moderate pain, and then strong opioids (e.g. morphine) for intractable or moderate to severe pain, until the patient is pain free (WHO, 2010). One of the strengths of the analgesic ladder is the use of combinations of treatments and adjuvants to analgesics.

Clearly nurses have a vital role in both direct administration of analgesics, monitoring their effectiveness, and in educating patients regarding their drug regime. The importance of assessment and acting on patients' reports of pain cannot therefore be underestimated. In acute settings patients often rely on nurses for pain relief although they may be reluctant to ask. For many the use of patient controlled analgesia (PCA) can overcome some of these issues, but not all neuroscience patients have either the cognitive ability or manual dexterity to be able to manage PCA and nurses must therefore be especially vigilant in monitoring for the effects and side-effects of analgesics.

Pharmacological interventions for neuropathic pain

Anti-depressants and anti-convulsants

Anti-depressants and anti-convulsants are the front line management for neuropathic pain (NICE, 2010). Tricyclics are more effective than other anti-depressants, but usually result in more side-effects (Bennett, 2006) so may not be well tolerated by patients. There is clear evidence of the effectiveness of tricyclic anti-depressants, although they are not licensed for treatment of neuropathic pain (NICE, 2010). The role of SSRIs is unclear and there is no evidence of whether these drugs have a role in the prevention of neuropathic pain (Saarto and Wiffen, 2007). There have been very few trials comparing anti-depressants with anti-convulsants (Bennett, 2006).

Opiates and other drugs

There is some evidence for the effectiveness of tramadol in treating neuropathic pain, but a significant proportion of patients who take this drug will suffer from side-effects, such as nausea and vomiting (Duehmke *et al.*, 2006). Opioids are often avoided over fears of addiction. There is little evidence of the effectiveness of opioids in treating neuropathic pain in the short-term, but they do seem to be effective in the longer-term (Eisenberg *et al.*, 2006). Local anaesthetics administered via intravenous infusion have also been used in some trials and have been shown to be as effective as anti-convulsants and opiates (Challapalli *et al.*, 2005), although this is unlikely to be used in clinical practice.

Complementary therapies and other interventions

Distraction

It is recognised that pain involves a psychological component and demands attention from the individual, involving activation of the anterior cingulate gyrus (Frankenstein *et al.*, 2001). We are all aware that when we are in pain at night or when alone it feels worse than when activity is going on around us. Distraction is a valid form of pain relief and moving attention away from a painful stimulus is known to reduce perception of pain (Frankenstein *et al.*, 2001) by modulating activity within the anterior cingulate gyrus and focusing attention on other attention-demanding activities. Nurses should facilitate distraction as an adjuvant to promote pain relief, for example encouraging patients to watch television or engage in conversation.

Massage

Massage has been used for pain relief, often for pain of muscular origin such as low back pain. While there is some evidence that the therapy may be beneficial, there are insufficient trials on which to base conclusive advice (Ernst, 1999). Massage may be more effective when combined with patient education and exercise for low back pain (Furlan *et al.*, 2008).

Trancutaneous electrical nerve stimulation (TENS)

TENS has been shown to be effective for both somatic and neuropathic pain and the analgesic effects occur rapidly (Johnson, 2006). TENS involves the application of an electrical current through the skin from a portable stimulator attached to surface electrodes and is thought to work by selectively stimulating non-noxious large diameter sensory (A-beta) fibres and thereby closing the gate at the spinal level. Prolonged use is also thought to encourage endorphin release. Nurses need to assist patients in learning to use the device, and where to place the electrodes to achieve maximum effectiveness from this therapy. The electrodes should be placed on an unaffected area of skin along the path of major nerves and proximal to the site of pain. As the effects of TENS stop when the device is turned off, patients should be advised to leave the electrodes in place and to use the device periodically throughout the day as pain relief is required (Johnson, 2006).

Acupuncture

Acupuncture is an ancient remedy and part of the practice of traditional Chinese medicine. It is based on the principle that needles placed through the skin will stimulate the flow of Qi (pronounced Chi) or energy through energy channels called meridians. Acupuncture has been shown in functional MRI studies to modulate nociceptive input and to have an influence on the limbic system within the brain (Asghar *et al.*, 2010). Acupuncture has also been shown to be effective for neuropathic and other pain, with the effects lasting longer than with TENS, although it is often not effective immediately (Johnson, 2006). NICE has recommended acupuncture as an evidence-based intervention with the publication of the guidance (NICE, 2009) on low back pain.

SUMMARY

Nurses are central to effective management of pain for people with neurological conditions and need to be knowledgeable about a variety of interventions. Pain and anxiety are mediated through similar systems, so psychological support and education regarding pain and pain management for patients is as vital as administering analgesia. Patient-centred care should take account of the views and preferences of patients regarding pain management.

REFERENCES

Abbey J, Piller N, De Bellis A *et al.* (2004) The Abbey Pain Scale. A 1-minute numerical indicator for people with late-stage dementia. *International Journal of Palliative Nursing* 10:6–13.

Aponte JC, Deantonio R (2006) Muscle relaxants versus placebo for tension-type headache prophylaxis (Protocol). *Cochrane Database of Systematic Reviews* Issue 3. Art. No.: CD006144. DOI: 10.1002/14651858.CD006144

Asghar AUR, Green G, Lythgoe MF (2010) Acupuncture needling sensation: The neural correlates of deqi using fMRI. *Brain Research* 1315(22):111–118.

Baer E, Davitz LJ, Lieb R (1970) Influences of physical pain and psychological distress: in relation to verbal and non-verbal patient communication. *Nursing Research* 19(5):388–392.

Bennett M (2001) The LANSS pain scale: the Leeds Assessment of Neuropathic Symptoms and Signs. *Pain* 92:147–157.

Bennett M (2006) *Neuropathic Pain.* Oxford: Oxford University Press.

Bennett MH, French C, Schnabel A *et al.* (2008) Normobaric and hyperbaric oxygen therapy for migraine and cluster headache. *Cochrane Database of Systematic Reviews* Issue 3. Art. No.: CD005219. DOI: 10.1002/14651858. CD005219.pub2.

Bennett MI, Smith BH, Torrance N *et al.* (2005) The S-LANSS score for identifying pain of predominantly neuropathic origin: validation for use in clinic and postal research. *Journal of Pain* 6:149–158.

Bjorn RM (2004) Epidemiology and genetics of cluster headache. *Lancet Neurology* 3(5):279–283.

Bouhassira D, Attal N, Alchaar H *et al.* (2005) Comparison of pain syndromes associated with nervous or somatic lesions and development of a new neuropathic pain diagnostic questionnaire (DN4). *Pain* 114:29–36.

Bouhassira D, Attal N, Fermanian J *et al.* (2004) Development and validation of the Neuropathic Pain Symptom Inventory. *Pain* 108:248–257.

Bourbonnais F (1981) Pain assessment: development of a tool for the nurse and the patient. *Journal of Advanced Nursing* 6(4):277–282.

Brønfort G, Nilsson N, Haas M *et al.* (2004) Non-invasive physical treatments for chronic/recurrent headache. *Cochrane Database of Systematic Reviews* Issue 3. Art. No.: CD001878. DOI: 10.1002/14651858.CD001878.pub2.

Busch V, Gaul C (2008) Exercise in migraine therapy – is there any evidence of efficacy? A critical review. *Headache* 48:890–899.

Cady R, Farmer K, Beach ME *et al.* (2007) Nurse-based education: an office-based comparative model for education of migraine patients. *Headache* 48:564–569.

Challapalli V, Tremont-Lukats IW, McNicol ED *et al.* (2005) Systemic administration of local anesthetic agents to relieve neuropathic pain. *Cochrane Database of Systematic Reviews* Issue 4. Art. No.: CD003345. DOI: 10.1002/14651858.CD003345.pub2.

Chronicle EP, Mulleners WM (2004) Anticonvulsant drugs for migraine prophylaxis. *Cochrane Database of Systematic*

Reviews Issue 3. Art. No.: CD003226. DOI: 10.1002/14651858.CD003226.pub2.

Craig AD (2003) Pain mechanisms: Labeled lines versus convergence in central processing. *Annual Review of Neuroscience* 26:1–30.

Craig AD (2010) *Mapping pain in the brain.* Available from: http://www.wellcome.ac.uk/en/pain/microsite/science2.html Accessed July 2010

Davitz LJ, Sameshima Y, Davitz J (1976) Suffering as viewed in six different cultures. *American Journal of Nursing* 76(8):1296–1297.

Dickenson AH (2002) Gate control theory of pain stands the test of time. *British Journal of Anaesthesia* 88(6):755–757.

Dodick D (2009) Medication overuse headache. In: MacGregor and Frith *ABC of Headache.* Oxford: Wiley-Blackwell.

Dodick DW, Capobianco DJ (2001) Treatment and management of cluster headache. *Current Pain and Headache Reports* 5:83–91.

Donaldson L (2008) *150 Years of the Annual Report of the Chief Medical Officer.* London: Department of Health.

Duehmke RM, Hollingshead J, Cornblath DR (2006) Tramadol for neuropathic pain. *Cochrane Database of Systematic Reviews* Issue 3. Art. No.: CD003726. DOI: 10.1002/14651858.CD003726.pub3.

Dworkin RH (2002) An overview of neuropathic pain: syndromes, symptoms, signs and several mechanisms. *Clinical Journal of Pain* 18(6):343–349.

Ebersberger A (2001) Physiology of meningeal innervation: aspects and consequences of chemosensitivity of meningeal nociceptors. *Microscopy Research and Technique* 53:138–146.

Eisenberg E, McNicol ED, Carr DB (2006) Opioids for neuropathic pain. *Cochrane Database of Systematic Reviews* Issue 3. Art. No.: CD006146. DOI: 10.1002/14651858. CD006146.

Ene KW, Nordberg G, Bergh I *et al.* (2008) Postoperative pain management: The influence of surgical ward nurses. *Journal of Clinical Nursing* 17:2042–2050.

Ernst E (1999) Massage therapy for low back pain: a systematic review. *Journal of Pain and Symptom Management* 17(1):65–69.

Fernandez-de-las-Penas C (2008) Physical therapy and exercise in headache. *Cephalalgia* 28(Suppl 1):36–38.

Fernandez-de-las-Penas C, Alonson-Blanco C, Cuadrado ML *et al.* (2006) Are manual therapies effective in reducing pain from tension-type headache ? A systematic review. *Clinical Journal of Pain* 22:278–285.

Frankenstein UN, Richter W, McIntyre MC *et al.* (2001) Distraction modulates anterior cingulate gyrus activations during the cold pressor test. *NeuroImage* 14(4):827–836.

Fricke B (2001) Current concepts of meningeal innervation: An introduction. *Microscopy Research and Technique* 53:93–95.

Fricke B, Andres KH, During MV (2001) Nerve fibres innervating the cranial and spinal meninges: morphology of nerve fibre terminals and their structural integration. *Microscopy Research and Technique* 53:96–105.

Friedman BW, Greenwald P, Bania TC *et al.* (2007) Randomized trial of IV dexamethasone for acute migraine in the emergency department. *Neurology* 69:2038–2044.

Fullarton A (2002) Examining the comfort of the unconscious patient. *European Journal of Palliative Care* 9(6):232–233.

Furlan AD, Imamura M, Dryden T *et al.* (2008) Massage for low-back pain. *Cochrane Database of Systematic Reviews* Issue 4. Art. No.: CD001929. DOI: 10.1002/14651858.CD001929.pub2.

Galer BS, Jensen MP (1997) Development and preliminary validation of a pain measure specific to neuropathic pain: the Neuropathic Pain Scale. *Neurology* 48:332–338.

Gelinas C, Johnston C (2007) Pain assessment in the critically ill ventilated patient: validation of the Critical-Care Pain Observation Tool and physiologic indicators. *Clinical Journal of Pain* 23(6):497–505.

Gelinas C, Fillion L, Puntillo KA *et al.* (2006) Validation of the Critical-Care Pain Observation Tool in adult patients. *American Journal of Critical Care* 15(4):420–428.

Goadsby P (2003) Migraine: diagnosis and management. *International Medicine Journal* 33:436–442.

Goadsby P (2007) Emerging therapies for migraine. *Neurology* 3(11):610–619.

Goadsby PJ, Edvinsson L (1994) Human in vivo evidence for trigeminovascular activation in cluster headache. Neuropeptide changes and effects of acute attack therapies. *Brain* 117(3):427–434.

Godfrey H (2005) Understanding pain. Part 1: Physiology of pain. *British Journal of Nursing* 14(16): 846–852.

Halfens R, Evers G, Abu-Saad H (1990) Determinants of pain assessment by nurses. *International Journal of Nursing Studies* 27(1):43–49.

International Association for the Study of Pain (2010) IASP *Pain terminology.* Available from: http://www.iasp-pain.org/AM/Template.cfm?Section=General_Resource_Links&Template=/CM/HTMLDisplay.cfm&ContentID=3058#Pain Accessed July 2010.

International Headache Society (2010) *IHS classification ICDH-II* Available from: http://ihs-classification.org/en/02_klassifikation/ Accessed July 2010.

Johnson MI (2006) Transcutaneous electrical nerve stimulation (TENS) and acupuncture. In: Bennett M *Neuropathic Pain.* Oxford: Oxford University Press.

Kelman L (2006) Pain characteristics of the acute migraine attack. *Headache* 46:942–953.

Kelman L (2007) The triggers or precipitants of the acute migraine attack. *Cephalalgia* 27:394–402.

Kernick D, Goadsby PJ (2009) *Headache: A Practical Manual.* Oxford: Oxford University Press.

Köseoglu E, Akboyraz A, Soyuer A *et al.* (2003) Aerobic exercise and plasma beta endorphin levels in patients with migrainous headache without aura. *Cephalalgia* 23:972–976.

Krause SJ, Backonja MM (2003) Development of a neuropathic pain questionnaire. *Clinical Journal of Pain* 19:306–314.

Leiderman-Davitz L, Davitz JR (1978) Black and white nurses' inferences of suffering. *Nursing Times* 74(17):708–710.

Lenberg CB, Burnside H, Davitz LJ (1970) Inferences of pain and psychological distress: (iii) in relation to length of time in the nursing education programme. *Nursing Research* 19(5):399–401.

Linde K, Allais G, Brinkhaus B *et al.* (2009a) Acupuncture for migraine prophylaxis. *Cochrane Database of Systematic Reviews* Issue 1. Art. No.: CD001218. DOI: 10.1002/14651858.CD001218.pub2.

Linde K, Allais G, Brinkhaus B *et al.* (2009b) Acupuncture for tension-type headache. *Cochrane Database of Systematic Reviews* Issue 1. Art. No.: CD007587. DOI: 10.1002/14651858.CD007587.

Mann E (2008) Neuropathic pain: could nurses be more involved? *British Journal of Nursing* 17(19):1208–1213.

May A (2008) Hypothalamic deep-brain stimulation: target and potential mechanism for the treatment of cluster headache. *Cephalalgia* 28:799–803.

McCaffrey M, Ferrell B (1991a) Patient age: Does it affect your pain control decisions? *Nursing91* 21(9):44–48.

McCaffrey M, Ferrell B (1991b) How would you respond to these patients in pain? *Nursing91* 21(6):34–37.

McCaffrey M, Ferrell B (1992a) How vital are vital signs? *Nursing92* 22(1):43–46.

McCaffrey M, Ferrell B (1992b) Does life-style affect your pain-control decisions? *Nursing92* 22(4):58–61.

McCaffrey M, Ferrell B (1992c) Does the gender gap affect your pain-control? *Nursing92* 22(8):48–51.

McCaffery M, Ferrel BR, Pasero C (2000) Nurses' personal opinions about patients' pain and their effect on recorded assessment and titration of opioid doses. *Pain Management Nursing* 1:79–87.

McClean WJ (2003) Identifying and managing pain in people with dementia. *Nursing and Residential Care* 5(9):428–430.

McCrory DC, Gray RN (2003) Oral sumatriptan for acute migraine. *Cochrane Database of Systematic Reviews* Issue 3. Art. No.: CD002915. DOI: 10.1002/14651858.CD002915.

Melzack R (1987) The short-form McGill Pain Questionnaire. *Pain* 30:191–197.

Melzack R, Wall PD (1965) Pain mechanisms: a new theory. *Science* 150(699):971–979.

Menken M, Munsat TL, Toole JF (2000) The global burden of disease study – implications for neurology. *Archives of Neurology* 57:418–420.

Merskey H, Bogduk N (1994) *Classification of Chronic Pain.* (2nd edition). Seattle: IASP Press.

Messlinger K, Ellrich J (2001) Meningeal nociception: electrophysiological studies related to headache and referred pain. *Microscopy Research and Technology* 53:129–137.

Mett A, Tfelt-Hansen P (2008) Acute migraine therapy: recent evidence from randomized comparative trials. *Current Opinion in Neurology* 21(3):331–337.

Moja L, Cusi C, Sterzi R *et al.* (2005) Selective serotonin re-uptake inhibitors (SSRIs) for preventing migraine and tension-type headaches. *Cochrane Database of Systematic Reviews* Issue 3. Art. No.: CD002919. DOI: 10.1002/14651858.CD002919.pub2.

Mørch CD, Hu JW, Arendt-Nielsen L *et al.* (2007) Convergence of cutaneous, musculoskeletal, dural and visceral afferents onto nociceptive neurons in the first cervical dorsal horn. *European Journal of Neuroscience* 26:142–154.

Morinan A (2000) Neurobiological mechanisms in pain control. *Nursing and Residential Care* 2(6):280–282.

National Institute for Health and Clinical Excellence (2009) *Low Back Pain*. London: NICE.

National Institute for Health and Clinical Excellence (2010) *Neuropathic Pain: the pharmacological management of neuropathic pain in adults in non-specialist settings.* London: NICE.

Novakovic S, Tzoumaka E, McGivern J *et al.* (1998) Distribution of the tetrodotoxin-resistant sodium channel PN3 in rat sensory neurons in normal and neuropathic conditions. *Journal of Neuroscience* 18:2174–2187.

Oftedal G, Straume A, Johnsson A *et al.* (2008) Mobile phone headache: a double-blind, sham-controlled provocation study. *Cephalalgia* 27:447–455.

Passero C, McCaffery M (1999) *Pain: Clinical Management.* St Louis: Mosby.

Price DD, McGrath PA, Rafii A *et al.* (1983) The validation of visual analogue scales as ratio scale measures for chronic and experimental pain. *Pain* 17(1):45–56.

Radat F, Swendsen J (2004) Psychiatric co-morbidity in migraine: a review. *Cephalalgia* 25:165–178.

Rowe BH, Colman I, Edmonds ML *et al.* (2007) Randomized controlled trial of intravenous dexamethasone to prevent relapse in acute migraine headache. *Headache* 48:333–340.

Saarto T, Wiffen PJ (2007) Antidepressants for neuropathic pain. *Cochrane Database of Systematic Reviews* Issue 4. Art. No.: CD005454. DOI: 10.1002/14651858.CD005454.pub2.

Schafheutle E, Cantrill J, Noyce P (2004) The nature of informal pain questioning by nurses – a barrier to postoperative pain management. *Pharmacy World and Science* 26(1):12–17.

Schestatsky P, Kumru H, Valls-Solé J *et al.* (2007) Neurophysiologic study of central pain in patients with Parkinson disease. *Neurology* 69:2162–2169.

Short L, Burnett ML, Egbert AM *et al.* (1990) Medicating the post-operative elderly: How do nurses make their decisions? *Journal of Gerontological Nursing* 16(7):12–17.

Sloman R, Rosen G, Rom M *et al.* (2005) Nurses' assessment of pain in surgical patients. *Journal of Advanced Nursing* 52:125–132.

Solomon P (2001) Congruence between health professionals' and patients' pain ratings: a review of the literature. *Scandinavian Journal of Caring Sciences* 15:174–180.

Stephan MM (2005) Signals from the frontline. *The Scientist* 19(Suppl 1):20–23.

Stovner LJ, Hagen K, Jensen R *et al.* (2007) The global burden of headache: a documentation of headache prevalence and disability worldwide. *Cephalalgia* 27:193–210.

Strassman AM, Weissner W, Williams M *et al.* (2004) Axon diameters and intradural trajectories of the dural innervation in the rat. *Journal of Comparative Neurology* 473:364–376.

Sudlow CLM, Warlow CP (2001). Posture and fluids for preventing post-dural puncture headache. *Cochrane Database of Systematic Reviews* Issue 2. Art. No.: CD001790.

van Iersel T, Timmerman D, Mullie A (2006) Introduction of a pain scale for palliative care patients with cognitive impairment. *International Journal of Palliative Nursing* 12(2):54–59.

Warden V, Hurley A, Volicer L (2003) Development and psychometric evaluation of the pain assessment in advanced dementia PAINAD scale. *Journal of American Medical Directors Association* 1:9–15.

White FA, Jung H, Miller RJ (2007) Chemokines and the pathophysiology of neuropathic pain. *Proceedings of the National Academy of Sciences* 104(51):20151–20158.

Williamson A, Hoggart B (2005) Pain: a review of three commonly used pain rating scales. *Journal of Clinical Nursing* 14(7):798–804.

Williamson DJ, Hargreaves RJ (2001) Neurogenic inflammation in the context of migraine. *Microscopy Research and Technique* 53:167–178.

World Health Organisation (2010) *WHO's Pain Ladder* Available from: http://www.who.int/cancer/palliative/painladder/en/ Accessed July 2010

Young J, Siffleet J, Nikoletti S *et al.* (2006) Use of a behavioural pain scale to assess pain in ventilated, unconscious and/or sedated patients. *Intensive and Critical Care Nursing* 22:32–39.

18

Assessment and Management of Bladder and Bowel Problems

Mandy Wells, Deborah Yarde and Sue Woodward

INTRODUCTION

Urinary and faecal incontinence are prominent features of neurological disorders, such as stroke, multiple sclerosis, spinal cord injuries and inflammation, brain injuries, Parkinson's disease and dementias, and can have a major impact on psychological and social wellbeing. Due to the complex neurological control of micturition, patients with neurological damage anywhere along the pathway can present with bladder dysfunction. The nature of the presenting problem depends on where in the pathway the nerve damage has occurred. Incontinence has three main aetiological mechanisms: disorders of the bladder and its local spinal network, central nervous system lesions and cognitive disorders, and impaired functional abilities. One might therefore expect a high incidence of incontinence in patients with neurological problems. Depending on the specific neurological condition, prevalence of bladder and bowel problems may affect as many as 75% of patients. NICE guidelines for incontinence in neurological disease are in development.

PHYSIOLOGY OF MICTURITION

The lower urinary tract (LUT), which is comprised of the ureters, bladder and urethra, is innervated by three sets of peripheral nerves. Parasympathetic nerves, which arise at the sacral level of the spinal cord (S2–S4), excite the bladder and relax the urethra. Lumbar sympathetic nerves

(T10–L2) inhibit the bladder body and excite the bladder base and urethra. Pudendal nerves control the external urethral sphincter and associated mechanisms of the pelvic floor. All these nerves contain afferent (sensory) axons as well as efferent pathways. The peripheral innervation of the bladder passes through the cauda equina and sacral plexus, but is centrally controlled and coordinated by micturition centres in the pons and the frontal lobe (Fowler, 1999).

Bladder filling

It is thought that tension receptors within the wall of the detrusor muscle are stimulated as it is stretched during bladder filling. More recently it has been suggested that the urothelium releases chemical stimuli when stretched and that this mechanism, rather than tension receptors, stimulates afferent impulses that convey the sensation of bladder fullness (Fry, 2005). Impulses generated during filling are transmitted to the sacral micturition centre (S2–S4) where a reflex response sends an impulse back to the bladder. This results in the detrusor muscle relaxing, so that pressure does not build up within the bladder, and the external urethral sphincter contracting to maintain closure at the bladder neck during filling. As this phase is controlled by sacral spinal reflexes, an individual is unaware of bladder filling at this stage.

During filling, messages are also sent via the spinothalamic tract towards the brain, but it is not until the bladder is approximately two thirds full that these messages reach the frontal lobes and perception of the

Neuroscience Nursing: Evidence-Based Practice, 1st Edition.
Edited by Sue Woodward and Ann-Marie Mestecky
© 2011 Blackwell Publishing Ltd

sensation of bladder fullness takes place. The bladder is constantly either filling and storing urine, or emptying (micturition). The pontine micturition centre switches between these two states, under the influence of the frontal micturition centre (Fowler, 1999). The storage phase of the urinary bladder can be switched to the voiding phase either involuntarily when bladder capacity is reached, e.g. in babies and some patients with dementia, or voluntarily and influenced by social norms and perception of bladder fullness (Fowler, 1999).

Voiding

Adults normally void approximately 4–500 ml of urine six or seven times daily, depending on fluid intake, although the detrusor muscle can stretch to hold a significantly larger amount than this optimum capacity. Normal micturition requires the detrusor muscle to contract simultaneously with relaxation of the external urethral sphincter to enable a pressure to build up inside the bladder at the same time as the resistance at the bladder neck is reduced (Fry, 2005).

The pontine micturition centre directly excites bladder motor neurones in the sacral cord during micturition causing the detrusor to contract; at the same time, it inhib-its the external urethral sphincter motor neurones, causing the sphincter to relax (Blok, 2002). Contraction of the detrusor muscle is maintained until the bladder is emptied fully.

URINARY SYMPTOMS AND INCONTINENCE

The International Continence Society (ICS) defines urinary incontinence as 'the complaint of any involuntary leakage of urine' (Abrams *et al.*, 2002). Urinary incontinence is one of a number of lower urinary tract symptoms (LUTS) that may be identified during patient assessments and affects approximately 25% of females and 10% of males among the general population in the UK at any given time. The prevalence among patients with neurological disorders is much higher.

The ICS has attempted to standardise the terminology used by clinicians throughout the world for many years. The terminology is updated periodically as understanding of bladder physiology develops. LUTS have also been defined and divided into either storage, voiding or post-micturition symptoms (Abrams *et al.*, 2002) (Table 18.1).

There are several distinct types of urinary incontinence (Abrams *et al.*, 2002) (Table 18.2).

Table 18.1 Urinary symptoms.

Main problem	Symptoms
Storage symptoms	• Increased daytime frequency: voiding more than eight times per day • Nocturia: waking once or more at night to void • Urgency: a sudden compelling desire to pass urine which is difficult to defer • Urinary incontinence
Voiding symptoms	• Slow stream: perception that urinary flow is reduced compared to previous performance • Splitting or spraying of the urinary stream • Intermittent stream: urine flow which stops and starts • Hesitancy: difficulty in initiating micturition • Straining: muscular effort used to initiate, maintain or improve the urinary stream • Terminal dribble: a prolonged final part of micturition, when the flow has slowed
Post-micturition symptoms (experienced immediately after micturition)	• Feeling of incomplete emptying • Post-micturition dribble: the involuntary loss of urine immediately after finishing passing urine

Adapted from Abrams *et al.*, 2002.

Table 18.2 Types of urinary incontinence.

Type	Signs and symptoms
Stress urinary incontinence	Leak on exertion, e.g. coughing, sneezing. Normal voiding pattern
Urge urinary incontinence/overactive bladder	May experience urgency without incontinence (overactive bladder dry) or involuntary leakage associated with urgency (overactive bladder wet) Frequency Nocturia
Mixed urinary incontinence	Involuntary leakage on exertion associated with urgency
Acute/chronic urinary retention (with overflow incontinence)	Hesitancy Slow stream Straining to void Patient may or may not have overflow incontinence Frequency Significant post-void residual >300 ml
Reflex incontinence/terminal detrusor overactivity	Incontinence when the bladder reaches capacity and a single, sustained detrusor contraction empties the bladder fully
Continuous urinary incontinence	Complaint of continuous leakage

NEUROLOGICAL CONDITIONS AND BLADDER DYSFUNCTION

Sometimes the term 'neurogenic bladder' is used to describe bladder dysfunction in patients with neurological conditions, but this simply means that the bladder dysfunction is of neurological origin, rather than referring to a specific type of bladder problem. Table 18.3 identifies the type of problem that is likely to be associated with different neurological disorders.

Damage to the lower motor neurone

Abrams (2006) identifies that damage to the lower motor neurone causes lost bladder sensation, absent detrusor contractility, reduced bladder compliance, reduced sphincter function, and patients often need to void by straining. Damage to the sacral micturition centre (T12/L1 and below) will result in the detrusor losing its nervous innervation and losing tone. The detrusor does not contract and the bladder cannot empty. This will result in the development of a high residual volume within the bladder and is commonly seen in patients with lower spinal and peripheral lesions.

Damage to the upper motor neurone

Damage to the upper motor neurone causes lost bladder sensation, detrusor overactivity and reduced bladder compliance (Abrams, 2006). Sphincter function is normal during filling but may be overactive during voiding. If the lesion is above T12/L1, the detrusor muscle still receives impulses from the sacral micturition centre, but these are not being coordinated by the brain. The bladder may empty and overactive bladder or detrusor–sphincter dyssynergia can result. Unfortunately for many patients following spinal injury, it cannot be determined on the basis of the neurological level of the injury whether the upper or lower motor neurone is affected (Doherty *et al.*, 2002).

Detrusor–sphincter dyssynergia

This potentially dangerous condition is characterised by lack of coordination of the contractions of the detrusor muscle and external urethral sphincter. Contraction of the detrusor, urethral sphincter and urethral tissue occurs simultaneously resulting in a high pressure building up inside the bladder. This can ultimately cause a retrograde flow of urine up the ureters towards the kidneys, leading to upper urinary tract dilatation and renal impairment (Abrams, 2006).

ASSESSMENT OF BLADDER FUNCTION

Lower urinary tract symptoms cannot be used to make a definitive diagnosis and a thorough bedside assessment is required followed, if necessary, by urodynamic investiga-

Table 18.3 Common types of urinary incontinence associated with neurological disorders.

Type of bladder dysfunction	Causes
Stress urinary incontinence	Pregnancy and childbearing, menopause, pelvic floor or urethral sphincter dysfunction (the incontinence is not necessarily related to the neurological condition) Weak urethral sphincter following spinal damage below T12/L1 affecting the sacral micturition centre
Overactive bladder/urge urinary incontinence	Sensory causes: UTI, indwelling urethral catheters, bladder irritants (e.g. caffeine/alcohol) Motor causes: multiple sclerosis, Parkinson's disease, head injuries, stroke
Chronic urinary retention – with or without detrusor sphincter dyssynergia	Outflow obstruction: Constipation and faecal impaction, blocked urinary catheter, urethral strictures Neurogenic causes: multiple sclerosis, spinal cord injury, Guillain–Barré syndrome, other peripheral neuropathies, e.g. diabetic neuropathy
Reflex incontinence/terminal detrusor overactivity	Dementias, acute confusional disorders, unconscious and sedated patients
Continuous urinary incontinence	Usually due to a vesico-vaginal or vesico-rectal fistula. Rarely seen and not usually due to neurological problems May occur in multi-system atrophy

tions. The nurse has a pivotal role in the recognition, assessment and subsequent management of urinary incontinence (DH, 2000; RCN, 2006). Urinary incontinence is a symptom and should be investigated like any other symptom by taking a detailed history, followed by physical examination and investigations.

There is a lot of stigma and embarrassment for patients surrounding incontinence and they may be reluctant to discuss the problem. Trigger questions (Box 18.1) should be asked during routine assessment to identify patients who might have a bladder or bowel problem (DH, 2003). If a patient responds positively to a trigger question then further in-depth assessment, using appropriate continence assessment tools, is crucial if an accurate diagnosis is to be made. It is important to remember that patients are partners in all care delivery strategies and part of the assessment must include their perception of the problem and their views as to how they would like to see the problem managed.

History taking

Ideally a continence assessment tool should be used as this provides an aide memoir for the assessor as well as facilitating accurate documentation, but there are a number of essential components required for every continence assess-

---

Box 18.1   Trigger questions

- How often do you go to the toilet to empty your bladder during the day?
- How often are you woken at night by the desire to pass urine?
- Do you ever feel an urgent need to rush to the toilet? If so do you make it in time?
- How often do you open your bowels?
- Do you ever feel like you are not emptying your bladder fully?
- Do you ever feel like you are not emptying your bowel fully?

---

ment (Table 18.4). If no continence specific assessment tools are available within the practice area, the nurse should ensure that all of these components are assessed in detail. After taking the patient's history in detail, further physical examination is needed and simple investigations may be required (Box 18.2). All of these, except urodynamics are considered an essential part of continence assessment and should be undertaken by nursing staff.

There are a number of internationally recognised valid and reliable tools for the assessment of urinary inconti-

Table 18.4 Key components of continence assessment.

Aspect of assessment	Questions to consider
General health history	• Identification of reversible conditions that contribute to urinary incontinence (e.g. arthritis, obesity, smoking) • Impact of incontinence and how the problem is currently managed • Patient's and carer's views of treatment options
Past medical, surgical and obstetric history	Include obstetric history, pelvic surgery, prostatectomy, hysterectomy, diabetes as well as neurological history
Diet and fluid intake	• Volume and type of fluid intake (note bladder irritant fluids, e.g. caffeine, alcohol) • Diet intake (including fibre)
Drug history	Check for common medications that have effects and side-effects on the bladder (e.g. diuretics, sedatives, anti-cholinergics). Many medications have effects on the bladder that are not routinely recognized
History of incontinence and urinary symptoms	• Use an assessment checklist as discussed above. • Identify most bothersome symptoms • Reassessment of patients with neurological disability/disorder is important as their disease progresses
Bowel habit	Bowel frequency, constipation, faecal incontinence
Functional abilities (including disabilities)	• Manual dexterity • Mobility • Cognitive function
Quality of life for patient and family	• Reducing social contact • Impact on relationships • Evidence of depression
Environment	• Access to toilet facilities • Laundry facilities

---

Box 18.2 Examination and investigation of urinary incontinence

• Abdominal examination
• Pelvic floor, perineal and rectal examination
• Urinalysis
• Post-void residual urine measurement
• Frequency/volume charting
• Urodynamics

---

nence, LUTS and impact on quality of life that have been developed by the International Consultation on Incontinence (ICIQ) (Avery *et al.*, 2004). None of the ICIQ questionnaires have been developed specifically for use with patients with a neurological diagnosis, although one is currently in development. Woodward (2006) found a paucity of assessment tools designed for this specific patient group and developed an assessment tool that was found to be valid and reliable and should be considered for the nursing assessment of patients with neurological conditions.

Physical examination and investigations

Physical examination

Physical examination is imperative, but patients are rarely examined in both primary and secondary health care settings (RCP, 2006). Abdominal palpation should be carried out to detect a full bladder or constipation. Perineal skin condition may reveal maceration or excoriation due to sitting in a wet environment. The nurse should also observe for obvious vaginal or rectal prolapse. Pelvic floor assessment should only be undertaken by those with the competence to do so and is beyond the scope of this chapter, but interested readers are referred to Haslam and Laycock (2007). Rectal examination should be performed to check for amount and consistency of stool and to exclude constipation/faecal impaction.

Investigations
Urinalysis

Urinalysis must be undertaken. Haematuria may suggest urinary tract infection (UTI), stones, or cancer, while glucosuria may cause polyuria and exacerbate symptoms. The nurse should use dipsticks that test for leucocytes and nitrites, indicative of UTI. If the urine tests positive for nitrites and leucocytes and the patient is symptomatic, a mid-stream urine should be sent for culture and sensitivities and a course of antibiotics should be prescribed pending results (NICE, 2006).

Post-void residual volume

This should preferably be estimated by using portable ultrasound equipment, but may be assessed by in–out catheterisation. A residual volume up to 100 ml should be considered within normal limits in someone with a neurological disability (Fowler *et al.*, 2009) although some expert clinicians will argue that it can be higher than this. There is no research or even expert consensus on what is the norm in various disease processes or across various age groups.

Frequency–volume charting

Detailed description of the pattern of frequency, volume of voiding, and fluid intake should be obtained through three day frequency–volume chart. Charting will provide more objective information on the number of incontinent episodes, the frequency of micturition and functional bladder capacity. Charting for three days allows for sufficient detail to be collected, while ensuring patient compliance (NICE, 2006).

Urodynamics

Urodynamic investigations aim to reproduce the patient's symptomatic complaints and to provide a pathophysiological explanation by correlating the patient's symptoms with the urodynamic finding. Patients are normally treated conservatively and urodynamic investigations are only recommended if this fails (NICE, 2006), as they are invasive and can lead to the patient developing UTI. Such investiga-

tions have not been shown to influence outcomes if carried out before initial treatment. Referral for urodynamics should be considered if the diagnosis is uncertain, the patient has failed to respond to conservative management or if there is other complicating co-morbidity.

Urodynamics are more likely to be necessary for patients with neurological disease than for those without. It is usual to perform urodynamic investigations following spinal cord injury after spinal shock has resolved. These baseline urodynamics establish whether there is a detrusor contraction in response to bladder filling and whether or not detrusor–sphincter dyssynergia has developed. They may also be used to assess the effects of disease progression on the lower urinary tract, e.g. for people with multiple sclerosis.

MEDICAL AND NURSING MANAGEMENT OF URINARY INCONTINENCE
Stress incontinence

Stress incontinence is initially treated conservatively with a three month course of pelvic floor exercises. There are no studies that have examined the use of pelvic floor exercises in people with neurological disease, but there is evidence that pelvic floor muscle training is both safe and effective (Hay-Smith and Dumoulin, 2006; NICE, 2006). The exercises should be performed three times a day and may take six months or longer to have their optimal effect (Herbert, 2008). Nurses are ideally placed to teach pelvic floor exercises, but consideration needs to be given to the neurological patient's sensory perception around the saddle area (perineum) as the patient must be able to feel the pelvic floor move to perform the exercises. If a patient lacks sensation referral to a specialist continence physiotherapist or nurse may be indicated for electrical stimulation and/or biofeedback treatment.

Urge urinary incontinence/overactive bladder

The pathophysiology of the overactive bladder is complex. Increased afferent activity, decreased capacity to process afferent information, decreased suprapontine inhibition, and increased sensitivity to contraction-mediating transmitters are all potential causes of an overactive bladder (Andersson, 2004). Conservative management with bladder training or pharmacological interventions is recommended initially, but other interventions (e.g. botulinum-A toxin injections, sacral nerve stimulation and posterior tibial nerve stimulation) are emerging treatments. Obvious sensory triggers (see Table 18.3) should be treated or eliminated. Some patients experience overactive bladder symptoms in conjunction with voiding inefficiently. It is then important that a regime of intermittent catheterisation (see below: Clean intermittent self catheterisation) is commenced in addition to any other treatment.

Bladder training

Bladder training aims to increase the time interval between voids and there is some evidence that this is effective (Wallace *et al.*, 2004) in the absence of medication, although the mechanism of action is unclear. It is thought that by stretching the detrusor, the effects of unstable contractions may be reduced and bladder capacity increased (Wilson *et al.*, 2002), but effects may be psychological, i.e. patients learn not to empty their bladder 'just in case' and develop better bladder habits. To be successful patients need to be cognitively able, motivated and encouraged to perform the technique as it can be uncomfortable and in the short term could increase the number of incontinence episodes. The importance of ongoing support usually from a suitably trained nurse is vital in sustaining the patient through the process. Using a bladder diary during the programme provides a permanent record for baseline and subsequent evaluation of symptoms (Robinson *et al.*, 1996) and provides feedback, aiding motivation.

Fluid manipulation

People with urge incontinence tend to reduce their fluid intake in order to reduce the severity of the symptoms (Pearson and Kelber, 1996). A fluid intake of 1.5–2 litres a day should be maintained and patients should reduce/avoid bladder irritant fluids such as caffeine and alcohol. Although the evidence underpinning fluid manipulation in patients with urinary incontinence is limited there is mounting evidence that the restriction of caffeinated fluids (Tomlinson *et al.*, 1999, Bryant *et al.*, 2002), including fizzy drinks containing caffeine, has a beneficial effect on bladder symptoms. It is important that caffeine is reduced gradually to avoid withdrawal effects such as headache.

Antimuscarinic medication

Antimuscarinic (anticholinergic) drugs are the mainstay treatment for overactive bladder (NICE, 2006). A number of antimuscarinic medications are available, but the most common preparations are oxybutynin and tolterodine. It is generally accepted that no one product is better than the others, although tolterodine has a lower side-effect profile than oxybutynin and sustained-release preparations also cause fewer side-effects (e.g. dry mouth, blurred vision, dyspepsia and constipation) compared with immediate release preparations (Hay-Smith *et al.*, 2005). A more recent Cochrane review has determined that there is no

evidence of benefit in using antimuscarinics for patients with multiple sclerosis, and that there was a high rate of adverse events (drug side-effects) in included trials (Nicholas *et al.*, 2009).

Desmopressin (DDAVP)

The use of DDAVP is becoming more frequent for patients who have nocturia, especially in patients with neurological conditions such as multiple sclerosis, although this use is not currently licensed in the UK. DDAVP is a synthetic anti-diuretic hormone which stops the patient from producing urine at night and is most commonly used for children with bedwetting (enuresis) (Glazener and Evans, 2002). It appears to be safe in middle-aged people with neurological conditions and can be beneficial if the patient gets up frequently at night and is losing sleep (Bosma *et al.*, 2005; NICE, 2006). In the older person there is a risk that the patient might develop hyponatraemia and therefore urea, electrolyte and creatinine levels are assessed before and after commencement of treatment.

Botulinum toxin-A (Botox-A)

Botox-A is a potent neurotoxin derived from the bacterium *Clostridium botulinum* and is known to block the release of acetylcholine and temporarily paralyse any muscle into which it is injected. The precise mechanism of action when injected into the detrusor muscle is unknown (NICE, 2006). Patients who have failed other treatments for their overactive bladder symptoms may be offered Botox-A (Neel *et al.*, 2007; Popat *et al.*, 2005). Intravesical injections are carried out via cystoscopy and last for an average of 6–9 months, so they do have to be repeated if found to alleviate the patient's symptoms. These repeat injections have so far been found to be safe and have shown beneficial outcomes for the patients (Reitz *et al.*, 2007). This treatment is thought to be promising for refractory urge urinary incontinence, but there is little trial evidence supporting its use (Duthie *et al.*, 2007) and longer term studies have yet to report.

Sacral nerve stimulation (SNS)

SNS, also known as sacral modulation, is an innovative treatment for refractory overactive bladder symptoms. It is thought that appropriate electrical stimulation of the sacral reflex pathway will inhibit the reflex behaviour of the bladder (Abrams *et al.*, 2003). Permanently implantable sacral root stimulators have been developed to stimulate the S3 nerve roots. Patients first undergo a percutaneous nerve evaluation (PNE) in which a needle is inserted through the sacral foramina under local anaesthetic. This is connected to an external pulse generator and left in place for a few days. Those who show satisfactory response to the PNE may then proceed to a permanent implant, with a programmable pulse generator inserted in the abdomen. Approximately two-thirds of patients achieve continence or substantial improvement in symptoms with SNS (Herbison and Arnold, 2009), and the available data show that beneficial effects appear to persist for up to three to five years after implantation.

Percutaneous posterior tibial nerve stimulation (PTNS)

More recently PTNS, in which a current is applied through an acupuncture needle inserted into the posterior tibial nerve just above the ankle, has been researched. The stimulus travels from here to the S3 nerve route and is thought to have a neuromodulation effect on bladder function, although the mechanism of action is not completely understood. To date there is only one published randomised controlled trial of this therapy. This study suggests that the therapy has benefit for many patients whose overactive bladder symptoms have not been relieved by antimuscarinics (Peters *et al.*, 2009). PTNS is currently the subject of a NICE review, but this guidance is yet to be published.

Urinary retention/overflow incontinence

Urinary retention in patients with neurological disease is normally chronic in nature and it is the resulting overflow incontinence which causes the patient to seek help. Trauma to the spinal cord can cause acute retention and, in the conscious patient, this is easily differentiated from chronic retention by the supra-pubic pain it causes. If acute retention is likely to recur following catheterisation, the treatment regime would be the same as for chronic retention. A residual volume in excess of 100 ml is clinically significant and the bladder needs to be drained (Fowler *et al.*, 2009).

Non-neurological causes (outflow obstruction) must be excluded and treated if possible before concluding that the retention is due to the neurological disorder. The commonest cause of outflow obstruction is constipation and faecal impaction, but other causes include prostatic enlargement, urethral structure, bladder tumours and calculi, which may necessitate a urology referral.

Clean intermittent self-catheterisation (CISC)

CISC is effective in managing urinary retention and is considered to be the gold standard treatment (Winder, 2008). Patients performing CISC have a significantly reduced risk of UTI compared with patients who have indwelling catheters (Turi *et al.*, 2006), preserving

the upper urinary tract. Rates of other complications are also lower (Weld and Dmochowski, 2000). Many patients find CISC has a positive impact on quality of life, but it is not completely free of complications, including urethral perforation, stricture formation and neoplastic changes (Pomfret and Winder, 2007). Not all patients will be able to perform CISC due to cognitive impairment, poor manual dexterity or inability to accept the procedure psychologically (Woodward and Rew, 2003) and failure to catheterise frequently enough can lead to incontinence and damage to the upper urinary tract, so careful patient assessment is required. Nurses are ideally placed to introduce the concept to patients and to teach the technique.

The frequency of CISC is individualised and depends on how quickly the residual volume recollects within the bladder, but may be necessary every 3–6 hours. Most catheters in use are single-use hydrophilic/coated catheters, aimed at reducing trauma and easing insertion. There is a lack of reliable evidence to show that these products have benefit over multiple-use or non-coated catheters and further research is urgently required (Moore *et al.*, 2007). CISC is preferably performed by patients themselves, but if this is not possible it may be performed by a relative or care-giver, although again there is a lack of evidence of the impact of this on infection rates (Moore *et al.*, 2007). Some catheters are also available with an integrated drainage bag, which many patients find useful especially when learning the technique. For patients with dexterity problems a variety of handles are also available.

Indwelling urinary catheters

Indwelling urinary catheters should be used only after alternative methods of management have been considered, due to serious risks of long-term complications and infection, which could lead to septicaemia and death (NICE, 2003). Catheter associated UTI accounts for the highest incidence of all health care acquired infections (Pratt *et al.*, 2007) and an evidence-based catheter care bundle has been developed as part of the Saving Lives Campaign (DH, 2007). For patients with neurological conditions either short (<28 days) or long-term (>28 days) urinary catheterisation may be indicated (Table 18.5), although there is no high quality evidence supporting specific catheter policies for adults with neurological bladder disorders (Jamison *et al.*, 2004). Informed consent must always be obtained, if feasible, prior to catheterisation.

Catheter selection

Catheters should be selected carefully taking into consideration the size, length and duration of catheterisation.

Table 18.5 Indications and contraindications for catheterisation.

Indications	Contraindications
• Urinary retention • Accurate fluid balance/acutely ill • Assessment/ investigations (e.g. urodynamics) • Management of incontinence – as a last resort!	• Competent patient has not consented • No permission from medical staff • Two failed attempts at catheterisation – refer on to more experienced practitioner

Table 18.6 Catheter Materials.

Short-term materials (up to 3 weeks)	Long-term materials (up to 12 weeks)
• Latex • PTFE coated latex • Siliconised latex • PVC	• Silicone elastomer • Hydrogel coated latex • Silver alloy coated latex • 100% silicone • Hydrogel coated 100% silicone

Female length catheters (26 cm) can only be used for women, while standard length (43 cm) catheters must be used for male catheterisation. Obese women and those who are very immobile may achieve better drainage with a standard length catheter. Smaller Charriere sizes (10–14 Ch) with a 10 ml balloon are recommended to reduce trauma (NICE, 2003), which can result in inflammation within the urethra and bypassing. Choice of catheter material is influenced by the necessary duration of catheterisation (Table 18.6). There is some evidence that bacteria and encrustation are less likely to adhere to catheters with a hydrogel coating, but there is little evidence of difference in outcomes between coated latex and silicone catheters (NICE, 2003). More recently silver alloy catheters have been introduced and shown to reduce infection in short-term catheterisation (up to one week), after which there is no evidence of significant difference in infection rates (Schumm and Lam, 2008). There is also some suggestion that hydrogel-coated latex catheters are better tolerated than silicone catheters (Jahn *et al.*, 2007) and silicone catheters have a tendency to 'cuff' on deflation, which can cause injury on removal (NICE, 2003). However silicone catheters must be used if there is any suggestion of latex allergy.

Drainage systems

Patients who are given the opportunity will often express a preference for a catheter valve over a drainage bag and there is no evidence of increased infection rates when using a valve (NICE, 2003). However patients must first be assessed for their manual dexterity, cognitive ability and preferences for night-time drainage before using a valve (Medical Devices Agency, 1997). If a valve is unsuitable the catheter is continuously drained through a closed drainage system to reduce infection (Pratt *et al.*, 2007). For mobile patients a leg bag is attached to the catheter and is changed according to the manufacturer's instructions (normally every 7 days) (NICE, 2003). Each night a larger capacity single-use night bag is attached to the leg bag so that urine drains through one to the other. This night bag is removed in the morning, the urine emptied down a toilet and the bag discarded.

Suprapubic catheterisation

The suprapubic route should be the first choice of route for long-term catheterisation in patients who are wheelchair bound or sexually active. Although initial insertion of a suprapubic catheter is a surgical procedure, sometimes requiring a general rather than local anaesthetic, this route is preferable for women with neurological conditions. Reduced mobility means that they are unable to change position easily when sitting which in turn puts pressure on the catheter possibly causing erosion of the urethra and bladder neck. Access to a suprapubic site is also easier for hygiene purposes (Getliffe, 2003).

Whichever catheter system is being used, nurses must ensure that patients receive information on how to care for the catheter and accessories, identify infection and other catheter related complications and whom to contact if problems occur.

Reflex incontinence

Behavioural methods of management of reflex incontinence can work, such as habit training in which an individual toileting regime is planned to coincide with the patient's pattern of voiding, but this is not always successful.

Containment

If continence cannot be achieved for people with reflex or other types of incontinence then the urine voided must be contained and skin integrity maintained. Containment may be achieved by utilising products such as urinary sheaths,

Bioderm device or pads with pants (reusable and disposable). The same types of pads can be used for the containment of urine and faeces and are funded through health authority budgets and usually provided by community health services. The smallest pad possible that will contain the urine loss should be selected and these should be fitted according to the manufacturer's instructions. Other urological products (catheters, drainage bags, sheaths) are prescription-only items and may be prescribed by suitably qualified nurses. Sheaths must be correctly measured and fitted according to manufacturers' instructions, and the Bioderm device can be particularly useful for men with retracted anatomy (Woodward, 2007). Patients and carers must be advised to ensure frequent skin care is maintained and about appropriate use of barrier creams.

PHYSIOLOGY OF DEFECATION

Normal defecation takes place when faeces move through the rectum, distending it and increasing the anorectal angle that is maintained by the puborectalis muscle. The internal anal sphincter which is under autonomic control relaxes, and if it is convenient to evacuate the bowel the external sphincter can be voluntarily relaxed for defecation to take place (Coggrave, 2005). If it is not convenient the external sphincter, which is normally contracted at rest, can voluntarily be contracted further for a short period. This will allow the faeces to move back up in to the rectum and delay defecation until it is more convenient (Emmanuel, 2004).

The desire to defecate is termed 'call to stool' and a repeated inhibition of this desire can lead to constipation. It is often at its strongest after a meal, particularly breakfast, or after exercise when the gastrocolic response is at its strongest and peristalsis increases. This reflex reaction in the gut results in mass movement of faeces through the colon (Woodward, 2010). Lack of mobility will delay this action resulting in slow transit constipation, and this is often seen in patients with neurological conditions (Barrett, 2002).

Emptying the bowel should be a painless procedure requiring little or no effort. It is aided by correct positioning on the toilet, i.e. with feet firmly planted on the floor or a stool with the forearms resting on the thighs, and by relaxing the pelvic floor so that it descends. Evacuation of the bowel cannot occur without causing odour and patients should be allowed to do this sitting comfortably on the toilet whenever possible: privacy cannot be over emphasised.

NEUROLOGICAL CONDITIONS AND BOWEL DISORDERS

Faecal incontinence and constipation are common among people with neurological conditions, as a result of cognitive

---

> **Box 18.3   Prevalence of bowel problems**
>
> - Stroke – faecal incontinence (23%)
> - Multiple sclerosis – constipation and/or faecal incontinence (39–73%)
> - Spinal cord injury (95%)
> - Parkinson's disease – constipation (50%)
> - Diabetic neuropathy – constipation (<88%), faecal incontinence (20%)
>
> Adapted from Wiesel and Bell, 2004.

impairment, reduced mobility, loss of control of pelvic floor muscles, loss of ano-rectal and pelvic floor sensation, or altered colonic motility. Neurogenic bowel refers to constipation or faecal incontinence associated with a neurological condition (Wiesel and Bell, 2004). Box 18.3 identifies the prevalence of bowel problems associated with common neurological conditions. Treatment of one problem can often precipitate another (Coggrave *et al.*, 2006).

Constipation

Defecation normally occurs between three times a day and once every three days. Constipation is defined as 'unsatisfactory defecation characterised by infrequent stools, difficult stool passage, or both. Difficult stool passage includes straining, a sense of difficulty passing stool, incomplete evacuation, hard/lumpy stools, prolonged time to stool, or need for manual manoeuvres to pass stool' (Brandt *et al.*, 2005). Chronic constipation is further defined as the presence of these symptoms for at least six months and affects many patients with neurological disease.

Two sub-types of constipation have been distinguished: slow transit constipation and functional outlet obstruction (evacuation disorder). Impairment of rectal emptying is thought to be due to abnormal use of a normal pelvic floor. During straining, the puborectalis muscle contracts instead of relaxing and the anal canal remains closed, preventing defecation. It has also been suggested that instead of this non-relaxing pelvic floor, in some patients the problem is due to insufficient propulsive force being generated in the pelvis (Koutsomanis *et al.*, 1995). An evacuation disorder may occur concurrently with slow gut transit. Slow transit constipation is the result of a failure to move faecal material through the colon at a normal rate. The aetiology of slow transit constipation is unknown, but is likely to be multifactorial.

Patients with neurological problems are at risk of developing both forms of constipation for a variety of reasons. Constipation may be mechanical, with slow gut transit being most common cause (Norton, 2006) (see Box 18.4). Decreased mobility will reduce the movement of faeces through the gut and in patients reliant on others to help them use the toilet this can be further compounded by poor facilities and lack of privacy. Constipation can also be compounded by an inability to take sufficient dietary fibre or fluids and by the side-effects of medication used to treat many neurological problems.

Faecal incontinence

Patients with neurological conditions could present with faecal incontinence (FI) which is involuntary leakage of solid or liquid faecal material, or anal incontinence which is involuntary passing of flatus. The volume of faecal material passed is variable and may involve only a light soiling on underwear, but may be equally distressing to patients and severely impacts on the quality of life. FI is often cited as the reason for admission to nursing home care (Whitehead *et al.*, 2001).

To remain continent patients need to be able to sense when the rectum is filling, to distinguish its contents, to store the faeces for a period of time, and to prevent unwanted leakage of solid, liquid or gas from the anus. Faecal incontinence has many causes and contributing factors among people with neurological conditions (Box 18.5).

Box 18.4   Neurological causes of constipation

- Spinal cord injury or trauma
- Cerebrovascular disease
- Parkinson's disease
- Multiple sclerosis
- Autonomic neuropathy

Box 18.5   Causes of faecal incontinence (FI) in neurological disorders

- Impaired puborectalis function resulting in loss of ano-rectal angle
- Pudendal nerve damage resulting in impaired pelvic floor function caused by nerve root compression
- Faecal impaction with faecal fluid overflow
- Loss of motivation to maintain continence or cognitive decline
- Decreased rectal sensation due to neuropathy
- Neurological disorders affecting spinal nerve roots/ability to have voluntary control

---

ASSESSING BOWEL FUNCTION

A history of co-existing medical conditions, diet and fluid intake, prescribed and over-the-counter medication/laxatives, as well as specific bowel symptoms (Box 18.6) should be taken (Norton and Barrett, 2002). Assessment of stool consistency is aided by using the Bristol Stool Form Scale (Lewis and Heaton, 1997). Bowel symptom diaries may also be completed by patients for seven days and can be particularly helpful in assessing patients who have difficulty recalling symptoms.

There are a number of published constipation rating scales, but none have been developed specifically for assessing patients with neurological conditions. If nurses wish to use an assessment tool for FI, this needs to include elements that bother patients the most, including psychological and quality of life issues, such as unpredictability and coping strategies (Cotterill *et al.*, 2008). The faecal incontinence assessment tool of choice, along with user

---

Box 18.6   Nursing assessment of bowel symptoms

General bowel symptoms:
- Bowel frequency
- Presence/absence of urge to defecate
- Stool consistency
- Bleeding (on wiping/in toilet)
- Abdominal pain
- Any recent changes
- Effect on quality of life and relationships

Constipation symptoms:
- Difficulty emptying bowel (incomplete evacuation)
- Painful evacuation
- Straining
- Passing mucus
- Bloating
- Need to digitate (anally/vaginally)

Faecal incontinence symptoms:
- Frequency of bowel accidents/leakage. Are these linked to stool consistency or activities?
- Type of leakage (solid/liquid/mucus/wind)
- Amount of leakage (small stain on underwear/complete bowel evacuation)
- Passive soiling
- How is the problem currently managed

Adapted from Norton and Chelvanayagam, 2004.

guides, is available from the ICIQ website, together with the assessment tools for urinary incontinence.

BOWEL MANAGEMENT PROGRAMMES

Patients with neurological conditions need to have an individualised, planned bowel management programme rather than dealing with problems as they occur. Any bowel programme should provide predictable and effective elimination of stool using a combination of conservative, pharmacological and/or assistive methods (Wiesel and Bell, 2004). Bowel management needs to take place in a safe, but pleasant environment. While independent bowel care is the ideal, this is not always achievable and consent from the patient must be obtained before carers engage in bowel care, particularly if the patient requires digital removal of faeces. The involvement of the patient's partner or family is inappropriate in most cases.

Bowel management should ideally be scheduled after a meal to capitalise on the gastro-colic reflex, although there is some evidence that this reflex might be reduced in patients who have suffered spinal cord injury (SCI) and multiple sclerosis (MS) (Wiesel and Bell, 2004). Assistive techniques, such as abdominal massage, seating position and the Valsalva manoeuvre have been used by patients to empty the rectum, but little research has been undertaken. Spinal cord injured patients report finding evacuation easier when sitting than lying in bed (Nelson *et al.*, 1993). Prolonged straining should be avoided as haemorrhoids and rectal prolapse may result. Specific bowel management guidelines have been produced for patients with SCI (SCI Centres of the UK & Ireland, 2009).

Digital ano-rectal stimulation

This technique can be used by patients following spinal injury at T12 or above in whom reflex bowel function is still present. This should be performed by inserting a lubricated, gloved finger into the rectum and slowly rotating against the rectal mucosa (Wiesel and Bell, 2004) (see Box 33.6). This should stimulate peristalsis in the left colon, relaxation of the rectal wall and passage of flatus and stool. Stimulation in this way should be performed for no longer than one minute and repeated every 5–10 minutes until evacuation is complete (Wiesel and Bell, 2004). This technique may be helpful in other neurological conditions, such as stroke, but is unproven as yet.

Management of constipation

Patients with neurological conditions are at risk of developing constipation if a bowel management programme is unsuccessful or for other reasons (see Box 18.3). Most cases of constipa-

tion are successfully treated with simple non-pharmacological measures. Medication with constipating side-effects should be reviewed and discontinued if possible.

Diet, fluid and lifestyle changes

Simple measures start with a trial of increased fibre, fluid intake, exercise and lifestyle changes. Adequate fibre intake needs to be maintained as this will normally reduce transit time and increase frequency of defecation. There is little evidence that increasing dietary fibre is effective in the management of severely constipated patients and this may induce symptoms such as abdominal distension and flatulence, particularly in those patients with a slow gut transit. There is some evidence that increasing dietary fibre will increase gut transit time and reduce frequency of defecation in some patients with neurological conditions (e.g. Parkinson's disease and SCI), but fibre intake is often inadequate and patients should take the amount required to achieve a stool of a consistency that they can easily pass (Coggrave, 2008). There is also no evidence that stool consistency and constipation can be affected by increasing fluid intake or exercise (Müller-Lissner *et al.*, 2005), but if the patient is dehydrated then increasing fluid intake may help. Lifestyle changes around a toileting routine (Box 18.7) to instil good defecatory habits may help.

Laxatives

Oral and/or rectal laxatives may be necessary to treat constipation and should be tried according to the patient's preferences and assessment findings (Wiesel and Bell, 2004). Laxatives should be rotated every couple of months,

---

Box 18.7   Recommended toileting routine

- Attempt defecation regularly (e.g. 20–30 minutes after breakfast to capitalise on the gastro-colic reflex)
- Unhurried defecation, about 10 minutes, to ensure defecation is complete
- Don't ignore the urge to defecate
- People with limited mobility should have help to get to the toilet
- Supported seating if the person is unsteady on the toilet
- Adopt a good functional position for defecation (knees flexed and above hips – put feet up on a footstool if necessary to achieve this, lean forward with elbows resting on knees and relax)
- Adequate privacy

otherwise they lose their effectiveness. The lowest effective dose of a laxative should be used, and should be reduced as soon as symptoms begin to resolve. Treatment may begin with a bulk-forming laxative (e.g. Fybogel), unless the patient has slow transit. If stools remain hard then the prescription may include or change to an osmotic laxative (e.g. movicol or lactulose). If stools are soft, but difficult to pass, or defecation is incomplete, an oral stimulant laxative may be added (e.g. senna). Rectal stimulants may be required (e.g. glycerine or bisacodyl suppositories) and patients who have poor manual dexterity and wish to maintain their bowel care independently may find a suppository inserter helpful. Should the constipated stool be beyond the reach of the examining finger, then enemas are the next step, but large volume enemas (e.g. phosphate) should be a last resort.

Biofeedback

Gut directed biofeedback training has become an established therapy for constipation and involves patients being taught to defecate effectively by using bracing of the abdominal wall muscles and effective relaxation of the pelvic floor muscles (Emmanuel and Kamm, 2001). Balloon systems or electrical stimulation can be used as forms of biofeedback, but both rely on the patient learning to recognise appropriate relaxation of the pelvic floor. One study has shown the effectiveness of this intervention for some people with bowel problems as a result of MS (Wiesel *et al.*, 2000).

Transanal irrigation (Peristeen)

Transanal irrigation has been used to treat both intractable constipation and faecal incontinence (Christensen *et al.*, 2006). The patient sits on the toilet and instils between 750 ml to a litre of water via a specially lubricated short rectal catheter with an integral balloon to keep it in place. Although the initial research was undertaken in a group of patients with SCI, it is now being more widely used by specialist nurses with patients with other neurological conditions, e.g. MS. The Peristeen Anal Irrigation System (Coloplast Ltd) has been licensed for transanal irrigation in the UK.

Digital removal of faeces (DRF)

DRF, also known as manual evacuation, should only be used when required, with patient consent and by a skilled individual. The technique involves inserting a lubricated, gloved finger to break up and hook the stool out (see Box 33.6). This noxious stimulation may trigger autonomic dysreflexia (see Chapter 33) in patients following SCI and anaesthetic lubricant can help to reduce this. Patients with an areflexic bowel following SCI at L1 or below rely on DRF to evacuate their bowel and there is no alternative. Nurses must ensure that they are competent to undertake this procedure (RCN, 2008; NPSA, 2004).

Management of faecal incontinence

There is little evidence underpinning prevention and management of FI and guidance has developed from expert consensus (NICE, 2007). Treatment options for FI remain limited and under-researched. A treatment programme combining a regular planned bowel management routine using dietary manipulation, pharmacological treatments to control stool consistency and behavioural techniques is often helpful. The aim of management is often to reduce the volume of stool produced, alter the consistency to a more solid, formed stool and then use suppositories/ enemas to evacuate the bowel. This enables the patient to deal with their bowel management at a time and place that suits them and reduces the fear of unpredictable leakage or accidents.

Pharmacological interventions

Several drugs are used in the pharmacological management of FI to either induce constipation, bulk the stools or aid defecation (Box 18.8). These drugs are often used as an adjunct to other behavioural or surgical interventions. Constipating agents are used to reduce the volume of the stool produced and firm up the consistency of liquid stools, although they are not licenced for treatment of FI. Loperamide may be useful for liquid stools once the cause has been established. It is taken regularly before meals and can be an effective treatment for faecal incontinence, but side-effects include constipation (Cheetham *et al.*, 2002).

Some patients, particularly those with spinal and other neurological problems, may require bowel evacuation using suppositories, enemas or digital removal of faeces if

---

Box 18.8 Commonly used drugs used to manage faecal incontinence

Constipating agents:
- Loperamide
- Codeine phosphate

Bulking agents:
- Ispaghula husk
- Bran
- Methylcellulose

constipating agents are used, and care must be taken to ensure that the patient does not become impacted. Use of a constipating agent in combination with an evacuation aid makes bowel evacuation more predictable and enables it to be planned at a time to suit both the patient and carers. This may be a particularly important factor to consider when planning a bowel management programme for patients requiring nursing assistance in the community.

Biofeedback for FI

Stimulation to the rectum, either using air (in a balloon) or an electric current, assists the patient in identifying and improving tone and contraction in the external anal sphincter. Evidence to support the use of biofeedback compared to conservative management remains limited (Norton *et al.*, 2006), but there is some evidence that patients with mild to moderate MS might find it helpful for FI (Wiesel *et al.*, 2000). A recent Cochrane review of the role of biofeedback and/or sphincter exercises did not provide conclusive evidence of the effectiveness of the therapy, although there was some evidence that elements of biofeedback may have had some therapeutic effect (Norton *et al.*, 2006).

Electrical stimulation

Electrical stimulation has been used to treat urinary incontinence for many years and more recently has been increasingly used for faecal incontinence, although once again there is extremely limited evidence of effectiveness (Hosker *et al.*, 2007). Electrical stimulation aims to enhance voluntary anal sphincter contraction or sensation. It is unclear how frequently this needs to be applied and for how long a period of time or where the electrodes are best placed, in order to be effective.

Anal plugs

Anal plugs can also be an effective form of management for some, but tend to be better tolerated by patients with poor ano-rectal sensation. Other patients find the plug uncomfortable to wear (Norton and Kamm, 2001), but they do allow patients a certain amount of freedom to go about activities of daily living without fear of an episode of FI. Many patients will use plugs on 'special occasions', when they need to be sure that they will not have a bowel accident while out.

Anal plugs are inserted into the rectum and sit above the sphincters. These plugs come wrapped in a water soluble film, so vaseline must be used for insertion, rather than a water-based lubricant. If water soluble lubricants are used, the covering of the plug will begin to dissolve, causing the plug to open prematurely and making insertion difficult. On contact with the natural moisture in the rectum the plug expands to form a barrier to faecal leakage. It can stay in position for up to 12 hours and is permeable to flatus. Removal is achieved by pulling gently on a gauze 'tail' which hangs from the anus.

SUMMARY

Bladder and bowel problems are common and have a significant impact on quality of life for people with neurological conditions. It is imperative that an interdisciplinary approach is taken to assessment and management, but nursing staff are ideally placed to coordinate care and initiate simple interventions. This can also be done in conjunction with specialist nurses in continence care.

REFERENCES

Abrams P (2006) *Urodynamics*. (3rd edition). London: Springer Ltd.

Abrams P, Blaivas JG, Fowler CJ *et al.* (2003) The role of neuromodulationin the managementof urinary urge incontinence. *British Journal of Urology International* 91(4):355–359.

Abrams P, Cardozo L, Fall M *et al.* (2002), The standardisation of terminology of lower urinary tract function: Report from the Standardisation Sub-Committee of the International Continence Society. *Neurourology and Urodynamics* 21:167–178.

Andersson KE (2004), Mechanisms of disease: central nervous system involvement in overactive bladder. *Nature Clinical Practice Urology* 1(2):103–108.

Avery K, Donovan J, Peters T *et al.* (2004) ICIQ: a brief and robust measure for evaluating the symptoms and impact of urinary incontinence. *Neurourology and Urodynamics* 23(4):322–330.

Barrett J (2002), Pathopathology of constipation and faecal incontinence in the elderly. In: *Bowel Care in Older People* Potter J, Norton C, Cottenden A (ed). London: Royal College of Physicians pp 5–22.

Blok BF (2002) Central pathways controlling micturition and urinary continence. *Urology* 59(5 Suppl 1):13–17.

Bosma R, Wynia K, Bahlikova E *et al.* (2005) Efficacy of desmopressin in patients with multiple sclerosis suffering from bladder dysfunction: a meta-analysis. *Acta Neurologica Scandinavica* 112(1):1–5.

Brandt LJ, Prather CM, Quigley EM *et al.* (2005) Systematic review on the management of chronic constipation in North America. American *Journal of Gastroenterology* 100(Suppl 1):S5–S21.

Bryant CM, Dowell CJ, Fairweather G (2002) Caffeine reduction education to improve urinary symptoms. *British Journal of Nursing* 11(8):560–565.

Cheetham MJ, Brazzelli M, Norton C *et al.* (2002) Drug treatment for faecal incontinece in adults. *Cochrane Database of Systematic Reviews* Issue 3 Art no.:CD 00216 DOI:10.1002/14651858Cd002116.

Christensen P, Bazzocchi G, Coggrave M *et al.* (2006) A randomised, controlled trial of transanal irrigation versus conservative bowel management in spinal cord-injured patients. *Gastroentererology* 131(3):738–747.

Coggrave M (2005) Management of neurogenic bowel. *British Journal of Neuroscience Nursing* 1(1):6–13.

Coggrave M (2008) Neurological continence. Part 3: Bowel management strategies. *British Journal of Nursing* 17(15):962–968.

Coggrave M, Wiesel P, Norton CC 2006 Management of faecal incontinence and constipation in adults with central neurological diseases. *Cochrane Database of Systematic Reviews* Issue 2. Art. No.: CD002115. DOI: 10.1002/14651858.CD002115.pub3.

Cotterill N, Norton C, Avery KNL *et al.* (2008) A patient-centred approach to developing a comprehensive symptom and quality of life assessment of anal incontinence. *Diseases of the Colon and Rectum* 51:82–87.

Department of Health (2000) *Good Practice in Continence Services*. London: DH.

Department of Health (2003) *The Essence of Care*. London: DH.

Department of Health (2007) *High Impact Intervention No 6: Urinary Catheter Care Bundle*. London: DH.

Doherty JG, Burns AS, O'Ferrall DM *et al.* (2002) Prevelance of upper motor neuron vs lower motor neuron lesions in complete lower thoracic and lumbar spinal cord injuries. *Journal of Spinal Cord Medicine* 25(4):280–292.

Duthie JB, Herbison GP, Wilson DI, Wilson D 2007 Botulinum toxin injections for adults with overactive bladder syndrome. *Cochrane Database of Systematic Reviews* Issue 3. Art. No.: CD005493.

Emmanuel A (2004) The physiology of defecation and continence. In: Norton C and Chelvanayagam S *Bowel Continence Nursing*. Beaconsfield: Beaconsfield Publishers.

Emmanuel AV, Kamm MA (2001) Response to a behavioural treatment, biofeedback, in constipated patients is associated with improved gut transit and autonomic innervation. *Gut* 49: 214–219.

Fowler CJ (1999) Neurological disorders of micturition and their treatment. *Brain* 122:1213–1231.

Fowler CJ, Panicker JN, Drake M *et al.* (2009) A UK consensus on the management of the bladder in multiple sclerosis. *Journal of Neurology, Neurosurgery and Psychiatry* 80:470–477.

Fry C (2005) The physiology of micturition. *Women's Health Medicine* 2(6):53–55.

Getliffe K (2003) Catheters and catheterisation. In: Getliffe K, Dolman M *Promoting Continence: A clinical research resource* (2nd edition). London: Bailliere Tindall.

Glazener CMA, Evans JHC (2002) Desmopressin for nocturnal enuresis in children. *Cochrane Database of Systematic Reviews* Issue 3 Art no.:Cd002112 Doi:10.1002/14651858CD002112.

Haslam J, Laycock J (2007) *Therapeutic Management of Incontinence and Pelvic Pain: Pelvic organ disorders*. (2nd edition). London: Springer.

Hay-Smith EJC and Dumoulin C (2006) Pelvic floor muscle training versus no treatment, or inactive control treatments, for urinary incontinence in women. *Cochrane Database of Systematic Reviews* Issue 1. Art.No:CD005654.

Hay-Smith J, Ellis G, Herbison GP (2005) Which anticholinergic drug for overactive bladder symptoms in adults. *Cochrane Database of Systematic Reviews* Issue 3. Art. No.: CD005429.

Herbert J (2008) The importance of the pelvic floor muscles. *Continence Essentials* 1:82–84.

Herbison GP, Arnold EP (2009) Sacral neuromodulation with implanted devices for urinary storage and voiding dysfunction in adults. *Cochrane Database of Systematic Reviews* Issue 2. Art. No.: CD004202.

Hosker G, Cody JD, Norton CC (2007) Electrical stimulation for faecal incontinence in adults. *Cochrane Database of Systematic Reviews* Issue 3. Art. No.: CD001310. DOI: 10.1002/14651858.CD001310.pub2.

Jahn P, Preuss M, Kernig A, Langer G, Seifert-Huehmer A (2007) Types of indwelling urinary catheters for long-term bladder drainage in adults. *Cochrane Database of Systematic Reviews* Issue 3. Art. No.: CD004997.

Jamison J, Maguire S, McCann J (2004) Catheter policies for management of long term voiding problems in adults with neurogenic bladder disorders. *Cochrane Database of Systematic Reviews* Issue 2. Art. No.: CD004375.

Koutsomanis D, Lennard-Jones JE, Roy AJ *et al.* (1995) Controlled randomised trial of visual biofeedback versus muscle training without a visual display for intractable constipation. *Gut* 37:95–99.

Lewis SJ, Heaton KW (1997) Stool form scale as a useful guide to intestinal transit time. *Scandinavian Journal of Gastroenterology* 32(9):920–924.

Medical Devices Agency (1997) *Catheter Valves: A multi-centre comparative evaluation A22*. London: HMSO.

Moore KN, Fader M, Getliffe K (2007) Long-term bladder management by intermittent catheterisation in adults and children. *Cochrane Database of Systematic Reviews* Issue 4. Art. No.: CD006008. DOI: 10.1002/14651858. CD006008.pub2.

Müller-Lissner SA, Kamm MA, Scarpignato C *et al.* (2005) Myths and misconceptions about chronic constipation. *American Journal of Gastroenterology* 100:232–242.

National Institute for Health and Clinical Excellence (2003) *Infection Control: Prevention of health care associated infection in primary and community care*. London: NICE.

National Institute for Health and Clinical Excellence (2006) *Urinary Incontinence: The management of urinary incontinence in women*. London: RCOG Press.

National Institute for Health and Clinical Excellence (2007) *Faecal Incontinence*. London: NICE.

National Patient Safety Agency (2004) *Improving the Safety of Patients with Established Spinal Injuries in Hospital*. London: NPSA.

Neel KF, Soliman S, Salem M *et al.* (2007) Botulinum-A toxin: solo treatment for neuropathic non-complaint bladder. *Journal of Urology* 178(6):2593–2597.

Nelson A, Malassingne P, Amerson T *et al.* (1993) Descriptive study of bowel care practices and equipment in spinal cord injury. *Spinal Cord Injury Nursing* 10(2):65–67.

Nicholas RS, Friede T, Hollis S, Young CA (2009) Anticholinergics for urinary symptoms in multiple sclerosis. *Cochrane Database of Systematic Reviews* Issue 1. Art. No.: CD004193.

Norton C (2006) Constipation in older patients: effects on quality of life. *British Journal of Nursing* 15(4):188–192.

Norton C, Barrett J (2002) Assessing the individual. In: *Bowel Care in Older People*. Potter J, Norton C, Cottenden A (eds) London: Royal College of Physicians.

Norton C, Chelvanayagam S (2004) *Bowel Continence Nursing*. Beaconsfield: Beaconsfield Publishers Ltd.

Norton C, Hosker G, Brazzelli M (2006) Biofeedback and/or sphincter exercises for the treatment of faecal incontinence in adults. *Cochrane Database of Systematic Reviews* 2000(2): CD002111 DOI:10.1002/4651858 CD002111.pub2.

Norton C, Kamm MA (2001) Anal plug for faecal incontinence. *Colorectal Disease* 3:323–327.

Pearson BD, Kelber S (1996) Urinary incontinence: treatments, interventions, and outcomes. *Clinical Nurse Specialist* 10(4):177–182.

Peters KM, MacDiarmid SA, Wooldridge LS (2009) Randomized trial of percutaneous tibial nerve stimulation versus extended-release tolterodine: results from the overactive bladder innovative therapy trial. *Journal of Urology* 182(3):1055–1061.

Pomfret I, Winder A (2007) The management of intermittent catheterisation: assessing patient benefit. *British Journal of Neuroscience Nursing* 3(6):266–271.

Popat R, Apostolidis A, Kalsi V *et al.* (2005) A comparison between the response of patients with idiopathic detrusor overactivity and neurogenic detrusor overactivity to the first intradetrusor injection of botulinum-A toxin. *Journal of Urology* 174(3):984–989.

Pratt RJ, Pellowe CM, Wilson JA *et al.* (2007) National evidence-based guidelines for preventing health care-associated infections in NHS hospitals in England. (EPIC2). *Journal of Hospital Infections* 65S;S1–S64.

Reitz A, Denys P, Fermanian C *et al.* (2007) Do repeat intra-detrusor botulinum toxin type A injections yield valuable results? Clinical and urodynamic results after five injections in patients with neurogenic detrusor overactivity. *European Urology* 52(6):1729–1735.

Robinson D, McClish D, Wyman J (1996) Comparison between urinary diaries completed with and without intensive patient instructions. *Neurological Urodynamics* 15(2):143–148.

Royal College of Nursing (2006) *Improving Continence Care for Patients: The role of nurses*. London: RCN.

Royal College of Nursing (2008) *Bowel Care: Including digital rectal examination and manual removal of stool. Guidance for nurses*. London: RCN.

Royal College of Physicians (2006) *Audit of Bladder and Bowel Care in the Elderly*. London: RCP.

Schumm K, Lam TBL (2008) Types of urethral catheters for management of short-term voiding problems in hospitalised adults. *Cochrane Database of Systematic Reviews* Issue 2. Art. No.: CD004013.

Spinal Cord Injury Centres of the UK & Ireland (2009) *Guidelines for the Management of Neurogenic Bowel Dysfunction after Spinal Cord Injury*. Peterborough: Coloplast Ltd.

Tomlinson BU, Dougherty MC, Pendergast JF *et al.* (1999) Dietary caffeine, fluid intake and urinary incontinence in older rural women. *International Urogynaecology and Journal of Pelvic Floor Dysfunction* 10(1):22–28.

Turi MH, Hanif S, Fasih Q *et al.* (2006) Proportion of complications in patients practising clean intermittent self-catheterisation (CISC) vs indwelling catheter. *Journal of the Pakistan Medical Association* 56(9):401–404.

Wallace SA, Roe B, Williams K *et al.* (2004) Bladder training for urinary incontinence in adults. *Cochrane Database of Systematic Reviews* Issue 1. Art. No.: CD001308.

Weld KJ, Dmochowski RR (2000) Effect of bladder management on urological complications in spinal cord injured patients. *Journal of Urology* 163(3):768–772.

Whitehead WE, Wald A, Norton NJ (2001) Treatment options for faecal incontinence. *Diseases of the Colon and Rectum* 44:131–142.

Wiesel PH, Bell S (2004) Bowel dysfunction: assessment and management in the neurological patient. In: Norton C, Chelvanayagam S *Bowel Continence Nursing*. Beaconsfield: Beaconsfield Publishers Ltd.

Wiesel PH, Norton C, Roy AJ *et al.* (2000) Gut focused behavioural treatment (biofeedback) for constipation and faecal incontinence in multiple sclerosis. *Journal of Neurology, Neurosurgery and Psychiatry* 69(2):240–243.

Wilson PD, Bo K, Hay-Smith J *et al.* (2002) Conservative treatment in women. In: Abrams P, Cardozo L, Khoury S, Wein A editor(s). *Incontinence: 2nd International Consultation on Incontinence, July 1–3, 2001*. Plymouth: Health Publication Ltd.

Winder A (2008) Intermittent catheterisation. *Journal of Community Nursing* 22(5):42–47.

Woodward S (2006) Development of a valid and reliable tool for assessment of urinary incontinence in people with neurological problems. *British Journal of Neuroscience Nursing* 2(5):247–255.

Woodward S (2007) Urinary incontinence in Parkinson's disease. *British Journal of Neuroscience Nursing* 3(3):92–95.

Woodward S (2010) Bowel physiology. *British Journal of Neuroscience Nursing* (in press).

Woodward S, Rew M (2003) Patients' quality of life and clean intermittent self-catheterisation. *British Journal of Nursing* 12(18):1066–1074.

Section III
Neurological Investigations and Neurosurgical Procedures

19

Neurological Investigations

Jane Connor and Kirsty Andrews

INTRODUCTION

Advances in technology have led to the replacement of many investigations that less than a decade ago were commonplace in neurological practice, e.g. myelography. More sophisticated technology now enables more rapid diagnosis by less invasive means.

In clinical practice it is the nurse who will almost certainly prepare and offer explanation of the neurological investigation to the patient. It is essential that the nurse is conversant with the investigation and potential contraindications and where appropriate, have knowledge of the specific pre and post-investigation care. This chapter provides an overview of some of the most commonly employed neurological investigations.

STRUCTURAL NEUROIMAGING: CRANIAL STRUCTURES

Conventional radiography (x-ray)

An x-ray film is created when x-rays are projected on to a photographic plate through the body's organs. Bone allows fewer x-rays to penetrate it than fat and skin thus generating a shadow on the photographic plate. The denser the tissue the less penetration of x-rays, therefore air will show up as black, bone as white and muscle, fat and fluid as different shades of grey.

X-rays may be ordered to determine if the skull has been fractured following trauma. The need for x-rays has been dramatically reduced in the light of contemporary procedures such as computed tomography (CT) and magnetic resonance imaging (MRI).

Neuroscience Nursing: Evidence-Based Practice, 1st Edition.
Edited by Sue Woodward and Ann-Marie Mestecky
© 2011 Blackwell Publishing Ltd

Computed tomography (CT)

CT is a non invasive technique that uses x-rays to produce a cross-sectional image of internal structures of the body. CT images of the head can show the differences and boundaries between brain tissue, bone, blood, cerebrospinal fluid (CSF) and air. Although modern CT scanners can differentiate between different types of brain tissue, i.e. grey and white matter, MRI is far superior at doing so. CT is the most common form of neuroimaging used. It is the method of choice to demonstrate intracranial haemorrhages and hydrocephalus.

There is no specific preparation for patients to undergo a CT. During the procedure the patient lies on a padded table with their head in the doughnut shaped ring of the scanner which contains x-ray emission and detection apparatus. Following positioning of the patient, a CT of the head usually takes less than 5 minutes.

Contrast agents can be used to enhance images; Figure 19.1 is a CT scan of the brain with contrast and Figure 19.2 is without contrast. Contrast is used most commonly to provide better visualisation of intracranial tumours and abscesses. Contrast agents are contraindicated where patients are known to have allergies to contrast agents or in patients who have renal dysfunction.

Magnetic resonance imaging (MRI)

MRI is considered a chief tool in neuroscience diagnostics. MRI scanning uses a powerful magnetic field, pulses of radio waves and a computer to produce detailed images of the internal structures of the body. The human body is largely water which contains an abundance of hydrogen protons. In a magnetic environment protons act like magnets and align parallel with the magnetic field. Radiofrequency pulses are then introduced. This has the

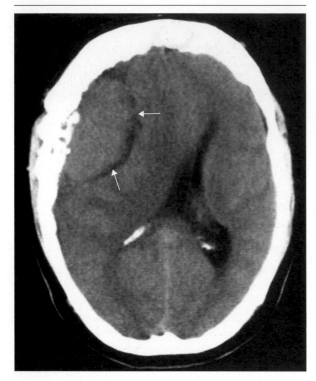

Figure 19.1 Meningioma. Pre contrast CT scan showing that the density of the meningioma (arrows) is slightly greater than the brain substance. Reproduced from Peter Armstrong, Martin Wastie, Andrea G. Rockall, *Diagnostic Imaging 6e*, Wiley-Blackwell, with permission.

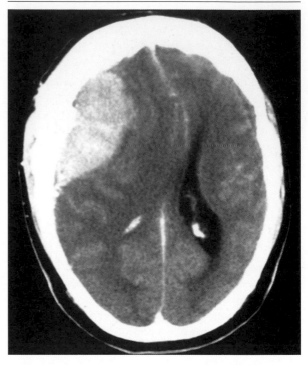

Figure 19.2 Meningioma. Enhanced scan showing marked contrast enhancement of the tumour. Note the thickening of the overlying bone. Reproduced from Peter Armstrong, Martin Wastie, Andrea G. Rockall, *Diagnostic Imaging 6e*, Wiley-Blackwell, with permission.

effect of giving the protons energy and moves them out of their alignment. When the radiofrequency pulses stop, the protons return to align with the magnetic field losing their energy in the process. As the protons move they emit a signal that can be detected, which is used to form an image.

By altering the time of the radio frequency pulses the image can be changed or weighted, referred to as T1 and T2 weighting. The contrast or brightness of tissues imaged is dependent on the parameters of T1 and T2 weighting and proton density (i.e. the amount of water in the tissues). The ventricles appear dark and the grey matter appears darker than white matter on a T1 weighted image (low signal); this can be seen in Figure 19.3. This produces images which show clear anatomical structures. On T2 weighted images (high signal) the ventricles appear white and grey matter is lighter than white matter, T2 allows for the identification of pathological changes, see Figure 19.4. MRI provides more detailed images of tissue characteris-

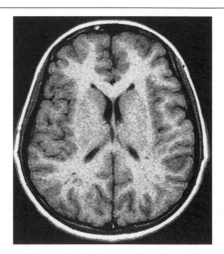

Figure 19.3 Normal brain MRI. Axial section at the level of the lateral ventricles. T1-weighted image. Reproduced from Peter Armstrong, Martin Wastie, Andrea G. Rockall, *Diagnostic Imaging 6e*, Wiley-Blackwell, with permission.

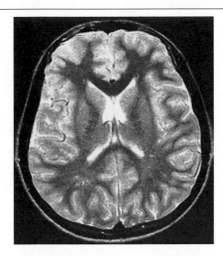

Figure 19.4 Normal brain MRI. Axial section at the level of the lateral ventricles. T2-weighted image. Reproduced from Peter Armstrong, Martin Wastie, Andrea G. Rockall, *Diagnostic Imaging 6e*, Wiley-Blackwell, with permission.

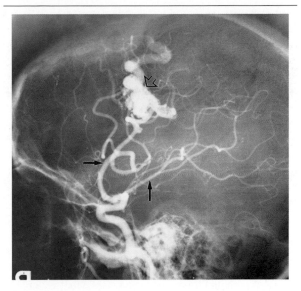

Figure 19.5 Arteriovenous malformation. Carotid angiogram showing a collection of large abnormal vessels (large open arrow) supplied by the middle cerebral artery (horizontal arrow.) On this injection the posterior cerebral artery (vertical arrow), but not the anterior cerebral artery, has filled. Reproduced from Peter Armstrong, Martin Wastie, Andrea G. Rockall, *Diagnostic Imaging 6e*, Wiley-Blackwell, with permission.

tics than CT and is therefore more sensitive in diagnosing tumours and demyelination.

Because MRI involves a magnetic field, patients and staff are asked to remove all metallic items, as patient safety may be compromised and metal may distort images. Those patients with fixed internal metallic devices may be unsuitable for MRI and arrhythmia has been reported in patients with pacemakers. Patients who are particularly apprehensive about lying in the MRI tunnel or who are claustrophobic, will usually have a light sedative prior to the scan. The patient lies on a padded table that moves through the scanner. The scan is noisy and can last up to 45 minutes. MRI is not thought to be harmful, however it has not been proven to be safe for use during pregnancy.

See also the discussion below under: Functional MRI (fMRI).

Angiography

Cerebral angiography is an invasive procedure that provides images of the vasculature of the brain. A catheter is inserted under a local anaesthetic into the femoral artery and a contrast medium is injected via the catheter to highlight cerebral blood vessels. X-rays are taken during this procedure at 5–20 second intervals to trace the contrast moving through the blood vessels. Advances in magnetic resonance angiography (MRA) may eventually make this procedure redundant.

Angiography can provide detail of the anatomical structure of vascular malformation and aneurysms (Figure 19.5 shows an arteriovenous malformation). It can also be used to identify stenosis, thrombus and spasm of vessels.

Pre-procedure preparation for cerebral angiography includes a baseline set of neurological observations, completing local pre-procedure policy and marking pedal pulses to make assessment post-procedure easier. Metformin should be temporarily discontinued as it can cause renal impairment in the presence of certain contrast media. A groin shave may be carried out in the angiography suite, however, there is little evidence to support this practice. Occasionally a light sedation may be given.

Following the procedure and removal of the catheter, pressure is applied to the groin site using manual pressure or with a pressure device such as a Femostop. The patient remains supine in bed for two hours, with the head of the bed at 30 degrees or less, to reduce the risk of haemorrhage at the groin site (Pope, 2002). Thereafter the patient can slowly be raised in bed and mobilised after four hours, if their condition allows. Post-angiography, patients can develop puncture site haematoma, transient or, in rare cases, permanent neurological deficit, a reaction to the contrast medium, and groin or cervical vessel dissection (Dawkins *et al.*, 2007). Neurological observations are completed quarter hourly for the first hour to detect any neurological change and then reduced to half hourly. Bilateral pedal pulses and monitoring of the colour, temperature and sensation of the lower limbs should be undertaken, with neurological observations, to examine for vascular interruption. It is vital that the groin site is checked for possible haemorrhage or haematoma formation every 15 minutes for at least the first hour, followed by half hourly checks. Consumption of fluids should be encouraged to aid removal of the contrast agent from the body more speedily.

Magnetic resonance angiography (MRA)

Advances in MRA may eventually make traditional invasive angiography redundant. MRA uses MRI technology to visualise the intracranial vasculature. MRA is a non invasive form of angiography (see: Angiography) which can visualise intracranial arterial and venous circulations. It is used to evaluate the blood vessels feeding vascular tumours and to provide detail of the anatomical structure of vascular malformations and aneurysms. It has obvious advantages over angiography; the risks of arterial puncture and those associated with catheterisation of the vasculature, i.e. thromboembolic events, are avoided. MRA is not as sensitive as angiography at detecting vessel stenosis.

STRUCTURAL NEUROIMAGING: SPINAL STRUCTURES

X-ray

Anterior/posterior (AP), lateral and oblique views can highlight structural abnormalities of the vertebral column such as stenosis of the vertebral foramen, spondylosis or spondylolisthesis (see Chapter 34). Patients with metastases of the vertebral column will show abnormalities on plain x-rays, particularly in the vertebral body and bony pedicles, with vertebral collapse, wedge fractures or dislocation being particularly evident.

Following spinal trauma the vertebral column is examined in the first instance using x-rays. The standard series consists of AP, lateral and open mouth to view the odontoid peg. If the lateral film cannot clearly visualise the cervicothoracic junction (C7–T1), a swimmer's view is taken. However, because of the difficulty in adequately imaging the spine in this way, many emergency departments now prefer to routinely CT the whole spine instead.

Spinal CT

A CT scan can highlight the vertebrae in more detail than an x-ray; it is useful in detecting bony abnormalities, fractures and herniated discs. However, spinal cord, soft tissue and ligament injuries are best differentiated using MRI scan (Wee *et al.*, 2008). Where the patient has a penetrating injury to the spinal cord, CT scan and CT angiography may be used to identify the direction of the penetrating object.

MRI

MRI produces good quality imaging across sagital, axial and coronal plains. It is used to examine soft tissue including the spinal cord, nerves and disc integrity and is able to distinguish between extradural, intradural, extramedullary or intramedullary lesions (see Chapter 34). MRI has superseded myelography as the investigation of choice to identify nerve root compression. Where spinal instability of the vertebral column is suspected the patient should be treated as having an unstable spine and moved accordingly (see Chapter 33).

Myelography

MRI has superseded the need for a myelogram, but a myelogram may be performed when patients are especially claustrophobic, if MRI is contra-indicated, or if CT or MRI have not provided adequate detailed information. Myleography is a diagnostic procedure whereby a radio-opaque, water soluble contrast is injected intrathecally. The patient is placed on a moveable x-ray table that is tilted during the procedure to move the contrast medium through the spinal subarachnoid space. This part of the process can be distressing for patients and may cause nausea, especially when the patient is tilted head-down.

Myelography can identify root compression caused by stenosis of the intervertebral foramen, disc prolapse or tumour.

Myelography is contraindicated in pregnancy, due to risk to the unborn child. Local pre-procedure policy should be completed in preparation for myelography. The patient should not eat for three hours pre-test, however oral fluids are encouraged, as hydrating the patient helps to prevent a post-procedure headache. A review of medication should be undertaken to ensure that a drug reaction with a contrast medium does not occur. Anti-coagulants may be temporarily suspended to reduce the risk of haemorrhage.

Patients should be prepared that the procedure can be uncomfortable and that neck and back pain may be felt during and after the test. Post-procedure care is similar to that of lumbar puncture. In addition, the patient's head should be raised for at least 12 hours and consumption of fluids should be encouraged in order to remove the contrast agent from the body.

FUNCTIONAL NEUROIMAGING

The aim of functional neuroimaging is to explore regional cerebral functions and to precisely localise specific functional areas.

Functional MRI (fMRI)

fMRI is an adaptation of MRI that measures the haemodynamic response that accompanies increases in brain activity. Deoxygenated blood and oxygenated blood produce different magnetic signals; the resultant local increase in oxyhaemoglobin, relative to deoxyhaemoglobin, in activated brain tissue leads to magnetic signal variation that can be detected using an MRI scanner (Frackowiak and Turner 2000). fMRI is extremely useful in locating the precise location of functional areas of the brain; this information is vital to neurosurgeons when they are planning surgery to remove lesions near to eloquent functional areas. During the scan the patient will be asked to perform a series of tasks. What these are will be dependent on the area being mapped; for example, to detect the speech area the patient would be required to perform a series of tasks involving speech during the scan. fMRI is also being used to further our understanding of the physiological basis for specific cognitive functions. The advantage of fMRI over positron emission tomography (PET) and single photon emission computed tomography (SPECT) (see below) is that it does not require the use of radioactive isotopes to construct images and imaging time is considerably reduced.

Positron emission tomography (PET)

Before fMRI was available, functional neuroimaging was performed with PET scanners or more rarely with SPECT scanners. PET and SPECT are generally used for research and are not widely available for use in clinical practice. PET and SPECT use radioactive isotopes to produce three-dimensional colour pictures of functional areas of the brain. By tagging glucose or oxygen with a positron emitting isotope (radionuclides) blood flow to the tissues can be visualised. The more metabolically active the tissue, the higher the demands for glucose and oxygen, and therefore blood flow. The patient is injected or inhales a positron emitting radioactive isotope. As the radioactive substance expires, positrons are released which react with electrons,

annihilation occurs and energy is released. The PET scanner detects this energy and it is computed into 3D images.

PET scanning is contraindicated in pregnancy. It is important that the patient keeps still during the scan, so the patient must be prepared for this as it can take up to one hour to complete. Substances that could alter the brain's metabolic activity should not be taken for 24 hours prior to the scan, e.g. caffeine, alcohol and nicotine. Intravenous (IV) infusions of dextrose should not be administered for six hours prior to the scan.

The patient will receive the IV radioisotope one hour prior to the scan. At the end of this hour, the patient's head is placed in a PET scanner. To localise specific functional areas of the brain, the patient will be asked to perform a series of tasks, the nature of these tasks will depend on the functional area being explored. At the end of the procedure the patient is encouraged to drink plenty of fluids to clear the radio isotope from the circulation. Special precautions are usually unnecessary when handling bodily fluids post-procedure. Normal infection control procedures should be followed when disposing of bodily fluids. Patients can use toilet facilities normally.

Single photon emission computed tomography (SPECT)

A pharmaceutical which is labeled with a radioactive isotope (radiopharmaceutical) is either injected, ingested, or inhaled. Similar to PET, the radiopharmaceutical concentrates in areas of the brain with the highest blood flow, i.e. those that are the most metabolically active. However unlike PET, as the radioactive isotope decays, gamma rays are emitted which are detected immediately by a gamma camera. The information is processed by a computer and 3-dimensional images are reconstructed of the distribution of the radiopharmaceutical in the brain.

SPECT is sensitive in diagnosing Alzheimer's disease (AD) and differentiating vascular dementias from AD.

The scan itself can take between 20 and 60 minutes. The patient will be injected with the radiopharmaceutical 20 minutes prior to the scan. The patient is required to lie still throughout the scan as movement can interfere with the images.

It is rare for the radiopharmaceutical to cause an adverse reaction and in most cases it is a mild skin reaction. However, post-procedure, the patient should be observed for hives, itching, or shortness of breath. Adrenaline should be prescribed in the 'as required' section of the drug chart in case of an adverse reaction. Radiopharmaceuticals are eliminated in the urine, faeces, and other bodily fluids.

It is therefore advisable to encourage patients to drink plenty of fluids after a SPECT scan (Hinkle, 2002). Special precautions are usually unnecessary when handling bodily fluids post-procedure. Normal infection control procedures should be followed when disposing of bodily fluids. Patients can use toilet facilities normally.

NEUROPHYSIOLOGY

Neurophysiology is concerned with diagnosis and monitoring of disease by measurement of the electrical activity of the brain, the spinal cord, nerves and muscles.

Electroencephalography (EEG)

Hans Berger first introduced the EEG in 1929 (Wallace *et al.*, 2001). Berger found that human scalp recordings showed continuous, rhythmic oscillations that were not dependent on stimuli (sound, light and touch). EEG is non-invasive and the electrical activity of the brain is recorded using 10–20 electrodes, which are placed on the scalp in standard, internationally agreed, positions. The electrodes are connected to a computer which enables the electrical signal to be recorded on the EEG tracing as wavy lines, representing the fluctuations in electrical activity from moment to moment. Normal rhythms include the alpha, beta, delta, and theta rhythms.

The main use of the EEG is in the diagnosis of epilepsy and to define the patient's epilepsy syndrome e.g. partial or generalised (see Chapter 30). Specific EEG patterns are also associated with encephalitis, Creutzfeldt–Jakob disease and coma, so it can be a useful tool to assist in the diagnosis of these conditions. Prior to epilepsy surgery, the precise location of seizure generation has to be determined, which often requires the patient to be monitored for prolonged periods. Video recordings of the patient are made throughout the period to capture the physical manifestations of the seizure (telemetry). Video telemetry is also used to differentiate psychogenic non-epileptic seizures (pseudoseizures) from genuine epileptic activity.

A routine clinical EEG normally takes one-and-a-half hours. The EEG is recorded with the patient's eyes open and closed, and several methods may be used to enhance the sensitivity of the technique, which routinely include forced hyperventilation and stroboscopic photic stimulation (Fuller and Manford, 2000). Hair needs to be clean and dry for the procedure to enable the electrodes to be fixed to the scalp, and patients may need assistance to wash the electrode glue from their hair following the EEG.

Patients undergoing resective surgery for epilepsy (see Chapter 30) will have intracranial EEG monitoring (electrocorticography – ECOG) prior to surgery, which can localise the seizure focus more accurately. The electrodes can be placed via a burr hole if they are being placed on the surface of the brain (subdural electrodes). A craniotomy is required if the electrodes are being positioned to record activity from deeper structures of the brain, for example the hippocampus (depth electrodes).

Visual evoked potentials (VEPs)

VEPs test the function of the visual pathway from the retina to the occipital cortex. This is done by measuring the time taken for a visual impulse to travel the length of the visual pathway. A computer generates the visual stimulus, e.g. a patterned chequerboard. When the impulse reaches the visual cortex it is detected by scalp electrodes positioned over the region of the occipital lobes. The electrodes record the patient's response to the visual event. Each eye is tested separately and the results compared with the normal range. Damage to the pathway will result in reduced conduction velocity.

VEPs are used in the diagnosis of optic neuritis, optic tumours, retinal disorders, and demyelinating diseases such as multiple sclerosis (Lindsay and Bone, 2004).

Auditory evoked potentials (AEPs)

Auditory evoked potentials test the function of the auditory pathway from the outer ear to the auditory cortex. They are performed using a similar method to VEPs, but the stimulus is a series of computer-generated clicks played through headphones and the electrodes are positioned over the temporal lobes. The results of the AEPs assist in differential diagnosis and in estimating central auditory function. There is no specific pre- or post-procedure care indicated for evoked potential studies.

Electromyography (EMG)

The EMG evaluates and records the electrical activities of a muscle when at rest and while contracting (Lindsay and Bone, 2004). A resting healthy muscle produces little or no electrical activity, it is electrically silent. Electrical rhythms are produced when muscles contract. The EMG records the presence, size, and shape of these rhythms, to ascertain if muscle weakness is caused by nerve, muscle, or neuromuscular junction problems (Lawrence and Tasota, 2003). Electrical activity is measured in motor unit action potentials (MUAPs). In primary muscle disease, MUAPs are low amplitude, with frequent irregular discharges. In peripheral nerve disorders, MUAP amplitude is increased, with isolated, irregular discharges. In neuro-muscular disorders, such as myasthenia gravis, MUAPs are initially normal but progressively diminish in amplitude with sustained or repeated contractions (Lawrence and Tasota, 2003).

An EMG test lasts for approximately 1 hour. A needle electrode is inserted into a muscle and the electrical activity of the muscle under investigation is displayed on an oscilloscope (Lindsay and Bone, 2004). The needles used are thin, fine and about one and a quarter inches long. The needle is usually inserted in the relaxed muscle and moved inside gently in order to record the muscle activity. The patient may feel pain when the needle is first inserted through the skin because pain receptors are located in this area. Once inside the muscle, the sensation is usually perceived as discomfort or pressure rather than pain. The needle probe is used only as a recording device.

In preparation for an EMG, it is recommended that the patient should avoid caffeine and tobacco products for 3 hours before the test, as these substances can affect test results (Lawrence and Tasota, 2003). Medications, such as muscle relaxants should be discontinued prior to the EMG. Haematomas can form at EMG needle insertion sites so it should be regularly assessed after the procedure. Patients may experience some aching or bruising post-procedure, which is normally relieved with simple analgesia.

Nerve conduction studies (NCS)

NCS can evaluate the motor and sensory function of specific nerves. NCS can measure the speed of nerve conduction and also the amplitude of the impulse (action potential). Motor NCS are performed by first electrically stimulating a peripheral motor nerve. The velocity of nerve conduction is determined by measuring and recording the time it takes for the impulse to travel from the site of stimulation, i.e. the start of a peripheral motor nerve, to the recording site, which is the muscle supplied by the nerve. Sensory nerve conduction studies are performed by electrical stimulation of a peripheral nerve at one point along the nerve, e.g. the finger, and recording the time it takes for the impulse to be conducted to a site further along the same nerve, e.g. the wrist. The conduction speed and amplitude of the action potential can be measured.

NCS can assist in the diagnosis of neuropathies and can establish the pattern of peripheral nerve involvement, i.e. whether it is focal (e.g. carpel tunnel syndrome), or generalised (e.g. demyelinating neuropathy).

Normal body temperature needs to be maintained because low body temperature slows nerve conduction. It is important to ascertain if the patient has a pacemaker or a deep brain stimulator as precautions will need to be taken during the procedure. All jewellry should be removed prior to the NCS.

BIOPSIES

Muscle biopsy

A muscle biopsy is undertaken using either a needle or open surgery, the latter being the most effective method (Lynn *et al.*, 2004). During needle muscle biopsy, the area may be anaesthetised, a needle is inserted into the muscle and a small sample of muscle is removed. The wound site does not usually require suturing. Open surgery for muscle biopsy requires that the local area is anaesthetised, an incision is made and small sections of muscle are removed. In this instance, biopsy is usually taken from the calf, thigh, upper arm or shoulder and the incision requires suturing. Laboratory examination may include one or more of the following: histology, histochemistry and immunohisto-chemistry. A muscle biopsy is indicated in order to distinguish between a myopathy and a neuropathy, and in the diagnosis of specific myopathies.

The patient is prepared for the procedure in line with local pre-procedure policy and may be prescribed a sedative. Post-procedure the wound site should be observed for bleeding. Other risks associated with muscle biopsy include haematoma formation, pain and infection. The patient should be advised to limit heavy use of the biopsy limb for a number of days after the procedure (Lynn *et al.*, 2004).

Nerve biopsy

A nerve biopsy is the extraction of a portion of nerve. The nerve that is most often biopsied is the sural nerve which is located on the lateral aspect of the ankle, as it is less sensitive than other nerves. During the procedure, which is undertaken is an operating theatre, the local area is anesthetised and approximately 1 cm of the nerve is dissected from a cut made around 25 cm above the heel (Lynn *et al.*, 2004). Analysis of nerve fibres can be complicated and lengthy (Lauria and Lombardi, 2007), making nerve biopsy a rare course of action. A nerve biopsy is indicated in order to distinguish between demyelination and axon degeneration and in the diagnosis of neuropathies.

Nerve biopsy is contraindicated in patients with diabetes mellitus and peripheral vascular disease due to the risk of infection and poor wound healing (Lynn *et al.*, 2004). The patient should be prepared according to pre-procedure policy and sedation may be prescribed. Post-procedure vital signs are recorded and the wound site monitored for bleeding. The most common complication of a nerve biopsy is paresthesia which can occur for up to 48 hours after the procedure. The patient may complain of pain at the surgical site which can last a few weeks.

LUMBAR PUNCTURE (LP)

A lumbar puncture is a medical procedure whereby a needle is inserted into the lumbar subarachnoid space to attain CSF. The needle is usually inserted between the 3rd and 4th lumbar vertebrae, to prevent accidental puncturing of the spinal cord, which terminates between L1 and L2. A lumbar puncture is performed for either diagnostic or therapeutic purposes. Analysis of CSF can assist in the diagnosis of some polyneuropathies, multiple sclerosis, subarachnoid haemorrhage, meningitis and encephalitis. A lumbar puncture is contraindicated in the presence of raised intracranial pressure (ICP) as herniation can occur. CSF pressure can be measured at the time of LP using a manometer. The normal characteristics and constituents of CSF are detailed in Chapter 2.

Lumbar puncture is either performed at the patient's bedside or in a dedicated clinical room. To ensure that valid consent is gained, the procedure is discussed with the patient and questions answered by the health care professional. The patient is required to lie on his/her side with knees drawn upwards towards the chest (see Figure 19.6), to widen the space between the vertebrae. Alternatively the patient may be positioned sitting at the side of the bed, leaning over a bed table and supported by pillows if their conditions allows.

To minimise the risk of infection the surrounding lumbar area is draped and the skin cleansed using an antiseptic product. The LP is carried out using an aseptic technique and universal precautions. The subcutaneous tissue is anaesthetised using lidocaine to minimise pain. Once the local anaesthetic has worked, usually between three and five minutes, an atraumatic spinal needle can be introduced from L2/3 downwards. An atraumatic spinal needle has been found to reduce the incidence of post lumbar puncture headache (Thomas *et al.*, 2000).

Once the spinal needle is in place a manometer set can be attached and CSF pressure measured, and CSF collected for testing. Following the procedure the patient can rest or mobilise as able. Confinement to bed does not determine whether a patient complains of post lumbar puncture headache (Teece and Crawford, 2002).

Headache following an LP is usually the result of CSF leakage and usually occurs within 48 hours of the LP. The headache is usually self limiting, but may last for up to one week. In most cases it responds to analgesia, rest and fluids (Ahmed *et al.*, 2006). If the headache does not resolve, the patient may benefit from an epidural blood patch. This involves the interlaminar injection of 12–15 ml of blood, which should be infused as close as possible to the original puncture site (Slipman *et al.*, 2005). A blood patch seals the puncture site thus preventing the leakage of CSF. The patient should be encouraged to rest for one to two hours post epidural blood patch. Increased fluid intake has no effect on CSF manufacture and does not prevent the occurrence of post-lumbar puncture headaches (Ahmed *et al.*, 2006).

A nurse should be available to offer the patient support and reassurance throughout the procedure. Post LP care requires the nurse to monitor the patient's LP site for evidence of CSF leak and to assess the patient for post-lumbar puncture headache.

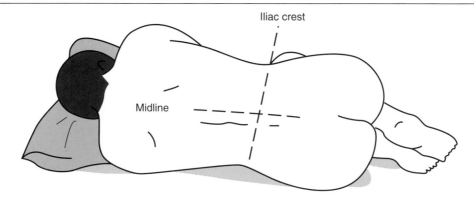

Figure 19.6 Position for lumbar puncture. Head is flexed onto chest and knees are drawn up. Reproduced from Lisa Dougherty and Sara Lister *The Royal Marsden Hospital Manual of Clinical Nursing Procedures 7e*, Wiley-Blackwell, with permission.

SUMMARY

Advances in neuroimaging have led to significant improvements in the early detection and treatment of many neurological conditions and to a better understanding of neuroanatomy. For many patients undergoing a neurological investigation is the first step to finding out a diagnosis and patients are therefore often anxious and fearful of the unknown. Nurses play a vital role in providing support, reassurance and information before, during and after the investigations.

REFERENCES

Ahmed SV, Jayawarna C, Jude E (2006). Post lumbar puncture headache: diagnosis and management. *Postgraduate Medical Journal* 82(973):713–716.

Dawkins AA, Evans AL, Wattam J *et al.* (2007) Complications of cerebral angiography: A prospective analysis of 2,924 consecutive procedures. *Neuroradiology* 49(9):753–759.

Frackowiak SJ, Turner R (2000) *Functional imaging of the nervous system. In: Neurosurgery: The Scientific Basis of Clinical Practice* (3rd edition). Crockard A, Hayward R and Hoff JT (eds) Oxford: Blackwell Science.

Fuller G, Manford M (2000), *Neurology: An illustrated colour text*. Edinburgh: Churchill Livingstone.

Hinkle JL (2002) SPECT: A powerful imaging tool: Illuminating the brain's physiology. *American Journal of Nursing* 102(3):24A–24G.

Lauria G, Lombardi R (2007). Skin biopsy: a new tool for diagnosing peripheral neuropathy. *British Medical Journal* 334:1159–1162.

Lawrence BL, Tasota FJ (2003) Detecting neuromuscular problems with electromyography. *Nursing* 33(4):82.

Lindsay KW, Bone I (2004) *Neurology and Neurosurgery Illustrated*. (4th edition). Edinburgh: Churchill Livingstone.

Lynn DJ, Newton HB, Rae-Grany AD (2004). *The 5-Minute Neurology Consult*. Philadelphia: Lippincott Williams and Wilkins.

Pope WL (2002) Cerebral vessel repair with coils and glue: Dentler on the mind. *Nursing* 32(7):46.

Slipman CW, El A, Omar H, Bhargava A (2005) Transforaminal cervical blood patch for the treatment of post-dural puncture headache. *American Journal of Physical Medicine and Rehabilitation* l84(1):76–80.

Teece S, Crawford I (2002) Bedrest after lumbar puncture. *Emergency Medicine Journal* 19:432–433.

Thomas SR, Jamieson DRS, Muir KW (2000). Randomised controlled trial of atraumatic versus standard needles for diagnostic lumbar puncture. *British Medical Journal* 321:986–990.

Wallace BE, Wagner AK, Wagner EP *et al.* (2001) A history and review of quantitative electroencephalography in traumatic brain injury *The Journal of Head Trauma Rehabilitation* 16(2):165–190.

Wee B, Reynolds JH, Bleetman A (2008) Imaging after trauma to the neck. *British Medical Journal* 336:154–157.

20

Common Neurosurgical Procedures

Anne Preece

INTRODUCTION

Neurosurgery encompasses a variety of surgical procedures to treat primarily brain, spinal cord and peripheral nerve disorders. Approximately 110 neurosurgical procedures per 100,000 population are carried out annually (SBNS, 2000). The nature of this major surgery instils anxiety and apprehension, so it is vital that every aspect of the patient's pathway is managed efficiently. This chapter will explain some of those procedures and the measures that are utilised to minimise post-operative complications.

GENERAL PRE-OPERATIVE NURSING MANAGEMENT

A complete pre-operative assessment is essential for all patients undergoing a neurosurgical procedure. It is common practice for patients to be seen in nurse-led pre-operative assessment clinics, usually two to four weeks prior to elective surgery. Suitably trained nurses have been shown to perform as well as preregistration house officers in assessing patients pre-operatively (Kinley *et al.*, 2002). Kinley and colleagues also showed that medical staff ordered twice as many unnecessary tests as the nurses. Table 20.1 summarises the essential components of pre-operative assessment and nursing management.

IMMEDIATE PRE-OPERATIVE PREPARATION

On admission the pre-assessment requires re-checking to ensure that everything is completed and that there are no

new developments. In particular the patient must be apyrexial. MRSA screening on admission is mandatory for any patient undergoing an invasive neurosurgical procedure (DH, 2006).

There is now evidence that inadvertent perioperative hypothermia can increase the risk of surgical site infections (NICE, 2008). Patients should therefore be kept warm in hospital pre-operatively by remaining dressed and only changing into a hospital gown at the last minute, or by wearing a dressing gown prior to elective procedures. Any patient undergoing a procedure lasting 30 minutes or longer should be warmed in theatre using forced-air warming devices and given warmed fluids perioperatively. The patient's temperature should not be allowed to fall below 36°C (DH, 2006).

Neurosurgical procedures are associated with an increased risk of developing a deep vein thrombosis (DVT) or pulmonary embolus (PE) due to immobility and venous stasis during the procedures. DVT prophylaxis includes thigh-length, sequestrated anti-embolic stockings (NICE, 2007a), but generally heparin will not be given pre-operatively. Patients are advised to continue wearing the stockings for up to 6 weeks post-operatively (Williams, 2007).

Hair shaving is no longer carried out pre-operatively. Normally a minimal amount of hair is shaved along the incision line in theatre, although more might be removed in an emergency. Hair does not increase the risk of post-operative wound infections (Bekar *et al.*, 2001).

Informed consent must be obtained prior to surgery. Consent should be obtained by a practitioner who is competent to perform the procedure the patient will undergo and the patient must be allowed time to ask questions and

Neuroscience Nursing: Evidence-Based Practice, 1st Edition.
Edited by Sue Woodward and Ann-Marie Mestecky
© 2011 Blackwell Publishing Ltd

Table 20.1 Components of preoperative assessment.

Assessment	Rationale
Detailed nursing history to include discharge planning	Discharge planning commences at pre-assessment. Patients need awareness of diagnosis, treatment, hospital routine, pain control, personal responsibilities and possible changes in life style to optimise recovery Providing sufficient information has been shown to decrease anxiety, post-operative complications and to shorten length of stay (DH, 2003) Identify family support structure
Neurological observations	To provide a baseline of any abnormalities prior to surgery
Cardiovascular assessment: record pulse, blood pressure, ECG	To identify any problems and provide a baseline. Unknown hypertension is often picked up at this stage. A history of existing problems such as transient ischaemic attacks, vascular disease and claudication will not necessarily preclude anaesthetic but will require more intensive peri- and post-operative monitoring
Respiratory assessment: chest x-ray, SaO2	To identify any problems and provide a baseline. Patients are requested to stop smoking prior to an anaesthetic. Patients who have existing respiratory problems will require detailed assessment by an anaesthetist and physiotherapist. Any anatomical oral or dental problems are noted in order to pre-empt any difficult intubations
Nutrition assessment	To serve as a baseline and for early detection of those at risk of malnutrition: surgery increases metabolic rate
Pressure area risk assessment	To serve as a baseline for early detection of those at risk of pressure sores
Height, weight, BMI	To facilitate calculation of drug doses
Detailed mental and physical neurological examination	To provide baseline of patient's condition and assess suitability for anaesthetic. Opportunity to provide health education on issues related to smoking, alcohol abuse, weight loss and nutrition
Previous operations/ anaesthetics	Any problems identified, e.g. nausea and vomiting previously – ensure anti-emetic is prescribed
Allergies	Note any allergies
Check current medications	Some medications need to be stopped prior to surgery, especially anticoagulants and non-steroidal analgesia. Insulin dependent diabetics will need to be admitted a few days before surgery to stabilise and actively manage glucose levels
Full blood count, anticoagulation profile, urea and electrolytes, glucose, group and save, C-reactive protein, calcium and liver function tests	To provide a patient profile, baseline and identify any abnormalities
Imaging	Relevant to patient's pathology
Patients' require informed consent	Not always possible due to the nature of neurological conditions. Ensure that family/ appropriate others understand the procedure. Under normal circumstances only the patient can consent to treatment. If the patient can't consent the final decision rests with the medical staff as to what is in the patient's best interest (DH, 2005) (see Chapter 36)

to reach a decision (DH, 2001). The medical staff must ensure that the patient has the mental capacity to consent (see Chapter 36) and understands the extent of surgery, the risks of anaesthesia and the possible complications such as haemorrhage, permanent disability, loss of function and independence.

Patients undergoing an anaesthetic are required to remain nil-by-mouth to reduce the risk of perioperative aspiration. The length of time that patients fast pre-operatively is often unnecessarily long and puts patients at undue risk (Mestecky, 2006). There is no evidence that drinking clear fluids up to a few hours prior to surgery increases the risk of aspiration (Brady *et al.*, 2003) and the RCN (2005) recommends the '2 and 6' rule for healthy adults undergoing elective surgery. Water may be drunk up to 2 hours before surgery, allowing the continuation of oral medication, particularly antiepileptic drugs. Solid food should be stopped 6 hours prior to surgery, including any milk and nasogastric feeds. Anaesthetists will consider further interventions for high risk patients on an individual basis (RCN, 2005).

OVERVIEW OF SURGICAL PROCEDURES

Burrhole

A burrhole is a small opening made in the skull. It consists of a 3 cm incision made through the skin, temporal fascia and periosteum on the affected side. Any bleeding is controlled with electrical cautery. A 2 cm burrhole is made using a drill (see Figure 20.1) and then a conical burr is used to carefully enlarge the hole. Minimal pressure must be used to avoid slipping into the brain tissue (Greenberg 2006).

Burrholes are most commonly used to:

- Drain chronic subdural haematomas
- Insert external ventricular drains
- Facilitate the removal of bone flaps during craniotomy
- Biopsy brain tissue (e.g. suspected tumours), using stereotactic techniques

Burrholes are insufficient to drain an extradural or acute subdural haematoma (Lindsay and Bone, 2004). Extradural haematomas are most commonly associated with trauma, where the middle meningeal artery is ruptured with a subsequent rapid build up of blood between the dura mater and skull (see Chapter 32). A burrhole and craniectomy may be positioned centrally over the haematoma if the patient is deteriorating rapidly, but this will rarely provide sufficient decompression and a craniotomy will be needed (Lindsay and Bone, 2004).

Post-operative complications

The two main complications following burrhole surgery are:

- Bleeding/re-collection of the haematomas
- Infection

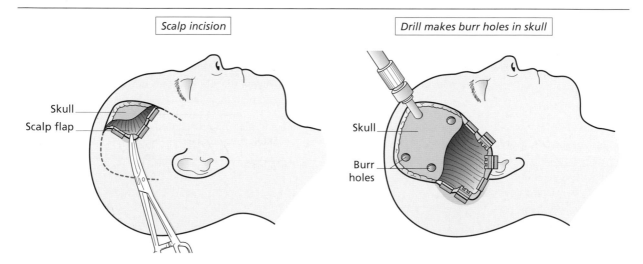

Figure 20.1 Creation of burr holes for a craniotomy. Redrawn from image provided by Medtronic Sofamor Danek USA.

If a burrhole biopsy of a vascular tumour has been performed, bleeding can lead to rising intracranial pressure and rapid deterioration (see Chapter 7).

Craniotomy

A craniotomy is a surgical incision in the skull to facilitate surgery on the brain. A circular series of burrholes are performed, soft wire is inserted between two burrholes to saw through the bone and raise a bone flap (Figure 20.2). The bone is re-secured with wires following surgery (Greenberg, 2006). A craniotomy might be performed to gain access to the supratentorial region (frontal, parietal, temporal and occipital lobes) to:

- Remove/debulk tumours
- Remove vascular malformations
- Remove extradural, subdural or intracerebral haematomas
- Drain cerebral cysts, abscesses or empyemas
- Remove frontal, temporal or parietal lobes following trauma to reduce intracranial pressure
- Clip cerebral aneurysms

Although most aneurysms are now treated by endovascular coil embolisation there are occasions where some aneurysms will require clipping because they are too difficult to embolise or coiling has failed (see Chapter 23).

Awake-craniotomy enables the surgeon to test the patient's functions, such as movement, sensation or speech during the surgery, which reduces the risk of damage to functional areas of the brain. Testing of regional cortical function may also be refined by cortical stimulation using electrodes, and of the underlying white matter tracts by using sub-cortical stimulation. Some patients are awake throughout the procedure and receive local anaesthetic to the scalp for the incision. Other surgical teams may wake the patient up only when invasive surgery has begun. Patients tend to become tired and are usually anaesthetised for the end of surgery and the closing of the skull and scalp.

Post-operative complications

Complications following craniotomy include:

- Bleeding into tumour site, especially from large metastatic lesions
- Cerebral oedema
- Infarction due to inadvertent compression of arteries intraoperatively
- Seizures – approximately 40% occur with tumours in the frontal, temporal and parietal lobes. Prophylactic phenytoin 300 mg nocte is given to patients undergoing tumour surgery (Lindsay and Bone, 2004)
- Infection

Stereotaxis

Stereotactic surgery uses a system of three-dimensional coordinates with an external frame to precisely locate a site to be operated on through a burrhole (Figure 20.3). Image-guided frameless stereotaxis is now more

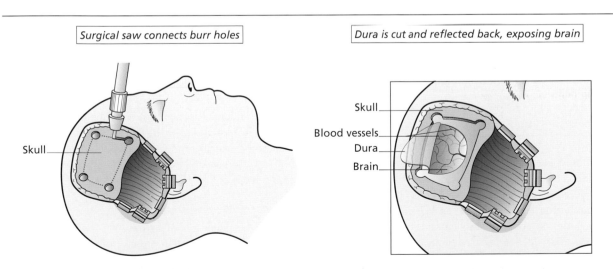

Figure 20.2 Opening of craniotomy. Redrawn from image provided by Medtronic Sofamor Danek USA.

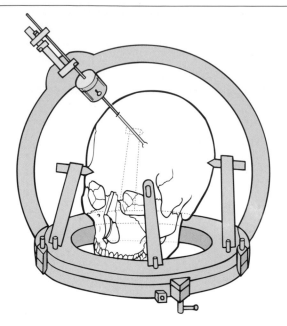

Figure 20.3 Schematic diagram of stereotactic biopsy of cerebral tumour using the Cosman–Roberts–Wells (CRW) system. Reproduced from Andrew H. Kaye, *Essential Neurosurgery*. Wiley-Blackwell, with permission.

Box 20.1   Indications for stereotaxis

- Brain biopsies
- Treatment of movement disorders (e.g. tremor, dystonia – see Chapter 26)
- Pain disorders – particularly intractable pain
- Abscess and cyst drainage
- Radioisotope placement in tumour beds (brachytherapy)
- Cortical mapping for tumours in eloquent areas
- Somatosensory evoked potentials recorded during surgery under GA to assess the relationship between the motor strip and lesion to be resected

---

commonly used (see: Neuronavigational systems). Stereotaxis tends to be confined to minimally invasive procedures (Box 20.1) as the frame is cumbersome and unpleasant for the patient to wear. It is particularly useful for targeting tumours in eloquent areas (e.g. motor strip, sensory and speech areas) to minimise damage (Duffau *et al.*, 2005).

The frame is applied on the same day as the surgery. CT and MRI compatible frames then allow scans to be taken.

Three dimensional coordinates are plotted prior to surgery taking place and an x-ray guided probe is passed through the burrhole. Lesions in the posterior fossa region are difficult to target and the frame restricts access to the surgical field. Guidance tends to be restricted to a single target as changing targets and realigning measurements during surgery is cumbersome and time consuming and, as a result, inaccurate (Duffau *et al.*, 2005).

Some patients need to be awake for part or all of the surgery, so particular care has to be taken to ensure that they are properly prepared and supported throughout the procedure. There is little evidence documented about patients' experiences during surgery, but it is generally well tolerated by most (Palese *et al.*, 2008). Patients tended to focus on keeping their emotions in check pre- and post-operatively, whilst during surgery they became involved with the task and felt they had a degree of control.

Post-operative complications

Complications are uncommon from this type of surgery and the patient is normally home within a few days. There is a very small risk of seizures or bleeding at the biopsy site.

Decompressive craniectomy

A craniectomy involves the surgical removal of a portion of the skull to facilitate treatment. A bone flap is raised in the same way as for a craniotomy and then removed completely. The defect is repaired at a later date (see Cranioplasty). The most common indication is for the reduction of intracranial pressure (ICP) following a head injury.

The use of craniectomy is controversial and currently two major trials are in progress to evaluate the effectiveness of this treatment. The RESCUE ICP trial is a UK-based international randomised controlled trial to determine the effectiveness of a decompressive craniectomy compared to medical management alone to treat brain injury (Corteen *et al.*, 2007). Craniectomy is also being considered for patients with malignant middle cerebral artery infarction. Again this would be performed to reduce ICP but there have been insufficient randomised trials to evaluate the efficacy of this procedure (Vahedi *et al.*, 2005).

Post-operative complications

One of the major complications that used to occur was brain herniation through the craniectomy and a subsequent infarct. It is now recommended to perform a large bi-frontal craniectomy (≥12 cm diameter) to avoid this (Corteen *et al.*, 2007).

Cranioplasty

A cranioplasty is a surgical repair of a defect or deformity of the skull. Over the centuries many materials have been used including coconut shells, bones from human and non-human donors, gold, silver, titanium and biosynthetic materials such as resins, ceramics and acrylic (Li *et al.*, 2008). The most common indications are to replace a portion of skull following craniectomy and to repair a deformity following trauma, infection, growth abnormality or tumour erosion.

Following craniectomy, the bone flap used to be stored in a surgical pouch inside the patient's abdominal wall until it was required, keeping it in a safe, sterile environment. This practice is no longer carried out except on rare occasions when a patient may have had emergency surgery abroad and is then repatriated. Bone flaps are now cleaned, sterilised and stored until they are required to help fashion a replacement titanium plate. Once this is done they are discarded (Tazbir *et al.*, 2005; Li *et al.*, 2008).

The process of making a plate involves using 3-D images from CT scan slices of the required section of the skull and feeding these into a 3-D workstation. This then produces a computer generated image of the skull clearly delineating the defect. From this a prosthesis can be fashioned using a mirror section of the opposite side of the skull, enabling the correct contours to be obtained for the best possible fit to the defect. A mould is prepared from the plan and the anodised titanium plate is pressed directly from the mould. The advent of these modern imaging facilities has greatly improved the cosmetic outcome for this group of patients, particularly those left with very deep depressions to which plates were previously difficult to fit (Li *et al.*, 2008).

Post-operative complications

The two most common complications are:

- Haematomas developing under the plate
- Infections

Sometimes patients complain of headaches or tightness around the plate site initially but these symptoms usually resolve. If they become too severe the plate might have to be removed (Li *et al.*, 2008).

Posterior fossa craniectomy

Posterior fossa craniectomy involves the removal of a bone flap to access infratentorial or high cervical lesions. It is not essential to replace the bone flap following surgery as the neck muscles provide adequate protection (Lindsay and Bone, 2004). Indications for posterior fossa craniectomy include:

- High cervical:
  - Chiari malformations
  - Decompression of syringomyelia
- Infratentorial:
  - Intrinsic tumours occurring in the cerebellar hemisphere (metastatic lesions, primary tumours such as a haemangioblastoma, cysts and abscesses)
  - Extrinsic tumours (acoustic neuromas/schwannomas)
  - Lesions in the brain stem

(Lindsay and Bone, 2004)

The aim of surgery for patients with acoustic neuromas (see Chapter 21) is to remove the tumour and preserve facial nerve function. Monitoring the facial nerve during surgery, via brain stem auditory responses (the facial nerve runs parallel to the acoustic nerve), has improved outcome and is now considered mandatory (BAO-HNS 2002). Surgery doesn't improve hearing on the affected side but residual hearing may be saved (Koerbel *et al.*, 2005). Total removal is achieved in up to 97% of patients, with a 1% mortality (BAO-HNS 2002).

Post-operative complications

Post-operative complications can be severe for this group of patients due to the disturbance in the cerebellar and brain stem region (see Chapter 3). Swelling or compression of the cerebellum will cause both damage to the spinocerebellar pathways leading to ataxia, loss of motor skills, loss of balance, and damage to the vestibular nuclei leading to nystagmus, vertigo, loss of balance, nausea and vomiting (Lindsay and Bone, 2004).

Damage to the corticobulbar pathway, including the nuclei of the glossopharyngeal and vagus nerves (IX and X cranial nerves respectively) situated in the medulla, leads to dysphagia and dysarthria (difficulty articulating speech (Lindsay and Bone, 2004)) (see Chapter 12). Swelling in this region may also lead to obstructive hydrocephalus due to compression of the cerebral aqueduct. The facial nerve (VII) may be damaged during acoustic neuroma surgery, which results in an inability to close the eye properly, a drooping mouth and an inability to clench the teeth.

Transphenoidal hypophysectomy

Transphenoidal hypophysectomy is a means of surgically accessing the pituitary gland through the nasal cavity via the sphenoid sinus. The pituitary gland may also be accessed via the transcranial route, depending on the size of the tumour (see Chapter 21). Where possible, the transphenoidal route (Figure 20.4) is advocated as it is associated with a lower complication rate (NICE, 2003).

There are essentially three possible routes:

- Trans-nasal via a small incision at the back of the nose, directly into the sphenoid sinus
- Via an incision along the front of the nasal septum and tunnelled back to the sphenoid sinus

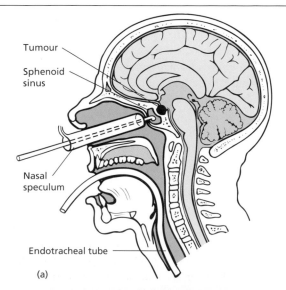

Tumour

Sphenoid sinus

Nasal speculum

Endotracheal tube

(a)

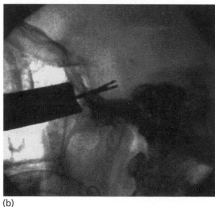

(b)

Figure 20.4 (a) Diagram of operative exposure in transsphenoidal resection of pituitary tumour. A self retaining retractor is inserted and the anterior wall of the sphenoid sinus is removed. (b) Intra-operative x-ray showing the retractor in position and the forceps in the pituitary fossa. Reproduced from Andrew H. Kaye, *Essential Neurosurgery.* Wiley-Blackwell, with permission.

- Via an incision under the lip through the upper gum, entering the nasal cavity and thence the sphenoid sinus (NICE, 2003)

All three approaches use a minimally invasive fibre optic endoscope (4 mm), which is passed through the incision to maximise visualisation of the tumour, and a specially designed angled lens allows for a panoramic view of the tumour to aid resection (NICE, 2003). A port attached to the endoscope enables aspiration or biopsy of the lesion assisted by neuronavigation. The tumour bed is then packed with fatty tissue (usually the patient's own from the abdomen) if there is any evidence of a CSF leak following the procedure. Nasal packs are inserted post-operatively and are usually removed after two to three days (NICE, 2003). The standard procedure is to follow-up surgery with radiotherapy to minimise tumour re-growth (Frank *et al.*, 2006).

The trans-nasal route is becoming more popular as the route of choice as this is the least invasive and uses the natural nasal passages. This route is less painful and nasal packs are not usually required. It results in lower incidence of CSF leaks and shorter lengths of hospital stay (Frank *et al.*, 2006).

Post-operative complications

Transphenoidal hypophysectomy carries with it a lower risk of complications compared with conventional surgery. Length of hospital stay is also reduced from an average of four to ten days down to two to five days (NICE, 2003). There are, however, several post-operative complications to be aware of following this procedure including:

- CSF leak
- Bleeding into the nasal or adenoma cavity
- Diabetes insipidus
- Underactive pituitary

Bleeding can cause increasing pressure on the optic nerve or optic chiasm resulting in deterioration in visual acuity and visual field defects. Bitemporal hemianopia is the most likely defect that will occur and is a loss of vision in both temporal fields, i.e. in the outer half of each eye (Mestecky, 2010). It is essential, therefore, to assess visual fields each time observations are performed (see Chapter 13) and any defect should be reported to medical staff immediately (Levy, 2004).

Damage to the posterior pituitary can result in diabetes insipidus, characterised by excessive thirst and urine output. This is due to insufficient secretion of ADH (see Chapter 16) and is usually self-limiting, resolving within 12–36 hours (Lindsay and Bone, 2004).

Trans-oral surgery or maxillotomy

The trans-oral route is via the mouth and is used primarily to access the anterior aspect of the brain stem, the base of the skull and the C1/C2 vertebrae, whilst avoiding unnecessary manipulation of the brain stem, cranial nerves and spinal cord (NHNN, 2004). Access to this area of the CNS is limited by the extent to which the patient can open their mouth. To improve access a maxillotomy is performed. This involves the surgical sectioning of the maxilla, which allows movement of all or part of the maxilla into the desired position to expose the central skull base (Govender, 2005).

The trans-oral approach can be used to access a number of tumours including meningiomas, anterior chordomas or abscesses by removing all or part of the clivus. This is a shallow depression in the occipital bone which supports the upper part of the pons (Govender, 2005). This procedure can also be used for patients with rheumatoid arthritis who have developed subluxation of C1/C2 and require atlanto-axial or occipito-axial fusion to stabilise the spine. It is also utilised in treating trauma patients who have a high cervical fracture or a fractured odontoid peg (Govender, 2005).

Trans-oral maxillotomy is carried out as a joint procedure by a head and neck surgeon and a neurosurgeon. The head and neck surgeon will expose the maxilla and then split the hard and soft palate to expose the clivus. At this point the neurosurgeon will take over and complete the surgery (Tamaki *et al.*, 2001).

Endoscopic trans-oral surgical techniques are being developed which do not require a maxillotomy, thereby reducing the risk of post-operative complications (de Divitiis *et al.*, 2004).

Post-operative complications

The immediate post-operative complications may include:

* Oedema
* Haematomas
* Lower cranial nerve deficits
* CSF leaks

Shunting

Shunting is the movement of fluid from one compartment to another. In this case it involves the surgical removal of CSF from the ventricles due to hydrocephalus and is discussed in Chapter 25.

Neuronavigational systems

The term neuronavigation is used to describe the computer-assisted technologies used by neurosurgeons to guide them to operate more accurately, particularly on deep-seated lesions and skull based surgery where access is difficult (Rampling *et al.*, 2004; Willems *et al.*, 2006).

Stereotaxis enables precise location and treatment of lesions within the brain, but the need for an external frame secured to the patient's head is both cumbersome and restrictive. Neuronavigation is a frameless stereotactic procedure relying on a number of techniques to create a link between a CT/MRI image, the patient, and the surgical instruments. It generates a three-dimensional real time image of a tumour on a computer screen. A pre-operative CT or MRI scan is taken and special markers or fiducials are placed on the patient's scalp. The systems currently use infrared light sources fixed to the surgical instruments which enable the patient to be linked to the previously acquired CT or MRI image on the computer screen. The position of the surgical instrument is then visible on the screen throughout the surgical procedure. This enables 3-D orientation with the aim of making surgical interventions more precise and less traumatic (Willems *et al.*, 2006).

Neuronavigation is not without its own challenges. The main one is 'brainshift' error, as the intracranial structures move on opening the skull and dura, resulting in loss of accuracy in identifying surgical targets. There is a potential added problem of further tissue displacement during surgery due to oedema, fluid drainage, compliance of tissue, etc. Therefore, to maintain accuracy for effective surgery, coordinates need to be updated constantly. So far the use of intraoperative MRI with neuronavigation has shown encouraging results, particularly for the radical resection of intracerebral neoplasms (Rampling *et al.*, 2004; Willems *et al.*, 2006).

Neuronavigational assisted craniotomies can be performed for:

* Biopsy and/or resection of tumours – partial or radical
* Drainage of abscesses, cysts
* Insertion of chemotherapy directly into tumour bed
* Arteriovenous malformations
* Epilepsy

The accuracy of the surgery depends on the quality of the equipment being used and the experience of the neurosurgeon using it. To date no randomised controlled trials have been performed to assess the benefits of its use compared with other methods. The decision to use neuronavigation for certain conditions depends on whether the neurosurgeon believes it is the most beneficial course of action (Willems *et al.*, 2006).

POST-OPERATIVE NURSING MANAGEMENT FOR ALL NEUROSURGICAL PATIENTS

Most patients undergoing major neurosurgery will be admitted to a critical care area for a period of time (Douglas and Rowed, 2005). In 2000 a review of critical care services categorised patients according to the level of care required rather than the patient location (Table 20.2) (DH, 2000). Most major neurosurgical cases fall into the level 2 category, with a decreased conscious level being considered a 'single organ failure', and so require admission to a critical care facility at least overnight for intensive observation. Patients undergoing minor neurosurgical procedures may be managed by suitably trained nurses in a level 1 facility (ward).

Neurological observations

Regular neurological observations on post-operative patients will rapidly identify signs of deterioration, and will facilitate appropriate action. Where nurses have been trained to undertake such assessments, particularly in specialised units, patient outcome is improved (Patel *et al.*, 2005; Mestecky 2007). The frequency with which the Glasgow Coma Scale (GCS – see Chapter 8) should be recorded is not clearly defined in the literature, but the risk

of rapid deterioration is known to be higher in the first six hours following injury or surgery (Frank *et al.*, 2006; NICE, 2007a; Sahuquillo and Arikan, 2006). Table 20.3 provides an expert consensus from a number of neuroscience units on the frequency of performing GCS assessments. NICE guidelines for acute head injuries are also available (NICE 2007b). This is only a guide however, and there is no substitute for clinical decision making based on individual assessment of a patient's condition.

Any deterioration in level of consciousness (LOC, limb movements or pupil reaction should be reported to a member of the medical staff immediately. Assessment of consciousness should always be recorded concurrently with vital signs, pupil responses and limb movements. Serial assessments will demonstrate trends which can be compared to the baseline observations (see Chapter 8).

Vital signs

Cardiovascular system

Pulse and blood pressure should be monitored. Patients may exhibit signs of reduced circulating volume (tachycardia, low blood pressure, shallow and rapid respirations, reduced urine output) due to general fluid loss during surgery, particularly if they have been given osmotic diuretics such as mannitol (Cook, 2005). Low circulating fluid volume should be treated with 0.9% sodium chloride in the first instance. Dextrose 5% should be avoided as it is predominantly water and has a propensity to increase cerebral oedema (Cook, 2005) (see Chapter 8).

Blood pressure should be maintained and realistic parameters must be set to guide intervention post-operatively based on the pre-operative baseline. Severe hypertension can cause bleeding in a tumour bed (Rampling *et al.*, 2004). Hypotension can lead to hypoperfusion, ischaemia and infarct. Arrhythmias may be seen due to the effects of anaesthesia, which causes increased sympathetic discharge. It should also be noted that systemic changes may accompany neurological deterioration as a late sign accompanying rising ICP (Cook, 2005; Mestecky, 2007) (see Chapter 8).

Respiratory system

Hypoxia must be avoided and oxygen saturation maintained $\geq 95\%$. Hypoxia leads to a reduced cerebral blood flow which in turn can very quickly lead to cerebral ischaemia and infarcts (Patel *et al.*, 2005; NCEPOD, 2007). Respiratory rate, depth and pattern should be observed and compared with the baseline pattern documented for the patient. Patients with decreased level of consciousness who are unable to protect their airway are at risk of aspiration pneumonia. Respiratory complications and

Table 20.2 Classification of critical care patients.

Level 0	Patients whose needs can be met through normal ward care in an acute hospital
Level 1	Patients at risk of their condition deteriorating, or those recently relocated from higher levels of care, whose needs can be met on an acute ward with additional advice and support from the critical care team
Level 2	Patients requiring more detailed observation or intervention, including support for a single failing organ system or post-operative care and those 'stepping down' from higher levels of care
Level 3	Patients requiring advanced respiratory support alone or basic respiratory support together with support of at least two organ systems. This level includes all complex patients requiring support for multi-organ failure

Source: Department of Health, 2000.

Table 20.3 Frequency of neurological observations following surgery.

Head injury obs (see NICE, 2007b)	Craniotomy for space occupying lesion (SOL)	Craniotomy for aneurysm, post fossa surgery
Perform neuro obs half hourly until GCS is 15 When GCS is 15 perform neuro obs: • half hourly for two hours, then • hourly for four hours, and • two hourly thereafter If patient deteriorates after the initial two hours revert to half hourly observations	Perform neuro obs: • half hourly for four hours, then • hourly for four hours, and • two hourly for four hours Thereafter as patient condition and clinical judgement dictate	Perform neuro obs: • half hourly for six hours, then • hourly for six hours, and • two hourly for six hours Maintain SaO$_2 \geq 95\%$ Reduce observations as patient and clinical judgement dictate NB Blood pressure may be monitored hourly for first 24 hrs

Table 20.4 Classification of post-operative pain by surgical procedures.

Major pain	Moderate pain	Mild pain
– Complex spinal surgery – Cervical/lumbar laminectomy – Foramen magnum decompression – Posterior fossa craniectomy – Sacral nerve stimulator	– Craniotomy/cranioplasty – Posterior fossa craniectomy – Transsphenoidal hypophysectomy – Ventriculoperitoneal shunt – Anterior cervical decompression – Lumbar microdiscectomy – Spinal cord stimulator – Deep brain stimulation – Carotid endarterectomy	– ICP bolt insertion – Burr hole biopsy – Trigeminal thermocoagulation – Drainage of chronic sub-dural haematoma – Carpal tunnel decompression – Ulnar nerve transposition – Muscle biopsy

Adapted from National Hospital for Neurology and Neurosurgery, 2002.

signs of potential aspiration should be monitored (see Chapter 12).

Temperature

Normothermia should be maintained post-operatively. A 1°C increase in temperature causes a 10% increase in the cerebral metabolic rate. Metabolic responses such as this can have a deleterious effect on the patient's neurological recovery (Mestecky, 2006) (see Chapter 14).

Pain relief

Regular pain assessment (see Chapter 17) and interventions to prevent pain developing is more effective than treating established pain (Thibault *et al.*, 2007). Pain relief and antiemetic cover is normally commenced intra-operatively about an hour before the anaesthetic is due to be reversed (Thibault *et al.*, 2007).

The best method for managing pain relief following cranial surgery has been debated for some time (Maxwell *et al.*, 2007). Two significant misconceptions exist: namely, that there is a low incidence of pain following craniotomy surgery, and that opioids can cause respiratory depression and distort pupillary signs so masking potential patient deterioration post surgery (Sudheer *et al.*, 2007). There is a distinct lack of evidence to support either of these claims. Studies have shown that up to 50% of patients undergoing craniotomies reported moderate to severe pain which was poorly controlled, while 90% of neuroanaesthetists still prescribed codeine phosphate as first line analgesia (Roberts, 2005). An audit at one neurosurgical centre found similar results (NHNN, 2002) and led to a new classification of the degree of post-operative pain (Table 20.4).

Thibault and colleagues (2007) found that post-operative pain following craniotomy was influenced more by the surgical incision through the muscle, and subsequent spasm caused by muscle retraction, than from manipulation of the brain or meningeal tissue. Consequently occipital and posterior fossa approaches produced the most intensive pain. Frontotemporal and frontoparietal approaches were associated with moderate to severe pain, and frontal craniotomies, where there is the least muscle, were associated with less pain. Overall, 76% of patients experienced moderate to severe pain (Thibault *et al.*, 2007).

In post-craniotomy patients Sudheer *et al.* (2007) trialled morphine (via patient controlled analgesia (PCA)) vs tramadol (via PCA) vs codeine phosphate (by four hourly injections of 60 mg). Vomiting occurred in 50% of patients with tramadol, 20% with morphine and 29% with codeine phosphate. The patients receiving morphine were the most satisfied with their analgesia, followed by the patients receiving codeine phosphate. Even though the patients receiving codeine phosphate suffered from peaks and troughs in their pain control this was preferable to increased nausea (Sudheer *et al.*, 2007). Those receiving tramadol were the least satisfied due to unsatisfactory pain control and nausea.

Nausea and vomiting is a common adverse effect following the administration of tramadol (Roberts, 2005). As vomiting raises the ICP it can be argued that this may significantly increase the risk of developing post-operative neurological dysfunction. Studies have also shown that giving ondansetron concurrently to reduce nausea actually reduces the analgesic effect of tramadol considerably. Tramadol is also known to interfere with some antiepileptic drugs such as phenytoin (Roberts, 2005).

Although opioids have little effect in low doses, rises in cerebral metabolic rate and cerebral blood flow have been reported following administration of high doses (Gupta and Summons, 2001), however, these effects have not been shown to have any adverse influence on patient outcomes to date. Patient controlled morphine has been shown to be both effective and safe and should be the drug of choice for moderate to severe pain (Roberts, 2005). Table 20.5 summarises the drugs most commonly used in the control of pain following neurosurgery.

Wounds and drains

Not all neurosurgical procedures require drains postoperatively. They are used most commonly to drain residual blood following tumour resection and for drainage of subdural haematomas. Two types of drain are commonly used: either a gravity drain or a closed suction drain. They can either be attached to a plain drainage bag to act as a gravity drain or have a pre-vacuumed plastic bottle attached to provide low pressure suction. Drains are **never** attached to a wall suction unit as aggressive suction will tear small vessels on the brain's surface causing haemorrhages (Gazzeri *et al.*, 2007). It is important to state on the observation chart where the drains are placed and what type they are.

Suction drains would be used to drain tumour beds but would not be put in place if the patient had had chemotherapy wafers inserted (Rampling *et al.*, 2004). Suction drains or gravity drains may be used for subdural haematomas, depending on the extent of the bleed. Weigel *et al.* (2003) demonstrated that gravity drains are effective for draining chronic subdural haematomas, reducing the risk of recurrence without additional complications. Subgaleal gravity drains (galea aponeurotica is a tough layer of fibrous tissue above the periosteum and below the skin) are effective at draining pockets of CSF that can collect near a craniotomy flap. As they are less invasive they have also been shown to be effective with suction to drain chronic subdural haematomas in high risk patients (Gazzeri *et al.*, 2007).

Wounds and/or drain sites need to be observed for signs of oozing or CSF leaks. The amount of drainage needs to be recorded on a fluid balance chart. Wounds usually only have a small dressing over the site for 24 hours and are then left exposed and dry once the drain, if used, has been removed. Wounds should be monitored for signs of infection such as redness, pain, warmth to touch, swelling or discharge. There is no definitive evidence to determine when clips/sutures should be removed, but the scalp has a good blood supply and heals quickly enabling supratentorial sutures/clips to be removed at 3–5 days. Posterior fossa surgery involves dissection of the overlying muscles, so removing the clips/sutures at 7–10 days allows more time for the muscle to recover. This practice varies between neurosurgical centres and tends to be influenced by the surgeon's preference.

Elimination

Patients undergoing major neurosurgical procedures will all have indwelling urethral catheters post-operatively to accurately measure urine output. These must be inserted and managed aseptically and removed as soon as they are no longer required (DH, 2006).

Particular attention needs to be paid to bowel movements as codeine phosphate and tramadol are known to cause constipation. Excessive straining may raise ICP and should be avoided. Assessment of bowel function and management of constipation is discussed in detail in Chapter 18.

Table 20.5 Common drugs used for pain and nausea management post-neurosurgery.

Drug	Action	Dose
Codeine phosphate	Weak opioid for mild to moderate pain	30–60 mg 4 hourly orally or intra muscularly. Maximum dose: 240 mg/24 hr
Paracetamol	Non-opioid for mild to moderate pain	1 g 4 hourly oral or IV. Maximum dose: 4 g/24 hr
Tramadol	Synthetic opioid for moderate pain	50–100 mg 4–6 hourly Maximum dose: 600 mg/24 hr
Morphine sulphate	Opioid with high affinity for μ receptors	PCA: 100 mg morphine, made up to 50 ml with 0.9% sodium chloride – Initial bolus of 2 mg (1 ml) – Duration of injection 1 min – 10 min lockout – No background infusion – Infusion 60 mg/60 ml, titrated to patient requirements Maximum dose: 30 mg in 4 hours Alternatively: 5–10 mg 4 hourly IM, or oramorph 5–20 mg 2–4 hourly
Cyclizine (antihistamine)	Blocks histamine receptors in the chemoreceptor trigger zone in the medulla. Helps control nausea, vomiting, motion sickness	50 mg TDS oral, IM, IV
Ondansetron (serotonin receptor antagonist)	Blocks serotonin receptors in the gastrointestinal tract and medulla For post-operative nausea	8 mg 1 hour preoperatively, then 8 mg at 8 hourly intervals post-operatively for 24 hr Can be used for breakthrough nausea/vomiting, together with cyclizine: 8 mg/8 hourly

Hydration and nutrition

Patients should commence oral fluid intake as soon as this is tolerated, unless they have reduced level of consciousness, impaired swallowing or have undergone posterior fossa surgery (RCN, 2005). If oral fluid intake is not possible, patients should receive 0.9% sodium chloride as first line fluid replacement (Cook, 2005) (see Chapter 16).

Systemic metabolic responses that occur following surgery/injury include: hypermetabolism, hypercatabolism and hyperglycaemia, the consequences of which are malnutrition, reduced immunocompetence, accelerated visceral protein depletion and impaired healing (Mestecky, 2007). There can be an increase of up to 60% in basal metabolic rate (BMR) in the first 48 hours following head injury or major surgery, particularly in patients who are agitated.

Gastro-intestinal prophylaxis may be required if the patient is unable to take oral fluids and/or diet. Omeprazole or ranitidine are the drugs of choice and are effective in reducing gastric acid by blocking histamine H2 receptors in the gastrointestinal tract, thereby reducing the risk of bleeding from gastroduodenal erosions (Garrett *et al.*, 2003).

Nausea and vomiting may be problematic following surgery and need to be controlled with anti-emetics. The risks of nausea, retching and vomiting are fluid and electrolyte imbalance, a compromised airway, aspiration pneumonia, malnutrition, disruption of the surgical site, venous hypertension. A subsequent increase in ICP can pose a severe threat to post-operative recovery (Garrett *et al.*, 2003; Neufeld and Newburn-Cook, 2008). The choice of antiemetic depends on the aetiology of the vomiting. The vomiting centre in the medulla oblongata can be triggered either directly (from the cerebral cortex – fear, anticipation; the somatosensory cortex – smell; vestibular nuclei – motion sickness) or indirectly (by anaesthetia or surgical manipulation) (Garrett *et al.*, 2003).

Antihistamines such as cyclizine are effective in the initial treatment of post-operative nausea and vomiting which may be caused by the anaesthetic or the surgical site involved. It is particularly good for vertigo and motion sickness symptoms which patients can complain of following posterior fossa surgery and disturbance of the cerebellum or brain stem (Neufeld and Newburn-Cook, 2008). Nurses should ensure that a second anti-emetic has been prescribed in case the first one does not work within an hour. Ondansetron is a useful adjunct to cyclizine, blocking serotonin receptors in the gastrointestinal tract and medulla and can be administered within in an hour of cyclizine if required (see Table 20.5).

Mobilisation

Early mobilisation is essential to avoid complications of bed rest and reduced mobility, such as chest infections and pneumonia, deep vein thrombosis and pulmonary emboli, and pressure sores.

Evidence based prevention of DVT and pressure sores have been discussed in Chapter 8. Management of bladder and bowel complications is discussed in Chapter 18.

SPECIFIC POST-OPERATIVE NEUROSURGICAL NURSING CARE

As well as providing the general care described above for all neurosurgical patients, some patients who have undergone certain procedures have specific additional care and requirements.

Post-craniotomy

Many patients take a while to return to their pre-operative level of consciousness following craniotomies, due to the effects of the anaesthesia and brain manipulation. Modern anaesthetic agents enable patients to recover quickly, but there may be temporary changes in their mental state for the first few hours with or without new focal signs (Gupta and Summons, 2001; Douglas and Rowed, 2005). These usually resolve within the first few hours, but it is important to have clear instructions from the surgeons as to what is acceptable. Any deviation from the patient's baseline needs to be discussed with the surgical team as a matter of urgency. Further CT or MRI scans may be required to delineate the problem.

It is also important that these patients are well hydrated, but care must be taken not to overload those who have had tumour surgery, as they have a propensity to develop postoperative cerebral oedema. As a general rule 2 litres per 24 hours is sufficient (Rampling *et al.*, 2004). Patients who have had aneurysmal surgery will require at least 3 litres per 24 hours to maintain an adequate circulating volume, prevent vasospasm and maintain adequate cerebral perfusion (see Chapter 23).

A daily urinalysis for glucose should be undertaken for patients who are receiving dexamethasone (patients with tumours). If the urinalysis is positive for glucose the blood glucose should be monitored. Hyperglycaemia disrupts the blood brain barrier increasing cerebral oedema (Lindsay and Bone, 2004). Insulin may be required to reduce the blood glucose levels to within normal levels.

Post-craniectomy

Particular attention must be paid to the site of bone flap removal: this should be clearly documented in the patient's notes and tight bandages should be avoided. Patients who have had a hemicraniectomy should not be positioned on the same side as the missing bone flap for the first 48 hours. This could push intracranial contents inward, increasing ICP (Tazbir *et al.*, 2005). The patient should be turned every two hours, but the head should always rest on the solid side of the cranium. The craniectomy site should be observed for changes in appearance, such as bulging (a sign of increased pressure), inflammation, and for CSF leakage. Any change in appearance of or drainage from the incision should be reported to the medical staff immediately.

For small craniectomies the patient does not require any special protection but both the patient and family need to be aware of the bony defect on discharge. For larger craniectomies, especially those over the temporo-parietal region, a temporary protective helmet may be required prior to discharge. Cranioplasty should then be performed within six months (Tazbir *et al.*, 2005).

Posterior fossa surgery

Particular attention needs to be paid to assessment of respiratory function due to risk of dysphagia and aspiration. Swallowing assessment (see Chapter 12) is required before allowing oral fluids. If there is a delay in this assessment the patient should continue on IV fluids and commence nasogastric feeding to avoid aspiration pneumonia.

If there is any facial nerve deficit, particular attention needs to be paid to eye care. Due to tear deficiency eye drops will be required. Hypromellose is most commonly used and may be required as frequently as hourly to reduce soreness. Long acting ointment is used to lubricate the eye at night to prevent frequent wakening of the patient. A clear bubble shield is advocated for night wear to protect the cornea from abrasions. It must not be worn all the time as the warm moist environment that develops underneath can precipitate infections (BAO-HNS 2002). The patient should receive education on eye care prior to discharge. Protective eye wear without prescription lenses will protect the eye from dust when outdoors. If the facial weakness is more severe a temporary tarsorrhaphy (suturing of the outer aspect of the upper and lower eyelids) may be required. In extreme circumstances this may be permanent (Koerbel *et al.*, 2005).

Post-transsphenoidal hypophysectomy

Prophylactic hydrocortisone is commenced either on induction of anaesthesia or post-operatively to avoid hypo-adrenalism. Cortisol levels are checked at three/four days post-operatively and, if high, the hydrocortisone will be discontinued. If hydrocortisone is continued levels need to be checked regularly as an outpatient.

Patients need to be advised of the signs of CSF rhinorrhoea, i.e. a post-nasal drip, a drip on moving their head forward and a salty taste in their mouth, and instructed to advise nursing staff should this occur. The presence of CSF can be confirmed using a urinalysis dip stick which will react positively for glucose. CSF leaks must be monitored carefully due to the risk of infection and subsequent meningitis. Persistent leaks may need to be treated with a temporary lumbar drain to encourage the CSF to follow its normal path. In extreme cases a dural graft may be required.

Accurate recording of fluid balance is essential as transient diabetes insipidus is a common post-operative problem. If urine output exceeds 200 ml/hr for two consecutive hours (if catheterised), or over 800 ml in four hours, and is dilute with a specific gravity of <1.005, a serum and urine sample should be sent to determine the osmolality and sodium levels which will enable a diagnosis of diabetes insipidus (see Chapter 16).

Post-transoral surgery

These patients will be nursed in a level 3 facility post-operatively (DH, 2000). Trans-oral patients may be nasally intubated or have an elective tracheostomy, and maxillotomy patients will have an elective tracheostomy. Both groups of patients will be ventilated for at least 24–48 hours (Tamaki *et al.*, 2001; NHNN, 2004). Post-operative re-intubation may be difficult due to anatomical problems or instability of the neck and also the danger of compromising the integrity of the trans-oral wound (NHNN, 2004).

Patients will have a nasogastric tube post-operatively, regardless of whether they are ventilated or not, to ensure adequate nutrition during the first five days as swelling subsides, allowing the surgical incision to heal (Tamaki *et al.*, 2001). Specific attention needs to be paid to mouth care. Regular mouthwashes are advocated as well as the use of soft toothbrushes to avoid mucosal damage (Lowery, 1999).

A lumbar drain is usually inserted during surgery to minimise CSF leaks post-operatively and removed at five days as long as there are no complications (Tamaki *et al.*, 2001). Patients must be told not to blow their nose for up to 10 days post-operatively. This can induce or exacerbate a CSF leak but can also push air from the sinuses under the skin and cause swelling around the eyes (Tamaki *et al.*, 2001).

SUMMARY

Neurosurgical procedures are many and varied with different levels of complexity. New procedures are being developed all the time with the purpose of making the patient pathway as easy and safe as possible. Endoscopic procedures combined with modern imaging techniques are moving neurosurgery on from craniotomies to much less invasive techniques. These techniques are improving outcomes for patients and reducing levels of morbidity. However this group of patients still rely heavily on the expert knowledge and skills of the neuroscience nurse (Mestecky, 2007).

REFERENCES

Bekar A, Korfali E, Dogan S *et al.* (2001) The effect of hair on infection after cranial surgery. *Acta Neurochirurgica* 143(6):533–536.

Brady M, Kinn S, Stuart P (2003) Preoperative fasting for adults to prevent perioperative complications. *Cochrane Database of Systematic Reviews* Issue 4. Art. No.: CD004423. DOI: 10.1002/14651858.CD004423.

British Association of Otorhinolaryngologists Head and Neck Surgeons (2002) *Acoustic Neuromas: Clinical effectiveness guidelines*. London: BAO-HNS Royal College of Surgeons.

Cook N (2005) Fundamentals of fluids and hydration in the nursing of the neuroscience patient. *British Journal of Neuroscience Nursing* 1(2):61–66.

Corteen E, Timofeev I, Kirkpatrick P, Hutchinson P (2007) The RESCUEicp study of decompressive craniectomy: implications for practice. *British Journal of Neuroscience Nursing* 3(9):428–433.

De Divitiis O, Conti A, Angileri FF *et al.* (2004) Endoscopic transoral-transclival approach to the brainstem and surrounding cisternal space: anatomical study. *Neurosurgery* 54(1):125–130.

Department of Health (2000) *Comprehensive Critical Care: A review of adult critical care services.* London: DH.

Department of Health (2001) *Good Practice in Consent Implementation Guide: Consent to examination or treatment.* London: DH.

Department of Health (2003) *The Community Care Act: Guidance for implementation.* London: DH.

Department of Health (2005) *Mental Capacity Act.* London: DH.

Department of Health (2006) *Saving Lives: Reducing infection, delivering clean and safe care.* High impact intervention: No. 4 Care bundle to prevent surgical site infection; No. 6 Urinary catheter care bundle. London: DH.

Douglas M, Rowed S (2005) The implementation of a postoperative care process on a neurosurgical unit. *Journal of Neuroscience Nursing* 37(6):329–333.

Duffau H, Lopes M, Arthuis F *et al.* (2005) Contribution of intraoperative electrical stimulations in surgery of low grade gliomas: a comparative study between two series without (1985–1996) and with (1996–2003) functional mapping in the same institution. *Journal of Neurology, Neurosurgery and Psychiatry* 76:845–851.

Frank G, Pasquini E, Farneti G (2006) The endoscopic versus the traditional approach in pituitary surgery. *Neuroenocrinology* 86(3–4):240–248.

Garrett K, Tsuruta K,Walker S (2003) Managing nausea and vomiting: current strategies. *Critical Care Nurse* 23(1):31–52.

Gazzeri R, Galarza M, Neroni M (2007) Continuous subgaleal suction drainage for the treatment of chronic subdural haematoma. *Acta Neurochirurgica* 149(5):487–493.

Govender S (2005) Outcome of transoral surgery. *Journal of Bone and Joint Surgery* 87(111): 283.

Greenberg MS (2006) *Handbook of Neurosurgery.* (6th edition). New York: Thieme Medical Publishers.

Gupta AK, Summons A (2001) *Notes in Neuroanaesthesia and Critical Care.* Cambridge: Cambridge University Press.

Kinley H, Czoski-Murray C, George S (2002) Effectiveness of appropriately trained nurses in preoperative assessment: randomised controlled equivalence/non-inferiority trial. *British Journal of Medicine* 325:1323–1326.

Koerbel A, Gharabaghi A, Safawi-Abbasi S (2005) Evolution of vestibular schwannoma surgery: the long journey to current success. *Neurosurgery Focus* 18(4):1–6.

Levy A (2004) Pituitary disease: presentation, diagnosis and management. *Journal of Neurology, Neurosurgery and Psychiatry* 75:47–52.

Li G, Wen L, Zhan RY *et al.* (2008) Cranioplasty for patients developing large cranial defects combined with post-traumatic hydrocephalus after head trauma. *Brain Injury* 22(4):333–337.

Lindsay KW, Bone I (2004) *Neurology and Neurosurgery Illustrated.* (4th edition). Edinburgh: Churchill Livingstone.

Lowery R (1999) A case report: maxillotomy for removal of a clival chordoma. *Journal of Neuroscience Nursing* 31(5):303–308.

Maxwell SRJ, Bateman DN, Myles PS *et al.* (2007) Choice of opioid analgesics in postoperative care. *The Lancet* 369:9578.

Mestecky AM (2006) Metabolic responses after severe head injury and how to optimise nutrition: a literature review. *British Journal of Neuroscience Nursing* 2(2):73–79.

Mestecky AM (2007) Management of severe traumatic brain injury: the need for the knowledgeable nurse. *British Journal of Neuroscience Nursing* 3(1):7–13.

Mestecky AM (2010) Managing primary pituitary tumours: assessments and complications. *British Journal of Neuroscience Nursing* 6(5):222–226.

National Confidential Enquiry into Patient Outcome and Death (2007) *Trauma: Who cares?* London: NCEPOD.

National Hospital for Neurology and Neurosurgery (2002) *Acute Pain Management Guidelines.* London: NHNN.

National Hospital for Neurology and Neurosurgery (2004) *Management of Patients Following Trans-oral Surgery or Maxillotomy.* London: NHNN.

National Institute for Health and Clinical Excellence (2003) *Endoscopic Transspenoidal Pituitary Adenoma.* London: NICE.

National Institute for Health and Clinical Excellence (2007a) *Guideline 46: Venous Thromboembolism: Reducing the risk of venous thromboembolism in inpatients undergoing surgery.* London: NICE.

National Institute for Health and Clinical Excellence (2007b) *Head Injury: Triage, assessment, investigation and early management of head injury in infants, children and adults.* London: NICE.

National Institute for Health and Clinical Excellence (2008) *Management of Inadvertent Perioperative Hypothermia in Adults.* London: NICE.

Neufeld SM, Newburn-Cook CV (2008) What are the risk factors for nausea and vomiting after neurosurgery – a systematic review. *Canadian Journal of Neuroscience Nursing* 30(1):23–34.

Palese A, Skrap M, Fachin M *et al.* (2008) The experience of patients undergoing awake craniotomy: in the patients' own words. A qualitative study. *Cancer Nurse* 31(2):166–172.

Patel HC, Bouamra O, Woodford M *et al.* (2005) Trends in head injury outcome from 1989 to 2003 and the effect of neurosurgical care: an observational study. *The Lancet* 366(9496):1538 –1544.

Rampling R, James A, Papanastassiou V (2004) The present and future management of malignant brain tumours:

surgery, radiotherapy, chemotherapy. *Journal of Neurology, Neurosurgery and Psychiatry* 75(2):24–30.

Roberts GC (2005) Post-craniotomy analgesia: current practices in British neurosurgical centres – a survey of post-craniotomy analgesic practices. *European Journal of Anaesthesiology* 22(5):325–327.

Royal College of Nursing (2005) *Clinical Practice Guidelines: Perioperative fasting in adults and children.* London: RCN.

Sahuquillo J, Arikan F (2006) Decompressive craniectomy for the treatment of refractory high intracranial pressure in traumatic brain injury. *Cochrane Database of Systematic Reviews* Issue 1. Art. No. CD003983.

Society of British Neurological Surgeons (2000) *British Neurosurgical Workforce Plan 2000–2015.* London: SBNS.

Sudheer PS, Logan SW, Terblanche C *et al.* (2007) Comparison of analgesic effect and respiratory effects of morphine, tramadol and codeine after craniotomy. *Anaesthesia* 62(12):1294–1295.

Tamaki N, Nagashima T, Ehara K (2001) Surgical approaches and strategies for skull based chordomas. *Neurosurgical Focus* 10(3):E9.

Tazbir J, Marthaler MT, Moredich C *et al.* (2005) Decompressive hemicraniectomy with duraplasty: a treatment for large-volume ischaemic stroke. *Journal of Neuroscience Nursing* 37(4):194–199.

Thibault M, Girard F, Moumdjian R *et al.* (2007) Craniotomy site influences postoperative pain following neurosurgical procedures: a retrospective study. *Canadian Journal of Anaesthesia* 54(7):544–548.

Vahedi K, Benoist L, Kurtz A *et al.* (2005) Quality of life after decompressive craniectomy for malignant middle cerebral artery infarction. *Journal of Neurology, Neurosurgery and Psychiatry* 76:1181–1182.

Weigel R, Schmiedek P, Krauss JK (2003) Outcome of contemporary surgery for chronic subdural haematoma: evidence based review. *Journal of Neurology, Neurosurgery, Psychiatry* 74:937–943.

Willems PWA, van der Sprenkel JW, Tulleken CA *et al.* (2006) Neuronavigation and surgery of intracerebral tumours. *Journal of Neurology* 253:1123–1136.

Williams M (2007) Cutting edge neurosurgery. *The Journal of Perioperative Practice* 17(12):577–582.

Section IV
Management of Patients with Intracranial Disorders and Disease

21

Management of Patients with Intracranial Tumours

Emma Townsley

INTRODUCTION

Brain tumours cause a significant burden to patients and their families and carers. Patients most often face progressive deterioration in their physical, cognitive and psychosocial functioning, which has a deleterious effect upon their quality of life. The patient pathway from diagnosis to treatment and follow-up is frequently complex. Without a committed and experienced multidisciplinary team (MDT) the care and management can become fragmented, exacerbating the difficulties experienced. Nurses have a key role to play in ensuring that patients and their carers are adequately supported and are provided with sufficient information to allow them to make informed choices about their care and management. This chapter will provide the reader with the necessary knowledge required to manage the care of patients with brain tumours, and to educate and support the patient and their families.

The specific medical management of different tumour types is presented in the first part of the chapter which is followed by nursing assessment, care and management.

Particular emphasis will be given to the document *Improving Outcomes for Brain and Other CNS Tumours* (NICE, 2006a), which provides evidence-based guidance on the key aspects of service provision in order to achieve the best outcomes for patients with brain tumours.

EPIDEMIOLOGY

Primary brain tumours are rare, accounting for as little as 1.6% of cancer in England and Wales (NICE, 2006a); they are however the second largest cause of neurological related death after stroke (Rees, 2004).

The reported incidence of primary central nervous system (CNS) tumours is 15–16 per 100,000 population (NICE, 2006a), however it is likely to be nearer to 20 per 100,000 (Pobereskin and Chadduck, 2000). The incidence of metastatic brain tumours is increasing as many patients are living longer with primary cancer. The specific epidemiology of each tumour type will be discussed below.

PATHOPHYSIOLOGY

Tumours are divided into two distinct categories: benign and malignant. Benign tumours are comprised of cells that are well differentiated, resembling the normal cells from which they arise. Benign tumours tend not to infiltrate into surrounding tissues and are considered to be non-life threatening. Malignant tumour cells however show significant abnormalities, including: nuclear atypia, frequent mitosis and necrosis. They are associated with rapid growth and will invade surrounding tissues (Kearney and Richardson, 2006). Malignant tumours can also metastasise, i.e. cells detach from the primary tumour, are transported in the bloodstream, lymphatic system or cerebrospinal fluid, and proliferate at the metastatic site.

Neuroscience Nursing: Evidence-Based Practice, 1st Edition.
Edited by Sue Woodward and Ann-Marie Mestecky
© 2011 Blackwell Publishing Ltd

Tumours arise when cells begin to grow and divide in an unregulated fashion. Uncontrolled cell growth is thought to be caused by genetic changes that transform a normal cell into a malignant cell (Gabriel, 2007). Mutation in genes occurs as a result of errors in the replication of deoxyribonucleic acid (DNA) (Corner and Bailey, 2001). Three types of genes are involved: oncogenes, tumour suppressor genes, and DNA repair genes (Gabriel, 2007). Oncogenes are genes that promote cell birth and growth; if they mutate, excessive cell multiplication can occur. Tumour suppressor genes are the gatekeepers of the cell cycle; their role is to inactivate cell proliferation. DNA repair genes normally function by repairing DNA damage; the loss of this function allows accumulation of DNA mutation and eventually tumour formation. In summary, benign and malignant tumours arise when the normal growth and differentiation of cells is disrupted.

AETIOLOGY

The cause of most primary brain tumours is unknown. The only definite risk factors are previous exposure to ionising radiation, or a genetic predisposition. Cranial radiation, even at low therapeutic doses, has been shown to increase the relative risk of meningiomas and gliomas (Ron *et al.*, 1988). These tumours typically occur in areas previously subjected to radiation and may take many years to develop following treatment. A number of known genetic disorders predispose patients to develop brain tumours, although these comprise a small minority in terms of overall tumour incidence (Table 21.1).

There is currently no evidence to suggest that lifestyle factors influence the development of a primary brain tumour. Although there has been much media interest in the role of mobile phones in the development of brain tumours, extensive follow-up data over 10 years do not support a link between mobile phone use and the incidence of brain tumours (Hepworth *et al.*, 2006).

OVERVIEW OF TUMOUR TYPES AND CLASSIFICATION

Brain tumours can be classified or differentiated in a number of ways: by their tissue of origin, their location, or their rate of growth. Primary brain tumours are those that arise from the brain tissue. The most frequently occurring are those arising from glial cells (glial tumours or gliomas), which comprise 50% of primary brain tumours. Primary tumours can also arise from neuroembryonic cells, the meninges, nerve sheaths and pituitary cells. Secondary tumours are those that have spread to the brain from a primary site of disease.

Table 21.1 Genetic disorders and associated tumours.

Syndrome	Associated tumours
Neurofibromatosis type 1	Neurofibromas, malignant nerve sheet tumour, optic nerve glioma, astrocytoma
Neurofibromatosis type 2	Bilateral acoustic schwannomas, multiple meningiomas, astrocytomas, glial hamartomata
Von Hippel–Lindau syndrome	Haemangioblastoma
Tuberous sclerosis	Subependymal giant cell astrocytoma, cortical tubers
Li–Fraumeni	Astrocytomas/primitive neuroectodermal tumour
Cowden's disease	Dysplastic ganglioma of the cerebellum
Turcot's syndrome	Medulloblastoma, glioblastoma
Gorlin syndrome	Medulloblastoma

Adapted from National Institute for Health and Clinical Excellence, 2006a.

Intra-axial tumours arise within the brain, i.e. the cerebral hemispheres, brain stem and cerebellum. Extra-axial tumours grow outside of the brain but within the cranium, for example, within the cranial nerves, pituitary gland and meninges. Further distinction can be made between tumours which grow infratentorially and supratentorially. For example, 70–80% of paediatric tumours occur in the cerebellum (infratentorial), whereas most adult tumours are found in the cerebral hemispheres (supratentorial) (Rampling, 2003).

The terms benign and malignant are considered to lack validity when applied to intracranial tumours in the clinical setting for the following reasons:

- The cranium is a rigid structure, therefore all tumours have the potential to increase intracranial pressure (ICP), which can be fatal
- Tumours that grow slowly can compress or infiltrate normal brain tissue, causing neurological deficits or interfering with vital brain stem functions

- Some slow growing tumours can undergo malignant transformation into more aggressive forms

(NICE, 2006a)

For these reasons, the *Improving Outcomes Guidance for Brain and Other CNS Tumours* document (NICE, 2006a) classifies tumours as either high-grade or low-grade. These terms are in keeping with the World Health Organisation (WHO) tumour classification system. Gliomas are graded I–IV: grade I tumours are the slowest growing of the four grades and Grade IV tumours are the fastest. Grades I and II are referred to as low-grade gliomas and grades III and IV are high-grade tumours.

The most commonly used system for classifying brain tumours is the WHO classification, which identifies as many as 120 different tumour types. An adapted and abridged version of the WHO classification (see Table 21.2) demonstrates a cross section of cell types that give rise to tumours and includes the likely anatomical locations for some tumours. The table also includes tumours that are not included in the WHO classification, such as metastases.

COMMON TYPES OF TUMOUR: GLIOMA, MENINGIOMA AND METASTASES

Gliomas

The most commonly occurring primary brain tumours are gliomas, which account for over 50% of all tumours within the brain. Gliomas arise from glial cells including astrocytes, oligodendrocytes and ependymal cells. Gliomas can be fast growing (high-grade, malignant) (see Figure 21.1) or slow growing (low-grade, benign) (see Figure 21.2). Generally, the higher the grade, the more diffuse and infiltrative the tumour. High-grade malignant gliomas are defined as cancer, a definition which tends not to be applied to low-grade gliomas, even though grade II gliomas almost always undergo malignant transformation eventually.

Astrocytoma

This is the most common type of glioma, and develops from the astrocyte. The least aggressive form is the grade II or diffuse low-grade astrocytoma. They grow slowly, but can undergo malignant transformation to a grade III or IV lesion, resulting in a mean survival of between five and seven years (Rees, 2002). Grade III or anaplastic astrocytomas are high-grade and contain more rapidly dividing cells, resulting in a median survival time of between two and three years. The most aggressive type of astrocytoma is the grade IV glioma or glioblastoma multiforme (GBM).

These contain poorly differentiated cells, grow rapidly and contain regions of necrosis. The prognosis is poor: only 20% of patients survive for more than two years. Grade III and IV gliomas can arise *de novo,* or by transformation from a lower-grade tumour.

Oligodendroglioma

Five per cent of brain tumours arise from oligodendrocytes. They are also graded according to their rate of growth and cell behaviour. Studies have demonstrated that oligodendrogliomas behave more benignly than astrocytomas; this is thought to be due to their sensitivity to treatments such as radiotherapy and chemotherapy (Cairncross *et al.*, 1998). The average survival time for a low-grade (grade II) oligodendroglioma is nine years. High-grade forms are known as anaplastic oligodendrogliomas (grade III); 30–38% of people with this diagnosis will live for five years.

Mixed glioma

'Mixed gliomas' or oligoastrocytomas, contain varying proportions of astrocytic and oligodendroglial elements, and tend to show behaviour intermediate to that of the 'pure' tumour types.

Ependymoma

Tumours arising from ependymal cells account for 5% of brain tumours in the adult population. The ependymal cells line the ventricle walls and therefore ependymomas often arise in the ventricles, but can occur in other locations within the cerebral hemispheres. They are graded from I – III. Grade III ependymomas are considered to be malignant. Less is known about how the grade of the ependymoma correlates to prognosis. Survival at five years is thought to be about 50% for all grades.

Meningioma

Tumours which arise from the meningeal cells are called meningiomas, and account for 25% of primary brain tumours (Rampling, 2003). They are extra-axial tumours that can arise anywhere on meningeal surfaces, over the cerebral convexities, around the skull base and, rarely, within the ventricles (Figure 21.3). The vast majority of meningiomas arise spontaneously, although they can occasionally result as a late complication of radiotherapy. Most meningiomas grow slowly and are non-infiltrative. They may cause reactive thickening ('hyperostosis') of overlying bone. The commonest form is a grade I meningioma, which is not infiltrative and is often removed with surgery.

Table 21.2 An adapted and abridged version of the WHO classification.

Neuroepithelial tumours			
Cell origin	Types	WHO grade	Anatomical locations
Astrocytic cells (glial cell)	Pilocytic astrocytoma	I	Cerebral hemispheres
	Diffuse astrocytoma	II	Brain stem
	Anaplastic astrocytoma	III	Optic tracts
	Glioblastoma multiforme	IV	
	Giant cell glioblastoma and Gliosarcoma		
	Subependymal giant cell astrocytoma		
	Pleomorphic xanthoastrocytoma		
Oligodendroglial cells (glial cell)	Oligodendroglioma	II	Cerebral hemispheres
	Anaplastic oligodendroglioma	II	Brain stem
Ependymal cells (glial cell)	Ependymoma	I & II	Cerebral hemispheres
	Anaplastic ependymoma	III	Intraventricular
	Myxopapillary ependymoma		
	Subependymoma		
Mixed glial cell tumours (glial cell)	Oligoastrocytoma	II	Cerebral hemispheres
	Anaplastic oligoastrocytoma	III	Brain stem
Choroid plexus	Choroid plexus papilloma		Intraventricular
	Choroid plexus carcinoma		Cerebellopontine angle
Neuronal/mixed glial– neuronal cells	Gangliocytoma		Cerebral hemispheres
	Ganglioglioma		
	Dysembryoplastic neuroepithelial tumour (DNET)		
	Central neurocytoma		
Pineal parenchyma	Pineocytoma		Pineal region
	Pineoblastoma		
	Mixed		
Embryonic cells	Medulloblastoma		Cerebellum (paediatric)
	Primitive neuroectodermal tumour (PNET)		and cerebral hemispheres (adults)

Adapted from: Kleihues and Cavanee (2000); Abrey and Warren (2003).

Metastases

These are tumours that have spread to the brain from a primary site of malignancy outside the CNS, and account for 20% of brain tumours. They occur in 20–40% of patients with a variety of cancers, and are particularly common in those with primary disease in lung and breast. They may occur in brain parenchyma (intra-axial) or in the meninges and skull base (extra-axial). Lesions can be solitary or multiple. They generally carry poor prognoses, which are determined by both the effects of the brain metastases themselves and the presence of disseminated malignancy elsewhere in the body.

CLINICAL SIGNS AND SYMPTOMS

Intracranial tumours present with a variety of symptoms and clinical signs. The clinical presentation will be dependent upon the tumour's location within the brain, its rate of growth and its pathology, i.e. whether it infiltrates sur-

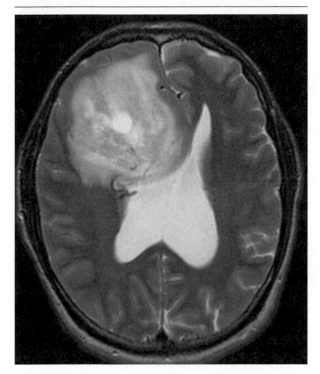

Figure 21.1 T2 image of a high-grade anaplastic astrocytoma with a heterogeneous appearance. Note enlarged vessels at posterior aspect of mass. Reproduced from C. Clarke *et al.*, *Neurology: A Queen Square Textbook.* Wiley-Blackwell, with permission.

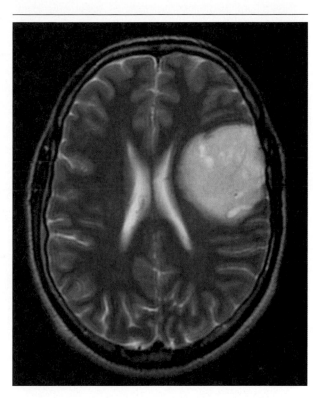

Figure 21.2 T2 image of a homogeneously appearing right frontal low-grade astrocytoma. Reproduced from C. Clarke *et al.*, *Neurology: A Queen Square Textbook.* Wiley-Blackwell, with permission.

rounding brain tissue, or is non-invasive. Symptoms associated with brain tumours include headaches, seizures, changes in cognitive function and mood, and progressive focal neurological deficit, e.g. limb weakness or numbness, problems with vision or speech (Grant, 2004). However, most of these are not exclusive to brain tumours. Headache, mood changes and seizures are commonly seen in general practice. A GP will on average see one adult patient who has a primary brain tumour every 7 years (Humphreys, 2005).

DIAGNOSIS

Clinical examination

A clinical history and neurological examination needs to be undertaken when patients present with symptoms indicative of an intracranial lesion. These examinations should include: an assessment of conscious level (Glasgow Coma Scale), mental test score, fundoscopy, assessment of visual fields, assessment of eye movements and focal deficits.

Diagnostic imaging

Cross sectional imaging with computed tomography (CT) or magnetic resonance imaging (MRI) is used to identify, localise and characterise tumours within the brain. There are features on imaging which give an indication as to the underlying nature of the tumour (Table 21.3). Imaging is also used to monitor the effects of treatment and to guide decisions about further therapy.

TREATMENT

The main treatment modalities used for brain tumours are surgery, radiotherapy and chemotherapy. Anatomical position, tumour pathology and patient performance score are the key prognostic indicators and influence treatment options (NICE, 2006). The purpose of treatment and ongoing follow-up is to increase survival and to maximise the patient's quality of life by managing any symptoms or side-effects of treatment (NICE, 2006).

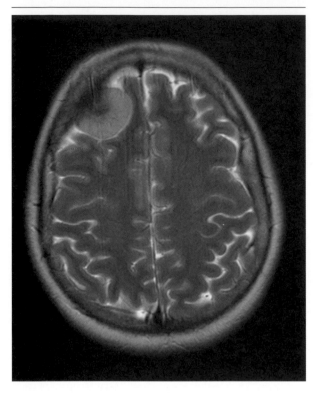

Figure 21.3 Sagittal contrast enhanced axial T2 images demonstrating a grey matter iso-intense mass displacing the frontal lobe with hyperostosis but no associated oedema. Reproduced from C. Clarke *et al.*, *Neurology: A Queen Square Textbook.* Wiley-Blackwell, with permission.

Surgery

Surgery plays an essential role in the management of almost all brain tumours, although the aim and type of procedure varies depending on the nature and site of the lesion. Obtaining tissue for histological diagnosis (biopsy) is usually imperative.

Tumour tissue taken during biopsy or debulking procedures currently provides the definitive diagnosis of tumour type and grade. Frozen sections may be examined during surgery to guide immediate decisions regarding the extent of excision. A number of additional techniques may be used to characterise the tumour tissue, including immuno-histochemistry, electron microscopy, cell culture and molecular genetics.

Surgery is also undertaken to reduce the mass effect of tumours (debulking), and the number of tumour cells (cytoreduction), which can increase the efficacy of subsequent cytotoxic therapy. It may be feasible to remove some tumours completely (curative resection), although this is usually only possible with extra-axial lesions such as meningiomas, schwannomas and some low-grade parenchymal tumours. Surgical resection may also help to control tumour related seizures.

Brain tissue which is deemed to be eloquent, e.g. the motor strip or Broca's area, requires careful consideration prior to undergoing surgery in order to ensure that new neurological deficits are not caused by the surgery itself.

Table 21.4 summarises the surgical procedures and techniques used for investigating, treating and palliating tumours. Refer to Chapter 20 for further detail of each surgical procedure and for the pre- and post-operative care and management.

Table 21.3 Typical imaging features for glioma, metastases and meningioma.

High-grade glioma	Low-grade glioma	Metastases	Meningioma
• Intra-axial • Irregular 'ring' or patchy enhancement with surrounding oedema (low attenuation on CT, high signal on MRI) • Usually marked mass effect on surrounding brain See Figure 21.1	• Intra-axial • Usually non-enhancing • Low attenuation/density on CT, high signal on MRI • Sometimes calcified • Relatively little mass effect for size of tumour See Figure 21.2	• Often intra-axial but can be meningeal • Almost all enhance • Often have large surrounding oedema (low attenuation on CT, high signal on MRI) and mass effect for enhancing lesion size	• Extra-axial • Can be over convexities or skull vault • Dense pre-contrast on CT, often same intensity as brain on MRI • Enhance homogeneously • Sometimes calcified • May show oedema in adjacent brain See Figure 21.3

Radiotherapy

Radiotherapy involves using ionising radiation which causes cellular damage, most significantly to DNA, and results in cell death. Radiotherapy is a focused treatment and does not affect cells that are not in the field of treatment. In most cases it is given as an adjunct to surgical treatment. It is rarely aimed at cure, but can prolong survival and palliate symptoms. The aim of radiotherapy is to damage the tumours cells whilst minimising the damage that occurs to the surrounding normal brain tissue. The success of the treatment depends upon the tumour's sensitivity to radiation and the tolerance of the surrounding tissues (Corner and Bailey, 2001). Radiotherapy can be delivered in a number of ways. Factors influencing the delivery of radiotherapy include: the type of tumour, the likely response to treatment, and the fitness of the patient to tolerate the treatment.

Fractionated radiotherapy

Fractionated radiotherapy involves delivering the treatment in divided doses over a number of weeks. Because of the toxic effects of radiotherapy upon the surrounding brain, the total dose of radiotherapy to the brain is limited to 50–60 Gy. The dose is then divided into daily fractions of between 1.6 and 2.0 Gy per day. Dividing the dose over a longer period of time enables the normal tissues to withstand the treatment and gives them an opportunity to recover.

Stereotactic radiotherapy

Stereotactic radiotherapy enables more accurate tumour localisation by immobilising the patient using a stereotactic frame. It is suitable for treating small volumes, such as residual tumour following surgery. Fractionated stereotactic radiotherapy enables treatment of irregular lesions and is given in smaller, but multiple doses.

Intensity modulated radiotherapy (IMRT)

IMRT also targets the tumour volume and enables more accurate shaping of the fields of radiotherapy to the shape of the tumour. It can be used to treat larger areas and improves the accuracy of the target volume.

Table 21.4 Summary of the surgical procedures and techniques used for investigating, treating and palliating tumours.

Surgical procedure	Purpose of surgery
Stereotactic biopsy Frameless stereotaxy Open biopsy	Used to obtain tissue sample for histopathology
Excision – total surgical resection	Performed on non-infiltrating and easily accessible tumours, e.g. meningioma
Resection and debulking Awake craniotomy Lobectomy	Performed to reduce the tumour bulk and mass effect
Ventriculo-peritoneal shunt	For emergency decompression and management of tumours obstructing the ventricles, e.g. ependymoma
Insertion of reservoir (see Chapter 25)	Used to palliate cystic lesions which can give rise to neurological signs or raised intracranial pressure, e.g. oligodendrogliomas
Cystoperitoneal shunt	If a cyst requires frequent drainage involving repeated skin puncture and risk of infection, the cystic fluid is shunted via a peritoneal shunt
Carmustine implants: biodegradable polymer wafers that contain chemotherapy called carmustine (Gliadel)	The wafers are inserted into the surgical cavity and slowly dissolve over a number of weeks enabling the cytotoxic (tumour killing agent) to affect the abnormal cells locally

Whole brain radiotherapy (WBRT)

WBRT is generally used in a palliative context and involves lower doses of radiation to the whole brain.

Stereotactic radiosurgery (SR)

SR is used to treat small volumes of tumour using a stereotactic positioning as with surgery. High doses of radiation can be delivered precisely, often in a single fraction. Use of SR is restricted to tumours smaller than 4 cm in diameter, which are well defined. It is well tolerated by patients and does not require repeated visits for planning and treatment.

Chemotherapy

Chemotherapy can be administered either orally, intravenously, intrathecally or implanted surgically. Chemotherapy acts upon the DNA of the cell, either damaging the DNA or preventing it from repairing during the cell cycle; therefore chemotherapy drugs are most effective when cells are rapidly dividing (Corner and Bailey, 2001). Chemotherapy will inhibit cell division in all cells, not just tumour cells. Therefore, a number of generic side-effects are prevalent (see Table 21.5)

The effectiveness of chemotherapy in the management of brain tumours is limited. The brain is protected from chemotherapy by the blood–brain barrier (BBB) which prevents many chemotherapy drugs from entering the brain (Graham and Cloughesy, 2004). Some tumours result in the breakdown of the BBB, theoretically enabling the agents to access the tumour. The doses of chemotherapy used are often limited by the toxicities caused to the body, and when the BBB has broken down toxic drug concentrations occur within the normal brain tissue also (Guerrero, 1998).

The timing of treatment and agents used will depend upon the sensitivity of the tumour to chemotherapy and the stage of the disease. *Neoadjuvant chemotherapy* is given prior to surgery or radiotherapy, *concomitant chemotherapy* is given at the same time as radiotherapy and *adjuvant chemotherapy* is used after surgery/radiotherapy to damage as many residual tumour cells as possible.

Steroids

Cerebral oedema is common in patients with brain tumours and is one of the contributing factors causing neurological deterioration, which results in impaired quality of life (Kaal and Vecht, 2004). Corticosteroids are used to treat oedema at various stages in order to control the effects of cerebral oedema (Guerrero, 1998).

Dexamethasone is the corticosteroid most frequently used for treating cerebral oedema (Kaal and Vecht, 2004). In current practice, doses can vary from 16 mg per day to

Table 21.5 Chemotherapy commonly used to treat intracranial tumours and the side-effects.

Generic side-effects	Drug name (route)	Specific side-effects
Myelosuppression • Anaemia • Neutropenia • Thrombocytopenia Gastrointestinal • Nausea • Vomiting • Constipation • Diarrhoea Reproductive system • Amenorrhoea • Infertility Fatigue	Temozolomide (oral) Procarbazine (oral) CCNU (oral) Vincristine (IV) Methotrexate (oral, IV, intrathecal) Etoposide (oral, IV) Carmustine (Wafers) Carboplatin (IV) Cisplatin (IV) Doxorubicin (IV)	Headache Flu-like symptoms Peripheral neurotoxicity Mucositis No generic side-effects Wound infection

Sources: Guerrero, 1998; Corner and Bailey, 2001; McAllister *et al.*, 2002; Kearney and Richardson, 2006; www.cancerbackup.org.uk Accessed July 2010.

0.5 mg per day. The effect of dexamethasone on cerebral oedema and consequently on neurological function, can improve performance status. The patient's response to corticosteroid therapy is usually measured against their neurological status (Nahaczewski *et al.*, 2004). Steroids can produce an improvement within the first 8–48 hours of administration. The side-effects associated with dexamethasone administration can contribute to a reduced level of functioning and affect quality of life. Table 21.6 provides a summary of the side-effects of dexamethasone.

Palliative and supportive care

For some patients in the advanced stages of disease, palliative care may be the most appropriate management. At the early stages of diagnosis and treatment patients' symptoms will be managed by the neurosurgeon or oncologist. Once symptom control becomes complex, or the disease progresses and treatment options are limited, specialist palliative care may be required. Specialist palliative care teams manage complex symptoms and provide emotional support to patients in addition to supporting relatives and carers (NICE, 2006).

SPECIFIC TREATMENT FOR EACH TYPE OF TUMOUR

High-grade gliomas

Surgery

In the case of diffuse and infiltrating tumours such as high-grade gliomas, it is not possible to totally excise the lesion. The tumour is resected or 'debulked' in order to collect a tissue sample (biopsy) and to reduce the mass effect of the tumour, providing symptomatic relief from raised ICP. Debulking the tumour enables cyto-reduction and, although surgery is not curative in the case of malignant tumours, reduction of the mass can prove advantageous in terms of reducing ICP, improving symptoms and maximising the effect of adjuvant treatment such as radiotherapy and chemotherapy. Such surgery can also be undertaken to provide palliative relief at the time of disease recurrence.

Due to the infiltrative nature of glial tumours and the underlying malignant nature of high-grade gliomas, surgery is not curative. Multidisciplinary decisions regarding the safety of biopsy verses debulking are discussed by relevant team members. Often such decisions are based upon the location of the tumour and the patient's performance status. Patients of a younger age with a high functional performance score as measured by the Karnofsky Performance Score (KPS) or the World Health Organisation performance status are more likely to benefit from debulking surgery.

Table 21.6 Side-effects of dexamethasone.

Organs and systems involved	Effect
Immune system	Increased susceptibility to infections
	Masks sign of infection
	Delayed healing
Dermatologic	Acniform rash
	Skin thinning
	Striae (stretch marks)
	Hair thinning
	Flushing & night sweats
Renal and urinary	Polyuria
	Polydipsia
	Nocturia
Metabolic and endocrine	Impaired glucose tolerance
	Hyperglycaemia – diabetes
	Inhibit thyroid stimulating hormone secretion (TSH)
	Appetite stimulant
	Weight gain
	Cushing's syndrome: truncal obesity, moon face
	Potassium wasting
	Adrenal insufficiency on withdrawal
	Menstrual irregularities
Gastrointestinal	Dyspepsia
	Gastrointestinal ulceration
	Candidiasis (thrush)
Neurobehavioral	Insomnia
	Agitation
	Hyperactivity
	Irritability
	Psychosis (rare)
Musculoskeletal	Proximal myopathy: weakness of the upper arms and thighs
	Osteoporosis: risk of vertebral body fractures

Source: Guerrero, 1998; McAllister *et al.*, 2002; Nahaczewski *et al.*, 2004.

Radiotherapy

Radiotherapy post surgery is standard treatment for high-grade gliomas. Median survival improves for patients undergoing radiotherapy treatment of doses around 60 Gy (Walker *et al.*, 1978). For patients with a good performance score, survival can be improved from 5–6 months to a median survival of 9–12 months. Because of the infiltrative nature of these tumours, the volume or area of brain treated needs to include a 2–3 cm margin beyond the evident radiological abnormality (Gregor, 1997). The treatment consists of 30 fractions of radiotherapy, meaning that 30 doses of radiation are delivered to the tumour. The total dose delivered for radical radiotherapy is between 55 and 60 Gy; dividing these doses into daily fractions of treatment means that the patient undergoes approximately 6 weeks of treatment. It is usually given on an outpatient basis and the patient attends the department on week days. The treatment itself takes as little as 10 minutes per day.

For those patients who are less well, palliative radiotherapy will be given. The dose of radiotherapy delivered in each fraction is higher, but the overall dose is usually 30 Gy. Treatment is given over two weeks, every other day of the week. Such regimes result in fewer side-effects, less time spent undergoing treatment and there is some evidence to suggest that it is equivalent to conventional radical radiotherapy. Radiotherapy can usually only be given once so is not a treatment option at the time of disease recurrence.

Chemotherapy

Recent developments have paved the way for more effective use of chemotherapy in the case of anaplastic oligodendroglioma and newly diagnosed glioblastoma multiforme (GBM).

A recent randomised controlled trial has demonstrated a survival benefit for patients with GBM who are treated with temozolomide chemotherapy concomitantly with their radiotherapy. This regime was followed by a further 6 months of adjuvant chemotherapy. When compared to standard treatment of radiotherapy alone overall survival in the chemoradiation group increased from 12.1 months to 14.6 months. Two years following treatment 26% were still alive, compared with only 10% for those patients who received radiotherapy alone (Strupp *et al.*, 2005). Following a technical appraisal by NICE (2007), radiotherapy with concomitant temozolomide is now standard treatment for patients diagnosed with a GBM who have a good performance score and are likely to tolerate the side-effects of combined treatment. Similar studies are currently being undertaken to establish whether concurrent

chemoradiation would have a similar survival benefit for patients with grade III gliomas.

Chemotherapy is also considered at the time of disease recurrence. Responses rates for chemotherapy are poor: as little as 30% of recurrent gliomas respond to treatment (Rampling, 1997). Response is measured in terms of symptomatic relief and radiological improvement. There is no evidence that chemotherapy improves overall survival but it can increase the time to further progression.

Surgical implant of chemotherapy

An international randomised controlled phase III study compared carmustine wafers with placebo wafers (Westphal *et al.*, 2003); all patients went on to receive adjuvant radiotherapy. Median survival was 13.8 months in the carmustine implant group, and 11.6 months for patients in the placebo group. Further subgroup analysis demonstrated that those patients diagnosed with glioblastoma (GBM) who had undergone a resection of 90% or more, showed a median survival gain of 2.15 months in the carmustine group compared to the placebo group.

The NICE guidelines have licensed the use of carmustine wafers in patients with GBM for whom 90% resection is achievable. Surgery must be undertaken by specialist neurosurgeons who spend at least 50% of their time dedicated to neuro-oncology surgery, and management decisions should be made pre-operatively following discussion and agreement by the multidisciplinary team (NICE, 2007)

Low-grade gliomas

Surgery

In the case of low-grade gliomas, the role of debulking surgery is less clear. Because these tumours cause few symptoms for a number of years prior to transformation, the timing of treatment poses a dilemma (Whittle, 2004; Mason, 2005). There have been no prospective randomised controlled trials comparing timing and extent of surgery in terms of survival advantage (Mason, 2005) or biopsy against tumour excision or expectant ('watch and wait') management (Whittle, 2004). Retrospective studies have indicated that there may be a role for surgical resection in that it can reduce tumour-related morbidity such as epilepsy. If the tumour is in a non-eloquent area of the brain, surgical debulking is sometimes regarded as a first-line treatment, however many are in eloquent regions where excision would result in significant morbidity (Rees, 2002).

Following advances in functional imaging and intra-operative electrical stimulation Duffau and colleagues (2005) suggested that resection of low-grade glioma can be carried out more safely and may improve survival, however only 25% of low-grade gliomas are completely resectable in the hands of an experienced neurosurgeon.

Radiotherapy

The timing of treatment for slow growing low-grade gliomas is less defined than for high-grade gliomas. A multicentre study demonstrated that early radiation treatment following initial surgery does not improve overall survival. However, the time it takes for the tumour to progress to a higher grade increased from 3.4 years to 4.8 years for those patients who receive radiotherapy early (Karim *et al.*, 2002). Time to progression can be prolonged; however those patients receiving treatment early may be more likely to experience late side-effects such as long-term cognitive decline (Taphoorn and Klein, 2004).

Patients at higher risk of disease progression should receive radiotherapy early in the treatment pathway. Such patients include: those over 40, when the largest diameter of the tumour is equal to or greater than 6cm, tumours that cross the midline, and the presence of neurological deficit (Pignatti *et al.*, 2002). Patients who experience intractable seizures can benefit symptomatically from early radiotherapy. Van den Bent and colleagues (2005) reported that 25% of patients who had been irradiated had seizures at 1 year compared with 45% of those who had not been treated. The overall dose of radiotherapy is slightly less for low-grade glioma (50.4Gy) and it is delivered in fractions of 30.

Chemotherapy

Low-grade gliomas are slow growing; their cells divide slowly over time making them less chemosensitive. Treatment is usually reserved until the time that the tumour displays more aggressive characteristics, i.e. at the time the tumour is transforming to a higher grade. Studies to investigate survival advantages in high risk low-grade glioma patients, comparing early radiotherapy with chemotherapy are in the pipeline.

Meningioma

Surgery

Meningiomas tend to be treated surgically, and the degree of resection is determined by location and size of the tumour. Meningiomas on the convexities are usually more successfully excised than those at the skull base.

Radiotherapy

Radiotherapy is reserved for meningiomas which are of a high-grade, II or III. In some instances grade I meningiomas will also be irradiated if there is extensive invasion of other tissues, at second or subsequent relapse, or when surgery is contraindicated (NICE, 2006a). The aim of treatment is to reduce the risk of recurrence. Meningiomas are more discreet tumours which tend not to infiltrate. For this reason it is possible to treat with a smaller margin thus reducing the volume of normal brain included in the treatment field. Depending on the size and location of residual tumour stereotactic radiotherapy and intensity modulated radiotherapy (IMRT) can be used.

Chemotherapy

These tumours are not chemosensitive, and cytotoxic drug treatment plays no role their management. Some meningiomas express oestrogen receptors and treatment with hormonal modulation may have an effect on their growth.

Metastases

Surgery

Metastases may be excised in the case of solitary lesions or up to three lesions if surgically accessible and the systemic disease is well controlled. Such surgery is palliative and can provide symptomatic relief.

Radiotherapy

Whole brain radiotherapy (WBRT) has been used to palliate metastatic disease; usually a total dose of 20Gy is given in five fractions over a week. Stereotactic radiosurgery (SR) is used to treat small volumes of tumour.

Chemotherapy

If the primary cancer is chemosensitive, as is the case with small cell lung cancer, there is some evidence to suggest that systemic chemotherapy has a role to play in disease management (Gerrard and Franks, 2004). However chemotherapy tends to be used in circumstances where there is active disease outside of the CNS in patients who have not previously received multiple chemotherapy regimes.

LESS COMMON TYPES OF TUMOUR

PITUITARY TUMOURS

Marian Lanyon, Clinical Nurse Specialist: Pituitary, National Hospital for Neurology and Neurosurgery, London

Tumours arising from the pituitary gland are, in the main, pituitary adenomas and their causes remain largely unknown (Honegger *et al.*, 2008) (Figure 21.4). Most pituitary adenomas develop extremely slowly; patients may have experienced unexplained symptoms for many years. Carcinoma of the pituitary gland, accompanied or not by metastases, is extremely rare (Scheithauer *et al.*, 2001).

Pituitary adenomas may be classified as either 'functioning' or 'non-functioning' tumours. Functioning tumours produce excess pituitary hormones, causing hormonal symptoms. Non-functioning tumours are generally larger in size and cause pressure symptoms, i.e. headaches and, because of the close proximity to the optic chiasm, disturbances in vision. They also lead to underproduction of many of the pituitary hormones

FUNCTIONING PITUITARY TUMOURS

Functioning tumours are named either after the hormone that is secreted in excess, e.g. prolactinomas or growth hormone secreting adenoma, or by the disease that is caused by the excess of the circulating hormone, e.g.

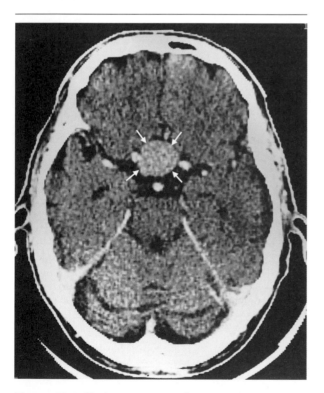

Figure 21.4 Pituitary tumour. Computed tomography scan after contrast shows a mass in the pituitary fossa which enhances vividly (arrows). Reproduced from Peter Armstrong, Martin Wastie, Andrea G. Rockall, *Diagnostic Imaging 6e*, Wiley-Blackwell, with permission.

Cushing's disease. It may be helpful to refer to Chapter 3 for an overview of the pituitary gland and the functions of each of the hormones it produces, which will enable the reader to better understand the specific signs and symptoms of each of the functioning tumours.

Prolactinoma

Hypothalamic dopamine controls the production of prolactin by the pituitary gland, the positive feed-back mechanism is interrupted by the presence of the tumour. The excess production of prolactin, or hyperprolactinaemia, stimulates breast milk production and galactorrhoea. Women will have oligomenorrhoea or amenorrhoea due to the excess of prolactin affecting other hormones produced by the pituitary, i.e. luteinising hormone and follicle stimulating hormone. Men will have reduced libido and impotence. Headaches and visual disturbances are also commonly experienced by the patient if the tumour is >10 mm in diameter. Prolactinomas are the most common of the functioning pituitary tumours. They can be classified as *micro*prolactinomas that measure <10 mm in diameter and *macro*prolactinomas that are >10 mm in diameter (Powell *et al.*, 2003).

Investigations

The elimination of other causes of hyperprolactinaemia is required before a diagnosis is made. Raised prolactin blood levels can be caused by commonly-prescribed tranquillisers and anti-emetics, venepuncture stress, pregnancy and primary hypothyroidism (Powell *et al.*, 2003). Pituitary function blood tests, visual function and MRI of the pituitary gland are arranged.

Medical treatment

Most prolactinomas will respond to medication; surgery is rarely performed. Dopamine agonists, bromocriptine and caberlogine trigger the pituitary receptors resulting in the reduction of prolactin blood levels (dopamine inhibits the synthesis and release of prolactin from the pituitary) and effecting shrinkage of the tumour (Mah and Webster, 2002). In addition, visual function is often improved.

Transphenoidal surgery (see Chapter 20) is employed for those patients who do not respond to dopamine agonist therapy, for those with severe visual symptoms, and for patients who are unable to tolerate dopamine agonists (Verhelst and Abs, 2003).

Growth hormone secreting pituitary adenoma

Growth hormone (GH) secreting adenomas produce and secrete GH in excessive amounts over a number of years.

This causes the very rare acromegaly, which, if untreated, results in a shortened life-span. The excess GH causes a gradual thickening of cartilage and excessive growth of soft tissues leading to enlargement of facial features, particularly the nose and the jaw as well as increase in hand and foot size. These changes occur very gradually. Other symptoms include excessive perspiration, sleep apnoea, colon polyps, carpal tunnel syndrome, hypertension and diabetes mellitus (Powell *et al.*, 2003).

Investigations

GH does not have a direct effect on many of the cells in the body; rather its actions are mediated by insulin like growth factor -1 (IGF-1), which is secreted from the liver under the control of GH. The level of IGF-1 and GH are both used as a measure of disease activity.

Pituitary function blood tests, visual function assessment and MRI of the pituitary gland are also arranged. Most patients will be found to have a pituitary macroadenoma (larger than 10 mm) and some of the tumour may reach into the cavernous sinus or impinge on other structures.

Transphenoidal surgery

Surgery is curative in about two thirds of patients (Powell *et al.*, 2003). The soft tissues, if cured, will start to shrink days after the surgery. A post-surgical growth hormone suppression test and IGF-1 level determine the likelihood of cure (Nomikos *et al.*, 2005).

Medical treatment

Somatostatin analogues work by mimicking somastatin, which is the hypothalamic hormone that suppresses the release of GH. The reduction of GH and IGF-1 levels improves the patient's symptoms. These somatostatin analogue preparations are used for patients awaiting surgery and for those undergoing radiotherapy treatment which can take several years for the full effect to be felt.

Radiotherapy

Radiotherapy is employed for acromegalic patients who have a residual tumour after surgery. As it can take many years for the GH and IGF-1 levels to reduce to normal limits after radiotherapy (Castinetti *et al.*, 2008), medical treatment will also be employed in the meantime. Hypopituitarism, or loss of the pituitary hormones, can develop as a consequence of radiotherapy. Close medical monitoring is required so that timely pituitary hormone replacement can be initiated if required (Powell *et al.*, 2003).

Adrenocorticotrophic hormone (ACTH) secreting pituitary adenoma

ACTH secreting adenomas produce and secrete excess ACTH. The consequence of excess ACTH is the overstimulation of the adrenal glands and excess secretion of cortisol, resulting in Cushing's disease. The signs and symptoms of the disease are:

- Increased fat deposition: moon face, central obesity, buffalo hump
- Increased bruising, scarring, thinning of skin, slow wound healing
- Insulin resistance
- Muscular weakness
- Abdominal striae
- Hypertension
- Hirsutism, acne
- Hypogonadism: loss of libido, irregular periods
- Psychological disturbances: anxiety, depression, mania
(Nussey and Whitehead, 2001).

Investigations

Serum and urinary cortisol levels will be elevated. An MRI scan of the pituitary gland is performed.

Transphenoidal surgery

The high cure rate makes this the treatment of choice. Ketoconazole or metyrapone medication to block excess cortisol production is used pre-operatively for several weeks.

Post-operatively, the patient will require steroid replacement and long-term surveillance (Atkinson *et al.*, 2005). Radiotherapy is employed for patients in whom surgery was unsuccessful.

NON-FUNCTIONING PITUITARY TUMOURS

Hypopituitarism

Most of these tumours are macroadenomas and due to their size will compress the surrounding pituitary tissue causing a reduction in many of the pituitary hormones (hypopituitarism). The hormones are not equally depressed: growth hormone, corticotrophin, gonadotrophin and thyroid stimulating hormone are the most affected. The symptoms of hypopituitarism may include:

- Lethargy
- Oligomenorrhoea or amenorrhoea
- Reduced libido

Headache may have been experienced for many years and confused with cluster or migraine headache. The patient will have decreased peripheral vision due to pressure on the optic chiasm.

Investigations

Blood tests will be performed to determine the levels of each of the pituitary horrmones and visual field tests will determine the degree of visual field loss. An MRI will determine the site and size of the lesion.

Surgical treatment

Transphenoidal hypophysectomy will usually produce recovery of vision immediately (Powell *et al.*, 2003). The patient's vision often continues to improve over months. Most patients will require long term hormone replacement therapy and regular monitoring by an endocrinologist.

Radiotherapy

Radiotherapy is performed in some cases to reduce the possibility of recurrence.

RARE TUMOURS INVOLVING THE PITUITARY GLAND

Craniopharyngioma

These rare lesions, originating from within the remnant of embryonal cells, are to be found between the pituitary and the hypothalamus and can be solid or cystic (Levy and Lightman, 1997). They produce symptoms of hypopituitarism, headache and visual dysfunction.

Pre- and post-operative care of patients undergoing transsphenoidal surgery is detailed in Chapter 20.

VESTIBULAR SCHWANNOMA – ACOUSTIC NEUROMA

Vestibular schwannomas are benign slow growing tumours of the vestibulo-cochlear nerve (VIII cranial nerve), more commonly referred to as acoustic neuromas. They typically grow within the internal auditory canal but as they increase in size they enlarge into the cerebellopontine region and compress the brain stem.

The tumour arises from the Schwann cells (the cells which form the myelin sheath surrounding peripheral nerves) of the vestibular portion of the vestibulo-cochlear nerve hence the name vestibular schwannoma. Vestibular schwannomas represent around 6% of all intracranial tumours (NICE, 2006a).

Clinical signs and symptoms

Ninety percent of patients with acoustic neuroma present with hearing loss and up to 70% will experience tinnitus (BAO, 2002). Any patient presenting with a history of unilateral hearing loss or tinnitus should be investigated. In cases where the tumour has grown into the cerebello-pontine angle patients can present with balance problems, impaired facial sensation (due to compression of the trigeminal nerve) and in rare cases, raised ICP as the tumour obstructs the flow of CSF causing obstructive hydrocephalus. The facial nerve runs parallel to the vestibulo-cochlear nerve in the confined space of the internal auditory canal which, as the tumour grows, leads to the facial nerve being compressed. Despite this, facial paralysis is an uncommon presenting sign.

Diagnosis

Audiological tests will be performed in the first instance followed by an MRI, which is the most sensitive test for identifying acoustic neuromas.

Treatment

Treatment decisions are determined by size and position of the tumour, age of the patient, overall health, and the need to preserve hearing. There are three main management options, which are as follows.

Interval scanning

If the tumour is small, causing no symptoms and shows no evidence of growth, interval scans or 'watchful waiting' is an appropriate management option (Tschudi *et al.*, 2000). This course of treatment is more likely to be undertaken in patients who are over 65.

Surgical removal

The objective of surgery is to preserve residual hearing and facial nerve function. The introduction of microsurgical techniques has resulted in increasing degrees of precise anatomical and functional preservation of the facial and cochlear nerves (Koerbel *et al.*, 2005). 96% of acoustic neuromas that are amenable to microsurgery, can be totally removed (Yamakami *et al.*, 2003).

A number of different surgical approaches are used depending upon the location of the tumour. The suboccipital (retrosigmoid) approach is used when hearing preservation is attempted (Kondziolka *et al.*, 2003). The translabyrinthine approach destroys hearing but provides direct exposure to the tumour. There is less chance of causing damage to the facial nerve with this approach. The middle fossa approach is less frequently employed; it is performed via a temporal craniotomy and requires elevation of the temporal lobe to expose the auditory canal from above (Kondziolka *et al.*, 2003). Hearing can be preserved with this approach and it is usually chosen for patients with tumours confined to the internal auditory canal.

Facial paralysis is the greatest single source of disability following surgery. Such complications are a greater risk for patients with large neuromas (BAO, 2002). Even patients with minimal disturbances to facial nerve function experience personal distress post surgery (Cross *et al.*, 2000).

Pre- and post-operative management of patients undergoing such surgery is detailed in Chapter 20. Specific care of cranial nerve impairments is detailed in Chapter 13.

Stereotactic radiosurgery/stereotactic radiotherapy

Patients with small tumours, residual tumours, or bi-lateral tumours with a risk of total hearing loss may be referred for radiotherapy treatment. The radiotherapy is either delivered in a single dose (radiosurgery) or fractionated. There are long term risks associated with radiotherapy (see: Care of the patient undergoing radiotherapy). In the case of benign tumours, patients are likely to live long enough to experience these side-effects; therefore patients continue to be followed up and to have serial scanning indefinitely.

RARE TUMOURS: INCIDENCE OF LESS THAN 1–2 PER MILLION PER YEAR

Overall, in the case of rare tumours such as medulloblastoma, pineal region tumours and optic nerve gliomas, the evidence base for clinical practice and service provision is limited (NICE, 2006a). Table 21.7 provides an overview of tumour types.

SERVICE GUIDANCE FOR THE MANAGEMENT OF PATIENTS WITH BRAIN TUMOURS

A key document that guides the provision of services for patients with brain tumours is *Improving Outcomes for People with Brain and Other CNS Tumours* (Brain and CNS Improving Outcomes Guidance (IOG) – NICE, 2006a,b). The documents provide key recommendations to ensure a coordinated and MDT approach to the care and management of brain tumour patients. The key recommendations are summarised in Box 21.1.

NURSING CARE AND MANAGEMENT

Neuroscience nurses have a key role to play in addressing the needs of this patient group, and can contribute greatly to improving quality of life for patients and their carers. Enhancing patients' understanding of their symptoms, diagnosis, treatment and side-effects is essential to meeting their supportive care needs. The IOG (NICE, 2006a,b) outlines a number of specific nursing skills, many of which will be addressed in the following section.

Nursing management of generic patient problems such as epilepsy, physical disability, cognitive impairment, and speech and language difficulties are described in Chapters 30, 11, 9 and 12 respectively. Similarly, the care of patients undergoing diagnostic investigations, and immediate pre- and post-operative care are discussed in Chapters 19 and 20, so this will not be discussed in the following section.

The supportive care needs of patients and their carers

The term 'supportive care' has been described in key documents such as *Improving Supportive and Palliative Care for Adults with Cancer* (NICE, 2004) and the *National Service Framework for Long Term Conditions* (DH, 2005). *The IOG for Brain and Other CNS Tumours* (NICE, 2006a) describes supportive care as an umbrella term which encompasses the care of patients and their carers throughout their disease pathway. Supportive care is delivered by a range of health care professionals, depending upon the patient's care needs. Sensitive communication and provision of information are key components of good supportive care (Davies and Higginson, 2003; NICE, 2006a).

The need for supportive care in this patient and carer group is reported as being greater than other cancer populations (Janda *et al.*, 2008). One of the frequently unmet needs of patients and carers is support to deal with 'uncertainty about the future'. Patients reporting high unmet support needs were most interested in receiving help to improve their lifestyle, reduce stress, maintain social networks, and manage difficult behaviour. Carers expressed interest in receiving more support to help them improve their lifestyle, interact with health services effectively, manage stress, and manage difficult patient behaviours (Janda *et al.*, 2008).

Existential questions about the meaning and purpose of life, death and disability can be challenging for nurses to address; however, existential support is an important aspect of care. Strang *et al.* (2001) undertook a qualitative study investigating nurses, patients and carers' opinions of existential support. The nurses felt that it was difficult to address the existential concerns of patients due to lack of time, knowledge and confidence. Patients and carers expressed a desire to have the opportunity to talk about death and disability. However, they perceived the staff to be under stress, afraid and unskilled. Prerequisites for effective existential support include: being able to talk openly and in an atmosphere of trust, with staff that were not afraid, and who had the courage to remain with the

Table 21.7 An overview of tumour types.

Tumours of cranial nerves			
Cell origin	Types	WHO Grade	Anatomical locations
Schwann cells	Schwannoma Neurofibroma Malignant peripheral nerve sheath tumour		Cerebellopontine angle Skull base Acoustic nerve
Tumours of the meninges			
Meningeal cells	Meningioma – many variants Atypical meningioma Anaplastic (malignant) meningioma	I II III	Cerebral hemispheres Intraventricular Cerebellopontine angle Sellar region Pineal region Skull base
Other central nervous system tumours			
Germ cell	Germinoma Embryonal carcinoma Teratoma Yolk sac tumour		Sellar region
B cells (90%) Primary disease cell, e.g. breast, lung, colon, melanoma	Primary cerebral lymphoma Metastatic tumours		Cerebral hemispheres Cerebral hemispheres (80%) Cerebellum (15%) Brain stem (5%) Cerebellopontine angle Sellar region Skull base
Tumours of the sellar region			
	Pituitary adenoma Pituitary carcinoma Craniopharyngioma		Sellar region
Extra dural tumours			
	Chordoma Chondrosarcoma Paraganglioma		Skull base

patient. Existential needs are not prioritised and this can to some extent be due to time constraints. In order to provide support, nurses need to make time to listen to patients, and let patients express their uncertainty and anxieties about the future (Strang *et al.*, 2001).

In a busy neurosurgical unit there are many demands on the nurse's time, but it is important to remember that the psychological care of patients is as important as any other aspect of their care. Listening to patients' and carers' concerns is central to assessing and identifying their support

---

Box 21.1 Key recommendations of Improving Outcomes for People with Brain and other CNS Tumours (NICE, 2006a, b)

1. The care of all patients to be co-ordinated through MDT and to include:
   a. a designated lead in every acute trust
   b. MDT members at the neuroscience centre and the cancer centre
   c. an appropriate key worker.
2. Cancer networks to set up local mechanisms to ensure that patients with imaging that suggests a CNS diagnosis are discussed at the neuroscience MDT members.
3. Neuropathology and radiology services to provide appropriate diagnostic investigations pre-operatively, intra-operatively and post-operatively.
4. Ready access to neurosurgical service. Pre-operative discussions should take place at neuroscience MDT members to determine optimum surgical approach and the processing of tissue, including intra-op histological evaluation.
5. Health care professionals should have face-to-face communication with patients at critical points in the care pathway. High-quality written information material should be made available to patients/carers and other professionals as needed.
6. Clinical nurse specialists should be core members of the team, often functioning as the key-worker.

Patients should have ready access to specialist health care professionals, e.g. neuropsychology/psychiatry, occupational therapy, speech and language therapy, and physiotherapy.
7. Palliative care specialists should be included as members of the neuroscience and cancer network MDTs.
8. Rapid access to allied health professional (AHP) assessment and rehabilitation services. Immediate access to specialist equipment.
9. Data collection systems in place that allow entry of information on all patients with a radiologically or histologically confirmed CNS tumour. This data to be made available to health care professionals.
10. The National Cancer Research Institute Clinical Studies Group encouraged to develop an extended portfolio of trials. Cancer networks need to ensure trials are supported and patients entered into trials.
11. National tumour groups for rare CNS tumours should be established to coordinate the approach to care. They should also maintain a national register of all these cases.

Source: NICE, 2006a, b.

---

needs. Once support needs have been identified, appropriate referrals to relevant members of the MDT can be made promptly; this may include psychologists, clinical nurse specialists, community nurses and palliative care teams.

Communication of diagnosis and other significant information

Patients may have received some information about their possible diagnosis prior to attending the neuroscience centre. It is extremely important to establish what the patient has been told and what they have understood. They may have been told that a tumour is suspected, that there is abnormal tissue, a growth, or a lesion. When the diagnosis is confirmed, it is important to establish what patients understand by the term 'tumour'. Some will assume that a tumour is cancer; others assume that a tumour is not cancer. Terms such as benign and malignant can be confusing and require clarification. In the case of patients who have a reduced conscious level, cognitive impairment or

speech and language deficits, it will be necessary to clarify this information with the family/friends.

Buckman (1992) defines bad news as any news that will drastically and negatively alter the person's view of his or her future. Neuroscience nurses are often responsible for reiterating bad or significant news. In some instances, patients and relatives may not have had the opportunity to ask additional questions at the time of diagnosis. Patients and carers value face-to-face communication with skilled health care professionals who are able to:

> 'engage with patients on an emotional level, to listen, to assess how much information a patient wants to know, and to convey information with clarity and sympathy'
> (Bristol Royal Infirmary Inquiry 2001, cited in NICE 2004:p 56.).

The *Improving Outcomes Guidance for Patients with Brain and Other CNS Tumours* recommends that:

'Health care professionals should have face-to-face communication with patients, their relatives and carers at critical points in the care pathway to discuss diagnosis, prognosis, treatment options (including no treatment), recurrence and end-of-life care'.

(NICE 2006a:p101)

Advanced communication skills training is a prerequisite for neuro-oncology clinical nurse specialists and is recommended for other members of the MDT who are involved in breaking bad news.

Advanced communication skills training is also useful for ward based neuroscience nurses and may be accessed via the local cancer network or palliative care teams. Communicating significant news best practice guidelines for health care professionals are available within most neurosurgical and oncology settings.

Recommendations from the supportive and palliative care guidance stipulates that:

Teams should ensure that patients and carers are able to discuss information with a health or social care professional in a private environment, with support where needed to cope with its emotional impact. Patients' attention should also be drawn to other sources of assistance to understand and interpret information, such as helplines and support groups. Contact details should be provided in writing, if requested.

(NICE, 2004:p68)

Prior to discharge neuroscience nurses should ensure that patients and their carers have been provided with sufficient information regarding: their diagnosis, future treatment plans and outpatient appointments, medications and side-effects, driving restrictions, seizure management, and the contact details of their key-worker. Information should also be available regarding community based support services such as: benefits advice, local support and information organisations. Table 21.8 includes sources of patient information, advice and support organisations.

Table 21.8 Sources of patient information, advice and support.

Brain and Spine Foundation www.brainandspine.org.uk	Information and support Helpline staffed by health care professionals
Cancer Research UK www.cancerhelp.org.uk	Information and support Helpline staffed by cancer information nurses
Cancerbackup www.cancerbackup.org.uk	Information and support Helpline staffed by oncology nurses
Macmillan Cancer Support www.macmillan.org.uk	Practical, medical, emotional and financial support. Information centres, support groups and internet discussion forums • Information about living with cancer • Information about cancer types and treatment Helpline staffed by health care professionals and trained volunteers
The Pituitary Foundation www.pituitary.org.uk	Information and advice for patients, carers and health care professionals Gives general advice and is staffed by endocrine nurse specialists
Samantha Dickson Brain Tumour Trust www.braintumourtrust.co.uk Telephone: 0845 130 9733	Provides support and funds research. Umbrella for many smaller brain tumour charities who fundraise for the charity Information helpline and regional support groups
Meningioma UK www.meningiomauk.org	Information and support Regional support group information
British Acoustic Neuroma Association (BANA) www.bana-uk.com	Library of information and equipment Regional support groups and members forum

Key worker involvement

The importance of key working, care co-ordination and person centred care is highlighted within *The National Service Framework for Long Term Conditions* (DH, 2005) and the IOG for brain and other CNS tumours (NICE 2006a).

The IOG states that:

> *The key worker should promote continuity of care and manage transitions of care. This is achieved by assessing patients' needs, ensuring care plans have been agreed with patients and that findings from assessments and care plans are communicated to others involved in a patient's care*
>
> (NICE 2006a p32).

It is likely that a clinical nurse specialist will take on the role of key worker in the early stages of the patient pathway, providing supportive care and promoting continuity of care. However, the key worker role is transferred to the most appropriate health care profession as the patient's needs change.

Neuroscience nurses can aid patients by ensuring that the key worker is aware of the patient's admission to hospital, and by updating any changes in care. In the case of patients who have not yet been allocated a key worker, it is important for neuroscience nurses to work with the MDT to identify an appropriate key worker.

CARE OF THE PATIENT UNDERGOING RADIOTHERAPY

Once a patient is diagnosed and the treatment plan explained, it may be a week before they meet with an oncologist to discuss the treatment in depth. It is helpful to give patients and carers a rough idea of the timescales of future appointments and planned treatment. Overall there is a paucity of research regarding cranial radiotherapy side-effects and nursing management. Some symptom management approaches can be extrapolated from cancer related research into hair loss, fatigue management and skin changes. The section below will describe the experiences of patients undergoing treatment including side-effects and how to manage these.

Radiotherapy planning

The patient will undergo a number of appointments in the radiotherapy department prior to commencing treatment. The planning of the radiotherapy requires that the patient's head be immobilised to ensure that the patient is in the same position for each treatment, enabling accuracy for the delivery of the radiation. A thermoplastic mould is made (Figure 21.5). Depending on the location of the tumour the patient will either be positioned prone or supine, both of which can be very daunting, particularly for those patients with claustrophobia. Once the mask or shell is made, a planning CT is taken with the patient in the mask. The planning CT is then compared with the CT scan taken either before or after surgery and detailed planning of the radiotherapy field is undertaken. The planning process may take up to four weeks. Palliative radiotherapy does not require as much detailed planning and can usually be commenced within two weeks. Stereotactic radiosurgery can be performed on a single occasion. An immobilising frame is attached to the patient's head and imaging is undertaken with the frame *in situ*. The treatment is administered in a single dose.

Side-effects of cranial radiotherapy

Worsening symptoms during radiotherapy treatment can occur early on in treatment (acute reaction) or as the treatment progresses. See Table 21.9 for a summary of the side-effects of cranial radiotherapy. Patients may experience an exacerbation of their presenting symptoms, i.e. focal neurological deficits, headaches and seizures. Such symptoms are thought to be a consequence of cerebral

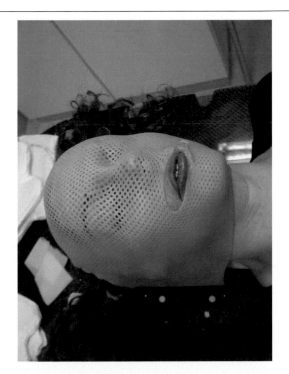

Figure 21.5 Thermoplastic mould.

Table 21.9 Summary of the side effects of cranial radiotherapy.

Cranial radiotherapy (RT) side-effects	Acute reactions – within days of treatment	Early delayed reactions – weeks to 6 months	Late delayed reactions – years after treatment
Symptoms	• Exacerbation of presenting symptoms • Headaches • Worsening neurology or seizures • Symptoms are usually transient	• Alopecia • Skin reactions, i.e. erythema/desquamation • Exacerbation of presenting symptoms • Fatigue • Somnolence	• Cognitive impairment – dementia • Increased risk of stroke • Neoplasia – radiotherapy-induced tumours • Endocrine dysfunction
Cause	• Cerebral oedema	• Dividing cells in the field of RT • Cerebral oedema • Neuronal toxicity	• Radionecrosis of white matter that can be indistinguishable from tumour progression • DNA damage – carcinogen • Damage to small vessels • Hypothalamic radiation
Management	• Reassurance • Steroids if indicated	• Prepare and inform patient • Aqueous cream to skin • Steroids and reassurance • Physiotherapy/occupational therapy	• Informed consent • Stress the relevance for patients likely to survive their tumour by a number of years • Monitor changes in neuropsychometry and provide ongoing support • Long-term endocrine follow-up and hormone replacement • Treatment of secondary tumours (excluding further radiotherapy)

oedema and understandably cause concern to patients, as symptoms mimic disease progression. Patient information and advice should include these potential side-effects. Reassurance and support should be given when such symptoms do occur (Guerrero, 2002).

Patients experiencing marked neurological deterioration may be offered a course of steroids to help reduce the oedema. Headaches are managed with analgesia, such as paracetamol or codeine based drugs if required. Headaches that do not resolve with regular analgesia may respond to steroid therapy or a combination of both. Managing seizures in these circumstances involves reassuring the patient of the underlying cause of increasing seizures. For those taking anti-epileptic drugs (AEDs), it is important to ensure that the patient is concordant with medications and if necessary check their blood levels. Patients who have not previously taken AEDs or have sub-therapeutic blood levels will require review by a neurologist.

Fatigue

Fatigue is commonly experienced. The aetiology of radiation induced fatigue is not fully understood. The effect of fatigue is cumulative and increases during the treatment (Kearney and Richardson, 2006). During a six week course of radiotherapy, tiredness and fatigue may become increasingly evident around weeks three and four, and may reach its peak two to three weeks following treatment (Guerrero, 2005). There are no medical interventions that can treat fatigue; steroid therapy is reserved for patients who experience worsening neurology or signs of raised ICP. The management of fatigue during treatment is limited. Travelling to and from the radiotherapy department can contribute to fatigue leaving little time for patients to engage with wider support strategies for managing fatigue (Faithfull, 2006). For some patients, fatigue can be a considerable problem and may last for months after the treatment. Somnolence is a term used to describe fatigue which is severe and lasts over a number of weeks. The long duration and severity of fatigue symptoms can lead to anxiety as patients fear that the fatigue is an indication that the tumour has not been controlled by the radiotherapy (Faithfull and Brada, 1998; Guerrero, 2005). Patients require reassurance that fatigue can be long lasting and that it has no bearing upon the effectiveness of the radiotherapy treatment.

A Cochrane review concluded that there is limited evidence that psychosocial interventions are effective at reducing fatigue during active treatment (Goedendorp *et al.*, 2009). Interventions specifically intended to relieve treatment related fatigue such as: educating patients about fatigue, teaching self-care and coping techniques, activity management and learning to balance between activity and rest, may be of some benefit (Goedendorp *et al.*, 2009). In order to ensure that patients in the community are accessing advice and support to manage their fatigue, referral for occupational therapy can be useful.

Hair loss

The roots of the hair have a high mitotic rate and are therefore susceptible to radiation damage. Hair loss tends to occur approximately three weeks into treatment. Hair may re-grow within three to six months depending on the total dose of radiation received to the scalp. The texture and thickness of the hair may vary and areas that received a higher dose will remain sparsely populated with hair or be bald. It is important to advise patients of the likely timescale of hair loss.

Patients express little concern about hair loss around the time of diagnosis and first oncology consultation. Often the threat of the tumour and shock of diagnosis will take precedence. However, as the treatment approaches, and during treatment, concern about hair loss becomes more evident. For many patients there may be no obvious physical signs of disease prior to hair loss. It can for many patients be associated with feelings of vulnerability, mortality, shame, powerlessness and a loss of sexuality (Freedman, 1994; Kearney and Richardson, 2006).

Nurses need to provide sufficient information and education about hair loss and teach strategies to cope with emotions associated with hair loss (Batchelor, 2001). Patients undergoing cranial radiotherapy are entitled to a wig on NHS prescription. A wig fitting can be arranged prior to hair loss occurring.

Skin changes

During treatment the dermal and epidermal layers of the skin are damaged. Skin changes occur when the epidermis fails to proliferate and the repopulation of normal cells is inhibited (Kearney and Richardson, 2006). Erythema is described as dry, red, warm, sensitive skin and is sometimes described as 'tight' (Corner and Bailey, 2001). It occurs within two to three weeks of commencing treatment and healing occurs once treatment has ceased. Dry desquamation can occur toward the end of treatment and last for a couple of weeks after treatment: skin is dry, itchy and may peel or flake. Less commonly patients may experience moist desquamation resulting in skin blisters and slough. It can occur behind the ears when they are within the radiotherapy field and is more likely to be a problem if the patient wears glasses and the skin is regularly disturbed when glasses are taken on and off (Guerrero, 1998).

A structured literature review by Glean *et al.* (2001) revealed a lack of consistency in the research undertaken and the applied practical management of radiotherapy skin reactions. Despite this, the main aims in caring for impaired skin include: maximising comfort, minimising trauma, preventing infection and proctecting against further damage (Guerrero, 1998). This may be achieved by the application of simple moisturising cream such as aqueous cream and advising patients to protecting their skin from sunlight. To minimise irritants to the skin, patients are advised to use a mild shampoo, use the cool setting on the hairdryer, and refrain from dyeing hair until the skin has recovered. Unnecessary anxiety can be reduced by educating the patient about the cause of skin reactions, the likely course of skin reactions and how to manage these.

Less common side-effects
Nausea and vomiting

Many patients assume that radiotherapy is emetogenic, however unless the cerebellum or brain stem is being treated, nausea is an uncommon side-effect. Pre-treatment information should highlight that nausea and vomiting is not a common side-effect unless caused by an underlying raised intracranial pressure (Guerrero, 2005). When patients are symptomatic, antiemetics are prescribed and their effectiveness is monitored.

Some patients experience anxiety induced nausea; the mask may cause some patients to feel claustrophobic and anxious. Relaxation techniques can be useful, and some radiotherapy departments are able to play music in the treatment room which can be of comfort to patients.

Sensitivity to taste and smell

Some patients report that they can smell the radiotherapy treatment; others report hypersensitivity to smell and alterations in taste (Guerrero, 2005). This is thought to be due to stimulation of the olfactory nerve endings during treatment. Changes in taste can lead to reduced dietary intake. It is important to discuss diet and appetite with patients to ensure that they receive adequate nutrition during treatment.

Problems with hearing

During the course of treatment patients may report unilateral hearing loss or irritation in the ear canal. This is caused by radiation-induced erythema along the external auditory meatus and is called otitis externa. Oedema can also cause inflammation and obstruction of the eustachian tube resulting in secretory otitis media. These symptoms usually resolve approximately between four and six weeks after treatment is completed (Guerrero, 2005).

CARE OF THE PATIENT UNDERGOING CHEMOTHERAPY

Chemotherapy is administered in the oncology setting as an inpatient, or more commonly as an outpatient. Chemotherapy nurses are responsible for ensuring that the patient receives the appropriate chemotherapy, the correct dose, and via the correct route, as with all medications. In addition chemotherapy nurses are responsible for patient safety and providing side-effect support (Kearney and Richardson, 2006). Neuroscience nurses encounter patients who are due to be undergoing chemotherapy following surgery, or who have been previously treated with chemotherapy and may be experiencing side-effects.

The chemotherapeutic treatment options vary depending upon tumour type. The generic side-effects of chemotherapy are summarised in Table 21.5. Drug specific information is provided at the oncology centre; many centres in the UK use patient information provided by Cancerbackup (www.cancerbackup.org.uk). Patients and carers can access this information via the internet, or request printed copies from the organisation.

Some patients have preconceived ideas about chemotherapy; they may know somebody who has undergone treatment. It is important to stress to patients that there are many different chemotherapy agents and the side-effects vary depending upon the type and dose of drug. A common concern is hair loss. However, the most commonly used chemotherapeutic agents (temozolomide and PCV combination) do not cause alopecia.

Nurses are involved with monitoring side-effects and instigating appropriate management of symptoms, i.e. anti-emetics, laxatives, strategies to manage fatigue.

In addition to explaining how chemotherapy affects patients, neuroscience nurses should ensure that they have an understanding of patients' experiences of chemotherapy, be aware of the strong and varied emotions that patients may need to express, and enable the patient to feel understood (Corner and Bailey, 2001). Treatment is associated with psychological distress including anxiety, depression, distress and mood swings (Kearney and Richardson, 2006).

CARE OF THE PATIENT UNDERGOING STEROID THERAPY

Corticosteroid agents such as dexamethasone are similar to the natural corticosteroids produced by the adrenal glands and are often prescribed to brain tumour patients (Nahaczewski *et al.*, 2004). Peritumoral and vasogenic oedema can occur at various time points throughout the disease process: at diagnosis, prior to surgery, around the time of surgery, during radiotherapy, at the time of disease recurrence, and in the terminal phase of a disease. Symptoms caused by oedema that respond to steroid therapy include: raised intracranial pressure, headaches, motor deficits, cognitive impairment, and speech and language dysfunction (Gerrard and Franks, 2004; Lovely, 2004; Nahaczewski *et al.*, 2004).

For treatment of cerebral oedema the British National Formulary (2007) recommends an initial (loading) dose of 10 mg, followed by 4 mg every 6 hours for 2–10 days. The rationale for this dosing regimen is unclear. There is no evidence base to support a maximum dose of 16 mg, or divided doses throughout the day. These regimes have been decided upon empirically.

There has only been one randomised controlled trial investigating dosing regimes and functional outcome for dexamethasone. The results of the study demonstrate that a 4 mg dose of dexamethasone produces the same effect on functional performance scores as 16 mg (Vecht *et al.*, 1994). Side-effects increased with the duration and dose of dexamethasone treatment. This suggests that there is a net benefit in using lower dose dexamethasone when compared to higher dose dexamethasone. Table 21.6 lists the side-effects of dexamethasone.

The care required for in-patients undergoing steroid therapy is detailed in Box 21.2. Unless taken over a short period of time (less than 3 weeks), corticosteroids should not be stopped abruptly: the adrenal glands cease producing cortisol when synthetic steroids are ingested. Sudden withdrawal of steroids can result in the body having a deficiency of cortisol which when severe, can cause a potentially fatal condition, called Addisonian crisis. Symptoms of cortisol deficiency include: weakness, tiredness, weight loss, vomiting, diarrhoea, abdominal pain,

Box 21.2   Care plan for patients undergoing steroid therapy

Goal: To ensure that the patient understands the purpose and side-effects of steroid medication

Actions
- Assess patient's level of understanding
- Explain reason for steroid medication
- Provide information and explanation of potential side-effects
- Ensure patient and/or carer understand medication dose at discharge
- Ensure patient and/or carer can identify side-effects at discharge
- Provide written information to patient and/or carer

Goal: Safe administration of steroids

Actions
- Administer medication as prescribed
- Administer prescribed gastric protection medication as prescribed
- Ensure steroids taken with food

Goal: Identify side-effects

Actions
- Perform daily urinalysis
- Monitor and record blood glucose as appropriate
- Observe for changes in behaviour – anxiety, insomnia, euphoria
- Observe for signs of infection – monitor vital signs
- Encourage patient to report side-effects
- Inform medical team of significant side-effects

Intracranial tumours: patient perspective

In 2001, I was diagnosed with a 3rd ventricular pilocytic astrocytoma, and was very sick at the time as a result of its large size and position, and consequential severe hydrocephalus. I was 19 at the time, and in hindsight had been suffering detrimental effects from the tumour for at least five years. My friends were in the first or second year of university and beginning their adult lives, while I was dependant on my parents and living at home. I felt completely alone, and that cognitive deficits had made my life not worth living. In particular, my antero-grade memory was very bad, while my retrograde memory was very clear, and this trapped me into ruminating over long-distant memories.

Though grateful that my tumour was 'so-called' benign and was low grade, it took me many years to feel any enjoyment in my life and look forward to the future. I became resentful when well-meaning friends and family would tell me everything was ok, and that they could see no change in my personality or functioning. I felt that I had died at 19, and in the time since had inherited a second, greatly diminished life barely worth living.

In 2003, I underwent further surgery for residual tumour. Throughout the process, I was struck by the lack of information provided to brain tumour patients, and in particular, information on the services available for their treatment. I was very fortunate in understanding my treatment options, but this only came about because medical connections in my family helped me to navigate the system.

To help me cope, I look to longstanding medical professionals, researchers, and advocates for inspiration. I also try to eat well and exercise regularly. When stressed or down, I try to think about other people, the environment, and broader issues rather than my own problems.

My greatest wish is that there is a cure for all brain tumours. Also, that upon diagnosis, patients receive a comprehensive information package containing information about the relevant type of brain tumour, the area of brain affected, possible cognitive and emotional changes to expect, treatment options, support groups in their area, and online and telephone contacts where they can receive more information. I would also hope for a widespread understanding by the wider community about the disease, and the difficulties faced by patients and caregivers living with it.

dizziness and fainting. To minimise the withdrawal symptoms, and the risk of Addisonian crisis, steroid doses are reduced gradually over time and patients should be educated about the signs of cortisol deficiency.

The provision of written information regarding steroids, side-effects and management of side-effects is essential; over time patients will tend to regulate their steroid doses depending upon symptoms and side-effects. Neuroscience units should have a policy for the use of steroids to ensure that clear instructions about dose alterations have been given (Davies *et al.*, 1996). Written information may be available locally and pharmacy will issue patients with a 'steroid card'. Cancerbackup (www.cancerbackup.org.uk) provide generic information about steroids for patients with cancer.

SUMMARY

Brain tumours are relatively rare, but make up a large proportion of the workload of neuroscience centres. The symptoms and effect of the tumour is dictated more by the location of the tumour than by its cell origin or name. There are many types of tumour giving rise to a variety of symptoms which include physical and cognitive impairment. Treatment options comprise surveillance, surgery, radiotherapy, chemotherapy, rehabilitation and palliation. In order to meet the care needs of patients with brain tumours it is important to be aware of the variety of treatment options, their effects and side-effects. In addition, provision of supportive care by neuroscience nurses is essential to improving the experience of patients and their carers, who face the physical, cognitive, psychological and social problems associated with living with a brain tumour.

REFERENCES

Abrey LE, Warren PM (2003*) Brain Tumours*. Oxford: Health Press Limited.

Atkinson AB, Kennedy A, Wiggam MI *et al*. (2005). Long-term remission rates after pituitary surgery for Cushing's disease: the need for long-term surveillance. *Clinical Endocrinology* 63(5):549–559.

Batchelor D (2001) Hair and cancer chemotherapy: consequences and nursing care – a literature study. *European Journal of Cancer Care* 10(3):147–163.

British Association of Otorhinolaryngologists – Head and Neck Surgeons (2002) *Clinical Effectiveness Guidelines: Acoustic neuroma (vestibular schwannoma) BAO-NHS Document 5*. London: Royal College of Surgeons of England. Available from: http://www.entuk.org/members/publications/ceg_acousticneuroma.pdf Accessed July 2010.

Buckman R (1992) *How to Break Bad News*. London: Macmillan

Cairncross JG, Ueki K, Zlatescu MC *et al*. (1998) Specific genetic predictors of chemotherapeutic response and survival in patients with anaplastic oligodendrogliomas. *Journal of the National Cancer Institute* 90:1473–1479.

Castinetti F, Morange I, Dufour H *et al*. (2008) Radiotherapy and radiosurgery in acromegaly. *Pituitary*. Jan 4 [Epub ahead of print].

Corner J, Bailey C (2001) *Cancer Nursing: Care in context*. Oxford: Blackwell Science Ltd.

Cross T, Sheard CE, Garrud P *et al*. (2000) The impact of facial paralysis on acoustic neuroma patients. *Laryngoscope* 110(9):1539–1542.

Davies E, Clarke C, Hopkins A (1996) Malignant cerebral glioma II. Perspectives of patients and relatives on the value of radiotherapy. *British Medical Journal* 313: 1512–1516.

Davies E, Higginson I (2003) Communication, information and support for adults with malignant cerebral glioma: a systematic review. *Supportive Care in Cancer* 11:21–29.

Department of Health (2005) *National Service Framework for Long Term Conditions*. London: DH. Available from: www.dh.gov.uk

Duffau H, Lopes M, Arthuis F *et al*. (2005) Contribution of introperative electrical stimulations in surgery of low grade gliomas: a comparative study between two series without (1985–96) and with (1996–2003) functional mapping in the same institution. *Journal of Neurology and Neurosurgery and Psychiatry* 76:845–851.

Faithfull S (2006) In: Kearney N, Richardson A. *Nursing Patients with Cancer: Principles and practice*. Edinburgh: Churchill Livingstone.

Faithfull S, Brada M (1998) Somnolence syndrome in adults following cranial irradiation for primary brain tumours. *Clinical Oncology* 10:250–254.

Freedman TG (1994) Social and cultural dimensions of hair loss in women treated for breast cancer. *Cancer Nursing* 17(4):334–341.

Gabriel J (2007) *The Biology of Cancer*. England: John Wiley & Sons, Ltd.

Gerrard GE, Franks KN (2004) Overview of the diagnosis and management of brain, spine and meningeal metastases. *Journal of Neurology Neurosurgery and Psychiatry* 75:ii37.

Glean E, Edwards S, Faithfull S *et al*. (2001) Intervention for acute radiotherapy induced skin reactions in cancer patients: the development of a clinical guideline recommended for use by the college of radiographers. *Journal of Radiotherapy in Practice* 2:75–84.

Goedendorp MM, Gielissen MF, Verhagen CA *et al*. (2009) Psychosocial interventions for reducing fatigue during cancer treatment in adults. *Cochrane Database of Systematic Reviews* Issue 1. Art. No.: CD006953. DOI: 10.1002/14651858.CD006953.pub2.

Graham CA, Cloughesy TF (2004) Brain tumour treatment: chemotherapy and other new developments. *Seminars in Oncology Nursing* 20:260–72.

Grant R (2004) Overview: Brain tumour diagnosis and management/Royal College of Physicians Guidelines. *Journal of Neurological and Neurosurgical Psychiatry* 75:(Suppl II:37–42).

Gregor A (1997) *Radiotherapy*. In: Davies EH and Hopkins A. *Improving Care for Patients with Malignant Glioma*. London: Royal College of Physicians pp 53–61.

Guerrero D (ed) (1998) *Neuro-Oncology for Nurses*. London: Whurr Publishers Ltd.

Guerrero D (2002) Neuro-oncology: a clinical nurse specialist perspective. *International Journal of Palliative Nursing* 8(1):28–29.

Guerrero D (2005) Understanding the side effects of cranial irradiation and informing patients and carers. *British Journal of Neuroscience Nursing* 1(3):118–121.

Hepworth SJ, Schoemaker MJ, Muir KR *et al.* (2006) Mobile phone use and risk of glioma in adults: case-control study. *British Medical Journal* 332:883–887.

Honegger J, Zimmerman S, Psaras T *et al.* (2008) Growth modelling of non-functioning pituitary adenomas in patients referred for surgery. *European Journal of Endocrinology* 158(3):287–294.

Humphreys C (2005) Health needs assessment: adults with tumours of the brain and central nervous system in England and Wales. National Institute for Health and Clinical Excellence. *Improving Outcomes in Brain and other Central Nervous System Tumours*. London: The Stationery Office.

Janda M, Steginga S, Dunn J *et al.* (2008). Unmet supportive care needs and interest in services among patients with a brain tumour and their carers. *Patient Education and Counseling* 71:251–258.

Kaal EC, Vecht CJ (2004) The management of brain edema in brain tumors. *Current Opinion in Oncology* 16:593–600.

Karim AB, Afra D, Cornu P *et al.* (2002) Randomized trial on the efficacy of radiotherapy for cerebral low-grade glioma in the adult: European Organization for Research and Treatment of Cancer Study 22845 with the Medical Research Council study BRO4: an interim analysis. *International Journal of Radiation Oncology, Biology, Physics* 52:316–324.

Kearney N, Richardson A (2006) *Nursing Patients with Cancer: Principles and practice*. London: Elsevier Churchill Livingstone.

Kleihues P, Cavanee WK eds. (2000) *World Health Organisation Classification of Tumours: Vol 1. Pathology and genetics of tumours of the nervous system*. Lyon: IARC Press.

Koerbel A, Safavi-Abbasi S, Tatagiba M *et al.* (2005) Evolution of vestibular schwannoma surgery: the long journey to current success. *Neurosurgical FOCUS* 18 (4):1–6.

Kondziolka D, Lunsford D, and Flickinger J, (2003) Comparison of management options for patients with acoustic neuromas. *Neurosurgical FOCUS* 14 (5): 1–7.

Levy A, Lightman S (1997) *Endocrinology*. Oxford: Oxford University Press.

Lovely MP (2004) Symptom management of brain tumour patients. *Seminars in Oncology Nursing* 20(4):273–283.

Mah PM, Webster J (2002) Hyperprolactinaemia: aetiology, diagnosis, and management. *Seminars in Reproductive Medicine* 20(4):365–374.

Mason W P (2005) Advances in the management of low grade gliomas. *The Canadian Journal of Neurological Sciences* 32:18–26.

McAllister LD, Ward JH, Schulman SF *et al.* (2002) *Practical Neuro-oncology: A guide to patient care*. USA: Butterworth-Heinemann.

Nahaczewski AE, Fowler SB, Hariharan S (2004) Dexamethasone therapy in patients with brain tumours – a focus on tapering. *Journal of Neuroscience Nursing* 36(6):340–343.

National Institute for Health and Clinical Excellence (2004) *Improving Supportive and Palliative Care for Adults with Cancer. NICE service guidance*. Available from: www.nice.org.uk/csgsp. Accessed July 2010.

National Institute for Health and Clinical Excellence (2006a) *Improving Outcomes in Brain and Other Central Nervous System Tumours. The Manual*. London: The Stationery Office.

National Institute for Health and Clinical Excellence (2006b) *Improving Outcomes in Brain and Other Central Nervous System Tumours. The Evidence Review*. London: The Stationery Office.

National Institute for Health and Clinical Excellence (2007) *Carmustine Implants and Temozolomide for the Treatment of Newly Diagnosed High Grade Glioma*. London: The Stationery Office.

Nomikos P, Buchfelder M, Falbusch R (2005) The outcome of surgery in 668 patients with acromegaly using criteria of biochemical 'cure'. *European Journal of Endocrinology:* 152(3):379–387.

Nussey SS, Whitehead SA (2001) *Endocrinology: An integrated approach*. Oxford: BIOS Scientific pp 126–128.

Pignatti F, Van Den B M, Curran D *et al.* (2002) European Organization for Research and Treatment of Cancer Brain Tumour Cooperative Group, and European Organization for Research and Treatment of Cancer Radiotherapy Cooperative Group. Prognostic factors for survival in adult patients with cerebral low-grade glioma. *Journal of Clinical Oncology* 20:2076–2084.

Pobereskin LH, Chadduck JB (2000) Incidence of brain tumours in two English counties: a population based study. *Journal of Neurology, Neurosurgery, and Psychiatry* 69:464–471.

Powell MP, Lightman SL, Laws Jr ER (2003) *Management of Pituitary Tumours: The clinician's practical guide*. (2nd edition). Totowa, New Jersey: Humana.

Rampling R (1997) Chemotherapy: determining the appropriate treatment. In: Davies EH and Hopkins A (eds). *Improving care for Patients with Malignant Glioma*. London: Royal College of Physicians.

Rampling R (2003) *Brain and other central nervous system tumours* UK: Cancer Research UK publication. Available from: http://www.cancerresearchuk.org/ Accessed July 2010.

Rees JH (2002) Low-grade gliomas in adults. *Current Opinion in Neurology* 15:657–661.

Rees J (2004). Neurological oncology. *Medicine* 32(10):75–79.

Ron E, Modan B, Boice J *et al.* (1988) Tumors of the brain and nervous system following radiotherapy in childhood. *New England Journal of Medicine* 319:1033–1039.

Scheithauer BW, Fereidooni F, Horvath E *et al.* (2001) Pituitary carcinoma: an ultrasoundal study of eleven cases. *Ultrastructural Pathology* 25(3):227–242.

Strang S, Strang P, Ternestedt BM (2001) Existential support in brain tumour patients and their spouses. *Supportive Cancer Care* 9:625–633.

Strupp R, Mason WP, van den Bent *et al.* (2005) European Organization for Research and Treatment of Cancer Brain tumour and Radiotherapy Groups; National Cancer Institute of Canada Clinical Trials Group. Radiotherapy plus concomitant and adjuvant temozolomide for glioblastoma. *New England Journal of Medicine* 352:987–996.

Taphoorn MJB, Klein M (2004) Cognitive deficits in adult patients with brain tumours. *The Lancet* 3:159–168.

Tschudi DC, Linder T, Fisch U (2000) Conservative management of unilateral acoustic neuromas. *American Journal of Otology* 21:722–728.

Van Den Bent M J, Afra D, Schraub S *et al.* (2005) Long term efficacy of early versus delayed radiotherapy for low-grade astrocytoma and oligodendroglioma in adults: the EORTC 22845 randomised trial. *Lancet* 366:985–990.

Vecht CJ, Hovestadt A, Verbiest HBC *et al.* (1994) Dose-effect relationship of dexamethasone on Karnofsky performance in metastatic brain tumors: a randomized study of doses of 4.8 and 16 mg per day. *Neurology* 44:675–680.

Verhelst J, Abs R (2003) Hyperprolactinemia: pathophysiology and management. *Treat Endocrinology* 2(1):23–32.

Walker MD, Alexander E Jr, Hunt WE *et al.* (1978) Evaluation of BDCN and/or radiotherapy in the treatment of anaplastic gliomas. *Journal of Neurosurgery* 49:333–343.

Westphal M, Hilt DC, Bortey E *et al.* (2003) A phase 3 trial of local chemotherapy with biodegradable carmustine (BCNU) in patients with primary malignant glioma. *Neuro-Oncology* 5:79–88.

Whittle I R (2004) The dilemma of low grade glioma. *Journal of Neurology Neurosurgery and Psychiatry* 75(suppl II):ii31–ii36.

Yamakami I, Uchino Y, Kobayashi E *et al.* (2003) Conservative management, gamma-knife radiosurgery, and microsurgery for acoustic neuromas: a systematic review of outcome and risk of three therapeutic options. *Neurological Research* 25:682–690.

22

Management of Patients with Stroke and Transient Ischaemic Attack

Jane Dundas, Beverley Bennett and Julia Slark

INTRODUCTION

Stroke is a preventable and treatable disease, and has only recently been perceived to be a high priority within the NHS (RCP, 2008). The publication of the National Stroke Strategy (DH, 2007) has led to a national drive for the prevention of stroke, and major improvements in both acute and long-term stroke care in the United Kingdom (UK). This strategy is to be implemented over the next ten years to address health inequalities and secure stroke service improvements in line with evidence-based quality markers and the recently published clinical guidelines (RCP, 2008; NICE, 2008).

DEFINITIONS

Stroke is defined as:

> *...a clinical syndrome of rapidly developing clinical signs of focal (or global in case of coma) disturbance of cerebral function, with symptoms lasting twenty-four hours or longer or leading to death with no apparent cause other than of vascular origin.*
>
> World Health Organisation (1988)

A transient ischaemic attack (TIA) is defined as signs and symptoms of stroke which resolve within 24 hours, although TIA symptoms normally resolve in a few minutes or hours. If neurological symptoms persist for longer it should be assumed that the person has had a stroke (RCP,

2008). The term *brain attack* has also been used to describe a neurovascular event, which emphasises the level of urgency with which stroke and TIA should be treated (NAO, 2005; RCP, 2008).

EPIDEMIOLOGY

Stroke is the third most common cause of death worldwide after coronary heart disease and all types of cancer combined (Warlow *et al.*, 2008). It also causes a greater range of disabilities than any other condition and is the leading cause of long-term disability in the developed world (Adamson *et al.*, 2004). Two-thirds of stroke deaths occur in developing countries and, as a result of an increase in the proportion of older people and the predicted effects of current smoking patterns in developing countries, it is expected that stroke mortality will have almost doubled by 2020 (Warlow *et al.*, 2008).

Incidence

Each year approximately 130,000 people in England and Wales will have a stroke of which 87,700 are first strokes and 53,700 recurrent strokes (Office of National Statistics, 2001). This is roughly the equivalent of someone having a stroke every five minutes. Nearly three quarters of cases occur in people over the age of 65 and half in those over the age of 75. If they live to their 85th year, one in four men and one in five women can expect to have a stroke (Sudlow and Warlow, 1997). The incidence of TIAs is more difficult to establish, since they may not be reported due to their sometimes fleeting nature. The number of TIAs occurring each year in England alone is estimated to be 20,000 (NAO, 2005).

Neuroscience Nursing: Evidence-Based Practice, 1st Edition.
Edited by Sue Woodward and Ann-Marie Mestecky
© 2011 Blackwell Publishing Ltd

Mortality

Stroke causes over 60,000 deaths each year in the UK and in 2004 stroke caused 8% of deaths in men and 12% of deaths in women (Allender *et al.*, 2006). Approximately two-thirds of deaths occur within the first week after a stroke, most commonly due to neurological consequences, e.g. raised ICP and acute obstructive hydrocephalus. For older patients about half of all deaths are due to the complications of immobility, e.g. pneumonia or pulmonary embolism, usually after the first week (Bamford *et al.*, 1990).

In recent years stroke mortality and incidence has declined at varying rates across Japan, North America and Western Europe (Thorvaldsen *et al.*, 1999), but the proportion of deaths from stroke has remained constant. Reasons for this international fall in stroke mortality rate remain unclear although they could include advances in detection by neuro-imaging or improvements in management (Thorvaldsen *et al.*, 1999). The Oxfordshire Community Stroke Project (OCSP, 1981–1986) (Bamford *et al.*, 1990) indicated a higher mortality rate for primary intracerebral haemorrhage (PICH). The overall 30-day case fatality rate was 19% (10% infarction: 50% PICH); the 1-year case fatality rate was 31% (23% infarction: 62% PICH).

Burden of stroke

At one year after stroke approximately 30% of patients will be dead, and 40% of survivors will be dependent on others (Warlow *et al.*, 2008). In the UK it has been estimated that one in five acute hospital beds and a quarter of places in residential or long-term care are occupied by patients with stroke. The costs of direct care are £2.8 billion a year; £1.8 billion is lost from reduced productivity and disability, while informal care costs £2.4 billion – a total of £7 billion a year (DH, 2007). Patients who survive a stroke or transient ischaemic attack (TIA) are at particularly high risk of subsequent cardiovascular events, including recurrent stroke, myocardial infarction (MI) and death from vascular causes (Hankam and Spence, 2007); survivors are also more likely to be left with a major disability (Rothwell, 2007).

AETIOLOGY

About 85% of strokes result from ischaemia and infarction of brain tissue caused by diminished blood flow due to thrombotic or embolic complications of atheroma. Risk factors for ischaemic stroke are detailed in Table 22.1. The remaining 15% of strokes are caused by a primary intracerebral haemorrhage (PICH) (Figure 22.1).

Table 22.1 Risk factors for ischaemic stroke.

Risk factors	Relative risk
Modifiable	
Hypertension	2.3
Diabetes mellitus	2–3
Atrial fibrillation	5
Smoking	2
Alcohol (> 30 units/week)	2.5–4
Physical inactivity	0.3–0.5
Obesity	1–2
Hyperhomocysteinaemia	5–7
Life events (malnutrition)	2
Serum albumin <42 g/l	0.6
Non-modifiable	
Age (per decade)	2.2
Male sex	1.4
Ischaemic heart disease	2.5
Social class	1.6–3.5
Peripheral vascular disease	2
Previous stroke	9–15
Previous TIA	7
Ischaemic heart disease	2.5
Heart failure	2.5–4.4
Family history	1.4–2
Ethnicity	(see text)

Adapted from MacWalter and Shirley, 2003.

Ischaemia

Ischaemia is a term used to refer to a reduction in blood supply, whereby there is a mismatch between blood flow and the requirements of the cerebral tissue for substrates to maintain normal cellular functions. *Infarction* refers to irreversible damage and death of tissue (necrosis) caused by ischaemia.

Atherosclerosis

Atherosclerosis is the most common cause of ischaemic stroke. It is believed that atheroma begins to develop as a result of an inflammatory response, leading to the gradual deposit of lipid compounds within the arterial wall. These may fibrose leading to the formation of plaque. This process is accelerated by factors such as hypertension, diabetes, cigarette smoking and hyperlipidaemia and the arterial walls may become necrotic, ulcerated or calcified. Atherothrombotic plaque may build up within the arterial lumen causing a critical stenosis. The development of ath-

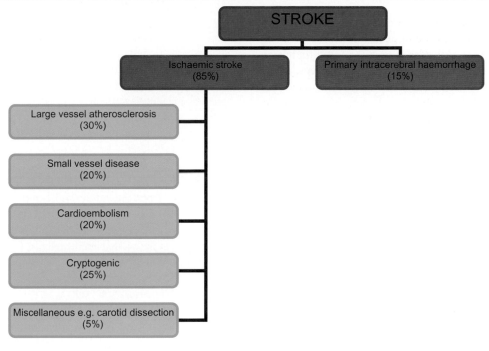

Figure 22.1 Stroke aetiology.

eromatous plaque may also excite platelet activity thus causing thrombus to develop within the arterial wall. Atherothrombotic material may then fragment (embolise) leading to arterial occlusion within the brain. The most common sites for build up of plaque affecting the cerebral circulation are at places of arterial branching, e.g. the carotid bifurcation and the vertebral arteries. Extracranially, the aortic arch and carotid arteries are the most common sites.

Cardio-embolic stroke

Cardiogenic emboli are the second most common cause of ischaemic stroke. Single or multiple emboli may arise from the heart, most commonly as a result of atrial fibrillation (AF) or damage to the myocardium (e.g. post MI). About 20% of all ischaemic strokes are embolic (Warlow *et al.*, 2008). Symptoms vary depending on the site (or sites) of occlusion; blockage of a major vessel such as the internal carotid artery may cause a total anterior circulation infarct whereas microscopic particles may cause a TIA. Most commonly the route of the embolus is via the extracranial carotid arteries but emboli may also occlude branches of either the vertebral or basilar arteries. The clinical priority is to find the possible source of the embo-

lism, for example: recent myocardial infarction, valvular disease (or prosthetic valves), infective endocarditis, or patent foramen ovale (PFO).

Intracranial small vessel disease (SVD)

This is a condition caused by widespread changes in the small arteries and arterioles of the brain predominantly in older age groups and usually in the presence of diabetes and hypertension; changes occur within the vessel walls, which thicken and become less elastic. Lacunar infarcts make up about 20% of ischaemic strokes and are thought to be caused by SVD although debate continues (Warlow *et al.*, 2008). Vasculitis and cerebral amyloid angiopathy are rare causes of SVD. Other rare causes of ischaemic stroke are detailed in Box 22.1.

RISK FACTORS

Age

Although stroke can occur in children or young adults, it is predominantly a disease of older people. The Framingham study (Wolf *et al.*, 1992) indicated that the incidence of stroke increases dramatically with age, approximately doubling in successive decades.

Ethnicity

Although it is widely accepted that the rates of cardiovascular disease and stroke mortality and morbidity are higher in black and minority ethnic groups, the causes of this are not fully understood and these groups have been under-represented in research (Lip *et al.*, 2007). Socio-economic factors may exert an influence.

Hypertension

Chronic hypertension is the greatest modifiable risk factor for both ischaemic and haemorrhagic stroke independent

---

> **Box 22.1   Rare causes of ischaemic stroke**
>
> - Head injury (see Chapter 32) and neck trauma
> - Arterial dissection
> - Connective tissue or inflammatory disorders, e.g. systemic lupus erythematosus (SLE), vasculitis
> - Migraine associated vasospasm
> - Haematological disorders, e.g. polycythaemia, sickle cell disease, antiphospholipid syndrome
> - Infection, e.g. tuberculosis, syphilis, human immunodeficiency virus (HIV)
> - Damage to intra or extracranial arteries following cancer, irradiation and chemotherapy
> - Substance abuse, e.g. cocaine, ecstasy
> - Perioperative stroke particularly during cardiac or vascular procedures
> - Rare genetic conditions, e.g. Fabry's disease, homocystinuria, and cerebral autosomal dominant arteriopathy with subcortical infarcts and leukoencephalopathy (CADASIL)
> - Oral contraceptives, hormone replacement therapy (HRT), pregnancy

---

of age or gender (Warlow *et al.*, 2008). Risk increases with the degree of hypertension and risk factors may also be inter-related, e.g. blood pressure is affected by diet and alcohol. Traditionally greater significance has been attributed to the diastolic rather than the systolic blood pressure, but the opposite is probably true (Wolf, 2003). Prolonged hypertension causes structural changes in the vessel walls such as arteriolar thickening, fibroid necrosis, formation of aneurysms and the build up of atheroma in the large vessel walls (Poulter *et al.*, 2000).

Cholesterol

Recently the Stroke Prevention with Aggressive Reduction of Cholesterol Levels (SPARCL) trial has demonstrated the relationship between serum cholesterol levels and stroke and has shown that statins reduce risk of stroke and overall cardiovascular risk (Amarenco *et al.*, 2006).

Causes of primary intracerebral haemorrhage (PICH)

The main cause of PICH is hypertension. Aneurysms and arteriovenous malformations are less common causes and are presented in Chapter 23. Table 22.2 lists other causes of PICH.

PATHOPHYSIOLOGY

Ischaemic stroke

The critical level for ischaemia to develop is when cerebral blood flow falls below 18 ml/100 g/min; lethal levels are below 10 ml/100 g/min (Dirnagl and Pulsinelli, 1990). When CBF falls below 15 ml/100 g per minute, electrical activity of the affected neurones ceases due to insufficient energy substrates being delivered to fuel the sodium–potassium adenosine triphophate (Na^+/K^+) pumps (see Chapter 1) but structural integrity is retained. If reperfu-

---

Table 22.2 Causes of primary intracerebral haemorrhage.

Anatomical	Haemodynamic	Haemostatic	Other

- Structural abnormalities, e.g.
  ◦ AVM
  ◦ Cerebral aneurysm
- Cerebral amyloid angiopathy
- Small vessel disease
- Haemorrhage from ischaemic infarct
- Intracranial venous thrombosis
	- Chronic hypertension
	- Acute hypertension, e.g.
	  ◦ Eclampsia in pregnancy
	  ◦ Renal failure
		- Anticoagulants
		- Haematological disorders, e.g.
		  ◦ Haemophilia
		  ◦ Thrombocytopenia
		  ◦ Myeloid leukaemia
		- Thrombolysis
			- Intracerebral tumours
			- Alcoholism
			- Cocaine and other drug use

sion occurs quickly, it is possible for the cells in the affected zone to recover (Brodal, 2004). This zone has been termed the ischaemic penumbra (Touzani *et al.*, 2001), and is derived from the Latin *paene* 'almost'+*umbra* 'shadow'. The penumbra region may recover completely if good cerebral blood flow is re-established, e.g. following thrombolysis. This highlights the importance of rapid recognition and treatment" (NAO, 2005). It remains unclear how long the window for therapeutic intervention may be; it may be as little as three hours. If reperfusion does not occur the affected area will infarct.

In addition to vascular occlusion (thrombotic or embolic) ischaemia can be caused by prolonged or significant hypotension. The elderly are particularly vulnerable as with increasing age autoregulation becomes less effective. The resultant reduction in cerebral blood flow usually causes hypoperfusion in areas between two major cerebral arteries and these events are termed 'watershed infarcts'.

Symptoms of neurological dysfunction arise from the specific area of the brain which has been affected. The most widely accepted method of stroke classification is the Oxford Stroke Classification, also known as the Bamford classification (Bamford *et al.*, 1991). With this system strokes are divided into four categories (Box 22.2). This system of classification is relatively straightforward and uses clinical information to determine underlying pathology. Examples of clinical signs for each classification are shown in Table 22.3

Haemorrhagic stroke

The small penetrating end-vessels (perforators) that supply the deep grey and white matter of the basal ganglia, internal capsule, thalamus, cerebellum and brain stem are most affected by hypertension. Chronically raised blood pressure causes degenerative changes in these vessels which

may eventually rupture causing subsequent haemorrhage. Bleeding into the brain tissue results in a mass of blood being formed which raises intracranial pressure and can cause significant brain damage. Intracranial pressure is discussed in Chapter 7.

Venous stroke

Venous stroke is a rare disorder resulting from thrombosis of the venous sinuses or intracerebral veins. The most common location for thrombosis is the superior sagittal sinus (70–80% of cases). Venous stroke accounts for only 0.5% of all strokes; it can affect any age group and has often been associated with poor outcomes. Morbidity is estimated at 15–25%, with mortality at 10–50% (Baker *et al.*, 2001). The severity of the symptoms at outset determines the outcome; the more severe cases are nearly always fatal. The most common presenting symptoms are headache, nausea, focal neurological deficits, seizures, altered consciousness or papilloedema.

The patient must be monitored closely for signs of rising intracranial pressure (see Chapter 7). Diagnosis is confirmed using MRI with MR venography or CT with CT venography. Imaging may reveal a variety of lesions including haemorrhages, oedema and infarctions. Medical management may appear contradictory since the presence of haemorrhage does not preclude treatment with anticoagulation therapy; in fact evidence supports the use of early anticoagulant therapy, with a reduction in death and dependency (RCP, 2008).

CLINICAL SIGNS AND SYMPTOMS OF STROKE

The clinical features of stroke (Box 22.3) depend on the location and extent of brain damage; no two patients will display identical symptoms. Differentiation between haemorrhagic and ischaemic stroke on clinical signs alone is not straightforward. Urgent CT scanning is necessary to determine a management plan, particularly if thrombolysis is to be considered, but also with a view to the prescription of anti-platelet medication where there may be risk of further haemorrhage.

DIAGNOSIS

Immediate clinical assessment and treatment are vital to optimise outcomes. Outside hospital, the use of a simple reminder of the symptoms of stroke such as the FAST test (Facial weakness, Arm weakness, Speech disturbance, Time to call 999) is advocated as a method of rapidly screening patients for stroke or TIA (DH, 2007). For people who are admitted to accident and emergency it is

---

Box 22.2   Classification of stroke

TAC – Total anterior circulation stroke
LAC – Lacunar stroke
PAC – Partial anterior circulation stroke
POC – Posterior circulation stroke

An additional code is added as the last letter:
(S) – Syndrome: uncertain pathogenesis prior to imaging
(I) –   Infarct (e.g. TACI)
(H) – Haemorrhage (e.g. TACH)

Table 22.3 Clinical signs for stroke classification.

Stroke classification	Clinical signs	
TACI (Total anterior circulation stroke – infarct)	All of these symptoms: • Dysphasia • Visuo-spatial impairment • Homonymous hemianopia • Motor/sensory deficit (more than two of: face/arm/leg)	
PACI (Partial anterior circulation stroke – infarct)	Either: Two out of three signs as TACI: • Dysphasia • Visuo-spatial impairment • Homonymous hemianopia • Motor/sensory deficit (more than two of: face/arm/leg) Or: Cortical dysfunction alone Or: Mild motor/sensory deficit	
POCI (Posterior circulation stroke – infarct)	Any of the following features: • Isolated homonymous hemianopia • Cerebellar dysfunction without ipsilateral motor or sensory deficit • Eye movement dysfunction • Bilateral motor or sensory deficit • Cranial nerve palsy and contralateral motor/sensory deficit	
LACI (Lacunar stroke – infarct)	Any one of the following: • Pure motor stroke (more than two of: face/arm/leg) • Pure sensory stroke (more than two of: face/arm/leg) • Sensorimotor stroke (more than two of face/arm/leg) • Ataxic hemiparesis	None of these: • New dysphasia • New visuo-spatial deficit • Proprioceptive sensory loss only • No vertebrobasilar features

---

Box 22.3 Signs and symptoms of stroke

• Motor deficits: facial weakness, focal limb weakness, loss of fine finger movement
• Altered sensation: numbness, tingling
• Disturbance of conscious level
• Acute memory impairment
• Altered higher cerebral function: orientation
• Disorders of speech and language
• Visuo-spatial dysfunction: neglect, inattention
• Apraxia (loss of the ability to perform learned movements)
• Visual disturbance: diplopia, homonymous hemianopia, loss of vision
• Disturbance of hearing
• Loss of balance, vertigo
• Ataxia: poor co-ordination
• Nausea, vomiting
• Headache

recommended that diagnosis is made using a detailed validated tool such as Recognition of Stroke in the Emergency Room (ROSIER) (RCP, 2008). However it should be noted that some strokes (e.g. posterior circulation) may not be picked up using these tools. Patients suspected of having had a stroke should be assessed by either a neurologist or a physician with a special interest in stroke to establish an accurate clinical diagnosis and the best course of treatment as rapidly as possible (RCP, 2008). Other differential diagnoses that may present with focal cerebral symptoms of sudden onset (Box 22.4) must be excluded.

Diagnostic tests

Computerised tomography (CT) scan

All patients displaying symptoms of a stroke should be scanned as soon as possible within 24 hours of initial onset of the event. When clinically indicated, urgent scans must be available within one hour of admission, e.g. indications for thrombolysis, severe headache, or patients on anticoagulation therapy (RCP, 2008). CT is the most accurate method of demonstrating cerebral haemorrhage within the first week and it is identifiable almost immediately. It is possible to detect early ischaemia on CT within two hours of stroke, although usually signs of infarction develop over the first one to seven days (Figure 22.2). A normal scan does not mean that the patient has not had a stroke. CT may also be used to detect subarachnoid blood (see Chapter 23) and to identify other neurological disease which may be confused with stroke.

Magnetic resonance imaging (MRI)

About 50% of infarcts never become visible on CT, therefore a scan using diffusion weighted magnetic resonance imaging may be indicated to detect small infarcts, particularly lesions occurring in the brain stem. Recent guidelines (NICE, 2008) recommend MRI for all patients following TIA.

Electrocardiogram (ECG)

This should be carried out for all patients following a stroke. Cardiac arrhythmias are a cause of cardio-embolic stroke and should be treated; ventricular hypertrophy or cardiomyopathy may indicate previously undiagnosed chronic hypertension. Acute myocardial infarction (with or without pain: the so-called 'silent' infarct) may occur at onset of stroke and remain otherwise undetected.

> **Box 22.4   Conditions which may mimic stroke**
>
> - Migraine
> - Epilepsy
> - Structural intracranial lesions, e.g. brain tumour
> - Central nervous system infections
> - Multiple sclerosis
> - Metabolic and toxic disorders
> - Transient global amnesia
> - Benign postural vertigo and other labyrinthine disorders
> - Psychological disorders
> - Neuromuscular disorders

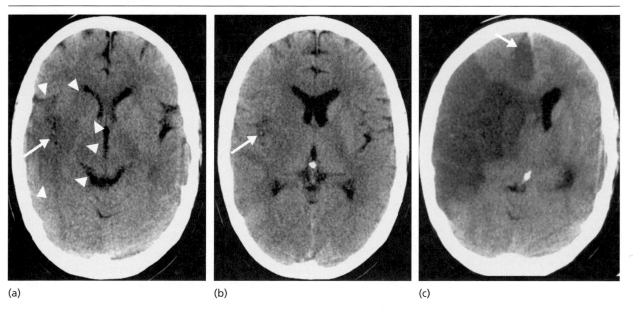

(a)   (b)   (c)

Figure 22.2 Unenhanced CT brain scan 4 h after stroke onset (a,b). There is hypoattenuation of the right caudate and lentiform nuclei, insular and temporal cortex (*arrowheads*) and a hyperattenuated (blocked) sylvian branch of the right middle cerebral artery (MCA) (*arrow*). (c) Follow-up scan at 48 h shows an extensive, hypoattenuated, and swollen right hemisphere infarct involving most of the MCA territory and also the territory of the right anterior cerebral artery (*arrow*) (ACA). The ACA involvement is probably because of compression of the ACA by the infarct mass effect. Reproduced from Charles P. Warlow *et al.*, *Stroke: Practical Management 3e*, Wiley-Blackwell, with permission.

Echocardiography is used to screen for cardiogenic causes of emboli, e.g. thrombus, vegetation or patent foramen ovale (PFO).

Ultrasound studies

Doppler or duplex sonography of the major extracranial arteries (particularly the carotid arteries) may be used to identify stenosis or occlusion which may require surgical intervention, e.g. carotid endarterectomy.

Laboratory tests

Blood is screened for haematological and clotting abnormalities, inflammatory and infection markers and electrolytes; renal and hepatic chemistry and vitamin deficiency will be checked. Most underlying haematological disorders will be identified through routine investigations, but other more rare conditions may require specific screening, e.g. anti-phospholipid syndrome (APS) (Woodward, 2007). Younger female patients with symptoms of stroke or TIA should be screened for APS by checking for the presence of anticardiolipin antibodies and lupus anticoagulant, particularly if there is a history of recurrent miscarriages or migraine.

Transient ischaemic attack (TIA)

Early identification and diagnosis of TIA is imperative since effective intervention may dramatically reduce the risk of completed stroke (RCP, 2008). Risk of subsequent stroke should be assessed using a validated scoring system such as the $ABCD^2$ score (Johnston *et al.*, 2007) (Box 22.5). People with crescendo TIAs (two or more in a week) should be treated as high risk whatever their $ABCD^2$ score.

MEDICAL MANAGEMENT OF STROKE AND TIA

The aims of medical treatment following stroke and TIA are to optimise survival, prevent recurrent stroke or other serious vascular events and to prevent complications, such as aspiration pneumonia.

In addition to the management of neurological symptoms, the medical management of patients following stroke includes cardiac and respiratory care, metabolic and fluid management and blood pressure control.

Thrombolysis and hyperacute management

Thrombolysis with alteplase is the recommended treatment for acute ischaemic stroke (NICE, 2008). It has been shown to significantly improve outcomes in patients meeting the criteria for administration within three hours

---

Box 22.5 $ABCD^2$ score: presenting within 7 days of symptoms

	Score
Age ≥60 years	1
Blood pressure systolic > 140 or diastolic ≥ 90	1
Unilateral weakness	2
Speech disturbance (no weakness)	1
Duration ≥60 minutes	2
Duration 10–59 minutes	1
Diabetes	1

Patients with a score ≥4 must be assessed and investigated within 24 hours of symptom onset. Those at lower risk, with an $ABCD^2$ score ≤3, should receive specialist assessment and treatment within seven days. Source: Royal College of Physicians, 2008.

---

of onset of symptoms (Wardlaw *et al.*, 2003). However the national guidelines (RCP, 2008) recommend that it should only be administered in centres which have sufficient infrastructure to provide a well-organised stroke service, namely: staff specifically trained in the delivery of thrombolysis and in monitoring for associated complications, nursing staff with specialist training in stroke and thrombolysis, immediate access to imaging and staff trained to provide accurate interpretation of images, and access to neurosurgery for the treatment of raised ICP.

Secondary prevention of stroke and TIA

Patients who have suffered a stroke remain at a 30–40% increased risk of a further stroke within five years. Measures for secondary prevention should be commenced as soon as a diagnosis of stroke or TIA is confirmed. Patients found to have causal factors such as carotid stenosis may benefit from early interventions such as carotid endarterectomy and those found to have a cardiac cause may require anticoagulation to reduce their risk of having a large completed stroke.

Antiplatelet medications

The national guidelines (RCP, 2008) recommend the introduction of aspirin 300 mg daily for the first two weeks after an ischaemic stroke unless contra-indicated. Discussion of individual risk factors should be incorporated into the plan of care. Patients who suffer from aspirin intolerance or dyspepsia may be prescribed an alternative antiplatelet agent such as clopidogrel 75 mg or a proton pump inhibitor such as omeprazole in addition to aspirin. Aspirin is not effective in preventing stroke or TIA in those who have no history of such events.

Anticoagulation

The national guidelines (RCP, 2008) recommend delaying the consideration of anticoagulation for patients following disabling ischaemic stroke in the context of atrial fibrillation for up to two weeks due to the risk of haemorrhagic transformation.

Management of hypertension

Numerous treatment trials have demonstrated that the risk of stroke is substantially reduced when blood pressure is lowered (RCP, 2008). Following a TIA or stroke, hypertension should be tightly controlled using anti-hypertensive medications such as diuretics, ACE inhibitors and calcium channel blockers. Blood pressure targets should be set at 140/80 mmHg or less in this patient population (Williams *et al.*, 2004).

Statin treatment

Recommended targets for cholesterol levels in this patient population are <3.5 mmol (RCP, 2004). Simvastatin, 40 mg, is the initial drug of choice, however recent evidence suggests that statin treatment may increase the risk of haemorrhagic extension or transformation in the acute phase and therefore should not be prescribed either in the hyperacute stage or for haemorrhagic stroke (RCP, 2008).

Lifestyle modification

Evidence suggests that for every 43 patients provided with advice on smoking cessation, one stroke per year would be prevented (Hankey and Warlow, 1999). Reducing alcohol intake to less than two units per day is recommended since excess alcohol contributes to hypertension (Williams *et al.*, 2004). Health promoting behaviours such as exercise, weight loss and the introduction of a healthy diet (five portions of fruit and vegetables per day) should also be encouraged. Patient's compliance with changes to their lifestyle will require ongoing advice, monitoring, encouragement and reinforcement (Birns and Fitzpatrick, 2005).

Diabetes mellitus

Diabetes is an independent risk factor for stroke or TIA, and hyperglycaemia is also a risk factor for death and increased disability. No hard evidence has been found from limited studies in this area but the consensus of opinion is that the recommended treatment target for blood glucose concentration for patients following acute stroke is between 4.0 and 11 mmol/l (RCP, 2008).

SURGICAL MANAGEMENT OF STROKE AND TIA

Carotid endarterectomy

Carotid endarterectomy (CEA) is a surgical procedure used to clear plaque from a blocked artery and is usually carried out under local anaesthetic. CEA is the treatment of choice for patients with symptomatic carotid stenosis of 70–99% according to the European Carotid Surgery Trial (ECST) criteria (Rothwell *et al.*, 2003) or 50–99% according to the North American Symptomatic Carotid Endarterectomy Trial (NASCET) criteria (Rothwell *et al.*, 2004). Carotid angioplasty or stenting is sometimes used as an alternative to CEA, although there is limited research to compare the efficacy and safety of stenting to CEA (RCP, 2008).

Decompressive craniectomy

Malignant middle cerebral artery infarction is a rare, life-threatening complication of stroke where space occupying brain oedema presents within two to five days of stroke onset. This usually occurs in younger people without brain atrophy. It is essential that this is treated rapidly before damage becomes irreversible; patients should be referred within 24 hours of onset and treated within a maximum of 48 hours (RCP, 2008). Decompressive craniectomy is discussed in Chapter 20 and Chapter 7.

Surgical treatment of acute intracerebral haemorrhage

There is little evidence to establish the efficacy of surgical evacuation of haematoma at the acute stage. Patients should be monitored for the development of symptomatic hydrocephalus in specialist neuroscience or stroke units. The current recommendations state that previously fit patients should be considered for neurosurgical intervention if they have hydrocephalus (RCP, 2008).

EVIDENCE-BASED NURSING MANAGEMENT

A holistic and multiprofessional approach

The *National Service Framework for Older People* (DH, 2001 p65) stipulated that all patients should be treated by 'specialist stroke teams within designated stroke units'. This was reinforced by the *National Clinical Guidelines for Stroke* (RCP, 2008). A collaborative multidisciplinary or interdisciplinary team approach to stroke care is considered essential, as no single profession is able to manage the care of the patient following a stroke. A collaborative approach facilitates an individualised treatment programme, with members of the team working closely together to assess and identify the needs of patients and their families throughout the stroke illness trajectory.

Nurses are integral to the stroke multidisciplinary team (Figure 22.3) and the range of knowledge, skills and competencies required for effective stroke nursing is continually expanding (McMahon *et al.*, 2003). Health care policy and professional developments in stroke care have added impetus to the growth in specialist stroke nursing roles. Indeed, the increasingly specialised nature of stroke nursing has been recognised in the foundation of the National Stroke Nursing Forum (NSNF); one of its aims being to identify and develop the knowledge and skills required by nurses working in stroke services (McMahon *et al.*, 2003; Perry *et al.*, 2004).

A key attribute of stroke nursing is its holistic approach and many nursing interventions are informed by other members of the multiprofessional stroke team, such as physiotherapists, occupational therapists and speech and language therapists. This is evident in the aspects of stroke

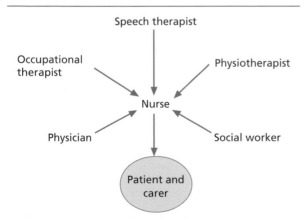

Figure 22.3 The model of care or rehabilitation that can be adopted on a geographically defined stroke unit, in which each member of the multidisciplinary team influences the nursing input to the patients and carers, as well as having direct interaction with them. Reproduced from Charles P. Warlow *et al.*, *Stroke: Practical Management 3e*, Wiley-Blackwell, with permission.

nursing which have received most research attention and which represent crucial elements of stroke management that require a skilled, consistent approach across the multiprofessional team; for example, patient positioning and mobilising, swallowing assessment and nutritional management, and an awareness of cognitive and perceptual problems. Stroke nurses are increasingly involved in identifying stroke and TIA, undertaking acute assessments of eligibility for thrombolysis on admission to hospital and fast-tracking patients into an acute stroke bed. By initiating investigations and treatment without having to wait for medical staff, nurses can positively influence patient outcomes. Other key elements of the stroke nurse's role include physiological monitoring, pain management, facilitating rehabilitation through emotional support, motivation and education, and the support of families. In addition, end of life care has been recognised as a new and challenging aspect of stroke care. Each of these elements is addressed here, with reference to the current evidence base.

Monitoring the acutely ill stroke patient

Physiological monitoring of the acutely ill stroke patient is vital in order to reduce the risk of death and disability (Jones *et al.*, 2007). As most deaths following a stroke arise from complications associated with the clinical symptoms, continuous physiological monitoring is a priority in at least the first 24 hours. Nurse-led physiological monitoring can ensure the early detection of complications, resulting in faster interventions and improved stroke survival (Jones *et al.*, 2007).

Particularly dangerous neurological sequelae of stroke are:

- Raised intracranial pressure (see Chapter 7)
- Cerebral oedema
- Hydrocephalus (see Chapter 25)

Serial neurological assessment is therefore vital in the first hours and days following stroke (see Chapters 7 and 8).

Blood pressure

In acute stroke, autoregulation is impaired so that blood flow to the ischaemic brain becomes dependent on systemic blood pressure. A rapid fall may result in decreased blood flow to an already underperfused brain (Hyde and Dowell, 2002). High blood pressure could, therefore, play a major role in maintaining blood flow in the acute stroke patient so it should not be pharmacologically treated. Only in hypertensive emergencies involving cerebral oedema or cerebral haemorrhage, or if the patient is a candidate for thrombolysis, should a reduction of blood pressure to 185/110 mmHg or lower be effected (RCP, 2008).

Respiratory

Hypoxia will exacerbate ischaemic brain damage so it is crucial to monitor respiratory function. Current recommendations suggest that oxygen saturation levels should be maintained above 95%, either by sitting the patient up as soon as their condition permits (RCP, 2008), or by oxygen therapy. Oxygen therapy should only be administered if blood saturation levels drop below 95% (RCP, 2008).

Respiratory assessment and management is presented in Chapter 15.

Blood glucose

Between 10 and 20% of acute stroke patients are hyperglycaemic on admission and high blood glucose levels can increase neuronal damage within the ischaemic penumbra; potentially impacting on stroke outcome. Blood glucose should be maintained within normal limits (RCP, 2008) and close monitoring in the acute phase is required, to detect changes in plasma glucose concentrations (Jones *et al.*, 2007).

Body temperature

Pyrexia following stroke is common, due either to infection or the effect of the stroke on central temperature regulation. As a strong link has been established between pyrexia and poorer stroke outcomes, temperature monitoring and treatment with antipyretic medication are recommended (Jones *et al.*, 2007; RCP, 2008).

In addition to physiological monitoring, nurses also undertake specific risk assessments relating to: moving and handling, nutrition, pressure sores, falls and deep vein thrombosis (DVT) (Cross, 2008). However, the acutely ill stroke patient requires assessment by all members of the stroke team who can also intervene to prevent complications and promote recovery.

STROKE REHABILITATION

Preventing complications and promoting recovery

Early mobilisation

Although the exact association between positioning and neurological recovery has yet to be established, correct positioning of a patient following stroke (see Figure 22.4) is important in preventing potential complications arising from impaired movement. These include skin breakdown, muscle spasticity, urinary tract infections, chest infections, mobility-related falls, shoulder pain and deep vein thrombosis (RCP, 2004; Arias and Smith, 2007) (see also Chapters 8 and 11).

Nurses' ability to position patients correctly following a stroke is essential and improvements in nursing practice have been achieved through a multiprofessional, collaborative stroke training programme reported by Dowswell *et al.* (1999) and Forster *et al.* (1999a,b). However, this was tempered by the fact that there were no significant improvements in patient outcomes and in a larger, multisite study, Jones *et al.* (2005) were unable to demonstrate any impact on patient outcomes following a teaching intervention to improve nurses' positioning of patients following a stroke.

There is no standard definition of what constitutes early mobilisation, but it would appear to include sitting the patient up, being out of bed within 24 hours, being assessed by a physiotherapist between eight and 24 hours after admission, and training in transfer, sitting and walking between 24 and 72 hours (Arias and Smith, 2007). Early mobilisation can be facilitated by appropriately trained nurses or a physiotherapist. Early mobilisation is particularly important in preventing venous thromboembolism (VTE), a common complication for patients with weak or paralysed legs which can result in deep venous thrombosis (DVT), or the most serious consequence of DVT: pulmonary embolism (Harvey, 2003). Although antithrombotic medication should be avoided in patients with haemorrhagic stroke, aspirin and the use of graduated elastic compression stockings (GECS) are recommended in the NICE guidelines (NICE, 2008). More recently published findings from the *Clots in Legs Or sTockings after Stroke* (CLOTS) trial 1, provide insufficient evidence for the routine use of GECS in patients with acute ischaemic stroke. Findings showed that GECS can even present a greater risk to patients of skin breaks, blisters, ulcers and skin necrosis (CLOTS Trial Collaboration, 2009).

Another potential complication of stroke which can be prevented by careful positioning and early mobilisation is spasticity. It has been estimated to occur in 19% of patients and, although the clinical presentation will vary between patients, spasticity is associated with pain and interferes with rehabilitation interventions (McCrea *et al.*, 2008). Accurate assessment and careful management are essential (Jarrett, 2006) (see Chapter 11). Pharmacological interventions with anti-spasmodics are widely used but the evidence base has yet to be established (McCrea *et al.*, 2008). Local botulinum toxin injections do appear to be

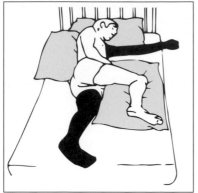

Lying on affected side
No backrest. One or two pillows for head.
Affected shoulder moved well forward.
Place good leg forward on a pillow.
Pillow placed behind back.

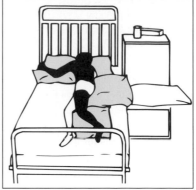

Lying on unaffected side
No backrest. One or two pillows for head.
Affected shoulder forward with arm
 on pillow.
Place affected leg backward on a pillow.
Pillow placed behind back.

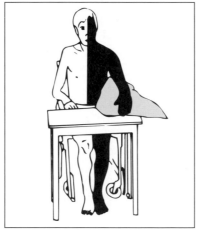

Sitting up
Sitting well back and in centre of chair.
Affected arm placed well forward on
 table or pillow.
Feet flat on floor.
Knees directly above the feet.

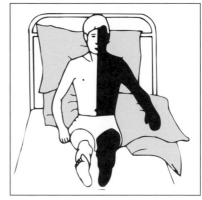

Sitting in bed
Sitting in bed is not desirable.
Affected arm placed on pillow.
Legs are straight.
Sitting upright and well supported.

Figure 22.4 The typical chart used to guide the positioning of stroke patients with hemiplegia (shown in black) whilst in bed. Reproduced from Charles P. Warlow *et al.*, *Stroke: Practical Management 3e*, Wiley-Blackwell, with permission.

effective in reducing spasticity, in combination with a range of motion exercises and splinting (RCP, 2004; Ozcakir and Sivrioglu, 2007).

Dysphagia, nutritional management and hydration
Dysphagia occurs in 64–90% of people affected by a stroke and, because all patients with swallowing difficul-

ties are at risk of developing aspiration pneumonia, their swallowing should be screened on admission by a dysphagia trained professional (RCP, 2008). Malnutrition is also a significant risk and is associated with slower recovery and a poorer outcome for the patient (RCP, 2008). All patients should have their nutritional status assessed within 48 hours of admission, using a validated screening method

(RCP, 2004) (see Chapter 16). The assessment and management of dysphagia is discussed in Chapter 12.

The nutritional management of a person with dysphagia involves close liaison with both the speech and language therapist (SLT) and dietitian, but nurses are responsible for the patient's ongoing assessment, weight monitoring, providing assistance for patients who cannot eat and drink unaided and for managing alternative methods of feeding. The maintenance of a patient's oral hygiene is also important (RCP, 2004), as this is not only essential for the patient's comfort, but there is also an established link between poor oral hygiene and an increased risk of pneumonia (Brady *et al.*, 2006). Evidence is lacking regarding oral care interventions in hospital (Brady *et al.*, 2006), but adherence to local practice standards should be expected (see also Chapters 8 and 12).

In the event of a patient being unable to swallow safely, particularly in the early days, all nurses will need to be able to pass a nasogastric (NG) tube following local clinical guidelines (Best, 2007), although ensuring that the NG tube remains in place is challenging (Horsburgh *et al.*, 2008) (see Chapter 16). In addition, nurses also need to ensure that medication is administered in the most appropriate form. Crushing tablets and opening capsules to facilitate medication administration via enteral feeding tubes is generally unsafe and liquid preparations should be used whenever possible (Morris, 2005; Wright *et al.*, 2006).

Bowel and bladder management

Between 40 and 60% of patients with moderate to severe stroke experience urinary and faecal incontinence in the initial stages. Detrusor overactivity can result in frequency, urgency and urge urinary incontinence (Thomas *et al.*, 2008). The persistence of these problems can present a significant challenge to carers on discharge from hospital. The quality of the continence care that a person receives following stroke can impact on their overall quality of life, therefore, the management of bowel and bladder problems are essential activities in stroke acute care and rehabilitation. *The National Clinical Guideline for Stroke* (RCP, 2008) recommend that established assessment and management protocols for urinary and faecal incontinence and constipation should be in place, that these conditions should be actively managed from admission and that all nurses should be able to assess incontinent patients. A structured approach and input from specialist continence nurses are recommended (Thomas *et al.*, 2008).

Enabling a person to regain continence following stroke will need to be individualised but general principles include the avoidance of catheterisation which should only

be used after alternative management methods have been considered (RCP, 2004). Early mobilisation and taking a person to the toilet as soon as they are stable can assist a person to regain a sense of control (Nazarko, 2007a) and independence in toileting has been identified as important in avoiding both the need for assistance and the feelings of decreased self-esteem (Clark and Rugg, 2005). Management of bladder and bowel problems is discussed in detail in Chapter 18.

Communication difficulties

Around one-third of people who are affected by a stroke will experience some degree of dysphasia or aphasia (Parr *et al.*, 1997). Dysarthria, caused by damage to the muscles involved in speaking; and dyspraxia, difficulty in co-ordinating the movements required to produce speech, also challenge the communication abilities of people affected. Unfortunately, even in health care settings, people with communication difficulties are often excluded from decision-making, or from social conversation, because health care professionals lack the knowledge and skills to engage them effectively (Knight, 2005). Assessment by a SLT is essential so that appropriate communication strategies can be identified and taught to both staff and relatives (RCP, 2004) (see Chapter 12).

For people who have difficulty understanding and following verbal conversation or written language, a visual format is more easily processed and enables them to control what they wish to communicate (Murphy and Cameron, 2005). A particularly helpful and comprehensive visual aid to communicating essential clinical information has been developed by Cottrell and Davies (2006). Connect, the communication disability network (www.ukconnect.org), offers a range of interactive programmes which are extremely helpful in promoting confidence in the use of 'total communication' strategies; particularly as practical sessions are led and evaluated by people with aphasia (Fursland, 2005).

Cognitive, perceptual and sensory deficits

Cognitive and perceptual impairments include hemi-inattention/neglect, memory, attention, praxis, and executive function deficits, which can significantly affect both a person's ability to engage with rehabilitation following stroke and their longer term recovery. Despite such impairments, patients can still derive significant benefit from participating in rehabilitation (Rabadi *et al.*, 2008). Sensory impairments, particularly visual changes, can also impact on motor and functional recovery (Patel and Taylor, 1999; Nazarko, 2007b). Although no specific strategies have been identified as being more successful than others in the management of these often 'invisible' effects of stroke (Bowen and Lincoln, 2007; Nair and Lincoln, 2007), nurses need to be aware of their potential impact on rehabilitation and to incorporate appropriate techniques, wherever possible, into their interventions with patients and their families.

Neglect/inattention

A stroke affecting the right hemisphere (more specifically the parietal lobe) can affect a person's awareness of the space around them and can cause difficulty with attending to one side of space, usually the left (see also Chapter 11) (Bowen and Lincoln, 2007). This can result in 'neglect' of a person's left arm and a failure to attend to things positioned on the left (RCP, 2004), causing difficulty with tasks such as washing, dressing and eating, which in turn restricts independence (Bowen and Lincoln, 2007). Visual scanning and 'retraining' patients to attend to the neglected field by using visual, verbal and tactile cues are described as the mainstay of current therapy (Bowen and Lincoln, 2007). For example a patient may be taught to turn their plate one quarter turn after each mouthful until the complete meal is eaten.

Memory

Memory can be affected in a number of ways following a stroke, such as when learning new information or skills, or remembering and retrieving information. Prospective memory, i.e. remembering to do something in the future, can also be impaired (RCP, 2004). Using techniques which capitalise on preserved ability, or compensatory strategies such as notebooks, diaries and electronic organisers, memory training and participation in rehabilitation, are all recommended in the absence of evidence for specific techniques (RCP, 2008; Nair and Lincoln, 2007).

Attention

Focusing and sustaining attention on a task are essential for many cognitive and motor functions, and impairments can negatively impact on rehabilitation. Careful planning of nursing and therapy sessions to minimise the demands placed on patients with attention deficits, and avoidance of background distractions are recommended (RCP, 2008) (see Chapter 9). Lincoln *et al.* (2000) suggest that training may improve alertness and sustained attention.

Praxis

Apraxia, or dyspraxia affects a person's ability to organise the actions required to perform a skilled activity such as

dressing (Walker *et al.*, 2003). The effects of dyspraxia can be seen in assessment, when a patient may put on clothes in a disorganised manner: upside-down or back-to-front (Walker and Walker, 2001). How dyspraxia influences a person's ability to relearn to dress remains unclear, but in aspects of patient care such as washing and dressing there is a clear indication that nurses require awareness and understanding of facilitation techniques to support patients with dyspraxia (Booth *et al.*, 2001; Booth *et al.*, 2005).

Executive function

Frontal lobe damage can result in impairments to executive functioning, specifically affecting a person's ability to initiate behaviour, such as planning and problem-solving; and the ability to self-monitor social behaviour. Executive function deficits are common in stroke patients and incorporating executive function rehabilitation into patient interventions can provide opportunities for training in problem-solving and information processing (Struder, 2007) (see Chapter 9).

Sensory deficits – visual changes

Around 60% of patients affected by a stroke will experience visual problems and they are more common in those who have had right hemisphere strokes (Nazarko, 2007b). Blurred or double vision can often be remedied with corrective lenses, prisms, or eye patches and nystagmus can be treated pharmacologically (Nazarko, 2007b). However, hemianopia, a sensory impairment resulting in loss of half of the visual field, presents a significant barrier to motor and functional recovery following stroke. As it often co-exists with visuo-spatial neglect, the two conditions can be difficult to distinguish (Patel and Taylor, 1999) (see Chapter 11). Compensatory strategies such as scanning the environment or placing things on the person's affected side are helpful and spectacles with built-in prisms can also help (Nazarko, 2007b). As many visual problems following stroke can be easily corrected or can improve with interventions, patients would benefit from formal screening for visual problems.

Pain and fatigue

Physical barriers to engagement in rehabilitation following a stroke include pain and fatigue, both of which may be overlooked as symptoms of stroke, but they are common, potentially treatable and need to be addressed (Appelros, 2006). Pain can be a particular problem following a stroke, affecting recovery and rehabilitation, but it is often not recognised and is poorly managed. Two particular causes

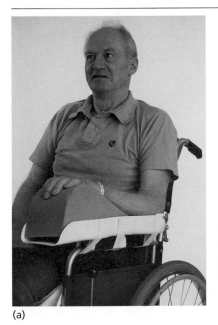
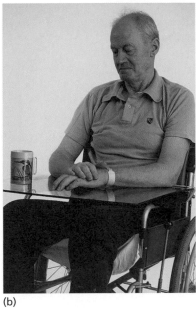
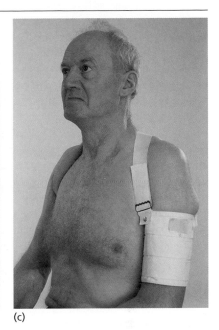

(a)　　　　　　　　　　　　(b)　　　　　　　　　　　　(c)

Figure 22.5 By supporting the weight of the arm, glenohumeral subluxation can be reduced. This may be achieved when the patient is sitting using an arm support (a) which attaches to the chair or wheelchair or, alternatively, a perspex tray (b) which, because it is transparent, allows the patient to check on the position of their feet. Both are better than pillows which invariably end up on the floor. Several designs of sling (c) are available to reduce subluxation when patients are upright. Reproduced from Charles P. Warlow *et al.*, *Stroke: Practical Management 3e*, Wiley-Blackwell, with permission.

of pain deserve specific consideration because of the difficulty they present in their effective management; these are hemiplegic shoulder pain and neuropathic (central post-stroke) pain.

Hemiplegic shoulder pain

Hemiplegic shoulder pain, or post-stroke shoulder pain, occurs in at least 30% of patients (RCP, 2004); although another estimate placed it at 70% (Bender and McKenna, 2001). Post-stroke shoulder pain can adversely affect both length of in-patient rehabilitation and overall functional outcome (Pomeroy *et al.*, 2001). Yet, contrary to the established belief that it results from subluxation, the relationship remains unclear and incorrect handling is more likely to be a contributing factor in both its development and exacerbation (RCP, 2004). Because the causes have not been clearly identified, post-stroke shoulder pain is difficult to define (Bender and McKenna, 2001) but four categories of pain have been identified, including joint pain caused by an incorrectly aligned joint, muscle pain, altered sensitivity resulting from CNS damage,

and shoulder–hand syndrome (Bender and McKenna, 2001).

Effective interventions and strategies for the prevention and management of post-stroke shoulder pain have not been conclusively established; but strapping the shoulder might reduce the incidence of pain (Figure 22.5). The use of foam supports, correct positioning and education of staff and carers regarding correct handling of the hemiplegic arm are essential (Bender and McKenna, 2001).

Neuropathic pain

Post-stroke, neuropathic pain is caused by damage to the central or peripheral nervous system, or both. It differs from physiological pain in both its complexity and the approaches to its management (Pasero, 2004). The frequency of neuropathic pain following stroke has been estimated between 5 and 20% (RCP, 2008) and approaches to management involve the use of anticonvulsant or antidepressant medication (see also Chapter 17).

Fatigue

In addition to pain, fatigue can be a common and persistent problem following a stroke and can prevent a person's full participation in rehabilitation, delay their functional improvement and accentuate their physical and cognitive symptoms (Michael, 2002). Therefore, nurses need to assess the presence and severity of fatigue and to identify the potential causes, such as underlying nutritional or metabolic deficiencies and physiological co-morbidities such as anaemia or cancer. Several fatigue assessment scales are available (Mead *et al.*, 2007) and in both the short and longer terms, developing structured daily routines and strategies to conserve energy can help (Michael, 2002). Strategies for the management of fatigue following stroke are similar to those used with people with multiple sclerosis (see Chapter 28).

Supporting the process of rehabilitation: emotional well-being, motivation and education

Once a person's condition has stabilised, their needs and those of their carers become essentially educational. Successful adjustment and adaptation depend upon how well they acquire the new knowledge and skills that they need in order to get on with their lives. The challenge for the rehabilitation team is how to help them to learn. However, the suddenness of a stroke can be emotionally overwhelming and a person's ability to engage in the rehabilitation process, particularly in the early stages, can be inhibited or delayed because emotional and psychological needs may be a greater priority. A person may need time to grieve for the losses incurred by the stroke before they can get on with their physical rehabilitation, and nurses need to be aware of this.

In the context of rehabilitation, readiness to change needs to be assessed, in order to prepare the patient for the work ahead of them and, according to Dalton and Gottlieb (2003), nurses have a key role in assessing and supporting the patient during this transitional phase. This can be achieved by acknowledging the patient's concerns, listening to their perspective and valuing their opinions about what needs to change. Dalton and Gottlieb (2003) identify a number of factors in a person which may trigger this readiness, including:

- Perceiving that their health concern is not going to resolve
- The change in their physical condition taking on a new significance
- Feeling able to manage their stress
- Having sufficient energy

- Perceiving that they have adequate support in undertaking change

Motivation also plays a vital role in determining patient outcomes (Maclean *et al.*, 2000a). However, the concept of motivation is poorly understood, and labeling patients who fail to engage in a rehabilitation programme as lazy (Maclean *et al.*, 2000b) or apathetic (Resnick, 1998) is not only unhelpful but also fails to recognise the role that professionals play in supporting patients through what is often a long and difficult process. Indeed, it has been suggested that motivation is more to do with the way in which a patient evaluates their chances of successful rehabilitation and that this is influenced by social or external factors; suggesting that there are factors which can positively or negatively affect a person's motivation. Strategies that are likely to enhance motivation include setting clear and revisable goals, making the patient feel that their views are valid and welcome, and acceptance of the patient's idiosyncrasies and avoiding clashing with the patient's value system.

In addition, a warm, approachable and competent manner are valuable and reminding the patient that goals exist beyond the ward setting (Maclean and Pound, 2000). It is most important to avoid placing the responsibility for motivation and recovery solely on the individual patient. Nurses play a key role in identifying barriers to rehabilitation and enhancing the patient's readiness to learn.

Education

The provision of information and patient and carer education are essential in improving knowledge of stroke, enhancing satisfaction with services and reducing emotional distress (Smith *et al.*, 2008), and the content, timing and method of presentation are all important (Wachters-Kaufmann *et al.*, 2005). Garrett and Cowdell (2005) identified that initially, the focus for information may be on understanding the diagnosis, the results of investigations and likelihood of recovery. Whilst medical staff are normally approached, information about the control of symptoms is sought from nurses and nurses can assist in identifying and accessing the most appropriate sources of information (Garrett and Cowdell, 2005). Over time, information needs become more diverse and wide ranging, and include reducing the chance of another stoke, and longer-term issues such as financial matters and social services.

The means by which information is provided also requires careful consideration and it should be made available in a range of formats and languages. Verbal information should be supported by written sources, although the readability and suitability of written information should not be assumed (Hoffmann *et al.*, 2004; Tooth and Hoffmann, 2004). Pictorial formats, models, videos, audiotapes and web-based sources of information can be provided to accommodate individual learning needs and abilities, and education strategies should aim to actively involve patients and carers (Garrett and Coldwell, 2005).

End of life care

Although improvements in early treatment and rehabilitation have significantly reduced the numbers of people who die following a stroke, it is estimated that around 20% of people affected will die within one month of the event (Rogers and Addington-Hall, 2005). Many of these deaths will occur in hospital, including acute stroke wards and stroke rehabilitation units, where the needs of dying patients may not be fully acknowledged. In recognition of this, the *National Clinical Guidelines for Stroke* (RCP, 2008) recommend staff training in the principles and practice of palliative care and access to specialist palliative care expertise. The development of a model of service interaction, relating neurology, rehabilitation and palliative care (neuropalliative rehabilitation), should present opportunities to enable nurses to successfully embed palliative care principles into stroke care (Sutton, 2008).

Transfer of care and long-term management

Whilst the roles of stroke nurse specialists tend to focus on acute stroke services, the consultant and coordinator roles are more diffuse, often working across the stroke care continuum, from primary prevention to long-term care. Once the acute recovery phase has passed, continuing rehabilitation and longer term management are essential. The role of family caregivers should be considered from the outset and their needs for support must not be neglected (RCP, 2008).

The psychosocial effects of stroke

Personal accounts of stroke highlight the intense emotional distress experienced and the ensuing struggle to cope during the period of rehabilitation and beyond and it is not surprising that mood disorders following stroke are common.

Emotionalism

Although mood disturbances following stroke have been generally well-documented, emotionalism – characterised by difficulty controlling crying or laughing – has been relatively neglected (House *et al.*, 2004). However, in the first six months following stroke, between 20 and 25% of people will experience emotionalism and report crying or laughing 'in situations that would have not previously have provoked such behaviour' (House *et al.*, 2004). These emotional outbursts can be sudden and unpredictable; causing distress and embarrassment. They can negatively impact on contact with family and friends and lead to social avoidance. Emotionalism is also associated with an increase in depressive symptoms, although, fortunately, the majority of people affected do not experience diagnosable depression (House *et al.*, 2004).

Therapeutic interventions for emotionalism have tended to focus on pharmacological approaches. Numerous clinical trials with antidepressant medication have been reported and the use of antidepressants is recommended (Stroke Association, 2006; RCP, 2008). However, no specific antidepressant has been identified as the most effective and House *et al.* (2004) concluded that further data are required before recommendations can be made regarding the pharmacological treatment of post-stroke emotionalism. Other approaches have sought to explore the interpersonal dimensions of emotionalism and the ways in which emotional displays are managed by those closest to the person affected, but again no specific strategies have been identified as more successful than others (Manzo *et al.*, 1998). Acknowledging that the behaviour is due to the stroke is important and empathy and understanding are essential. Advice for relatives and friends focuses on distraction, or treating an emotional display as 'a minor inconvenience' and continuing with the conversation that may have provoked the emotionalism (Stroke Association, 2006). With time, the frequency and severity of emotionalism declines.

Anxiety

Anxiety can be provoked by specific activities or events, or might occur without provocation. Whatever the cause, anxiety can exert seriously adverse effects on daily functioning, personal relationships and the quality of life for a person affected by a stroke. Anxiety following stroke might also be associated with post-traumatic stress disorder (PTSD) and can be characterised by intrusive memories or flashbacks to the traumatic event of the stroke (McCoy, 2006). The person may feel that they are re-experiencing the stroke event and do not want to think about what happened because of the unpleasant feelings this generates (McCoy, 2006). For both generalised anxiety disorder and PTSD, psychological therapies might be of value; possibly in combination with benzodiazepines or antidepressant medication (RCP, 2004)

Depression

Whilst emotionalism and anxiety are undeniably distressing, depression has received most attention from researchers and practitioners. This is justifiable because it is the most debilitating mood disturbance following stroke, and is associated with increased morbidity, delayed rehabilitation, longer periods of hospitalisation and generally poorer outcomes for the person affected (Turner-Stokes and Hassan, 2002). Estimates of depression following stroke vary radically. O'Rourke *et al.* (1998) suggests that 23–60% of stroke survivors will experience depression and Lincoln *et al.* (2003) indicated an even wider range of 25–79%. However, Hackett *et al.* (2005) suggest a pooled estimate of 33% for all stroke survivors who experience depression.

Depression can occur in response to any life-changing event where a person has experienced a catastrophic loss of independence, self esteem and perceived status in society; and not everyone is equipped to cope with the grieving and adjustment processes (Rochette *et al.*, 2007). There is also an increased risk of stroke-related mood disturbance in patients who are unable to process loss events due to a decrease in cognitive ability (Rickards, 2005) It has been proposed that areas of the brain responsible for the control of mood may be damaged by a stroke, causing a neurochemical imbalance resulting in mood disturbance (Robinson *et al.*, 1990), but systematic reviews of the literature have identified no conclusive evidence for this theory (Aben *et al.*, 2001; Carson *et al.*, 2000).

Reported risk factors for the development of depression include previous history of depression or psychiatric illness, living alone, lack of social support and social isolation (Ouimet *et al.*, 2001). In females, the estimated risk of developing depression following stroke is 7–10% greater than in males (Paolucci *et al.*, 1999). A person experiencing depression following a stroke is more likely to die over the course of 5 years, than a non-depressed person (Jorge *et al.*, 2003) and there is also a significantly increased risk of suicide, particularly in people under the age of 60 and in females (Teasdale and Enberg, 2001).

Screening for anxiety and depression should occur within the first month following a stroke, together with keeping the patient's mood under review. However, although there is widespread agreement that the early recognition and management of depression following stroke are essential, consensus regarding the most appropriate assessment tools, diagnostic criteria and effective interventions for the prevention and treatment of depression following stroke has yet to be reached. The Hospital Anxiety and Depression Scale (HADS) remains a popular screening tool, possibly because it can be administered by nurses and other members of the multiprofessional team. For patients with communication impairments, the Stroke and Aphasia Depressions Questionnaire is more appropriate (Bennett and Lincoln, 2006).

Supporting carers

It is important to recognise that the emotional costs of providing long-term care to a person affected by a stroke can also be great, and that carers are more prone to the development of depression than the wider population (Wyller *et al.*, 2003). Informal caregivers provide indispensable support following a person's return home and their ability to manage this caring role is crucial (Ski and O'Connell, 2007). However, it has been identified that the greater the care giving burden, the greater the level of emotional distress for carers and interventions to support carers are essential in maintaining their emotional wellbeing (Brereton *et al.*, 2007).

Ensuring that appropriate support is available to a person experiencing a stroke and their carers has been highlighted as a 'key area of challenge' in the *National Stroke Strategy* (DH, 2007). Emotional support features highly in nursing interventions within the context of community-based stroke services (Burton and Gibbon, 2005; Bennett and Greensmith 2007) as well as in hospital-based contexts (Dundas, 2006; Bennett *et al.*, 2007). For patients with severe or persistent depression, psychological therapies or antidepressant medication might be considered (RCP, 2008)

SUMMARY

Care of patients following stroke is complex and requires skilled and knowledgeable nurses to coordinate care of the patient with other members of the multidisciplinary team. While several guidelines have been produced addressing stroke care, there is still a paucity of evidence supporting some aspects of care and further research is required. The profile of stroke and TIA care has been raised and developments in hyperacute care and thrombolysis mean that patients who suffer from stroke should now benefit from improved outcomes providing symptoms are recognised and acted upon as a medical emergency.

Stroke: patient perspective

I am 62 years old and I am a window fitter by trade. On the morning of my stroke I got up early to ring my bosses to let them know I was unable to come into work again that day. I made a cup of tea for my wife and when I took it downstairs, I was unable to carry the cup without spilling the tea on each step. I did feel peculiar, but was unaware that I had had a stroke. My wife noticed instantly that my face was drooping on the right side and thought something serious had happened. She arranged an emergency appointment with the doctor who then told us to go to the hospital immediately since my heart rate was 130 and I was in atrial fibrillation.

By this stage, I was confused and unsure of what was happening around me and I had lost power in my right arm. After some initial tests in A&E, I was admitted to the Stroke Unit. By the following day, the power had returned to my arm and I was feeling less confused but my speech was still affected and I had difficulties with numbers and telling the time.

Therapy

My occupational therapist helped me with my measurements and we worked on some drawings and site plans to obtain accurate measurements for the buildings. I found this much more difficult as it was something I took for granted prior to my stroke. I had an ability to know measurements by sight before and when I looked at an architect's drawing, my mind had the ability to understand immediately what size windows would be needed and where they would go without hardly thinking about it. After my stroke, I stared at architect's drawings for hours and they made little or no sense. I still find it difficult now to work out measurements when doing DIY for example. I have to keep checking and re-checking that I have the correct measurements.

I have found that when I am tired, my speech is not as fluent as it is when I am well rested. I did also suffer some side effects from my medication and I found that I was easily depressed about my condition. I become impatient and frustrated and wanted everything to go back to how it was before my stroke.

The Future

I am hopeful that I can return to work soon. I may not be able to do the same work as before as I have dizzy spells, which is obviously dangerous on a building site. I still feel impatient sometimes when things don't go right or if I cannot say what I want to say. However, I am a lot better than I was so I am grateful for that.

For further examples of stroke survivor's experiences please refer to the Different Strokes website available at: www.differentstrokes.co.uk

REFERENCES

Aben I, Verhey F, Honig A *et al.* (2001) Research into the specificity of depression after stroke: a review on an unresolved issue. *Progress in Neuropsychopharmacology and Biological Psychiatry* 25:671–689.

Adamson J, Beswick A, Ebrahim S (2004) Is stroke the most common cause of disability? *Journal of Stroke and Cerebrovascular Diseases* 13(4):171–177.

Allender S, Colquhoun D, Kelly P (2006) Competing discourses of workplace health. *Health (London)* 10(1):75–93.

Amarenco P, Bogousslavsky J, Callahan A *et al.* (2006) High-dose atorvastatin after stroke or transient ischaemic attack. *New England Journal of Medicine* 355:549–559.

Appelros P (2006) Prevalence and predictors of pain and fatigue after stroke: a population-based study. *International Journal of Rehabilitation Research* 29(4):329–333.

Arias M, Smith L (2007) Early mobilization of acute stroke patients. *Journal of Clinical Nursing* 16:282–288.

Baker M, Opatowsky M, Wilson J *et al.* (2001). Rheolytic catheter thrombolysis of dural venous sinus thrombosis: A case series. *Neurosurgery* 48(3):487–494.

Bamford J, Sandercock P, Dennis M *et al.* (1990) A prospective study of acute cerebrovascular disease in the community: the Oxfordshire Community Stroke Project 1981–1986. 2. Incidence, case fatality rates and overall outcome at one year of cerebral infarction, primary intracerebral and subarachnoid haemorrhage. *Journal of Neurology, Neurosurgery and Psychiatry* 53:16–22.

Bamford J, Sandercock P, Dennis M *et al.* (1991) Classification and natural history of clinically identifiable subtypes of cerebral infarction. *Lancet* 22 337(8756):1521–1526.

Bender L, McKenna K (2001) Hemiplegic shoulder pain: defining the problem and its management. *Disability and Rehabilitation* 23(16):698–705.

Bennett B, Barnston S, Smith R (2007) Emotional support after stroke, part 1: Two models from hospital practice. *British Journal of Neuroscience Nursing* 3(1):19–23.

Bennett B, Greensmith C (2007) Emotional support after stroke, part 2: A community practice model. *British Journal of Neuroscience Nursing* 3(2):61–64.

Bennett H, Lincoln N (2006) Potential screening measures for depression and anxiety after stroke. *International Journal of Therapy and Rehabilitation* 13(9):401–406.

Best C (2007) Nasogastric tube insertion in adults who require enteral feeding. *Nursing Standard* 21(40):39–43.

Birns J, Fitzpatrick M (2005) secondary prevention of *stroke. British Journal of Neuroscience Nursing* 1(1):32–37.

Booth J, Davidson I, Winstanley J *et al.* (2001) Observing washing and dressing of stroke patients: nursing intervention compared with occupational therapists. What is the difference? *Journal of Advanced Nursing* 33(1):98–105.

Booth J, Hillier V, Waters K *et al.* (2005) Effects of a stroke rehabilitation education programme for nurses. *Journal of Advanced Nursing* 49(5):465–473.

Bowen A, Lincoln N (2007) Cognitive rehabilitation for spatial neglect following stroke. *Cochrane database of Systematic Reviews* (2):CD003586.

Brady M, Furlanetto D, Lewis S *et al.* (2006) Staff-led interventions for improving oral hygiene in patients following stroke. *Cochrane Database of Systematic Reviews* (4):CD003864.

Brereton L, Carroll C, Barnston S (2007) Interventions for adult family carers of people who have had a stroke: a systematic review. *Clinical Rehabilitation* 21(10):867–884.

Brodal P (2004) *The Central Nervous System: Structure and function.* (3rd edition). Oxford: Oxford University Press.

Burton C, Gibbon B (2005) Expanding the role of the stroke nurse: a pragmatic clinical trial. *Journal of Advanced Nursing* 52(6):640–650.

Carson A, MacHale S, Allen K *et al.* (2000) Depression after stroke and lesion location: a systematic review. *Lancet* 356(9224):122–126.

Clark J, Rugg S (2005) The importance of independence in toileting: the views of stroke survivors and their occupational therapists. *British Journal of Occupational Therapy* 68(4):165–171.

CLOTS Trial Collaboration (2009) Effectiveness of thigh-length graduated compression stockings to reduce the risk of deep vein thrombosis after stroke (CLOTS trial 1): a multicentre, randomised controlled trial. *The Lancet* 373(9679):1958–1965.

Cottrell S, Davies A (2006) *Stroke Talk: A communication resource for hospital care.* London: Connect Press.

Cross S (2008) Stroke care: a nursing perspective. *Nursing Standard* 22(23):47–56.

Dalton C, Gottlieb L (2003) The concept of readiness to change. *Journal of Advanced Nursing* 42(2):108–117.

Department of Health (2001) *National Service Framework for Older People.* London: DH.

Department of Health (2007) *National Stroke Strategy.* London: DH.

Dirnagl U, Pulsinelli W (1990) Autoregulation of cerebral blood flow in experimental focal brain ischaemia. *Journal of Cerebral Blood Flow and Metabolism* 10:327–336.

Dowswell G, Forster A, Young J *et al.* (1999) The development of a collaborative stroke training programme for nurses. *Journal of Clinical Nursing* 8:743–752.

Dundas J (2006) An evaluation of use of the HADS scale to screen for post-stroke depression in practice. *British Journal of Neuroscience Nursing* 2(8):399–403.

Forster A, Dowswell G, Young J *et al.* (1999a) Effects of a physiotherapist-led stroke training programme for nurses. *Age and Ageing* 28:567–574.

Forster A, Dowswell G, Young J *et al.* (1999b) Effect of a physiotherapist-led training programme on attitudes of nurses caring for patients after stroke. *Clinical Rehabilitation* 13:113–122.

Fursland E (2005) Finding the words. *Nursing Standard* 20(1):24–25.

Garrett D, Cowdell F (2005) Information needs of patients and carers following stroke. *Nursing Older People* 17(6):14–16.

Hackett M, Yapa C, Parag V *et al.* (2005) Frequency of depression after stroke: a systematic review of observational studies. *Stroke* 36(6):1330–1340.

Hankam D, Spence D (2007) Combining multiple approaches for the secondary prevention of vascular events after stroke. *Stroke* 38:1881–1885.

Hankey GJ, Warlow CP (1999) Treatment and secondary prevention of stroke: evidence, costs, and effects on individuals and populations. *Lancet* 354(9188):1457–1463.

Harvey R (2003) Prevention of venous thromboembolism after stroke. *Topics in Stroke Rehabilitation* 10: 61–69.

Hoffmann T, McKenna K, Worrall L *et al.* (2004) Evaluating current practice in the provision of written information to stroke patients and their carers. *International Journal of Therapy and Rehabilitation* 11(7):303–310.

Horsburgh D, Rowat A, Mahoney C *et al.* (2008) A necessary evil? Interventions to prevent nasogastric tube-tugging after stroke. *British Journal of Neuroscience Nursing* 4(5):230–234.

House A, Hackett M, Anderson C *et al.* (2004) Pharmaceutical interventions for emotionalism after stroke. *Cochrane Database of Systematic Reviews* (2):CD0033690.

Hyde S, Dowell M (2002) Acute stroke management: the importance of vital signs. *Nurse 2 Nurse* 2(12):10–12.

Jarrett L (2006) The nurse's role in assessing and measuring spasticity. *Nursing Times* 102(15):26–28.

Johnston SC, Rothwell PM, Nguyen-Huynh MN *et al.* (2007) Validation and refinement of scores to predict very early stroke risk after transient ischaemic attack. *Lancet* 369(9558):283–292.

Jones A, Tilling K, Wilson-Barnett J *et al.* (2005) Effect of recommended positioning on stroke outcome at six months: a randomised controlled trial. *Clinical Rehabilitation* 19:138–145.

Jones S, Leathley M, McAdamm J *et al.* (2007) Physiological monitoring in acute stroke: a literature review. *Journal of Advanced Nursing* 60(6):577–594.

Jorge R, Robinson R, Arndt S *et al.* (2003) Mortality and post-stroke depression: a placebo-controlled trial of antidepressants. *American Journal of Psychiatry* 160(10):1823–1829.

Knight G (2005) *Better Conversations: A guide for relatives.* London: Connect – the Communication Disability Network.

Lincoln N, Majid M, Weyman N (2000) Cognitive rehabilitation for attention deficits following stroke. *Cochrane Database of Systematic Reviews* (4):CD002842.

Lincoln N, Nicholl C, Flannaghan T *et al.* (2003) The validity of questionnaire measures of assessing depression after stroke. *Clinical Rehabilitation* 17(8):840–846.

Lip GY, Barnett AH, Bradbury A *et al.* (2007) Ethnicity and cardiovascular disease prevention in the United Kingdom: a practical approach to management. *Journal of Human Hypertension* 21(3):183–211.

Maclean N, Pound P (2000) A critical review of the concept of patient motivation in the literature on physical rehabilitation. *Social Science and Medicine* 50:495–506.

Maclean N, Pound P, Wolfe C *et al.* (2000a) The concept of patient motivation. A qualitative analysis of stroke professionals' attitudes. *Stroke* 33(2):444–448.

Maclean N, Pound P, Wolfe C *et al.* (2000b) Qualitative analysis of stroke patients' motivation for rehabilitation. *British Medical Journal* 321(7268):1051–1054.

MacWalter RS, Shirley CP (2003) *Managing Strokes and TIAs in Practice.* London: Royal Society of Medicine Press Ltd.

Manzo J, Heath R, Blonder L (1998) The interpersonal management of crying among survivors of stroke. *Sociological Spectrum* 18:161–184.

McCoy K (2006) Even a minor stroke might lead to stress and anxiety. *Neurology* 66:15–16.

McCrea J, Langhorne P, Pandyan A *et al.* (2008) Systemically-acting pharmacological interventions for spasticity after stroke (Protocol). *Cochrane Database of Systematic Reviews* (3):CD006874.

McMahon A, Irwin P, Redehan E (2003) Identifying priorities for strengthening and developing the nursing contribution in the field of practice: A case study in stroke care. *Nursing Times Research* 8(3):202–212.

Mead G, Lynch J, Greig C *et al.* (2007) Evaluation of fatigue scales in stroke patients. *Stroke* 8(7):2090–2095.

Michael K (2002) Fatigue and stroke. *Rehabilitation Nursing* 27(3):89–94,103.

Morris H (2005) Administering drugs to patients with swallowing difficulties. *Nursing Times* 101(39):28–30.

Murphy J, Cameron L (2005) *Talking Mats: A resource To enhance communication.* Stirling: University of Stirling.

Nair R, Lincoln N (2007) Cognitive rehabilitation for memory deficits following a stroke. *Cochrane Database of Systematic Reviews* (3):CD002293.

National Audit Office (2005) *Reducing Brain Damage: Faster access to better stroke care.* London: The Stationery Office.

National Institute for Health and Clinical Excellence (2008) *Stroke: national clinical guidelines for diagnosis and initial management of acute stroke and transient ischaemic attack (TIA).* London: Royal College of Physicians.

Nazarko L (2007a) Stroke and continence: The benefits of assessment. *Nursing and Residential Care* 9(5):203–206.

Nazarko L (2007b) Visual impairment in stroke sufferers. *Nursing and Residential Care* 9(3):109–111.

Office of National Statistics (2001) Stroke incidence and risk factors in a population-based cohort study. In: *Office of National Statistics Health Statistics Quarterly* (12) Winter.

O'Rourke S, MacHale S, Signorini D *et al.* (1998) Detecting psychiatric morbidity after stroke: comparison of the GHQ and the HAD Scale. *Stroke* 29(5):980–985.

Ouimet M, Primeau F, Cole M (2001) Psychosocial risk factors in poststroke depression: a systematic review. *Canadian Journal of Psychiatry* 46:819–828.

Ozcakir S, Sivrioglu K (2007) Botulinum toxin in poststroke spasticity. *Clinical Medicine and Research* 5(2):132–138.

Paolucci S, Antonucci G, Pratesi L *et al.* (1999) Poststroke depression and its role in rehabilitation. *Archives of Physical Medicine and Rehabilitation* 80:985–990.

Parr S, Byng S, Gilpin S (1997) *Talking About Aphasia: Living with loss of language after stroke.* Buckingham, Open University Press.

Pasero C (2004) Pathophysiology of neuropathic pain. *Pain Management Journal* 5(4):(Suppl 1):3–8.

Patel S, Taylor L (1999) Only half of the world: hemianopia or neglect. *British Journal of Therapy and Rehabilitation* 6(7):327–329.

Perry L, Brooks W, Hamilton S *et al.* (2004) Exploring nurses' perspectives of stroke care. *Nursing Standard* 19(12):33–38.

Pomeroy V, Niven D, Barrow S *et al.* (2001) Unpacking the black box of nursing and therapy practice for post-stroke shoulder pain: a precursor to evaluation. *Clinical Rehabilitation* 15:67–83.

Poulter N, Thorn S, Kirby M (2000) *Shared Care for Hypertension.* London: Isis Medical Media.

Rabadi M, Rabadi F, Edelstein L *et al.* (2008) Cognitively impaired stroke patients do benefit from admission to an acute stroke unit. *Archives of Physical Medicine and Rehabilitation* 89(3):441–448.

Resnick B (1998) Motivating older adults to perform functional activities. *Journal of Gerontological Nursing* 24(11):23–30.

Rickards H (2005) Depression in neurological disorders: Parkinson's disease, multiple sclerosis and stroke. *Journal of Neurology, Neurosurgery and Psychiatry* 76(Suppl 1):148–152.

Robinson R, Morris P, Fedoroff J (1990) Depression and cerebrovascular disease. *Journal of Clinical Psychiatry* 51(7)Suppl:26–31.

Rochette A, Bravo G, Desrosiers J *et al.* (2007) Adaptation process, participation and depression over six months in first-stroke individuals and spouses. *Clinical Rehabilitation* 21:554–562.

Rogers A, Addington-Hall J (2005) Care of the dying stroke patient in the acute setting. *Journal of Research in Nursing* 10(2):153–167.

Rothwell P (2007) Making the most of secondary prevention. *Stroke* 38(6):1726.

Rothwell P, Eliasziw M, Gutnikov S *et al.* (2004). Endarterectomy for symptomatic carotid stenosis in relation to clinical subgroups and timing of surgery. *The Lancet* 363(9413):915–924.

Rothwell PM, Gutnikov SA, Warlow CP for the European Carotid Surgery Trialists' Collaboration (2003) Reanalysis of the final results of the European Carotid Surgery Trial. *Stroke* 34:514–523.

Royal College of Physicians (2004) *National Clinical Guidelines for Stroke.* (2nd edition). London: RCP.

Royal College of Physicians (2008) *National Clinical Guidelines for Stroke* (3rd edition). London: RCP.

Ski C, O'Connell B (2007) Stroke: the increasing complexity of carer needs. *Journal of Neuroscience Nursing* 39(3):172–179.

Smith J, Forster A, House A *et al.* (2008) Information provision for stroke patients and their caregivers. *Cochrane Database of Systematic Reviews* (2): CD001919.

Stroke Association (2006) *Psychological Effects of Stroke* Fact sheet 10 Available from: www.stroke.org.uk

Struder M (2007) Rehabilitation of executive function: to err is human, to be aware – divine. *Journal of Neurologic Physical Therapy* 31(3):128–134.

Sudlow CL, Warlow CP (1997) Comparable studies of the incidence of stroke and its pathological types: results from an international collaboration. International Stroke Incidence Collaboration. *Stroke* 28(3):491–499.

Sutton L (2008) Addressing palliative and end-of-life care needs in neurology. *British Journal of Neuroscience Nursing* 4(5):235–238.

Teasdale T, Enberg A (2001) Suicide after stroke: a population study. *Journal of Epidemiology and Community Health* 55(12):863–866.

Thomas L, Cross S, Barrett J *et al.* (2008) Treatment of urinary incontinence after stroke in adults. *Cochrane Database of Systematic Reviews* (1):CD004462.

Thorvaldsen P, Davidsen M, Brønnum-Hansen H *et al.* (1999) Stable stroke occurrence despite incidence reduction in an aging population: stroke trends in the danish monitoring trends and determinants in cardiovascular disease (MONICA) population. *Stroke* 30(12):2529–2534.

Tooth L, Hoffmann T (2004) Patient perceptions of the quality of information provided in a hospital stroke rehabilitation unit. *British Journal of Occupational Therapy* 67(3):111–117.

Touzani O, Roussel S, MacKenzie ET (2001) The ischaemic penumbra. *Current Opinions in Neurology* 14(1):83–88.

Turner-Stokes L, Hassan N (2002) Depression after stroke: a review of the evidence base to inform the development of an integrated care pathway. Part 1: Diagnosis, frequency and impact. *Clinical Rehabilitation* 16(3):231–247.

Wachters-Kaufmann C, Schuling J, Hauw T *et al.* (2005) Actual and desired information provision after a stroke. *Patient Education and Counseling* 54:211–217.

Walker C, Walker M (2001) Dressing ability after stroke: a review of the literature. *British Journal of Occupational Therapy* 64(9):449–454.

Walker C, Walker M, Sunderland A (2003) Dressing after a stroke: a survey of current occupational therapy practice. *British Journal of Occupational Therapy* 66(6):263–268.

Wardlaw JM, del Zoppo G, Yamaguchi T *et al.* (2003) Thrombolysis for acute ischaemic stroke (Cochrane review). *Cochrane Database of Systematic Reviews* Issue 3. Review updated in Issue 4 (2008).

Warlow C, Dennis M, van Gijn J *et al.* (2008) *Stroke: A practical guide to management.* (3rd edition). Oxford: Blackwell Publishing.

Williams B, Poulter N, Brown M *et al.* (2004) Guidelines for management of hypertension: report of the fourth working party of the British Hypertension Society. *Journal of Human Hypertension* 18:1991–1994.

Wolf P (2003) Cerebrovascular risk. In: Izzo J and Black H (eds) *Hypertension Primer: The essentials of high blood pressure.* (3rd edition). Philadelphia: Lippincott, Williams and Wilkins.

Wolf PA, D'Agostino RB, O'Neal MA *et al.* (1992) Secular trends in stroke incidence and mortality: the Framingham Study. *Stroke* 23:1551–1555.

Woodward S (2007) Antiphospholipid (Hughes) syndrome. *British Journal of Neuroscience Nursing* 3(1):16–18.

World Health Organisation (1988) World Health Organisation MONICA Project (monitoring trends and determinants in cardiovascular disease): a major international collaboration. *Journal of Clinical Epidemiology* 41:105–141.

Wright D, Chapman N, Foundling-Miah M *et al.* (2006) *Consensus Guideline on the Medication Management of Adults with Swallowing Difficulties.* London: Medendium Group Publishing.

Wyller T, Thommessen B, Sødring K *et al.* (2003) Emotional well-being of close relatives to stroke survivors. *Clinical Rehabilitation* 17(4):410–417.

23

Management of Patients with Intracranial Aneurysms and Vascular Malformations

Ann-Marie Mestecky

INTRODUCTION

Cerebral aneurysms and vascular malformations are anomalies of the cerebral vasculature. They can cause intracranial haemorrhages with devastating consequences for some patients; for others the clinical manifestation can be relatively minor and recent developments in medical treatment can for some lead to swift recovery. Rupture of intracranial aneurysms most commonly causes bleeding into the subarachnoid space and is referred to as aneurysmal subarachnoid haemorrhage (ASAH). ASAH is one the most common neurological emergency conditions treated in specialist neuroscience units. Vascular malformations are less common and most often present with intracranial haemorrhage. The management and care of patients with aneurysms and vascular malformations is often complex and challenging and requires a multidisciplinary approach by a specialist team of health care professionals.

ANEURYSMS

Aneurysms are small thinned walled blisters protruding from the arteries of the Circle of Willis or its near branches (Hankey and Wardlaw, 2008) (Figure 23.1). Aneurysms that rupture are usually small, between 5 and 15 mm in diameter. The deposition of thrombus within larger aneurysms (>2 cm) actually strengthens the wall of the aneurysm and makes them less prone to rupturing. The majority

of aneurysms have a narrow neck which widens into a small sac (Figure 23.2) and are called saccular or berry aneurysms. The walls of the aneurysm are continuous with those of the parent vessel. However there is an absence of the normal muscular and internal elastic layers within the wall of the aneurysm.

INCIDENCE OF ANEURYSMS

Incidence of aneurysms is 6–8 per 100,000 person years (Hankey and Wardlaw, 2008). According to angiographic and autopsy studies, intracranial aneurysms have a prevalence of between 0.5 and 6% (Linfante and Wakhloo, 2007). For the majority, aneurysms are asymptomatic for life and therefore go undetected. Those that become symptomatic most commonly present with ASAH.

AETIOLOGY OF ANEURYSMS

The mechanism by which intracranial aneurysms form and rupture is not fully understood. It is evident however that genetic and environmental factors contribute to their pathogenesis, in addition to haemodynamic forces. Environmental factors such as smoking and excessive drinking are the most important risk factors (Feigin *et al.*, 2005). Chronic hypertension will almost certainly contribute to degeneration of the vessel wall at the points where aneurysms most commonly occur (bifurcation points along the circle of Willis). In approximately 8% of those that rupture there is a familial link which suggests a genetic influence. It is probably the interaction of these and many more factors, e.g. age, which leads to eventual

Neuroscience Nursing: Evidence-Based Practice, 1st Edition.
Edited by Sue Woodward and Ann-Marie Mestecky
© 2011 Blackwell Publishing Ltd

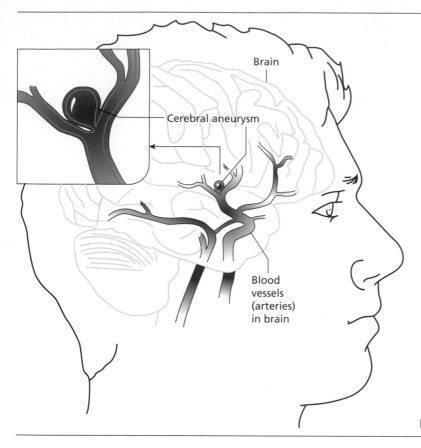

Figure 23.1 Cerebral aneurysm.

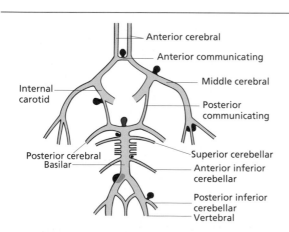

Figure 23.2 Usual sites of cerebral aneurysms. Reproduced from Andrew Kaye, *Essential Neurosurgery*, Wiley-Blackwell, with permission.

rupture. Many patients at the time of the bleed are partaking in activities that increase blood pressure, e.g. physical exercise and sexual intercourse.

OTHER CAUSES OF SPONTANEOUS SUBARACHNOID HAEMORRHAGE (SAH)

Ruptured aneurysms are the most common cause of spontaneous SAH, accounting for approximately 80% of all cases. Arteriovenous malformations account for 5% and are discussed in detail later in this chapter. A further 5% are due to non-aneurysmal perimesencephalic haemorrhage. In this subset of SAH patients, blood is seen only in the perimesencephalic cisterns which lie anterior to the midbrain. There is no risk of rebleeding and life expectancy is not affected (Greebe *et al.*, 2007).This patient population has a benign clinical course and does not have a significant reduction in quality of life, although they can still have fatigue and headaches for a period of time following the SAH. Other rare causes include: bleeding disorders, CNS infections, CNS tumours and cocaine abuse.

The incidence of spontaneous SAH is approximately 9 per 100,000 of the population per annum, with higher rates in Finland and Japan and in non-white ethnic groups (de Rooij *et al.*, 2007). SAH can occur at any age, but the incidence increases with age with a reported peak incidence in the sixth decade (Pobereskin, 2001). SAH has a female preponderance but this gender distribution varies with age. At younger ages there is a higher incidence in men, while after the age of 55 years, the incidence is higher in women (de Rooij *et al.*, 2007).

SIGNS AND SYMPTOMS OF ANEURYSMAL SAH

The haemorrhage occurs abruptly, causing a sudden severe headache which is often described as the 'worst headache imaginable'; some may have the sensation of something bursting, seconds prior to the headache. The signs and symptoms following the initial rupture will depend on the severity of the bleed. For 10–15% of patients with SAH, the bleed will be catastrophic resulting in death either at the time of the bleed or during transportation to hospital (Huang and van Gelder, 2002).The severity of a SAH is graded according to the World Federation of Neurological Surgeons (WFNS) grading system, which considers Glasgow Coma Scale (GCS) score on admission and the presence or absence of motor deficits. Those that suffer a poor grade SAH (grade 4 and 5), will undoubtedly have an increase in intracranial pressure (ICP) due to the volume of the bleed, with a subsequent drop in cerebral perfusion pressure and level of consciousness. Patients with a better grade SAH (grades 2–3) may experience a transient loss of consciousness, but rapidly recover to GCS 13–14. Those with a grade 1 SAH present with a GCS of 15 and diagnosis for these patients is not always straightforward (see: Diagnosis).

The force of the SAH can also cause bleeding into the brain parenchyma with the subsequent formation of an intracerebral haematoma, or into the ventricular system resulting in an intraventricular haemorrhage, either of which is most likely to occur in those with a grade 4 or 5 SAH. Early focal signs, e.g. dysphasia, are indicative of focal brain damage caused by an intracerebral haematoma. Approximately 6–10% will have one or more seizures at the time of the bleed and approximately a thirdof patients will have a seizure at some stage following the bleed (Mayberg *et al.*, 1994). Most patients will have a reactive hypertension on admission which may serve to protect the brain against ischaemia when ICP is raised. It probably results from the reflex response to raised ICP and an increase in circulating catecholamines. The reactive hypertension generally settles within 3–5 days. As the blood circulates in the CSF it causes meningeal irritation, the symptoms of which become apparent within a few hours

of the bleed and may include neck rigidity, photophobia, irritability and low fever. Blood can also irritate the lumbar and sacral nerve roots causing sciatica and lower back pain. Nausea and vomiting are also common symptoms.

Not all patients with a symptomatic aneurysm present with a SAH. Less than 10% of patients will present with pressure symptoms due to the mass effect of the aneurysm, the clinical manifestation of which will depend on the site of the aneurysm. The most common instance of this is a posterior communicating artery aneurysm producing a nerve palsy of the oculomotor nerve (cranial nerve III).

DIAGNOSIS

Patients with a suspected SAH will have a full neurological examination followed by a computed tomography (CT) scan. Third generation CT scanners have a sensitivity of 98% in the 24 hours following the SAH. Blood is typically seen in the area of aneurysm rupture in the basal cisterns (Figure 23.3). For a small number of patients with SAH the CT will be negative. This is for one of two reasons: either the SAH is too small in volume to be detected, or there is a delay in the patient seeking medical advice following the SAH (typically a grade 1 SAH). The sensitivity of CT rapidly decreases with the passage of time, after 24 hours it falls to 93% (Sames *et al.*, 1996).

In CT negative cases where the clinician suspects that a SAH is probable based on clinical history, a lumbar

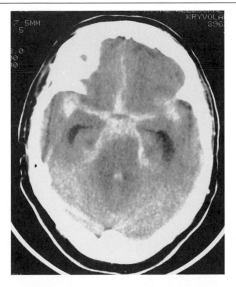

Figure 23.3 Blood in the Sylvian fissure and basal cisterns indicative of subarachnoid haemorrhage. Reproduced from Andrew Kaye, *Essential Neurosurgery*, Wiley-Blackwell, with permission.

puncture (LP) is performed. An LP will only be performed once the possibility of a raised ICP has been ruled out for fear of herniation (refer to Chapter 19 for further detail on LP). The CSF is visually inspected for xanthochromia (a yellow discolouration indicating the presence of bilirubin, which is released from red blood cells as they haemolyse). Xanthochromia will not be present until approximately 8 hours following the SAH. This test has poor sensitivity and can result in false negative and positive results. It is therefore recommended that the cerebrospinal fluid (CSF) is sent to the biochemistry laboratory for further testing using spectrophotometry (UK NEQAS, 2003).

Following confirmation of SAH the source of the bleed has to be identified. In specialist centres invasive cerebral angiography (refer to Chapter 19) has largely been replaced by CT angiography (CTA) or magnetic resonance angiography (MRA) which are non-invasive and can be performed immediately following a positive CT scan. CTA or MRA will provide information of the location and the anatomy of the aneurysm. Where there is high suspicion of an aneurysm despite a negative CTA, invasive cerebral angiography will be performed as this is regarded as the gold standard and is the most sensitive test for identifying aneurysms. There is a very small risk of permanent neurological complication associated with angiography in patients with SAH, reported as 0.07% (Cloft *et al.*, 1999). Multiple aneurysms are found in 20% of cases.

NURSING AND MEDICAL MANAGEMENT OF THE PATIENT WITH AN ANEURYSMAL SAH

Patients need to be closely monitored in the acute period as there are a number of secondary complications that can occur, which can result in further deterioration in the neurological condition of the patient. The nurse needs to be vigilant for early signs of deterioration and be aware of the specific management for each complication that can arise. It is therefore imperative that patients are nursed in an appropriate area where they can be closely monitored; the degree to which this will be required will depend on the grade of the SAH. The patient's neurological observations need to be monitored frequently in addition to respiratory and cardiovascular observations and fluid balance. Patients with a poor grade SAH will be nursed in a critical care unit and will have additional invasive monitoring as required. Common neurological and systemic complications of SAH include: rebleeding, hydrocephalus, vasospasm, raised ICP, hypo/hypernatraemia and cardiac arrhythmias. These complications, with the exception of

rebleeding, can all occur before or after the aneurysm has been treated. Where the care or management discussed is specific to either the pre- or post-treatment phase this will be clearly stated. The specific nursing and medical management for each complication is discussed below. Table 23.1 shows a summary of the nursing management.

Rebleed

The peak time for rebleeding to occur is within the first 24 hours. The risk of a rebleed remains a possibility until the aneurysm is treated. Without intervention to occlude the aneurysm 40% will rebleed within one month (Locksley, 1966). A rebleed occurs more commonly in the early hours following the initial bleed because the fibrin platelet plug that covers the point of rupture is very fragile, which makes it more vulnerable to disturbance with changes in arterial blood pressure. A rebleed occurring days after the initial SAH is thought to occur due to dissolution of the clot by natural fibrinolytic activity (Roos *et al.*, 2003). Antifibrinolytics can prevent this from occurring however they have not been found to improve outcome. The benefits are offset by the increase in poor outcome caused by cerebral ischeamia as a result of treatment with antifibrinolytics (Roos *et al.*, 2003).

A rebleed is usually more severe than the initial bleed and is often fatal. An experienced neuroscience nurse can usually recount experiences of talking to a patient coherently one minute and the next resuscitating the patient following a significant rebleed. Until such time as the aneurysm is treated the nurse should be alert to the possibility of a rebleed.

Ideally the patient is nursed in a quiet environment. A noisy environment for a patient who is already stressed with a headache would almost certainly elevate their blood pressure. Every effort should be made to reduce auditory stimuli such as unnecessarily loud monitor alarms and phone ring tones.

Sufficient analgesia to keep the patient pain free is essential. Often headache can be severe and can be a cause of agitation and distress for the patient. The severity of headache should be assessed regularly and analgesia prescribed based on the individual need of the patient. The most commonly used analgesics are paracetamol, codeine based analgesia, morphine and occasionally tramadol. Patients with severe headache may require two or more of these as regular analgesia. It is essential to have additional analgesia prescribed on the 'as required' side of the drug chart to reduce the time patients have to wait for analgesia, which can be an additional cause of distress and anxiety for the patient. Constipation is a common side-effect of

Table 23.1 Summary of the nursing management of patients with subarachnoid haemorrhage.

General risk	Nursing management
Airway – possible risk of airway obstruction due to reduced conscious level Breathing – possible risk of respiratory compromise	• Close monitoring of respiratory rate, depth and symmetry. Listen for sounds that may indicate partial airway obstruction, i.e. snoring, gurgling • Frequent monitoring of SpO_2 • Ensure suction is set up and ready to use and appropriate sized Guedel airways are available at bedside • Encourage regular deep breathing exercises. Liaise with physiotherapist to optimise respiratory care
Cardiovascular – risk of arrhythmias	• Close monitoring of rate, rhythm and volume of pulse. Grade 3 SAH and above require continuous cardiac monitoring • Monitor for arrhythmias. Refer to Chapter 14 for specific management of arrhythmias and pulmonary oedema
Pain	• Regular assessment of pain. Administer analgesia as required • Offer airline eyeshields • Nurse in a quiet darkened area • Regular reassurance and support
Neurological	• Frequent assessment of neurological observations • Inform medical and senior nursing colleagues of any deterioration in condition • Maintain bedrest with the head between 0 and 30° to optimise cerebral perfusion pressure. If known to have raised ICP maintain head at 30°
Specific complications Rebleeding	• Ensure blood pressure is maintained within set parameters • Nurse in a quiet environment and reduce noxious stimuli that could increase blood pressure • Avoid constipation – maintain adequate hydration, administer aperients • Offer regular support and reassurance
Vasospasm Prophylactic treatment Symptomatic vasospasm	• Nimodipine 60 mg PO every 4 hours for 21 days • Maintain a strict fluid balance chart, ensure a positive fluid balance • Triple H therapy when the aneurysm has been secured
Raised ICP	• See Chapter 7
Acute hydrocephalus	• See Chapter 25 for management of an EVD
Seizures	• Appropriate measures to maintain patient safety if seizure should occur • Administer AEDs (if prescribed)
Hyponatraemia	• Monitor electrolytes at least daily • Determine cause of hyponatraemia • Treat SIADH and CSW (see Chapter 16)
Fever	• Keep temperature <37°C • Refer to Chapter 14 for specific management
Hyperglycaemia	• Monitor blood glucose levels • Hyperglycaemia in those with poor clinical condition should be managed with an insulin infusion as per local protocol to keep the blood glucose levels within normal levels
Deep vein thrombosis	• Thigh-length anti-embolism stockings until fully mobile • Intermittent pneumatic compression devices may be used as an alternative or in addition to stockings (NICE, 2007)

AEDs – antiepileptic drugs; BP – blood pressure; CSW – cerebral salt wasting; EVD – external ventricular drain; SAH – subarachnoid haemorrhage; SIADH – syndrome of inappropriate antidiuretic hormone.

opioid analgesics which should be managed before it becomes a problem by ensuring adequate hydration, a balanced diet and the use of prophylactic aperients. Non-steroidal anti-inflammatory drugs (NSAIDs) are very effective, once the aneurysm has been excluded, for controlling pain. They help reduce the cerebral irritation caused by the inflammation to the meninges.

There is no evidence to suggest that bedrest reduces the incidence of a rebleed in patients with a low grade SAH. Most surgeons prefer patients to be on bedrest to prevent significant alterations in blood pressure. Patients with a grade 1 SAH, will usually have toilet privileges as it probably poses less of a risk than straining on a bedpan. Aperients (stool softeners) are prescribed to limit straining. Patients are nursed flat to 30 degrees; patients with poorer grade SAH who have raised ICP will usually require head elevation to 30° to lower ICP (refer to Chapter 7 for more detail), whereas patients with symptomatic cerebral vasospasm may be nursed flat to improve cerebral arterial blood flow (see: Delayed cerebral vasospasm).

Patients who are alert are informed about their condition and the possible risks of the intervention to secure the aneurysm; this elicits fears and anxiety in nearly all patients. Nurses need to make time to sit and listen to the patient's fears and to allay them where possible. It is always reassuring for patients to hear of others who have recently been successfully treated and discharged from hospital.

Management of blood pressure prior to the aneurysm being treated

Nursing management to reduce the risk of a rebleed is aimed at reducing the factors that could contribute to sudden changes in blood pressure (BP). Management of BP prior to the aneurysm being treated is not straightforward as the risk of a rebleed must be balanced with the need to maintain an adequate cerebral perfusion pressure (CPP) in patients with raised ICP.

There is no consensus on the ideal BP. Some clinicians advocate maintaining systolic BP (SBP) <160 mmHg to reduce the risk of a rebleed. However, reducing the BP could precipitate or accentuate cerebral ischaemia (Wiebers *et al.*, 2006). van Gijin *et al.* (2007) suggest that BP should only be treated if mean arterial pressure (MAP) is >130 mmHg. Wiebers *et al.* (2006) make a similar recommendation of treating BP if MAP >130 to 140 mmHg. If lowering of BP is required it is recommended that intravenous antihypertensives are used, e.g. labetolol (Wiebers *et al.*, 2006). This will enable a more controlled lowering of the BP, preventing a sudden drop that could be detrimental to cerebral tissue. The patient will require continuous monitoring of arterial BP and should be nursed in an appropriate environment to facilitate this. Parameters for BP should be agreed with the clinician based on the patient's baseline and their clinical condition, i.e. whether the patient has a significantly raised ICP. Management of BP following the aneurysm being treated is presented under the section on 'triple H therapy'.

Hydrocephalus

Acute hydrocephalus will occur within 24 hours in 10–20% of patients. Blood in the subarachnoid space congeals in and around the arachnoid villi (where CSF is reabsorbed) obstructing the CSF outflow. The obstructive hydrocephalus will result in raised ICP with a subsequent deterioration in the patient's neurological status. Deterioration in the patient's condition should be reported promptly to enable early intervention. Following a CT scan an external ventricular drain (EVD) will be inserted to divert the flow of CSF until such time as the CSF is clear of blood and normal flow can occur. For care of an EVD refer to Chapter 25.

Subacute hydrocephalus (within 7 days of the SAH) and delayed hydrocephalus (after 10 days of the SAH) are causes of delayed neurological deterioration.

Delayed cerebral vasospasm (DCV)

Delayed cerebral vasospam (DCV) is the narrowing of the lumen of cerebral vessels. The resultant increased cerebrovascular resistance in the affected arteries reduces the cerebral blood flow to cerebral tissue, which can result in cerebral ischaemia and can progress to infarction. It is proposed that DCV is caused by the release of a high concentration of certain substances from the erythrocytes of the blood clot as they disintegrate (Dietrich and Ralph, 2000), which occurs 3–4 days post SAH. The substance most implicated in the pathogenesis of DCV is oxyhaemoglobin which is thought to act as a spasmogen (Dietrich and Ralph, 2000). Others suggest that localised inflammatory responses, including the release of cytokines, may lead to the hamodynamic changes (Fassbender *et al.*, 2001). It is likely that the pathogenesis of DCV is multifactorial.

Delayed cerebral vasospasm occurs most commonly between days 3 to 10 after the SAH, with a peak at day 7 and usually subsides around day 14. It can have devastating consequences for the patient; 13–14% of patients will either die or have severe disabilities (Kassel *et al.*, 1990) and many more will have moderate long-term neurological impairment. Although 60% of patients with ASAH have angiographic evidence of vasospasm, approximately only

30% will become symptomatic, i.e. will develop ischaemic deficits.

The ischaemia that ensues from the DCV generally occurs over a few hours, presenting as an evolving ischaemic stroke, so it is imperative to be vigilant for early signs. Twenty-five percent of symptomatic patients will have a reduction in level of consciousness, 25% will have focal deficits involving the affected hemisphere and 50% will have both (Hijdra *et al.*, 1986). The spasm is usually most severe in the arteries closest to the ruptured aneurysm. As most aneurysms are of the internal carotid, anterior cerebral and middle cerebral arteries, these vessels are most commonly affected. The focal deficits that will ensue if spasm is symptomatic in these vessels is presented in Table 23.2.

Patients with poor grade SAH tend to have diffuse spasm. Owing to the possible number of differential diagnoses for the signs and symptoms of DCV, i.e. hydrocephalus and cerebral oedema, it is necessary to perform a CT to eliminate other intracranial causes. Hyponatreamia can also result in reduced consciousness and is a common problem following SAH, so serum sodium should also be checked. A transcranial doppler (TCD), which is a noninvasive measure of CBF that can be performed at the bedside, is sometimes used to assist with the diagnosis. It can detect increases in blood flow velocity which indicate the narrowing of vessels. A mean velocity of CBF of more than 120 cm per second in major vessels is indicative of vasospasm.

Nimodipine

Nimodipine has been found to significantly reduce morbidity and mortality rates associated with DCV (Rinkel *et al.*, 2005), however it does not prevent DCV from occurring. The dose is 60 mg four hourly, orally, for 21 days. Hypotension is problematic for some patients for whom 30 mg, two hourly, may be considered. When patients are unable to absorb via the oral route, IV nimodipine is administered via a central line, initially at a rate of 1 mg/hr because of the risk of profound hypotension. Continuous monitoring of arterial BP is essential and allows for early detection of hypotension. The infusion is increased to 2 mg/hr if BP is not compromised.

It is posited that nimodipine blocks calcium influx into the ischaemic neurones, and acts as a neuroprotecter, preventing further damage to the ischaemic cerebral tissue. It is likely that it also promotes collateral circulation by dilating minute cerebral arteries and so improving cerebral tissue perfusion (Rinkel *et al.*, 2005). Cerebral angiography has failed to demonstrate that nimodipine dilates the large cerebral vessels as was once thought.

Triple-H therapy: hypertension, hypervolaemia and haemodilution

The aim of triple –H therapy for DCV is to improve cerebral blood flow by increasing the BP, expanding the blood volume (hypervolaemia) and reducing blood viscosity (haemodilution)(Origitano *et al.*, 1990). Autoregulation is often impaired in the arteries that are affected by vasospasm and therefore blood flow through these affected vessels should respond passively to changes in systemic BP.

Administration of crystalloids and colloids will increase the intravascular volume (hypervolaemia) which will augment cardiac output and increase BP. Where volume expansion alone fails to achieve the required BP, noradrenaline is often prescribed. The administration of crystalloids reduces the viscosity of the blood (haemodilution) which is indicated by the fall in haematocrit. Lower haematocrit levels improve oxygen delivery to brain tissue (Wiebers *et al.*, 2006). This treatment is contraindicated if the aneurysm is untreated, due to the high risk of rebleeding, therefore early obliteration of the aneurysm is advocated when the clinical condition allows (Egge *et al.*, 2001).

There are no large prospective randomised trials to prove the effectiveness of this treatment and hence no

Table 23.2 Characteristic ischaemic deficits for the most commonly affected arteries

Arterial territory	Deficits
Anterior cerebral artery	• Contralateral hemiparesis (leg greater than the arm) • Apathy • Withdrawn • Incontinence • Expressive dysphasia (dominant hemisphere only)
Middle cerebral artery	• Contralateral hemiparesis and hemisensory loss (arm and face greater than the leg) • Expressive dysphasia (dominant hemisphere only) • Contralateral homonymous hemianopia
Internal carotid artery	• Symptoms and signs of middle cerebral and anterior cerebral arteries

agreed protocol of triple-H therapy. Most SAH patients are treated to some degree prophylactically by ensuring that they have a positive fluid balance. The administration of three litres of intravenous fluid in 24 hours (usually isotonic saline, 0.9%) is the norm with adjustments as needed depending on body size, haemodynamic measurements and electrolytes (Wiebers *et al.*, 2006). Maintaining a positive fluid balance and avoiding hypovolaemia is paramount and it is the nurse's responsibility to take appropriate measures to ensure adequate filling for the duration of the acute period (see Chapter 16 for assessment of fluid status).

If the patient develops symptomatic vasospasm, then more invasive measures to achieve triple-H are implemented expeditiously. Patients need invasive monitoring to guide treatment which requires the patient to be nursed in a critical care area. Parameters for BP, central venous pressure (CVP) and haematocrit should be set on an individual patient basis taking account of the patient's baseline BP and any co-morbidities that could predispose the patient to the complications associated with triple H therapy, i.e. pulmonary oedema and congestive cardiac failure (Egge *et al.*, 2001). Generally CVP is maintained between 8 and 12 mmHg and blood pressure 20–50 mmHg above baseline (Wiebers *et al.*, 2006). A vasopressor (most commonly noradrenaline) is often administered to achieve the latter following adequate filling with intravenous fluids.

Other measures to treat DCV

Dilatation of the affected vessels by cerebral angioplasty is performed by a skilled neuroradiologist in some specialist centres. Vasodilating drugs can be administered into the affected vessels during the procedure which can target the smaller vessels not accessible to mechanical angioplasty. Papaverine has been used for this purpose, however this drug has many side-effects and there is a need to find a safer more effective drug (Smith and Enterline, 2000). Preliminary studies using alternative drugs have demonstrated effective reversal of DCV by, e.g. intra-arterial milrinone, a phosphodiesterase III inhibitor which has vasodilating and inotropic properties (Arakawa *et al.*, 2001), and intrathecal sodium nitroprusside (SNP), a nitric oxide donor (Kumar *et al.*, 2003). Further studies are awaited to determine if the reversal in DCV translates into improved patient outcomes.

Magnesium is known to dilate cerebral arteries and to block N-methyl-D-aspartate (NMDA) receptors in injured neurones. In a subgroup analysis in the Cochrane review of all randomised clinical trials of calcium antagonists in SAH, magnesium was found to reduce the occurrence of delayed cerebral ischaemia (DCI) and that of poor outcome (van den Bergh, 2009). However the authors of the review concluded that further trials were required before conclusions could be drawn (Dorhout *et al.*, 2007). The results from a phase III randomised, placebo-controlled, double-blinded, multi-centre trial (MASH) are awaited (see also van den Bergh on behalf of MASH, 2005).

Raised intracranial pressure (ICP)

Patients with poor grade SAH (4 and 5) are likely to have an immediate and prolonged raised ICP. All patients are at risk of developing a delayed rise in ICP due to brain oedema and obstructive hydrocephalus. Management of ICP is presented in Chapter 7.

Seizures

Seizures are not uncommon following SAH particularly in patients with associated intracerebral haematoma. There are no controlled trials to establish whether the prophylactic administration of antiepileptic drugs (AEDs) reduces seizures. There is no consensus as to whether all SAH patients should receive prophylactic AEDs. Some suggest that prophylactic AEDs should be used for one week following SAH in all patients (Suarez *et al.*, 2006) on the basis that a seizure could lead to a rebleed before treatment. Whereas Wiebers *et al.* (2006) and Ropper *et al.* (2004) suggest administering AEDs only if the patient has a seizure. There is no evidence to suggest that seizures persist in those that have had a seizure/s in the acute period following SAH.

EXTRACRANIAL COMPLICATIONS ASSOCIATED WITH SAH

Neurogenic cardiac arrhythmias

Cardiac arrhythmias are common after a SAH. The cause and management of these cardiac arrhythmias are discussed in detail in Chapter 14.

Neurogenic pulmonary oedema (NPE)

Poor grade SAH patients may develop neurogenic pulmonary oedema. The cause and management of NPE are discussed in detail in Chapter 14.

Fever

Temperatures >38°C are common following a SAH, the causes of which are multifactorial. A source of infection can be identified in a large number of patients (Oliveira-Filho *et al.*, 2001), but for others no cause is found. Fever has been found to be associated with increased risk of symptomatic cerebral vasospasm and with poorer outcomes (Oliveira-Filho *et al.*, 2001). As with any acute injury to the brain, fever puts additional metabolic demands on the brain and can further compromise cerebral function. Despite little evidence from randomised controlled trials to support cooling, the general consensus is that appropriate management to reduce the temperature to normal levels should be taken (Wartenberg and Mayer, 2006). Refer to Chapter 14 for a detailed discussion of the possible causes and management of pyrexia.

Hyperglycaemia

Hyperglycaemia is commonly seen following all types of acute acquired brain injuries, and SAH is no exception. The severity of the disruption to normal glucose control is relative to the severity of the initial bleed and is attributed to the hypermetabolic and stress responses that occur following severe insults to the brain. Hyperglycaemia following SAH has been found to be a significant predictor of poor functional outcome (Sarrafzadeh *et al.*, 2004; Wartenberg and Mayer, 2006). Strict glucose control has been reported to improve outcomes in critically ill patients in intensive care (van den Berghe *et al.*, 2005). Whilst control of blood glucose levels with an insulin infusion is recommended (Feigin and Findlay 2005; Suarez *et al.*, 2006), there are no large clinical trials to support the safety and efficacy of this treatment for patients with SAH (Warternberg and Mayer, 2006).

Hyponatraemia

Hyponatraemia is the most common electrolyte disturbance following SAH. Two causes of hyponatraemia are cerebral salt wasting (CSW) and syndrome of inappropriate production of antidiuretic hormone (SIADH). It is essential that the cause is determined as the treatment is different for each of the causes. The management of both is discussed in Chapter 16. Daily monitoring of electrolytes in the acute period is essential. Utmost care must be taken when treating SIADH as restriction of fluids could predispose the patient to cerebral ischaemia.

Deep vein thrombosis

When the aneurysm has been secured the patient should be commenced on low molecular weight heparin (LMWH) (NICE, 2010). Until such time thigh-length antiembolism stockings should be used; intermittent pneumatic compression devices may be used as an alternative or in addition to stockings (NICE, 2010). Patients who are alert should be encouraged to perform regular foot exercises.

TREATMENT OF THE ANEURYSM

The aim is to secure the aneurysm to prevent a bleed/rebleed from occurring. Securing the aneurysm can be done either by surgical clipping or by endovascular coiling. For patients who are in good clinical condition, treatment of the aneurysm is performed at the earliest possible time and most certainly within 72 hours of the bleed to minimise the risk of rebleed and to enable treatment of symptomatic vasospasm. The treatment of patients in a poor clinical condition is largely dependent on the physician's assessment of probable outcome.

Traditionally craniotomy and clipping of the aneurysm was standard treatment, however the 1990s saw a radical change in the treatment of aneurysms. With the development of the guglielmi detachable coil in 1991, there was a gradual move towards interventional neuroradiologsts treating more aneurysms by endovascular coiling. A large randomised international subarachnoid aneurysm trial (ISAT) (n=2,143) compared the traditional clipping with coiling primarily in good grade patients (Molyneux *et al.*, 2002). Outcomes at one year were significantly more favourable for the group that had had coiling. Although the ISAT results are well accepted in the management of aneurysms, the main criticism of the ISAT is that the population in the study were largely young, had a good grade and involved aneurysms of the anterior circulation. This reduces the ability to generalise findings to all SAH patients. It is also acknowledged that not all aneurysms are suitable for coiling because of their shape and location.

It is generally agreed that close liaison between a practitioner who is experienced with endovascular techniques and a vascular neurosurgeon is required to determine the best treatment for individual patients (Suarez *et al.*, 2006).

Endovascular coiling

Coiling is performed in the angiography suite usually under general anaesthesia. A microcatheter is passed into the cerebral arteries via a femoral arterial sheath. Soft detachable coils, soldered onto a stainless steel delivery wire are introduced through the microcatheter into the sac of the aneurysm (see Figure 23.4). When positioned at the neck of the aneurysm the coils are advanced out of the catheter and into the fundus of the aneurysm. A low voltage current is applied to the delivery wire which dissolves the uninsulated connection between it and the platinum coil, leaving the coil situated in the fundus of the aneurysm. The guiding wire is removed. The positively charged coil is thought to attract the negatively charged blood elements thus inducing thrombosis within the aneurysm. A number

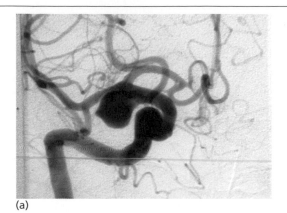

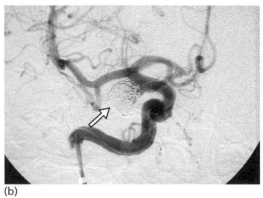

Figure 23.4 (a) Endovascular treatment of internal carotid artery aneurysm. (b) shows the aneurysm excluded from the circulation following the endovascular insertion of coils. Reproduced from Andrew Kaye, *Essential Neurosurgery*, Wiley-Blackwell, with permission.

of coils maybe required to pack the aneurysm depending on its size. The coiling reduces the pulsatile flow within the fundus and seals the weak part of the wall of the aneurysm. Over time further thrombus forms within the aneurysm and endothelialisation of the neck occurs.

The main limitation of coiling is that complete occlusion is only achieved in approx 70% of cases following the first attempt. However there is only a very small possibility that the aneurysm will rebleed; 0.016% in the ISAT trial rebled within the year following coiling. A follow-up angiogram is indicated at 6 months following the endovascular coiling to determine if the aneurysm has been completely occluded. Further elective endovascular coiling may be required to obliterate the aneurysm.

Complications post endovascular coiling

There is a very small risk that the aneurysm could rupture during the procedure which is associated with high mortality and morbidity rates. More commonly microthrombi can become dislodged during and following the procedure which make their way into the cerebral circulation distal to the aneurysm causing a thromboembolic event. The neurological deficits that ensue will depend on the size of the artery that has been affected. The subsequent cessation or reduction in blood flow can rapidly lead to ischaemia of the affected area. The patient is heparinised during the procedure to reduce the possible risk of thromboembolic events. Heparin infusion maybe continued after the procedure for 24 hours if there is thought to be a risk of microthrombi, with the aim of maintaining the activated partial thromboplastin time (APPT) at 2–3 times normal level. When coil loops are protruding into parent vessels then heparinisation is often used for 24–48 hours. Aspirin may also be prescribed for a number of weeks following the procedure. When coil loops are moving within the parent vessel stents may be used to wedge the coil loop into the aneurysm.

Migration of the coil from the aneurysm into the cerebral circulation is a rare complication however there is an increased risk with wide neck aneurysms.

SPECIFIC NURSING MANAGEMENT TO MONITOR/TREAT FOR POST-COILING COMPLICATIONS

Close monitoring of neurological condition is required post procedure, patients are generally nursed in a critical care area for at least 24 hours. The femoral puncture site should be checked at regular intervals for signs of bleeding, and circulation observations should be performed at each check to ensure that the limb is well perfused. If the patient is receiving a continuous heparin infusion post procedure then close monitoring of APTT is required, with the aim of maintaining the APTT at 2–3 times normal level. The heparin dose should be titrated accordingly.

The length of time that flat bedrest is required post procedure will depend on the patient's clinical condition and whether post procedure and/or complications of SAH, e.g. symptomatic vasospasm are present.

The nurse should alert the clinician immediately to any new focal neurological deficits that might indicate a thromboembolic event. If this is suspected then an urgent CT is warranted. If no other cause is detected on the CT that accounts for the deterioration, e.g. hydrocephalus, then a thromboembolic event is most likely. ABCIXIMAB

(Reopro®), a IIb/IIIa inhibitor which prevents platelet aggregation, may be given.

Clipping

Coiling is not always appropriate for all aneurysms, e.g. because of their shape. Unlike coiling, clipping offers a permanent secure aneurysm in most cases. Early surgical intervention is preferable to reduce the risk of a rebleed, however surgery may be delayed in patients with a poor clinical condition. Similarly to coiling close monitoring is required in a critical care area to allow for early detection of deterioration. In addition to monitoring for all possible complications associated with SAH (listed above) deterioration can occur post surgery as a result of brain oedema and haemorrhage. Refer to Chapter 20 for post craniotomy care.

PROGNOSTIC FACTORS

Rosengart *et al.* (2007) reported the non-modifiable predictors of unfavourable outcome (those present on admission) as: increasing age, high WFNS grade on admission, greater SAH thickness on CT, intraventricular and intracerebral haemorrhage and history of hypertension. Variables present during hospitalisation associated with poor outcome were: symptomatic vasospasm, infarction and temperature >38°C on the 8th day (Rosengart *et al.*, 2007).

OUTCOMES

Despite advances in management strategies for SAH, the mortality rate remains high. Hop *et al.* (1997) reviewed 21 studies between the years 1960 and 1992, and found that the mortality rates varied between 32 and 67%. The case fatality during this period decreased by 0.5% per year. There are no current data of a similar size SAH population to determine whether the number of deaths has continued to decrease at the same rate.

The outcomes for SAH survivors are less well studied than the traumatic head injury population, however there are similarities between the patient populations in the patterns of physical and neuropsychological deficits that follow.

Hackett and Anderson (2000) conducted a follow-up study of a large well defined SAH population. One year following SAH (n = 432), 56% of the population were alive. Many patients continued to experience significant reductions in quality of life; 46% of survivors reported an incomplete recovery, 50% had ongoing memory problems, 39% had disturbances in their mood, 10% had self-care problems and 14% had speech problems. These impairments in neuropsychological and physical functioning significantly impacted on the individuals to perform their social roles in the family or the workplace. This study reported that two thirds of survivors returned to paid employment whereas an earlier study had reported a less favourable outcome, of only one third (Hellawell *et al.*, 1999).

Physical impairments are more easily identified than subtle changes in cognitive function and behaviour. Ogden *et al.* (1993) reported that patients who were regarded as having a 'good outcome' by a neurologist had high level deficits in memory and cognitive functioning identified by neuropsychological examination. This highlights the importance of testing such functions by the appropriate professionals prior to discharge. Impairments in some patients may be subtle and only recognised by those closest to the patient. Concerns expressed by family members should be taken seriously and assessments by the occupational therapist and neuropsychologist should be conducted prior to discharge from hospital to allow early institution of appropriate therapy. Symptoms such as headache, fatigue, sleep disturbance and irritability are also common problems that can persist.

Following discharge, early follow-up by either the clinical nurse specialist (CNS) or the medical team is important to address any cognitive or behavioural problems that were not identified until the patient returned home.

Effect on family members

Family members are also significantly affected as most of the ongoing care, which is often long-term, falls to those closest to the patient (Mezue *et al.*, 2004). The high personal and emotional cost to the carer has been highlighted in recent studies (Pritchard *et al.*, 2001; Mezue *et al.*, 2004). These findings are especially significant since SAH affects a younger population and could indirectly affect the long-term recovery of the patient in addition to leading to the breakdown of the family. It is imperative that ongoing support is available to patient and family. Follow up by a multiprofessional team is essential to monitor ongoing problems and to offer expert advice. The clinical nurse specialist can be an invaluable source of help in hospital and following discharge.

The Brain and Spine Foundation (www. brainandspine.org.uk) is a good source of information and advice for family members. The Brain Aneurysm Foundation (www.bafound.org) is an American website but provides valuable information and advice for patients and family.

ARTERIOVENOUS MALFORMATIONS

Arteriovenous malformations (AVM) are congenital lesions. They are composed of a complex tangled amalgamation of veins and arteries with an absence of capillaries. They generally have several torturous arterial feeding vessels winding around a vascular knot of tortuous vessels called the 'nidus'. Due to the absence of capillaries, blood flows under high pressure from the nidus into large draining veins creating a high intraluminal pressure, resulting in the veins being dilated and aneurysmal in appearance and puts them at risk of rupture. A number of patients will have aneurysms of the arteries feeding the nidus, of the nidus itself or of vessels remote from the AVM. There are often small areas of haemorrhage and calcification within the AVM.

AVM lesions are graded before treatment according to the Spetzler–Martin grading system (Spetzler and Martin, 1986); the system is useful in predicting the outcome of therapeutic treatment. It considers the size and location, i.e. whether it is situated near to functional areas of the brain (eloquent), of the lesion, and whether or not it has deep venous drainage. Grade I AVMs are small, superficial, and located in non-eloquent areas of the cortex whereas grade V AVMs are large, deep, and situated near eloquent areas of the brain (see Figure 23.5). The higher the grade the more risk involved in treating the lesion.

INCIDENCE

AVMs are relatively uncommon. It is difficult to know what their exact prevalence is as many remain symptomless and therefore go undetected. It is estimated to be approximately 0.01% of the general population (Friedlander,

2007). The sexes are equally affected. Haemorrhage from AVMs accounts for approximately 2% of all strokes (Friedlander, 2007). In a population based study in Minnesota, the detection rate for symptomatic cases was 1.2 per 100,000 person-years (Brown *et al.*, 1996).

AETIOLOGY

No genetic or environmental risk factors for cerebral AVM have been clearly identified. AVMs are congenital and are thought to have a long developmental period. They are not regarded as familial (Friedlander, 2007).

PRESENTATION SIGNS AND SYMPTOMS

Those that become symptomatic usually do so in the second to fourth decade. The most common presentation is an intracerebral haemorrhage (ICH) and less commonly a SAH or intraventricular haemorrhage, depending on the position of the AVM. Approximately 20–25% of patients present with seizures, this presentation is more common if the AVM is situated near the cortex. Patients may also present with headache or with a progressive neurological ischaemic deficit, e.g. hemiparesis or intellectual impairment. The ischaemic deficits arise because of the 'steal phenomenon'. Due to the rapid flow of blood through the arteriovenous shunts of the AVM, blood is diverted or 'stolen' from adjacent normal brain which results in the area becoming ischaemic.

Assessment of the lesion

An MRI and MRA will provide detail of the AVM in relation to surrounding structures. An invasive cerebral angiography is the gold standard to determine the anatomy of

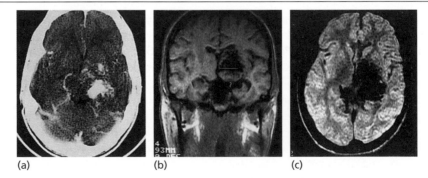

(a)   (b)   (c)

Figure 23.5 (a) The arteriovenous malformation enhances vividly on the CT scan after intravenous contrast and the major dilated feeding vessels can be seen. (b) The MRI shows the position of the malformation in coronal and axial planes and further information about the feeding vessels and draining veins (c). Reproduced from Andrew Kaye, *Essential Neurosurgery*, Wiley-Blackwell, with permission.

the AVM, i.e. the size, which vessels are feeding and draining the nidus and whether there are aneurysms present.

TREATMENT

AVMs can be treated by surgical excision, endovascular embolisation, radiosurgery, or by a combination of these. The possible benefits versus risks are assessed for each individual patient as to which treatment would be most effective.

If haemorrhage is the presenting sign there is not the same urgency to treat the AVM as there is for aneurysms owing to the fact that AVMs are not associated with the high rate of rebleeding as aneurysms. The patient will usually be given time to recover prior to undergoing treatment of the AVM

There is currently no agreement on how best to treat patients that have a diagnosed unruptured AVM. Because the annual haemorrhage rate for this population is relatively low at 2–4% per annum (Mast *et al.*, 1997), some argue that it may be better not to treat the AVM, particularly in older patients. There are however, a number of features of the AVM that are regarded as high risk for haemorrhage. These include deep location, deep venous drainage, and those with arterial aneurysms, and would be taken into consideration when making a decision about whether to treat or not. Each patient is assessed on an individual basis and the risks of intervening are assessed against the risks of leaving the AVM untreated. Following haemorrhage the risk of a rebleed in the following 12 months increases threefold, but decreases to 2–4% in successive years.

To determine how best to manage patients with unruptured AVMs, a randomised trial of unruptured brain arteriovenous malformations (ARUBA) is being conducted in the United States, Canada, Europe, and Australia. A total of 800 patients in 90 centres will be randomly assigned to invasive therapy (endovascular, surgical, and/or radiation therapy) versus medical management alone. Patients will be followed for a minimum of 5 years and a maximum of 7.5 years (mean, 6.25 years) from randomisation. Final study results will be available in 2012 (Wiebers *et al.*, 2003).

Craniotomy and surgical resection

AVMs are excised by microsurgical techniques with the operating microscope (Ogilvy *et al.*, 2001). Complete resection is usually possible for most grade I, II and III AVMs. Grade III are usually treated with embolisation prior to surgical excision (see: Embolisation). Surgical resection for grade I, II and III AVMs is associated with a high success rate with very low mortality and morbidity (Hamilton and Spetzler, 1994). Grade IV and V AVMs are associated with a high risk of operative mortality and morbidity that exceeds the risks associated with the natural history of the lesion (Fiorella *et al.*, 2006), therefore these lesions are rarely treated by surgical resection.

Embolisation

Patients will either have the embolisation under general anaesthetic or under deep sedation, the latter allows for intermittent testing of neurological status. There is no evidence to suggest that complication rates are lower for one or the other (Ogilvy *et al.*, 2001). Embolisation is most frequently used to reduce the size of the AVM prior to radiosurgery or surgical resection. The main feeding vessels are embolised, i.e. an embolic agent is infused into the vessels via a microcatheter to interrupt the blood flow to the lesion thus reducing the surgical risk of haemorrhage. For many patients more than one embolisation is required prior to resection. In a small number of patients with small AVMs, embolisation may be a successful cure.

Advancements in the development of microcatheter technology and liquid embolic agents have enabled small vessels deep in cerebral structures to be treated that were previously inaccessible (Linfante and Wakhloo, 2007). If surgical resection is to follow embolisation it is usually performed within a few days of the final embolisation. Palliative embolisation is sometimes offered to those with inoperable AVMs (grade IV and V) who have progressive neurological deficits. The aim is to reduce the flow through the AVM in the hope of reducing the 'steal effect' and thereby limiting further neurological deterioration (Ogilvy *et al.*, 2001).

Ledezema *et al.* (2006) reported outcomes of 295 embolisation procedures in 168 patients. Excellent or good outcomes (Glasgow Outcome Scale ≥ 4) were achieved in 152 (90.5%) patients; unfavorable outcomes (Glasgow Outcome Scale 1 to 3) were 3.0% at discharge with a 1.2% mortality related to the procedure. The majority of the embolisations were performed as an adjunct to surgery or radiosurgery. Predictors of unfavourable outcomes were: deep venous drainage, Grade III to V and periprocedural haemorrhage (Ledezma *et al.*, 2006).

Stereotactic radiosurgery (radiotherapy)

Radiosurgery is a sharply localised, single dose of high radiation (Zabel Du –Bois *et al.*, 2006). It can be delivered by one of two machines: a gamma knife or the linear accelerator (LINAC). A CT scan and cerebral angiogram are undertaken with a stereotactic frame in place. Using the frame and coordinates, the location of the nidus can be plotted. The aim of treatment is to completely obliterate the AVM with minimal injury to the surrounding brain tissue. The effects of the radiation occur gradually over months to three years. It is thought that the walls of the vessels thicken and eventual closure of the lumens occur (Tu *et al.*, 2006). Patients remain at the same risk of haemorrhage within the latency period as they would if the AVM had been untreated and this is therefore not the treatment choice for those who present with a haemorrhage.

Seizures may become more frequent in the days and weeks following treatment. Nausea, vomiting and headaches may also be problematic in the early post-treatment phase, although these complications are rare. Delayed complications are more serious and include radiation necrosis and cerebral oedema. Radiation necrosis occurs in approximately 10% of patients. The oedema that accompanies the radiation necrosis is treated with corticosteroids, or in some patients it can resolve spontaneously. However, in the minority of cases it may be necessary to resort to surgical resection of the affected area so as to improve functional and neurological outcome (Massengale *et al.*, 2006).

Radiosurgery is recommended when the AVM is less than 3 cm in diameter and is located in an eloquent area where resection is likely to cause neurological deficits (Ogilvy *et al.*, 2001, Friedlander, 2007). Treatment of grade IV and V AVMs with radiosurgery is associated with very significant risks of morbidity and mortality and is therefore not recommended (Han *et al.*, 2003).

NURSING MANAGEMENT

The nursing management of patients with AVMs presenting with an ICH will be the same as for patients who have had an ICH from other causes (refer to Chapter 22 for nursing management). Those presenting with a SAH from an AVM will have a more benign clinical course than aneurysmal SAH patients because vasospasm and rebleeds are rare. Therefore there is no urgency to treat the AVM, generally patients will recover from the initial bleed before treatment commences.

The post-operative nursing management following craniotomy and surgical resection of AVM is the same as for any post-operative craniotomy procedure and is presented in Chapter 20. Complications that may occur are haemorrhage and cerebral oedema.

Recommendations from the special writing group of the Stroke Council (Ogilvy *et al.*, 2001) recommend that patients are monitored in a neurological intensive care for a minimum of 24 hours. Normotension and euvolaemia are recommended with the exception of a minority of

cases, where tight control of blood pressure may be prescribed to reduce the risk of post-operative haemorrhage (see: Post-operative nursing management following embolisation) (Ogilvy *et al.*, 2001). A post-operative check angiogram is routinely performed to ensure the AVM has been completely excised.

The post-operative nursing management following embolisation

The patient is closely monitored for potential neurological deterioration which can arise due to haemorrhage or ischaemia. Venous occlusion with embolic agents can lead to outflow obstruction with subsequent haemorrhge. Less commonly following embolisation of large AVMs, as a result of reduction in arteriovenous shunting, the CPP may suddenly increase in the surrounding brain tissue resulting in acute post-embolisation haemorrhage. If this is a perceived risk following the procedure then hypotensive treatment may be prescribed post-operatively to maintain a low systolic blood pressure (Fiorella *et al.*, 2006). The parameter for the BP will be decided on an individual basis taking account of the baseline BP. Ischaemia can occur for the same reason as it does for aneurysms, i.e. catheter-induced thrombotic emboli.

Anticoagulant is not usually given post procedure unless a venous thrombosis arises as a complication of the procedure or if venous outflow is sluggish. In such cases a heparin infusion will be administered (see: Specific nursing management to monitor/treat for post-coiling complications).

Patients are generally maintained on bedrest overnight until they are reviewed by the neuroradiologist.

OUTCOMES

The outcomes for patients following AVM haemorrhage are better than for those caused by aneurysms, which is partly due to the younger age of patients and because AVMs are not associated with as many severe complications. Haemorrhage from an AVM is associated with a 5–10% risk of death and approximately 30% risk of a permanent or disabling neurological deficit (ApSimon *et al.*, 2002).

Although the outcome for the majority of patients with AVMs is more favourable than for those with aneurysms, the minority can suffer similar longterm disabilities to those associated with SAH.

OTHER VASCULAR MALFORMATIONS

Much less common vascular abnormalities are cavernous malformations and venous malformations.

Cavernous malformations

Cavernous malformations are small in size; they vary from a few millimetres to 3 centimetres. Their shape resembles that of a raspberry. They consist of a cluster of abnormal dilated blood vessels and can be found anywhere within the brain. Patients will either present with seizures, a progressive neurological deficit or intracranial haemorrhage (<25%). If and when these malformations become symptomatic they are usually surgically treated and less commonly treated with radiosurgery.

Venous malformations

Venous malformations are composed of abnormal veins that drain into a dilated venous trunk. They are usually situated deep in cerebral white matter. Haemorrhage is rare and their clinical importance is unclear. Venous malformations are usually treated conservatively as there is almost no risk of haemorrhage. In the rare cases where haemorrhage does occur and surgery is performed a cavernous malformation that wasn't previously identified is usually found to have caused the haemorrhage (Wiebers *et al.*, 2006).

SUMMARY

Despite the significant advances in endovascular embolisation and treatments for cerebral vasospasm, ASAH is still associated with substantial morbidity and mortality. The secondary complications that arise contribute significantly to the poor outcomes associated with ASAH. Nursing patients following ASAH can be challenging as there are numerous complications that patients can develop which can significantly hamper their clinical progress. Skilled and knowledgeable nurses play an essential role in detecting and acting upon early changes in the patient's neurological condition and ensuring that medical management is implemented expeditiously.

Although the outcome for the majority of patients with AVMs is more favourable than for those with aneurysms, the minority can suffer similar long term cognitive, physical, emotional and behavioural impairments. Collaborative working with other allied health professionals to identify and appropriately manage individual problems is paramount to enable optimal recovery.

Subarachnoid haemorrhage: patient perspective

Subarachnoid haemorrhage is traumatic – sudden and shocking – but it was several weeks after leaving hospital, that its impact dawned on me. At the time, I was extraordinarily calm. Having been told all the possible risk factors of surgery, I simply accepted that I had no option but to sign the consent form.

Care on the ward helped me to cope. Once diagnosed, I felt confident that I was in good and knowledgeable hands. Being regularly monitored and looked after by kind and reassuring nurses, I felt very safe and was happy to let the 'professionals' take charge.

As well as the specialist neuro nursing care, I recall other seemingly small but important things – being fed when I was too weak to feed myself; and a wonderful bed bath after yet another sleepless night. Although the ward was busy, the calm atmosphere helped me to remain calm as well. The 'compulsory' rest hour after lunch when visitors were excluded, and the lights turned down was very welcome.

Close friends and family had a rather different experience, having been (not surprisingly) extremely worried and upset when I was very ill. I welcomed their visits, although some of them found visiting a 'brain surgery' ward rather daunting; one or two people later admitted they simply hadn't been able to face coming in.

In hospital, I found it difficult to retain much information. A specialist nurse drew a picture of an aneurysm and explained about forfeiting my driving licence. A 2-page handout on SAH and recovery was useful, though rather general. More detailed written information and advice would have been good.

Moving back to the hospital from which I'd been admitted, communication between the two was poor. Staff on the noisy general medical ward seemed to have little or no understanding of SAH.

Back home, I gradually realised that recovery would be lengthy. Despite being 'neurologically intact' [GOS 1], I still had some cognitive difficulties, persisting significant mental fatigue, depression, anxiety, and loss of self-confidence. Hospital care was excellent but post-discharge support was non-existent, other than outpatient follow-up with the neurosurgeon. I would have welcomed a support group, a phone number for the ward for my specific queries, and some psychological support (for cognitive and emotional difficulties). My GP offered to see me – six weeks after I left hospital! My main lifelines were good friends and a telephone helpline (Brain and Spine Foundation).

REFERENCES

ApSimon HT, Reef H, Phadke RV *et al.* (2002) A population-based study of brain arteriovenous malformation: long-term treatment outcomes. *Stroke* 33:2794–2800.

Arakawa Y, Kikuta K, Hojo M *et al.* (2001) Milrinone for the treatment of cerebral vasospasm after subarachnoid haemorrhage: Report of seven cases. *Neurosurgery* 48:723–728.

Brown RD, Wiebers DO, Torner JC *et al.* (1996), Incidence and prevalence of intracranial vascular malformations in Olmsted County, Minnesota, 1965–1992. *Neurology* 46:949–952.

Cloft, HJ, Gregory J, Dion JE (1999) Risk of cerebral angiography in patients with subarachnoid hemorrhage, cerebral aneurysm, and arteriovenous malformation: a meta-analysis. *Stroke* 30:317–320.

de Rooij NK, Linn FHH, van der Plas JA *et al.* (2007) Incidence of subarachnoid haemorrhage: a systematic review with emphasis on region, age, gender and time trends. *Journal of Neurology, Neurosurgery and Psychiatry* 78:1365–1372.

Dietrich HH, Ralph GD (2000) Molecular keys to the problems of cerebral vasospasm. *Neurosurgery* 46(3):517–530.

Dorhout Mees S, Rinkel GJE, Feigin VL *et al.* (2007) Calcium antagonists for aneurysmal subarachnoid haemorrhage. *Cochrane Database of Systematic Reviews* Issue 3. Art. No.: CD000277. DOI: 10.1002/14651858.CD000277. pub3.

Egge, A, Waterloo K, Sjoholm H *et al.* (2001) Prophylactic hyperdynamic postoperative fluid therapy after aneurysmal subarachnoid haemorrhage: a clinical, prospective, randomised, controlled study. *Neurosurgery* 49(3):593–606.

Fassbender K, Hodapp B, Rossol S *et al.* (2001) Inflammatory cytokines in subarachnoid haemorrhage: association with abnormal blood flow velocities in basal arteries. *Journal of Neurology, Neurosurgery and Psychiatry* 70:534–537.

Feigin VL, Findlay M (2005) Advances in subarachnoid haemorrhage. *Stroke* 37:305–313.

Feigin VL, Rinkel GJE, Lawes CM *et al.* (2005) Risk factors for subarachnoid haemorrhage. An updated systematic review of epidemiological studies. *Stroke* 36:2773–2780.

Fiorella D, Albuquerque FC, Woo HH *et al.* (2006) The role of neuroendovascular therapy for the treatment of brain arteriovenous malformations. *Neurosurgery Online* 59(5):S3-163–S3-177.

Friedlander RM (2007) Arteriovenous malformations of the brain. *The New England Journal of Medicine* 356:2704–2712.

Greebe P, Gabriel RN, Rinkel MD (2007) Life expectancy after perimesencephalic subarachnoid haemorrhage. *Stroke* 38:1222–1224.

Hackett ML, Anderson CS (2000) Health outcomes 1 year after subarachnoid haemorrhage *Neurology* 55:658–662.

Hamilton MG, Spetzler RF (1994) The prospective application of a grading system for arteriovenous malformations. *Neurosurgery* 34:2–7.

Han P, Ponce FA, Spetzler RF *et al.* (2003) Intention-to-treat analysis of Spetzler-Martin Grades IV and V arteriovenous malformations: natural history and treatment paradigm. *Journal of Neurosurgery* 98:3.

Hankey G, Wardlaw J (2008) *Clinical Neurology* (2nd edition). London: Manson Publishing.

Hellawell D, Taylor R, Pentland B (1999) Persisting symptoms and carer views of outcome after subarachnoid haemorrhage. *Clinical Rehabilitation* 13: 333–340.

Hijdra A, van Gijin J, Stefano S *et al.* (1986) Delayed cerebral ischaemia after aneurismal subarachnoid haemorrhage: clinicoanatomic correlations. *Neurology* 36:329–333.

Hop JW, Rinkel GJ, Algra A *et al.* (1997) Case fatality rates and functional outcome after subarachnoid haemorrhage: a systematic review. *Stroke* 28:660–664.

Huang J, van Gelder JM (2002) The probability of sudden death from rupture of intracranial aneurysms: a meta-analysis. *Neurosurgery* 51:1101–1105.

Kassel NF, Torner JC, Haley EC *et al.* (1990) The international cooperative study on the timing of aneurysm surgery: Part 1 – Overall management results. *Journal of Neurosurgery* 73(1):18–36.

Kumar R, Pathak A, Mathuriya SN *et al.* (2003) Intraventricular sodium nitroprusside therapy: A future promise for refractory subarachnoid haemorrhage-induced vasospasm. *Neurology India* 51(2):197–202.

Ledezma CJ, Hoh BL, Carter J *et al.* (2006) Complications of cerebral arteriovenous malformation embolisation: multivariate analysis of predictive factors. *Neurosurgery Online* 58(4):602–611.

Linfante I, Wakhloo AK (2007) Brain aneurysms and arteriovenous malformations advancements and emerging treatments in endovascular embolization. *Stroke* 38:1411–1417.

Locksley HB (1966) Natural history of subarachnoid haemorrhage, intracranial aneurysms and arteriovenous malformations. Based on 6368 cases in the cooperative study. *Journal of Neurosurgery* 25:321–368.

Massengale J, Levy R, Marcellus M *et al.* (2006) Outcomes of surgery for resection of regions of symptomatic radiation injury after stereotactic radiosurgery for arteriovenous malformations. *Neurosurgery* 59(3):553–560.

Mast H, Young WL, Koennecke HC *et al.* (1997) Risk of spontaneous haemorrhage after diagnosis of cerebral arteriovenous malformation. *Lancet* 350:1065–1068.

Mayberg MR, Batjer HH, Dacey R (1994) Guidelines for the management of aneurysmal subarachnoid haemorrhage: a statement for healthcare professionals from a special writing group of the Stroke Council, American Heart Association. *Stroke* 25:2315–2318.

Mezue W, Mathew B, Draper P *et al.* (2004) The impact of care on carers of patients treated with aneurismal subarachnoid haemorrhage. *British Journal of Neurosurgery* 18(20):135–137.

Molyneux AJ, Kerr RS, Stratton I *et al.* (2002) International Subarachnoid Aneurysm Trial (ISAT) of neurosurgical clipping and endovascular coiling in 2143 patietns with ruptured aneurysms: a randomised trial. *Lancet* 360:1267–1274.

National Institute for Health and Clinical Excellence (2010) *Guideline 46: Venous Thromobembolism: Reducing the risk of venous thromboembolism in inpatients undergoing surgery.* London: NICE.

Ogden JA, Mee EW, Henning M (1993) A prospective study of impairment of cognition and memory and recovery after subarachnoid hemorrhage. *Neurosurgery* 33:572–587.

Ogilvy CS, Stieg PE, Awad I *et al.* (2001) AHA Scientific Statement. Recommendations for the management of intracranial arteriovenous malformations: a statement for healthcare professionals from a special writing group of the Stroke Council, American Stroke Association. *Stroke* 32:1458–1471.

Oliveira-Filho J, Ezzeddine MA, Segal AZ *et al.* (2001) Fever in subarachnoid haemorrhage. Relationship to vasospasm and outcome. *Neurology* 56:1299–1304.

Origitano TC, Wascher TM, Reichman H *et al,* (1990) Sustained increased cerebral blood flow with prophylactic hypertensive hypervolaemic hemodilution (Triple-HTherapy) after subarchnoid haemorrhage. *Neurosurgery* 27(5):729–774.

Pobereskin LH (2001) Incidence and outcome of subarachnoid haemorrhage: a retrospective population based study. *Journal of Neurology, Neurosurgery and Psychiatry* 70:340–344.

Pritchard C, Foulkes l, Lang DA *et al.* (2001) Psychosocial outcomes for patients and carers after aneurysmal subarachnoid haemorrhage. *British Journal of Neurosurgery* 15:456–463.

Rinkel GJE, Feigin VL, Algra A *et al.* (2005) Calcium antagonists for aneurysmal subarachnoid haemorrhage. *Cochrane Database Systematic Reviews* 1:CD000277.

Roos YB, Rinkel GJE, Vermeulen M *et al.* (2003) Antifibrinolytic therapy for aneurysmal subarachnoid haemorrhage. *Cochrane Database of Systematic Reviews* Issue 2. Art. No.: CD001245. DOI: 10.1002/14651858.CD001245.

Ropper AH, Gres D, Dienger M *et al.* (2004) *Neurological and Neurosurgical Intensive Care* (3rd edition). Philadelphia: Lippincott Williams and Wilkins.

Rosengart AJ, Schulthesis K, Tolentino J *et al.* (2007) Prognostic factors for outcome in patients with aneurysmal subarachnoid haemorrhage. *Stroke* 38(8):2315–2321.

Sames TA, Storrow AB, Finkelstein JA *et al.* (1996) Sensitivity of new generation computed tomography in subarachnoid haemorrhage. *Academic Emergency Medicine* 3:16–20.

Sarrafzadeh A, Haux D, Kuchler I *et al.* (2004) Poor grade aneurysmal subarchnoid haemorrhage: relationship of cerebral metabolism to outcome. *Journal of Neurosurgery* 100:400–406.

Suarez JI, Tarr RW, Selman WR (2006) Aneurysmal subarachnoid haemorrhage. *New England Journal of Medicine* 354:387–396.

Smith T, Enterline D (2000) Endovascular treatment of cerebral vasospasm. *Journal of Vascular and International Radiology* 11(5):547–559.

Spetzler RF, Martin NA (1986) A proposed grading system for arteriovenous malformations. *Journal of Neurosurgery* 65:476–483.

Tu J, Stoodley M, Morgan M *et al.* (2006)Responses of arteriovenous malformations to radiosurgery: ultrastructural changes. *Neurosurgery Online* 58(4):749–758.

UK National External Quality Assessment Scheme (NEQAS) for Immunochemistry Working Group (2003) National guidelines for analysis of cerebrospinal fluid for bilirubin in suspected subarachnoid haemorrhage. *Annals of Clinical Biochemistry* 40:481–488.

van den Berghe G, Schoonheydt K, Becx P *et al.* (2005) Insulin therapy protects the central and peripheral nervous system of intensive care patients. *Neurology* 64:1348–1353.

van den Bergh WM on behalf of the MASH Study Group (2005) Magnesium sulfate in aneurysmal subarachnoid haemorrhage: A randomised controlled trial. *Stroke* 36:1011–1015.

van den Bergh WM (2009) Magnesium in subarachnoid haemorrhage: proven beneficial? *Magnesium Research* 22(3):121–126.

van Gijin J, Kerr RS, Rinkel GJ (2007) Subarachnoid haemorrhage. *Lancet* 369:306–318.

Wartenburg KE, Mayer SA (2006) Medical complications after subarachnoid haemorrhage: new strategies for prevention and management. *Current Opinion in Critical Care* 12(2):78–84.

Wiebers DO, Feigin VL, Brown RD (2006) *Jr Handbook of Stroke.* (2nd edition). Philadelphia: Lippincott Williams & Wilkins.

Wiebers DO, Whisnant JP, Huston J *et al.* (2003) International Study of Unruptured Intracranial Aneurysms Investigators. Unruptured intracranial aneurysms: natural history, clinical outcome, and risks of surgical and endovascular treatment. *Lancet* 362:103–110.

Zabel-Du Bois A, Milker-Zabel S, Huber P *et al.* (2006) Stereotactic LINAC-based radiosurgery in the treatment of cerebral arteriovenous malformations located deep, involving corpus callosum, motor cortex, or brainstem. *International Journal of Radiation Oncology, Biology and Physics* 64:1044–1048.

24

Management of Patients with Central Nervous System Infections

Ava Easton, Stephen Pewter, Huw Williams, Leann Johnson, Ed Wilkins and Ann-Marie Mestecky

ACUTE BACTERIAL MENINGITIS

Ann-Marie Mestecky

Meningitis is inflammation of the meninges; more specifically the arachnoid and pia membranes and the intervening subarachnoid space. Bacterial meningitis is inflammation caused by bacterial infection. It is associated with high morbidity and mortality and requires urgent medical intervention to minimise the impact of the disease. Viral meningitis generally has a more benign clinical course and rarely requires hospitalisation. Meningitis can also be caused by other pathogens, e.g. fungi or parasites, however these are rare and most often affect people who are immunocompromised.

AETIOLOGY AND EPIDEMIOLOGY

The most common causes of acute community acquired bacterial meningitis are *Neisseria meningitidis* and *Streptococcus pneumoniae*. *Mycobacterium tuberculosis* meningitis has a more chronic presentation and is presented at the end of the section on meningitis.

Neisseria meningitidis (meningococcus) is the most common cause of acute bacterial meningitis in the UK. It mainly affects babies and children under five years. Older teenagers are the second most at risk group. There are a

number of known serogroups (strains) of meningococcal bacteria, the most common of which are *Neisseria meningitidis* serogroup B and C. The introduction of the MenC vaccine has led to a decline in the number of cases of serogroup C and consequently the majority of cases are now caused by MenB (Meningitis Research Foundation, 2009). A meningococcal group B vaccine is currently going through phase III trials.

Meningococci are spread through the exchange of saliva and other respiratory secretions during coughing, sneezing and intimate kissing. Close prolonged contact is usually required to transmit the bacteria (Health Protection Agency, 2009). People harmlessly carry meningococci in the nasopharynx and it is not known why some people develop the disease. Factors such as a compromised immune system can provide an opportunity for the bacteria to overcome the body's immune defences to cause disease. Meningococci can cause meningitis and/or septicaemia. Most people will have symptoms of both. When meningococci cause meningitis and/or septicaemia it is called meningococcal disease. Meningococcal disease affects around 2,000 people in the UK and Ireland every year (Meningitis Research Foundation, 2009).

The bacterium *Streptococcus pneumoniae* (pneumococcus) is the second most common cause of meningitis in the UK, but accounts for the majority of cases in adults. There are 90 serotypes of this bacterium. Similar to meningococci, these bacteria can live in the nasopharynx usually without causing disease. A compromised immune system, e.g. HIV, alcoholism, splenectomy, chronic otitis media,

Neuroscience Nursing: Evidence-Based Practice, 1st Edition.
Edited by Sue Woodward and Ann-Marie Mestecky
© 2011 Blackwell Publishing Ltd

sickle cell disease, are particular factors that predispose people to pneumococcal meningitis.

The pneumococcal conjugate vaccine was introduced to the childhood immunisation programme in the UK in September 2006 (Donovan and Blewitt, 2009). It protects against seven of the most common serotypes and has led to a subsequent reduction in childhood cases. The efficacy of the vaccine has not been proven in older adults (Hayderman *et al.*, 2003).

A CSF leak due to head injury or neurosurgery allows direct invasion of the meninges by bacteria. *Staphylococcus aureus* is the most common cause following craniotomy. *S. pneumoniae* and gram negative bacilli such as *Escherichia coli* (*E. coli*), *Pseudomonas* spp and *Klebsiella* spp are the most common pathogens to cause meningitis following a recent open skull fracture (Hankey and Wardlaw, 2008).

Less common causes of acute bacterial meningitis

Before the introduction of the *Haemophilus influenzae* type b (Hib) vaccine in the 1990s, Hib was the most common cause of meningitis in children under four years. It is now a rare cause in all age groups. The Hib vaccine is being introduced in developing countries, however the number of cases world wide and associated deaths still remains unacceptably high. As a consequence of routine vaccination programmes in the developed world, e.g. Hib and MenC, the incidence of meningitis in babies has decreased, therefore increasing the proportion of patients that are adults (Bonthius and Karacay, 2002).

Listeria monocytogenes is an uncommon cause of meningitis, but occurs especially during pregnancy and in immunosuppressed older adults >55 years. It accounts for less than 5% of cases in adults.

Viral meningitis

Viral meningitis is more common than bacterial, but most cases of viral meningitis are unreported because the disease is often mild and does not require hospitalisation (Donovan and Blewitt, 2009). The most common viruses to cause meningitis are mumps, cytomegalovirus and enteroviruses.

PATHOPHYSIOLOGY

Micro-organisms can enter the cerebrospinal fluid (CSF) directly via the sinuses or through a fracture in the skull. More commonly they enter by the indirect route: the blood stream. The upper respiratory tract is the most common site of colonisation, from where the bacteria overcome the immune defence mechanisms to enter the blood stream. It is not well understood how the bacteria penetrate the blood–brain barrier but once they have entered the CSF the bacteria rapidly multiply because the CSF does not contain the necessary defences to fight bacterial invasion, e.g. immunoglobulins and complement components. The bacteria or their toxins induce a potent inflammatory reaction by the meninges, the ventricles and the brain parenchyma (Boss, 2006). The inflammatory response causes vasodilation and migration of neutrophils into the subarachnoid space. A purulent exudate accumulates in the subarachnoid space which affects the reabsorption of CSF. The exudate blocks the arachnoid villi resulting in communicating hydrocephalus. Inflammation of the outer layer of the brain (cerebritis) typically occurs and abscess formation can result when a localised area of the brain tissue becomes affected. Purulent exudate can also spread into the sheaths of the spinal and cranial nerves. Infection may spread through the walls of blood vessels (vasculitis) causing thrombosis and possible infarction of brain tissue.

The inflammatory response often results in loss of the integrity of the blood–brain barrier with leakage of fluid from the intravascular compartment into the brain (vasogenic oedema) causing an increase in intracranial pressure (ICP). Raised ICP can also occur as a consequence of hydrocephalus.

In meningococcal disease septicaemia can occur with or without meningitis. Septicaemia occurs when the bacteria invade the blood stream and release endotoxins. In such cases shock rapidly occurs. Septicaemia will not be covered in this chapter. Adam and Osborne (2005) comprehensively present the management and nursing care of the patient with septicaemia.

CLINICAL SIGNS AND SYMPTOMS

Early identification is essential to reduce mortality and morbidity (van de Beek *et al.*, 2004) as meningitis can cause death within hours of presentation. However, in the very early stage of meningitis and septicaemia (the prodromal stage) the symptoms may be similar to flu, i.e. headache, pyrexia, nausea, painful joints and lethargy. Symptoms can progress over one to two days but usually develop rapidly, i.e. within a couple of hours. A large prospective study found that the classic triad of stiff neck, fever and altered consciousness were only found to be present in 44% of patients (van de Beek *et al.*, 2004). However 95% of patients presented with at least two signs and symptoms of headache, fever, neck stiffness and alterations in consciousness.

Kernig's sign and Brudzinski's sign are present in about half of adults. A positive Kernig's sign is present when pain is felt in the neck, back and the legs when the examiner flexes the patient's hip and extends the knee whilst in the supine position. Brudzinski's sign is when the hips flex to lift the legs in response to the examiner flexing the patient's neck. Both are indicative of meningeal irritation.

Signs of raised ICP may be present due to hydrocephalus and or cerebral oedema. Altered consciousness may also be a late sign of shock which will occur in meningococcal septicaemia. Seizures develop in approximately 20% of patients. A petechial/purpuric non-blanching rash, i.e. a rash that does not fade when pressure is applied is indicative of meningococcal septicaemia. A glass is used so that the rash can be seen when the pressure is applied. The rash is typically purpuric, (purplish patches or spots caused by extravasation of blood into the skin), and diffuse. A rash is not present in all patients with meningococcal disease. A rash may or may not be present in meningitis caused by other bacteria.

DIAGNOSIS

If, following a thorough physical examination, there is suspicion of meningitis the clinician will perform a lumbar puncture (LP), providing there are no signs suggestive of raised ICP or other contraindications, e.g. bleeding disorders. Performing a LP in a patient with signs of raised ICP is contraindicated as the LP could cause brain herniation (see Chapter 19). When the diagnosis is uncertain a CT scan may be done to exclude other causes and to ensure that it is safe to do a LP. In such cases blood cultures should be taken and empiric antibiotics administered prior to the scan being performed (see: Medical management/treatment). Identification of the causative organism on CSF culture is possible in 70–85% of cases (Hankey and Wardlaw, 2008). CSF findings are of a raised white cell count, raised protein and low glucose level; glucose and protein are relatively normal in cases of viral meningitis. A blood glucose should be sent at the same time as the CSF for comparison. Blood cultures and swabs from the throat and any septic sites should also be sent for culture.

MEDICAL MANAGEMENT AND TREATMENT

Studies have shown that patient outcomes are less favourable when there are delays in the administration of antibiotics (Miner *et al.*, 2001). An algorithm for the early management of bacterial meningitis and meningococcal meningitis was published jointly by the Meningitis Research Foundation (MRF) in collaboration with the British Infection Society (Hayderman *et al.*, 2003). It rec-

ommends that patients presenting to a GP with suspected meningitis should receive benzylpenicillin before urgent transfer to an accident and emergency department.

On presentation of any patient to A&E with suspected meningitis, empirical antimicrobial treatment should be administered as soon as the lumbar puncture has been performed and immediately in those who present in a critical condition. Empirical treatment includes ceftriazone or cefotaxime bd and for patients who have an anaphylactic history with penicillins or a rash with cephalosporins, chloramphenicol is used. Amoxicillin 2g 4 hourly is given in addition to ceftriazone to patients suspected of having meningitis caused by Listeria monocytogenes, i.e. patients who are immunosuppressed and those over the age of 55 years. Once the causative organism has been identified from CSF culture the antimicrobial agent may be changed and will be determined by the pathogen that has been isolated. The microbiology services are instrumental for giving advice on the antimicrobial treatment of the disease. Antibiotics are given for a period of 7–14 days, depending on the causative organism and the clinical response to treatment.

Dexamethasone is the only adjunctive therapy to significantly reduce the mortality and morbidity for meningitis (van de Beek *et al.*, 2007). A systematic review (Cochrane review) concluded that dexamethasone should be administered in conjunction with the first dose of antibiotics for all cases of community acquired bacterial meningitis (van de Beek *et al.*, 2007). The algorithm recommends a 4-day course of dexamethasone 0.15 mg/kg, six hourly, commencing with or before the initial dose of antibiotic is given to all patients with acute bacterial meningitis.

NURSING MANAGEMENT

Patients need to be closely monitored in the acute period. There are a number of secondary complications that can result in further deterioration of the neurological condition of the patient, e.g. hydrocephalus, cerebral oedema, cerebral infarction. The nurse needs to be vigilant for early signs of deterioration and to be aware of the specific management for the complications that can arise. It is therefore imperative that patients are nursed in an appropriate area where they can be closely monitored; the degree to which this will be required will depend on the clinical presentation of the individual patient. Some patients will require urgent transfer to intensive care if they have presented with severe shock and or coma. Other patients may be diagnosed early allowing for early treatment with antibiotics, and the clinical presentation is such that the patient does not at that time require monitoring in an ICU. However all patients are at risk of neurological deterioration and the nursing care discussed in the following section is relevant to all patients. The evidence for the nursing management of raised ICP has been presented in Chapter 7.

Airway and breathing

Immediate assessment and maintenance of a clear airway is the first priority. Patients who are deteriorating rapidly or who present with a Glasgow Coma Scale (GCS) of 8 or less will require intubation and respiratory support. Patients who are breathing spontaneously should be assessed regularly for an adequate depth and rate of breathing to allow for effective clearance of CO_2. Patients who are drowsy are at risk of partial airway obstruction and hypoventilation which could lead to retention of CO_2, which will increase ICP. Oxygen should be administered if necessary to maintain optimal oxygen saturations, i.e. >96%.

Patients who are able to follow commands should be encouraged to do regular deep breathing exercises to reduce the risk of respiratory complications.

Circulation

The patient should be regularly assessed for early signs of shock, i.e. rise in heart rate, prolonged capillary refill time, increase in respiratory rate, and reduced urine output. Hypotension is a late sign of shock. Blood pressure (BP) should be maintained to ensure a cerebral perfusion pressure (CPP) >60 mmHg (see Chapter 7).

Patients presenting with shock will require inotropic and vasopressor support to maintain CPP and perfusion to other vital organs. All patients should have continuous cardiac monitoring because of the risk of cardiac arrhythmias. Antipyretics should be administered regularly and cooling measures should be employed to reduce the temperature (see Chapter 7).

Neurology

In the acute stage the patient needs to be closely monitored for potential neurological deterioration. A minimum of half hourly neurological observations should be performed. All patients are at risk of developing a rise in ICP due to brain oedema and obstructive hydrocephalus. Signs and symptoms of raised ICP and management of ICP is presented in Chapter 7. Patients are also at risk of neurological deterioration due to cerebral infarction.

Seizures occur in approximately 17% of patients and are most likely to occur in the first 48 hours of hospitalisation (Wang *et al.*, 2005). Appropriate safety measures should be in place to protect the patient in case a seizure should occur. If seizure activity occurs, rapid control is required to prevent ischaemic damage which can rapidly ensue due to the increased metabolic demands of the brain. Patients should be commenced on phenytoin and receive an initial loading dose of intravenous phenytoin 18 mg/kg following the first seizure. Intravenous lorazepam 4 mg should also be prescribed as required in case subsequent seizures occur.

Pain management

It is imperative to keep the patient comfortable and to reduce noxious stimuli. In the ward setting codeine based analgesia and paracetamol (acetaminophen) are administered for headache, whereas in the critical care setting the opioids fentanyl and morphine sulphate are commonly used. Opioid analgesics can compromise blood pressure so careful monitoring is required, particularly in patients who are haemodynamically unstable. Constipation is a common side-effect of opioid analgesics which should be managed before it becomes a problem by ensuring adequate hydration, a balanced diet and the use of prophylactic aperients. There is insufficient evidence for recommendations to be made about which analgesics are the most effective and have the least undesirable side-effects.

Fluid management

The aim is to maintain normovolaemia. Hypovolaemia can result in hypotension and a fall in cerebral perfusion pressure, which can predispose the brain to ischaemia; hypervolaemia can potentially exacerbate cerebral oedema. Frequent assessment of the patient's hydration status and a strict fluid balance are necessary to inform decisions on fluid replacement. Patients with meningitis can develop syndrome of inappropriate production of antidiuretic hormone (SIADH). The patient will have dilutional hyponatramia and may require fluid restriction. However this must be done with the utmost caution so as not to compromise cerebral perfusion pressure.

Intravenous fluids containing dextrose should be avoided. Dextrose solutions will lower plasma osmolality; the hypo-osmolar state will cause water to move by osmosis across the BBB and will contribute further to cerebral oedema. Refer to Chapter 16 for further detail on the management of fluids and electrolytes and SIADH.

General nursing care

All patients with meningitis will either have raised ICP or are at risk of increased ICP, therefore general nursing care should aim to prevent and reduce possible elevations in the patient's ICP (see Chapter 7).

TRANSMISSION

Community-acquired bacterial meningitis and meningococcal septicaemia are notifiable diseases. The consultant in communicable disease control or consultant in public health medicine should be notified promptly (Meningitis Research Trust, 2002). All close patient contacts are offered prophylactic antibiotics which will be coordinated by the public health team.

Patients with community acquired bacterial meningitis should be nursed in a side room for 24 hours; following this time there is no longer a risk of spread of meningococci. Health care workers who come into contact with patients with meningococcal meningitis do not require prophylactic antibiotics, however in the rare instance of the nose or mouth being splattered with droplets from the patient's respiratory tract, e.g. during suctioning, prophylaxis should be considered. Appropriate precautions should be taken to prevent such contamination.

PROGNOSIS

Mortality and morbidity depends on the type of bacteria, the age of the patient and neurological condition at initial presentation. *Streptococcus pneumoniae* meningitis is associated with a mortality of 19%, *N. meningitidis* 13%, and *H. influenzae* 3% (Hankey and Wardlaw, 2008). Patients presenting with severe neurological impairments at presentation have very poor outcomes. Although associated with high mortality and morbidity the majority of patients who develop meningitis will go on to lead normal lives.

Viral meningitis

Viral meningitis is usually a very mild illness and the majority will make a full recovery and not require medical attention. A very small percentage of people with viral meningitis can make a slow recovery and have long term problems, such as persistent headaches, lethargy and memory impairments.

PHYSICAL, COGNITIVE AND PSYCHOSOCIAL IMPAIRMENTS FOLLOWING MENINGITIS

The risk of long term impairments is greatest in, but not confined to, those who experience neurological complications at the time of their acute illness.

Hearing loss

Cochlear damage can occur due to the direct effect of bacterial toxins which can lead to sensorineural deafness in approximately 20% of patients. Hearing loss can be mild to profound and can affect one or both ears. An early assessment of hearing should be performed to determine the degree of loss and to assess whether the patient is a candidate for cochlea implants. Alternative forms of communication such as lip reading and sign language may have to be learned (Donovan and Blewitt, 2009).

Patients should be given details of the Royal National Institute for Deaf People (RNID), which is a voluntary organisation that offers support and advice.

Cranial nerve palsies

One or more cranial nerve palsies occurs in 30% of patients, most commonly cranial nerves III, IV, VI, VII and VIII. See Chapter 13 for the specific care and management of cranial nerve impairments.

Epilepsy

Patients can continue to have seizures or go on to develop epilepsy following the acute period of the disease. It is important that patients and relatives are given appropriate information on antiepileptic drugs and what to expect during a seizure (refer to Chapter 30).

Cognitive impairments

The effect of memory loss can vary. Many people experience short-term memory loss, or find it hard to concentrate following meningitis. This can make everyday tasks very difficult and can cause problems when returning to work (The Meningitis Trust, 2002). Refer to Chapters 9 and 29 for strategies to manage memory loss.

Fatigue

Patients may experience fatigue for weeks or months following the disease. Management of fatigue is discussed in Chapter 28.

SUPPORT

The Meningitis Trust is a charity organisation in the UK that offers support, advice, counselling and financial support grants, and puts people in contact with others who have had similar experiences. It has a 24 hour nurse led helpline.

SUBACUTE MENINGITIS

Mycobacterium tuberculosis is a significant cause of meningitis in the UK. Approximately 2% of tuberculosis (TB) cases develop meningitis (Meningitis Trust, 2008). Unlike other types of meningitis it is rare for TB meningitis to present as an acute neurological emergency, rather there is a chronic presentation. Most commonly the patient has a history of weight loss, fever, night sweats and malaise. Anti-TB drugs are given for six to nine months depending on the severity of the disease and the response to treatment. Table 24.1 lists the initial anti-TB drugs and their adverse effects, which are numerous. Patient education and support is essential to optimise adherence. Liver function tests are performed at regular intervals; isoniazid is stopped if symptoms of hepatitis are present. Streptomycin can be used instead of rifampicin, and ethambutol can be substituted for pyrazinamide if adverse effects become a problem (Hankey and Wardlaw, 2008). Dexamethasone 12 mg is given for three weeks and then tapered for a further three weeks. Neurological impairments persist in 20–30% (Hankey and Wardlaw, 2008) and are similar to those for other types of bacterial meningitis.

ENCEPHALITIS

Ava Easton, Stephen Pewter,
Huw Williams

Encephalitis is inflammation of the brain tissue. It can occur at any age, in any part of the world. It is caused by either an infection (usually viral, but can be bacterial, fungal or parasitic) or by autoimmune disease. The initial stage of the illness commonly manifests as serious, acute and potentially life-threatening. Many patients are left with an acquired brain injury, although the degree and severity of permanent brain injury varies among those affected (Easton *et al.*, 2006).

EPIDEMIOLOGY AND AETIOLOGY

Very few epidemiological studies of encephalitis exist and the disorder is probably under-reported. Beghi *et al.* (1984) reported the US annual incidence as 7.4 people per 100,000 and, more recently, Khetsuriani *et al.* (2002) reported 7.3 hospitalisations per 100,000 population. There are no statistics for the UK, but based on the US figures it can be estimated that the incidence in the UK is about 4,000 cases per annum.

The most commonly identified infective cause in the UK is herpes simplex. Other commonly identified causes are herpes zoster, Epstein–Barr virus, mumps, measles and enteroviruses.

There are three broad types of encephalitis: acute infective encephalitis, post-infectious encephalitis (also known as acute disseminated encephalomyelitis or ADEM), which is an autoimmune process following infection elsewhere in the body, and finally auto-immune responses to other conditions in the body such as tumour or when antibodies block sites on nerve cells in the brain, preventing them from functioning normally. Examples include voltage-gated potassium channel antibody encephalitis

Table 24.1   Initial anti-TB treatment.

Drug	Dose	Adverse effects
Rifampicin	600 mg OD	• Skin rash • Nausea and vomiting • Hepatitis • Saliva and urine turns orange-red
Pyrazinamide	30–50 mg/kg OD	• Fever • Urticaria • Flushing • Nausea and vomiting
Isoniazid	5 mg/kg OD	• Skin rash • Nausea and vomiting • Confusional and psychotic states • Arthralgia • Hepatitis • Peripheral neuropathy
Pyridoxine (given to prevent peripheral neuropathy associated with the use of isoniazid)	20–50 mg OD	

Source: Hankey and Wardlaw, 2008; Joint Formulary Committee, 2009.

(VGKCaE) or anti-N-methyl-D aspartate receptor encephalitis (Anti-NMDAR encephalitis). The latter of these three types of encephalitis is of some significance since with early diagnosis and treatment, patients can recover well from some auto-immune encephalitides.

PATHOPHYSIOLOGY

Clinical manifestations are caused by cell dysfunction from direct infective invasion and associated inflammatory change (Hankey and Wardlaw, 2008) or by a secondary immune response to infection or immunisation. Inflammation may be widespread throughout the brain, often accompanied by inflammation of the meninges (meningo-encephalitis), or it may be localised, for example to the limbic system or the brain stem. Cerebral blood vessels become surrounded by lymphocytes and plasma cells, known as perivascular cuffing, which is characteristic of inflammatory processes.

Some viruses have a predilection for particular parts of the brain. Herpes simplex virus causes inflammation and haemorrhagic necrosis in the frontal and temporal lobes. Rabies virus tends to involve the medial temporal lobes, and varicella-zoster virus involves the cerebellum.

Infections are most commonly transmitted to the brain via the bloodstream (haematogenous spread). The infectious agent – often a virus introduced into the body by an insect bite – is present in the blood (viraemia) and crosses the blood–brain barrier into the brain. Infected neurones may rupture and subsequently the immune response causes inflammation and cerebral oedema, leading to raised intracranial pressure.

Some infections, such as rabies and herpes encephalitis, travel directly along neurones into the brain and some, such as herpes simplex and varicella zoster, may establish a persistent presence in sensory ganglia, which may lead to disease at a later stage. It has been known since the 1920s that the herpes virus can travel from its first site of entry into the body to the sensory ganglion cells and then on into the central nervous system (Goodpasture and Teague, 1923).

The most commonly identified non-infectious encephalitis is acute disseminated encephalomyelitis (ADEM) (Garg, 2006). In ADEM, there is widespread demyelination in the white matter of the brain and spinal cord. In developed countries, ADEM is now most often seen following mild upper respiratory infections. In developing countries other infections, such as measles, rubella and varicella, are more common causes of ADEM. Acute haemorrhagic leucoencephalitis (AHLE) is a more severe variant of ADEM and is often fatal (Garg, 2006). There is

a characteristic necrotising vasculitis, often with areas of haemorrhage around blood vessels.

CLINICAL SIGNS AND SYMPTOMS

Onset is commonly insidious; patients often have a several day history of malaise, myalgia and headache. 90% of patients will have a fever on presentation (Howard and Manji, 2009). Seizures frequently occur with acute infective encephalitis. Patients can also present with nausea, vomiting and signs of meningeal irritation (see: Clinical signs and symptoms). Reduced level of consciousness and raised ICP may also be present. Behavioural and speech disturbances may also be present.

DIAGNOSIS

The symptoms of encephalitis are shared with other illnesses, so differential diagnosis can be difficult (Whitley and Gnann, 2002). The presence of focal seizures and focal neurological signs can differentiate encephalitis from other encephalopathology (Chaudhuri and Kennedy, 2002). CT scanning is usually performed to rule out mass lesions and other pathology as well as to evaluate cerebral oedema when MRI is not available (Steiner *et al.*, 2005; Solomon *et al.*, 2007). CT scanning may also be used to rule out any mass effects before conducting a lumbar puncture. Where it is safe to do so, a lumbar puncture is an essential tool in the diagnosis and treatment of encephalitis and may be performed to assess CSF pressure and to obtain samples for infection screening. The diagnosis can be confirmed by the polymerase chain reaction (PCR) test for infections within the CSF (Chaudhuri and Kennedy, 2002; Solomon *et al.*, 2007). MRI may be able to detect other abnormalities early in the disease (Chaudhuri and Kennedy, 2002; Steiner *et al.*, 2005).

A good algorithm regarding the diagnosis and treatment of encephalitis in the immunocompetent patient has been developed by the Liverpool Brain Infections Group (Solomon *et al.*, 2007).

MEDICAL MANAGEMENT

Viral encephalitis is a medical emergency and, if suspected, treatment with anti-viral agents should be initiated without delay (Solomon *et al.*, 2007). The earlier that treatment is commenced, the less the risk of long-term complications. There is no specific therapy for most forms of viral encephalitis (Chaudhuri and Kennedy, 2002), with the exception of acyclovir for herpes simplex encephalitis and varicella-zoster encephalitis, however other anti-viral agents continue to be evaluated (Steiner *et al.*, 2005). Younger patients below 30 years of age (Whitley and

Gnann, 2002) and those in whom the duration of encephalitis was two days or less when acyclovir was started, have been shown to have better outcomes (Raschilas *et al.*, 2002) , although even with treatment the mortality from this disease remains high at 20–30% (Kennedy and Chaudhuri, 2002).

Acyclovir is administered intravenously three times daily (in the relevant dosage for the patient's bodyweight) for 14 days in immunocompetent patients, and for up to 21 days where the PCR remains positive, or the patient continues to be febrile (Solomon *et al.*, 2007) to prevent relapse. It may be discontinued if an alternative diagnosis is identified. Acyclovir selectively inhibits viral DNA in infected cells, thereby preventing viral reproduction and spread, while healthy cells are unaffected (Kennedy and Chaudhuri, 2002). Patients with herpes simplex encephalitis who are treated with acyclovir early, before they become comatose, have reduced morbidity and mortality (Steiner *et al.*, 2005). Side-effects include headache, nausea and vomiting and diarrhoea and more rarely hallucinations and liver failure.

High dose steroids have also been tried, but there is little evidence of effectiveness (Steiner *et al.*, 2005), although dexamethasone may be used for cerebral oedema. Symptomatic relief should also be initiated, such as intravenous phenytoin to control seizure activity, and antipyretics to reduce fever.

Secondary neurological complications include cerebral infarction, cerebral venous thrombosis, SIADH (see Chapter 16), and aspiration pneumonia (Steiner *et al.*, 2005).

NURSING MANAGEMENT

The acute nursing management is the same as for meningitis with the exception of the need for isolation. It is not uncommon for patients to be agitated and aggressive; strategies to manage these behaviours are presented in Chapter 10.

PROGNOSIS

Mortality resulting from infection by the herpes virus (the most common identified cause of viral encephalitis) is 20–30% with treatment. If encephalitis is left untreated, the mortality rate is about 70% (Schott, 2006).

PHYSICAL, COGNITIVE AND PSYCHOSOCIAL IMPAIRMENTS FOLLOWING ENCEPHALITIS

Encephalitis can have lasting repercussions for a person's day to day functioning. In a large survey, 69% of adult respondents reported that their illness had left them unable to return to their premorbid lifestyle, and 20% had suffered a breakdown in marriage following the illness (Dowell *et al.*, 2000). The effects of encephalitis upon an individual's quality of life and interpersonal relationships clearly persist beyond the acute period of neurological infection (Easton *et al.*, 2006).

One of the primary goals of rehabilitation is to facilitate the patient's return to living, working and socialising independently (Rössler and Haker, 2003; Wilson, 2003). Nurses need to consider not only to the neuro-anatomical foundations and neurological effects of an illness, but also the psycho-social aspects, incorporating cognitive, emotional, behavioural and social factors (Williams and Evans, 2003; Wilson, 2003). Cognitive impairment can negatively impact on recovery.

Cognitive impairment

The most severe deficits to cognition are usually associated with herpes simplex type-1 encephalitis. These can present with pervasive amnesia covering new material and/or existing memories (Hokkanen and Launes, 2000; Pewter *et al.*, 2007), communication problems such as incorrectly naming items (Okuda *et al.*, 2001) and impairment of executive functions such as attention and planning ability (Pewter *et al.*, 2007).

While, on the whole, non-herpetic encephalitis does not result in the same degree of cognitive impairment, amnesic and other cognitive deficiencies may occur, highlighting the importance of assessing patients on a case-by-case basis (Hokkanen and Launes, 2000; Pewter *et al.*, 2007). Hokkanen and Launes (2000) also note the occurrence of behavioural indications of executive impairment, including: impulsive, disinhibited actions, rigid behaviour, and lacking in initiative. Situationally inappropriate actions and speech have also been reported (Evans, 2003; Godefroy, 2003) even in the absence of evidence on formal testing. Recently, subtle deficits in tasks requiring executive function have been found across a wide range of patients with various aetiologies of encephalitis (Pewter *et al.*, 2007). These problems may, therefore, be widespread and may contribute to the behavioural difficulties and fatigue experienced by encephalitis patients.

Depression and anxiety

In addition to problems with cognition, encephalitis can result in lasting depression, anxiety and psychiatric illness (Pewter *et al.*, 2007). Difficulties with emotional adjustment are common and can be pervasive and severe regardless of the severity of cognitive and neuroanatomical damage (Kreutzer *et al.*, 2001). The presence or absence of insight into one's condition is thought to be an important mediator between cognitive impairment and psychological distress (Fleminger *et al.*, 2003). While awareness is often disturbed early in the course of recovery, improving insight during the months and years following injury can lead to reactive depression as the patients find themselves aware of their acquired limitations (Godfrey *et al.*, 1993). Since disturbance of insight is more resilient in more severely brain-injured cases, the presence of greater cognitive and psychosocial difficulties in this population can produce less subsequent depression, as patients may be less aware of the change in their abilities. Emotional dysfunction may, therefore, be equally or more problematic in patients with seemingly milder neurological injury.

Despite the role of emerging insight in triggering depression, accurate self-appraisal may be beneficial to the long-term adjustment, as greater self-awareness may produce greater motivation and ability to compensate for acquired difficulties and patients may find themselves less frustrated by attempting activities which are beyond their current capability (Ownsworth and Fleming, 2005). This is supported in one study of post-acute encephalitis patients which found that realistic self-appraisal was associated with a lesser degree of depression (Pewter *et al.*, 2007).

Socialising and employment

Little is currently known about the impact of encephalitis upon socialisation. However, individuals with a brain injury do tend to receive fewer visitors and to socialise less than the normal population, relying upon the immediate family for social contact (Elsass and Kinsella, 1987; Marsh *et al.*, 1990). This reliance upon the family can place additional strain upon relationships as the parents (Hooper *et al.*, 2007) and carers (Pewter, 2007) of encephalitic patients frequently report emotional distress relating to the neurobehavioural symptoms displayed by their relative. Subsequently, carers of a brain injured person report increased instances of alcoholism, tranquiliser usage, attendance of counselling for mental health problems, marriage breakdown, anxiety, depression and distress (Hall *et al.*, 1994; Kreutzer *et al.*, 1994). Nurses must be vigilant for distress among family members and offer support. The Encephalitis Society (2003; 2010) also provides support for patients, their families and carers and nurses should ensure that their contact details are passed on (www.encephalitis.info).

The workplace is another avenue for social contact. Between 26 and 70% of encephalitic patients successfully return to work, depending upon the aetiology and severity of their encephalitis (Hokkanen and Launes, 1997; Kaplan and Bain, 1999). While cognitive problems are in themselves a barrier to employment (Dikmen *et al.*, 1993), Andrewes and Gielewski (1999) report the case of one patient who was unable to remember which of her work colleagues had acted in a friendly manner towards her, making it difficult to maintain amicable relationships with colleagues.

Clinical neuropsychology/neuropsychiatry involvement

Given the breadth of socio-emotional problems faced by survivors of brain injury, the patient must be referred for clinical neuropsychology and/or neuropsychiatry assessment. Nurses are ideally placed to ensure timely and appropriate referrals. As noted above, anxiety and depression are very common and there is a corresponding threefold increase in the risk of suicide (Fleminger *et al.*, 2003). There is some provision for the treatment and management of brain injury and nurses need to ensure that such services are made clearly available for encephalitis patients (Easton *et al.*, 2006). For example, biological and bio-psychosocial treatment for depression and suicidal ideation are available through clinical psychology services (Fleminger *et al.*, 2003). In addition, anxiety-related disorders such as obsessive-compulsive behaviour can be distressing to post-encephalitis patients (Pewter *et al.*, 2007), but evidence from some cases has shown that cognitive behaviour therapy can help (Williams, 2003).

Fatigue

Fatigue can be a considerable problem following encephalitis, as compensating for any residual cognitive deficits can be stressful and tiring even when such compensation is successful enough to allow outwardly normal autonomous functioning (Greve *et al.*, 2002). Management of fatigue is discussed in Chapter 28.

Epilepsy and seizures

Epilepsy can be a significant problem for people after encephalitis, with nearly a quarter of people affected by encephalitis as an adult going on to experience seizures, and nearly half of all those affected as a child (Dowell *et al.*, 2000). See Chapter 30 for the management of seizures.

Headaches and bodily pain

Changes in sensation, headaches and pain in other parts of the body can last for several weeks after the acute illness, and sometimes may continue for some time after the acute phase. These may be made worse by lack of rest, having to concentrate hard, and/or bright lights. Dizziness also may occur, especially with sudden or rapid movement and may be accompanied by feeling nauseated. While stress and tension are usually the main causes, a doctor should always check persistent headaches or pain and referral to a pain clinic may be necessary where these problems persist (The Encephalitis Society, 2010).

Sensory changes

Vision, hearing, taste, smell, temperature and touch can all be affected by encephalitis. Problems can range from the complete loss of a sense to variations in sensitivity from one day to the next.

Hearing problems can occur for a number of reasons. Tinnitus is experienced as noise, commonly like a buzzing, hissing or ringing in the ears. Auditory agnosia is impaired recognition of non-verbal sounds and noises, but intact language function. In some cases the person can be extremely sensitive to certain noises, pitches, or where there is more than one sound at a time. They may be unable to tolerate many environments we take for granted (for example shopping centres and pubs).

Encephalitis: patient perspective

It locks you away
inside your mind
inside your head
it keeps you alone
and different

Deep down you know
what the difference is
who you used to be
the person you once were
But who are you now?

Try and explain it to others
can they really understand
Try saying "I feel different"
Folks politely ask me why?

Its simple,
my mind is like treacle
(the extra sticky kind)
that pulls out all your fillings
and causes your teeth to grind

My head is like a vacuum. …
of the cleaning type
that sucks up bits and pieces
clears away in one full swipe.

My memory is shot to pieces
my arms and legs are weak
my balance is non existent
held up by two left feet.

There's my vision too
my eyes – mere shadows
of their former selves
Two friends who find it hard to
work
although they can with help.

Some mornings I find it hard to
wake
My brain's been left behind
It's vanished, gone the night before
Looking for things I cannot find.

I feel like something's got me
Something weird form outer space.
Am I a "Stepford wife", a "zombie"?
Am I part of the Human Race?

It doesn't feel like it.

Do they tell you about the head pain,
The pressure building up,
The depression and the mood swings,
Desperation fills my cup.

My tendency to drop things
through my fingers light and weak
How many pairs of trousers torn
from falling off my feet.

Its changed my personality
every ailment caused by you
And so the list continues
my life revolves around –

trying to get over this
dreadful illness.

**Encephalitis,
it changes life,
it changes you.**

Source: The Encephalitis Society. Reproduced by kind permission of the Encephalitis Society.

FURTHER INFORMATION

Further information for patients and professionals can be obtained from the encephalitis society (www.encephalitis.info).

CEREBRAL ABSCESS

AETIOLOGY AND EPIDEMIOLOGY

An abscess is a localised collection of pus within the brain parenchyma. In the UK the prevalence is 2–3 cases per million (Fitzpatrick and Gan, 1999). A cerebral abscess develops as a result of spread of infection from adjacent structures, i.e. the middle ear or paranasal sinuses; following post-operative infections or penetrating trauma; or haematogenous spread of infection from teeth, pulmonary abscess or bacterial endocarditis. The most common causative organisms are *Staphylococcus aureus* (following trauma), *Streptococcus pneumoniae* and *Streptococcus milleri*. More than one organism can be isolated particularly when dental infection is the cause.

PATHOPHYSIOLOGY

The initial stage of abscess formation is focal inflammation and oedema of the periphery of the brain (cerebritis). The cerebritis evolves into a cerebral abscess which has a central core of necrotic tissue and pus forms in the abscess cavity. A collagen capsule surrounds the abscess.

CLINICAL SIGNS AND SYMPTOMS

Headache, fever, reduced consciousness, seizures and focal neurological signs are the most common presenting signs and symptoms.

DIAGNOSIS AND MEDICAL MANAGEMENT

Diagnosis can be confirmed with a CT with contrast, or by MRI. The original source for the infection is usually apparent from the medical history, e.g. long standing untreated dental infection. Small abscesses can be treated with intravenous antibiotics for the specific causative organism (Howard and Manji, 2009). Antibiotic therapy is usually required for several weeks. Large abscesses may require surgery in the form of craniotomy and excision or stereotactic guided aspiration to reduce ICP. In some cases the latter is performed to determine the causative organism.

NURSING MANAGEMENT

The acute nursing management is the same as for meningitis, with the exception of the need for isolation. See Chapter 20 for post-operative nursing management.

PROGNOSIS

Prognosis is poor in patients who have impaired consciousness and neurological impairments on admission, but is excellent for those who are fully conscious (Howard and Manji, 2009).

NEUROLOGICAL COMPLICATIONS OF HUMAN IMMUNODEFICIENCY VIRUS (HIV)

Leann Johnson and Ed Wilkins

EPIDEMIOLOGY OF HIV

The acquired immunodeficiency syndrome (AIDS) was first recognised in 1981 and is caused by the human immunodeficiency virus (HIV-1). HIV-2 causes a similar illness to HIV-1 but is less aggressive and is restricted mainly to Western Africa. The viruses originated from the closely related African primate simian immunodeficiency viruses, and sequence analysis has led to the estimate that HIV-1 was introduced into humans in the early 1930s (Holmes, 2001).

AIDS has grown to be the second leading cause of disease burden worldwide. It is now recognised that the immune deficiency is a consequence of continuous high-level HIV replication, leading to virus and immune-mediated destruction of the key immune effector cell, the CD4 lymphocyte. HIV affects 33.2 million people in the world with 2.5 million new cases and 2.1 million deaths as estimated by the World Health Organisation in 2007, indicating a levelling off of the global epidemic. Sub-Saharan Africa has the greatest burden of disease.

In the UK in 2006, 7093 new cases occurred, with an estimated overall prevalence of 73,000 (Health Protection Agency, 2007); approximately 21,600 of these are undiagnosed as calculated using population estimates and anonymous linked testing. The epidemic in many industrialised nations is changing, with heterosexual transmission becoming the dominant route and racial and ethnic minorities representing an increasing fraction. Worldwide, the major route of transmission (> 75%) is heterosexual; 5–10% of new HIV infections are in children and more than 90% of these are infected during pregnancy, birth or breastfeeding (WHO, 2007). The incidence in injecting drug users varies widely from country to country. It is relatively low in the UK being <1% in most areas, although in other areas of the world (e.g. Eastern Europe, Vietnam, North-East India and China) it accounts for the majority of infections.

HIV-2 differs from HIV-1 in that patients have lower viral loads, slower CD4 decline, lower rates of vertical transmission, and slower progression to AIDS. The economic and demographic impact of HIV infection in developing countries is profound as it affects the most economically productive and fertile ages and is also eroding the health and economic advances made in the last few decades. Access to antiretroviral (ARV) therapy for patients with HIV-related illness in resource-poor nations has improved significantly over the last few years with over 2 million receiving treatment, which represents approximately 28% of those estimated to require treatment.

Modes of transmission

HIV infection occurs by transmission of the virus to an uninfected individual by exposure to infected fluids. This can be by contact with blood, bodily fluids, sexual contact, and through breast milk. Likelihood of infection is dependent on the integrity of the exposed site, the type and volume of body fluid, and the viral load.

PATHOPHYSIOLOGY

HIV is a single-stranded RNA retrovirus from the lentivirus family. Following mucosal exposure, HIV is transported to the lymph nodes via dendritic, CD4 or Langerhans cells, where infection becomes established. Free or cell-associated virus is then disseminated widely through the blood with seeding of 'sanctuary sites', such as the CNS and testes, as well as latent CD4 cell reservoirs. With time, there is gradual attrition of the CD4 cell population resulting in increasing impairment of cell-mediated immunity with consequent susceptibility to opportunistic infections and certain cancers (Palella *et al.*, 2003). It has been calculated that each day more than 10^{10} virions are produced and 10^9 CD4 cells destroyed.

As CD4 cells are pivotal in orchestrating the immune response, any depletion in numbers renders the body susceptible to opportunistic infections (e.g. mycobacterium tuberculosis) and oncogenic virus-related tumours. The reduction in the number of CD4 cells circulating in peripheral blood is tightly correlated with the amount of plasma viral load. Both are monitored closely in patients and are used as measures of disease progression. The further a CD4 cell count falls below $200 \, \text{cells/mm}^3$ the more likely the patient is to develop an opportunistic infection.

CLINICAL SIGNS AND SYMPTOMS

As a neurotropic virus, HIV causes complex disease and usually infects the central nervous system early in infection (Kumar, 2007). Therefore neurological disease is a common feature of HIV infection and may present as part of an acute HIV seroconversion, or as a chronic process related to immunosuppression, or as a direct result of chronic viral infection.

Acute HIV infection/seroconversion

HIV seroconversion describes the process of conversion from HIV antibody negative to antibody positive. Most patients with HIV are diagnosed in the latent rather than acute stage of disease hence a substantial proportion of people are asymptomatic or mildly symptomatic at acute infection. As well as a transient flu like illness, patients may report a variety of symptoms including fever, rash, generalised lymphadenopathy, pharyngitis, diarrhoea, myalgia, arthralgia or headache. As a result of a rapid drop in CD4 T-lymphocyte cells during this phase of infection patients may be at risk of developing opportunistic infections such as *Pneumocystis jirovecii* pneumonia (PCP), although this is rare (Vento *et al.*, 1993).

Potential neurological manifestations of acute HIV infection include aseptic meningitis and rarely, a self limiting encephalopathy, Guillain–Barré syndrome, transverse myelitis, facial palsy, polyradiculitis and peripheral neuropathy.

Cryptococcal meningitis

The yeast *Cryptococcus neoformans* is the most common cause of meningitis associated with late stage HIV (CD4 $<50 \, \text{cells/mm}^3$). Many of the typical signs and symptoms of meningitis are absent. Most patients present with several weeks history of headache, fever and malaise. Focal neurology and seizures are rare but mild confusion is often a feature. Death occurs in 5–12% of patients within the first 2 weeks of diagnosis (Robinson *et al.*, 1999).

Toxoplasmosis

Toxoplasma gondii is a protozoan parasite carried by domestic and non-domestic animals with the final host being the cat. Humans become exposed through contact with the faeces of an infected cat or through eating undercooked contaminated meat. In the immunocompetent individual toxoplasmosis is rarely symptomatic (except during pregnancy where issues of miscarriage and foetal abnormalities arise). However in those infected with HIV the risk of developing toxoplasma-related pathology is high once the CD4 cell count falls below $100 \, \text{cells/mm}^3$. At this stage the patient is at risk of reactivating disease or developing acute infection as a result of primary exposure to the parasite. In the presence of HIV infection there is a > 30% risk of a previously infected individual reactivating their disease.

Although it may manifest itself in other organs, toxoplasmosis most commonly presents with encephalitis. It may cause widespread microscopic lesions and brain abscesses. Patients give a short history of headache, fever and drowsiness, which is rapidly followed with confusion, seizures and focal neurology. The areas of the brain most commonly infected include the parietal and frontal lobes, thalamus, basal ganglia and corticomedullary junction. Lesions are difficult to differentiate from CNS lymphoma.

Primary CNS lymphoma (PCNSL)

This haematological malignancy (a tumour of lymphocytes or lymphoblasts confined to the CNS) normally complicates late stage HIV when the CD4 cell count has fallen below 50 cell/mm^3. It occurs in approximately 5% of AIDS patients.

There are usually multifocal mass deposits in the brain. At the initial presentation lesions of PCNSL are often difficult to differentiate from those of toxoplasmosis due to similarity in clinical signs and symptoms, as well as presentation at the same advanced stage of HIV disease. However the duration of illness tends to be less rapid and may progress over weeks to months. Patients may present with headache, personality change, seizures, confusion or dulling of intellect and focal neurological signs correlating to the affected region within the brain.

Progressive multifocal leucoencephalopathy (PMFL)

This is a rapidly progressing demyelinating disease of the central nervous system caused by JC virus, which is usually fatal. It is normally associated with advanced stage HIV where the CD4 count is <50 cells/mm^3, however it has been described in patients with CD4 higher than 200 cells/mm^3. It is thought to be due to reactivation of latent JC virus, which the majority of the population are exposed to in childhood or early adulthood when an asymptomatic primary infection occurs. Patients present with focal deficits in 80% of cases, visual field defects and ataxia; seizures are not usually a feature.

Cytomegalovirus (CMV) encephalitis

CMV encephalitis is a rare presentation of CMV disease, which more commonly presents with retinopathy or colitis. Central nervous system disease presents with headache, neck stiffness and confusion.

Central nervous system tuberculosis

Co-infection with HIV and *Mycobacterium tuberculosis* is common. CNS tuberculosis includes tuberculous meningi-

tis, tuberculoma and spinal TB. In HIV positive patients with TB, pulmonary disease is more prevalent in those with a relatively preserved immune system (CD4>200 cells/mm^3); however with more advanced disease extrapulmonary infection, including tuberculous meningitis, becomes more common. In both the HIV and non-HIV setting the presentation of TB meningitis is similar and it carries a high degree of mortality and morbidity. However mortality is significantly greater in the HIV-infected group whereas morbidity is the same. Patients typically present with a prolonged insidious illness including fever, headache, meningism, focal CNS signs (see: Subacute meningitis). Patients are often slow to respond to therapy and may clinically and neurologically deteriorate before they begin to improve.

Other

A predominantly distal sensory neuropathy affecting the lower limbs is found in 30% of HIV-infected patients and is associated with lower CD4 counts (<200 cells/mm^3), high viral loads and older age. It results from axonal degeneration especially in unmyelinated nerve fibres. Hyperaesthesia, paraesthesia and pain or burning in the feet are common features. Diminished pinprick, light touch and vibration sense in association with loss of ankle reflexes is found. Certain anti-retroviral drugs are implicated in this pathology especially didanosine (ddI), stavudine (d4T), hydroxyurea and zalcitabine (ddC). With advances in HIV research newer drugs have been developed that are less likely to cause peripheral neuropathy and therefore the drugs implicated with this condition are now avoided where other options are available.

DIAGNOSIS AND INVESTIGATIONS

Diagnosis of HIV-related pathologies is often complicated and the time from presentation to diagnosis may be weeks to months. In all cases an accurate and detailed clinical history and examination is required in combination with laboratory investigations. When the pathology involves the central nervous system, neuro-imaging is essential with MRI scans providing more detailed information to aid the diagnosis. CT scan is often used as a screening tool, outside of normal working hours, to rule out acute pathology that warrants urgent action as well as helping the clinician to decide if it is safe to perform a lumbar puncture. At times electrophysiological studies may be helpful, such as EEG with suspected encephalopathy or nerve conduction studies in the presence of a peripheral neuropathy.

All patients with HIV-related central neurological disease require a lumbar puncture unless contraindicated.

This allows assessment of intracranial pressure and cerebrospinal fluid protein, glucose (compared to blood glucose), cell count, and specific stains, typically Gram, Ziehl–Neelsen (to diagnose tuberculosis) and India ink (to diagnose cryptococcal infection). Standard and extended (TB and fungal) culture should be performed as well as qualitative molecular (PCR) tests for TB, toxoplasma, CMV, JC virus, EBV, herpes simplex and varicella zoster viruses. Quantitative tests may be indicated for HIV (dementia/encephalopathy), JC virus (PMFL), and EBV (PCNSL).

On occasions despite extensive investigation the diagnosis remains unclear. At this stage neurosurgical opinion should be sought concerning a brain biopsy as tissue histology and microbial detection often help and may be the only method of coming to a conclusive diagnosis.

MEDICAL MANAGEMENT AND DRUGS

Antiretroviral treatment

The naïve patient

The decision to start therapy is a major one. It is dependent upon the symptom status of the patient, the CD4 count (and/or CD4%) and how quickly the level falls, the presence of co-morbidities, and the wishes of the patient. The risk of HIV-related disease and treatment-related toxicity increases as the CD4 falls and the likelihood of immunological recovery decreases. Nevertheless, successive surveys have demonstrated that up to one-third of patients do not present with their HIV until they are at an advanced stage when morbidity and mortality are not insignificant. Current practice is to recommend commencing treatment when the CD4 count falls below 350 cells/mm^3, above which the patient is rarely symptomatic (Gazzard *et al.*, 2008).

There are three major classes of drugs: nucleoside reverse transcriptase inhibitors (NRTI), non-nucleoside reverse transcriptase inhibitors (NNRTI) and protease inhibitors (PI). A potent combination (highly active antiretroviral therapy; HAART) should always be used and consists of three or more drugs: two NRTIs and either an NNRTI or a ritonavir-boosted PI. When starting treatment many factors need to be considered including: the potential drug interactions (e.g. anti-tuberculosis therapy), the presence of viral resistance, and patient lifestyle and wishes (e.g. a preference for once daily). Commencing antiretroviral therapy is not an emergency and there is always time to decide with the patient their optimum regimen thereby maximising adherence to the combination. All patients should have a viral resistance test performed prior to commencing therapy as there is a 5–10% incidence of primary viral resistance.

The treatment-experienced patient

A change in antiretroviral therapy may be necessary because of drug side-effects (early or late), difficulties in adherence, or virological failure. In a patient with a previously undetectable virus load (VL) (virus load is the measure of severity of viral infection) virus rebound is usually the first evidence of treatment failure.

With increasing time on a failing regimen, the VL rises towards baseline levels, resistance mounts, the CD4 count falls and clinical progression occurs. In essence, most early failures are related to adherence difficulties and most late failures are a result of virological resistance.

A new combination is decided upon based mainly on the result of a resistance test and prior drug exposure. Recent pharmacological developments have led to the introduction of two major new drug classes: entry inhibitors (fusion and chemokine receptor), and integrase inhibitors. These are of major advantage in treatment experienced patients who have extensive resistance to the standard therapies. These new drugs offer the patient treatments that are potent against their virus and can help them attain an undetectable viral load once again.

Cryptococcal meningitis

In addition to the management outlined under Acute bacterial meningitis/Medical management and treatment there are three phases in the management of cryptococcal meningitis: induction, maintenance, and secondary prophylaxis.

First-line induction treatment for cryptococcal meningitis is amphotericin B (0.7–1 mg/kg/day) with flucytosine (100 mg/kg/day), although the advantage of additional flucytosine is debatable. Standard amphotericin B should be used but this may be associated with renal toxicity, in which case liposomal amphotericin should be used. In patients with good prognostic factors, fluconazole (400 mg/day) is an alternative; itraconazole (400 mg/day) is less active than fluconazole and should only be used if other agents are contraindicated (Pukkila-Worley and Mylonakis, 2008).

Maintenance therapy and prophylaxis follows two weeks of induction therapy or CSF sterility. The patient should be switched to maintenance therapy with oral fluconazole 400 mg daily which is continued for a further six to eight weeks after which the dose is dropped to 200 mg daily. This represents secondary prophylaxis and should be continued until the CD4 count is >200 cells/mm³ and there is HIV viral undetectability.

All patients with cryptococcal disease should receive HAART and this should be commenced when it is safe to do so, usually at around two weeks when the patient is being switched from induction to maintenance therapy. When HAART is commenced immune responses are restored, an adverse consequence of this can be preexisting opportunistic infections clinically deteriorate which is referred to as immune reconstitution disease (IRS). There is a 10–20% occurrence of IRS which most commonly presents as culture-negative 'relapse' of meningitis.

Toxoplasmosis

Despite the characteristic imaging, it is often impossible to distinguish toxoplasma encephalitis from PCNSL with confidence. However, the response to a trial of anti-toxoplasma therapy is usually diagnostic, with clinical improvement occurring within the first week and significant reduction in the size of their lesions on imaging in the second week in over 90% of patients with toxoplasmosis. Treatment is divided into three phases: induction, maintenance, and prophylaxis. In addition, awareness of raised intracranial pressure from mass effect and the timing of HAART and complications of immune restoration are important considerations.

First line treatment is pyrimethamine (initial daily loading dose of 100–200 mg for two days followed by 50–100 mg daily) and sulphadiazine (1 to 2g qds) given for six weeks: pyrimethamine is given with folinic acid 15 mg daily. Dexamethasone (4 mg qds) should be given if there is significant mass effect (Montoya and Liesenfeld, 2004), however this may make it harder to differentiate between toxoplasmosis and PCNSL as the latter will also respond to steroids. The steroid dose should be tapered with clinical improvement over the ensuing two to four weeks.

Following successful induction, maintenance with pyrimethamine and either sulphadiazine or clindamycin should be continued at lower doses until the patient is successfully established on HAART with a CD4 count >200 cells/mm³. Co-trimoxazole 960 mg is an alternative, and is the preferred primary prophylactic in patients seropositive for toxoplasma. Failure to respond clinically and radiologically to therapy indicates the need for an urgent brain biopsy. All patients with cerebral toxoplasmosis should receive HAART and this is usually commenced around two weeks when the patient is being switched from induction to maintenance therapy. There is a small risk of immune reconstitution disease (IRS) which most com-

monly presents as paradoxical enlargement of the toxoplasma mass lesions.

Primary CNS lymphoma

Treatment is usually palliative with dexamethasone and symptomatic relief. Occasional responses to HAART have been reported but chemotherapy (methotrexate is the treatment of choice) and radiotherapy rarely produce much prolongation of survival which is usually 3–6 months.

Progressive multifocal leucoencephalopathy (PMFL)

There remains no specific treatment for PMFL outside of commencing or optimising antiretroviral drug treatment. HAART improves prognosis if commenced or optimised at time of diagnosis; however, mortality rate remains at 50% by one year. Some patients enter true remission of disease with stabilisation of neurological morbidity and the development of atrophy and gliosis on MRI.

Cytomegalovirus (CMV) encephalitis

Treatment for CMV is split into two phases: induction for two weeks followed by maintenance until there is sufficient immunological recovery (usually >200 cells/mm³), loss of CMV viraemia in blood and CSF, and clinical and neuroimaging features have regressed or stabilised. Therapy can then be discontinued. Ganciclovir IV is recommended for the induction therapy of CMV encephalitis and/or retinitis (Kedhar and Jabs, 2007). Foscarnet or cidofovir are two alternative second line agents though they have potential toxicities. Valganciclovir may be preferred if patient circumstances make IV administration inappropriate and it is the preferred choice for maintenance therapy after 2 weeks. Prophylaxis is not indicated.

TB meningitis and tuberculoma

As immune function falls, the likelihood of non-pulmonary tuberculosis, including both focal cerebral and meningeal disease, increases significantly. Therapy is split into two phases: induction and maintenance. In addition, awareness of the possibility of TB mass lesions (tuberculomas) developing or enlarging and the timing of HAART and complications of immune restoration are important considerations.

Induction therapy for known or presumptive fully sensitive mycobacterium tuberculosis is standard quadruple therapy, consisting of rifampicin, isoniazid, ethambutol, and pyrazinamide given for two months (with supplemental pyridoxine to prevent isoniazid neurotoxicity) (see: Subacute meningitis). Induction is followed by a 10 month maintenance phase with rifampicin and isoniazid. Fixed-dose combinations of drugs simplify the administration of therapy, improve adherence, and facilitate directly observed therapy (DOT) on a daily or three times weekly basis. Corticosteroids should be used in a decremental regimen as described for HIV-negative patients (Thwaites *et al.*, 2004). Choice of HAART is complicated due to drug interactions. IRS occurs in up to 20% of patients. This usually occurs 4–8 weeks after initiation of TB-therapy and is most common in those with a nadir CD4 <50 cells/mm^3 and a brisk CD4 response to HAART. It may present as focal disease away from the original site and reflects immune activation to dead or dying mycobacteria, or previously unrecognised tuberculosis; treatment with non-steroidal anti-inflammatory agents or corticosteroids is usually successful.

NURSING MANAGEMENT

The nursing management of patients infected with HIV is identical to those uninfected. However there are several other considerations that must be addressed which are not exceptional to HIV though arise more often in this setting.

Confidentiality

Unfortunately there remains a large stigma attached to the diagnosis of HIV and a patient's wish to maintain confidentiality about the diagnosis to themselves and their family must be respected at all times. Where the clinical condition of the patient does not allow for informed consent to counsel for an HIV antibody test, the decision to perform this test should be made by the senior physician after careful assessment as to how the knowledge of the result will affect management. The patient's relatives or partner should not be approached.

Medication adherence

Antiretroviral therapy is effective so long as the patient adheres to the medication. When admitted to hospital it is essential that a detailed list of the patient's medication and dosages is obtained and subsequently administered at the correct time. Omission of dosages of antiretrovirals encourages both resistance in the virus and poor adherence by giving the patient the wrong message that it is safe to miss medication. Where feasible for adherent patients, self-medication should be encouraged.

Control of infection

Standard infection control procedures should be followed for all patients, however when carrying out a procedure on an infected patient such as nasopharyngeal aspiration, it is important to wear a mask and eye protection to protect from splashes. However if a needle stick injury or mucosal splash occurs, medical advice concerning post-exposure HIV prophylaxis should be sought immediately (and ideally should be commenced within two hours of exposure). Aseptic non-touch technique (ANTT) should be used in the management of all invasive lines.

Disclosure

Patients newly diagnosed with HIV will require a lot of emotional support. The diagnosis invariably comes as a shock and patients may find it difficult to disclose to family and friends, however it is important that with time they are encouraged to do so particularly when individuals may have been at risk of acquiring the infection (sexual partners, children of an HIV positive mother, previously shared needles or razors). If the hospital HIV services have not already been involved, an urgent referral should be made to allow post-test counselling and specialist HIV input to be given as well as access to other support services.

SUMMARY

Despite the advances in diagnosis, pharmacological therapy and neurosurgery, CNS infections are associated with high morbidity and mortality. Successful management requires early intervention with pharmacological therapy and vigilance for early signs of complications.

REFERENCES

Adam SK, Osborne S (2005) *Critical Care Nursing Science and Practice* (2nd edition). Oxford: Oxford University Press.

Andrewes D, Gielewski E (1999). Work rehabilitation of a herpes simplex encephalitis patient with anterograde amnesia. *Neuropsychological Rehabilitation* 9(1):77–99.

Beghi E, Nicolosi A, Kurland L *et al.* (1984) Encephalitis and aseptic meningitis. Olmstead County, Minnesota, 1950–1981: I. Epidemiology. *Annals of Neurology* 16:283–94.

Bonthius DJ, Karacay B (2002) Meningitis and encephalitis in children. An update. *Neurologic Clinics* 20:1013–1038, vi–vii.

Boss B (2006) Alterations of neurologic function. In: Mccance K and Huether S (eds) *Pathophysiology: The Biologic Basis for Disease in Adults and Children* (5th edition). Mosby St. Louis: Elsevier.

Chaudhuri A, Kennedy PGE (2002) Diagnosis and treatment of viral encephalitis. *Postgraduate Medical Journal* 78:575–583.

Dikmen S, Machamer J, Temkin N (1993) Psychosocial outcome in patients with moderate to severe head injury: 2-year follow-up. *Brain Injury* 7(2):113–124.

Donovan C, Blewitt J (2009) An overview of meningitis and meningococcal septicaemia. *Emergency Nurse* 17(7):30–36.

Dowell E, Easton A, Solomon T (2000) *Consequences of Encephalitis*. Malton: The Encephalitis Society.

Easton A, Atkin K, Dowell E (2006) Encephalitis, a service orphan: the need for more research and access to neuropsychology. *British Journal of Neuroscience Nursing* 2(10):488–492.

Elsass L, Kinsella G (1987) Social interaction following severe closed head injury. *Psychological Medicine* 17(1):67–78.

Encephalitis Society (2003) *Encephalitis*. Malton: The Encephalitis Society.

Encephalitis Society (2010) *The after effects and social consequences of encephalitis* Available from: (http://www.encephalitis.info/images/iPdf/Research2/ProjectSummary.pdf) Accessed April 2010.

Evans JJ (2003) Rehabilitation of executive deficits. In: BA Wilson (ed) *Neuropsychological Rehabilitation: Theory and Practice*. Lisse: Swets and Zeitlinger.

Fitzpatrick M, Gan P (1999) Contrast enhanced CT in the early diagnosis of cerebral abscess. *British Medical Journal* 319(7204):239–240.

Fleminger S, Oliver D, Williams WH *et al.* (2003) The neuropsychiatry of depression after brain injury. *Neuropsychological Rehabilitation* 13(1–2):65–87.

Garg RK (2006) Acute disseminated encephalomyelitis. In: H Morris (ed) *Neurology Update*. Oxford: Radcliffe Publishing Ltd.

Gazzard B G, Anderson J *et al.* (2008) British HIV Association guidelines for the treatment of HIV-1-infected adults with antiretroviral therapy. *HIV Medicine* 9(8):563–608.

Godefroy O (2003) Frontal syndrome and disorders of executive functions. *Journal of Neurology* 250(1):1–6.

Godfrey HP, Partridge FM, Knight RG, Bishara S (1993) Course of insight disorder and emotional dysfunction following closed head injury: a controlled cross-sectional follow-up study. *Journal of Clinical and Experimental Neuropsychology* 15(4):503–515.

Goodpasture EW, Teague O (1923) Transmission of the virus of herpes labialis along nerve in experimentally infected rabbits. *Journal of Medical Research* 44:139–184.

Greve KW, Houston RJ, Adams D *et al.* (2002) The neurobehavioural consequences of St. Louis encephalitis infection. *Brain Injury* 16(19):917–927.

Hall KM, Karzmark P, Stevens M *et al.* (1994) Family stressors in traumatic brain injury: a two-year follow-up. *Archives of Physical Medicine and Rehabilitation* 75(8):876–884.

Hankey G, Wardlaw C (2008) *Clinical Neurology*. London: Manson Publishing.

Hayderman RS, Lambert HP, O'Sullivan I *et al.* on behalf of the British Infection Society (2003) The early management of suspected bacterial meningitis and meningococcal septicaemia in adults. *Journal of Infection* 46:75–77.

Health Protection Agency (2007) *HIV and other sexually transmitted diseases in the UK, A health protection report*. Available from: http://www.hpa.org.uk/hpr/archives/2007/news2007/news4707.htm#hiv Accessed July 2010.

Health Protection Agency (2009) *Background information – meningitis /meningococcal*. Available from: http://www.hpa.org.uk/webw/HPAweb&HPAwebStandard/HPAweb_C/1195733829169?p=1191942172840 Accessed July 2010.

Hokkanen L, Launes J (1997) Cognitive recovery instead of decline after acute encephalitis: A prospective follow up study. *Journal of Neurology, Neurosurgery and Psychiatry* 63(2): 222–227.

Hokkanen L, Launes J (2000) Cognitive outcome in acute sporadic encephalitis. *Neuropsychology Review* 10(3):151–167.

Holmes EC (2001) On the origin and evolution of the human immunodeficiency virus (HIV). *Biological Reviews* 76(2):239–254.

Hooper L, Williams WH, Wall SE *et al.* (2007) Caregiver distress, coping and parenting styles in cases of childhood encephalitis. In: BK Dewar, W H Williams (eds) *Encephalitis: Assessment and Rehabilitation Across the Lifespan* (Vol 17). Hove: Psychology Press.

Howard R, Manji H (2009) Infections in the nervous system. In: Clarke C, Howard R, Rossor M *et al.* (eds) *Neurology A Queen Square Textbook*. Oxford: Wiley-Blackwell.

Joint Formulary Committee (2009) *British National Formulary* (edition 58). London: BMJ Publishing group and RPS Publishing.

Kaplan C P, Bain K (1999) Cognitive outcome after emergent treatment of herpes simplex encephalitis with acyclovir. *Brain Injury* 13(11): 935–941.

Kedhar SR, DA Jabs (2007) Cytomegalovirus retinitis in the era of highly active antiretroviral therapy. *Herpes* 14(3):66–71.

Kennedy PGE, Chaudhuri A (2002) Herpes simplex encephalitis. *Journal of Neurology, Neurosurgery and Psychiatry* 73:237–238.

Khetsuriani N, Holman RC, Anderson LJ (2002) Burden of encephalitis-associated hospitalizations in the United States, 1988–1997. *Clinical Infectious Diseases* 35:175–182.

Kreutzer JS, Gervasio AH, Camplair PS (1994). Patient correlates of caregivers' distress and family functioning after traumatic brain injury. *Brain Injury* 8(3):211–230.

Kreutzer JS, Seel RT, Gourley E (2001) The prevalence and symptom rates of depression after traumatic brain injury: a comprehensive examination. *Brain Injury* 15(7):563–576.

Kumar AM (2007) Human immunodeficiency virus type 1 RNA Levels in different regions of human brain: Quantification using real-time reverse transcriptase–

polymerase chain reaction. *Journal of Neurovirology* 13:210–224.

Marsh NV, Knight RG, Godfrey HP (1990) Long-term psychosocial adjustment following very severe closed head injury. *Neuropsychology* 4:13–27.

Meningitis Research Trust (2002) *Meningococcal Meningitis and Meningococcal Septicaemia: Guidance notes*. (3ʳᵈ edition). Bristol: MRF.

Meningitis Research Foundation (2009) *Meningococcal disease*.   http://www.meningitis.org/assets/x/50114 Accessed July 2010.

Meningitis Trust (2008) *Tuberculous meningitis: the facts.* Available from: http://www.meningitis-trust.org/images/pdfs/TB-Meningitis.pdf Accessed July 2010.

Miner JR, Heegaard W, Mapes A *et al.* (2001) Presentation, time to antibiotics and mortality of patients with bacterial meningitis at an urban county medical centre. *Journal of Emergency Medicine* 21:387–392.

Montoya JG, Liesenfeld O (2004) Toxoplasmosis. *Lancet* 363(9425): 1965–1976.

Okuda B, Kawabata K, Tachibana H *et al.* (2001) Postencephalitic pure anomic aphasia: 2-year follow-up. *Journal of the Neurological Sciences* 187(1–2):99–102.

Ownsworth TL, Fleming J (2005) The relative importance of metacognitive skills, emotional status, and executive function in psychosocial adjustment following acquired brain injury. *Journal of Head Trauma Rehabilitation* 20(4): 315–332.

Palella F, Deloria-Knoll M, Chmiel J *et al.* (2003) Survival benefit of initiating antiretroviral therapy in HIV-infected persons in different CD4 cell strata. *Annals of Internal Medicine* 138:620–626.

Pewter SM (2007) *Neuropsychological impariment profiles and psychosocial outcome in acute encephalitis in adults*. Exeter: Unpublished Ph.D. Thesis, University of Exeter.

Pewter SM, Williams WH, Haslam C *et al.* (2007). Neuropsychological and psychiatric profiles of acute encephalitis in adults. In: BK Dewar, WH Williams (eds) *Encephalitis: Assessment and Rehabilitation Across the Lifespan* (Vol 17) Hove: Psychology Press.

Pukkila-Worley R, Mylonakis E (2008) Epidemiology and management of cryptococcal meningitis: developments and challenges. *Expert Opinions in Pharmacotherapeutics* 9(4):551–560.

Raschilas F, Wolff M, Delatour F *et al.* (2002) Outcome of and prognostic factors for herpes simplex encephalitis in adult patients: results of a multicenter study. *Communicable Infectious Diseases* 35(1):254–260.

Robinson PA, Bauer M, Leal MA *et al.* (1999) Early mycological treatment failure in AIDS-associated cryptococcal meningitis. *Clinic of Infectious Diseases* 28(1):82–92.

Rössler W, Haker H (2003) Conceptualising psychosocial interventions. *Current Opinion in Psychiatry* 16(6):709–712.

Schott J (2006) Limbic encephalitis: a clinician's guide. *Practical Neurology* 6:143–153.

Solomon T, Hart I *et al.* (2007) Viral encephalitis: a clinician's guide. *Practical Neurology* 7:288–305.

Steiner I, Budka H, Chaudhuri A *et al.* (2005) Viral encephalitis: a review of diagnostic methods and guidelines for management. *European Journal of Neurology* 12:331–343.

The Encephalitis Society (2010) *The after effects and social consequences of encephalitis*. Available from: http://www.encephalitis.info/images/iPdf/Research2/ProjectSummary.pdf Accessed July 2010

Thwaites GE, Chau T, Lan N *et al.* (2004) Dexamethasone for the treatment of tuberculous meningitis in adolescents and adults. *New England Journal of Medicine* 351(17):1741–1751.

van de Beek D, de Gans J, McIntyre P, Prasad K (2007) Corticosteroids for acute bacterial meningitis. *Cochrane Database of Systematic Reviews*, Issue 1. Art. No.: CD004405. DOI: 10.1002/14651858.CD004405.pub2.

van de Beek D, de Gans J, Spanjaard L *et al.* (2004) Clinical features and prognostic factors in adults with bacterial meningitis. *New England Journal of Medicine* 351:1849–1859.

Vento S, Di Perri G, Garofano T *et al.* (1993) Pneumocystis carinii pneumonia during primary HIV-1 infection. *Lancet* 3;342(8862):24–25.

Wang KW, Chang WN, Chang HW *et al.* (2005) The significance of seizures and other predictive factors during the acute illness for long term outcome after bacterial meningitis. *Seizure* 14: 586–592.

Whitley RJ, Gnann JW (2002) Viral encephalitis: Familiar infections and emerging pathogens *Lancet* 359:507–513.

Williams WH (2003) Neuro-rehabilitation and cognitive behaviour therapy for emotional disorders in acquired brain injury. In: BA Wilson (ed) *Neuropsychological Rehabilitation: Theory and practice*. Lisse: Swets and Zeitlinger.

Williams WH, Evans JJ (2003) *Biopsychosocial Approaches in Neurorehabilitation: Assessment and management of neuropsychiatric, mood and behavioural disorders*. Hove: Psychology Press.

Wilson BA (2003) *Neuropsychological Rehabilitation: Theory and practice*. Lisse: Swets and Zeitlinger.

World Health Organisation (2007) *Global HIV prevalence has levelled off*. Available from: http://www.who.int/mediacentre/news/releases/2007/pr61/en/index.html Accessed July 2010.

25
Management of Patients with Hydrocephalus

Stuart Hibbins

INTRODUCTION

The word hydrocephalus comes from the Greek for water (hydro) on the head (cephalus). Hydrocephalus is caused by any abnormality which affects the production, circulation or reabsorption of CSF. It is a condition which occurs in a variety of congenital and acquired disorders and can be found in all age groups. This chapter aims to provide an overview of hydrocephalus, a description of its causes and treatments and of the specific nursing care required.

Hydrocephalus can be described as the progressive dilatation of the ventricular system due to increased pressure of cerebrospinal fluid which results in an imbalance between CSF production and its re-absorption (see Chapter 2 for a review of CSF and its pathways). In the majority of cases hydrocephalus will result from either the obstruction of the CSF pathways (obstructive hydrocephalus) or the impairment of absorption of CSF (communicating hydrocephalus). However, a small number of cases result as a consequence of overproduction of CSF, as in choroid plexus papillomas.

EPIDEMIOLOGY

Establishing an accurate incidence of hydrocephalus is complicated by the heterogeneous nature of the condition (the causes are varied and can be particularly complex) and the difficulty in obtaining and collating statistical data from a wide range of institutions. However, the incidence of hydrocephalus has been reported as between 3 per 1000 live births in the USA and 0.66 per 1000 live births in Sweden (Persson *et al.*, 2007).

Also, in the USA it has been estimated that:

* There are at least 127,000 people with a shunt
* Each year there are approximately 70,000 new cases of hydrocephalus
* Over 36,000 of new cases will require shunt operations and 40% of these will need shunt revisions (Shafron, 2004)

In the UK the incidence of hydrocephalus has reduced in recent times due to the increase in the number of elective abortions and more in-depth antenatal screening. These factors have had the effect of reducing the number of infants born with hydrocephalus due to congenital conditions such as spina bifida. However, the number of infants born with hydrocephalus due to intraventricular haemorrhage has increased due to the improved care of premature neonates.

AETIOLOGY AND PATHOPHYSIOLOGY

Any abnormality affecting the circulation or reabsorption of CSF may result in hydrocephalus. The causes can be classified as either non-communicating hydrocephalus (an anatomical obstruction within the ventricular system), or as communicating hydrocephalus (functional obstruction to the arachnoid villi, the primary site of CSF absorption).

Neuroscience Nursing: Evidence-Based Practice, 1st Edition.
Edited by Sue Woodward and Ann-Marie Mestecky
© 2011 Blackwell Publishing Ltd

Where the cause of hydrocephalus is known it can be further classified as either congenital or acquired.

Hydrocephalus usually develops during the first decade of life, particularly in infants under one year where hydrocephalus is commonly associated with congenital abnormalities or intraventricular haemorrhage. Examples of various types of hydrocephalus in a paediatric population are given in Table 25.1 which shows cases admitted to a paediatric neurosurgical unit during a three year period. Hydrocephalus can however also develop during adolescence or adulthood. In older children and adults hydrocephalus develops as a result of a number of aetiologies, such as: trauma, infection, haemorrhage, brain tumours, or altered pathology associated with ageing.

Table 25.1 The aetiology of 78 cases of childhood hydrocephalus admitted to a regional paediatric neurosurgical unit (Hibbins, 2001).

Congenital conditions	35
Intraventricular haemorrhage	21
Meningitis	3
Trauma	1
Complication post-epilepsy surgery	2
Tumour	12
Other	2
Unknown	2
Total	78

The specific causes of hydrocephalus are now discussed.

Myelomeningocele

Myelomeningocele is the most common congenital defect of the nervous system (Shafron, 2004) and is associated with spina bifida cystica (the most severe form of spina bifida). It is a neural tube defect in which some of the vertebrae fail to form properly during early pregnancy. This results in the formation of a myelomeningocele, a sac which is visible at birth, containing CSF, nervous tissue and part of the spinal cord. There is often paralysis below the level of the myelomeningocele. Eighty-five to ninety per cent of cases go on to develop hydrocephalus and most of these will require a shunt (Shafron, 2004).

There has been a worldwide decline in incidence of myelomeningocele in recent times, due to improved screening, increased rates of elective abortion and the use of periconceptual folic acid (Shafron, 2004). Patients with myelomeningocele have abnormal anatomical features of the posterior fossa commonly associated with Chiari (type II) malformation (Arnold–Chiari malformation). The abnormal features include a small posterior fossa where the cerebellum, brain stem and fourth ventricle extend through the foramen magnum, frequently as far as the midcervical region (Figure 25.1). These abnormalities, depending on their severity, can compromise the CSF circulation, particularly at the cerebral aqueduct and the outlets of the fourth ventricle, resulting in hydrocephalus. Hydrocephalus may develop following surgery to close the myelomeningocele and it is important to observe for early signs of raised intracranial pressure as well as signs of life threatening brain stem compression, such as stridor, lower cranial nerve palsies or upper limb

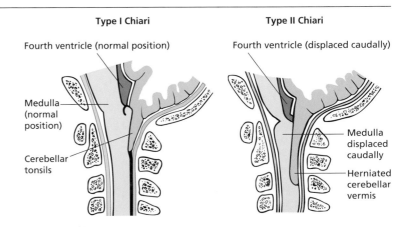

Figure 25.1 Major features of Chiari types I and II malformation. Reproduced from Andrew Kaye, *Essential Neurosurgery*, Wiley-Blackwell, with permission.

weakness (Thompson, 2004). Children with Chiari II malformation have a relatively poor prognosis in terms of intellectual outcome.

It is unlikely that a patient with shunted hydrocephalus due to myelomeningocele will ever be shunt independent (Thompson, 2004). Therefore it is important that young patients with shunted hydrocephalus due to myelomeningocele receive support and regular follow up throughout the transition from childhood to adulthood and beyond. This is because a past study of adults, all with spina bifida and shunted hydrocephalus, reported a significant number of sudden deaths occurring as a result of shunt malfunction (Tomlinson and Sugarman, 1995). It was also evident that some of the patients had received poor follow-up care during their transition from paediatric to adult services.

In Chiari (type I) malformation (CM I) the degree of hindbrain herniation is less profound than that seen in Chiari II malformation (Figure 25.1), however hydrocephalus still occurs in approximately 10% of cases (Lindsay and Bone, 2004). This is because the herniation of the cerebellar tonsils (which often lie below the level of the foramen magnum) is enough to cause obstruction to the CSF pathways at both the tentorial hiatus and basal cisterns. Patients with CM I can often be asymptomatic for many years before becoming symptomatic in adulthood, however with the advent of MRI this disorder is being diagnosed much earlier.

Aqueduct stenosis

Failure of the cerebral aqueduct (aqueduct of Sylvius) to develop during foetal growth will result in a narrowed, blocked or forked lumen known as aqueduct stenosis. It occurs in 10% of childhood cases of hydrocephalus and may present later in life during adulthood (Thompson, 2004). Because of its narrow lumen the aqueduct of Sylvius is also vulnerable to obstruction by several congenital and acquired pathologies such as infection, haemorrhage or by tumours in adjacent structures. Hydrocephalus in this instance is characterised by the presence of enlarged lateral and third ventricles with a normal size fourth ventricle, clearly visible by either CT or MRI. With MRI scanning it is now possible to differentiate between different types of aqueduct stenosis such as those caused by posterior fossa tumours or Chiari malformations.

Dandy Walker syndrome

Dandy Walker syndrome is a congenital brain malformation which is often associated with hydrocephalus. Patients have a cystic dilatation of the fourth ventricle due to the absence of the foramina of Luschka and Magendie. Hydrocephalus usually develops after birth and exists in seventy-five per cent of cases by the age of three months (Thompson, 2004). The dilated fourth ventricle can either be in communication with the rest of the ventricular system, or is encysted and separate from the ventricular system, and this will determine the method of treatment.

Intraventricular haemorrhage in infants

The germinal matrix is a highly vascularised region in the premature infant's brain which is vulnerable to injury during birth and the first few days of life. This is because premature infants lack the ability to autoregulate cerebral blood pressure leaving them susceptible to sudden changes in systemic blood pressure. In conditions of hypertension the fragile germinal matrix vessels can rupture resulting in intraventricular haemorrhage (IVH). Approximately 45% of newborn premature infants weighing less than 1500 grams develop an IVH due to germinal matrix haemorrhage. Most of these infants will remain asymptomatic, but 20% develop hydrocephalus and require a shunt (Thompson, 2004).

Brain tumours

Tumours growing in the midline of the brain (e.g. posterior fossa, the pineal area or the suprasellar region) will often cause obstructive hydrocephalus and raised ICP before the principal effects of the expanding tumour size (Chumas and Tyagi, 2005). However, hydrocephalus is cured by tumour removal in up to 80% of cases and the need for a permanent shunt is often avoided (Drake and Sainte-Rose, 1995). Hydrocephalus resulting from the overproduction of CSF is associated with tumours of the choroid plexus, however these tumours are extremely rare.

Meningitis

Infection or products of inflammatory processes within the CSF pathways can interrupt the absorption of CSF causing a communicating type of hydrocephalus. The subarachnoid spaces are particularly vulnerable to blockage by inflammatory exudates during the acute phase of meningitis. Successful treatment with antibiotics usually means that the hydrocephalus will resolve, however it may occur some months or years later due to scarring of cortical subarachnoid spaces. It is therefore important to monitor post-meningitic patients for signs of raised ICP. The probability of hydrocephalus is greater if the treatment of meningitis has been sub-therapeutic or is delayed (Thompson, 2004).

Head injury

Brain herniation (e.g. midline shift) due to the presence of an intracranial haematoma can obstruct the lateral ventricles by occluding the third ventricle. Alternatively a posterior fossa haematoma can compress the fourth ventricle and cause an obstruction to the CSF pathways (Selladurai and Reilly, 2007). Patients recovering from severe head injury are also at risk of developing a communicating type of hydrocephalus due to the effects of post-inflammatory processes and subsequent fibrosis of the subarachnoid spaces.

Subarachnoid haemorrhage in adults

Hydrocephalus occurs in approximately 20% of patients following subarachnoid haemorrhage (SAH) and usually presents during the first few days of the initial bleed. The presence of blood clots circulating in the CSF can obstruct the narrower parts of the CSF pathways and the presence of blood in the CSF will compromise the function of the arachnoid villi. About 10% of patients will develop hydrocephalus several months or years after the haemorrhage (Lindsay and Bone, 2004) and this is thought to be due to scarring within the subarachnoid spaces.

Normal pressure hydrocephalus

Normal pressure hydrocephalus (NPH) can occur in elderly patients and often presents with symptoms of memory impairment, gait disturbance and incontinence, and radiological evidence of enlarged ventricles. There are two types: NPH which is secondary to other pathologies (e.g. SAH, meningitis and head injury) and NPH which is idiopathic (unknown cause). It is thought that in both types an underlying pathology disturbs the CSF pathways and causes hydrocephalus. Compensatory mechanisms such as reduced CSF production help to reduce CSF pressure. However the ventricles remain enlarged and the patient is left with symptoms. NPH should be distinguished from those patients whose ventricular dilatation is secondary to brain atrophy associated with ageing.

Idiopathic intracranial hypertension (IIH)

Previously known as benign intracranial hypertension (BIH). IIH is characterised by the presence of raised ICP with no alteration of consciousness and there is no radiological evidence of ventricular enlargement. Although it can develop at any age, it usually occurs in adults during the third and fourth decade of life, affecting more women than men. There is no single known cause, however it is associated with various medications, metabolic and endocrinological disorders (Thompson, 2004). It is also associated with pregnancy and weight gain (Lindsay and Bone, 2004) and patients can present with severe intractable headaches and visual disturbances. Close ophthalmological observation is extremely important in these cases as permanent visual problems can result. IIH is a self limiting disease which in severe cases can be treated with medications such as acetazolamide, by repeated lumbar punctures (LPs) or by inserting a lumboperitoneal shunt.

Arrested hydrocephalus

Arrested hydrocephalus is where the neurological status of the patient is stable in the presence of enlarged ventricles. It is thought that compensatory mechanisms and an improvement in CSF circulation during growth may explain the absence of intracranial hypertension in these patients.

CLINICAL SIGNS AND SYMPTOMS

The clinical signs and symptoms of hydrocephalus will depend on the age of the individual at presentation, the underlying cause and the speed at which the obstruction to CSF flow occurs. The infant's skull, with its greater pliability, allows the head to expand before signs of raised ICP occur. In contrast to the infant skull, the older child and adult have rigid skulls and their condition will rapidly deteriorate as ventricular distension and increased ICP develop. The clinical signs and symptoms seen in various age groups are summarised in Table 25.2. Refer to Chapter 7 for a detailed account of the signs and symptoms of raised ICP.

INVESTIGATIONS

Cranial ultrasound

The use of cranial ultrasound in the infant with an open fontanelle is a safe and relatively easy method of imaging because it avoids the use of irradiation and can be performed within the ward environment. Cranial ultrasound can evaluate the supratentorial ventricular system (the lateral and third ventricles) for intraventricular haemorrhage and other causes of hydrocephalus common in infants.

CT and MRI

CT images enable the clinician to evaluate the whole ventricular system as well as the precise areas of CSF obstruction. For instance, a CT image showing enlarged lateral ventricles, a dilated third ventricle and a normal fourth ventricle would suggest an obstructive type of hydroceph-

Table 25.2 Clinical signs and symptoms of hydrocephalus according to age group.

Age group	Clinical signs and symptoms
Infants (1 year and under)	Early clinical symptoms (can be subtle): • Increasing head circumference • Tense or bulging fontanelle • Open cranial sutures • Prominent scalp veins • Sun-setting eyes • Lethargy • Feeding intolerance • Vomiting Late signs: • Critical signs of raised ICP • Changes to muscle tone (decreased, normal or increased) • Visual disturbances and papilloedema (can occur but more common in older age group)
Adults and older children	Acute onset: • Signs of raised ICP Gradual onset: • Change in behaviour • Poor concentration • Increasing drowsiness (sleeping more) • Visual disturbances • Papilloedema
Elderly	Acute onset: • Signs of raised ICP Gradual onset (over weeks or months): • Memory impairment • Gait ataxia • Headache • Incontinence These symptoms can be confused with signs of the aging process

alus, e.g. aqueduct stenosis (Figure 25.2), whereas a widespread dilatation of the ventricular system would suggest a communicating hydrocephalus.

As with cranial ultrasound, the use of MRI also avoids the use of irradiation and provides higher resolution images. This enables clinicians to visualise the CSF pathways and differentiate between various forms of obstructive hydrocephalus (particularly those due to tumours and Chiari malformations).

TREATMENT

Although many of the physiological principles which underpin modern surgical techniques were discovered in the early twentieth century (Pearce, 2003) it was not until the 1950s that two important developments revolutionised the treatment of hydrocephalus. Nulsen and Spiltz developed a valved shunt and Holter later used silicone rubber (a biocompatible material not previously used) to create an early version of today's shunt system. Previous to this

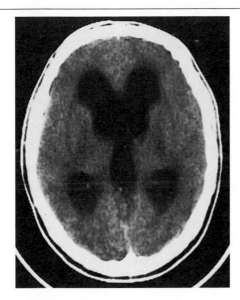

Figure 25.2 Hydrocephalus of the lateral and third ventricles due to aqueduct stenosis.
Reproduced from Andrew Kaye, *Essential Neurosurgery*, Wiley-Blackwell, with permission.

time there had been no reliable form of treatment and hydrocephalus was generally considered a fatal condition. However, despite this dramatic improvement in treatment, there continues to be a relatively high number of complications associated with modern shunting systems (Drake and Sainte-Rose, 1995).

MEDICAL MANAGEMENT

Treatment of hydrocephalus involves the redirection of CSF from the normal pathway to allow for absorption of CSF at an alternative site or the diversion of CSF past an obstruction. Once the underlying pathology is known the most appropriate treatment option is decided (see summary in Table 25.3). The surgical options available are:

- Insertion of a shunt. Most shunt systems work by draining CSF from the lateral ventricles to another part of the body via a hydrostatic pressure gradient (e.g. in a ventriculo-peritoneal (VP) shunt, CSF drains from the lateral ventricles to the peritoneal cavity where there is a lower hydrostatic pressure).
- An external ventricular drain (EVD). An EVD is a device used as a temporary measure to divert the flow

of CSF from a ventricle to an external receptacle. It is also used to as a temporary measure to treat raised ICP.
- Endoscopic third ventriculostomy (ETV). An ETV is performed to divert CSF past an obstruction within the ventricular system, usually by making an opening in the floor of the third ventricle using an endoscope (e.g. treatment of aqueduct stenosis).

Shunts

Ventriculo-peritoneal shunts (VP)

The insertion of a VP shunt is the standard treatment for patients with hydrocephalus (Shafron, 2004). VP shunts consist of a ventricular catheter, a valve, reservoir, and a distal catheter. The ventricular end is implanted into the ventricle via a burr hole and then connected to the reservoir which is placed on the surface of the mastoid bone, under the scalp (Figure 25.3). The reservoir contains a valve which prevents the backflow of CSF. The distal catheter is tunnelled through the subcutaneous tissues to the abdomen, and placed into the peritoneal cavity where the CSF is reabsorbed by the peritoneum. In children a long (at least 25cm) distal catheter is used to allow for future growth (Drake and Sainte-Rose, 1995).

Ventriculo-atrial shunts

In the past, areas such as the pleural cavity (ventriculo-pleural shunt) and right atrium (ventriculo-atrial shunt) were routinely used for the placement of the distal part of the catheter but these methods were associated with a high number of complications. Today these techniques are only used if the peritoneum cannot be used as the site of absorption (e.g. because of scarring from previous abdominal surgery or the presence of local infection). In the 1970s the VP shunt became the method of choice because it was a relatively easy procedure and had a higher success rate.

Lumbar peritoneal shunts

This method of CSF diversion is where the lumbar sub-arachnoid space is utilised for the proximal end of the shunt system and is sometimes the surgical option for patients with benign intracranial hypertension (BIH).

Shunt components

Valves

The valve is the part of the shunt which regulates the flow of CSF from the cerebral ventricles. There are various

Table 25.3 Summary of treatment options for hydrocephalus.

Cause of hydrocephalus	Treatment
Subarachnoid haemorrhage, intraventricular haemorrhage in infants, head injury	Not all patients will become permanently hydrocephalic therefore it is preferable to use an EVD or reservoir to allow clearing of the CSF during the acute phase, and proceed to VP shunt insertion if needed
Brain tumour	Hydrocephalus is often cured by tumour removal. During the acute phase an EVD can be utilised to temporarily divert CSF and a VP shunt can be inserted at a later date if needed (Marsh, 2007). A third of patients with a posterior fossa tumour will require a permanent shunt (Chumas and Tyagi, 2005)
Aqueduct stenosis	Endoscopic fenestration of the floor of the third ventricle (ventriculostomy). This allows communication between the third ventricle and the basal cistern and allows CSF to flow into the subarachnoid spaces
Dandy Walker syndrome or in patients with multiple arachnoid cysts which impair CSF flow (particularly those found in the suprasellar region, foramen magnum, and posterior fossa)	There are several surgical options and these include: • CSF diversion using a single shunt or a combination of shunts • Endoscopic fenestration of the cyst to allow communication with both the ventricular system and the subarachnoid spaces • A VP and (or) cysto-peritoneal shunt may be considered depending on the complexity of presentation
Chiari malformations type I and II	Insertion of ventricular peritoneal shunt for the treatment of hydrocephalus is performed prior to decompression surgery
Benign intracranial hypertension	If medical management with steroids, acetazolamide (a carbonic anhydrase inhibitor which decreases CSF production) is unsuccessful. Then repeated lumber puncture or lumboperitoneal shunt would be considered
Normal pressure hydrocephalus	Insertion of a ventricular peritoneal shunt improves the outcome of 50–70% of those patients with a known preceding cause (e.g. SAH). However only 30% of those of unknown cause improve after shunting (Lindsay and Bone, 2004)
Infection (e.g. meningitis)	Not all patients will become permanently hydrocephalic therefore it is preferable to treat with antibiotics and use an EVD to allow clearing of the CSF and proceed to VP shunt insertion if needed

designs of valves but no single design has proven to be better than any other (Drake and Sainte-Rose, 1995). Most valves are designed to open when a predetermined CSF pressure is reached and close when the CSF pressure falls. Valve designs are available in low, medium and high pressure types. There are also programmable valves where the opening pressure can be adjusted externally to suit the requirements of particular patients. MRI can alter the set-

tings of programmable shunts therefore the settings need to be checked after scanning.

Anti-siphon devices

A relatively large change in hydrostatic pressure occurs when an individual moves from a lying position to a standing position. Some patients are very sensitive to these changes in pressure and suffer symptoms such as

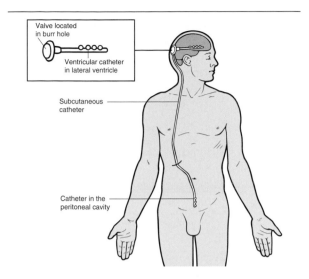

Figure 25.3 Diagram of ventriculo-peritoneal shunt. Reproduced from Andrew Kaye, *Essential Neurosurgery*, Wiley-Blackwell, with permission.

headaches and dizziness. The anti-siphon device is designed to reduce this problem by preventing the sudden 'over-drainage' of CSF by increasing the valve opening pressure. The problem of developing a shunt system that functions both in the horizontal and vertical position continues to elude shunt manufacturers.

Ventricular access devices

Ventricular access devices (also known as Ommaya reservoirs) are sometimes placed in the right frontal region to monitor ICP or treat infections. They consist of a ventricular catheter and a reservoir and can be used to perform percutaneous aspiration of CSF in situations of acutely raised ICP (Pople, 2002). They are often used in situations where the decision for definitive treatment (e.g. to insert a shunt) needs to be delayed.

External ventricular drain

This device allows the temporary relief of critically raised intracranial pressure (e.g. prior to tumour surgery) or it can be used to drain infected or bloodstained CSF, before definitive shunt surgery. Careful nursing management is necessary to avoid complications associated with their use (see: Nursing management).

Endoscopic third ventriculostomy

The use of endoscopic third ventriculostomy (ETV) to treat obstructive hydrocephalus has been well documented (Bergsneider *et al.*, 2006). In obstructive hydrocephalus it is thought that the cortical arachnoid villi are working normally (absorbing CSF) and that by making a hole in the floor of the third ventricle (using an endoscope) it is possible to bypass the site of obstruction. This allows the passage of CSF into the subarachnoid spaces where it can be absorbed by the arachnoid villi. The success of this method with obstructive hydrocephalus has encouraged its use in patient groups previously considered inappropriate, e.g. elderly patients with NPH (Pople, 2004). Cinalli (2004) reviewed a range of studies which used ETV in patients with obstructive hydrocephalus and reported a success rate of between 70 and 90%. There are also reports of success rates of 60% in adults with communicating hydrocephalus. Neuroendoscopy techniques are also used to fenestrate arachnoid cysts (e.g. in Dandy Walker syndrome).

Medical management

Certain drugs such as acetazolamide can be used to reduce CSF production and work by inhibiting the enzyme carbonic anhydrase. This enzyme is present in the choroid plexus epithelium and is essential for the production of CSF. Acetazolamide is often prescribed in patients with IIH.

Complications

Most studies show that approximately 40% of shunts will malfunction during the first year of insertion (Shafron, 2004). When shunts fail the existing shunt system is either partially or completely revised depending on the cause of the shunt malfunction. Mechanical failure may require a total or part revision of the shunt system. In cases of shunt infection, the existing shunt system is removed and an EVD sited. The patient is then treated with intravenous and intrathecal antibiotics. Daily CSF sampling is carried out to monitor for the presence of infection and when the CSF is clear a new shunt is inserted. A shunt which is over-draining can be modified by changing the valve type for one with a higher opening pressure. Alternatively an anti-siphon device or programmable shunt can be utilised. The causes of shunt malfunction are summarised in Table 25.4.

NURSING MANAGEMENT

Patients who arrive at the emergency department with a blocked shunt and signs of critically raised ICP will need prompt treatment (see Chapter 7). Once control of the airway, breathing and circulation is established, the use of osmotic diuretics such as mannitol may be considered,

Table 25.4 The causes and symptoms of shunt malfunction.

Type of malfunction	Symptoms
Obstruction: the most common site is the ventricular end, which can become embedded in the brain tissue or blocked with choroid plexus	Headaches, signs of raised ICP, infants may develop a subcutaneous CSF pouch around reservoir and tubing
Overdrainage: can be due to inappropriate valve	Low pressure headaches and subdural collections
Infection: usually occurs within several months of insertion. *Staphylococcus epidermis* (40%) and *Staphylococcus aureus* (20%) are the most common	Fever, irritability, signs of mechanical failure

particularly if there is a delay in organising definitive surgical treatment (Thompson, 2004). Alternatively the shunt can be tapped to remove a small amount of CSF to reduce ICP.

The treatment plan will depend on how acutely ill the patient is, the pathogenesis of hydrocephalus, and the patient's age (see Table 25.3). Prompt treatment of the raised intracranial pressure with a shunt or EVD will restore normal intracranial pressure and the patient should make a rapid recovery.

Preoperative care of the patient undergoing shunt insertion

In both the emergency and planned situation it is important for patients and their families to receive accurate information about their treatment and an opportunity to discuss this with a neurosurgeon. Information should be appropriate for a patient's age and level of understanding and could include the following:

- Diagrams of shunts and brain anatomy
- Literature from shunt manufacturers
- Information and advice from support groups (e.g. Association for Spina Bifida and Hydrocephalus)
- Use of anatomical manikins with shunts (dolls for children)
- Sample of a shunt device

The patient should not be overloaded with too much information at one time and should have access to all members of the interdisciplinary team throughout their hospitalisation.

Patients who are admitted to regional neurosurgical units with hydrocephalus are often a long way from their home and families and will require support from all members of the interdisciplinary team.

Local policy should be adhered to when preparing patients for surgery (see Chapter 20). Parents of infants, toddlers and young people should be encouraged to participate in all aspects of this care. If surgery is planned the patient will have more time to prepare for theatre. A shower prior to surgery is an effective way to minimise the risk of infection. Hair shaving is usually performed using an electrical hair clipper (in theatre) over the site of the craniotomy (to aid skin closure and prevent infection). It is important that this is discussed with the patient before surgery to avoid any distress post-operatively. Prophylactic antibiotics are usually administered at induction although the increased use of antimicrobial impregnated shunts may reduce the need for this in the future (Bayston, 2007).

Post-operative management of shunted patients

Once the patient has recovered from their anaesthetic and is breathing unaided, regular neurological assessment should be performed to detect early signs of haemorrhage or raised ICP. However signs of shunt malfunction are more likely to manifest several hours or days after surgery (it may take some time before CSF re-accumulates and causes raised ICP).

In the past, patients were initially nursed in the supine position and gradually elevated to the sitting position over one or two days after surgery to prevent over-drainage of the shunt and low pressure headaches. However, most modern shunt systems in use today require no special positioning considerations (Drake and Sainte-Rose, 1995). The exception to this is in infants and patients who are in a chronic state of deep coma (e.g. a persistent vegetative state) because they usually have high pressure valves inserted. These patients should be nursed in a slightly raised position (this increases the differential pressure gradient) to encourage the flow of CSF through the shunt system (Drake and Sainte-Rose, 1995). In infants this will avoid the risk of subcutaneous CSF leak around the ventricular catheter and the creation of a subcutaneous CSF pouch, which is difficult to treat. Infants are also at risk of developing a subcutaneous CSF leak due to the slackness of their skin, large ventricles, a thin rim of cortical mantle and their low ICP. The risk of developing a subcutaneous CSF pouch reduces with the formation of scar tissue which helps anchor the shunt system in place.

Once normal ICP is restored, particularly in patients who have undergone previous shunt insertions (or revisions), recovery from surgery should be relatively quick. Those patients who have undergone a primary shunt insertion may need more time to adapt to a new shunt device.

The prevention of skin problems around the valve site is achieved by avoiding any pressure to the scalp overlying the valve system. Patient groups most at risk of this occurring are infants and patients with disabilities. This means that parents and carers should be made aware of the importance of good patient positioning to avoid pressure areas developing over the site of the valve. There exists a common misconception amongst some patients that pumping the shunt reservoir assesses the shunt patency. On discharge from hospital patients and carers should be discouraged from pumping the valve chamber of the shunt as this has no diagnostic purpose (Thompson, 2007).

Post-operative management of the external ventricular drain (ETV) patient

Although ETV has the advantage of having fewer long-term complications than shunts, the procedure itself is not without risk. Serious haemorrhage from damage to the vascular structures adjacent to the site of the new ventriculostomy is a potential complication. Therefore vigilant neurological assessment for signs of intracranial haemorrhage is necessary during the acute post-operative period. Infection is also a complication which is more likely to manifest some time after surgery.

Patients are often encouraged to position themselves in a semi-upright position during the first couple of days following surgery to encourage the patency of the new ventriculostomy (May, 2004). However, because there is virtually no difference in the hydrostatic pressure between the third ventricle and the newly accessed subarachnoid spaces, this is not as effective as in shunted patients (where there exists a relatively large hydrostatic pressure gradient between the ventricles and the peritoneal cavity).

Nursing management of an external ventricular drain

CSF drainage via an EVD allows the temporary relief of hydrocephalus. An EVD is inserted in the lateral ventricles and connected to a closed collection system outside of the body (Figure 25.4). It can be used for continuous or intermittent CSF drainage and the measurement of CSF pressure. Indications for use include: temporary drainage for infected or blocked shunts, short-term treatment of raised ICP and the diversion of bloodstained or infected CSF.

The main role of the nurse caring for a patient with an EVD is the safe management of the EVD system and the accurate documentation of CSF drainage.

The neurosurgical team will give instructions on the pressure level (in cmH$_2$O) at which the CSF collection chamber is to be set or, alternatively, the volume of CSF to be drained each hour. The former requires the nurse to move the adjustable chamber to the specific pressure level requested by the neurosurgical team. The latter requires the nurse to frequently monitor the drainage and set the

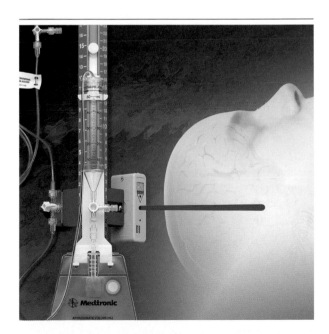

Figure 25.4 An external ventricular drain. Image provided by Medtronic Sofamor Danek USA.

pressure level of the chamber to achieve the volume of drainage required. The volume of CSF drainage should be recorded for each hour and its appearance noted for colour and clarity. There is a risk of ventricular collapse and subdural haematoma if excessive drainage of CSF occurs (approximately >25ml/hr). If excessive drainage should occur the nurse should turn off the drain, reassess the patient and inform the neurosurgical team immediately. Under drainage can lead to increased ICP and neurological deterioration. If under drainage occurs the patency of the drain can be checked by observing for a swing of CSF in the tubing or by lowering the chamber below the level that it was set and observing for CSF flow. If it appears to be blocked, i.e. there is no CSF flow and no swing of fluid in the tubing, the neurosurgical team should be informed immediately and the patient should be monitored more frequently.

During physiotherapy or interventions known to increase ICP, e.g. suctioning (see Chapter 7), the EVD should be either turned off for the duration of the intervention or the chamber should be raised by 5–10cmH$_2$0 above the prescribed level to prevent excessive drainage of CSF. The drain should be turned off when a patient needs to change their position (e.g. from lying down to sitting up in bed) and the zero level realigned with the foramen of Monro. During transportation the EVD should be kept in an upright position.

The zero level on the EVD must be consistently level with the position of the catheter in the ventricle, i.e. the foramen of Monro. The anatomical reference points most commonly cited with which to align the zero pressure mark of the EVD scale are the external auditory meatus or tragus of the ear (Pope, 1998; Ropper *et al.*, 2004). These points correspond with the bridge of the nose if the patient is in the lateral position. Local protocols should agree the anatomical reference point to ensure that all staff are consistently using the same point. The EVD should be aligned with the anatomical reference points using a laser or carpenter's level (Bisnaire and Robinson, 1997) to ensure accuracy of the leveling.

To minimise the risk of infection, the patient and carer should be encouraged to avoid touching the system. Most EVDs are designed to minimise the risk of infection, however access to the system is often necessary (e.g. to gain CSF samples, administer intrathecal drugs, change the drainage bag, etc.) therefore it is extremely important to maintain asepsis. All dressings should be changed if soiled or loose. The drainage bag should not be allowed to become too full or heavy and should be changed by the time it is three quarters full (Woodward *et al.*, 2002).

Discharge of shunted patients

The diagnosis and treatment of hydrocephalus will be a time of great anxiety for parents and patients, and it is the role of the nurse to provide reassurance and support.

Verbal and written information provided during the preoperative period should be reinforced prior to discharge. It is important to establish that as long as there are no complications, a person can lead a relatively normal life with a shunt device (see: Patient Perspective below).

There has been a greater awareness during recent times of the need for vigilant follow-up of shunted patients, however a small number of patients continue to suffer blindness or death as a result of undetected chronic shunt malfunction (Pople, 2004). Particular attention should be given to those patients who move from paediatric to adult services. The UK Association of Spina Bifida and Hydrocephalus (ASBAH) recommends the following:

- Patients should have a baseline scan when they are well, six to twelve months after shunt insertion. Patients should have their own copy of the scan, if they live far away from their neurosurgical unit
- Patients and carers should receive written instructions of what symptoms to look out for and when to contact their doctors
- Patients should also be given details of their valve type to inform the neurosurgical team on subsequent treatment
- Patients should be made aware of the potential dangers of programmable and external magnetic sources (e.g. will need to have their shunt valve checked or readjusted after MRI)
- All patients under 60 should have annual visual acuity checks by an optician and a three yearly check-up by a neurosurgeon or dedicated hydrocephalus outpatient clinic (dependant on local policy)

Discharge of ETV patients

ETV patients should be followed-up in a similar way as shunted cases. Regular checks of visual acuity should be made, and patients should be made aware of the signs of raised ICP. There should also be a regular check-up by a neurosurgeon or dedicated hydrocephalus outpatient clinic.

Although the success rate for ETV is relatively high, follow up after successful treatment is extremely important as late failure can occur in up to 40% of cases and sudden death as little as two years after apparent successful ETV (Pople, 2004).

Prognosis

Patients can expect near-normal life expectancy. However, their developmental prognosis depends on the underlying pathology of hydrocephalus. For instance, in the premature infant with hydrocephalus secondary to an IVH, there is a significant incidence of cerebral palsy, epilepsy and global developmental delay, whereas in the older patient there may be no long-term effects from hydrocephalus caused by a brain tumour (Thompson, 2007).

SUMMARY

Surgery is currently moving away from treatment with shunts and towards endoscopic treatments in cases where the underlying pathology makes it possible. While knowledge of hydrocephalus has advanced considerably during the course of time it is by no means complete (Bergsneider *et al.*, 2006).

Hydrocephalus: patient perspective

In the run up to both GCSEs and A Levels my shunt failed and my neurosurgeon tried various types before finding one – a programmable shunt – to suit me. My hydrocephalus affects me on a daily basis. I suffer from regular headaches, which can be remedied by taking paracetamol, but sometimes the headache niggles away all day. It's annoying, but I'm used to it now.

Going to university to study law was a daunting experience; moving away from home, leaving my friends, starting in a new city. Daunting, but exciting as well. It was the beginning of a new adventure and I could be my own person.

As I sometimes find it difficult to get my bearings I was worried that if I was in a big city, on my own, I would get horribly lost one day. The first few weeks there were weird. Finding my way round was probably the hardest thing. I'm not very good at directions. Life seemed a real emotional rollercoaster at times. But once I found a great group of friends, I had a great time. I have always been open about my condition, but I didn't tell my flatmates for a few weeks. When I did, I found that they'd never heard of hydrocephalus. They were very understanding, and didn't treat me any differently.

I always carry a shunt alert card and made sure my housemates and friends knew about the card and are aware of the warning signs of shunt failure.

My hydrocephalus isn't serious enough for me to need additional help from the university to help me complete my studies.

For me university was a great experience. I began my Bar Vocational Course, the barrister training course last September and I'm back living in halls of residence again. The course is the most difficult I have studied, but it's a great experience, and I know I am on the right path to get to where I want to be … a successful barrister.

So who knows? I may well be the next Lord Chancellor, or perhaps the next Tony Blair? One thing I can be sure of, I intend to be a major player within the judiciary system, so watch this space! Disability shouldn't get in our way, and I won't let it.

REFERENCES

Bayston R (2007) Bactiseal: A system to prevent catheter infections in shunts and external ventricular drains. *British Journal of Neuroscience Nursing* 3 (11):526–531.

Bergsneider M, Egnor M, Johnston M *et al.* (2006) What we don't (but should) know about hydrocephalus. *Journal of Neurosurgery* (3 Suppl Pediatrics) 104:157–159.

Bisnaire D, Robinson L (1997) Accuracy of leveling intraventricular collection drainage systems. *Journal of Neuroscience Nursing* 29(4):261–268.

Chumas P, Tyagi A (2005) Neurosurgical techniques. In: David A. Walker D, Perilongo G *et al.* (eds). *Brain and Spinal Tumors of Childhood*. Oxford: Hodder Arnold.

Cinalli G (2004) Endoscopic third ventriculostomy. In: Cinalli G, Maixner WJ, Sainte-Rose C (Eds) *Pediatric hydrocephalus*. Milan: Springer.

Drake J, Sainte-Rose C (1995) *The Shunt Book*. Oxford: Blackwell Science.

Hibbins S (2001) Data from 78 cases of hydrocephalus admitted to the Paediatric Neurosurgical Unit at King's College Hospital, London, between July 1996 and March 1999. Previously unpublished.

Lindsay K, Bone I (2004) *Neurology and Neurosurgery Illustrated*. (4th edition). Edinburgh: Churchill Livingstone.

Marsh H (2007) Brain Tumours. *Surgery* 25(12):526–529.

May L (2004) Neurosurgery. In: *The Surgical Nursing of Children*. Chambers M, Jones S (eds) Edinburgh: Butterworth-Heinemann.

Pearce J (2003) *Fragments of Neurological History*. London: Imperial College Press.

Persson E, Anderson S, Wiklund L *et al*. (2007) Hydrocephalus in children born in 1999–2002: epidemiology, outcome and ophthalmological findings. *Child's Nervous System* 23(10):1111–1118.

Pope W (1998) External ventriculostomy: A practical application for the acute care nurse. *Journal of Neuroscience Nursing* 30(3):185–190.

Pople I (2002) Hydrocephalus and shunts: What neurologists should know. *Journal of Neurology, Neurosurgery and Psychiatry* 73 (Suppl I): i17–i22.

Pople I (2004) Hydrocephalus. *Surgery* 22 (3):60–63.

Ropper AH, Gress DR, Diringer MN *et al*. (2004) *Neurological and Neurosurgical Intensive Care*. (4th edition). Philadelphia: Lippincott Williams and Wilkins.

Selladurai B, Reilly P (2007) *Initial Management of Head Injury: A comprehensive guide*. Australia: McGraw Hill.

Shafron D (2004) Paediatric neurosurgery. In: Layon A, Gabrielli A, Friedmann W (eds) *Textbook of Neurointensive Care* p285–335. Philadelphia: Saunders.

Thompson D (2004) Hydrocephalus and shunts. In: Moore A, Newell D (eds). *Neurosurgery Principles and Practice.* pp 430–442 New York: Springer.

Thompson D (2007) Hydrocephalus. *Surgery* 25(12): 522–525.

Tomlinson P, Sugarman I (1995) Complications with shunts in adults with spina bifida. *British Medical Journal* 311:286–287.

Woodward S, Addison S, Shah S *et al*. (2002) Benchmarking best practice for external ventricular drainage. *British Journal of Nursing* 11(1):47–53.

FURTHER INFORMATION FOR HEALTH PROFESSIONALS AND PUBLIC

Association for Spina Bifida and Hydrocephalus (ASBAH) http://www.asbah.org/

Section V
Management of Patients with Long-Term Conditions

26
Management of Patients with Common Movement Disorders

Liz Scott, Pauline McDonald and Rachel Taylor

PARKINSON'S DISEASE

INTRODUCTION

Parkinson's disease (PD) is predominantly a movement disorder affecting learned voluntary movement, but also features non-motor symptoms. It is a progressive condition caused by degeneration of the dopaminergic nigrostriatal pathways resulting in a depletion of dopamine. PD is the second most common neurodegenerative disorder (Thomas *et al.*, 2006) and is characterised by bradykinesia, rigidity and resting tremor. It manifests when 80% of dopaminergic neurones have been lost.

PD affects functional abilities such as handwriting, fine motor skills, communication, swallowing, mobility, postural stability and the ordering and sequencing of movements. Dopamine also contributes to cognitive functions such as the ability to concentrate, maintain motivation, mood, problem-solving, decision-making and visual perception. Exccutive dysfunction is common, as are anxiety and depression. There is wide variation in how individuals are affected.

EPIDEMIOLOGY

The UK incidence of PD is 10,000 cases per annum, with a total prevalence of around 120,000 (de Lau and Breteler, 2006). PD affects more men than women, the relative risk being 1.5 times greater. The difference is possibly due to greater exposure to toxins or head trauma in men, and the neuroprotection offered by oestrogen in women (Wooten *et al.*, 2007).

Onset of PD is related to age. It affects 1% of the population over 60 years and 4% over 80 years, but does not exclusively affect older people. Of the 120,000 sufferers in the UK 1 in 20 were diagnosed under the age of 40 years (Schrag and Schott, 2006). PD in people under 20 years is rare, usually genetic and referred to as juvenile PD. The average survival from diagnosis at the age of 62 years is approximately 20 years. Survival rates for other types of Parkinsonism such as multiple system atrophy (MSA) and progressive supranuclear palsy (PSP) are not so favourable (Birdie *et al.*, 2001).

AETIOLOGY

The cause of PD remains elusive, but both environmental (Box 26.1) and genetic factors may be crucial to the development of the disease.

Genetic factors

The chance of developing PD by the age of 80 is about 2%, increasing to 5–6% if a parent or sibling is affected. If both a parent and a sibling have PD then the risk increases to 20–40% (Lazzarini *et al.*, 1994), suggesting a genetic component. The study of the genetics of PD is complex as mutations have been identified in at least 10 different genes.

Head trauma

Evidence for head trauma as a causative factor for PD is conflicting, but more recent studies have shown increased risk following repeated loss of consciousness (Dick *et al.*, 2007) and that mild to moderate closed head injury may increase the risk of PD decades later (Goldman *et al.*, 2006).

Neuroscience Nursing: Evidence-Based Practice, 1st Edition.
Edited by Sue Woodward and Ann-Marie Mestecky
© 2011 Blackwell Publishing Ltd

Box 26.1   Environmental risk factors

- Occupational exposure to metals, e.g. manganese, copper, lead and iron
- Rural living, farming, exposure to herbicides, pesticides, well water drinking
- 1-methyl-4-phenyl-1,2,3,6-tetrahydropyridine (MPTP) exposure: synthetic type of pethidine produced illegally in early 1980s similar to herbicide paraquat

---

Box 26.2   Symptoms of Parkinson's disease

Motor symptoms
- Bradykinesia/hypokinesia
- Rigidity
- Resting tremor
- Postural instability
- Freezing
- Dystonia
- Dysphagia
- Communication difficulty
- Hypomimia (reduced facial expression)

Non-Motor Symptoms
Autonomic dysfunction
- Urinary dysfunction
- Constipation
- Sexual dysfunction

Neuropsychiatric symptoms
- Anxiety
- Apathy
- Depression
- Sleep disturbance

Other non-motor symptoms
- Restless legs
- Excessive daytime somnolence
- Pain

PATHOPHYSIOLOGY

The neuropathology of PD is dominated by the degeneration of the dopaminergic nigrostriatal pathways, but the first neurones to be affected are non-dopaminergic. The substantia nigra and striatum are affected later in the condition (Ahlskog, 2007). Post-mortem findings characteristic of PD include Lewy bodies, neuronal loss and loss of neuromelanin within the substantia nigra.

Lewy bodies

Lewy bodies are inclusion bodies found in some neurones in the substantia nigra and other structures affected in PD (e.g. cerebral cortex, thalamus, brain stem). Lewy bodies are thought to be related to the disposal of damaged proteins, but it is unclear whether Lewy bodies are harmful or protective (Harrower *et al.*, 2005).

Neuronal death

The pathology of PD starts in the brain stem and ascends towards the cortex. Motor symptoms arise because depletion of dopamine producing neurones in the substantia nigra results in inhibition of the direct pathway that facilitates movement and excitation of the indirect pathway that inhibits movement (see Chapter 3). Neuronal loss in olfactory nucleus, brain stem and myenteric plexus of the gastrointestinal tract for example, is associated with the non-motor symptoms of PD such as sensory disturbance, sleep disorders and autonomic symptoms affecting the gut. Later neocortical areas are affected and dementia develops.

Loss of neuromelanin

Loss of neuromelanin from the substantia nigra results in depigmentation so that the substantia nigra appears paler when compared with normal brains. The role of neuromelanin in the development of PD is unclear.

Oxidative stress

Oxidative stress is implicated in the pathogenesis of PD, occurring when there is excess production of free radicals (Grosset *et al.*, 2009). These can damage DNA, enzymes, cellular proteins and unsaturated fatty acids. The body responds with agents that destroy or mop up free radicals such as glutathione. In PD the levels of glutathione in the substantia nigra are reduced.

CLINICAL SIGNS AND SYMPTOMS

Bradykinesia and hypokinesia (slowness and poverty of movement) are diagnostic features, supported by either rigidity and/or resting tremor. PD has traditionally been classified as a motor disorder but it is now clear that significant non-motor symptoms are associated with the condition (Box 26.2).

DIAGNOSIS

The diagnosis is a clinical one and idiopathic PD needs to be differentiated from conditions that produce Parkinsonian symptoms (Box 26.3). If the condition is suspected the patient should be referred to a neurologist or geriatrican with a special interest in PD within six weeks and treatment should not be initiated in the primary care setting (NICE, 2006). Where the clinician is confident of the diagnosis and the patient has a good response to anti-Parkinson medication there is no need for further investigation. The diagnosis should be kept under review and reconsidered if atypical clinical features develop.

MEDICAL MANAGEMENT

Pharmacological therapy

The mainstay of treatment for PD is pharmacological. Treatment is symptomatic and does not slow disease progression. There is no universal first choice drug therapy for either early PD or for adjuvant drug therapy in later PD (NICE, 2006).

Monoamine oxidise type B (MAO-B) inhibitors

MAO-B inhibitors, selegiline (Eldepryl, Zelapar) and rasagiline (Azilect), inhibit the breakdown of dopamine so that it remains available in the synaptic cleft for longer. Selegiline is metabolised to amphetamine derivatives. It can increase alertness and is best avoided in the elderly or those who have a history of hallucinations or confusion. An oral fast-melt preparation, which is safer for elderly patients, is available.

Dopamine agonists

Dopamine agonists mimic the action of dopamine. Ergot-derived dopamine agonists, bromocriptine (Parlodel), pergolide (Celance) and cabergoline (Cabaser), are not widely used, with increasing evidence of serious and potentially life-threatening adverse events (e.g.cardiac valvulopathy and pulmonary fibrosis) (Grosset *et al.*, 2006). NICE guidelines (2006) recommend non-ergot-derived agonists including ropinirole (Requip), pramipexole (Mirapexin), rotigotine (Neupro) and apomorphine (Apo-Go).

Dopamine agonists can delay the development of dyskinesia (involuntary movements), dystonia and motor fluctuations (Hauser *et al.*, 2007) and are effective either as monotherapy or in combination with other drugs. Common side-effects include nausea and vomiting, postural hypotension, somnolence, confusion and hallucinations. They have also been associated with behavioural changes, such as impulse control disorders (Voon *et al.*, 2006). If nausea and vomiting are problematic, the only safe anti-emetic for people with PD is domperidone (Motilium). Metoclopramide (Maxalon) and prochlorperazine (Stemitil) are dopamine antagonists and occupy dopamine receptors, worsening symptoms.

Apomorphine

When patients experience motor complications of levodopa (discussed below), apomorphine is indicated. Apomorphine is a powerful non-ergot dopamine agonist, but cannot be taken orally, as it is lost through hepatic first pass metabolism. It is administered subcutaneously. Apomorphine acts within 5–35 minutes, with a duration of action of 45–100 minutes. It can be used as a single 'rescue' injection or may be infused during waking hours using the specifically designed APO-go pump. Long term studies do not indicate any significant tolerance to the anti-Parkinson effect (Deleu *et al.*, 2004).

Levodopa

Dopamine cannot cross the blood–brain barrier (BBB), but the precursor of dopamine, levodopa, can and is converted into dopamine by the enzyme dopa decarboxylase within the brain. To prevent peripheral conversion, levodopa is combined with a dopa decarboxylase inhibitor (DDCI) to form co-beneldopa (Madopar) or co-careldopa (Sinemet). Long-term administration is associated with escalating doses and the development of motor complications (see Box 26.4) within four to six years of taking levodopa (Ahlskog and Muenter, 2001). A strategy of delaying treatment with levodopa has developed, using dopamine

Box 26.4   Motor complications of levodopa

- End of dose wearing-off of medication effectiveness
- Unpredictable loss of symptom control
- Dyskinesia (drug induced writhing involuntary movements)
  - Peak dose dyskinesia
  - Diphasic dyskinesia (at start and end of each dose)
  - Dystonia (painful cramping of muscles)
- Psychiatric
  - Confusion
  - Hallucinations
  - Delusions
  - Illusions
  - Punding

Adapted from Clarke, 2006.

agonists or MAO-B inhibitors as first line treatment (Hauser *et al.*, 2007).

Problems with the absorption of levodopa contribute to motor fluctuations. Levodopa competes with protein for uptake from the gut. Gastric emptying times are slower in PD patients and this can also interfere with the absorption of levodopa. For this reason many people benefit from taking levodopa on an empty stomach at least 40 minutes before a meal.

A new system to deliver levodopa directly to the duodenum (Duodopa) via a PEG (percutaneous endoscopic gastrostomy) tube has recently been licensed. Aimed at people with advanced PD for whom the medication works, but causes problems with dyskinesia or prolonged, unpredictable off periods, Duodopa enables much lower doses of levodopa to be continuously infused. Funding (£30,000 per annum) for this treatment is currently via exceptional case committee submission for individual patients.

Catechol-O-methyltransferase (COMT) inhibitors

Despite the addition of DDCI to levodopa, only a small amount of the orally administered dose crosses the BBB. The rest is metabolised by the enzyme COMT. By inhibiting COMT more levodopa is available for longer to cross the BBB. There are currently two COMT inhibitors available: entacapone and tolcapone.

Entacapone (Comtess) leads to significant reduction in 'off' time and a reduction in levodopa dose (Deane *et al.*, 2004). A triple combination of levodopa, carbidopa and entacapone is now available (Stalevo). Tolcapone

(Tasmar) can cross the BBB and can only be used in patients where entacapone has failed, provided that liver function is carefully monitored. Treatment must be withdrawn if enzymes rise two to three times above the upper limit of normal.

Entacapone and tolcapone increase levodopa-associated side-effects. Diarrhoea is common and may require withdrawal of the drug. They also stain urine a dark reddish colour, so patients need to be warned.

Amantadine

Amantadine is an anti-viral agent, which was discovered to have an anti-Parkinson effect by chance. Amantadine is thought to reduce receptor activity and while evidence underpinning this is lacking (Crosby *et al.*, 2003), NICE (2006) recommends its use as an anti-dyskinesia agent. The most common side-effects are ankle oedema, livedo reticularis, confusion and hallucinations.

Anticholinergics

Anticholinergics inhibit central muscarinic acetylcholine receptors, restoring the balance between dopamine and acetylcholine, reducing overactivity in the thalamus and thereby reducing tremor. They cause extensive side-effects including: nausea, dry mouth, constipation, dizziness, blurred vision, urine retention, reduced short term memory and psychotic symptoms including confusion and hallucinations. Elderly people are particularly susceptible and anticholinergics should be avoided in people over 70 years.

Deep brain stimulation (DBS)

DBS is an effective treatment for people with PD whose symptoms are not adequately controlled by medication or who suffer severe dyskinesia (Breen and Heisters, 2007), but it is only suitable for 1.6–4.5% of people with PD (Morgante *et al.*, 2007). Selection criteria for DBS were established by NICE in 2003: patients must be generally fit, with no depression or dementia, responsive to levodopa and exhibit refractory motor symptoms.

Three sites are used for DBS. Stimulation of the thalamus provides partial or complete suppression of tremor in 80% of patients; stimulation of the globus pallidus interna (GPi) can benefit all motor symptoms, and stimulation of the subthalamic nucleus (STN) can benefit all motor symptoms of PD in 70–80% of patients (Rodriguez-Oroz *et al.*, 2005). STN stimulation is preferred over GPi in the UK, but it is not possible to say which target is superior or safer on the basis of current evidence (NICE, 2006).

An electrode is passed through a burr hole to the subthalamic nucleus stereotactically. The electrode is connected to a battery powered programmable pulse generator implanted just below the clavicle. Once programmed, the electrode produces a high frequency stimulation which suppresses abnormal activity in the target nucleus and reduces abnormal movements (Byrd *et al.*, 2000). For some patients the results of DBS can be disappointing. They may need to continue to take medication and may still experience fluctuations in their condition. DBS carries a small risk of stroke, loss of speech and haemorrhage. The battery for the stimulator will need to be changed every three to five years and patients should not go through security machines at airports, have an MRI, receive diathermy or deep heat treatment. The post-operative care of these patients is discussed in Chapter 20.

NURSING MANAGEMENT

MacMahon and Thomas (1998) have defined four stages of PD: diagnosis, maintenance, complex and palliative. In a hospital setting patients admitted with PD are likely to be in the complex or palliative stages (Table 26.1) of the disease.

Medication administration

Administering medication on time is vital. In hospital, drugs will need to be administered outside the normal drug round times. Failure to do this has many contributory factors (Box 26.5) and will result in poorly controlled PD, evidenced by loss of independent mobility and difficulty communicating, eating and swallowing, and often a longer stay in hospital (NICE, 2006).

Patients may become anxious and ask for medication repeatedly because they are aware of the problems that a delay will cause. This can make the patient appear difficult and demanding. One woman's experience is described:

'I received a phone call from the hospital telling me that my mother had had a stroke and was comatose. I rushed to the ward to find my mother in a Parkinson's freeze [off state] having had none of her routine Parkinson's drugs since the previous night'

(Parkinson's Disease Society, 2008)

Enabling patients to self-medicate can overcome these problems. If this is not possible every effort should be made to give the patient their medication on time. Nurses are uniquely placed to influence the medicine management of people with PD in hospital. Buxton (2007) has highlighted good practices from around the UK, including pill timers or alarm clocks to remind staff if medication is due outside normal drug round times.

Neuroleptic malignant syndrome (NMS)

Abrupt withdrawal of medication, e.g. if nil-by-mouth, may risk developing NMS and should be avoided. Symptoms include muscular rigidity, high fever, unstable blood pressure, agitation, delirium and eventually coma and death in 5–11% of cases (Stotz *et al.*, 2004). These symptoms may be misdiagnosed as infections and NMS can be missed. Left untreated, pneumonia, renal failure, seizures, arrhythmias and respiratory failure may develop. Restoring anti-Parkinson medication will aid recovery.

Dysphagia

Dysphagia (see Chapter 12) is common, occurs early in the course of the disease and between 50 and 80% of people with PD will eventually be affected (Marks *et al.*, 2001). Dysphagia is not always linked to disease severity and may not respond to increasing doses of levodopa, suggesting that the cause may be degeneration in non-dopaminergic pathways in the brain (Miller *et al.*, 2006). Thickened fluids and soft or pureed diets can reduce the risks, but early referral to the speech and language therapist (SLT) is required.

Alternative methods of administering anti-Parkinson medication should be explored. In hospital a naso-gastric

Table 26.1 Features of the complex and palliative stages of Parkinson's disease.

Complex	Palliative
• Increasingly complex drug regimens	• Inability to tolerate adequate dopaminergic therapy
• Increasing medication side-effects	• Unsuitable for surgery
• Increasing disability and complex symptom control	• Advanced co-morbidity

Adapted from MacMahon and Thomas, 1998.

Box 26.5 Factors contributing to failure to administer drugs on time

- Lack of understanding of ward staff
- Inflexible drug rounds
- Lack of staff
- Not listening to patients and carers
- No opportunity to self medicate

tube may be passed. Dispersible co-benyldopa can be administered via this route and can replace capsule/tablet medication. Amantadine syrup is available and dopamine agonist drugs may be administered via trans-dermal patch (rotigotine) or continuous infusion (apomorphine).

Sialorrhea (drooling) results from an inability to swallow saliva rather than increased production. On average 1.5–2 litres of saliva is produced daily, so poor lip seal and infrequent swallowing can lead to drooling. Treatment is difficult as most drugs used to dry the mouth, such as anticholinergic medications, can exacerbate mental confusion. Injections of botulinum toxin-A to salivary glands have been shown to be safe and effective at reducing drooling (Lagalla *et al.*, 2006). However, a simpler solution is to suggest chewing sugar free gum or sucking sugar free sweets, which helps to trigger frequent swallowing.

Communication

Hypomimia (reduced facial expression) can hinder communication as individuals appear less engaged in social interactions. The voice may become monotonous and the volume reduced. Speech becomes slurred and lacks articulation, so early referral to the SLT is important (see Chapter 12). If the voice is very soft and the person has good articulation, a voice amplifier may help or a pacing board can aid a patient to speak more slowly. Portable keyboards, such as the light writer, depend on good manual dexterity so may not be helpful. Writing can be particularly difficult. As the pen travels across the paper, writing gets smaller (micrographia). Printing and concentrating hard on writing slowly and deliberately can help.

Anaesthesia

Patients who are nil-by-mouth prior to surgery should be given medication up to 2 hours before the administration of an anaesthetic. If prolonged surgery is envisaged or the patient is to be nil-by-mouth post-operatively, an apomorphine pump can be used.

Monitoring symptoms

An on/off chart (Figure 26.1) may be used to record the patient's state at regular intervals. Completed correctly these charts inform changes in medication regimen.

Nursing management of patients undergoing apomorphine therapy

An 'apomorphine challenge' may be conducted by a Parkinson's disease nurse specialist (PDNS) to determine the patient's response, establish the optimum dose, and identify side-effects that might contra-indicate use.

Seventy-two hours prior to the challenge the patient will be prescribed domperidone (20 mg TDS) as apomorphine is a powerful emetic. On the morning of the challenge anti-Parkinson medication is withheld, mobility is assessed at baseline, and lying and standing blood pressure is recorded. Injections of apomorphine are given every 45 – 60 minutes until a response is seen. If no response is observed following a dose of 7 mg the challenge is discontinued and the patient is classed as a non-responder.

If the challenge is successful the patient and their carer are taught how to administer sub-cutaneous injections or site an apomorphine pump. About 25% of people with an apomorphine infusion can manage the treatment independently, 50% need family or carer help and 25% need district nurse input (Manson *et al.*, 2002).

Apomorphine infusions may cause formation of uncomfortable skin nodules, which can impede absorption. The manufacturer has produced advice for managing nodules (Box 26.6), but there is little published evidence to support these interventions. High or low frequency ultrasound has been used with some success, but has not been formally evaluated. Some patients find silicone gel patches helpful (McGee, 2002), but again there is no evidence to support this claim.

Diet and nutrition

A recent meta-analysis has suggested that vitamin E may play a role in reducing the risk of developing PD (Etminan *et al.*, 2005), but once symptoms of PD have emerged there is no evidence that anti-oxidants slow progression (Weber and Ernst, 2006). It has been proposed that the ketogenic diet may confer symptomatic and disease modifying activity in neurogenerative disorders such as PD and Alzheimer's disease (Gasior *et al.*, 2006). Ketones are used by cell mitochondria for ATP generation and may protect neurones from free radicals (VanItallie and Nufert, 2003). There is insufficient evidence of effectiveness and this may not be the best diet for people with PD as it requires high protein and fat intake.

Weight loss is common and can be due to reduced calorie intake, increased energy expenditure or a combination of both. Up to half of patients with PD will experience unintentional weight loss and many will experience eating difficulties of some sort (Palhagen *et al.*, 2005). Physical and social factors (Box 26.7) also contribute to weight loss and many patients require help with eating and drinking. Nurses should protect patient mealtimes and utilise red tray schemes in hospital. Small meals taken more regularly may be easier, timed after medication has been given.

Time	On with no side effects	On with dyskinesia (mild/moderate/severe)	Off	Sleeping
01.00				
02.00				
03.00				
04.00				
04.30				
05.00				
05.30				
06.00				
06.30				
07.00				
07.30				
08.00				
08.30				
09.00				
09.30				
10.00				
10.30				
11.00				
11.30				
12.00				
12.30				
13.00				
13.30				
14.00				
14.30				
15.00				
15.30				
16.00				
16.30				
17.00				
17.30				
18.00				
18.30				
19.00				
19.30				
20.00				
20.30				
21.00				
21.30				
22.00				
22.30				
23.00				
23.30				
24.00				

Figure 26.1 On/off chart.

A well balanced diet is advisable and nutritional supplements may be appropriate. Protein reduction or redistribution diets have been suggested to optimise the absorption of levodopa, but are not always a viable option in patients who are already struggling to maintain their weight and nutritional intake. Ensuring that levodopa is taken at least 30–40 minutes before a meal may reduce the interaction.

Some patients gain weight, associated with compulsive eating due to dopamine agonists (Nirenberg and Waters,

---

Box 26.6   Managing nodules

- Change the infusion site daily
- Use only the lower abdominal wall (below the umbilicus) and the upper outer aspect of the thighs to site the infusion
- Always dilute apomorphine with equal amounts of 0.9% w/v sodium chloride for injection
- Insert the needle at an angle of 45°. If the needle is inserted intra-dermally apomorphine will irritate the skin and may cause ulceration
- After removing the needle massage the site to help disperse the apomorphine
- Basic hygiene, such as washing hands and the area of skin where the needle is to be inserted, should be promoted. Microbial contamination can worsen nodules

---

Box 26.7   Factors influencing weight loss

- Anorexia – possibly related to changes in sense of smell
- Nausea – drug side-effect
- Dysphagia
- Ill-fitting dentures
- Cognitive decline
- Constipation
- Difficulty shopping for/preparing food
- Poor manual dexterity
- Slow eating – meals become cold and unappetising
- Motor fluctuations

2006). Weight gain has also been noted following DBS, possibly related to reduced energy expenditure because of reduction in dyskinesia and tremor (Tuite *et al.*, 2005). Referral to a dietician should be made if unexpected weight change is noted.

Mobility

Gait, balance and posture are all affected and contribute to mobility difficulties. Patients walk with reduced arm swing, shortened steps and a characteristic stooped posture, which may result in contractures and further compromise mobility (e.g. contractures of the plantarflexors make heel strike difficult). Poor posture also contributes to breathing, speech and swallowing problems and falls.

Impaired balance or postural instability will develop as the disease progresses. Loss of righting reflexes is proba-

bly caused by degeneration in the globus pallidus. Anticipatory postural reflexes are diminished or missing and, when combined with flexed posture, reduced muscle strength, slowness, freezing and axial rigidity, the risk of falling is greatly increased.

Festination is produced by a combination of stooped posture, weight centred on the balls of the feet and short steps leading to a progressively faster and faster pace. The person feels that their top half is moving faster than their legs so they have to run to stop themselves from falling. Festination often results in falls.

Freezing

Freezing is the inability to initiate movement or the sudden transient inability to move. This is a motor feature of PD and different from switching 'off', which is a drug effect. People describe it as though their feet are stuck to the floor and they are unable to take the next step. This typically happens when trying to initiate movement (start hesitation), when walking through a doorway or turning. Freezing does not respond to dopaminergic medication, can be exacerbated by anxiety and increases the risk of falling.

Nurses can use visual and auditory cueing strategies to enhance cortical mechanisms to activate and sustain movement via the pre-frontal regions of the brain. Some people place masking tape strips on the floor in places where they frequently freeze so that they can use them to step over. Laser walking sticks and frames are also available, which generate a beam of light to step over. Saying 'one, two, three, step' or chanting and using rhythm can also help. Stairs or steps rarely cause difficulty as the riser acts as a visual cue.

Falls

Falling is common in PD, due to multiple factors (Box 26.8). Once a person has experienced one fall their risk of having another increases and falls are often associated with hospital admission. NICE (2004) recommends that the person who has fallen undergoes a multi-factorial falls risk assessment. Nurses should identify patients who meet this criterion and refer on.

Postural (orthostatic) hypotension was found in 48% of people with PD (Allcock *et al.*, 2004) and is often a cause of falling. Patients complain of dizziness on standing, visual disturbances, fainting or falling, and should avoid sudden postural changes, large meals or quantities of alcohol, hot baths and straining during defaecation. Interventions include raising the head of the bed at night, increasing fluid and salt intake and wearing compression

Box 26.8 Factors contributing to falls

- Impaired balance
- Stooped posture
- Festinating gait
- Freezing
- Urinary urgency and incontinence
- Orthostatic hypotension due to:
  - Autonomic dysfunction
  - Side-effects of medication
  - Anti-hypertensives
  - Co-morbidity

stockings. Anti-Parkinson drugs may be reduced if the problem is severe. Fludrocortisone can be used to raise blood pressure but domperidone may have a greater effect (Schoffer *et al.*, 2007).

Nurses should record lying and standing BP for all PD patients. The patient should lie supine for at least 10 minutes before measuring the blood pressure. The reading should then be taken again within 3 minutes of standing. If the systolic pressure drops by more than 20 mmHg, or is less than 90 mmHg, orthostatic hypotension is diagnosed (Kaufmann, 1996).

Neuropsychiatric symptoms

Anxiety

Anxiety and depression may be pre-morbid symptoms of PD in some patients. Compared to other disease populations, people with PD tend to experience more generalised anxiety, panic disorder and social phobia, which are thought to affect 40% of patients (Richard, 2005).

Treatment for anxiety is usually with selective serotonin reuptake inhibitors (SSRI). Benzodiazepines may help, but long-term use should be avoided because of the risk of falls and sedation. Non-pharmacological interventions such as psychotherapy, cognitive behaviour therapy, relaxation, reassurance and exercise including yoga/tai chi may help. Insufficient research has been conducted into the management of anxiety in PD to provide evidence-based recommendations.

Panic attacks, characterised by breathlessness, palpitations and a sense of foreboding, are common and may be related to switching 'off' (Richard, 2005). Panic attacks affect up to 30% of patients (Nuti *et al.*, 2004), who often feel so unwell that they will call paramedics. Patients may feel that their medication will never work again and they will be stuck in the 'off' phase forever. These feelings are particularly acute when a person is not in control of their medication, e.g. when hospitalised. Treatment should be based on improving 'on' time and developing strategies to deal with panic attacks.

Managing panic attacks is difficult and the evidence base is limited. Nurses should reassure patients that the feeling will pass. Understanding the cause, i.e. that it is the imbalance of neurotransmitters in the brain, can help some patients. Listening to patients and helping them to devise their own coping strategies may be the most beneficial course.

Depression

Major depression occurs in 10% of patients while up to 50% will suffer from some form of depression during the course of the disease (Metman, 2006). It is not clear whether depression is caused by damage to the serotonergic neurotransmission system, limbic noradrenergic and dopaminergic systems or whether it is the result of the psychosocial effects of living with the disease, but depression often predates the diagnosis (Clarke, 2006). Dopaminergic replacement sometimes improves depression, but not reliably.

Assessing depression is problematic, as some markers of depression are also symptoms of PD, e.g. poor appetite, sleep disturbance, cognitive impairment, lethargy and restlessness. Depression is probably under-diagnosed in PD and many patients who meet the criteria for depression do not consider themselves depressed (Weintraub, 2004). Nurses need to listen to carers' descriptions of changes in mood and personality. The PDQ-39 (Jenkins *et al.*, 1997) is a questionnaire designed specifically for people with PD and measures the impact of the illness, the physical functioning and emotional well-being. It may be a more useful tool than generic depression rating scales.

There is insufficient evidence of the efficacy and safety of treatments for depression in PD and research is urgently needed (Ghazi-Noori *et al.*, 2004). SSRIs are widely used to treat depression, but must be avoided in patients taking MAO-B inhibitors. Electroconvulsive therapy can be used in severe cases of depression that have not responded to other treatments. Psychological approaches to treating depression in PD are popular, but there is little evidence published to endorse their use. Peer support is helpful and joining a local support group can be beneficial for both the patient and their partner/carer. Patients should also be encouraged to exercise, which may elevate mood, boost energy and improve sleep.

Apathy

Apathy is an absence of interest in aspects of social, emotional or physical life and is common in PD, affecting 32%

of patients (Kirsch-Darrow *et al.*, 2006). It is thought that apathy results from disease-related physiological changes rather than a psychological reaction to disability. It is closely related to cognitive impairment and can sometimes improve with the administration of cholinesterase inhibitors (Pluck and Brown, 2002). There are no published studies into the treatment of apathy in PD. Anti-depressants and stimulants (e.g. methylphenidate, modafinil) have been tried, but there is little indication as to how successful these treatments are.

Patients are commonly misunderstood, being labelled as lazy or difficult. Helping partners and carers to realise that it is the condition not the person who is to blame often helps. Psychological interventions, such as CBT, are unhelpful due to the nature of the condition, which is characterised by diminished engagement and motivation.

Sleep disturbance

Over 74% of people with PD experience sleep disruption, although this is often not recognised or treated (Dhawan *et al.*, 2006). It is thought to arise from degeneration of the sleep regulation centres in the brain-stem and thalamo-cortical pathway. Sleep disturbance is multifactorial (Box 26.9) and requires careful nursing assessment.

Sleep fragmentation

Patients are often tired and ready for bed at a relatively early hour, sleep for 2 or 3 hours and then wake, finding it difficult to go back to sleep. Nurses should assess why the patient wakes. Difficulty turning over in bed and nocturia are common problems and may be helped by long-acting dopamine agonists or levodopa. Many patients go to bed early and sleep from 9 pm to 3 am for example. Six hours sleep may be sufficient and patients should be advised to retire later, waking around 6 am.

Box 26.9 Contributory factors to sleep disorders

- Delayed sleep onset
- Sleep fragmentation
- Depression and anxiety
- Rapid eye movement (REM) behaviour disorder
- Vivid dreams and nightmares
- Hallucinations and confusion
- Restlessness
- Pain
- Excessive day time sleepiness

REM sleep behaviour disorder (RBD)

During RBD a person acts out dreams while sleeping; actions range from mild restlessness to getting out of bed, crying and shouting and can be unsettling for those sleeping in the same room. Approximately 33% of patients with PD have RBD and it may be a pre-morbid symptom in up to 40% of patients (Chaudhuri *et al.*, 2006). RBD is caused by the loss of normal skeletal atonia during REM sleep. Clonazepam has been shown to reduce the severity of RBD, although it is unclear how, and is the treatment of choice (Gugger and Wagner, 2007).

Vivid dreams, nightmares and hallucinations

Vivid dreams are common, but if nightmares cause distress avoiding dopaminergic medications at bedtime can help. If night time hallucinations or worsening confusion occur the diagnosis should be reviewed as it could indicate the development of dementia with Lewy bodies (DLB) (see Chapter 29) or Parkinson's disease dementia. If this proves to be the case treatment with an atypical neuroleptic drug such as quetiapine (Korczyn, 2006) or an acetylcholinestrase inhibitor such as rivastigmine can be beneficial.

Restless legs

Restless legs syndrome (RLS) is common in PD and again may be a premorbid symptom. It is characterised by an urge to move the legs to stop unpleasant sensations, but movement provides only temporary relief. The aetiology is unclear, but there is an association with dopamine levels or some drugs (Thomas and MacMahon, 2006), and differential diagnosis from other conditions (e.g. cramp, thyroid and vitamin B12 deficiency) is important. RLS is most noticeable at night and can impact on a person's ability to go to sleep, compounding daytime sleepiness.

Good sleep routines and education about the condition can help. Massaging the legs with creams can be soothing, and exercise, stretching and regular walks are beneficial. Short term use of benzodiazepines can promote sleep, but dopamine agonists are the treatment of choice. Studies have shown improvements in sleep, quality of life and anxiety with ropinirole and pramipexole (Ondo *et al.*, 2004).

Pain

Off period and early morning dystonia are common, painful and interfere with sleep as levodopa is not administered at night. Long-acting dopaminergic drugs can help. Arthritic pain can be exacerbated by rigidity and bradykinesia. Patients may also experience neuropathic pain. Assessment and management of pain is detailed in Chapter 17.

Excessive daytime sleepiness

Daytime sleepiness is common, affecting approximately 50% of patients, and is associated with dopamine agonist drugs and sometimes levodopa. As soon as the person is resting comfortably and not distracted they fall asleep. Patients are not sleeping because of tiredness and this can be prevented by engaging in activity. Modafinil may be used to improve alertness (NICE, 2006) and nurses should give advice for promoting sleep (Box 26.10).

Autonomic dysfunction

Degeneration of catecholaminergic, monoaminergic and serotoninergic nuclei result in autonomic dysfunction characterised by urinary dysfunction, constipation, sexual dysfunction, orthostatic hypotension, weight loss and excessive sweating. If autonomic dysfunction is an early prominent feature, the diagnosis should be reviewed to consider multiple system atrophy (MSA).

Urinary dysfunction

The most frequently reported urinary symptom is nocturia (frequency at night), which can cause fatigue and increase the risk of falls. Nocturia may be a symptom of infection, diabetes mellitus and heart disease and these should first be ruled out before any other treatment is commenced. As PD progresses the person may experience daytime urinary urgency and frequency (Woodward, 2007) because of detrusor overactivity caused by disinhibition of the pontine micturition centre. See Chapter 18 for management of urinary dysfunction.

Constipation

Constipation affects 50% of people with PD (Sakakibara *et al.*, 2003). Constipation has many contributory factors including Lewy bodies in the gut wall reducing gut motility and delaying colonic transit time, reduced physical mobility, inadequate dietary intake, or weak abdominal muscles and functional outlet obstruction (anal sphincter problems). Management of constipation is discussed in Chapter 18.

Sexual dysfunction

Erectile dysfunction and premature ejaculation are the most commonly reported sexual problems affecting up to 60% of men with PD (Singer, 1989). Other causes of erectile dysfunction (e.g. cardiovascular disease, diabetes, hypertension, hypercholesteroleamia, smoking, prostate cancer and psychiatric disorders) should be investigated before assuming that PD is the cause. Alcohol and some medications (e.g. beta blockers) can also cause impotence.

Women with PD are less satisfied with their sexual relationships and suffer difficulty with arousal, orgasm, dyspareunia and vaginismus (Welsh *et al.*, 2004). People with PD may also experience diminished libido because of low self esteem. These issues need to be carefully explored with a trained counsellor, but nurses are ideally placed to identify patients with sexual dysfunction and refer on.

Discussion of sexual issues should form part of a nurse's assessment. If erectile dysfunction is identified nurses should screen for underlying causes. If no underlying cause is identified, referral to an erectile dysfunction nurse specialist is warranted. Erectile enhancement methods include vacuum devices and injections of prostaglandin E. Most men prefer to use drugs to promote and sustain an erection and men with PD are able to obtain sildenafil (Viagra) and tadalafil (Cialis) on prescription. For women vaginal dryness can be problematic and vaginal lubrication can help. Using a vibrator may help to achieve orgasms. Night-time may not be the best time to have sexual intercourse because medication levels are reduced and patients may prefer a time of day when motor performance is optimum.

Box 26.10   General advice for promoting sleep

- Have a night-time routine, but avoid fixed bedtimes: missing them may provoke anxiety
- Optimise the environment, temperature, noise and light
- Get up at the same time each day
- Exercise regularly, but avoid exercise at least 4 hours before bedtime
- Avoid caffeine, smoking and alcohol before going to bed.
- Milky drinks before bed can help (dairy products contain tryptophan, which acts as a natural sleep inducer)
- Patients may experience 'sleep benefit' so an afternoon nap may help, but use an alarm clock to ensure the patient does not sleep too long
- Avoid long periods of inactivity
- Adequate exposure to morning sunlight helps maintain circadian rhythms
- Consider relaxation techniques, aromatherapy and massage

Adapted from Crabb, 2001.

Hypersexuality

Dopaminergic and dopamine agonist medications flood the brain with dopamine triggering reward seeking behaviours such as hypersexuality and sexual delusions (Rees *et al.*, 2007), causing distress and often relationship breakdown. Sexual impulses become more intense and loss of impulse control (see: Impulse control disorders) can become problematic. Many patients lack insight, making it difficult to tackle the behaviour because the person doesn't acknowledge the problem. Reducing anti-Parkinson medications can help, but may also reduce Parkinsonian control.

Nurses are often the first person to be alerted to this type of behaviour either by the patient or their partner. It is important that the type of sexual behaviour is identified as child protection may need consideration. An appointment with the neurologist managing the patients PD should be made as soon as possible. Failing this, advice should be sought about reducing medication.

Impulse control disorders (ICD), dopamine dysregulation syndrome (DDS) and punding

ICD including pathological gambling, compulsive eating and hypersexuality, affect approximately 14% of patients (Voon *et al.*, 2006). DDS involves compulsive taking of dopamine replacement therapy, exceeding prescribed doses. Punding (pointless, repetitive action) such as sorting of objects, or activities often associated with a previous occupation may also occur.

The aetiology of these behaviours is unclear, but may be due to stimulation of dopamine receptors in the limbic system by dopamine agonists, thereby influencing mood and behaviour. Young men or those with a previous history of a mood disorder, drug abuse, alcohol abuse or obsessive compulsive disorder are at greatest risk of developing ICD (Stamey and Jankovic, 2008). DDS can develop as patients strive for perfect Parkinson's control. The beneficial effect of medication can encourage an individual to exceed the prescribed dose, resulting in dyskinesia. Nurses should be alert to this as hospitalised patients may take their own drugs as well as those administered by nursing staff.

The psychosocial consequences of these behaviours can be devastating and both patients and families should be informed of their potential development. Nurses should enquire about these behaviours, bearing in mind that the person experiencing this behaviour may deny or try to hide it. These behaviours can sometimes be modified by a reduction in dose or withdrawal of dopaminergic drugs (Mamikonyan *et al.*, 2008).

Psychosocial aspects of PD

Employment

There may be financial implications around employment and the increasing costs of disability. Disability discrimination legislation requires employers to make reasonable adjustments to enable employees to continue working, which may be possible for some time. Specialist employment support workers, Job Centre Plus and associated agencies can offer advice. Disability can affect other family members and one in five earners leave employment to become carers (Burchardt, 2003).

Social isolation

Anxiety and depression make socialising stressful; consequently carers may find their social interactions curtailed. Day centres help patients acclimatise to going out and carers groups provide support and occasionally a sitting service. The Parkinson's Disease Society (PDS) has a network of local branches that offer the opportunity to meet others with PD and develop social networks. The Younger Parkinson's Network (YPN) is a volunteer group within the PDS and provides for the needs of patients under 65 years.

Care packages

Patients' needs are unpredictable and nurses must ensure timely multidisciplinary referrals and assessments are made. Increasing physical and mental disability means that many patients will eventually require residential care. Moving from home into institutional care is a trying time for both patients and families and they will need support.

PARKINSON PLUS DISORDERS

It is often difficult to distinguish Parkinson Plus disorders (multiple system atrophy, progressive supranuclear palsy and dementia with Lewy bodies) from PD initially. Clinicians are alerted by more rapid deterioration of function, increasing disability and a disappointing response to anti-Parkinson medication.

Multiple system atrophy (MSA)

MSA can be divided into 3 types: striatonigral degeneration (SND) characterised by Parkinsonism, olivopontocerebellar atrophy (OPCA) characterised by cerebellar symptoms such as gait and limb ataxia, and Shy Drager syndrome (SDS) characterised by autonomic symptoms (e.g. erectile dysfunction, urinary incontinence, postural hypotension and syncope). The cause of MSA remains unclear.

SND is most likely to be confused with PD. Symptom onset (see Table 26.2) is often bilateral, but may be unilateral. Mean age of onset is 54 years (Clarke, 2006). Initially some patients respond to dopaminergic drugs, but the effect is not sustained, diminishing after about two years. MSA progresses more quickly than PD, with a mean survival of around nine years from diagnosis (Schrag *et al.*, 2008). Most patients (80%) are disabled within five years of diagnosis, many requiring a wheelchair.

Progressive supranuclear palsy (PSP)

PSP presents with symmetrical symptoms, falls and postural instability. Falls within the first two to three years of developing symptoms strongly suggest PSP; people with PD tend to fall much later in the disease (Clarke, 2006). Patients also develop a supranuclear ophthalmoplegia which results in vertical then horizontal eye movements being lost. People with PSP seldom respond to levodopa. Mean survival is around seven years from diagnosis. The aetiology of PSP is unknown, but neurofibrillary tangles and atrophy in the cerebral cortex, striatum, substantia nigra and brain stem are found at post-mortem.

Managing MSA and PSP

There are no specific treatments for these conditions. The PSP Association suggests that amantadine and amitriptyline may help with movement, but there is no evidence to support this. Botulinum toxin can be used to relieve blepharospasm.

Patients, families and carers need a great deal of physical, emotional and psychological support to live with these devastating neurodegenerative conditions. It is important that patients are seen early and reviewed regularly by the multi-disciplinary team. Adaptations to the home may need to be made and special equipment can be ordered by the occupational therapist or district nurse. Early intervention is vital in preventing complications and carer burnout. Planning for end of life care is a sensitive issue but patients need to have the opportunity of writing an advance decision or establishing a Lasting Power of Attorney (see Chapter 36). This is important in both MSA and PSP as patients lose the ability to communicate in the final stages of the disease and in PSP dementia may rob them of the capacity to make decisions.

Table 26.2 Symptoms associated with Parkinson's Plus syndromes.

Multiple system atrophy (MSA)	Progressive supranuclear palsy (PSP)
• Heightened emotional response • Unintentional sighing • Dysphagia • Weak, quiet voice or complete loss of speech • Urinary incontinence • Constipation • Laryngeal stridor • Postural hypotension	• Postural instability/ frequent falls • Pseudobulbar palsy • Behavioural/cognitive impairment – mood swings, loss of insight • Neck dystonia • Dysarthria • Dysphagia • Visual disturbances – inability to look up or down • Blepharospasm – inability to open the eye lids

---

Parkinson's disease: patient perspective

13 years ago I was diagnosed with PD. Nothing could have prepared me for that moment and what was to follow over the next 13 years as the illness gradually worsened. When I am asked what it is like to live with Parkinson's disease it is easy to say how badly you feel and how humiliated you feel in the presence of other people and how your dignity has been whipped out from underneath you like a rug.

But living with Parkinson's is all about winning the battle everyday that you are given. It's about overcoming setback after setback, about chasing dreams that were shattered so long ago, about rebuilding your life in a way that is meaningful not only for you but also your friends and family.

During the 'honeymoon' period of my illness Parkinson's was no more than an irritation. It had caused my right arm and leg to slow down causing problems shaving and sometimes walking. While I knew it was an incurable disease, if it stayed this way for the rest of my life I would be contented. So in those two to three years

I maintained much of what I had been doing – walking, running, cycling, driving a car going out for meals with friends and family.

Four years after diagnosis I began to realise that the illness was much more serious than I had ever imagined. Walking was now problematic and I was experiencing the on/off fluctuation known to PD sufferers. My medication, Sinemet, had become less efficacious and I was experiencing up to five hours of complete immobility unable to do anything for myself, crawling on my hands and knees to the toilet. Telling my brain what I wanted to do: like putting one foot in front of the other, being fed my food because I could not hold the knife and fork.

The honeymoon had turned into a nightmare. When I did manage to go out in an 'on' state I was petrified of having an off period in an unfamiliar place and not being able to talk to anyone, so the panic attacks started, a terrible feeling of imminent death or catastrophe about to befall you.

Dealing with Parkinson's is really about attitude and getting the right mix of medication. That's what pulled me through those bad years and finally I met a person who cared enough to take time looking at my medication and get it just right.

Parkinson's is not only about the sufferer, but also about family members who are also caught up in the dragnet of this dreadful disease. It does not respect any life time dreams once shared with loved ones nor whether they get any rest or sleep because they are caring for you. It rides roughshod over everything you have planned to do or are doing. To reach a point of acceptance of this illness is not possible as it might be with the loss of a limb or other faculty. That is because it is constantly on the move, constantly and insidiously taking and stripping more and more of you every day, every month and every year. I call it a disease of pre-maturity because it takes so much from you long before its time.

It is hope, the hope of a cure one day, the hope of future with my life partner and children and grandchildren that keep me going for I know that it may be able to take my body, but it will never steal or quench the hope that I have.

I dedicate this to all those medical professionals who take time to listen and care about their patients.

DYSTONIA

Dystonia is characterised by sustained, repetitive muscle contractions that produce abnormal postures affecting the trunk, neck, face, or limbs (Tarsy and Simon 2006) and is thought to be a disorder of the basal ganglia. Primary (idiopathic) dystonia occurs without a recognised pathology and affects 152 people per million (ESDE, 2000). Dystonia may also occur secondary to other pathologies such as a stroke or toxins (Vitek, 2002). It affects each individual differently and can affect independence by disrupting mobility and the performance of tasks, which can impact on education, employment and relationships. This is a painful, embarrassing, poorly understood condition that patients and sometimes medical personnel struggle to deal with.

EPIDEMIOLOGY

While the exact incidence is unknown, there are an estimated 600 per million (Butler *et al.*, 2002) or a total of 38,000 people affected in the UK (DH, 2005). Studies from Europe and the USA demonstrate prevalence rates between 111 and 3,000 per million (Defazio *et al.*, 2004). Variation in prevalence and incidence rates are thought to be largely due to research methodologies used.

Age at onset of symptoms is significant and gives an indication as to whether or not the dystonia is likely to spread. Adult onset dystonias, diagnosed over the age of 28 years are more likely to be focal. Dystonias that develop in middle to late childhood usually start as a focal dystonia but are likely to spread to other areas of the body and follow a more severe course (Nemeth, 2002). In addition to age at onset, dystonia is commonly classified by distribution or aetiology (Table 26.3).

More women are affected with primary segmental and focal dystonia than men. The exception is of focal dystonia arising in a limb, including writer's cramp, where men predominate (Warner *et al.*, 1999).

AETIOLOGY

The aetiology of dystonia is dependent on type. Primary, idiopathic dystonia has no known cause and is unaccompanied by other neurological abnormalities except for tremor and occasionally myolconus. Genetic links have been identified in young onset primary dystonia where 70% of the patients will have a mutation of the DYT1 gene (Edwards and Bhatia, 2004) and there are now 16 genes associated with dystonia.

Secondary dystonias have a number of causes including metabolic abnormalities, drugs (Table 26.4), stroke, anoxia and trauma (Vitek, 2002). Dystonia–plus syndromes are idiopathic with no neurodegeneration (Edwards and

Table 26.3 Classification of dystonia.

Distribution	Aetiology
• Focal – affects one area of body • Segmental – affects two or more areas of body next to each other • Hemidystonia – affects ipsilateral leg and arm • Multifocal two or more non-contiguous parts • Generalised – affects legs and other areas of the body	• Primary – with possible genetic influence • Secondary • Heredodegenerative –symptom of a neurodegenerative disorder • Dystonia plus – occurs alongside another disorder, e.g. myoclonus or parkinsonism

Table 26.4 Causes of secondary dystonia.

Drugs	Toxins
• Antipsychotic • Levodopa • Dopamine agonists • Anticonvulsants • Serotonin reuptake inhibitors • Dopamine D2 receptor blocker	• Manganese • Carbon monoxide • Carbon disulphide

Bhatia, 2004). Dystonia may also be a feature of some hereditary neurological disorders (heredodegenerative dystonia).

Paroxysmal dystonia can occur following acquired brain injury and in several families a genetic linkage has been identified. It occurs intermittently with no neurological deficit noted between attacks and may be triggered by factors such as alcohol, caffeine and less commonly hunger, fatigue, nicotine and emotional stress (Nemeth, 2002). This type of dystonia can present as an epileptic attack or episodic ataxia so differential diagnosis is crucial (Tarsy and Simon, 2006).

PATHOPHYSIOLOGY

Dystonia is characterised by the involuntary contraction of agonist and antagonist muscles (Obeso *et al.*, 2002). Most cases occur in the absence of an identified structural lesion in the nervous system, but the structures of the basal ganglia or thalamus are commonly affected by focal lesions in secondary dystonia (Mink, 2003).

Electrophysiological data have demonstrated that there is altered neuronal activity within the basal ganglia (Vitek, 2002). Decreased firing of the globus pallidus neurones could ultimately lead to increased activity in the 'direct' pathway (see Chapter 3) leading to excessive inhibition of the globus pallidus and excessive disinhibition of motor cortical areas (Mink, 2003).

Some dystonias are associated with a depletion of dopamine (Mink, 2003), resulting in disruption of activity in the 'indirect pathway' (see Chapter 3). Dopamine receptors may be affected by drugs such as dopamine agonists or antipsychotics (Tarsy and Simon, 2006). Dystonia has also been reported following structural changes in the spinal cord, brain stem or peripheral nerves (Vitek, 2002).

Heredodegenerative dystonias are also associated with pathological abnormalities involving the basal ganglia. The dystonia is part of a more widespread neurodegenerative condition such as Farh disease, in which calcification is found in the putamen, caudate, thalamus and white matter (Nemeth, 2002).

SIGNS AND SYMPTOMS

Signs and symptoms of dystonia are presented in Table 26.5.

DIAGNOSIS

Diagnosis is primarily based on history and clinical presentation (Box 26.11). Some investigations may be indicated to exclude underlying pathology.

MEDICAL MANAGEMENT

Dystonia is a complex disorder to treat. Patient symptoms are variable as is their response to treatment. Treatment is initially pharmacological, but surgery may be indicated if symptoms are intractable to medical management. Anticholinergics are considered the first line treatment in generalised/segmental dystonia (Edwards and Bhatia, 2004), but other drugs may also be used (Box 26.12).

Focal dystonias have been successfully treated with botulinum toxin (Holmes, 2003) and this has been the first-line management for all focal dystonias as well as the most affected areas of generalised dystonias for some time. Botulinum toxin inhibits the release of acetylcholine across the neuromuscular junction, resulting in temporary reduction in muscle activity. The treatment is effective for approximately 12 weeks and requires repeated injections to maintain the effect. Neutralising antibodies can develop in response to botulinum toxin injections, most commonly in patients on higher doses or who have frequent top-up doses (Munchau and Bhatia, 2003). Treatment failure from

Table 26.5 Signs and symptoms of dystonia.

Dystonia type	Signs and symptoms
Blepharospasm	Repetitive forceful involuntary eye closure
Oromandibular dystonia	Involuntary jaw clenching, opening or deviation of jaw
Hemifacial spasm/ Miege's syndrome	Blepharospasm and oromandibular dystonia
Laryngeal dystonia	Adductor – strained or strangled voice Abductor – breathy, whispery voice
Cervical dystonia/ spasmodic torticollis	Involuntary twisting or turning of neck, often accompanied by tremor
Writer's cramp	Involuntary hand postures when writing
Musician's	Involuntary hand postures when playing instrument
Focal limb dystonia	Involuntary twisting flexion or extension postures of arms legs or digits
Camptocormia	Abnormal flexion of the trunk when standing or walking, disappears in the supine position
Paroxysmal	Dystonic episodes with no neurological symptoms in between
Myoclonus	Dystonia of arms, legs, trunk and bulbar muscles with brief myoclonic jerks

Source: Ben-Shlomo *et al.*, 2002; Edwards and Bhatia, 2004; Grant and Meager, 2005; Tarsy and Simon, 2006.

one toxin may successfully respond to a different toxin. Administration of botulinum toxin is contraindicated in pregnancy and breast feeding and caution is required when using it in patients with neuromuscular transmission disturbance such as myasthenia gravis (Munchau and Bhatia, 2003).

Acute drug induced dystonic reactions require prompt treatment with IV anticholinergics, such as benztropine, to

---

Box 26.11   Diagnosis of dystonia

- Clinical examination
- Symptom history
- Drug history
- Family history
- History of trauma prior to onset of symptoms
- MRI to exclude structural lesions
- Blood tests, e.g. to exclude Wilson's disease

Box 26.12   Pharmacological management of dystonia

- Anticholinergics
- Baclofen
- Benzodiazepines
- Levodopa (for dopa-responsive dystonia)
- Botox – focal dystonia, e.g. blepharospasm

---

prevent laryngeal and pharyngeal spasms from compromising the airway (Dressler and Benecke, 2005). These types of reactions most commonly occur in people under the age of 20 and symptoms include torticollis (wry neck) and opisthotonus (extreme arching of the spine and neck). Oculogyric crisis, in which the eyes roll upwards involuntarily, could also occur before airway problems develop.

Segmental, hemidystonia, multifocal and generalised dystonia may all be treated with medication, although this may not produce satisfactory results (Aziz and Yianni, 2002). In severe cases, where symptoms remain intractable to oral medication, an intrathecal baclofen pump may be considered.

Surgical treatment

Functional neurosurgical interventions (Box 26.13) are used for more widespread dystonias or those that do not respond well to medical treatment (Aziz and Yianni, 2002). DBS has proven effective for generalised dystonia and spasmodic torticollis (Bittar *et al.*, 2005).

NURSING MANAGEMENT

The goal of care is to promote independence and quality of life through an integrated process of education, assessment, care planning and service delivery.

Focal dystonia and use of botulinum toxin

Focal dystonias are often responsive to 'geste antagoniste', a sensory trick where a part of the body close to the dys-

---

Box 26.13   Surgical management

- Deep brain stimulation
- Pallidotomy/thalamotomy
- Peripheral denervation, i.e. cervical dystonia, where there has been no response to other treatments
- Microvascular decompression, i.e. hemifacial spasm where arteries may compress the facial nerve

---

Table 26.6 Symptoms of baclofen overdose and rapid withdrawal.

Overdose	Rapid withdrawal
Excess salivation	Itching
Dizziness	Low blood pressure
Insomnia	Light-headedness
Euphoria	Muscle rigidity
Raised blood pressure	Rare but severe
Depression	High temperature/fever
Confusion/anxiety	Altered mental state
Nausea/vomiting	Spasticity
Respiratory depression	Tingling sensation

Source: UK National ITB™ Forum (2006) Steering Group National Document – Version 1, with permission from Medtronic.

tonic area is touched lightly and the dystonia temporarily ceases, although this is not effective in all patients. Botulinum toxin is usually administered by a doctor, but suitably trained nurses are also able to administer it. The time that the patient is being injected with botulinum toxin presents an opportunity to offer support (Grant and Meager, 2005). This may also provide an opportunity for the nurse to identify if onward referral needs to be made for medication adjustments or counselling (Whitaker *et al.*, 2001).

The patient should be given information about the treatment as it can diffuse into muscles adjacent to those injected producing transient side-effects. Depending on the muscles injected, these may include dysphagia, excessive facial weakness, partial ptosis (rarely diplopia), hypophonia, hoarseness, aspiration and stridor. Nurses should be vigilant for such side-effects. Some muscle weakness, distant from the site of the injections, as well as occasional generalised weakness is also possible. This is very rare and may be due to the toxin spreading via the circulation (Munchau and Bhatia, 2003).

Caring for patients with an intrathecal baclofen pump

In rare cases intrathecal baclofen infusions are successful where dystonia is resistant to oral medication and botulinum toxin (Dykstra *et al.*, 2005). This involves the implantation of an intrathecal catheter and a small disc shaped infusion pump. Standard placement of the pump is in the lower abdominal wall less than an inch from the skin surface, as the pump must be accessible for refilling by placing a needle through the skin into a filling port in the centre of the pump (Hseich and Penn, 2006).

When a patient is being considered for intrathecal baclofen a nurse specialist is ideally placed to coordinate patient care. Following initial medical assessment, the patient is given a test dose of intrathecal baclofen before being considered for surgical placement of the infusion pump. The nurse will provide the patient and carer with education and support throughout this process (Ridley and Rawlins, 2006).

For the first 48 hours following infusion pump insertion, observation of vital signs, fluid balance and monitoring for depression of the CNS is required (UK ITB Steering Group, 2006). The patient should be nursed in a supine position to reduce the incidence of headache caused by loss of CSF for between three and seven days following surgery. There should be pressure dressings on the lumbar and abdominal wounds to help the pump to 'bed in'. Wounds should be inspected for bleeding, CSF leak and infection. The patient should be mobilised on the advice of medical staff (UK ITB Steering Group, 2006).

Discharge advice should be given regarding wound care, follow up appointments, pump titration and subsequent refills. The patient and carers should be aware of the signs of overdosing with baclofen or system failure (Table 26.6). Overdosing most commonly occurs due to human error when setting up the pump. Malfunction of the pump or catheter or missed refill will result in a rapid withdrawal of baclofen. The patient should be given advice about what to do in an emergency and specific information about the pump, such as the fact that they may set off alarms at airport security (Ridley and Rawlins, 2006).

Pain management

Patients with severe dystonia that crosses a joint are likely to experience three types of pain and require appropriate analgesia for each. Dystonic muscle pain is akin to severe cramp and is caused by an increased need for blood flow, for nutrients and oxygen and for removing waste due to the excessive muscle contraction. There is a reduced supply due to compressed blood vessels. Microscopic fibres also tear in the affected and opposing muscles.

Arthralgia occurs due to the excessive forces applied by the dystonic muscles and increased physical stress placed on the joint. The normal skeletal alignment is often deformed. Neuropathic pain also occurs due to compression of nerves as they pass through muscle tissue. Assessment and management of pain is discussed in Chapter 17.

Positioning and mobility

Physiotherapy may help with gait, transfers, strengthening and stretching exercises to prevent contractures. Occupational therapists can provide adaptations to maintain independence in the home (Tarsy and Simon, 2006). Nurses should ensure that appropriate and timely referrals are made. Dystonic postures may lead to some areas of skin being vulnerable to breakdown. Appropriate positioning and vigilance as well as good hygiene will help prevent this from occurring. It may be necessary to involve social services to arrange support in the home environment.

Paroxysmal dystonia

Nursing care focuses around avoiding triggers to these attacks and maintaining a safe environment whilst the person is affected by this condition. Episodes can last from five minutes to four hours and can occur several times per day (Nemeth, 2002).

Psychosocial care

Dystonia causes abnormal posturing which physically disfigures various parts of the body. High levels of psychological distress, such as low self esteem, negative self image, social isolation and fear of rejection in relationships, have been noted in patients with disfiguring conditions (Valente, 2004) with the majority of difficulties being related to social situations (Rumsey *et al.*, 2004). This can cause problems at work and often people withdraw from social situations because of embarrassment about their appearance.

Optimal medical treatment may reduce disease severity, however people with cervical dystonia report an impact on their quality of life that is comparable to some other serious neurological conditions such as multiple sclerosis, PD and stroke. Depression has been reported in 24% of patients with cervical dystonia and 75% experience pain. Cognitive or other types of treatment should be considered

as well as conventional drug treatment to overcome these problems (Ben-Shlomo *et al.*, 2002). Nurses are able to develop a rapport with patients with dystonia (Grant and Meager 2005) and offer opportunities to discuss and offer advice on how they can cope with such problems.

Dystonia: patient perspective

I have cervical dystonia, which affects the whole of my right shoulder and arm. It started with a slight rotation of the head to the left. I then developed a tremor in my right arm. It was at this point I was sent for neurological tests as up until then I was told it was stress. Dystonia was diagnosed, a word that I had never heard before and nor had my GP.

Slowly things got worse, by this I mean my head was constantly rotating. My head also dropped forward and pain became a major issue as my neck muscles went into spasm as they pulled my head over to the left.

Three years ago I was offered Botox injections. The first injections into three of my neck muscles gave me tremendous relief but only lasted for eight weeks and I had to get through another four weeks of pain until my next appointment. Although I was told that dystonia was not progressive, I have found that I am far worse than when it started.

The condition has had a huge impact on my life. I can no longer drive as I can't centralise my head. Shopping is an ordeal as I can't look up or see where I am going. Reading is impossible as the head tremor makes it impossible to focus. The dentist chair is agony as he always wants to work from my right hand side and my head points to the left. Hairdressers all have backward leaning sinks and this is impossible for me.

My right arm does not allow me to lift properly, which makes running my home difficult re: ironing, cooking, vacuuming etc. If I push and make myself do those things, it has a rebound effect with extra pain and tremors.

Emotionally I am wrecked, socially I am embarrassed and physically I am utterly frustrated and worn out. On a daily basis the pain is horrendous with little expectation of a change in the future.

When I was admitted into hospital, none of the staff had heard of dystonia. I was also treated with drugs that worsened my symptoms.

HUNTINGTON'S DISEASE (HD)

Huntington's disease is an autosomal dominant inherited neurodegenerative disorder, characterised by motor, cognitive and psychiatric symptoms, progressing over 15–20 years (Foroud *et al.*, 1999). Death occurs, not due to the disease itself, but causes associated with it. The most common age of symptom onset is between 30 and 50 years. There are currently no preventative or curative treatments so management aims to reduce symptoms and improve quality of life for patients and their families (Nance and Westphal, 2002)

EPIDEMIOLOGY

The prevalence of HD is highest in populations of Northern European origin and varies between different countries. HD has a worldwide prevalence of 1:20,000 and there are an estimated 6,500–8,000 affected individuals in the UK (Harper, 2005). Throughout Europe (excluding the UK), studies reveal fairly uniform prevalence estimates of 3–5 per 100,000 (Harper, 1992).

AETIOLOGY

HD is an autosomal dominant inherited condition. There is equal incidence in both sexes and equal transmission by both sexes. Affected individuals have a 50% risk of transmitting the gene to each of their children (Harper and Jones, 2002). The HD gene (ITI5) and disease-causing mutation were identified in 1993 (Huntington's Disease Collaborative Group, 1993). It encodes a large protein called Huntingtin, which appears to have some role in protein trafficking and cellular metabolism (Handley *et al.*, 2006). The disease-causing mutation is an abnormally long, repeated trinucleotide. In the normal gene, the number of repeats is between 7 and 27. An individual has the disease-causing mutation if they have a copy of the gene with 40 or more repeats.

PATHOPHYSIOLOGY

The most obvious pathology in HD occurs in the basal ganglia, although other areas of the brain are affected (Raunch and Savage, 1997). Post-mortem examinations of the brains of people with advanced disease reveal atrophy of the striatum (see Chapter 3), accompanied by an enlargement of the lateral ventricles. Such brains also weigh around 10–20% less than age-matched controls (Gutekunst *et al.*, 2002).

Degenerative changes also occur in other brain regions connected to the striatum as disease progresses, including the neocortex, thalamus, subthalamic nucleus, globus pal-

lidus, substantia nigra pars reticulate and hypothalamus (Handley *et al.*, 2006). Within the caudate nucleus, abnormalities result in the loss of inhibitory neurotransmitter GABA, acetylcholine (ACh), substance P and encephalins. There is relative sparing of dopamine. The significant loss of GABA and ACh, leads to a relative excess of dopamine activity in the basal ganglia and results in the abnormal movements that are the hallmark of the disease.

SIGNS AND SYMPTOMS

The main clinical features of HD are summarised in Table 26.7. Each individual will display some symptoms, but not others, and different symptoms occur at different stages of the disease (Kirkwood *et al.*, 2001), varying in severity.

Motor symptoms

Chorea (excessive, spontaneous movement) is the major movement abnormality, affecting approximately 90% of patients with adult onset HD (Kremer, 2002). The severity of chorea varies greatly, but normally increases with disease progression. Early on in the disease, patients will generally appear more fidgety and restless rather than displaying obvious choreic movements. In the late stages chorea usually decreases and is largely replaced by bradykinesia, rigidity and dystonia. Patients with advanced disease still experience choreic movements, although voluntary movements are few at this stage and the ability to maintain an upright head position is lost (Nance and Westphal, 2002).

Balance and co-ordination are also affected, with many patients having impaired postural reflexes. Gait disturbances in the early stages of the disease are generally subtle with patients experiencing difficulties with tandem walking and turning. As the disease progresses, walking becomes more problematic and falls are extremely common.

Cognitive changes

Cognitive impairment varies in severity from person to person and worsens over time. Cognitive deficits involve executive functions, i.e. the ability to plan, organise and monitor behaviour, be mentally flexible and adapt to new situations (Craufurd and Snowden, 2002). Memory is often impaired, although not completely lost. Semantic memory is fairly well preserved. Impairments in verbal fluency, visuospatial skills and the ability to sustain concentration can all also occur and as the disease progresses there is a slowing of all thought processes (Craufurd and Snowden, 2002).

Table 26.7 Signs and symptoms of Huntington's disease.

Motor	Cognitive	Psychiatric	OTHER
• Chorea • Impaired gait • Swallowing problems • Speech problems • Balance and coordination problems • Rigidity, dystonia, bradykinesia (usually later in disease) • Eye movement abnormalities	Increasing difficulties with: • Planning • Organisation • Multi-tasking • Judgement • Impulse control • Concentration • Memory	• Depression • Anxiety • Irritability • Aggression • Apathy • Obsessive compulsive disorder • Suicide • Disorders of sexual function • Psychosis	• Weight loss • Sleep disturbances • Incontinence (usually later in disease)

Even from early on cognitive changes can have a major impact on how a person is able to function in daily life. They may become impulsive, leading to reckless decision making and behaviour. Additionally low mood/depression is common and can have a major impact on cognitive functioning.

Psychiatric symptoms

Psychiatric symptoms may begin up to a decade before the onset of motor symptoms in many patients and often lead to considerable distress and difficulty for patients and their families/caregivers (Craufurd *et al.*, 2001). Psychiatric manifestations are strongly associated with stress, disability and placement decisions, i.e. whether a patient can be cared for in the community or requires institutional care.

Other symptoms

Weight loss is a common problem for people in the later stages of HD, but may occur at an earlier stage (Turner and Schapira, 2002). It was originally thought to be mainly related to the severity of chorea, but it is now known that a metabolic defect plays a role in weight loss that often goes unobserved (Myers *et al.*, 1991). Swallowing difficulties and problems with self feeding also contribute to weight loss, as do psychiatric symptoms, cognitive difficulties and financial hardship, which can lead to poor diet, dental problems and self neglect. Sleep disturbances are common, including reversal of the sleep-wake cycle, excessive daytime sleepiness and insomnia (Kremer, 2002), contributing to patient and caregiver anxiety and distress. A number of patients become incontinent of both urine and faeces in the later stages of the condition.

CLINICAL VARIANTS

Juvenile Huntington's disease (JHD)

Onset of the disease before the age of twenty is called juvenile Huntington's disease (JHD). Fewer than 10 percent of individuals develop JHD and it differs considerably from adult-onset disease (Nance, 2001), with bradykinesia and rigidity present early on. The earliest signs and symptoms of JHD are usually behavioural changes and school difficulties (Kremer, 2002). Psychiatric problems frequently present with a schizophrenia-like picture and patients are often misdiagnosed as having a primary psychotic illness. Children often have stiff, painful legs and walk on their toes. The earlier a child/young person develops the disease the less likely they are to have any choreic movements (Nance, 2001). Also around 25% of sufferers develop epileptic seizures whereas adult patients with HD show no greater frequency of epilepsy than the normal population.

Westphal variant

A small number of patients with adult onset HD present with rigidity and dystonia, rather than chorea, in a similar way to JHD. This is known as the Westphal variant and is usually seen in young adult patients – in their twenties and to a lesser extent, in their thirties (Kremer, 2002).

Late onset disease

Late onset disease (after seventy years) tends to be milder than typical adult onset disease. Chorea and voluntary motor abnormalities such as impaired gait, speech and swallowing are common (Gutekunst *et al.*, 2002).

Cognitive deterioration is generally less severe and psychiatric problems may or may not be present.

DIAGNOSIS

Before the discovery of the gene responsible, diagnosis was made on the basis of family history, progressive motor symptoms and cognitive/psychiatric problems (Kremer, 2002). Now diagnosis is confirmed via a simple blood test and those who have a known family history of the disease can undergo genetic testing to identify whether they carry the gene before the onset of symptoms. Such screening is not undertaken lightly, as there are huge possible psychological consequences to the individual and their family, and testing centres worldwide must adhere to guidelines developed in 1994 (IHA/WFN, 1994). Presymptomatic testing can only be carried out after the individual has undergone genetic counselling to ensure that the at-risk person is informed about the disease, its inheritance, risks to themselves and the practical and psychosocial implications of the test. Before the test is conducted informed consent must be given by the individual (Tibben, 2002).

Presymptomatic testing is carried out to to relieve uncertainty and facilitate informed choices about having children and planning for the future (Tibben, 2002). However finding out that at some unknown point in the future you will develop an incurable, progressive condition can be a huge burden and this is why the counselling process and continued psychological support is so crucial. Presymptomatic testing is not normally available to people under the age of 18.

Prenatal testing is possible for couples where one partner knows that they carry the gene. This involves testing the foetus via chorionic villus sampling (CVS) at around 11–12 weeks of pregnancy. An affected pregnancy would then be terminated. Preimplantation genetic diagnosis (PGD), which uses IVF techniques, is also available for some couples who do not wish to risk having a child who carries the HD gene.

MEDICAL MANAGEMENT

In spite of numerous interventions being tried a recent Cochrane review has revealed no evidence of effectiveness of any intervention in modifying the progression of the disease (Mestre *et al.*, 2009). Treatment is symptomatic and patients and their families/caregivers benefit most from a multidisciplinary care team (Haskins and Harrison, 2000). Symptom management is often a matter of trial and error as there is limited evidence to support specific interventions. However several groups, part of the European Huntington's Disease Network (www.euro-hd.net), are carrying out clinical trials into the management of the motor and psychiatric symptoms of the disease.

Chorea

There are a number of drugs which can be used to dampen chorea (Table 26.8), but many side-effects are more problematic than the chorea itself. It is essential therefore to assess the effect of the chorea on the patient's quality of life before considering medication.

Table 26.8 Medications used to manage chorea.

Class	Medication	Side-effects
Neuroleptics	Olanzapine	Sedation, parkinsonism, increased appetite, raised blood glucose and lipids leading to increased risk of stroke in older patients
	Risperidone	
	Quetiapine	As above, less effect on appetite
	Sulpiride	As above, less effect on lipids and glucose
	Haloperidol	Agitation, dystonia, sedation, akathisia, galactorrhoea and amenorrhea
		Sedation, parkinsonism, dystonia, akathasia, constipation, hypotension
Benzodiazepines	Clonazepam	Sedation, exacerbation of cognitive impairment, ataxia
	Diazepam	As above
Dopamine depleting agents	Tetrabenazine	Depression, sedation

Adapted from Rosenblatt *et al.*, 2008.

Rigidity and dystonia

Benzodiazepines, such as clonazepam or baclofen, can be helpful and anti-Parkinsonian medications such as levodopa are also used (Rosenblatt *et al.*, 2008).

Psychiatric symptoms

The psychiatric symptoms of HD are often under treated and yet they generally respond well to treatment. As the incidence of psychiatric symptoms is so high, with an increased risk of suicide, physicians should have a low threshold for actively treating these problems. An accurate assessment of the patient is crucial and the input of a neuropsychiatrist who can advise local community mental health teams is helpful. Patients who are depressed should be treated in the same way as any other person with depression and selective serotonin re-uptake inhibitors (SSRIs) such as citalopram, sertraline, paroxetine and fluoxetine are often used (Rosenblatt *et al.*, 2008). For people who are also experiencing insomnia with their depression, a more sedative antidepressant, such as mirtazapine, taken at night time can be helpful (Bonelli, 2003). Other psychiatric symptoms including obsessive compulsive disorder, psychosis and agitation should be treated according to current guidelines.

NURSING MANAGEMENT

Nurses play a key role in the care, management and support of the person with HD and their family. The goals of care are to improve function, reduce disability and improve quality of life.

Mobility and safety

Chorea, dystonia, rigidity, impaired balance and co-ordination and impaired postural reflexes result in gradually deteriorating mobility. Early referral to physiotherapy is required. Studies have demonstrated that physiotherapy interventions for people with early to moderately advanced disease not only help patients to maintain their mobility but also have a positive impact on other symptoms such as depression (Zinzi *et al.*, 2007; Busse *et al.*, 2008).

As the disease progresses, falls become more frequent and it becomes particularly difficult for patients to manage stairs, uneven and sloping surfaces. Walking sticks, rollators and walking frames may benefit people who are more rigid but can be unhelpful to people with chorea (Rosenblatt *et al.*, 2008). The environment needs to be regularly assessed to ensure that it is free from clutter.

Patients eventually become wheelchair bound and regular reassessments for wheelchair suitability by spe-cialists are essential. In the later stages of the condition, semi-reclining wheelchairs can reduce the need for restraints such as seat belts (Brown and Marder, 2001), which is desirable given that restraints can result in injuries to the limbs and chest. An occupational therapist can advise on suitable seating and how best to assist and move patients who have severe chorea. As patients become more rigid, passive stretching exercises help to prevent contractures and massage, hydrotherapy, and music therapy can help to promote relaxation (Brown and Marder, 2001). Careful attention should be paid to pressure area care to prevent skin breakdown.

Eating and drinking

Weight loss can be significant so early involvement of a dietician is essential. As the disease progresses, patients generally do better if they eat small meals often, as swallowing difficulties, problems with self feeding, poor concentration and fatigue can make large meals hard to manage and a frustrating experience for the patient. HD affects all the different stages of swallowing and patients need regular evaluation by a speech and language therapist so that appropriate modifications can be made (see Chapter 12).

People with HD find it hard to concentrate, so minimising distractions at mealtimes and making the environment as calm as possible is helpful. Some patients feel embarrassed about eating and drinking in public and taking time to find out a patient's food preferences is also crucial. Seating should promote posture that encourages safer swallowing and an occupational therapist can advise on aids for eating and drinking. Good oral hygiene and regular dental care are essential, particularly when patients are being encouraged to eat a high calorie, often sugary diet to prevent weight loss.

In the later stages of the condition, patients require pureed foods and thickened fluids and the issue of PEG feeding (percutaneous endoscopic gastrostomy tube) commonly arises. This is very much an individual decision (Brown and Marder, 2001) and if a patient is still able to communicate, it is imperative that their wishes regarding PEG feeding are explored if a valid advance decision has not been documented (see Chapter 36). Difficulties arise when the patient is unable to communicate their choices about PEG feeding or has lost capacity and then the multidisciplinary team must make the decision in partnership with the patient's family, taking into consideration the patient's prognosis, quality of life and any previous preferences they may have stated.

Communication

Communication difficulties occur frequently due to speech deterioration, cognitive and/or behavioural problems (see Chapters 9 and 10). Communication issues can lead to frustration for the patient which can result in temper outbursts and problems for carers. It is very important to allow the patient time to speak and, wherever possible, to ask simple questions that need only one word answers rather than open ended questions. Offering cues and prompts can also be helpful (Paulsen, 1999). Communicating in a calm manner, especially if the patient is becoming agitated, is helpful and the involvement of a SLT is beneficial. Some patients find communication aids helpful (Nance and Westphal, 2002).

Self care and elimination

As HD progresses, affected individuals become less able to meet their own care needs and require increasing assistance with washing, dressing, toileting, shopping, food preparation and household chores. Maintaining personal hygiene can be challenging as the cognitive and behavioural problems, coupled with chorea and coordination difficulties, can lead to patients becoming unable and/or unwilling to maintain their personal hygiene. Confrontation is rarely helpful and usually results in a worsening of the situation. Having a negotiated routine is more useful coupled with calm communication and clear explanations (Paulsen, 1999).

Incontinence can occur as reduced mobility and dexterity affects getting to the toilet and/or removing the necessary clothing in time. Regular reminders to go to the toilet can help, along with clothing with velcro fastenings, rather than buttons and zips. Any sudden changes in continence should be fully investigated to rule out other causes such as urinary tract infections (Paulsen, 1999) and the side-effects of medications. In the later stages of HD most people become incontinent although regular toileting can minimise this (Rosenblatt et al., 2008). Suitable continence products are important and the input of a continence advisor is helpful (see Chapter 18).

Sleep

A regular bedtime routine and having activities to do during the day can prevent daytime napping, which can affect sleep at night (Paulsen, 1999). Many of the medications prescribed to treat psychiatric symptoms help with sleep, but some patients require pharmacologic treatment for insomnia. Often patients will wake in the night due to hunger so ensure that snacks are easily available. A safe and comfortable bed is very important. Cot sides, even when padded, can cause injury to people with severe chorea (Busse et al., 2008). A number of other alternatives are available so that patients should not have to resort to sleeping on a mattress directly on the floor and an occupational therapist can assist with this. Pressure sensitive devices attached to mattresses, which sound when the patient is out of bed, can alert carers that a patient has either fallen from their bed or is out of bed and walking around (Brown and Marder, 2001).

Behaviour

A number of behavioural problems can occur in HD, varying from person to person and changing as the disease progresses. They can be extremely distressing for both the affected individual and their family and can present far more of a challenge than any of the other manifestations of the disease. Difficult behaviours include apathy, perseveration (getting 'stuck'), rigid thinking, lack of insight and denial, agitation, irritability and aggression, impulsivity and paranoia (Paulsen, 1999). These behaviours occur due to the changes within the brain, but can be exacerbated by triggers such as communication difficulties, frustration, hunger, over stimulation and noise, unfamiliar situations and the reactions and behaviours of others.

It is essential to be aware of triggers and to consider why an individual might be behaving in a certain way (See Chapter 10). Helpful strategies include: using routines, a consistent approach and giving plenty of warning about change of routine; keeping the environment as calm as possible; allowing time for the person to communicate and carry out tasks; using distractions; being positive and encouraging; keeping to promises and giving specific time limits; and avoiding confrontation (Rosenblatt et al., 2008).

Smoking

Smoking can present a problem, particularly in the later stages of the disease (Kremer, 2002). Changes in behaviour mean that people can be consumed by their desire to smoke to the point that they can become distressed, irritable and aggressive if they are not allowed to smoke on an almost continual basis. However, chorea and coordination problems, lack of awareness and insight make smoking particularly hazardous. Negotiating smoking routines, having designated areas in which the patient can smoke and using aids such as smoking aprons and specially adapted weighted ashtrays with flexible tubes can reduce the risk to the patient (Rosenblatt et al., 2008).

Family issues

Often family members will be caring for a person(s) with HD whilst knowing that they themselves are at risk of the condition or that their children/grandchildren are at risk. Carers may feel over-burdened by the demands that HD places on them or may experience guilt because they are no longer able to care for the person at home. Changes in an individual's personality, even fairly early on in the disease, can cause relationships to break down (Aubeeluck and Moskowitz, 2008). It is therefore important to always consider the situation of family members and the complexity of the issues that they face.

End of life issues

In the late stages of HD patients require 24 hour care and a significant number of people enter long term residential care, where they usually stay until death (Wheelock *et al.*, 2003). Where possible, the patient's preferences regarding place of care and death should be respected, although it is not always possible for a person to remain at home, even with a full and well planned care package. Management of symptoms such as agitation, pain and excess secretions is of the utmost importance and the input of palliative care specialists and use of tools such as the Liverpool Care Pathway for the Dying Patient are essential (Kristjanson *et al.*, 2006).

Huntington's disease: patient perspective

For me I think it started with depression about 2 or 3 years ago, I felt really unhappy at work, I couldn't really cope with it. Eventually I went to see the GP and he put me on some tablets. My husband started to notice the more physical aspects, me moving around, fidgeting, 'like ants in your pants', he said! On a visit to the GP about my depression he noticed it too and referred me to a neurologist for a brain scan. I found the tests the neurologist did a bit scary because I had no idea how terrible I would be at doing them. Things like remembering, he gave me a list of objects and then I had to remember them a bit later, I wasn't very good at it. He sent me for a genetic blood test, and the brain scan. Then we heard nothing for a couple of months.

Then on Friday the 22nd August – the date is burned in my brain – a letter came for me. I was at work so my husband opened it, we have no secrets and we assumed it was the 'nothing wrong' letter, otherwise they would tell you in person. So he opened it and it was a letter from the neurologist saying 'I'm terribly sorry to inform you that you've tested positive for Huntington's disease'. My husband describes reading that as like 'a massive kick to the stomach'. He was then charged with the horrible task of telling me. My first question was 'how long have I got left?'.

Shortly after my husband got in touch with the regional care advisor from the Huntington's Disease Association

and she has been absolutely wonderful; she has arranged everything for us. We have had a couple of visits to the consultant and at the last visit he seemed quite happy with my lack of progress! I am 59, so it has come to me late in life so the hope is that it will progress slowly. We don't have children but I have a brother. He decided not to be tested, but he is 63 and showing no signs so it seems he is clear. We didn't know about HD in our family, my mother died aged 86 so we think it is from my father's side but he died of cancer aged 63 showing no symptoms. We haven't had contact with his side of the family for over 20 years so we don't know if anyone else is affected.

So we are still going to carry on. I am not ill, I have a condition, there's a difference. It has not been a year yet, so it is still early days. We are trying our best to be as positive as we can, of course sometimes that can be difficult. I get frustrated when I can't do things, like fiddly buttons, or getting dressed if I am feeling a bit wobbly. It's a bit scary because you think that is such a simple thing to do, dressing yourself. It is not all the time, just occasionally, so I have to sit down and make myself calm down and try again, but it knocks your confidence. I retired from work straight away and I feel so much better now that I don't have to concentrate on that as well. Now we are just making the most of things, we go different places, go for walks, out for meals, and see friends.

SUMMARY

Movement disorders are highly complex conditions that impact significantly on the quality of life of patients and their families. The progressive nature of these disorders

means that patients need regular assessment and re-evaluation. All patients should have access to the support of a nurse specialist if possible. Treatment for these conditions is usually symptomatic and nurses must be mindful of patient needs, especially in acute settings, adapting ward routines to fit the needs of the patient, rather than expecting the opposite.

FURTHER INFORMATION

Further information regarding PD and Parkinson's Plus Syndromes can be obtained from the Parkinson's Disease Society (www.parkinsons.org.uk), the PSP Association (www.pspeur.org) and the Sarah Matheson Trust for MSA (www.msaweb.co.uk). Patients with dystonia should be made aware of opportunities for psychosocial support through support groups (www.dystonia.org.uk or www.actionfordystonia.co.uk). HD sufferers should be referred to the Huntington's Disease Association (www.hda.org.uk) or the Scottish Huntington's Association (www.hdscotland.org).

REFERENCES

Ahlskog JE (2007) Beating a dead horse: dopamine and Parkinson's disease. *Neurology* 69(17):1701–1711.

Ahlskog JE, Muenter MD (2001) Frequency of levodopa related dyskinesias and motor fluctuations estimated from cumulative literature. *Movement Disorders* 16:448–458.

Allcock LM, Ullyart K, Kenny RA et al. (2004). Frequency of orthostatic hypotension in a community acquired cohort of patients with Parkinson's disease. *Journal of Neurology, Neurosurgery and Psychiatry* 75:1470–1471.

Aubeeluck A, Moskowitz CB (2008) Huntington's disease Part 3: Family aspects of Huntington's disease. *British Journal of Nursing* 17(5):328–331.

Aziz T, Yianni J (2002) Recent advances in the surgical treatment of dystonia. *Advances in Clinical Neurology and Rehabilitation* 2(3):14–15.

Ben-Shlomo Y, Camfield L, Warner T (2002) What are the determinants of quality of life in people with cervical dystonia? *Journal of Neurology, Neurosurgery and Psychiatry* 72:608–614.

Birdie S, Rajput AH, Fenton M et al. (2001). Progressive supra nuclear palsy diagnosis and confounding features – report of 16 autopsied cases. *Movement Disorders* 17(6):1255–1264.

Bittar RG, Yianni J, Wang SY et al. (2005) Deep brain stimulation for generalised dystonia and spasmodic totricollis. *Journal of Clinical Neuroscience* 12(1):12–16.

Bonelli RM (2003) Mirtazapine in suicidal Huntington's disease. *Annals of Pharmacotherapy* 37(3):452.

Breen K, Heisters D (2007) A guide to deep brain stimulation surgery: A treatment for Parkinson's disease. *British Journal of Neuroscience Nursing* 3(12):554–559.

Brown MC, Marder K (2001) Palliative care for people with late-stage Huntington's disease. *Neurologic Clinics* 19(4):849–865.

Burchardt T (2003) *Professional's Guide to Parkinson's Disease*. London: The Parkinson's Disease Society.

Busse M, Khalil H, Quinn L et al. (2008) Physical therapy intervention for people with Huntington's disease. *Physical Therapy* 88(7):820–831.

Butler AG, Duffey POF, Hawthorne MR et al. (2002) An epidemiological survey of dystonia within the entire population of Northeast over the past nine years. *Movement Disorders* 17:1124–1125.

Buxton V (2007) How you can help people with Parkinson's 'get it on time'. *British Journal of Neuroscience Nursing* 3(4):140–144.

Byrd DL, Marks WJ, Starr PA (2000) Deep brain stimulation for advanced Parkinson's disease. *Journal of Neuroscience Nursing* 72(3):385–418.

Chaudhuri KV, Healy D, Schapira AHV (2006) Non motor symptoms of Parkinson's disease: diagnosis and management. *The Lancet* 5(3):235–245.

Clarke CE (2006) *Parkinson's Disease in Practice*. (2nd edition). London: Royal Society of Medicine Press Ltd.

Crabb L (2001) Sleep disorders in Parkinson's disease: the nursing role. *British Journal of Nursing* 10(1):42–47.

Craufurd D, Snowden J (2002) Neuropsychological and neuropsychiatric aspects of Huntington's disease. In: Bates G, Harper P, Jones L (eds). *Huntington's Disease* (3rd edition). Oxford: Oxford University Press.

Craufurd D, Thompson JC, Snowden JS (2001) Behavioural energy in Huntington's disease. *Neuropsychiatry, Neuropsychology and Behavioural Neurology* 14(4):219–226.

Crosby NJ, Deane KHO, Clarke CE (2003) Amantadine for dyskinesia in Parkinson's disease. *Cochrane Database of Systematic Reviews* Issue No 2.

Deane KHO, Spieker S, Clarke CE (2004) Catechol-O-methyltransferase inhibitors for levodopa-induced complications in Parkinson's disease. *Cochrane Database of Systematic Reviews* Issue 4.

Defazio G, Abbruzzese G, Livrea P et al. (2004) Epidemiology of primary dystonia. *Lancet Neurology* 3(11):673–678.

de Lau LM, Breteler MM (2006) Epidemiology of Parkinson's disease. *Lancet Neurology* 5:525–535.

Deleu D, Hanssens Y, Northway MG (2004) Subcutaneous apomorphine: An evidence based review of its use in Parkinson's disease. *Drugs and Ageing* 21(11):687–709.

Department of Health (2005) *National Service Framework for Long term Conditions*. Available from: www.dh.gov.uk/en/Publicationsandstatistics/Publications/PublicationsPolicyAndGuidance/DH_4105361 Accessed July 2010.

Dhawan V, Healy D, Pal S et al. (2006) Sleep related problems of Parkinson's disease. *Age and Ageing* 35:220–228.

Dick FD, de Palma G, Ahmadi A et al. (2007) Environmental risk factors for Parkinson's disease and Parkinsonism: The geoparkinson study. *Occupational and Environmental Medicine* 64(10):666–672.

Dressler D, Benecke R (2005) Diagnosis and management of acute movement disorders. *Journal of Neurology* 252:1299–1306.

Dykstra DD, Mendez A, Chappius D *et al.* (2005) Treatment of cervical dystonia and focal hand sydtonia by high cervical continuously infused intrathecal baclofen: A report of two cases. *Archives of Physical Medicine Rehabilitation* 86(4):830–833.

Edwards E, Bhatia K (2004) Dystonia. *Advances in Clinical Neurology and Rehabilitation* 4(2):20–24.

Epidemiological Study of Dystonia in Europe (ESDE) Collaborative Group (2000) A prevalence study of primary dystonia in eight European countries. *Journal of Neurology* 247(10):787–792.

Etminan M, Gill S, Samii A (2005) Intake of vitamin E, vitamin C, and carotenoids and the risk of Parkinson's disease: a meta-analysis. *Lancet Neurology* 4(6):362–365.

Foroud T, Gray J, Irashima J *et al.* (1999) Differences in duration of Huntington's disease based on age at onset. *Journal of Neurology, Neurosurgery and Psychiatry* 66:52–56.

Gasior M, Rogawski MA, Hartman AL (2006) Neuroprotective and disease-modifying effects of the ketogenic diet. *Behavioural Pharmacology* 17(5–60):431–439.

Ghazi-Noori S, Chung TH, Deane KHO *et al.* (2004) Therapies for depression in Parkinson's disease. *The Cochrane Library* Vol 1 Chichester: Wiley.

Goldman SM, Tanner CM, Oakes D *et al.* (2006) Head injury and Parkinson's disease risk in twins. *Annals of Neurology* 60(1):65–72.

Grant SA, Meager P (2005) The nurse's role in the management and treatment of dystonia. *Nursing Times* 101(19):50–51.

Grosset D, Grosset KA, Okun MS *et al.* (2009) *Parkinson's Disease – Clinician's Desk Reference*. London: Manson Publishing.

Grosset D, Schnachter M, Soar K *et al.* (2006) *Ergot Derived Drugs: A cross therapy evidence-based review*. London: Royal Society of Medicine Press.

Gugger J, Wagner M (2007) Rapid eye movement sleep behaviour disorder. *Annals of Pharmacotherapy* 41(11):1833–1841.

Gutekunst CA, Norhus F, Hersch SM (2002) The neuropathology of Huntington's disease. In: Bates G, Harper P, Jones L (eds). *Huntington's Disease* (3rd edition). Oxford: Oxford University Press.

Handley OJ, Naji JJ, Dunnett SB *et al.* (2006) Pharmaceutical, cellular and genetic therapies for Huntington's disease. *Clinical Science* 110:73–88.

Harper B (2005) Huntington's disease. *Journal of the Royal Society of Medicine* 98(12):550.

Harper PS (1992) The epidemiology of Huntington's disease. *Human Genetics* 89:365–376.

Harper PS, Jones L (2002) Huntington's disease: genetic and molecular studies. In: Bates G, Harper P, Jones L (eds). *Huntington's Disease* (3rd edition). Oxford: Oxford University Press.

Harrower TP, Michell AW, Barker RA (2005) Lewy bodies in Parkinson's disease: protectors or perpetrators? *Experimental Neurology* 195:1–6.

Haskins BA, Harrison MB (2000) Huntington's disease. *Current Treatment Options in Neurology* 2:243–262.

Hauser RA, Rascol O, Korczyn AD *et al.* (2007) Ten year follow up of Parkinson's disease patients randomised to initial therapy with ropinirole or levodopa. *Movement Disorders* 22(16):2409–2417.

Holmes S (2003) Botulinum toxin: a deadly substance with great therapeutic effect. *Professional Nurse* 19(2):85–87.

Hseich JC, Penn RD (2006) Intrathecal baclofen in the treatment of adult spasticity. *Neurosurgical Focus* 21(2):1–6.

Huntington's Disease Collaborative Group (1993) A novel gene containing a trinucleotide repeat that is expanded and unstable in Huntington's disease chromosomes. *Cell* 72:971–983.

International Huntington Association and the World Federation of Neurology Research Group on Huntington's Chorea (1994) Guidelines for the molecular genetics predictive test in Huntington's disease. *Journal of Medical Genetics* 31(7):555–559.

Jenkins C, Fitzpatrick R, Peto V *et al.* (1997) The Parkinson's Disease Questionnaire (PDQ-39): Development and validation of a Parkinson's disease summary index score. *Age and Ageing* 26:353–357.

Kaufmann H (1996) Consensus statement on the definition of orthostatic hypotension, pure autonomic failure, and multiple system atrophy. *Clinical Autonomic Research* 6:125–126.

Kirkwood SC, Su JL, Conneally PM *et al.* (2001) Progression of symptoms in the early and middle stages of Huntington's disease. *Archives of Neurology* 58(2):273–278.

Kirsch-Darrow L, Fernandez HH, Marsiske M *et al.* (2006) Dissociating apathy and depression in Parkinson's disease. *Neurology* 67(1):33–38.

Korczyn AD (2006) Management of sleep problems in Parkinson's disease. *Journal of the Neurological Sciences* 25 248(1–2):163–166.

Kremer B (2002) Clinical neurology in Huntington's disease. In: Bates G, Harper P, Jones L (eds). *Huntington's Disease* (3rd edition). Oxford: Oxford University Press.

Kristjanson LJ, Aoun SM, Oldham L (2006) Palliative care and support for people with neurodegenerative conditions and their carers. *International Journal of Palliative Nursing* 12(8):368–377.

Lagalla G, Millevolte M, Capecci M *et al.* (2006) Botulinum toxin type A for drooling in PD: a double blind, randomised placebo controlled study. *Movement Disorders* 21(5):704–707.

Lazzarini AM, Myers RH, Zimmerman TR Jr *et al.* (1994) A clinical genetic study of Parkinson's disease: evidence for dominant transmission. *Neurology* 44:499–506.

MacMahon DG, Thomas S (1998) Practical approach to quality of life in Parkinson's disease. *Journal of Neurology* 245(Suppl 1):S19–22.

Mamikonyan E, Siderowf AD, Duda JE *et al.* (2008) Long term follow-up of impulse control disorders in Parkinson's disease. *Movement Disorders* 23(1):75–80.

Manson AJ, Turner K, Lees AJ (2002) Apomorphine monotherapy in the treatment of refractory motor complications of Parkinson's disease: long term follow-up study of 64 patients. *Movement Disorders* 20(2):151–157.

Marks L, Turner K, O'Sullivan J *et al.* (2001) Drooling in Parkinson's disease: a novel speech and language therapy intervention. *International Journal of Language and Communication Disorders* 36(Suppl):282–287.

McGee P (2002) Apomorphine treatment: A nurse's perspective. *Advances in Clincial Neuroscience and Rehabilitation* 2:23–24.

Mestre T, Ferreira J, Coelho MM *et al.* (2009) Therapeutic interventions for disease progression in Huntington's disease. *Cochrane Database of Systematic Reviews* Issue 3. Art. No.: CD006455. DOI: 10.1002/14651858.CD006455.pub2.

Metman LV (2006) Epidemiology and clinical aspects of depression in Parkinson's Disease. *Parkinsonism and Related Disorders* 12(Suppl 1):10.

Miller N, Noble E, Jones D *et al.* (2006) Hard to swallow: Dysphagia in Parkinson's disease. *Age and Ageing* 35:614–618.

Mink JW (2003) The basal ganglia and involuntary movements. *Archives of Neurology* 60(10):1365–1368.

Morgante L, Morgante F, Moro E *et al.* (2007) How many Parkinsonian patients are suitable candidates for deep brain stimulation of subthalamic nucleus? Results of a questionnaire. *Parkinsonism and Related Disorders* 14(3):266–267.

Munchau A, Bhatia KP (2003) Use of botulinum toxin injection in medicine today. *British Medical Journal* 320:161–165.

Myers RH, Sax DS, Koroshetz WJ *et al.* (1991) Factors associated with slow progression in Huntington's disease. *Archives of Neurology* 48:800–804.

Nance M (2001) *The Juvenile HD Handbook. A guide for physicians, neurologists and other professionals.* New York: Huntington's Disease Society of America.

Nance MA, Westphal B (2002) Comprehensive care in Huntington's disease. In: Bates G, Harper P, Jones L (eds). *Huntington's Disease* (3rd edition). Oxford: Oxford University Press.

National Institute for Health and Clinical Excellence (2003) *Deep Brain Stimulation for Parkinson's Disease.* London: NICE.

National Institute for Health and Clinical Excellence (2004) *The Assessment and Prevention of Falls in Older People.* London: NICE.

National Institute for Health and Clinical Excellence (2006) *Parkinson's Disease: Diagnosis and management in primary and secondary care.* London: NICE.

Nemeth AH (2002) The genetics of primary dystonias and related disorders. *Brain* 125(4):695–721.

Nirenberg MJ, Waters C (2006) Compulsive eating and weight gain related to dopamine agonist use. *Movement Disorders* 21(4):524–529.

Nuti A, Ceravolo R, Piccinni A *et al.* (2004) Psychiatric co-morbidity in a population of Parkinson's disease patients. *European Journal of Neurology* 11(5):315–320.

Obeso JA, Rodríguez-Oroz MC, Rodríguez M *et al.* (2002) The basal ganglia and disorders of movement: pathophysiological mechanisms. *News in Physiological Science* 17(2):51–55.

Ondo W, Romanyshyn J, Dat Vuong K *et al.* (2004) Long term treatment of restless legs syndrome with dopamine agonists. *Archives of Neurology* 61:1393–1397.

Palhagen S, Lovefalt B, Carlsson M *et al.* (2005) Does L-dopa treatment contribute to reduction in body weight in elderly patients with Parkinson's disease? *Acta Neurologica Scandinavica* 111(1):12–20.

Parkinson's Disease Society (2008) *Life with Parkinson's Today – Room for Improvement.* London: PDS.

Paulsen JS (1999) *Understanding Behaviour in Huntington's Disease.* Ontario: Huntington Society of Canada.

Pluck G, Brown R (2002) Apathy in Parkinson's disease. *Journal of Neurology, Neurosurgery and Psychiatry* 73:636–642.

Raunch SI, Savage CR (1997) Neuroimaging and neuropsychology of the striatum. Bridging basic science and clinical practice. *Psychiatric Clinics of North America* 20:741–768.

Rees PM, Fowler CJ, Maas CP (2007) Sexual dysfunction 2: Sexual function in men and women with neurological disorders. *Lancet* 369(9560):512–525.

Richard IH (2005) Anxiety disorders in Parkinson's disease. *Advances in Neurology* 96:42–55.

Ridley B, Rawlins PK (2006) Intrathecal baclofen therapy: ten steps towards best practice. *Journal of Neuroscience Nursing* 38(2):72–82.

Rodriguez-Oroz MC, Obeso JA, Lang AE *et al.* (2005) Bilateral deep brain stimulation in Parkinson's disease: A multicentre study with 4 years follow up. *Brain* 128(10):2240–2249.

Rosenblatt A, Ranen NG, Nance MA *et al.* (2008) *A Physician's Guide to the Management of Huntington Disease.* (2nd edition). Ontario: Huntington Society of Canada.

Rumsey N, Clarke A, White P *et al.* (2004) Altered body image: the appearance-related concerns of people with visible disfigurement. *Journal of Advanced Nursing* 48(5):443–453.

Sakakibara R, Odaka T, Uchiyama T (2003) Colonic transit time and rectoanal videomanometry in Parkinson's disease. *Journal of Neurology, Neurosurgery and Psychiatry* 74:268–272.

Schrag A, Schott JM (2006) Epidemiological, clinical and genetic characteristics of early-onset Parkinsonism. *Lancet Neurology* 5(4):355–363.

Schrag A, Wenning GK, Quinn N *et al.* (2008) Survival in multiple system atrophy. *Journal of Neurology, Neurosurgery and Psychiatry* 79:232–234.

Schoffer KL, Henderson RD, O'Maley K *et al.* (2007) Non-pharmacological treatment, fludrocortisone and domperidone for orthostatic hypotension in Parkinson's disease. *Movement Disorders* 22(11):1543–1549.

Singer C (1989) Sexual dysfunction of men with Parkinson's disease. *Journal of Neurological Rehabilitation* 3:194–204.

Stamey W, Jankovic J (2008) Impulse control disorders and pathological gambling in patients with Parkinson's disease. *The Neurologist* 14(2):89–99.

Stotz M, Thummler D, Schurch M *et al.* (2004) Fulminant neuroleptic malignant syndrome after perioperative withdrawal of antiParkinsonian medication. *British Journal of Anaesthesia* 93(6):868–871.

Tarsy D, Simon DK (2006) Dystonia. *New England Journal of Medicine* 355(8):818–829.

Thomas S, MacMahon D (2006) Restless legs syndrome: A condition in search of recognition. *British Journal of Neuroscience Nursing* 2(5):222–226.

Thomas S, MacMahon DG, Maguire J (2006) *Moving and Shaping: A guide to commissioning integrated services for people with Parkinson's disease.* London: Parkinson's Disease Society.

Tibben A (2002) Genetic counselling and presymptomatic testing. In: Bates G, Harper P, Jones L (eds). *Huntington's Disease* (3rd edition). Oxford: Oxford University Press.

Tuite PJ, Maxwell RE, Ikramuddin S *et al.* (2005) Weight and body mass index in Parkinson's disease patients after deep brain stimulation surgery. *Parkinsonism and Related Disorders* 11(4):247–252.

Turner C, Schapira AHV (2002) Energy metabolism and Huntington's disease. In: Bates G, Harper P, Jones L (eds).

Huntington's Disease (3rd edition). Oxford: Oxford University Press.

UK ITB Steering Group (2006) *National Document – Version 1.* UK: Medtronic Ltd.

Valente SM (2004) Visual disfigurement and depression. *Plastic Surgical Nursing* 24(4):140–146.

VanItallie TB, Nufert TH (2003) Ketones: metabolism's ugly duckling. *Nutrition Reviews* 61(10):327–341.

Vitek JL (2002) Pathophysiology of dystonia: a neuronal model. *Movement Disorders* 17(Suppl 3):S49–S62.

Voon V, Hassan K, Zurowski M *et al.* (2006) Prospective prevalence of pathological gambling and medication associated with Parkinson's disease. *Neurology* 66(11):1750–1752.

Warner T, Camfield L, Marsden CD *et al.* (1999) Sex-related influences on the frequency and age of onset of primary dystonia. *Neurology* (53)8:1871–1873.

Weber CA, Ernst ME (2006) Antioxidants, supplements and Parkinson's disease. *Annals of Pharmacotherapy* 40(5):935–938.

Weintraub D (2004) Diagnosing and treating depression in patients with Parkinson's disease. *Psychiatric Annals* 34(4):299–304.

Welsh M, Hung L, Waters C (2004) Sexuality in women with Parkinson's disease. *Movement Disorders* 12(6):923–927.

Wheelock VL, Tempkin T, Marder K *et al.* 2003. The Huntington Study Group. Predictors of nursing home placement in Huntington disease. *Neurology* 60(6):998–1001.

Whitaker J, Butler A, Semlyn JK *et al.* (2001) Botulinum toxin for people with dystonia treated by an outreach nurse practitioner: a comparative study between a home and a clinic treatment service. *Archives of Physical Medicine and Rehabilitation* 82(4):480–484.

Woodward S (2007) Urinary incontinence in Parkinson's disease. *British Journal of Neuroscience Nursing* 3(3):92–95.

Wooten GF, Currie LJ, Bovbjerg VE *et al.* (2007) Are men at greater risk for Parkinson's disease than women? *Comment Journal of Neurology, Neurosurgery and Psychiatry* 78(8):905–906.

Zinzi P, Salmaso D, De Grandis R *et al.* (2007) Effects of an intensive rehabilitation programme on patients with Huntington's disease: a pilot study. *Clinical Rehabilitation* 21(7): 603–613.

27

Management of Patients with Motor Neurone Disease

Mary O'Brien

INTRODUCTION

Motor neurone disease (MND), is a rapidly progressive terminal neurodegenerative condition. The disease is referred to as amyotrophic lateral sclerosis (ALS) in North America and many other countries, however MND is regarded as an umbrella term comprising the four main classifications of disease: amyotrophic lateral sclerosis (ALS), progressive bulbar palsy (PBP), progressive muscular atrophy (PMA), and primary lateral sclerosis (PLS). MND results in weakness and wasting of muscles, loss of mobility and difficulty with speech, swallowing and respiration, often compounded by psychological effects. Oculomotor and sphincter muscles are usually unaffected. It was thought that intellect was unaffected; however, it is now known that some form of cognitive dysfunction occurs in 20–40% of cases (Abrahams *et al.*, 1996). There is also increasing evidence that MND is associated with fronto-temporal dementia (MND-D) in about 5% of cases (Leigh *et al.*, 2003).

EPIDEMIOLOGY

In most countries throughout the world the incidence of MND is in the region of 1–2 per 100,000 per year, resulting in a prevalence of around 6 per 100,000 at any one time (MND Association, 2007). The incidence of MND has been increasing, possibly due to better diagnostic procedures or because the disease is more common in older people and will continue to increase with an ageing population (MND Association, 2007). The mean age of onset is 56–63 years, but in those with a family history it is 47–52 years (Haverkamp *et al.*, 1995). Men are more commonly affected than women by a ratio of 1.6:1. More than 50% of patients die within three years of onset of their first symptom. Average survival from diagnosis is around fourteen months. Adverse prognostic indicators include bulbar or respiratory onset, short duration from first symptom to presentation, increasing age of onset, and male sex (Haverkamp *et al.*, 1995).

AETIOLOGY

The cause is largely unknown, but attempts have been made to determine if numerous environmental and toxic features, including exposure to heavy metals and the poliovirus, are risk factors for MND. To date proof of association has been scarce, but recently claims have been made of an increased risk amongst professional footballers (Chio *et al.*, 2005), possibly related to recurrent trauma or exposure to environmental toxins within fertilisers used on football pitches. Additionally, male military personnel were found to be 60% more likely to develop MND than those who had not served in the forces, however it is unclear how military service might increase risk (Weisskopf *et al.*, 2005).

The disease is sporadic in 90–95% of cases, but 5–10% of patients exhibit a positive family history, usually of an autosomal dominant inheritance. Despite recent advances, the genetic mutation in the majority of such cases remains unknown (Mitchell and Borasio, 2007). Extensive research into the cause of MND suggests that the disease may result from the complex interplay of a number of factors. Apart from the genetic factors already discussed, oxidative stress and excitotoxicity are the other main factors currently implicated.

Neuroscience Nursing: Evidence-Based Practice, 1st Edition.
Edited by Sue Woodward and Ann-Marie Mestecky
© 2011 Blackwell Publishing Ltd

Oxidative stress

Oxidative stress occurs when an excess of free radicals (highly reactive unstable molecules) triggers a cascade of biochemical reactions resulting in cell damage. The copper/zinc superoxide dismutase (SOD1) gene on chromosome 21 is crucial for antioxidant defence. Discovery of mutated forms of SOD1 in some familial cases (Rosen *et al.*, 1993) suggests that oxidative damage may have a role in motor neurone degeneration in MND.

Excitotoxicity

Excitatory neurotransmitters are essential for normal functioning of the nervous system. Excitotoxicity, a possible cause for motor neurone destruction, is thought to occur when the most abundant excitatory neurotransmitter, glutamate, becomes present at concentrations above that required for normal physiological function (van Cutsem *et al.*, 2005). This excess contributes to neuronal death by triggering an excessive calcium influx into the motor neurone resulting in a cascade involving free radicals which ultimately results in cell death.

PATHOPHYSIOLOGY

Degeneration of motor neurones occurs at all levels from the motor cortex of the brain to the anterior horn cells of the spinal cord. Clinical symptoms and disease classification are dependent on whether upper motor neurones (UMN), lower motor neurones (LMN) (see Chapter 4), or a combination of the two are affected. Distinction between types is not always clear and becomes less evident with disease progression.

CLINICAL SIGNS AND SYMPTOMS

The clinical features of MND result from progressive degeneration of both UMNs, leading to spasticity, hyperreflexia and weakness, and LMNs, resulting in flaccidity, hyporeflexia, fasciculations, muscle atrophy and weakness (Figure 27.1).

Amyotrophic lateral sclerosis (ALS)

ALS is the most commonly occurring type of the disease, accounting for approximately 65% of all cases. UMN and LMN involvement results in muscle weakness and wasting. Limb onset is the most common presentation in ALS occurring in approximately 70% of patients. Initially, upper limb distal weakness causes inability to perform fine finger movements such as fastening buttons; proximal weakness in the upper limbs can be manifest in difficulty raising the hands above the head. Wasting of the small muscles of the hands is common, as is fasciculation (muscle twitching), particularly in the proximal muscles (Evans and Shaw, 2001).

Lower limb onset can include vague initial symptoms such as fatigue following regular exercise, difficulty walking with increased tripping especially on uneven surfaces, and muscle cramps particularly at night. Proximal weakness can result in difficulty climbing stairs, while weak ankle dorsiflexion leads to foot drop. Profuse fasciculation can be noticed in the proximal muscles (Evans and Shaw, 2001).

Prognosis in ALS is normally two to five years from the onset of symptoms.

Progressive bulbar palsy (PBP)

PBP is an aggressive form of MND presenting with bulbar dysfunction causing dysarthria (slow, slurred speech) and/or dysphagia (difficulty swallowing). Muscles innervated by cranial nerves and corticobulbar tracts are predominantly affected. LMN (bulbar palsy) or UMN (pseudobulbar palsy) involvement can occur independently or together. Clinically, LMN involvement is reflected in facial weakness, poor elevation of the soft palate, and wasting, weakness and fasciculation of the tongue. UMN involvement manifests as pseudobulbar affect or emotional lability (pathological laughing/crying), brisk jaw jerk, and dysarthria. As speech problems worsen, dysphagia becomes more apparent. Initially swallowing difficulties may be limited to liquids, but eventually problems with chewing and coordination of swallowing result in repeated coughing and choking at mealtimes and even on saliva.

Prognosis in PBP is between six months and three years from the onset of symptoms (Evans and Shaw, 2001).

Respiratory onset in MND is rare, occurring as a result of the involvement of bulbar, cervical and thoracic motor neurones. Initial symptoms include dyspnoea on exertion and when prone (Evans and Shaw, 2001).

Progressive muscular atrophy (PMA)

PMA is thought to affect approximately 8% of people with MND. LMN are predominantly affected, resulting in wasting of the small muscles of the hands and fasciculations. Over time, those with PMA may develop some speech and swallowing difficulties and UMN involvement may become apparent.

Survival in PMA is usually in excess of five years from onset of symptoms (MND Association, 2007).

Primary lateral sclerosis (PLS)

PLS is a rare and relatively mild form of MND in which only UMN are affected. It is characterised by hyperreflexia

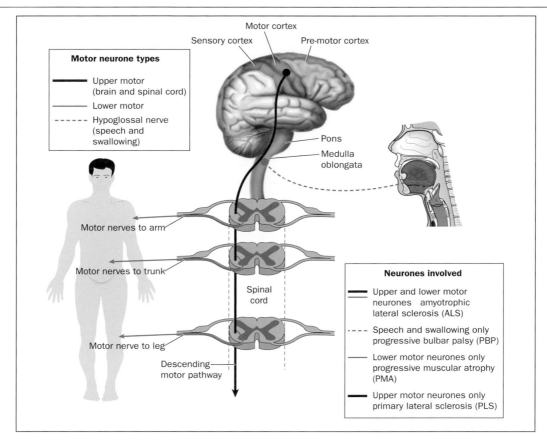

Figure 27.1 The various presentations of motor neurone disease and the neurones involved.
From Skelton J (2005) Nursing role in the multidisciplinary management of motor neurone disease. *British Journal of Nursing* **14**, 20–24. Reproduced with permission.

and a spastic gait. Sometimes a pseudobulbar syndrome develops. If the disease remains confined to UMN, those diagnosed with PLS can have a normal life-span, however LMN features can develop resulting in degeneration similar to that in ALS (MND Association, 2007).

DIAGNOSIS

The mean time from symptom onset to diagnosis is thirteen to eighteen months (Chio, 1999). There is no disease-specific test for MND; diagnosis is based differential diagnoses causing similar signs and symptoms.

A diagnosis of MND can be made if on clinical examination there is evidence of UMN and LMN involvement in three regions of the body over time and which cannot be attributed to other disease processes by electrophysiological or neuroimaging procedures, together with an absence of sensory signs. Depending on the extent of the clinical findings, the diagnosis can be further refined into

the categories of definite, probable, possible and suspected MND (Box 27.1).

MEDICAL MANAGEMENT

Guidelines for the management of some aspects of MND exist (Miller *et al.*, 1999, Andersen *et al.*, 2005; MND Association, 2005), and suggestions for best practice are available (Howard and Orrell, 2002; Leigh *et al.*, 2003). As randomised controlled trials do not exist for most aspects of MND care, many of these recommendations are based on evidence derived from consensus amongst experts.

The diagnosis

Patients suspected of having MND should be fast tracked through the health care system to avoid delays in obtaining a diagnosis (Leigh *et al.*, 2003; Andersen *et al.*, 2005). Telling the patient the diagnosis is a daunting prospect,

---

Box 27.1 Summary of revised El Escorial diagnostic criteria for MND

Definite
- Upper motor neurone signs and lower motor neurone signs in three regions

Probable
- Upper motor neurone signs and lower motor neurone signs in two regions

Probable with Laboratory Support
- Upper motor neurone signs and lower motor neurone signs in one region *or* upper motor neurone signs alone are present in one region and lower motor neurone signs defined by EMG are present in at least two regions

Possible
- Upper motor neurone signs and lower motor neurone signs (together) in only one region *or* upper motor neurone signs in two or more regions

Adapted from Leigh *et al.*, 2003.

---

with the potential to affect the future doctor–patient relationship if not handled sensitively (Andersen *et al.*, 2005). The diagnosis should be explained to the patient, accompanied by the person(s) of their choice, by a senior doctor preferably who has with experience of caring for people with MND (Howard and Orrell 2002; Leigh *et al.*, 2003; MND Association, 2005). Patient comprehension must be assessed and additional information offered appropriate to the person's needs (Andersen *et al.*, 2005). Patients should be referred to a specialised MND multidisciplinary team for ongoing follow up.

Disease modifying therapy

Although numerous potential disease-modifying therapies for MND have been the subject of clinical trials, to date only riluzole has been licensed. Riluzole, a glutamate release inhibitor, has been shown to increase survival by about three months. It is also thought to block sensitive sodium and calcium channels, thereby delaying neuronal damage. Guidelines for its use and monitoring have been published (NICE, 2001).

Symptomatic treatment

Symptoms experienced by patients can be directly or indirectly related to the disease processes. They should be treated as soon as they begin to interfere with the patient's quality of life. Evidence based and good practice guidelines on therapeutic interventions for common symptoms (Table 27.1) are available (Miller *et al.*, 1999; Oliver *et al.*, 2000; Andersen *et al.*, 2005).

EVIDENCE-BASED NURSING MANAGEMENT

The effects of MND on those diagnosed with the disease are diverse, complex and potentially overwhelming. It is claimed that coordinated multidisciplinary care enhances prognosis in MND (Traynor *et al.*, 2003). Multidisciplinary care should be made available to people with MND through attendance at an MND specialist centre on a two to three monthly basis (Andersen *et al.*, 2005; MND Association, 2005). Although the composition of the multidisciplinary team may vary slightly region by region, it is recommended that a core team includes the patient's GP, the district nursing team, clinical nurse specialists, occupational therapists (OT), physiotherapists, speech and language therapists (SLT), a supervising neurologist (preferably one with a specialist interest in MND), a palliative care team, a dietitian and a social worker.

The extent of each team member's involvement with the patient at any specific time will be determined by the nature of the problems being experienced. Involvement may increase and decrease over the duration of the disease, but the variable and often fast moving nature of the disease demands that patients are able to gain rapid access to team members without having to be re-referred.

Nursing involvement with people with MND occurs during all stages of the illness, from diagnosis to death. Skelton (2005) points to the nurse's role as one of monitoring the patient's condition, providing psychological support for both patient and carer and advising the patient and working with the medical team to control symptoms. Additionally, an awareness and understanding of the potential for the disease to impact on the psychological and social well-being of those affected will help nurses respond with sensitivity.

Ideally, a single point of contact should be established to coordinate all aspects of multidisciplinary care required by individual patients (Leigh *et al.*, 2003; Andersen *et al.*, 2005); MND nurse specialists frequently fill this position.

Communication

Up to 80% of people with MND will experience verbal communication difficulties at some point (Leigh *et al.*, 2003). These difficulties include increasing problems with articulation, slurred speech and a weak voice. Patients with bulbar onset illness can become anarthric within a few months of the onset of their dysarthria.

Table 27.1 Common symptoms: pharmacological and non-pharmacological management.

Symptom	Pharmacological recommendations	Additional/non-pharmacological suggestions
Sialorrhoea (saliva is produced that the patient is unable to swallow)	Hyoscine *(oral/trandermal)* Atropine drops *(sublingual)* Glycopyrrolate Amitriptyline	*If medication fails:* Botulinum toxin injections into parotid glands may help Irradiation of salivary glands Review doses of medication and fluid intake
Tenacious secretions	Carbocisteine Saline nebuliser	Cough assist taught by physiotherapist Mechanical insufflator-exsufflator (see Chapter 15)
Pseudobulbar affect (uncontrollable emotional lability)	Amitriptyline Fluvoxamine Citalopram	Advise patient that emotional lability is a physiological consequence of the disease, not a mood disorder
Cramps	Quinine sulphate Magnesium Carbamazepine Phenytoin Verapamil Gabapentin	Physiotherapy Physical exercise Hydrotherapy
Spasticity	Baclofen Tizanidine Dantrolene Diazepam	Physiotherapy Hydrotherapy (see also Chapter 11)
Depression	Amitriptyline SSRI	Psychological support Counselling
Anxiety	Diazepam *(tablets/suppositories)* Lorazepam *(sublingual)*	
Insomnia	Amitriptyline Hypnotics (e.g. zolpidem) Analgesia	Ensure comfort Explore causes, e.g. hypoventilation
Pain	Analgesia ladder (WHO 2010) Simple analgesia NSAIDs Weak opiates Strong opiates	Ensure comfort – elevate limbs Physiotherapy
Respiratory distress	Morphine *(oral, subcutaneous infusion)* Benzodiazepines *(sublingual, oral, suppositories)*	Assess respiratory function by vital capacity (VC) or sniff nasal pressure (SNP) Nocturnal pulse oximetry Non-invasive positive pressure ventilation (NIV) Invasive mechanical ventilation via tracheostomy (TV)
Terminal distress	Midazolam (relaxation/sedation) Morphine (pain/dyspnoea) Glycopyrronium (chest secretions) Buccal lorazepam (initial distress)	Advice available within the *Just in Case Kit* Available from the Motor Neurone Disease Association

Nurses should assess communication (see Chapter 12) and ensure timely referral to a SLT. Speech therapy should be initiated as soon as any alteration in speech or voice is observed. SLTs will provide advice on communication strategies and undertake assessment for and provision of communication aids. Patients with good articulation but a weak voice may benefit from using a voice amplifier. As the disease progresses it is necessary to employ alternatives to speech, often starting with writing and letter/picture boards and moving through increasingly technical solutions as disability worsens to include 'type to speak' devices and computerised speech synthesisers (Leigh *et al.*, 2003). Patients should be re-assessed every three to six months to monitor progression and review communication support needs (Andersen *et al.*, 2005).

Loss of, or difficulty with speech may also contribute to social isolation for patients with MND. Skelton (2005) highlights that patients with dysarthria can become isolated and withdrawn, becoming frustrated and embarrassed at the inability of others to comprehend what they are saying. Health care professionals, including nurses, may at times feel inadequate in their inability to understand a dysarthic patient (Skelton, 2005). Communicating with a dysarthric patient can be slow, difficult and frustrating for all concerned, therefore it is important that it takes place in a relaxed manner allowing sufficient time for meaningful interaction (Chapter 12) if patients are to be fully involved in decision making about their care. While the technical assessment and management of communication lies with the SLT, nurses are involved in reinforcing advice and monitoring the patient's condition.

Swallowing and nutrition

Nutritional status and weight loss are predictors of survival in MND (Desport *et al.*, 1999). Initial nutritional management includes modification of the texture and consistency of diet and fluids, use of dietary supplements and education of patients and carers regarding posture, head position and swallowing techniques (Miller *et al.*, 1999; Andersen *et al.*, 2005). It has been suggested that approximately 21% of MND patients are malnourished (Leigh *et al.*, 2003).

Bedside swallowing assessment by the nurse, incorporating careful history taking and observing the patient eating and drinking, can reveal the presence and severity of dysphagia (see Chapter 12). Early referral to a SLT and dietician is advocated (MND Association, 2005) and SLT assessment of swallowing may be supplemented by videofluoroscopy. Although regarded as the gold standard in the evaluation of dysphagia, it is not routinely used to monitor dysphagia in MND due to the risks associated with repeated exposure to radiation, costs and the practicalities of carrying out the procedure (Rio *et al.*, 2005). Following SLT swallowing assessment, advice on simple posture changes and swallowing techniques such as the double or triple swallow and the use of the 'chin tuck' (flexing the neck forwards on swallowing) may be given to ensure a safe swallow and protect the airway (Andersen *et al.*, 2005; MND Association, 2005).

Nutritional intake is not only inhibited by dysphagia; patients with hand and/or arm weakness eat more slowly than normal, are frequently exhausted by the effort of eating and often fail to finish meals. Many patients are reliant on the help of nurses or carers for their food and fluid intake. Where appropriate, patients should be referred to physiotherapy or occupational therapy for aids and advice regarding positioning at mealtimes (MND Association, 2005).

Dietary assessment is recommended using a variety of measures including dietary history and body mass index (BMI) (weight(kg) / height(m)^2) (Andersen *et al.*, 2005; MND Association, 2005). Recording a diet history provides details of meal patterns, the amount and type of food eaten and the time taken to complete a meal. Evidence of prolonged meal times, the need for assistance with eating and/or increasing difficulties manipulating and swallowing diet and/or fluids indicate a need to review nutritional status (Rio *et al.*, 2005). Supplements in the form of sip drinks, fortified foods, softened foods, high calorie powder and liquid products are routinely prescribed in an attempt to maintain nutritional status (Rio *et al.*, 2005). High protein and high calorie intake is encouraged, but should be tailored to the individual patient's requirements following an assessment by a dietician (MND Association, 2005).

Percutaneous endoscopic gastrostomy (PEG) (Figure 27.2) is the standard procedure for provision of enteral nutrition and fluids in MND (Andersen *et al.*, 2005) and is generally available in centres with endoscopic services (Rio *et al.*, 2005). Various factors influence the timing of PEG, including FVC (forced vital capacity), extent of dysphagia and the patient's overall condition (Miller *et al.*, 1999; MND Association, 2005). Additionally, weight loss of 10% or more of the baseline (pre-illness) weight is a prognostic indicator of malnutrition (MND Association, 2005) and should initiate consideration of PEG (Leigh *et al.*, 2003).

Careful patient education is vital to enable them to make an informed and timely decision about the intervention. Skelton (2005) recommends that nurses should involve the patient with early discussions about a possible need for PEG; Rio *et al.* (2005) stress the skill of the multidisciplinary team in patient education in this area, in offering a

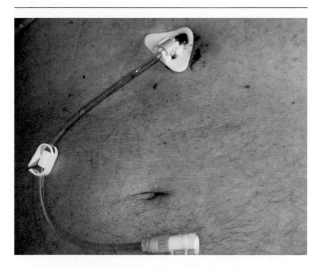

Figure 27.2 PEG tube in situ. From Kiernan, M.C. (2007) *The Motor Neurone Disease Handbook*, MJA, pages 188–189. © 2007 The Medical Journal of Australia. Reproduced with permission.

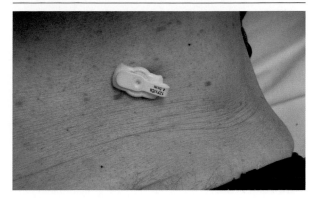

Figure 27.3 PRG tube in situ. From Kiernan, M.C. (2007) *The Motor Neurone Disease Handbook*, MJA, pages 188–189. © 2007 The Medical Journal of Australia. Reproduced with permission.

balanced view of the potential benefits and risks. It may be advantageous to introduce the patient to someone who has already undergone the procedure in an attempt to allay fears. Often, despite careful assessment and monitoring, patients are reluctant to undergo the procedure and delay making the decision to go ahead sometimes out of fear of being unable to continue with an oral intake following placement of the PEG. Patients should be reassured that oral intake may continue as long as their swallow remains safe.

Many patients use PEG feeding to supplement their oral intake, allowing them to continue to enjoy smaller meals without the need to meet their entire nutritional requirements via the oral route. PEG feeding can be achieved by bolus, drip or pump. There is no standard recommendation for the administration of PEG feeds. The type of feeding should be decided on an individual basis, taking the patient's specific circumstances into account, i.e. the amount of feeding required, the level of assistance required with feeding and the availability of suitable carers.

PEG placement, like any invasive surgical procedure, is not without risk; this is particularly so as placement requires sedation, increasing the potential for complications such as aspiration and respiratory depression. Risks associated with PEG may be reduced if tube placement is made before the patient's FVC falls below 50% of predicted (Mathus-Vliegen *et al.*, 1994). Patients with respiratory impairment and FVC <50% of predicted may feasibly have a PEG if non-invasive positive pressure ventilation

is administered (Gregory *et al.*, 2002), although this is not routinely performed in such patients. It has been claimed that PEG prolongs survival in MND by about eight months (Mazzini *et al.*, 1995), however, later studies have questioned this assertion (Forbes *et al.*, 2004).

Where PEG is not suitable, percutaneous radiologic gastrostomy (PRG), also known as radiologically inserted gastrostomy (RIG) is now a viable alternative. Rather than using an endoscope, a nasogastric tube is passed into the stomach to inflate it with air and the gastrostomy tube is then placed into the stomach under x-ray guided conditions. Figure 27.3 shows a PRG in situ. Evidence suggests that PRG is a safe and effective alternative to PEG (Chio *et al.*, 2004) with the advantage of not requiring sedation. It can be performed in patients at a more advanced stage of the disease and also in patients such as those with high-lying stomach as a result of diaphragm muscle weakness, in whom PEG placement would be difficult. PRG has been shown to have a greater procedural success rate than PEG (Thornton *et al.*, 2002), but is not currently as widely available.

Nasogastric tube feeding (NGT) is a less invasive procedure with fewer complications than PEG or PRG. It is generally only used as a short-term option enabling nutritional and fluid intake to continue while allowing non-invasive positive pressure ventilation (NIV, see Chapter 15) to be established so that patients with poor respiratory function can be stabilised prior to PEG or PRG placement. It may be used in those patients in whom PEG or PRG is not possible. Disadvantages that limit long-term use include the need to confirm the tube position on a daily basis, the unsightly appearance, increased oropharyngeal secretions, discomfort, nasal ulceration and erosion (Andersen *et al.*, 2005; Rio *et al.*, 2005).

Nurses caring for patients receiving enteral nutrition will need to ensure that patients and carers are provided with adequate instruction regarding the care of the PEG and the PEG site (see Chapter 16) prior to discharge and are fully aware of the procedures for re-ordering supplies and obtaining help should the tube become blocked or displaced (Skelton, 2005).

Respiratory management

Respiratory impairment in MND results mainly from respiratory muscle weakness and/or impaired bulbar function, leading to increased incidence of aspiration and bronchopneumonia (Howard and Orrell, 2002). Patients should be regularly assessed for symptoms of respiratory insufficiency, e.g. orthopnoea, dyspnoea on exertion, disturbed night time sleep with excessive daytime sleepiness, difficulty clearing secretions, morning headache, depression and poor appetite (Andersen *et al.*, 2005). Regular measurement of FVC (see Chapter 15) provides an indication of respiratory muscle strength and is recommended as a guide to respiratory management (Miller *et al.*, 1999; MND Association, 2005), but is not an accurate predictor of the need for assisted ventilation in MND (Leigh *et al.*, 2003).

Sniff nasal pressure (SNP) measures inspiratory muscle strength and is recommended particularly for monitoring those patients unable to perform FVC accurately due to facial muscle weakness (Andersen *et al.*, 2005; Leigh *et al.*, 2003). It is good practice to recommend vaccination against influenza and pneumonia and to treat any respiratory infection promptly. Patients with a weak cough who develop respiratory infections may benefit from using a cough assist device (see Chapter 15) (MND Association, 2005). Physiotherapy in the form of breathing exercises can increase lung capacity and cough assistance techniques can reduce the risk of chest infections thereby helping to delay the onset of respiratory difficulties (Bach, 1993).

For those patients affected by nocturnal hypoventilation, monitoring of overnight pulse oximetry is recommended (Andersen *et al.*, 2005). This is regarded as a more convenient cost effective and practical option than polysomnography (full sleep studies) (Leigh *et al.*, 2003). Non-invasive positive pressure ventilation, and the less frequently used invasive ventilation via tracheostomy (TV), are advocated for the relief of respiratory distress.

Figure 27.4 shows a MND patient with NIV in situ. NIV is utilised for symptomatic relief in chronic hypoventilation, while TV should be offered where long term survival is the goal (Miller *et al.*, 1999). However, Andersen *et al.*

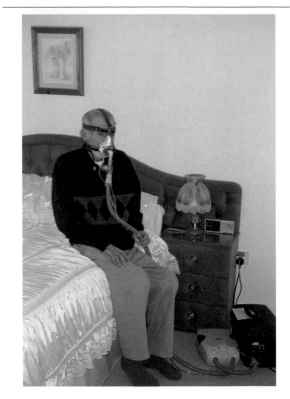

Figure 27.4 NIV in situ. Photo courtesy of Dr David Oliver.

(2005) highlight the lack of evidence regarding the timing and criteria for the use of NIV and TV in MND, with use varying across countries and cultures. NIV is regarded as a standard procedure in MND clinics in North America (Miller *et al.*, 1999) and in Japan most patients are offered ventilatory support, often via tracheostomy (Bourke and Gibson, 2004). A traditional reluctance to use mechanical ventilation amongst European neurologists (Borasio *et al.*, 1998) has gradually changed; nevertheless fewer than 5% of MND patients in Europe (including the UK) receive NIV (Bourke and Gibson, 2004).

It is recommended that FVC <50% of predicted should trigger discussions on NIV (Miller *et al.*, 1999). However, Leigh *et al.* (2003) regard this threshold as too low. Appearance of signs of respiratory insufficiency (see Chapter 15) should initiate discussions with the patient and carer regarding these treatment options and their long-term implications (Andersen *et al.*, 2005; MND Association, 2005). Evidence suggests that NIV improves survival and quality of life in MND (Bourke *et al.*, 2003) and should therefore be offered to suitable patients, particularly those with daytime symptoms of nocturnal hypoventilation and mild bulbar symptoms (MND Association, 2005). Leigh *et al.* (2003) suggest that the low uptake of NIV in the UK may reflect the limited resources available and concerns by care providers that it may be detrimental rather than beneficial to the patient's quality of life to prolong their life in this dependent manner.

Mechanical ventilation is not straightforward; there are frequently issues of compliance in severely disabled patients and increased burden is apparent for carers and relatives (Howard and Orrell, 2002; Andersen *et al.*, 2005; Mitchell and Borasio, 2007). Careful consideration and counselling is required when opting to pursue NIV; a planned approach based on recommendations is detailed in Box 27.2. While NIV may improve survival in MND, it does not have any effect on disease progression; ultimately a point will be reached when the breathing is no longer helped by NIV (Skelton, 2005).

Box 27.2   Planned approach to non-invasive positive pressure ventilation (NIV) in MND

- Monitor respiratory function and symptoms of hypoventilation
- Be alert to respiratory infections
- Begin discussions about respiratory support options with patient and carer before respiratory symptoms occur
- Assess the support available in the home
- Discuss both advantages and disadvantages of NIV with patient and carer
- NIV should be discussed in the wider context of palliative care
- Discuss end of life decisions, advanced directives, power of attorney, withdrawal of NIV and the pros and cons of TV
- Discuss the techniques and ensure patient and carer are familiar with equipment and procedures
- Instruct patient and carer about assisted cough techniques
- Initiate NIV, providing instruction for patient and carer(s); set up support system
- Periodically monitor NIV effectiveness by oximetry and assessment of symptomatic relief
- Assess patient and carer quality of life and carer strain periodically
- Agree a plan for NIV withdrawal with appropriate palliative measures

Adapted from Leigh *et al.*, 2003.

Pain and discomfort

Pain is a frequently occurring problem for a majority of people with MND. It commonly occurs in the early stages of the disease, often due to painful muscle cramps, but also affects a high proportion of patients in the later stages of the illness. Other causes include stiffness, spasticity, and pressure on the skin and joints from immobility. Physiotherapy, in the form of advice regarding gait, passive exercises and compensatory movements can help to avoid fatigue and maintain limb function, joint flexibility, and independence for as long as possible.

The WHO analgesic ladder (WHO 2010) should be followed and opiates used when non-narcotic analgesics fail (Miller *et al.*, 1999; Andersen *et al.*, 2005). Leigh *et al.* (2003) highlight the under use of opiates, despite their added advantage of relieving breathlessness and anxiety without necessarily shortening life. However, side-effects of both non-steroidal anti-inflammatory drugs (NSAIDS) and opiates must be considered and managed. It is recommended that side-effects are monitored, dosage is restricted to the minimum effective dose and that any resulting constipation is managed by ensuring adequate hydration, a balanced diet and the use of aperients (Leigh *et al.*, 2003; Oliver, 2002).

The use of a syringe driver for subcutaneous administration should be considered when there is a need for frequent medication. This is especially useful for patients with swallowing difficulties. On occasions it may be necessary to involve a pain management team (Leigh *et al.*, 2003). Attending to basic comfort using pressure relieving cushions and mattresses together with frequent changes of position can have a significant effect on pain resulting from immobility. Table 27.1 contains recommendations for the pharmacological and non-pharmacological management of pain (see also Chapter 17).

PSYCHOSOCIAL ISSUES

Psychosocial care comprises a wide range of concerns that are relevant not only to patients, but also frequently to their families and carers. Psychosocial issues can have a major effect on decisions regarding health care choices and yet this remains an area which is under-researched (McLeod and Clarke, 2007). The progressive nature of the disease means that those affected by MND face constant adaptation as their condition worsens. Often there is little time to adjust to a lost ability before it is superseded by another. The ability to adjust psychologically to these changes is seen as a prognostic indicator. Patients with high levels of anxiety, depression and feelings of helplessness tend to have shorter survival than those patients who attain psychological adjustment (McLeod and Clarke, 2007).

Oliver (2002) highlights that from the time of the diagnosis and often even before it has been made, patients (and their families) can experience a wide range of emotions, concerns and fears; fears of the diagnosis, the disease, dependency, disability, dying and death. Nurses should be aware of these possible concerns and be open with the patient and their family, and willing to discuss these issues if and when necessary (Oliver 2002; Oliver and Borasio, 2004). It is particularly important to enable discussion to take place before speech is badly affected, as trying to discuss sensitive issues via a communication aid can be particularly difficult and distressing for all involved (Oliver and Borasio, 2004).

Many patients have little understanding of what MND is when told their diagnosis. Faced with the unknown they and their families frequently seek out information in answer to their questions, often being mis-informed and distressed by media campaigns that seek to sensationalise. Unsolicited information may have a negative effect (O'Brien, 2004), as media campaigns often report bleak aspects of MND, such as helplessness and calls for assisted suicide, as well as misrepresenting modest advances as breakthroughs, falsely raising expectations (Leigh *et al.*, 2003).

It is vital that nurses caring for people with MND are knowledgeable about the condition to correct any misunderstandings. Fears of dependency and disability need to be addressed as many patients are anxious about loss of control and independence as their condition worsens. Occupational therapists have a vital role in maintaining independence and relieving the strain on carers by assessing for and providing aids for daily living and coordinating the provision of equipment such as wheelchairs and environmental controls. The emphasis on providing relief from the physical deterioration, while important, is somewhat limited and underestimates the significance of assessing and treating the psychological effects which are evident in most patients (McLeod and Clarke, 2007). Psychosocial support and an exploration of ways of developing coping strategies is vital (Oliver, 2002).

There is conflicting information regarding the extent of depression amongst MND patients (McLeod and Clarke, 2007). Depression and anxiety are frequently reported not only amongst patients but also amongst carers following a diagnosis of MND. It is vital that these issues are treated appropriately (see Table 27.1) and not regarded as unavoidable consequences of a progressive, terminal illness (Howard and Orrell, 2002).

Mitchell and Borasio (2007) point out that the family is the most important factor in quality of life amongst people with MND. Patients are part of a wider social network of family, carers and friends and there is generally a positive correlation between social support and the absence of depression (McLeod and Clarke, 2007). The stress associated with chronic illness can be moderated by the availability of good social support mechanisms.

While social support is protective against depression, and strongly associated with quality of life, the effects of the disabilities resulting from MND can inhibit patients' social activities (McLeod and Clarke, 2007). Reduced mobility means that patients can become increasingly housebound, while loss of speech and the ability to eat and drink mean the loss of normal socialising activities, which are vital to maintaining an active social support network. At the same time, previously clearly defined relationships change beyond recognition, with the loss of intimate relationships as spouses adapt to new roles as carers. Oliver and Borasio (2004) suggest that the wider family and social network may have similar concerns about the disease, death and dying as the patient. They may also have fears for the future without their loved one or about what they should tell children. The support of a psychologist or counsellor may be helpful (Oliver, 2002).

According to McLeod and Clarke (2007 p7) 'hope and hopelessness are important issues', as a diagnosis of MND forces changes, threatens stability and forces patients and their families to alter their life's plans. Hope is an important driver, helping to maintain psychological well-being and quality of life. Patients without hope are more likely to feel a sense of loss of control and to be prone to suicidal thoughts. Mitchell and Borasio (2007) recommend early assessment of hopelessness and the use of non-pharmacological interventions as the best approach to maintaining hope and meaning in life.

Hope may fuel desire to seek alternative treatments. Many patients explore complementary treatments which have no objective analysis of their efficacy, yet appear to be helpful and provide considerable psychological support (Leigh *et al.*, 2003). Patients report that seeking out alternative and complementary treatments is important to them because it increases their chances of finding something that might be beneficial to their condition. This is particularly pertinent as conventional medicine appears to have so little disease modification to offer.

Incredibly, many individuals experience hope and find meaning, while some even identify positive aspects to being diagnosed with MND. Writing in an online journal containing his thoughts hopes and fears, American Don Moore documents his progress through MND:

> *'I am trying to learn to focus on the positive aspects ... what in the world could be positive from having such a horrible disease? ... the opportunity to take advantage of what good time you have ... the opportunity to get affairs in order ... the opportunity to mend fences before you are on a death bed.'*

Many patients are able to maintain a positive approach to their illness and as a result they are less likely to be affected by depression and anxiety (McLeod and Clarke, 2007).

When faced with a terminal illness, it is only natural to begin to consider the deeper meaning of life and death (Oliver, 2002). This may involve the patient seeking solace within formal religious beliefs or seeking the opportunity to address concerns about the future. It can be difficult for nurses to enquire about a patient's spiritual needs, but there is a need to provide opportunities for patients and carers to discuss spiritual and cultural aspects of care.

Information needs

Some patients will cope with MND by seeking information about the disease to enable them to plan their life towards maximising functional ability and living life to the full. Active seekers of information in the study by O'Brien (2004) acquired information about MND from a variety of sources early in the course of the disease; when faced with an adverse event, they sought information in order to help them cope with it. Some people with MND cope on a day-to-day basis, selectively seeking information in a purposive way, about issues that concern them at that moment, feeling that it would be detrimental to have detailed general information about MND (O'Brien 2004). Additionally, some patients may not wish to know what will happen to them in the future. Information avoiders may cope by rejecting information about MND; anticipating future disabilities will do little to help with their current situation (O'Brien, 2004). It should be noted however, that patients can alter their information seeking behaviour as the disease progresses. Many patients use 'buffers' (friends or family members) to obtain information on their behalf. Buffers often shield patients from the full extent of information which may have a detrimental effect (O'Brien, 2004).

Nurses have traditionally taken on the role of patient educator, often assuming that they instinctively know what patients need to know and when they need to know it. It is vital that nurses understand the strategies adopted by people with MND regarding information about their condition and that the amount, type and timing of information they require at different phases in their illness will differ. They do not all want to have detailed information and many will want to be protected from it (O'Brien, 2004).

PALLIATIVE AND END OF LIFE CARE

Palliative care should be incorporated into all aspects of the management of MND, for patients and carers, and should ideally start at the time of the diagnosis (Borasio and Voltz, 1997). Mitchell and Borasio (2007) highlight that despite attempts to establish evidence-based guidelines, palliative care in MND still varies between countries and remains largely based on expert opinion. A recently developed care pathway addresses the palliative care needs of patients with a non-cancer diagnosis (Sutton, 2008).

Early referral to a local palliative care team to work in partnership with the MND multidisciplinary team is recommended (Andersen *et al.*, 2005); as is initiating discussions on end of life options whenever the patient asks, discussing issues around life sustaining options and revisiting the subject on a regular basis to take account of any changes to the patient's preferences. It is recommended that patient's views on life sustaining treatments are reviewed every six months (Andersen *et al.*, 2005). The UK Government's *End of Life Care Strategy* aims to improve choice and promote high quality care for all adults at the end of their lives (DH, 2008).

Hospices have often been viewed simply in terms of a place where people go to die. MND patients may resist attempts to encourage them to consider hospice care because of this association with death. However, the modern hospice approach focuses on the delivery of palliative care. Ideally palliative care in MND encompasses alleviating symptoms, offering emotional, psychological and spiritual support, removing barriers to a peaceful death and providing bereavement support, all with the aim of maximising quality of life for patients and their families (Oliver *et al.*, 2000). Often, attending a day hospice helps patients to experience the range of therapies, psychological and spiritual support available, building up a therapeutic relationship with hospice staff before taking up the option of respite care.

Terminal care

Media reports emphasising the most negative aspects of MND have helped to fuel fears amongst many patients that the final stages of the disease will involve choking, suffocation and pain. Patients should be reassured that good palliative care, addressing pain, dyspnoea and swallowing problems, contributes to maintaining quality of life and should result in a peaceful death; choking is very rare (Oliver and Borasio, 2004).

Death usually results from respiratory failure, often exacerbated by infection. Marked changes can occur in respiratory function over a few days; however even more rapid deterioration is common, 48–72% of patients deteriorate swiftly and die within 24 hours (Oliver and Borasio, 2004). The availability of medication and advice within the home reduces panic and allays fears of a distressing death. The MND Association developed the *Just in Case Kit* for just this purpose (MND Association 2010). The kit comprises a box containing medication prescribed by the GP for use under specific circumstances detailed in accompanying instruction leaflets. This ensures that health care professionals attending the patient at this time have immediate access to appropriate medication (see Table 27.1). Additionally, carers can administer medication to relieve anxiety whilst awaiting arrival of health professionals. Many patients prefer to be cared for at home at the end of life. With coordination of the multidisciplinary team through regular meetings together with good planning and support, this is possible (Oliver, 2002).

In preparation for the possibility of a rapid deterioration patients should be encouraged to discuss their preferences for end of life care. It is recommended that patients are assisted to formulate an advance decision or 'living will' to clarify their wishes regarding future care (Andersen *et al.*, 2005; Sutton, 2008; DH, 2008). Such documents are legally binding so long as they focus on the use of medical interventions for symptom control and not to end life prematurely (Skelton, 2005). They are also important for patients to document their choices regarding life sustaining interventions such as PEG, PRG and NIV/TV, in anticipation of a time when they may be unable to communicate their wishes. Advance decisions should be reviewed regularly to ensure that they continue to reflect the patient's views.

Bereavement

MND is a disease of continual losses; as a result family members often experience elements of bereavement from the time of the diagnosis onwards. It is important to acknowledge and recognise the potential mixture of emotions that can follow the death of the patient. Oliver (2002) highlights that there may be feelings of relief that the disease is over, mixed with feelings of guilt for having experienced the relief. Counselling and support for families may help to address these conflicting emotions; this may be provided by the palliative care team, but often

longer term help is required which would necessitate continuing domiciliary support (Howard and Orrell, 2002).

EXPERIMENTAL TREATMENTS/ CLINICAL TRIALS

Clinical trials in MND have tested many compounds that theoretically might affect disease progression, but which in reality have not (Leigh *et al.*, 2003). A summary of key clinical trials of putative disease modifying treatments in MND can be found in Mitchell and Borasio (2007). Research exploring the use of retrograde virus delivery of agents in animal models of MND has shown some encouraging findings with prolonged survival, but this has yet to be transferred into the human disease.

Stem-cell treatment

Considerable attention has been focused in recent years on the possible use of stem-cells as a treatment option in MND. As embryonic stem cells have the potential to develop into any type of cell within the body, scientists have wondered if it could be feasible to use them to repair cells damaged by disease. Reports indicate that, while there has been some success in generating neurones in animal testing, progress in human studies has been limited.

Apart from the technical challenges inherent in attempting to control the development of these stem cells, there are considerable ethical concerns regarding the destruction of blastocysts during harvesting of embryonic stem cells; sources of these blastocysts include unwanted embryos from in vitro fertilisation (IVF) and aborted embryos (MND Association, 2007). Measures suggested to increase the availability of embryos for research include the use of animal eggs as recipients for human DNA, however the use of such 'Chimeras' has raised public concern.

The availability of stem cell treatments in countries outside the UK has understandably been seized upon by patients eager for any treatment that might potentially affect the progression of their condition. It must be remembered however, that despite high financial costs to patients, these treatments are being offered without having been subjected to rigorous scientific evaluation of their safety or efficacy (MND Association, 2007). We are clearly at a very early stage in our understanding; before stem cell treatment can even be regarded as an experimental option, a considerable amount of work is needed (Mitchell and Borasio, 2007).

SUMMARY

MND results in profound limb weakness, speech, swallowing and breathing difficulties and has an average time from diagnosis until death of just 14 months. As a result those diagnosed with the condition have varied and complex needs, requiring input from a wide range of health, social and palliative care services. There is currently a dearth of studies providing a strong scientific evidence base for decisions regarding the care for people with the disease. Most recommendations are good practice points, which are based on consensus of experts in the MND field (Andersen *et al.*, 2005). The MND Association, Scottish MNDA and other international voluntary agencies are excellent sources of advice, information and support, for patients, their families and health professionals.

USEFUL CONTACTS

Motor Neurone Disease Association http://www.mndassociation.org

Motor Neurone Disease Scotland http://www.scotmnd.org.uk

ALS Association http://www.alsa.org

MND Australia http://www.mndaust.asn.au/

ALS Society of Canada http://www.als.ca

Motor neurone disease: patient perspective

After agreeing to write this, the patient's condition deteriorated so that typing became more difficult, hence he asked for questions so that he could focus his answers.

Q. What was the problem which initially made you see your doctor and how long had you been aware of this problem before seeking medical attention?

A. I fell flat on a 15 mile walk in Feb 2003 when right knee gave way. Got up and finished walk. Continued regular long walks through 2003 but developed sore knees which grew steadily worse. Climbing stairs became harder. Stumbles and falls increased in frequency espccially on rough ground. Soreness in feet developed. X-rays of knees taken in Oct. Arthritis suspected. By early 2004 trouble lifting right foot experienced. Increasing problems walking and climbing stairs. Dangerous to descend stairs. Sudden fits of rigidity to legs esp. on downhill slopes. A neurological ailment suggested in early 2004 but not MND and no definite diagnosis. Gradual worsening between mid 2004 and late 2005. Partial use of wheelchair outside became total by late 2005. In late 2005 voice began to fail.

Q. How long did your investigative period take before you were given a diagnosis?

A. MND not definitely confirmed until Summer 2006 when tests identified it. Earlier tests had identified a malfunctioning of my nervous system and MND was mentioned, but not positively identified.

Q. What was your experience of being given your diagnosis?

A. I was perfectly calm and not surprised. I knew I had something akin to MND from early 2004 and the medical staff were aware of my attitude.

Q. Was it handled well?

A. There was nothing to handle well or badly. The diagnosis confirmed the long known.

Q. What was your initial reaction to your diagnosis?

A. There was no shock or surprise as by the time the provisional diagnosis was confirmed I knew what I had. My reaction was to continue working, writing, organising conferences and editing. This I have done from early 2004 to the present.

Q. What level of support have you received since your diagnosis?

A. First rate support has been provided, beyond my most optimistic expectations.

Q. Have you received aids and equipment in a timely manner or have thcrc been delays?

A. Aids and equipment have been speedily supplied without unreasonable delays.

Q. How do you feel about using aids and equipment?

A. I use stairlifts, deltaframes, wheelchairs, etc., because they are essential to creative activity. I do not feel self-conscious about using disabled persons' equipment in public.

Q. How has the illness impacted on your work?

A. It has slowed down a programme of work which has developed over 40 years. I have had to abandon lecturing, give up overseas visiting lectureships, and greatly reduce the quantity of work done. Painting and sketching are no longer possible. Reading is hampered by inability to turn pages or to make notes, or to search through bookshelves.

Q. How do you feel about this?

A. Because MND advances slowly, there is time to match reduced abilities to curtailed activities and restricted ambitions. I am disappointed but that is all. The disease is a consequence of my own body malfunctioning. It is nobody's fault, and there is no malevolence in it. It is a physical process originating and ending in myself. Negative feelings, like bitterness, have no excuse.

Q. What impact has your illness had on your family and your family life?

A. My wife and I have no children as we married late in life. We shared many interests and spent much time together doing Salvation Army work; walking in the countryside; travelling abroad; visiting museums and art galleries; going to the theatre. All this has ended, but we still share everything. My wife spent her life in the Salvation Army looking after orphans and the old. She nursed my mother in her last years and now she nurses me without complaint. I feel keenly the burden I place on her.

Q. What does it mean to you to rely on others for assistance for your everyday needs?

A. It means no more and no less than any necessary reliance on specialist services such as are supplied by dentists, surgeons, firefighters, nurses or undertakers. The bodily indignities disappear once their necessity and purpose are recognised. A sense of humour helps.

Q. What are your thoughts about the future?

A. Difficult to answer at present because of recent developments. Until mid-2007 I was confident that I could surmount the physical restrictions which MND placed on me and thereby carry on working. I organised conferences in 2004, 2006 and planned one for 2008. I co-edited volume 1 of a planned series of books and compiled material for vols 2 and 3. Then, over a period of 3 months, my hands and arms grew severely disabled. My right arm and hand are virtually useless, and my left is much impaired. I am trying computer systems which dispense with keyboard and mouse but it is uncertain if I can attain that minimum output which is essential for meaningful progress.

REFERENCES

Abrahams S, Goldstein LH, Kew JJ *et al.* (1996) Frontal lobe dysfunction in amyotrophic lateral sclerosis. A PET study. *Brain: A Journal of Neurology* 119(6):2105–2120.

Andersen PM, Borasio GD, Dengler R *et al.* (2005) EFNS task force on management of amyotrophic lateral sclerosis: guidelines for diagnosing and clinical care of patients and relatives. An evidence-based review with good practice points. *European Journal of Neurology* 12:921–938.

Bach JR (1993) Mechanical insufflation-exsufflation: comparison of peak expiratory flows with manually assisted and unassisted coughing techniques. *Chest* 104(5):1553–1562.

Borasio GD, Gelinas D, Yanagisawa N (1998) Mechanical ventilation in amyotrophic lateral sclerosis: a cross-cultural perspective. *Journal of Neurology* 245:S7–12.

Borasio GD, Voltz R (1997) Palliative care in amyotrophic lateral sclerosis. *Journal of Neurology* 244:S11–7.

Bourke SC, Bullock RE, Williams TL *et al.* (2003) Noninvasive ventilation in ALS: Indications and effect on quality of life. *Neurology* 61:171–177.

Bourke SC, Gibson CJ (2004) Non-invasive ventilation in ALS: current practice and future role. *Amyotrophic Lateral Sclerosis* 5:67–71.

Chio A (1999) Survey: an international study on the diagnostic process and its implications in amyotrophic lateral sclerosis. *Journal of Neurology* 246 (Suppl 3):1–5.

Chio A, Benzi G, Dossena M *et al.* (2005) Severely increased risk of amyotrophic lateral sclerosis among Italian professional football players. *Brain* 128:472–476.

Chio A, Galletti R, Finocchiaro C *et al.* (2004) Percutaneous radiological gastrostomy: a safe and effective method of nutritional tube placement in advanced ALS. *Journal of Neurology, Neurosurgery, and Psychiatry* 75:645–647.

Department of Health (2008) *End of Life Care Strategy.* London: DH.

Desport JC, Preux PM, Truong TC *et al.* (1999) Nutritional status is a prognostic factor for survival in ALS patients. *Neurology* 53:1059.

Evans J, Shaw P (2001) Motor neurone disease: (1) Clinical features and pathogenesis. *The Pharmaceutical Journal* 267:681–683.

Forbes RB, Colville S, Swingler RJ & Scottish Motor Neurone Disease Research Group (2004) Frequency, timing and outcome of gastrostomy tubes for amyotrophic lateral sclerosis/motor neurone disease – a record linkage study from the Scottish Motor Neurone Disease Register. *Journal of Neurology* 251:813–817.

Gregory S, Siderowf A, Golaszewski AL, McCluskey L (2002) Gastrostomy insertion in ALS patients with low vital capacity: Respiratory support and survival. *Neurology* 58:485–487.

Haverkamp LJ, Appel V, Appel SH (1995) Natural history of amyotrophic lateral sclerosis in a database population.

Validation of a scoring system and a model for survival prediction. *Brain* 118:707–719.

Howard RS, Orrell RW (2002) Management of motor neurone disease. *Postgraduate Medical Journal* 78:736–741.

Leigh PN, Abrahams S, Al-Chalabi A *et al.* (2003) The management of motor neurone disease. *Journal of Neurology, Neurosurgery and Psychiatry* 74(Suppl 4):iv32–iv47.

Mathus-Vliegen LM, Louwerse LS, Merkus MP *et al.* (1994) Percutaneous endoscopic gastrostomy in patients with amyotrophic lateral sclerosis and impaired pulmonary function. *Gastrointestinal Endoscopy* 40:463–469.

Mazzini L, Corrà T, Zaccala M *et al.* (1995) Percutaneous endoscopic gastrostomy and enteral nutrition in amyotrophic lateral sclerosis. *Journal of Neurology* 242:695–698.

McLeod JE, Clarke DM (2007) A review of psychosocial aspects of motor neurone disease. *Journal of the Neurological Sciences* 258:4–10.

Miller RG, Rosenberg JA, Gelinas DF *et al.* (1999) Practice parameter: The care of the patient with amyotrophic lateral sclerosis (an evidence-based review): Report of the Quality Standards Subcommittee of the American Academy of Neurology. *Neurology* 52:1311.

Mitchell J, Borasio DG (2007) Amyotrophic lateral sclerosis. *The Lancet* 369:2031–2041.

Motor Neurone Disease Association (2005) *Evidence based reviews on respiratory management, nutritional management, making and communicating the diagnosis.* http://www.mndassociation.org/life_with_mnd/getting_more_information/publications/publications_1.html Accessed July 2010.

Motor Neurone Disease Association (2007) *Stem cells and motor neurone disease. Information sheet Q.* http://www.mndassociation.org/research/research_explained/stem_cells_and_mnd/index.html Accessed July 2010.

Motor Neurone Disease Association (2010) *Just in case kit.* Available from http://www.mndassociation.org/for_professionals/association_resources/jic_kit.html Accessed July 2010.

National Institute for Health and Clinical Excellence (2001) *Guidance on the Use of Riluzole (Rilutek) for the Treatment of Motor Neurone Disease.* London: NICE.

http://guidance.nice.org.uk/TA20/guidance/pdf/English Accessed July 2010.

O'Brien (2004) Information seeking behaviour among people with motor neurone disease. *British Journal of Nursing* 13(16):964–968.

Oliver D (2002) Palliative care for motor neurone disease. *Practical Neurology* 2:68–79.

Oliver D, Borasio GD (2004) Palliative care for patients with MND/ALS. *European Journal of Palliative Care* 11(5):185–187.

Oliver D, Borasio GD, Walsh D (eds)(2000) *Palliative Care in Amyotrophic Lateral Sclerosis.* Oxford: Oxford University Press.

Rio A, Ampong MA, Johnson J *et al.* (2005) Nutritional care of patients with motor neurone disease. *British Journal of Neuroscience Nursing* 1:38–43.

Rosen DR, Siddique T, Patterson D *et al.* (1993) Mutations in Cu/Zn superoxide dismutase gene are associated with familial amyotrophic lateral sclerosis. *Nature* 362:59–62.

Skelton J (2005) Nursing role in the multidisciplinary management of motor neurone disease. *British Journal of Nursing* 14:20–24.

Sutton L (2008) Addressing palliative and end-of-life care needs in neurology. *British Journal of Neuroscience Nursing* 4(5):235–238.

Thornton FJ, Fotheringham T, Alexander M *et al.* (2002) Amyotrophic lateral sclerosis: enteral nutrition provision – endoscopic or radiologic gastrostomy? *Radiology* 224:713–717.

Traynor BJ, Alexander M, Corr B *et al.* (2003) Effect of a multidisciplinary amyotrophic lateral sclerosis (ALS) clinic on ALS survival: a population based study, 1996–2000. *Journal of Neurology, Neurosurgery and Psychiatry* 74:1258–1261.

van Cutsem P, Dewil M, Robberecht W, van den Bosch L (2005). Excitotoxicity and Amyotrophic Lateral Sclerosis. *Neurodegenerative Diseases* 2:147–159.

Weisskopf MG, O'Reilly EJ, McCullough ML *et al.* (2005) Prospective study of military service and mortality from ALS. *Neurology* 64:32–37.

World Health Organisation (2010) *WHO's Pain Ladder.* Available from: http://www.who.int/cancer/palliative/painladder/en/ Accessed July 2010.

28

Management of Patients with Multiple Sclerosis

Vicki Matthews and Nikki Embrey

INTRODUCTION

Multiple sclerosis (MS) affects approximately 2.5 million people worldwide and is the most common cause of neurological disability among young adults (MacLurg *et al.*, 2005). Inflammation and demyelination of the CNS are the hallmarks of the disease, with the most common clinical course being acute inflammatory episodes superimposed on a background of progressive disability and impairment. It may exist at a sub-clinical level from fifteen years of age onwards, but what triggers the first symptomatic attack and classical course of the disease is not understood. MS predominately affects young people, can result in premature loss of productivity, reduced quality of life and pose a significant burden. The true economic cost remains difficult to ascertain because of variability in data collection (Kobelt, 2006).

EPIDEMIOLOGY

Epidemiological studies demonstrate a higher prevalence of 100–150/100,000 of the population in temperate regions, such as North America, Northern Europe and Australasia, than in tropical areas such as Africa. Generally speaking prevalence increases with distance from the equator. Scotland has levels as high as 1 in 500 (Zajicek *et al.*, 2007), while the rest of the UK has a prevalence of around 1 in 850 (Alonso *et al.*, 2007).

Migration can also influence the risk of developing MS. People who migrate before the age of fifteen from low to high prevalence countries acquire the same higher risk as the indigenous population. People who migrate after the age of 15 retain their original lower risk. The same occurs in reverse with acquisition of lower risk if migration is before 15 years from high to low (Paty and Ebers, 1998).

Presentation also varies between different ethnic populations and geographical regions (Miller *et al.*, 2003) with a greater frequency of relapsing-remitting MS (RRMS) in northern Europe. The overall incidence of MS is increasing, together with a sustained increase in prevalence of MS in women (MacLean and Freedman, 2009), although the reason for this increase is unclear.

The peak age for diagnosis is between the second and third decade, with diagnosis unusual after 55 years or before 15 years of age. While childhood MS is rare (Sevon *et al.*, 2000), approximately 5% of all MS patients experience onset of symptoms prior to the age of sixteen and most are diagnosed with RRMS (Tardieu and Mikaeloff, 2004).

AETIOLOGY

The aetiology of MS remains unknown, but it is thought to be an auto-immune mediated, inflammatory disease with the myelin sheath attacked by the body's own immune system. There is some evidence supporting this auto-immune aetiology (see Box 28.1). It is thought that an environmental agent affects genetically predisposed individuals at an early age, precipitating MS. The search continues to isolate the genetic markers, identify those who are predisposed to MS and determine the trigger that causes the disease. The role of infection as a trigger cannot be ruled out and there is some evidence to suggest that infection with Epstein–Barr virus (and cigarette smoking)

Neuroscience Nursing: Evidence-Based Practice, 1st Edition.
Edited by Sue Woodward and Ann-Marie Mestecky
© 2011 Blackwell Publishing Ltd

increases the risk of MS, whereas vitamin D may play a protective role (Munger and Ascherio, 2007).

PATHOPHYSIOLOGY

In genetically susceptible individuals a non-specific environmental trigger activates a dormant pool of auto-reactive T-lymphocytes resulting in an inflammatory cascade, with the oligodendrocyte cell misidentified as the target. The normally impermeable blood brain barrier (BBB) becomes 'leaky', allowing infiltration and attack by these auto-reactive T-cells with subsequent release of toxic inflammatory mediators. This results in myelin breakdown (Figure 28.1), axonal and glial injury, and conduction block. Relapses are the clinical expression of acute focal inflammation of the CNS, and progression is the likely consequence of diffuse neurodegeneration. Inflammatory events can also occur at a sub-clinical level without symptoms (Coles, 2003).

Box 28.1 Support for MS as an auto-immune condition

- Pathology studies have shown the influx of lymphocytes associated with demyelination around blood vessels, and compatible with autoimmunity
- Laboratory studies have induced an autoimmune inflammatory response that replicates MS
- Genetic studies have demonstrated associations with certain genetic types and in particular genes that are essential in the controlling immune responses

Source: Compston and Coles, 2002; Gold *et al.*, 2006.

Frequent relapse followed by repair, remyelination and restoration of conduction is a prominent feature of early MS. Each individual lesion will be at a different stage of inflammation, demyelination, remyelination and repair (Compston and Coles, 2002; Gold *et al.*, 2006).

Chronic inactive demyelinated plaques result in axonal loss, and repeated episodes result in overgrowth of astrocytes and scarring (Zajicek *et al.*, 2007). Permanent axonal loss is the most important factor in disability. There may also be complete or partial recovery from relapse, with likely accumulative disability over time. Debate continues surrounding the sequence of events and whether inflammation is secondary to programmed cell death, or the cause of cellular destruction, axonal degeneration and loss (Barnett and Prineas, 2004).

CLASSIFICATION/TYPES OF MS

The condition is classified by clinical course into four types (Figure 28.2).

- Relapsing remitting MS (RRMS)
- Secondary progressive MS (SPMS)
- Primary progressive MS (PPMS)
- Benign MS

The course of the disease for the majority of patients (85%) starts with RRMS (Thompson *et al.*, 2000). The first clinical episode is considered an inaugural event rather than a relapse. Some clinicians are now adopting the pragmatic approach of differentiating MS as either an active or inactive disease. Other terms used include 'malignant MS'; a rare, atypical and aggressive form of the disease usually affecting young adults and leading to early death (Burgess, 2002).

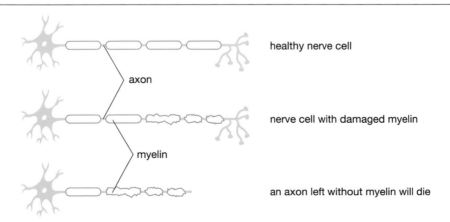

healthy nerve cell

axon

nerve cell with damaged myelin

myelin

an axon left without myelin will die

Figure 28.1 Demyelination. Reproduced with kind permission of the MS Trust.

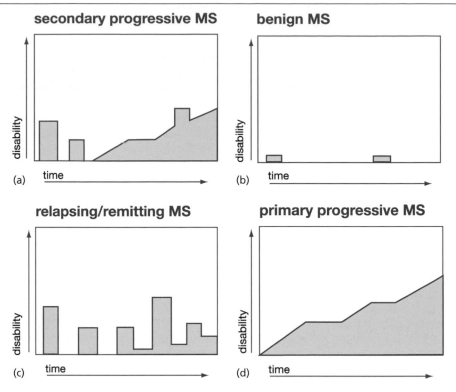

Figure 28.2 Progression of different types of MS. Reproduced with kind permission of the MS Trust.

Clinically isolated syndrome (CIS) defines a single clinical episode of demyelination in one specific location, so a diagnosis of MS is not made, but there is a risk that the patient may go on to develop MS. 60% of patients presenting initially with CIS will have lesions visible on MRI, with 20% of these developing MS in future years (Dalton *et al.*, 2002).

Relapsing-remitting MS

RRMS is typically diagnosed between the second and third decade after a sub-clinical course. Fifty per cent of this cohort will need to walk with the aid of a single stick after 10–15 years, and 75% will need help after 25 years (Thompson *et al.*, 2000), but it is important to remember that a quarter of patients will remain independently mobile all their life. The frequency of and interval between relapses is variable. The point at which a relapse will result in permanent axonal loss and disability is not completely understood or predictable, but up to 40% of relapses will leave permanent problems with accumulative impairment and disability (Lublin *et al.*, 2003).

Little is known about what initiates relapses or why some people have more frequent relapses. There is some

evidence of increased risk of relapse after systemic infection, with more systemic damage than spontaneous relapse (Polman *et al.*, 2006), and women are likely to relapse three months post-partum. Many patients diagnosed with RRMS will go on to develop SPMS, usually confirmed after a year or more of progressing disability, while others follow this remitting-relapsing course all of their lives.

Secondary progressive MS

SPMS is defined as progression of clinical disability (with or without relapses and minor fluctuations) after a relapsing-remitting onset, usually after ten years and not before three years from onset (Barnes, 2000). The system most affected earlier in the disease will be most affected at later stages. Visual dysfunction is likely to remain, but with significant reduction in acuity (McDonald and Compston, 2006). Symptoms become more chronic and can be superimposed with relapses.

Primary progressive MS

PPMS is diagnosed in about 10–15% of cases, often at an older age and with equal distribution amongst males and females (Bruck *et al.*, 2002). Patients typically present with greater spinal involvement, often more sparing of the cortex, but a more progressive disease from the outset. Less severe inflammatory processes are evident than in RRMS and SPMS, but progressive atrophy features highly with increasing loss of mobility. Three to five per cent of patients may also experience acute episodes superimposed on this progressive course (Tullman *et al.*, 2004).

Benign MS

Benign MS is characterised by mild, infrequent relapses (often affecting sensory functions) separated by long time intervals. It is thought to be a much slower form of RRMS (Sayao *et al.*, 2007) and the term is used to describe low levels of disease activity rather than the impact upon the individual.

CLINICAL SIGNS AND SYMPTOMS

The clinical course of MS evolves over time with progressing disability. Clinical signs and symptoms experienced may be primary, secondary or tertiary (see Box 28.2). Lesions produce a co-existence of sensory and motor symptoms, and include subtle, hidden problems of fatigue, pain, sexual dysfunction, cognitive, emotional and mood disorders. The onset of MS is often mono-symptomatic,

---

Box 28.2   Common signs and symptoms of MS

Primary symptoms
- Weakness
- Numbness
- Balance disturbance
- Visual problems
- Spasticity
- Fatigue
- Depression (? endogenous)

Secondary symptoms
- Depression (? reactive)
- Disuse weakness
- Bladder and bowel dysfunction
- Urinary infections
- Pressure sores
- Contractures
- Aspiration pneumonia

Tertiary symptoms
- Mood swings
- Social isolation
- Dependency

---

with evidence of a single CNS lesion in 45% of cases, although there may be symptoms indicating multiple lesions from onset (Compston and Coles, 2002). The frequency and severity of symptoms varies over time.

Optic tract lesions causing optic neuritis result in any or all of the following: blurring, dimming or 'fogginess of vision' with reduced visual acuity, dyschromatopsia (reduced colour perception) and painful eye movement. The long-term prognosis for visual function in patients with unilateral acute demyelinating optic neuritis is good; treatment with intravenous corticosteroids for the initial acute episode does not alter the long-term visual prognosis (Optic Neuritis Study Group, 2008).

Spinal cord lesions produce a range of symptoms that include limb weakness, bladder, bowel and sexual dysfunction. Spasticity, spasm, pain and sensory loss/ disturbance may also occur. Pain can be a frequent and disabling symptom for MS patients (Beiske *et al.*, 2008) and may be neuropathic or paroxysmal. Brain stem and cerebellar lesions may result in ataxia, tremor and loss of co-ordination, disturbance of ocular movement, intranuclear ophthalmoplegia, vertigo, dysarthria and dysphasia, trigeminal neuralgia, auditory disturbance (rare) and respiratory weakness (Ciccarelli and Toosy, 2006). Cerebral lesions produce a range of symptoms including hemisensory and motor symptoms and/or focal cortical deficits (rare) and cognitive impairment.

Debate continues regarding the nature and extent of cognitive dysfunction as a symptom of MS. Although about 50% of people with MS demonstrate cognitive deficits when formally evaluated, only 5–10% experience changes that significantly impact on daily living (Fischer *et al.*, 2000). Reported rates of depression range from 10% to 57% (Siegert and Abernethy, 2005). Depression is predominately affective and is the most common mental disorder in people with MS (Sadovnick *et al.*, 1996). Emotionalism or anxiety disorder may also occur (Bennett 2002).

DIAGNOSIS

MS remains a clinical diagnosis with no single diagnostic test able to confirm diagnosis, or sign or symptom specific to MS. A neurologist will combine accurate clinical history, neurological examination and assessment with application of diagnostic criteria to obtain a diagnosis. The standard criteria of two symptomatic episodes separated by time and space (Poser *et al.*, 1983) to confirm diagnosis are still used. Key diagnostic considerations are outlined in Box 28.3. Diagnostic tests (Table 28.1) are used to exclude other pathology/differential diagnoses and may be suggestive of a diagnosis of MS.

Table 28.1 Diagnostic tests and findings suggestive of MS.

Investigation	Findings in MS
Lumbar puncture (LP)	Oligoclonal bands present in CSF
Evoked potentials (VEP/AEP/SSEP) May be carried out if a patient is suspected to have PPMS or if differential diagnoses need to be excluded (Thompson *et al.*, 2000)	Delayed conduction velocity
PET scanning	Demonstrates potential relationship between cortical metabolic activity and sub-cortical lesions, but is used in limited centres (Bakshi, 2003)
MRI	Definite lesions in CNS on T2-weighted images

AEP – auditory evoked potentials; PET – positron emission tomography; PPMS – primary progressive MS; SSEP – somatosensory evoked potentials; VEP – visual evoked potentials.

Box 28.3   Key diagnostic considerations for MS

* Is the history compatible with MS?
* Are there multiple lesions in the CNS?
* Are the lesions demyelinating in nature?
* Is there an immunological abnormality in relation to the CNS?
* Are there alternative and more likely explanations?

Source: Miller *et al.*, 2006.

Magnetic resonance imaging (MRI)

MRI is probably the most common and useful diagnostic aid. Approximately 95% of patients with clinically definite MS have CNS lesions on T2 weighted brain MRI scans (Miller *et al.*, 2002). Normal brain MRI may be found in about 5% of people with mild, early onset MS

Box 28.4   Predictors of poor prognosis

* Older age; accumulation of disability may be age dependent (Confavreux *et al.*, 2003)
* Male
* High MRI lesion load (Rovaris *et al.*, 2003)
* Lack of recovery from first relapse
* High relapse rate (more than three per year) in the first five years
* Early cerebellar involvement
* Short intervals between relapses
* Early disability
* Insidious motor onset

(Palace, 2001). Two types of MR image may be taken (see Chapter 19). T1 weighted images provide better correlation between disability and 'black holes' of irretrievable axonal loss. T2 weighted images detect both new/active, and old lesions, showing mixed pathology and overall burden of disease. Gadolinium enhanced MRI identifies breaches in the BBB (signifying potential lesion evolution), significantly increasing the number of lesions detected in RRMS and SPMS (Koudriavtseva *et al.*, 1997).

Diagnostic criteria

The revised McDonald diagnostic criteria (Polman *et al.*, 2005) for clinically definite MS rely on MRI. Further criteria are set out for the diagnosis of primary progressive MS (Polman *et al.*, 2005). Patients may receive a diagnosis of clinically isolated syndrome (CIS) and subsequent risk of developing MS, or a confirmed diagnosis of not MS following investigation. The experience of the diagnostic process is central to subsequent adaptation (Wollin *et al.*, 2000).

STAGES OF MS

Life expectancy for people with MS is similar to the average population, with severe disability (as measured by the Expanded Disability Status Scale (EDSS) (Kurtzke, 1983) currently the highest risk factor for premature death (Pryse-Phillips and Costello, 2001). MS brings changing patterns of need and uncertainty about disability and impairment. Some potential early positive predictors include young onset, female, monoclonal optic neuritis as the first symptom, complete recovery of relapse versus gradual worsening of symptoms without recovery and sensory symptoms (Confavreux *et al.*, 2003). Negative predictors of poor outcomes with progressive and accumulative disability are identified in Box 28.4.

MEDICAL MANAGEMENT

The main therapeutic targets of treatment are to modulate or suppress the disease process, manage relapses appropriately and treat/alleviate symptoms.

Disease modifying therapies (DMTs)

Beta-interferons and copaxone

Interferon-beta 1a (Avonex, Rebif), interferon-beta 1b (Betaferon) and glatiramer acetate (Copaxone) are the three DMTs licensed in the UK. They have all been shown to positively impact on relapse rate, development of new MRI lesions and progression of disability (modest effect in some) in RRMS in large multi-centre randomised controlled trials (Burgess, 2005; Mutch, 2008). Patients with RRMS or SPMS are considered for treatment with DMTs, according to strict criteria, if they have had two or more significant relapses within two years (ABN, 2001).

DMTs all have a slightly different mode of action, but essentially work by reducing antibody/lymphocyte activity, reducing cytokine production and modifying the function of the immune system. Patients will be monitored by a neurologist with an interest in MS at least annually and under certain circumstances the DMTs may need to be stopped (Box 28.5). Patients receiving DMTs may experience side-effects including flu-like symptoms which ease over time, injection site reactions, muscle stiffness, insomnia, mood changes and alteration in menstrual patterns (Burgess, 2005).

Interferon-beta 1a and 1b are now licensed for treatment after a single clinical episode suggestive of MS. Interferon-beta may delay the time to second relapse in CIS. Patients with a single abnormal MRI scan at presentation may not have subsequent relapse in the early years. However, CIS patients developing MS according to the McDonald criteria at three months and at one year of follow up have a high (75–85%) probability of developing clinically definite MS within three years. It is recommended that treatment be initiated after the diagnosis of MS is made but only if this is within one year of the CIS and a high rate of further clinical relapses has been reported (ABN, 2007).

When DMTs were initially licensed in the UK there was significant controversy regarding their clinical and cost effectiveness, resulting in some patients not being able to receive the drugs due to differences in funding arrangements between geographical areas. Following extensive consultation and review via the National Institute of Health and Clinical Excellence (NICE) which resulted in a NICE recommendation not to fund DMTs through the NHS, the Department of Health developed a risk sharing scheme with the drug manufacturers to allow nominated prescribing centres throughout the UK to prescribe DMTs. Patients prescribed interferon-beta or Copaxone under the risk sharing scheme (DH, 2002) require annual review to monitor disease progression and the clinical and cost effectiveness of the treatment.

Natalizumab

When it was licensed in 2007, NICE Guidelines (2007) recommended the use of natalizumab (Tysabri) for rapidly evolving MS and active relapsing-remitting disease, characterised by two or more relapses a year. Tysabri is a recombinant monoclonal antibody against alpha 4 integrins. It acts by preventing the migration of immune cells across the blood brain barrier, which would result in inflammation and myelin destruction.

No DMT is effective for progressive disease, in the absence of relapses. Unfortunately the only treatment for PPMS or SPMS is symptomatic control.

Disease suppressing therapies

Immunosuppressants

Cochrane reviews of immuno-suppressants, mitoxantrone (Martinelli *et al.*, 2005) and azathioprine (Casetta *et al.*, 2007) suggest a role in the early inflammatory phase of the disease by inhibition of cell division and proliferation and suppression of white blood cells that induce the attack on the CNS. None are licensed specifically for the treatment of MS in the UK, but mitoxantrone is licensed in the US. Both must be prescribed following specific protocols and clinical guidelines (NICE, 2003). Mitoxantrone is a powerful immuno-suppressive agent, increasingly used to treat frequent, severe relapses, accumulative disability, non responders to interferon therapy, and to stabilise aggressive MS. Small clinical trials show benefits on dis-

---

Box 28.5   Indications for stopping disease modifying therapies (DMTs)

- Side-effects are intolerable or severe
- Two disabling relapses, defined by the examining neurologist, occur within a 12-month period
- Secondary progression with an increase in disability observable over 6 months
- Loss of ability to walk, with or without assistance, lasting for at least 6 months
- Pregnancy is planned (temporary cessation)

Source: Association of British Neurologists, 2007.

ability progression, MRI data and clinical exacerbations in RRMS and SPMS (Edan *et al.*, 1997; Millefiorini *et al.*, 1997; Hartung *et al.*, 2002).

Other therapies only occasionally used in MS include methotrexate, cyclophosphamide, cyclosporine, sulfasalazine and plasma exchange.

Intravenous immunoglobulin (IVIg)

IVIg is not used routinely in the treatment of MS, but may be prescribed for patients experiencing severe, frequent relapses for whom DMTs are contraindicated (ABN, 2005). A Cochrane review of two randomised trials using IVIg in patients with RRMS identified a reduction in relapse rate, but there was inadequate MRI and disability data to support a disease-modifying effect on the MS (Gray *et al.*, 2003).

Current trial therapies

Campath (alemtuzumab)

Campath is a humanised monoclonal antibody that acts by destroying T-cells that recognise myelin as foreign. It is licensed for use in B-cell chronic lymphocytic leukaemia and has been used in MS treatment since the 1980s. This treatment has beneficial effects in early aggressive MS on both MRI activity and relapse rate (Zajicek *et al.*, 2007). Side-effects include thrombocytopenia and other autoimmune conditions such as autoimmune renal disease.

Oral therapies

A number of oral therapies have completed, or are in final stages of clinical trial and undergoing licensing applications. They include fingolimod, cladribine and laquinimod (Kappos *et al.*, 2006).

Stem cells

Early trial results would suggest that high dose immunosuppression and stem cell transplantation may induce remission in aggressive RRMS and SPMS (Chandran *et al.*, 2007).

Complementary and alternative medicine (CAM)

People with MS are the most frequent users of CAM (Shinto *et al.*, 2006) as an adjunct to conventional western medicine and their use is acknowledged in the NICE Guidelines (NICE, 2003). Patients use CAM to attempt to impact on the course of the disease (e.g. dietary modification) or improve general health (e.g. yoga). Cannabis has been shown to provide effective pain relief and reduced spasticity (Rog *et al.*, 2005) and reflexology has been shown to improve bladder and bowel symptoms and reduce spasticity (Siev-Ner *et al.*, 2003) and improve quality of life (Mackereth *et al.*, 2009) in clinical trials.

Patients will also access a range of treatments, including hyperbaric oxygen, goat serum, bee venom, low dose naltrexone and unregulated stem cell transplants with little supportive evidence. Anecdotal evidence is plentiful for CAM, but there is little scientific research. Bowling (2000) provides a comprehensive and objective overview of CAM and MS.

NURSING MANAGEMENT IN THE DIAGNOSTIC PHASE

Self care and wellness

Traditional health care systems are inadequate for meeting all the needs of patients with long term conditions (DH, 2005a) and encourage dependency within that system (Nodhturft *et al.*, 2000). Early investment in self-care/management with positive health behaviours leads to better outcomes and improves quality of life (Lorig and Holman, 2003; Asra Warsi *et al.*, 2004). The terms self-care and self-management are used interchangeably, acknowledging that the patients' central role in self-management (DH, 2004; DH, 2005a; DH, 2005b) positively affects their ability to take control of, and manage their chronic illness (Donaldson 2001, Lorig and Holman, 2003). Self-management in MS requires knowledge, skills and understanding and encompasses a variety of activities (Box 28.6).

The concept of 'wellness' is promoted early in MS and patients are discouraged from perceiving themselves as ill (Burgess, 2002). Isolation, unpredictability, loss associ-

---

Box 28.6 Self-management activities

- Manage physical symptoms (self-efficacy)
- Adopt a healthy lifestyle
- Adhere to planned treatment
- Monitor the emotional and social impact of MS
- Problem solving/ planning/ taking action/ decision-making
- Utilise supportive resources
- Develop effective partnerships and joint decision-making with practitioners
- Self-monitor and interact with health care professionals
- Develop confidence and motivation to use own skills, information and professional services to 'take control' effectively

ated with functional limitations and unique experience of symptoms felt, together with levels of personal resilience, adaptability and social support, may have a profound impact on people's psychological and social functioning (McReynolds *et al.*, 1999).

Following a diagnosis of MS or CIS patients may envisage a future that assumes a life of accumulative disability and dependency upon a wheelchair. The unpredictability of MS can heighten anxiety and stress. Evidence suggests that stress exacerbates symptoms, increases risk of depression and reduces investment in self (Mohr *et al.*, 2000; Esposito *et al.*, 2001). Potential stressors may include fear of potential disability, risks to working role or relationships, lack of knowledge from 'experts' regarding the cause, lack of significantly effective treatments, and fear of isolation.

Timely and appropriate information, with repetition and clarification as necessary, mindful of anxieties, cognitive ability and sensitive to immediate need should be given within four weeks of diagnosis. This must be supported by practical contacts, support opportunities and creditable, relevant written or internet information which can be accessed at a time of personal choice. Early referral to a MS specialist nurse is essential.

MS specialist nurses may provide education programmes or 'courses' for newly diagnosed patients, often in collaboration with the voluntary sector. Newly diagnosed patients should be encouraged to understand their condition, recognising and avoiding triggers that exacerbate symptoms (Box 28.7). Patients with MS may also benefit from participating in an Expert Patient Programme (DH, 2001). Measurable improvements in patient outcomes through self-management programmes have been acknowledged extensively (DH, 2001).

Symptom management

Sensory disturbance is the presenting feature in 30–50% of cases (Zajicek *et al.*, 2007) with optic neuritis the most common visual problem. Blurring of vision, reduced colour vision, pain and photophobia or flashes of light may occur in the affected eye(s). High dose steroids are effective, but some patients may develop permanent visual loss.

Patients may describe burning, itching, crawling, heaviness, prickling, tingling, numbness, pins and needles, pressure, and hot and cold sensations. Sensations of chest tightness and pain (MS hug) are common due to spasm occurring within the intercostal muscles. Neck flexion/extension can provoke a sensation of electric shock down the spine and into limbs. The nurse must explain the mechanisms involved, assess daily activities for trigger factors and discuss useful medications such as anti-convulsants and anti-depressants that may help to alleviate these neuropathic symptoms (see Chapter 17).

Fatigue may be reported at onset and as an ongoing problem. The pathophysiology of fatigue is not understood, but patients report an overwhelming tiredness, and energy loss characterised by either focal muscle fatigability or a generalised sense of lassitude with a severity unlike the tiredness felt by healthy adults. Symptoms may include cognitive fatigue. Fatigue is one of the most disabling MS symptoms, significantly impacting on quality of life (QOL) and the most likely factor affecting ability to work. Onset can be rapid, associated with relapse and accompanied by other neurological symptoms, but fatigue may also be a chronic and fluctuating symptom.

Fatigue may be helped by amantadine (Symmetrel) 100 mg initially once daily increasing to twice daily (not after 2 pm). Modafinil (Provigil) 200–400 mg daily, may be helpful in treating excessive sleepiness in chronic conditions, but is used with caution and produces side-effects similar to MS symptoms through CNS stimulation. Nursing management of fatigue and other symptoms is discussed later in this chapter.

NURSING MANAGEMENT IN RELAPSE AND ACUTE EPISODE PHASE

Relapse management

Significant and common relapses include episodes of optic neuritis, transverse myelitis and brain stem events. A relapse is defined as an episode of neurological deterioration (in the absence of pyrexia) lasting more than 24 hours and attributable to the CNS (Leary *et al.*, 2005). It is now recognised that people with MS can have inflammation without clinical signs, or may experience deterioration with little to find in the neurological examination. Pseudo-relapses are a temporary worsening of existing symptoms, often from infection, illness or stress, and treatment of the trigger will resolve the symptoms without recourse to steroids. All patients should be screened for infection prior to commencing steroids. The patient is the expert in

---

Box 28.7   Triggers that exacerbate MS symptoms

- Heat and humidity
- Infection and general poor health
- Stress and anxiety
- Sleep deprivation and exhaustion

judging the significance of his/her relapse and specialist rapid access clinics provide assessment and treatment of early relapse.

Keeping the individual at the centre of shared decision-making during relapse will empower them at a time of further loss, uncertainty, chronic sorrow and repeated grieving. During relapse, altered mobility and sensation, mood, cognition, and steroid therapy can exacerbate existing problems such as urinary frequency and urgency, with episodes of incontinence for an individual who would maintain full control when well. The shock of diagnosis may reoccur with each relapse and psychological support at this stage is vital.

Steroid administration

Onset, duration and recovery of relapse are variable with each individual episode but evidence supports the use of high dose steroid therapy to hasten recovery of relapse without influencing long-term outcomes (Filippini *et al.*, 2002). Oral methylprednisolone 500 mg per day for five days or 1 gram IV per day for three days may be prescribed with Omeprazole 20 mg cover for previous history of gastric irritation or ulcer. Both may be administered at home if the patient's condition permits. A systematic review of oral versus intravenous steroids is underway to determine most effective treatment method (Burton *et al.*, 2008).

Patients must be fully informed, with realistic expectation about the role of steroids, mode of action and side-effects, which may include metallic taste, transient hyperglycemia, ankle oedema, urinary frequency, facial flushing, sleep disturbance, restlessness, mood change, mild euphoria and rarely, psychosis and avascular necrosis. Repeated steroid treatment is to be avoided.

Multidisciplinary care

A timely, multidisciplinary specialist neurological rehabilitation programme facilitates optimum functional recovery during and after relapse (NICE, 2003). Assessment of fitness and mobility with tailored exercise programmes to improve core stability, balance and positioning must be considered. Functional electric stimulation (FES) for drop foot of central neurological origin stimulates muscle contractions that mimic normal voluntary gait by applying electrical impulses to the common peroneal nerve (see Chapter 11). Orthotic splinting can maintain the patient's limbs in a correct functional position and minimise risk of drop foot as a secondary complication of prolonged poor positioning (NICE, 2009).

Home equipment and adaptation, aids to living, extended fatigue management and social and vocational advice/

support must be provided after relapse and reviewed at regular intervals. Rehabilitation and ongoing review is key to successful MS management and addresses the fluctuating, progressive nature of the condition.

NURSING MANAGEMENT IN PROGRESSIVE PHASE

In the progressive phase of the disease multiple symptoms (Box 28.8) can occur either independently, as co-dependents of each other, or as the sequelae of treatment. Multidisciplinary team working facilitates good symptom management and supports a positive response to life changes and adaptation necessitated by disease progression.

Pain

Prevalence of pain varies, but is experienced by up to 80% of patients at some stage of the disease (Khan and Pallant, 2007; Pöllmann and Feneberg, 2008). Patients commonly experience acute pain syndrome early in the disease trajectory and chronic pain in later stages, although acute pain can appear at any stage affecting 10% of MS patients (van den Noort and Holland, 1999). Acute paroxysmal pain such as trigeminal neuralgia results from abnormal axonal conduction. Sub-acute pain lasting days or weeks, such as in optic neuritis, is caused by demyelination. Chronic neuropathic pain may be directly related to the demyelination of sensory pathways in spino-thalamic tracts and posterior columns. Chronic musculoskeletal (somatic) pain, such as backache and painful leg spasms results from MS related symptoms rather than MS itself. Detailed pain assessment and treatment planning must be undertaken (see Chapter 17).

Fatigue

Primary fatigue is a lassitude of overwhelming tiredness unrelated to activity and is often at its worst during mid-afternoon when core body temperature is at its highest. Increased symptoms, including visual disturbance, persist

---

Box 28.8 Symptoms during progressive phase

- Pain
- Fatigue
- Bladder and bowel dysfunction
- Tremor
- Speech and swallowing difficulties
- Mobility difficulties
- Spasticity and spasm

until core body temperature returns to normal. Heat intolerance may sometimes be reported at onset, but more frequently later in the disease. Secondary fatigue as a common feature of chronic conditions and occurs for several reasons: reduced function and de-conditioning, increased effort to sustain activity, sleep disturbance, depression, poor general health and medication.

Assessment must include the nature, onset and duration of the fatigue, any contributing factors, the patient's previous/current activity and exercise levels, heat and environment, daily lifestyle, psychosocial issues and pain. The patient's understanding, strategies and coping behaviours, together with the impact of fatigue on other MS-related symptoms must also be assessed. Drug therapies that can exacerbate fatigue, such as anti-depressants, anti-spasmodics, night sedation and analgesics require review. Many factors are independent predictors of increased fatigue including mood and not working (Johansson *et al.*, 2008).

Energy-conservation strategies such as afternoon rest, pre-prepared meals, cooling showers in hot weather and pacing activities, together with adaptations to the home/work environment are among a number of self-management strategies (Box 28.9) that can reduce the impact of fatigue (Burgess, 2002). Body temperature should be controlled using cooling devices, air conditioning and avoiding temperature extremes. Factors that disturb sleep must be identified and appropriate interventions initiated. Clinical depression should be treated with a non-sedating anti-depressant. Positive lifestyle behaviours including aerobic exercise, and participation in fatigue programmes improve quality of life (Ennis *et al.*, 2006).

Box 28.9   Self-help strategies to manage fatigue

- Pace and spread activities over the day/week
- Prioritise and delegate appropriate activities
- Sit whenever possible
- Avoid hot baths and saunas
- Use home delivery/online shopping whenever practical
- Build quality time for self and family into daily routine
- Obtain a disabled badge
- Ensure some exercise is built into daily routine
- Use appropriate aids and adaptations
- Ask for help if needed

Adapted from Burgess, 2002.

Bladder dysfunction

Bladder dysfunction, although rare at onset, may present in acute relapse and is common later with 75–95% of patients with MS experiencing this symptom during the course of their disease (Nortvedt *et al.*, 2001, 2007). Two common types of bladder dysfunction are associated with MS. Failure to store urine is caused by uncontrollable bladder contractions (overactive bladder) and results in frequency, urgency and urge urinary incontinence. Failure to empty is caused by either atonic bladder, detrusor hyperreflexia with poorly sustained contractions, or detrusor–sphincter dyssynergia (lack of coordination of detrusor and external sphincter muscles); it results in retention, overflow incontinence, and frequent urinary tract infections with a characteristic post-void residual volume of urine of 100 ml or more. Some patients experience a combination of failure to store and failure to empty.

Bladder dysfunction can also be compounded by other contributory factors including concurrent medical conditions (e.g. urinary tract infection), medications, reduced mobility, poor cognition, reduced dexterity, spasticity, ataxia and/or tremor, nutrition and low fluid/high caffeine intake, and lifestyle issues. Detailed assessment is vital and both assessment and management are discussed further in Chapter 18. Consensus guidelines have recently been produced (Fowler *et al.*, 2009), which outline a simple algorithm for bladder management following urinalysis and assessment of post-void residual urine measurement. Antimuscarinic drugs may be indicated for overactive bladder symptoms, but if the patient's residual urine measurement exceeds 100 ml they should be taught clean intermittent self-catheterisation (Fowler *et al.*, 2009).

Bowel dysfunction

The neuro-pathophysiology of bowel dysfunction in MS is unclear. It is common in later MS with prevalence around 43–70% and is associated with disease duration. Patients may experience either constipation or faecal incontinence. Constipation occurs in approximately 50% of patients (DasGupta and Fowler, 2003) and contributory factors include medication, weakened abdominal muscles, spasticity, diet, and immobility. Faecal incontinence occurs weekly in approximately 25% of patients and less than monthly in approximately 51%. Contributory factors include constipation, causing rectal distension and overflow, diminished rectal sensation, sphincter dysfunction, medications and diet (van den Noort and Holland, 1999).

Assessment of patients' bowel dysfunction commences at diagnosis and continues throughout the patient's journey. Assessment and management of bowel dysfunction is detailed in Chapter 18. Referral to continence advisory services may be required.

Sexual dysfunction

The aetiology of sexual dysfunction in MS not understood, but problems appear more complex in women. A correlation between pontine atrophy and sexual dysfunction has been identified, and disease course, duration, disability, age and education factors are influential in the dysfunction experienced (Ward, 2005). Problems will include erectile dysfunction in men and altered genital sensation, lack of lubrication and loss of libido in women. There is a commonly held misconception that people with a disability do not engage in sexual activity or have sexual needs (Ward, 2005) and nurses are often reluctant to discuss such issues with patients, perceiving discussion to be too 'intrusive' or worrying that they will not be able to help. However patients often welcome the opportunity to discuss these issues, but may be too embarrassed to broach the subject.

Nursing assessment must be one of sensitive enquiry (Demirkiran *et al.*, 2006), but at the same time be structured. Minimally patients should be asked if their MS has affected their relationship. There are structured models of assessment for sexual dysfunction available to facilitate the assessment process and the Multiple Sclerosis Intimacy and Sexuality Questionnaire-19 (Sorgen-Sanders *et al.*, 2000) has been developed specifically for the assessment of people with MS.

Ward (2005) has discussed management of sexual dysfunction in women with MS in detail, but simple suggestions include using warmed water-soluble vaginal lubricant (K-Y jelly), use of a vibrator or other methods, such as oral sex, to increase clitoral stimulation and the likelihood of orgasm and watching adult movies to increase libido.

Tremor

Tremor (see Chapter 11) is described as one of the most disabling symptoms; even mild tremor makes simple tasks difficult to perform. Intention/action tremor associated with voluntary movement is the most common type of tremor seen in MS. Tremor amplitude increases as the patient reaches nearer to the target (e.g., when reaching for a cup) and is observed in finger-nose pointing using the index finger. The finger, as it approaches the target, becomes less coordinated. Postural tremor occurs whilst voluntarily sustaining a position with outstretched arms against gravity, or when the legs are crossed. It is common in MS, symptomatic of cerebellar dysfunction and includes titubation (swaying) of the head and neck. Maintaining an upright posture and specialised seating with good support

for the back and trunk and arm rests at an appropriate height can help. Patients will also require referral to physiotherapy and occupational therapy for help with managing this symptom.

Communication and swallowing

Communication disorders are more common than previously thought and affect between 40 and 50% of patients (Marchese-Ragona *et al.*, 2006). Brain stem lesions cause moderate to severe changes to normal speech patterns, such as dysarthria or dysphonia, and dysphagia, which may relapse and remit, increasing with disease progression.

Assessment is made to determine onset, duration, severity of problems, dysphagia symptoms, chewing difficulties and contributing factors such as fatigue, emotional upset, cognitive changes, and coexisting conditions. The impact of dysphagia on other aspects of health such as weight loss, malnutrition, dehydration, respiratory compromise, and sleep disturbances, changes in social and recreational activities must also be identified. Management of communication and swallowing problems is discussed in Chapter 12.

Mobility

Spasticity, tremor, ataxia, weakness, loss of balance, vertigo, pain, sensory or visual disturbance, and fatigue may all affect mobility. 50% of patients have difficulty with mobility within 15 years of diagnosis, requiring a walking aid or wheelchair (Zajicek *et al.*, 2007). The nature, onset and severity of the mobility problem must be assessed. Loss of balance, falling or inability to transfer or walk may be problematic and other factors contributing to altered mobility, such as environmental barriers, must also be identified.

Slow insidious worsening of motor function, permanent spasticity and spasms with progressive disability may leave the patient wheelchair dependent and at risk of secondary and tertiary complications. Formal assessment of the severity of altered mobility in MS is usually made with a timed walk (100metres) and the EDSS (Kurtzke, 1983). Multi-disciplinary rehabilitation with patient identified outcomes and shared goals is detailed in Box 28.10.

Spasticity

Spasticity is common in MS, due to damage to the upper motor neurones, accompanied by lower limb weakness, and either spasmodic or persistent stiffness (van den Noort and Holland, 1999). Spasticity may be exacerbated by numerous factors (Box 28.11). Assessment must consider

---

Box 28.10   Managing mobility problems

- Anti-spasticity drugs (see Chapter 11) with careful monitoring for side-effects and further weakness
- Gait assessment and retraining to avoid poor posture
- Provision of mobility aids to enable independent, safe mobility
- Stretching and strengthening exercises, balance training and relaxation exercises
- Energy-conservation training
- Environmental accessibility and adaptive equipment
- Wheelchair and seating services
- Prevention of pressure sores

Box 28.11   Factors that exacerbate spasticity in MS

- Temperature changes
- Infection
- Anxiety/stress
- Constipation
- Pain
- Immobility
- Disruption of skin integrity

---

causative or aggravating factors, onset, location and frequency, as well as the impact of spasticity on the patient.

Spasticity will restrict the patient's mobility, cause pain and risk secondary complications such as pressure sores. It could affect the individual's confidence to go out and impact on many activities of living. Treatment incorporating passive stretching of the affected joints alongside treatment of causative, aggravating factors such as pain and infection, may effectively manage mild spasticity. Physiotherapy can optimise posture and movement by focusing on strengthening exercises, stretching and balance, standing and weight-bearing. The maintenance of good functional positions can also be achieved by splinting limbs or through special or customised seating and by preventing factors that worsen spasticity and spasms (see Chapter 11). Severe spasticity requires treatment with muscle relaxants such as Baclofen, Tizanidine, dantrolene or gabapentin. Low and slow titration avoids side-effects such as weakness and drowsiness. Intrathecal baclofen pumps may be used for those who cannot tolerate oral baclofen (Jarrett *et al.*, 2002).

Intramuscular botulinum toxin may be considered for localised hypertonia or spasticity unresponsive to other treatments. Phenol injections may be given to motor points. All options must be aligned to neurophysiotherapy. Other medication may include clonazepam or diazepam which is effective at night, supporting sleep and reducing painful spasm. Further nursing management is discussed in Chapter 11.

NURSING MANAGEMENT FOR PEOPLE WITH ADVANCED MS

Many symptoms experienced by patients in the advanced stages of MS, including pain, spasms, fatigue, constipation or swallowing dysfunction have commonalities with cancer (Higginson *et al.*, 2006). Palliative care principles of a comprehensive multi-disciplinary team approach, symptom control, psychological and spiritual care are therefore applicable to people with MS. Death is often from secondary complications such as aspiration pneumonia, pulmonary embolism and opportunistic infections.

MS confronts all those involved in patient care with many challenges. Sensitive discussion about end of life care is a complex, demanding and important role. Innovative palliative care programmes can provide best practice, not only in MS but also in other long-term conditions (Embrey, 2008) and specialist palliative care services are developing expertise in managing progressive, advanced, neurological disease (NCPC, 2007).

Palliative care is a term often translated to mean 'terminal care' by patients (Burgess, 2002). Discussion about palliative and end of life care is initiated when the patient is receptive to this approach, not just when end of life may be near. Cognitive decline has implications for patients' capacity to consent and make treatment choices, and capacity regarding decision making must be assessed according to the mental capacity act (see Chapter 36).

Advance decisions may facilitate control over end of life care for the patient. Interventions will need sensitive, timely patient-led discussion in advanced MS and may include supra-pubic catheterisation, PEG feeding, use of baclofen pumps, antibiotics for recurring infections, and assisted ventilation and cardio-pulmonary resuscitation (UKMSSNA, 2006). Patients and their families require timely and appropriate information that supports the ability to discriminate between interventions that improve quality of life, and those that prolong life. Disease activity, lesion load and location, brain atrophy, emotional lability, side-effects to medications, reaction to increasing loss and disability can result in worsening mental health in advanced MS and suicide rates are high (Zajicek *et al.*,

2007). Depression, social isolation and distressing symptoms must be addressed to facilitate advance decision making.

ROLE OF THE MS SPECIALIST NURSE (MSSN)

The role of the MSSN is to act as clinical expert, educator and consultant in the management of care from pre-diagnosis through to end of life. Together with direct clinical care, the MSSN will provide evidence-based information and advice to any health and social care professional who is involved in patient care. The options available for people with MS are growing apace. No longer is it the case of 'diagnose and adios'; active management and the expectation to live well with MS is the philosophy of modern MS nursing care. Competencies for MSSN and other health professionals undertaking MS specialist roles have been developed (MS Trust *et al.*, 2009).

SUMMARY

Care of patients with MS requires the nurse to deal systematically with complex and often unpredictable problems. Patterns of disease are variable and each patient experiences a unique combination of symptoms at different rates. The nurse should acknowledge that the patient is the expert regarding their own disease and is often more informed and knowledgeable than many of those involved in their care. Detailed nursing management and guidance for MSSNs has been collated in the *UKMSSNA Clinical Management Manual* (2006), to which the reader is referred for further information.

Multiple sclerosis: patient perspective

'I'm sorry, but you have MS'. These few words, said to me, originally meant nothing. Then you start to think 'am I dying, will I be able to walk, can I continue with my job, is there a cure, there must be a cure surely in this day and age, isn't there?'

I was originally taken ill back in '95, where I was sent to hospital after losing the use of my arm; I spilt coffee down myself, having to go to sleep straight afterwards, and I woke up with a belting headache. Various tests were done with no conclusion.

In 2008, I had similar symptoms, and my GP sent me straight to the accident unit, as she thought I was having a stroke. So I had all the tests, MRI scans, lumber puncture, EFI tests etc. And this time they did conclude that I have MS.

What a difference this time. Emotions like fear, anger, depression, hate, why me, and others all came to mind. After leaving hospital, not having read all the documentation they provided, I got straight onto the internet reading things like miracle cures, all the things I should have done, like working in sunlight, moved closer to the equator, eaten blueberries, and fresh fish everyday, and all sorts of miraculous wizardry.

So now, I do things differently; a daily yoga routine, go on longer walks, play more golf (badly though I have to say), eat more fish, salads, vegetables, watch my weight. You know, the things that everyone should be doing.

I still have my 'down days' which I can put down to fatigue, memory wipe outs, being clumsy, balance problems, and little mishaps (on the bladder front) but at least I know what is causing them and I can deal with them.

The phrase 'USE IT OR LOOSE IT', was said to me at one of my yoga sessions. And it is very apt. I could sit around all day watching day time TV, doing very little, and that I think will guarantee that I will be in my wheelchair before I am fifty.

But my aim in life is not get to that stage.

So how am I now? It varies, and tomorrow I may have written this very differently. I have other challenges like I lost my job in March this year, not down to MS, but to the credit crunch (now that's a different story), but finding a new job isn't easy. (Maybe that is down to my MS, but who knows?)

A new emotion is more prevalent: Hope, that some day someone will find a cure, or at least a way to stop relapses, or if not limit them. There are some promising things going on with stem cell research, I just Hope that they can be in my life time.

REFERENCES

Alonso A, Jick SS, Olek Mj, *et al.* (2007) Incidence of multiple sclerosis in the United Kingdom. *Journal of Neurology* 254:1736–1741.

Asra Warsi BA, Wang PS, LaValley MP *et al.* (2004) Self-management education programs in chronic disease: a systematic review and methodological critique of the literature. *Archives International Medicine* 164:1641–1649.

Association of British Neurologists (2001) *Guidelines for the Use of Beta-interferon Glatiramer Acetate*. London: ABN.

Association of British Neurologists (2005) *Intravenous Immunoglobin in Neurological Diseases*. London: ABN.

Association of British Neurologists (2007) *Guidelines for Treatment of Multiple Sclerosis with Beta-interferon and Glatiramer Acetate*. London: ABN.

Bakshi R (2003) Fatigue associated with multiple sclerosis: diagnosis, impact and management. *Multiple Sclerosis* 9(3):219–227.

Barnes D (2000) *MS: Questions and Answers*. Weybridge: Merit Publishing International.

Barnett MH, Prineas JW (2004) Relapsing and remitting multiple sclerosis: pathology of the newlt forming lesion. *Annals of Neurology* 55:458–468.

Beiske AG, Pedersen ED, Czujko B *et al.* (2008) Pain and sensory complaints in multiple sclerosis. *European Journal of Neurology* 11(7):479–482.

Bennett F (2002) Psychosocial issues and interventions. In: Fraser RT, Clemmons DC and Bennett F (eds) *MS: Psychosocial and Vocation Interventions*. New York: Demos Medical Publishing.

Bowling AC (2000) *Alternative Medicine and Multiple Sclerosis*. New York: Demos Medical Publishing.

Bruck W, Lucchinetti C, Lassmann H (2002) The pathology of PPMS. *Multiple Sclerosis* 8:93–97.

Burgess M (2002) *Multiple Sclerosis: Theory and practice for nurses*. London: Whurr Publishers.

Burgess M (2005) The use of interferon beta-1b in multiple sclerosis and the MS nurse's role. *British Journal of Neuroscience Nursing* 1(3):132–138.

Burton JM, O'Connor PW, Hohol M *et al.* (2008) Oral versus intravenous steroids for treatment of relapses in multiple sclerosis. *Cochrane Database of Systematic Reviews* Issue 4 DOI: 10.1002/14651858.CD006921.

Casetta I, Iuliano G, Filippini G (2007) Azathioprine for multiple sclerosis. *Cochrane Database of Systematic Reviews* Issue 4. Art. No.: CD003982. DOI: 10.1002/14651858. CD003982.

Chandran S, Hunt D, Joannides A *et al.* (2007) Myelin repair: the role of stem and precursor cells in multiple sclerosis. *Philosophical Transactions Royal Society of Biological Sciences* 363:171–183.

Ciccarelli O, Toosy AT (2006) Mechanisms of disability and potential recovery in multiple sclerosis In: Thompson A (ed). *Neurological Rehabilitation of Multiple Sclerosis*. Abingdon: Informa Healthcare.

Coles A (2003) The immunology of multiple sclerosis. *Way Ahead* 7(2):4–5.

Compston A, Coles A (2002) Multiple sclerosis. *Lancet* 359:1221–1231.

Confavreux C, Vukusic S, Adeleine P (2003) Early clinical predictors and progression of irreversible disability in multiple sclerosis: an amnesic process. *Brain* 126(4):770–782.

Dalton CM, Brex PA, Miszkiel KA *et al.* (2002) Application of the new McDonald criteria to patients with clinically isolated syndromes suggestive of multiple sclerosis. *Annals of Neurology* 52:47–53.

DasGupta R, Fowler CJ (2003) Bladder, bowel and sexual dysfunction in multiple sclerosis: management strategies. *Drugs* 63(2):155–166.

Demirkiran M, Sarica Y, Uguz S *et al.* (2006) Multiple sclerosis patients with and without sexual dysfunction: are there any differences? *Multiple Sclerosis* 12(2):209–214.

Department of Health (2001) *The Expert Patient: a new approach to chronic disease management for the 21st Century*. London: DH.

Department of Health (2002) *Health Service Circular 2002/2004 Cost Effective Provision of Disease Modifying Therapies for People with Multiple Sclerosis*. London: DH.

Department of Health (2004) *Chronic Disease Management: A compendium of information*. London: DH.

Department of Health (2005a) *Supporting People with Long Term Conditions: An NHS and social care model to support local innovation and integration*. London: DH.

Department of Health (2005b) *Improving Care Improving Lives: Self-care – a real choice*. London: DH.

Donaldson L (2001) *The Expert Patient – a new approach to chronic disease management for the 21st Century*. London: DH.

Edan G, Miller D, Clanet M *et al.* (1997) Therapeutic effect of mitoxantrone combined with methylprednisolone in MS: a randomized multicentre study of active disease using MRI and clinical criteria. *Journal of Neurology, Neurosurgery and Psychiatry* 62:112–118.

Embrey N (2008) Exploring the lived experience of palliative care for people with MS 1: A literature review. *British Journal of Neuroscience Nursing* 4(11):9–16.

Ennis M, Thain J, Boggild M *et al.* (2006) A randomised controlled trial of a health promotion education programme for people with multiple sclerosis. *Clinical Rehabilitation* 20(9):783–792.

Esposito P, Gheorghe D, Kandere K *et al.* (2001) Acute stress increases permeability of the blood brain barrier through activation of brain mast cells. *Brain Research* 888:117–127.

Filippini G, Brusaferri F, Sibley WA *et al.* (2002) Corticosteroids or ACTH for acute exacerbations in multiple sclerosis. *Cochrane Database of Systematic Reviews* Issue 4. Art. No.: CD001331. DOI: 10.1002/14651858. CD001331.

Fischer JS, Priore RL, Jacobs LD *et al.* (2000) Neuropsychological effects of interferon beta-1a in relapsing multiple sclerosis. *Annals of Neurology* 48(6):885–892.

Fowler CJ, Panicker JN, Drake M *et al.* (2009) A UK consensus on the management of the bladder in MS. *Journal of Neurology, Neurosurgery and Psychiatry* 80(5):470–477.

Gold R, Linington C, Lassmann H (2006) Understanding pathogenesis and therapy of multiple sclerosis via animal models: 70 years of merits and culprits in experimental autoimmune encephalomyelitis research. *Brain* 129(8): 1953–1971.

Gray O, McDonnell GV, Forbes RB (2003) Intravenous immunoglobulins for multiple sclerosis. *Cochrane Database of Systematic Reviews* 2003, Issue 3. Art. No.: CD002936. DOI: 10.1002/14651858.CD002936.

Hartung HP, Gonsette R, Konig N *et al.* (2002) Mitoxantrone in progressive MS: a placebo controlled double-blind randomised multicentre trial. *Lancet* 364:1149–1156.

Higginson IJ, Hart S, Silber E *et al.* (2006) Symptom prevalence and severity in people severely affected by multiple sclerosis. *Journal of Palliative Care* 22:158–165.

Jarrett L, Nandi P, Thompson A (2002) Managing lower limb spasticity in multiple sclerosis: does intrathecal baclofen have a role? *Journal of Neurology Neurosurgery and Neuropsychiatry* 73(6):705–709.

Johansson S, Ytterberg C, Hillert J *et al.* (2008) A longitudinal study of variations in and predictors of fatigue in multiple sclerosis. *Journal of Neurology Neurosurgery and Psychiatry* 79:454–457.

Kappos J, Antel J, Comi G *et al.* (2006) Oral fingolimod (FTY720) for relapsing multiple sclerosis. *New England Journal Medicine* 355:1124–1140.

Khan F, Pallant J (2007) Chronic pain in multiple sclerosis: prevalence, characteristics, and impact on quality of life in an Australian community cohort. *Journal of Pain* 8(8):614–623.

Kobelt G (2006) Health economic issues in MS. *International MS Journal* 13:16–26.

Koudriavtseva T, Thompson AJ, Fiorelli M *et al.* (1997) Gadolinium enhanced MRI predicts clinical and MRI disease activity in RRMS. *Journal Neurology Neurosurgery and Psychiatry* 62:285–287.

Kurtzke JF (1983) Rating neurological impairment in multiple sclerosis; an expanded disability status scale. *Neurology* 33:1444.

Leary SM, Porter B, Thompson AJ (2005) Multiple sclerosis: diagnosis and the management of acute relapses. *Postgraduate Medical Journal* 81:302–308.

Lorig K, Holman H (2003) Self-management education, history, definition, outcome mechanisms. *Annals of Behaviour Medicine* 26(1):1–7.

Lublin FD, Baier M, Cutter G (2003) Effect of relapses on development of residual deficit in multiple sclerosis. *Neurology* 61:1528–1532.

Mackereth PA, Booth K, Hillier VF *et al.* (2009) Reflexology and progressive muscle relaxation training for people with multiple sclerosis: A crossover trial. *Complementary Therapies in Clinical Practice* 15(1):14–21.

MacLean HJ, Freedman MS (2009) Multiple sclerosis: following clues from cause to cure. *The Lancet Neurology* 8:6–8.

MacLurg K, Hawkins S, Evason E *et al.* (2005) A primary care-based needs assessment of people with multiple sclerosis. *British Journal of General Practice* 55(514):378–383.

Marchese-Ragona R, Restivo DA, Marioni G *et al.* (2006) Evaluation of swallowing disorders in multiple sclerosis. *Neurological Sciences* 4:335–337.

Martinelli I, Boneschi F, Rovaris M, Capra R, Comi GT (2005) Mitoxantrone for multiple sclerosis. *The Cochrane Database of Systematic Reviews* Issue 4. Art. No.: CD002127. DOI: 10.1002/14651858.CD002127.pub2.

McDonald I, Compston A (2006) The signs and symptoms of MS. In: Compston A, Confavreux C, Lassman H (eds). *McAlpine's MS.* (4th edition). Philadelphia: Churchill Livingstone.

McReynolds L, Koch C, Rumrill PD (1999) Psychosocial adjustment to multiple sclerosis: implications for rehabilitation professionals. *Journal of Vocational Rehabilitation* 12(2):83–91.

Millefiorini E, Gasperini C, Pozzilli C (1997) Randomised pleacebo controlled trial of mitoxantrone in RRMS; 24 month clinical and MRI outcome. *Journal of Neurology* 244:153–159.

Miller A, Johnson KP, Lublin F *et al.* (2002) *MRI in the Management of MS.* Beechwood, Ohio: Current Therapeutics, Inc.

Miller AE, Lublin F, Coyle PK (2003) *MS in Clinical Practice.* New York: Martin Dunitz.

Miller D, McDonald W, Smith K (2006) The diagnosis of MS. In: Compston A, Confavreux C, Lassman H *et al.* (eds) *McAlpine's MS.* (4th edition). Philadelphia: Churchill Livingstone.

Mohr DC, Goodkin E, Bacchetti P *et al.* (2000) Psychological stress and the subsequent appearance of new brain MRI lesions in MS. *Neurology* 55:55–61.

MS Trust, RCN, UK MS Specialist Nurse Association (2009) *Competencies for MS Specialist Services.* Letchworth Garden City: MS Trust.

Munger KL, Ascherio A (2007) Risk factors in the development of multiple sclerosis. *Expert Review of Clinical Immunology* 3(5):739–748.

Mutch K (2008) Glatiramer acetate (Copaxone) and its use in the management of relapsing-remitting MS. *British Journal of Neuroscience Nursing* 4(4):186–191.

National Council for Palliative Care (2007) *Addressing Palliative Care for People with Neurological Conditions.* London: NCPC.

National Institute for Health and Clinical Excellence (2003) *Multiple Sclerosis: Management of MS in primary and secondary care.* London: NICE.

National Institute for Health and Clinical Excellence (2007) *Natalizumab for the Treatment of Adults with Highly Active Relapsing–Remitting Multiple Sclerosis.* London: NICE.

National Institute for Health and Clinical Excellence (2009) *Functional Electrical Stimulation for Drop Foot of Central Neurological Origin*. London: NICE.

Nodhturft V, Schneider MA, Herbert P *et al.* (2000) Chronic disease self-management improving health outcomes. *Nursing Clinics of North America* 35(2):507–518.

Nortvedt MW, Riise T, Frugaard J *et al.* (2007) Prevalence of bladder, bowel and sexual problems among multiple sclerosis patients two to five years after diagnosis. *Multiple Sclerosis* 13(1):106–112.

Nortvedt MW, Riise T, Myhr KM *et al.* (2001) Reduced quality of life among multiple sclerosis patients with sexual disturbance and bladder dysfunction. *Multiple Sclerosis* 7(4):231–235.

Optic Neuritis Study Group (2008) Visual function 15 years after optic neuritis: a final follow-up report from the Optic Neuritis Treatment Trial. *Ophthalmology* 115:1079–1082.

Palace J (2001) Making the diagnosis of MS. *Journal of Neurology Neurosurgery and Psychiatry* 71(11 Suppl):ii3–ii8.

Paty DW, Ebers GC (1998) Clinical features. In: Paty DW, Ebers GC (eds) (1998) *Multiple Sclerosis*. Philadelphia: FA Davis Co.

Pöllmann W, Feneberg W (2008) Current management of pain associated with multiple sclerosis. *CNS Drugs* 22(4):291–324.

Polman CH, Reingold SC, Edan C *et al.* (2005) Diagnostic criteria for MS: 2005 revisions to the McDonald criteria. *Annals of Neurology* 56:840–864.

Polman CH, Thompson AJ, Murray JT *et al.* (2006) *Multiple Sclerosis: The guide to treatment and management*. (6th edition). New York: Demos Medical Publishing.

Poser C, Paty DW, Scheinberg L *et al.* (1983) New diagnostic criteria for MS: Guidelines for research protocols. *Annals of Neurology* 13:227–231.

Pryse-Phillips W, Costello F (2001) The epidemiology of MS. In: Cook SD. (ed) *Handbook of MS*. (3rd edition). New York: Marcel Decker.

Rog D, Turo B Nurmikko J *et al.* (2005) Randomized, controlled trial of cannabis-based medicine in central pain in multiple sclerosis. *Neurology* 65:812–819.

Rovaris M, Agosta F, Sormani MP *et al.* (2003) Conventional and magnetization transfer MRI predictors of clinical multiple sclerosis evolution: a medium-term follow-up study. *Brain* 126(10):2323–2332.

Sadovnick AD, Remick RA, Allen J *et al.* (1996) Depression and MS. *Neurology* 46:628–632.

Sayao AL, Devonshire V, Tremlett H (2007) Longitudinal follow up of 'benign' multiple sclerosis at 20 years. *Neurology* 68(7):496–500.

Sevon M, Sumelahti ML, Tienari P *et al.* (2000) MS in childhood and its prognosis. *International MS Journal* 8 (1):29–33.

Shinto l, Yadav V, Morris C *et al.* (2006) Demographic and health related factors associated with complimentary and alternative medicine (CAM) use in multiple sclerosis. *Multiple Sclerosis* 12(1):94–100.

Siegert R, Abernethy D (2005) Depression in MS: a review. *Journal of Neurology, Neurosurgery and Psychiatry* 76:469–475.

Siev-Ner I, Gamus D, Lerner-Geva L, Achiron A (2003) Reflexology treatment relieves symptoms of multiple sclerosis: a randomised controlled study. *Multiple Sclerosis* 9:356–361.

Sorgen-Sanders A, Foley FW, LaRocca NG *et al.* (2000) The Multiple Sclerosis Intimacy and Sexuality Questionnaire-19 (MSISQ-19). *Sexuality and Disability* 18:3–24.

Tardieu M, Mikaeloff Y (2004) MS in children. *International MS Journal* 11:36–42.

Thompson AJ, Montalban X, Barkhof F *et al.* (2000) Diagnostic criteria for primary progressive multiple sclerosis: a position paper. *Annals of Neurology* 47(6):831–835.

Thompson Miller AE, Lublin F *et al.* (2000) *MS in Clinical Practice*. New York: Martin Dunitz.

Tullman MJ, Oshinsky RJ, Lublin FD *et al.* (2004) Clinical characteristics of progressive relapsing MS. *Multiple Sclerosis* 10:451–454.

UKMSSNA (2006) *Clinical Management Manual*. Ledbury: UKMSSNA.

van den Noort S, Holland NJ (1999) *Multiple Sclerosis in Clinical Practice* (2nd edition). New York: Demos Medical Publishing Co. Inc.

Ward N (2005) Assessment and management of sexual dysfunction in women with multiple sclerosis. *British Journal of Neuroscience Nursing* 1(2):75–80.

Wollin J, Dale H, Spenser N *et al.* (2000) What people with newly diagnosed MS (and their families and friends) need to know. *International Journal of MS Care* 2:3–4.

Zajicek J, Freeman J, Porter B (2007) *Multiple Sclerosis Care* Oxford: Oxford University Press.

29
Management of Patients with Dementias

Katy Judd, Karen Harrison and Ian Weatherhead

INTRODUCTION

Dementia is an 'umbrella' term used to describe problems with cognition. There are many causes of dementia, although in approximately 75% of cases in the UK it is caused by either Alzheimer's disease (AD) or vascular dementia (Alzheimer's Society, 2007). Dementia costs the UK economy £17 billion per annum and costs are set to treble over the next 30 years as numbers of people affected are expected to double (DH, 2009). The costs of poor dementia care in hospital have been highlighted (Alzheimer's Society, 2009), both financially and the negative effect on the health of people with dementia due to longer lengths of stay.

With good multidisciplinary teamwork, symptoms can be managed, and the person with dementia and the carer helped to improve their quality of life. This chapter provides an overview of the diseases causing dementia, the investigations required to make a diagnosis, symptom management and the impact on family and carers.

EPIDEMIOLOGY

There are 700,000 people with dementia in the UK (DH, 2009), including 11,000 people from black and ethnic minority groups, and 18,500 people with an age of onset under 65 years. The well established prevalence rates for all dementias in the UK are shown in Table 29.1. The incidence of dementia is no greater in men or women (Cayton

et al., 1997), but more women have dementia because their life expectancy is greater and age is a risk factor.

Some people have a mixed picture, with both AD and vascular pathology. More rare causes of dementia include: unusual presentations of AD such as posterior cortical atrophy, movement disorders which cause dementia, such as Huntington's disease and progressive supranuclear palsy (see Chapter 26), corticobasal degeneration, multiple sclerosis (see Chapter 28) and variations of frontotemporal degeneration, prion diseases, alcohol-related dementia, HIV related dementia and Niemann–Pick disease. With the exception of potentially treatable causes, such as normal pressure hydrocephalus and cerebral vasculitis, dementia is a progressive, irreversible, neurodegenerative disease.

AETIOLOGY

For the majority of dementias the cause is unknown. It is likely to be multifactorial with age, genetic susceptibility, environmental factors, diet and general health being implicated. It is important to determine the disease causing the dementia in order to exclude depression or treatable causes, and to allow a trial of treatment with cholinesterase inhibitors for AD. It may be possible to slow progression in vascular dementia by controlling risk factors such as smoking, hypertension or cholesterol.

Genetics

Inherited dementias are rare. All genes that have been identified are inherited in an autosomal dominant way, although there may be 'susceptibility' genes as yet unknown. Genetic mutations in the amyloid precursor protein, or presenilin 1 or 2 genes are known to cause AD with a much earlier presentation (Growden and Rossor,

Neuroscience Nursing: Evidence-Based Practice, 1st Edition.
Edited by Sue Woodward and Ann-Marie Mestecky
© 2011 Blackwell Publishing Ltd

Table 29.1 Prevalence rates for dementia in the UK.

Prevalence by age	Proportion of dementia types
40–64 years: 1 in 400 65–69 years: 1 in 100 70–79 years: 1 in 25 80+ years: 1 in 6	Alzheimer's disease 55% Vascular dementia 20% Dementia with Lewy bodies 15% Frontotemporal dementia 5% Other causes 5%

Source: Alzheimer's Society, 2007.

2007). People with Down's syndrome are at increased risk of developing AD, perhaps because they have an extra copy of chromosome 21 which contains the gene for beta-amyloid protein production, although cholesterol levels may also be significant (Buckley, 2008). Familial forms of frontotemporal dementia, prion disease and a stroke syndrome called CADASIL (cerebral autosomal dominant arteriopathy with subcortical infarcts and leukoencephalopathy: see Chapter 22) also exist. Huntington's disease (see Chapter 26) also has cognitive and psychiatric symptoms due to a mutation in a DNA sequence.

If the family history is suggestive of a familial dementia, consent is taken to perform diagnostic testing for mutations, following discussion of the implications for siblings and children.

Creutzfeldt–Jacob disease (CJD)

CJD is a prion protein related disorder of the brain, often of an aggressive nature. Prion proteins are normally found in cell tissue. When they fold abnormally in the brain they form clusters and neuronal death occurs, giving a spongy appearance to the brain. Sporadic CJD has rapid onset and deterioration, with no clear cause. Familial CJD is inherited, the person having a genetic predisposition to develop abnormal prion proteins. Iatrogenic CJD occurs after having received contaminated blood/tissue. Variant CJD affects predominantly young people and is associated with eating infected meat products from cattle, commonly known as 'mad cow disease'.

CJD progresses more rapidly than other dementias. The average length of time a person will survive from diagnosis with sporadic CJD is four to six months, variant CJD one year, iatrogenic CJD approximately 1–2 years, and the disease course of inherited CJD depends on the mutation, but may be from months to years.

Korsakoff's syndrome and Wernicke's encephalopathy

Korsakoff's syndrome arises as a result of severe prolonged alcohol misuse and is caused by a lack of vitamin B1 (thiamine) due to poor diet and the body's inability to absorb vitamin B1 due to the effects of alcohol. Wernicke's encephalopathy can be a precursor to Korsakoff's syndrome if left untreated. Again, it is alcohol related, but can be reversed by aggressive treatment with vitamin B1.

Pick's disease

Pick's disease is a fronto-temporal dementia. Symptoms often include changes to personality and behaviour. Pick's bodies, which are unusual protein deposits, are identified within the brains of affected individuals.

Dementia with Lewy bodies (DLB)

DLB is often associated with Parkinson's disease (see Chapter 26) as many of the characteristics are the same. Lewy bodies, small protein deposits within neurones that cause cell dysfunction and commonly affect the neurotransmitters acetylcholine and dopamine, are also present in Parkinson's disease. Symptoms include confusion, memory loss, gait and movement difficulties. Affected individuals are highly sensitive to anti-psychotic drugs, which can make the illness worse or even prove fatal.

PATHOPHYSIOLOGY

Abnormal protein deposits (beta-amyloid, tau and alpha-synuclein) are present in post-mortem brain tissue in over 90% dementias (Goedert and Spillantini, 2007). Amyloid plaques and neurofibrillary tangles are seen in AD, particularly in the hippocampus which is important for memory. The neuropathology of frontotemporal dementias is increasingly complex as different clinical syndromes are being identified. Changes in brain structure are seen on imaging, with global cortical atrophy and enlargement of the ventricles seen in AD, focal atrophy in fronto-temporal dementia (which may be asymmetrical), and evidence of small vessel disease and sub-cortical infarcts in vascular dementia.

CLINICAL SIGNS AND SYMPTOMS

Dementia is defined as:

> a syndrome due to disease of the brain, ... in which there is a disturbance of multiple higher cortical functions, including memory, thinking, orientation, comprehension, calculation, learning capability, language and judgement

(WHO, 1992).

Consciousness is unimpaired.

The first symptom often reported is word finding difficulty. Problems with orientation to time and place, registration and recall, attention, calculation, naming, repetition, comprehension, reading, writing and drawing may be tested with the mini mental status examination (MMSE) (Folstein *et al.*, 1975) (see Chapter 9), which must be completed in full.

Specific symptoms depend on the area of the brain initially affected. For example: behavioural problems occur in frontal dementias such as Pick's disease, and speech and language problems occur in primary non-fluent aphasia and semantic dementias. All focal dementias progress to more global impairment over several years and abilities usually decline gradually. Symptoms are initially subtle and may be attributed to more common causes such as depression, particularly in younger people.

DIAGNOSIS

Diagnosis can be a prolonged process and often requires referral to specialist memory assessment services involving a neurologist or old age psychiatrist. Often, dementia and delirium are misdiagnosed; differential diagnosis is vital as early detection reduces morbidity (see Chapter 9). There is no single diagnostic test for the common dementias and medical investigations (see Table 29.2) are aimed at excluding treatable causes of cognitive impairment.

Structural imaging

Access to CT and MRI varies depending upon local protocols, patient tolerance, contraindications (see Chapter 19) and cost. Structural imaging will exclude an intracerebral lesion (e.g. tumours, or normal pressure hydrocephalus) as a cause for the cognitive impairment or aid subtype

Table 29.2 Comprehensive diagnosis.

Assessment/investigations	Rationale
Clinical history – from patient and independently from carer	To include educational and employment background (provides premorbid estimate of performance), past medical history (including psychiatric history), drug history, family history and cognitive history
Physical examination – general and neurological	To include a cardiac assessment, visual fields/disorientation, and primitive reflexes
Imaging	MRI brain unless contraindicated or unavailable (in which case a CT head will exclude a tumour). Will show the level of any atrophy, whether global or focal, and the presence of any vascular disease or infarcts
Neurophysiology (EEG)	EEG will distinguish between frontotemporal degeneration (in which alpha rhythm is usually normal) and Alzheimer's disease (in which alpha rhythm is usually reduced or absent), or identify subclinical temporal lobe spikes causing transient epileptic amnesia (see Chapter 30)
Neuropsychology	The full (30 questions) MMSE will give a basic guide to the domains affected. More detailed neuropsychological testing will cover verbal and performance IQ, verbal and visual memory, information processing, verbal fluency, literacy skills, naming, visual perception and executive (organisation and planning) function
Bloods	Biochemistry, haematology, treponemal serology (to detect untreated syphilis), B12, thyroid function, ESR and auto-antibodies are performed routinely. More rarely, HIV and genetic testing may be performed following appropriate counselling and consent
Other	More rarely – lumbar puncture, muscle, skin, bone marrow or cerebral biopsy may be performed

diagnosis, specifically differentiating AD from vascular dementia and frontotemporal dementia.

Functional imaging

SPECT and PET scanning (see Chapter 19) have been shown to improve the sensitivity and specificity of clinical criteria in diagnosing dementia (NICE, 2006).

Disclosure of the diagnosis

Disclosure of the emerging diagnosis is a sensitive task. Many nurses, particularly those working within memory assessment and neurological clinics, are key in providing post-diagnostic support and counselling to those newly diagnosed with dementia and their carers; this being one of the very specific remits of Admiral nurses. Whilst people may be seeking an explanation for their symptoms, many will find it hard to hear and accept the diagnosis.

MEDICAL MANAGEMENT

New approaches to the pharmacological treatment of dementia began in the 1980s and 1990s with the introduction of the acetylcholinesterase inhibitors (AChEIs), particularly in AD. AChEIs prevent the breakdown of acetylcholine, a neurotransmitter thought to be important in memory, thought and judgement. AChEIs used in clinical practice include rivastigmine, donepezil and galantamine. They are licensed in the UK for the symptomatic treatment of AD. In 2010 NICE guidelines recommended their use for the treatment of mild to moderate AD, overturning an earlier decision. AChEIs improve cognitive function and slow the decline for some (Birks, 2006). There is now considerable clinical experience of their use, but more robust trial evidence is required.

Anti psychotic and sedative medications

Antipsychotic medications are often used in managing dementia symptoms, such as wandering, in care home settings. NICE (2004) identified that one third of residents in care homes in the UK were receiving antipsychotic medication to manage dementia symptoms on a long-term basis. Memantine (Ebixa), a glutamatergic NMDA receptor antagonist, is now recommended for the treatment of moderate/severe AD (NICE, 2010). Anti-psychotic drugs have a role to play when prescribed appropriately, but they must always be considered as a last resort. A recent report (Alzheimer's Society, 2008), identifies the current unacceptably high level of use of antipsychotic medications in dementia, while NICE (2006) recommends that antipsychotics are prescribed and monitored by specialist mental health services. A detailed assessment must be carried out

so that other potential causes of behaviour change/challenging behaviour, such as changes in environment, infection, constipation, anxiety and depression (see Chapter 10) have been discounted. Agitation occurs in up to 70% of patients and while haloperidol has been used to manage aggression, it is associated with adverse effects and its effectiveness remains unclear (Lonergan *et al.*, 2002). There is no evidence to support routine use and treatment must be on an individual basis, while monitoring for adverse events. Anti-psychotic drugs must always and only ever be used for the benefit of the patient and not for the benefit of care staff (Weatherhead, 2009).

Future developments and current research

Stem cells

Stem cells research is underway to determine their potential for treatment of dementia. There is recent evidence that neural stem cells have improved memory in mice genetically engineered to have AD, by helping the brain to form new synapses (Blurton-Jones *et al.*, 2009).

Cannabinoids

Cannabinoids may regulate neurodegeneration by modulating excessive glutamate production, oxidative stress and neuroinflammation. Some studies have shown specific effects in interrupting the pathological process in AD, but there is a lack of robust clinical evidence of effectiveness and further research is required (Krishnan *et al.*, 2009).

NURSING MANAGEMENT

There are two very clear elements to good quality dementia care: the medical model/approach and the social model/approach. Both are inextricably linked and of distinct value to the care delivered to the person with dementia and their families. This has been the focus of recent policy and the National Dementia Strategy (NICE 2006; DH, 2009). Nursing management of dementia uses the 'social model' predominantly. Dementia affects the whole family, and people close to the person with dementia find themselves providing increasing amounts of care and support as the disease progresses.

Due to the cognitive difficulties, nurses must communicate with a main carer in addition to the patient in order that appropriate care and support is given. This can give rise to ethical and legal challenges such as disclosure of confidential health information, consideration of the patient's capacity for decision making, and potential disagreements among family members on the best interests of the patient. The nurse must therefore be aware of the Data Protection Act (1998), the Mental Capacity Act

(2005), Lasting Powers of Attorney, Advance Decisions, and the requirement to notify any illness impairing ability to drive to the Drivers and Vehicle Licensing Agency (DVLA) (For further information see: The Office of the Public Guardian http://www.publicguardian.gov.uk. See also Chapter 36).

Though it is argued that nursing care required by people with dementia will depend upon the causative disease and the stage of the illness, this is now seen as an approach that tends to be driven by the disease focused approach of the 'medical model'. With the pioneering approach of Tom Kitwood (1997) and the Bradford Dementia Group, a person-centred approach to care throughout the life-span of the disease, irrespective of the defined stages is now advocated.

Early on the purpose of diagnostic investigations, what they entail and how results will be given must be discussed. Nurses can establish a relationship with the patient and their family/carer, understanding the main problems from their perspective and liaising with other health and social care providers. Following the diagnosis nurses need to follow up on the consultant's discussions to check understanding, give advice on the next steps and continue liaison with local services. Later in the illness, nursing input will focus largely on symptom management.

Person centred care

All care should be delivered with a person centred approach. The term *person centred care* has its origins in the work of Carl Rogers (1961). It talks of seeing the *person* with dementia rather than dementia the disease first, i.e. the **PERSON** with dementia, rather than the person with **DEMENTIA** (Kitwood, 1997).

Person centred care (Box 29.1) takes into account the person's individual needs and preferences and seeks to respect their independence, autonomy and right to make their own choices; viewing each person with dementia as a unique individual, with a unique set of needs and requirements and with a rich past or life story.

Psychosocial interventions

'Psychosocial interventions' is an umbrella term for interventions to enhance quality of life, maximise the individual's functional performance (Yuhas *et al.*, 2006) and minimise the risks of future disability (Moniz-Cook and Manthorpe, 2009). A range of psychological interventions are currently provided for people with dementia, though availability varies greatly. In the early stages individual psychological treatment may be offered; this may focus on enhancing adjustment to the diagnosis or to mood, using

---

Box 29.1   Key features of person centred care

- Looks at care from the perspective of the individual
- Acknowledges each person as a unique individual with a rich history and their own memories, preferences, wishes and needs
- Respects the dignity, autonomy and independence of the person with dementia
- Focuses on the positive rather than the negative
- Focuses on strengths and abilities rather than weaknesses and disabilities
- Promotes well being
- Ensures care is planned around the individual not around the care system
- Acknowledges that there is usually a reason for a behaviour and views behaviours that challenge others as an expression of feelings and/or a means of communication
- Accepts the reality of the person with dementia and does not insist on bringing them into another reality that can cause them distress

---

cognitive behavioural therapy (CBT) (Scholey and Woods, 2003) or life review and strategies to improve memory such as cognitive stimulation therapy (Spector *et al.*, 2003). CBT has been shown to be effective in the early stages of dementia (Douglas *et al.*, 2004). In the later stages of dementia psychological interventions may include a variety of group activities, including many of those outlined in Table 29.3.

Psychosocial interventions fall into four major subgroups: communication techniques, behavioural strategies, environmental modifications and caregiver education, which will now be addressed.

Communication techniques

In later stages of dementia communication difficulties become increasingly evident due to shrinking vocabulary, decreased word fluency and receptive and expressive aphasias (see Chapter 12). Reading and writing skills are also progressively lost. Communication problems can be exacerbated by poor eyesight, hearing loss and even ill fitting dentures.

Poor communication often causes other difficulties for the person with dementia. Lack of understanding or awareness of what the patient is attempting to express, or lack of consideration and time constraints often play a key role

Table 29.3 Psychological interventions in dementia.

Intervention	What does this intervention involve?
Validation therapy	Validation therapy aims to restore dignity and prevent deterioration into a vegetative state (Holden and Woods, 1995), by having an empathic, non judgemental listener who can accept the person with dementia's view of reality, rather than trying to correct it by using a cognitive approach. Case example: Many people with dementia often talk about their children as if they are still children, rather than adults, a nurse may respond to the person's statement of '*I must get home to see to my children*' by stating '*you must love your children very much, would you like to tell me more about them..*'; rather than responding by simply saying '*your children are all grown up*'. Thus by using validation in this way it can aid stimulation and conversation with the person with dementia.
Reality orientation	Reality orientation (RO) is widely used in reminding people with memory loss of the here and now, i.e. day, date, name (Livingston *et al.*, 2005). This can often prove valuable, especially in the home environment, by keeping a large diary/wall chart to support reminders. RO was designed for people who are disorientated and have severe problems with memory (Holden and Woods, 1995). There are three principal types of RO: • 24 hr RO: The basic approach whereby all staff/carers constantly remind the person with dementia of time, date, day, place, etc. The environment should also be enhanced to support this approach, with the use of signs, clocks and calendars. • Group RO: Usually for three to six people, and lasting for around 30 minutes for up to six sessions. • Attitude RO: Entails all staff and carers using the same approach to an individual all the time, very personal for the individual, aimed at reducing conflict and confusion of messages and information.
Reminiscence therapy	Reminiscence involves the discussion of past activities, events and experiences, usually with aid of tangible prompts (i.e. photographs, familiar objects, music, etc.) and helps to retrieve memory from distant past (James, 2004). Traditionally reminiscence therapy has been used in a group setting. In today's multi-cultural society, it could be argued that this has limited value unless applied on a one to one basis.
Multi sensory therapy	Snoezelen provides sensory stimuli to stimulate the primary senses of sight, hearing, touch, taste and smell through the use of lighting effects, tactile surfaces, massage, music and the odour of relaxing essential oils (Chung *et al.*, 2002) and often in a specially equipped room (Burns cited in James, 2004). The costs of setting up a Snoezelen environment may make this a rare option for many in today's financially constrained market, even though evidence suggests it may have a therapeutic worth.
Cognitive stimulation therapy	Cognitive stimulation therapy uses themes from reality orientation aimed at information processing to enhance general cognitive and social functioning (Clare, 2003; Livingston *et al.*, 2005).
Life story	Life story work uses techniques of reminiscing and history taking, which recognises a person's present needs, wishes, likes and dislikes and makes a more positive interaction more likely. It aims to encourage better communication and relationships, more one to one time, it endeavours to see the person behind the illness, and aims to develop and shape person centred care (Hazell and Punshon, 2004). Using the principals of Kitwood (1997), focus is aimed at the person NOT the illness. Gubrium (2003) described the importance of a good life story in order to meaningfully engage with and understand a person with dementia's behaviour, and to try to make sense of the same.
Music therapy	Music in dementia care can be used as a means of improving memory, health and identity and can also be linked with reminiscence therapy. Music therapy can facilitate and enable communication through sound and movement (Aldridge, 2000).

in communication breakdown, which may result in behavioural changes as a direct consequence. Carers and nurses must understand the components of communication that are affected by dementia (Box 29.2). Many studies have identified similar strategies to aid communication with people with dementia (Goldsmith 1996; Yuhas *et al.*, 2006) (Box 29.3). Communication is discussed in further detail in Chapter 12.

Behavioural strategies

People with dementia often exhibit behaviour that can be described as 'unusual', or at times distressing, aggressive or disinhibited. There may be explanations for behavioural changes (Box 29.4), rather than it being a symptom suggesting progression of the illness. Goldsmith (1996) believes that a person's (with dementia) behaviour in whatever form is very often an attempt to express something they are unable to articulate verbally. Wandering or shouting may not simply be a function of the illness. Probably the most common behavioural change seen is aggression (Box 29.5) often towards carers, causing distress especially if this behaviour is uncharacteristic. Managing challenging behaviour is discussed in more detail in Chapter 10.

Environmental modifications

Considerable emphasis is placed on the living environment of the person with dementia. Even basic elements, such as noise, can have a profound effect and can be overwhelming, as the ability to process information slows. Nurses need to create a calming environment, where the television and radio are not competing with each other. Good lighting can help to reduce confusion in surroundings. As mobility can be affected, an environment free of obstacles is desirable. Clear labelling of doors, rooms, and cupboards can also help to reduce confusion and maintain a level of independent functioning (see also Chapter 10).

Assistive technology

Two thirds of dementia sufferers still live at home, many alone, so the use of assistive technology can help in maintaining independence. Dosette medication boxes with alarm reminders, movement sensors to switch lighting on at night, safety devices to turn the cooker off automatically if left on too long, bath and sink tap monitors and safety

---

Box 29.2   Communication difficulties experienced by people with dementia

- Difficulty following a conversation
- Slowness at responding
- Poor turn taking in conversation
- No initiation of conversation, only replies when someone else starts it
- Conversation wanders with frequent change of topic
- Speech is empty, conveys very little information
- Difficulty following the radio or television
- Failure to appreciate humour or sarcasm (linguistically)
- Difficulty remembering names of objects, people or places
- Using the wrong word
- Frequent repetition of the same phrase or topic
- Asks the same question again and again
- Mispronounces words
- Difficulty understanding written material although may still read aloud
- Difficulty writing (dysgraphia)
- Receptive dysphasia for the spoken word. Ability to take in written communication is often less impaired.
- Expressive dysphasia
- Aphasia

Box 29.3   Strategies to aid communication

- Use chosen name
- No discussion over person
- Validation rather than reality orientation
- Laughing with the person
- Use observation
- Mirroring

Box 29.4   Possible causes for behavioural changes

- Confusion
- Not understanding instructions
- Poor communication
- Environment
- Receptive/expressive dysphasia
- Depression
- Physical changes, i.e. pain, injury, delirium, infection, constipation
- Illness progression
- Frontotemporal dementia

See also Chapter 10.

Box 29.5 Possible causes of aggression

- Misunderstanding personal care; seeing it as intrusion into privacy
- The person has some insight into condition and is trying to cope and hide it from others
- Being unable to perform a particular task and becoming frustrated by the process
- Not being able to come to terms with an environment that may appear strange and be perceived as threatening
- Poor eyesight, hearing or interrupted sleep patterns may make a person prone to misunderstandings
- Aggressive behaviour occurs most often when the person is receiving intimate care, staff are more focused on the task rather than the individual (Cohen-Mansfield, 2005)
- Staffing may be perceived and experienced as being aggressive or threatening and provoke a defensive reaction
- The person may be expected to do or receive things which they perceive as being inappropriate
- Different carers having different approaches
- Noise and disturbance
- Physical restraint or inappropriate medication

Box 29.6 Content of carer information programmes

- Information/education about diagnosis and prognosis
- Opportunity to explore and understand behavioural changes associated with dementia and ways of coping with this
- An opportunity to share feelings of grief with others who are also in the grieving process
- Emotional support
- Help and guidance with decision-making
- Referral to community resources
- Physical and emotional well-being
- Socialisation
- Time for themselves
- Realisation that they are not alone

Source: Sarna and Thompson, 2008.

---

plugs, pressure sensor mats and door alarms to reduce the risk of walking out and getting lost can all be useful. Electronic 'tagging', though controversial, is seen as enabling and maximising independence and quality of life (Woods, 1999).

Caregiver education

Informal carers of people with dementia save the UK economy an estimated £6 billion a year and should be considered partners in care with health care professionals. Carer distress is common, whether living with the person with dementia or trying to maintain their independence when they are living alone. Nurses should provide education for the carer on the illness, symptoms, communication, managing behavioural concerns, finances, legal issues and future planning, which can help to reduce some anxieties around caring and ensure that the person with dementia and their carers are adequately supported.

NICE (2006) recommended a range of options for delivering carer education including individual or group psycho-education, peer support groups with other carers

and training courses on dementia. Carer education aims to reduce carer stress, improve the quality of the caring relationship, minimise the disruptive symptoms of dementia and help carers to recognise when homecare becomes unsafe or unfeasible (Yuhas *et al.*, 2006).

Family-centred therapeutic approaches and relationship-centred care have also been identified as beneficial (Hibberd *et al.*, 2008). For many families conflict can arise on deciding what is best for a loved one, and family-centred work can help to untangle and clarify differences and to provide a structure to help unite families in their approach, whilst still recognising individual values. Whether in group or individual sessions, nurses need to address a number of common themes with carers (Box 29.6) (Sarna and Thompson, 2008).

Carers should carry some form of identification with them which states that they are a carer. In case of accident, people will be alerted to the fact that they are caring for someone who may require assistance.

Community services

It can be hard to accept help after a lifetime of independence. Losing insight can be beneficial to the person with dementia, but of course makes providing external support in activities of daily living more difficult for the person to accept. It will be necessary for a carer to be present at any assessment by care providers; otherwise a person with dementia who lacks insight may decline offers of help.

A referral to the social services team should be initiated, or a community mental health team if behavioural and psychiatric symptoms are present. The Alzheimer's Society supports people with dementia of any cause and the nurse should provide details of the local branch of the Alzheimer's Society to both patients and families.

Social services

Social workers lead in undertaking a carer's assessment, which is a statutory right for all carers, and in the provision of an appropriate social care package. They can assist with benefit claims and provide information on day care centres, respite care, long-term care homes and voluntary organisations in the local area. They may also assist with referral to other health care professionals as required. Referral to social services may be made by nursing staff, via the patient's GP, or the person with dementia/carer can self refer by phoning the local social services department within the local council.

Admiral nurses

Admiral nurses (community psychiatric nurses who are allocated to the carer rather than the person with dementia) use a bespoke, comprehensive 17 point assessment schedule, to assess the impact of dementia on the carer and the person with dementia. A range of psychosocial interventions may be offered, or individuals may be directed to other services for advice and support.

Interventions including information, psycho-education, and practical advice and coping strategies may be offered through group and/or individual family contact. Admiral nurses also provide education, supervision, development and support to other professionals and service providers. There may be instances when the needs of the carer and those of the person with dementia may be in conflict with each other requiring each to receive their own support and or advocacy, which will require specific negotiation between professionals involved.

Admiral Nursing DIRECT (http://www.dementiauk. org/what-we-do/admiral-nursing-direct/), a telephone and email helpline, offers practical advice and emotional support to people affected by dementia and others in areas where there is no full Admiral nurse team.

Peer support

A growing peer support group is the Alzheimer Cafe. This often takes the form of a monthly gathering where people with dementia and/or their family and friends can be together in a safe, welcoming environment, in the company of other carers, volunteers and health care professionals, for the purpose of emotional support, education and social interaction. Talking with peers about the problems that dementia brings can help carers realise that they are not the only ones who feel powerless and distressed and can assist them to better manage their own situations (Hibberd *et al.*, 2008). It is thought that this also gives the person with dementia the feeling of being able to influence his/ her situation.

Physical activity programmes

There is some evidence that physical activity delays onset of dementia and slows cognitive decline in healthy older adults (Barnes *et al.*, 2007), but it is unclear whether exercise and physical activity can impact on cognition for people diagnosed with dementia. Some trials have been undertaken (Stevens and Killeen, 2006; Rolland *et al.*, 2007) which explore the impact of physical activity on cognitive function compared to usual care, but there is insufficient evidence to determine clinical effectiveness (Forbes *et al.*, 2008).

Complementary therapies

Use of complementary and alternative therapies is increasing, with concerns that patients are accessing therapies for which there is little evidence of effectiveness. A number of Cochrane reviews of complementary therapies for dementia have been undertaken. Readers should consider, however, that Cochrane reviews only consider large scale, high quality randomised controlled trials and that research into many complementary therapies is in its infancy. Lack of evidence of effectiveness from randomised controlled trials does not necessarily mean that there is evidence of no effectiveness, and many patients and carers will access complementary therapies in order to improve their sense of well-being and quality of life.

Aromatherapy and massage

One trial has shown benefit of aromatherapy on agitation and neuropsychiatric symptoms in people with dementia (Ballard *et al.*, 2002), but a recent Cochrane review has identified insufficient evidence to support this therapy and further research is required (Holt *et al.*, 2003).

It has been suggested that massage may counteract cognitive decline or reduce agitation and mood disorders, possibly mediated by the production of oxytocin. There is a consensus that the potential short-term effects of massage are more likely to impact on behaviour, mood and well-being (Hansen *et al.*, 2006), but of the 18 studies identified within this Cochrane review, all were of poor methodological quality.

Acupuncture

Acupuncture has been used for vascular dementia and, while 105 studies were identified on this subject in a Cochrane review, no high quality evidence or randomised controlled trials were found (Weina *et al.*, 2007).

Ginkgo bilboa

Ginkgo bilboa is commonly taken for memory and concentration, confusion, depression and anxiety. Evidence supporting ginkgo bilboa is conflicting, with one trial showing a large effect in favour of this therapy and others showing no benefit over placebo (Birks and Grimley Evans, 2009), but equally there was no evidence found of adverse effects.

Financial and legal issues

Benefits

There are extra costs associated with dementia, from travel costs for hospital visits to laundry costs if a person is incontinent. Such costs will have a greater impact for those living on a state pension, or who have had to give up work to provide full time care for example. Many older people are reluctant to claim benefits, seeing it as charity and somehow shameful, but they will have paid their National Insurance contributions and are entitled to claim. People with dementia and/or their carers may be entitled to a number of both means tested and non-means tested benefits (Box 29.7) and should be referred to their local social services department for help in navigating their way through the benefit system.

Lasting Power of Attorney

Discussion on Lasting Powers of Attorney (LPA) can be difficult, as it forces acknowledgement of potential future loss of capacity to make decisions. It may be easiest to discuss along the lines of 'hope for the best but plan for the worst'. There are two types of LPA that cover property and affairs or personal welfare. It is possible to apply for either or both and it is recommended that people ask a solicitor to make the arrangements. The property and affairs LPA gives the attorney(s) the power to make decisions about financial and property matters, such as selling a house or managing a bank account. The personal welfare LPA gives the attorney(s) the power to make decisions about health and personal welfare, such as day-to-day care, medical treatment, or where the person should live. A personal welfare LPA only ever takes effect when the donor lacks capacity to make decisions (see Chapter 36). A property and affairs LPA can take effect as soon as it is registered, even while the donor still has capacity, unless the donor specifies otherwise. For further information see: Office of the Public Guardian (www.publicguardian.gov.uk).

Driving

A person with dementia (or their carer) is legally required to inform the Driver and Vehicle Licensing Agency (DVLA) of their diagnosis. If they refuse, a medical practitioner may inform the DVLA directly. The driver's insurance company should also be informed of the diagnosis. It is usually possible for the DVLA to decide whether a person should be allowed to continue driving from the information provided by the person with dementia and the GP or hospital consultant, but it may be necessary to take a free driving test. While many have studied links between motor skills, driving behaviour and neuropsychological performance, a recent Cochrane review has not identified any studies that have examined the ability of cognitive testing or other driving assessment by drivers with dementia to predict driving ability or to reduce the incidence of accidents (Martin *et al.*, 2009). It may be possible to issue annual licences, renewed in consultation with the medical practitioner.

Third sector resources

Apart from the statutory services available for people with dementia and their carers, a valuable contribution to their support is provided by the third sector. Some of the more significant organisations that may be accessed by patients and their carers include: The Alzheimer's Society, Uniting Carers For Dementia, Carers UK and the Pick Disease Support Group.

End of life care

Dementia is a progressive neurodegenerative disease which significantly reduces survival (Neale *et al.*, 2001). The end of life care received by this group is often poor (Sampson *et al.*, 2006) and people with dementias have inequitable access to palliative care services (Hanrahan

---

Box 29.7   Possible benefits available

- Attendance allowance
- Incapacity benefit
- Disability living allowance
- Council tax reduction
- Severe disability premium
- Carer's allowance

and Luchins, 1995). Dementia care should incorporate a palliative care approach from the time of diagnosis until death. The aim should be to promote quality of life but also to enable people to die with dignity and in a place of their choosing, while supporting carers during their bereavement, which may both anticipate and follow death. Department of Health guidance calls for people with dementia to have the same access to palliative and specialist palliative care services as those that are cognitively intact. The National Council for Palliative Care (NCPC), through the work of its Dementia Project, identified best practice in the field across the UK and also developed guidance documents for those working in end of life care in dementia (see also Chapter 36).

SUMMARY

Providing good quality care to people with dementia and their carers can be challenging. Nursing has much to offer people with dementia and their carers throughout the 'journey' of the disease; from diagnosis through to death and beyond. People with dementia and their carers deserve the highest standards of care, support and technical expertise delivered within a relationship and person centred context. Nurses must rise to this challenge.

FURTHER INFORMATION

Admiral Nurse DIRECT Telephone helpline: 0845 257 9406

Dementia UK www.fordementia.org.uk; direct@fordementia.org.uk

Alzheimer's Society Telephone helpline: 0845 300 0336 www.alzheimers.org.uk

CJD Support Network Telephone helpline: 01630 673973

National Council for Palliative Care www.ncpc.org.uk

Office of the Public Guardian www.publicguardian.gov.uk/

Pick's Disease Support Group www.pdsg.org.uk

Alzheimer's disease: patient perspective

The following contribution was written by a man caring for his wife who has Alzheimer's disease.

Looking back, my wife has been ill for approximately 11 years, however the diagnosis was made around eight years ago. Six months ago my wife's mini mental test score was 9 (out of 30) and the doctor said she was technically in the severe stages of the disease. Now it is down to 5, although on casual acquaintance you might not think so.

We live on our own and I care for my wife at home. Clothes can be a problem, for example my wife kept on undoing zips on her trousers in places like restaurants. She refuses at present to wear skirts. So I bought trousers with elasticated waists. Toilets can be another problem. My wife has twice managed to get herself locked in toilets, so now in places we do not know we use a disabled toilet together, when available. Obtain a RADAR key from your Local Authority. Avoid toilets with two exits at all costs! I do the laundry and cooking. She still does simple tasks like peeling vegetables, makes our bed and helps with shopping. She does feed herself. She does undress and dress herself, but needs some supervision. I need to bath her now because she does not wash herself very well. I believe it is important that she is allowed to do what she can rather than to have it all done for her.

My wife is still in very good physical health, the progression of the disease is quite slow and we are still able to get out and enjoy life. I believe this is due to four things:

1. From the start the hospital and I ensured she was treated with donepezil (Aricept), which she still takes. I firmly believe that if my wife had been denied any drug treatment at all she would be in a nursing home at a cost 25 to 30 times of that paying for treatment. She might possibly even have passed away by now. As it is we are planning our golden wedding celebration with a party for family and friends next year.

2. With the knowledge of the hospital clinic we found another consultant who was prepared to provide a private prescription for memantine (Ebixa) on a trial basis. It was found to be effective and my wife is still taking the drug over three and a half years later.

3. Our GP and the hospital together prescribed sertraline, an antidepressant, which I believe has kept her calm and able to cope well with life in general. I am glad to say she is not aggressive in any way.

4. I ensure she eats a good diet and dietary supplements.

Helpful Activities

Avoid boredom. Getting out and about as much as possible is important for both the person with dementia and the carer. If you receive attendance allowance other savings follow including a 25% reduction in council tax, a disabled person's rail card and a cinema exhibitors association card. We go to the theatre and to local events. Lunch or afternoon tea at a garden centre is a cheap and pleasant way of filling in an afternoon. Family is important and we are lucky to have several grandchildren, many of whom live locally. They get on very well with my wife – children see the person rather than the dementia and they enjoy each others company, even though the children understand something is wrong. We still go away on holiday. If I tell people about the Alzheimer's disease they are very understanding and can be very helpful. I have not had any problems obtaining holiday insurance.

Accepting Help

We have a cleaner for three hours a week and a gardener for two hours once every two weeks, which helps me a great deal. So that I can play bowls once a week, my wife goes to a day sitting service run by volunteers on behalf of social services. This she thoroughly enjoys as they organise different events each week. We also make use of a sitting service called Breakaway which provides a free volunteer sitter if I have to go out. Being a carer can be demanding and cause stress at times. Some free time is important for both of us and I try to make sure I continue with my hobbies. I hope this has given you an idea of what is possible despite a diagnosis of Alzheimer's disease in a loved one.

REFERENCES

Aldridge D (2000) *Music Therapy in Dementia*. London: Jessica Kingsley.

Alzheimer's Society (2007) *Dementia UK: A report to the Alzheimer's Society on the prevalence and economic cost of dementia in the UK*. London: Alzheimer's Society.

Alzheimer's Society (2008) *Always a Last Resort: Inquiry into the prescription of antipsychotic drugs to people with dementia living in care homes*. London: Alzheimer's Society.

Alzheimer's Society (2009) *Counting the Cost: Caring for people with dementia on hospital wards*. London: Alzheimer's Society. Available from http://www.alzheimers.org.uk/site/scripts/news_article.php?newsID=579 Accessed July 2010.

Ballard CG, O'Brien JT, Reichelt K *et al.* (2002) Aromatherapy as a safe and effective treatment for the management of agitation in severe dementia: the results of a double-blind placebo-controlled trial with Melissa. *Journal of Clinical Psychology* 63(7):553–558.

Barnes D, Whitmer R, Yaffe K (2007) Physical activity and dementia: the need for preventative trials. *Exercise and Sports Science Reviews* 35(1):24–29.

Birks J (2006) Cholinesterase inhibitors for Alzheimer's disease. *Cochrane Database of Systematic Reviews* Issue 1 Art. No.: CD005593. DOI: 10.1002/14651858.CD005593.

Birks J, Grimley Evans J (2009) Ginkgo biloba for cognitive impairment and dementia. *Cochrane Database of Systematic Reviews* Issue 1. Art. No.: CD003120. DOI: 10.1002/14651858.CD003120.pub3.

Blurton-Jones M, Kitazawa M, Martinez-Coria H *et al.* (2009) Neural stem cells improve cognition via BDNF in a transgenic model of Alzheimer disease. *Proceedings of the National Academy of Sciences* 106(32):13594–13599.

Buckley F (2008) Cholesterol and Alzheimer type dementia among adults with Down's syndrome. *Down's Syndrome Research and Practice* 12(2):91–94.

Cayton H, Graham N, Warner J (1997) *Alzheimer's at Your Fingertips*. London: Class Publishing.

Chung JC, Lai CK, Chung PM *et al.* (2002) Snoezelen for dementia. *Cochrane Database of Systematic Reviews 4*, CD003152.

Clare L (2003) Cognitive training and cognitive rehabilitation for people with early-stage dementia. *Reviews in Clinical Gerontology* 13:75–83.

Cohen-Mansfield J (2005) Non pharmacological interventions for persons with dementia. *Alzheimer's Care Quarterly* 6(2):129–145.

Department of Health (2009) *Living Well with Dementia: A national dementia strategy*. London, DH.

Douglas S, James I, Ballard C (2004) Non-pharmacological interventions in dementia. *Advances in Psychiatric Treatment* 10:171–177.

Folstein MF, Folstein SE, McHugh PR (1975) 'Mini-mental state'. A practical method for grading the cognitive state of person with dementias for the clinician. *Journal of Psychiatric Research* 12:189–198.

Forbes D, Forbes S, Morgan DG *et al.* (2008) Physical activity programs for persons with dementia. *Cochrane Database of Systematic Reviews* Issue 3. Art. No.: CD006489. DOI: 10.1002/14651858.CD006489.pub2.

Goedert M, Spillantini M (2007) Tau protein and the dementias. In: Growden J, Rossor M (eds.) *The Dementias 2*. Philadelphia: Butterworth Heinemann Elsevier.

Goldsmith M (1996) *Hearing the Voice of People with Dementia*. London: Jessica Kingsley.

Growden J, Rossor M (eds.) (2007) *The Dementias 2*. Philadelphia: Butterworth Heinemann Elsevier.

Gubrium JF (2003) Generations: What is a good story? *American Society on Ageing* 27(3):21–24.

Hanrahan P, Luchins DJ (1995) Access to hospice programs in end-stage dementia: a national survey of hospice programs. *Journal of the American Geriatric Society* 43(1):56–59.

Hansen NV, Jørgensen T, Ørtenblad L (2006) Massage and touch for dementia. *Cochrane Database of Systematic Reviews* Issue 4. Art. No.: CD004989. DOI: 10.1002/14651858.CD004989.pub2.

Hazell J, Punshon C (2004) Successful life story work. *Psychologists Special Interest Group E (Working with Older People)* 85:32–34.

Hibberd P, Lemmer B, Keady J *et al.* (2008) A family-centred approach to dementia care. *Journal of Dementia Care* Sept/Oct:26–27.

Holden U, Woods RT (1995) *Positive Approaches to Dementia Care*. London: Churchill Livingston.

Holt FE, Birks TPH, Thorgrimsen LM *et al.* (2003) Aroma therapy for dementia. *Cochrane Database of Systematic Reviews* Issue 3. Art. No.: CD003150. DOI: 10.1002/14651858.CD003150.

James I (2004) Different forms of psychological interventions in dementia. *Nursing and Residential Care* 6(6):288–291.

Kitwood T (1997) *Dementia Reconsidered*. Buckingham: Open University Press.

Krishnan S, Cairns R, Howard R (2009) Cannabinoids for the treatment of dementia. *Cochrane Database of Systematic Reviews* Issue 2. Art. No.: CD007204. DOI: 10.1002/14651858.CD007204.pub2.

Livingston G, Johnston K, Katona C *et al.* (2005) Systematic review of psychological approaches to the management of neuropsychiatric symptoms of dementia. *American Journal of Psychiatry* 162:1996–2021.

Lonergan E, Luxenberg J, Colford JM *et al.* (2002) Haloperidol for agitation in dementia. *Cochrane Database of Systematic Reviews* Issue 2. Art. No.: CD002852. DOI: 10.1002/14651858.CD002852.

Martin AJ, Marottoli R, O'Neill D (2009) Driving assessment for maintaining mobility and safety in drivers with dementia. *Cochrane Database of Systematic Reviews* Issue 1. Art. No.: CD006222. DOI: 10.1002/14651858.CD006222.pub2.

Moniz-Cook E, Manthorpe J (2009) *Early Psychosocial Interventions in Dementia: Evidence based practice*. London: Jessica Kingsley.

National Institute for Health and Clinical Excellence (2004) *Dementia: management of dementia, including use of anti-psychotic medication in older people*. London: NICE.

National Institute for Health and Clinical Excellence, Social Care Institute for Excellence (2006) *Supporting People with Dementia and their Carers in Health and Social Care*. London: NICE/SCIE.

National Institute for Health and Clinical Excellence (2010) Alzheimer's disease – donepezil, galantamine, rivastigmine and memantine (review): appraisal consultation document [Online] available from: http://www.nice.org.uk/guidance/index.jsp?action=article&o=51047 accessed 11/10/10

Neale R, Brayne C, Johnson AL (2001) Cognition and survival: an exploration in a large multicentre study of the population aged 65 years and over. *International Journal of Epidemiology* 30(6):1383–1388.

Rogers C (1961) *On Becoming a Person*. Boston: Houghton Mifflin.

Rolland Y, Pillard F, Klapouszczak A *et al.* (2007) Exercise program for nursing home residents with Alzheimer's disease: a one year randomised, controlled trial. *Journal of the American Geriatrics Society* 55(2):158–165.

Sarna R, Thompson R (2008) Admiral nurses' role in a dementia carer's information programme. *Nursing Older People* 20(9):30–34.

Sampson EL, Gould V, Lee D *et al.* (2006) Differences in care received by person with dementias with and without dementia who died during acute hospital admission: a retrospective case note study. *Age and Ageing* 35:187–189.

Scholey KA, Woods B (2003) A series of brief cognitive behavioural therapy interventions with people experiencing both dementia and depression: a description of techniques and common themes. *Clinical Psychology and Psychotherapy* 10:175–185.

Spector A, Thotrgrimsen L, Woods B *et al.* (2003) Efficacy of an evidence based cognitive stimulation therapy programme for people with dementia: randomised control trial. *The British Journal of Psychiatry* 183:248–254.

Stevens J, Killeen M (2006) A randomised controlled trial testing the impact of exercise on cognitive symptoms and disability of residents with dementia. *Contemporary Nurse* 21(1):32–40.

Weatherhead I (2009) *Admiral nurses – still waiting for the promised DH urgent review of anti-psychotics 'the drug of last resort' for people with dementia*. Available from: Medical News Today http://www.medicalnewstoday.com/articles/160718.php Accessed July 2010.

Weina P, Zhao H, Zhishun L *et al.* (2007) Acupuncture for vascular dementia. *Cochrane Database of Systematic Reviews* Issue 2. Art. No.: CD004987. DOI: 10.1002/14651858.CD004987.pub2.

Woods B (1999) The person in dementia care. *Generations* 23(3):35–39.

World Health Organisation (1992) *International Classification of Diseases*. (10th edition). London: WHO.

Yuhas N, McGowan B, Fontaine T *et al.* (2006) Interventions for disruptive symptoms of dementia. *Journal of Psychosocial Nursing* 44(11):35–42.

30
Management of Patients with Epilepsy

Anthony Linklater

INTRODUCTION

Epilepsy is the most common serious chronic neurological condition. Epilepsy is characterised by a tendency to recurrent and unprovoked seizures of cerebral origin. The epileptic seizures themselves arise as a result of a transient disturbance of normal brain activity with abnormal excessive or synchronous discharging of cerebral neurons (Fisher *et al.*, 2005).

INCIDENCE

The overall incidence of epilepsy in the developed world has been found to be around 50 cases per 100,000 people per year (Hauser and Kurland, 1975) with a higher incidence found in those experiencing socioeconomic deprivation (Heaney *et al.*, 2002). The incidence of epilepsy varies with age, with a higher incidence found in childhood and also after the age of 65 years (Hauser *et al.*, 1991).

The prevalence of epilepsy is around 0.5–1% of the population (active epilepsy). It is estimated that there are around 450,000 people living with epilepsy in the UK (Macdonald *et al.*, 2000).

AETIOLOGY

Epilepsy is commonly thought of as a single condition, but there are many different types of epilepsy and various conditions can give rise to it. The specific cause of epilepsy may vary depending on the age at which the condition develops. In adolescents, idiopathic generalised epilepsies such as juvenile myoclonic epilepsy are more common. Most of the epilepsies developing in adulthood are focal epilepsies, with some due to structural lesions and others

arising as a result of head injury. Cerebrovascular disease is the most common cause of epilepsy in people developing the condition after the age of 60 years. For more than half of all adult patients who develop epilepsy, no specific aetiology can be identified although advances in neuroimaging are reducing this number as more focal abnormalities associated with epilepsy can now be identified.

PATHOPHYSIOLOGY

The clinical manifestation of a seizure will depend on the parts of the brain involved. In focal epilepsies, the synchronous discharges that occur during a seizure may begin in a discrete region of cortex and then spread to neighbouring regions. Focal epilepsies arise in the neocortex and limbic structures including the hippocampus and amygdala. Absence epilepsy is thought to arise from the thalamocortical system; the basic mechanisms of other generalised epilepsies are less well understood. Seizures of all types usually occur at unpredictable times and without warning, resulting in brief and stereotyped disturbances of awareness, behaviours, emotion, motor function and or sensation (ILAE, 1993). They interfere with daily life and can result in injury or even death (Hanna *et al.*, 2002).

SEIZURE CLASSIFICATION

Various specific seizure types have been identified and subsequently classified by the International League Against Epilepsy (ILAE, 1981). This system of classification recognises two broad types of epileptic seizures:

- Focal or partial seizures arising from epileptic foci in one region of cortex
- Generalised seizures characterised by discharges beginning diffusely throughout both hemispheres

Neuroscience Nursing: Evidence-Based Practice, 1st Edition.
Edited by Sue Woodward and Ann-Marie Mestecky
© 2011 Blackwell Publishing Ltd

Box 30.1 lists the ILAE classification of epileptic seizures.

Focal seizures

Simple partial seizures

When full awareness is preserved during a focal seizure, the seizure is categorised as a simple partial seizure. Simple partial seizures can occur with motor, somatosensory, autonomic, or psychic signs and symptoms, depending on the area of the cortex in which the seizure occurs. Simple partial seizures originating in the temporal lobe may produce symptoms such as an epigastric rising sensation, déjà or jamais vu, and autonomic changes. During these seizures there may be no visible clinical manifestation. If

the motor cortex is involved, then the seizure will consist of rhythmic motor activity contralateral to the focus.

Complex partial seizures

Complex partial seizures involve areas of the brain involved in determining consciousness such as the neocortex or limbic system. During the seizure there may be a partial or total loss of consciousness. Complex partial seizures may evolve from simple partial seizures or there can be impairment of consciousness from the onset of the seizure. The patient does not normally remember what occurs during the seizure. During these seizures, which usually last for between two and three minutes, automatic behaviours known as automatisms may occur. Automatisms take many forms and can include fumbling, fidgeting, fiddling, chewing, lipsmacking, swallowing, undressing, walking and running, and other repetitive motor actions. There is often a degree of confusion following the seizure and full recovery usually takes place over a period of around ten minutes. Complex partial seizures usually arise in the temporal and frontal lobes and are rarely seen in occipital and parietal lobe epilepsies (Duncan, 2007).

Complex partial seizures of temporal lobe origin

Around 60–70% of focal seizures originate in the temporal lobe and the commonest pathology is hippocampal sclerosis (Duncan, 2007). Hippocampal sclerosis is a condition in which there is atrophy of the hippocampus which can be detected with MRI. Complex partial seizures of temporal lobe origin often have a gradual onset and typically begin with an aura or simple partial seizure. There may be a blank spell with cessation of motor activity before a variety of automatisms occur as outlined above. Automatisms can sometimes persist for a prolonged period and the seizure will usually last for between two and ten minutes. Post-ictal confusion and headache are common.

Complex partial seizures of frontal lobe origin

Around 20 to 30% of partial seizures originate in the frontal lobes. They can be difficult to diagnose as the seizures may quickly spread to involve other areas of the brain changing the clinical presentation (Manford *et al.*, 1996). Complex partial seizures of frontal lobe origin typically have a sudden onset and are usually short in duration with a quick recovery. There may be motor manifestations with turning of the head and eyes and posturing of the limbs. They often occur from sleep and can occur in clusters.

Secondary generalised

The abnormal neuronal activity that underlies focal seizures can spread to involve both hemispheres, giving rise

---

> **Box 30.1　ILAE classification of epileptic seizures**
>
> **Focal (or Partial) Seizures**
> * Simple partial seizures (without impaired consciousness), with:
>   – Motor symptoms
>   – Somatosensory symptoms
>   – Autonomic symptoms
>   – Psychological symptoms
> * Complex partial seizures (with impaired consciousness):
>   – Simple partial onset followed by impaired consciousness
>   – Impaired consciousness at onset
> * Partial seizures evolving into secondarily generalised seizures
>
> **Generalised Seizures (Convulsive or Non-Convulsive)**
> * Absence seizures:
>   – Typical
>   – Atypical
> * Myoclonic seizures
> * Clonic seizures
> * Tonic seizures
> * Tonic clonic seizures
> * Atonic seizures
>
> **Unclassified Seizures**
>
> Source: International League Against Epilepsy, Commission on Classification and Terminology (1981).

to a generalised seizure. When this occurs, the seizure is categorised as being secondarily generalised.

Generalised seizures

Primarily generalised seizures involve widespread cortical involvement of both hemispheres from the beginning of the seizure, and usually a loss of awareness. There is a wide variation in clinical presentation. The ILAE classifies generalised seizures into:

* Absence seizures
* Atypical absence seizures
* Myoclonic seizures
* Clonic seizures
* Tonic seizures
* Tonic clonic seizures and
* Atonic seizures

Absence seizures

These seizures involve a sudden onset of staring with momentary impairment of consciousness which can last up to ten seconds. They often occur in children with childhood absence epilepsy and are a feature of other idiopathic generalised epilepsies (see: Classification of epilepsies). There may also be some mild clonic components.

Atypical absence seizures

These seizures also involve momentary impairment of consciousness but may be of a longer duration than typical absences and feature more pronounced changes in muscle tone. The onset and cessation can be more gradual than typical absence seizures.

Myoclonic seizures

These are characterised by sudden brief jerks often of the arms but they can involve any muscle group. When they involve limbs, they can be severe enough to result in falls. Even if there is no fall, injuries can occur if, for example, hot drinks are spilt.

Tonic seizures

These involve a sudden onset of stiffening of muscles resulting in increased tone often with impaired awareness and falls. A person having a tonic seizure will often fall backwards; injuries are common and can be severe in nature.

Atonic seizures

These seizures involve a sudden loss of muscle tone without warning causing a person to fall to the ground.

Injuries are common and often a person will fall forwards sustaining facial and other injuries.

Tonic clonic seizures

When there is a focal onset and the tonic clonic seizure occurs as a result of secondary generalisation, a simple partial seizure or aura may be experienced, which can serve as a useful warning, enabling the person to maintain their safety by alerting others or by lying down.

If the tonic clonic seizure is primarily generalised, it commences with a tonic phase. During this, the person may cry out as air is expelled from the lungs, the tongue or the inside of the cheek may be bitten and there may also be urinary or faecal incontinence. There may be apnoea secondary to laryngeal spasm. The heart rate and blood pressure will be elevated and there is excessive secretion of saliva. The tonic phase usually lasts between 10 and 20 seconds, followed by a clonic phase of rhythmic jerking of the limbs that is bilateral lasting for a variable duration, but usually less than 90 seconds. There is then a period of unconsciousness that gradually resolves with the individual experiencing a period of confusion. The person usually recovers full consciousness within anything from ten minutes to an hour. Afterwards they may complain of headache and aching muscles.

In recent years, the ILAE has been working towards a new system of classification. It has been argued, for example, that the distinction between focal and generalised seizures is not always immediately apparent and that the distinction between simple and complex partial seizures should be removed. The ILAE has also proposed changes to terminology such as introducing the term 'focal' to replace 'partial' when describing epileptic seizures (Engel, 2001). Some modification to the current 1981 seizure classification is expected as the ILAE views the process of classification as an ongoing dynamic process (Engel, 2006).

CLASSIFICATION OF EPILEPSIES

The ILAE has also developed a system of classification for the various epilepsies and epileptic syndromes (ILAE, 1989). This can allow for treatment decisions to be made appropriate for a particular syndrome and information about the likely prognosis to be discussed. In the current ILAE classification (ILAE, 1989), epileptic syndromes are classified according to whether the epilepsy features seizures with a generalised or focal onset. A second classification is made according to whether the underlying cause of the epilepsy is known. When the cause is known, the epilepsy is referred to as symptomatic. If the cause is not known, the epilepsy is classified as cryptogenic or idio-pathic. Idiopathic epilepsy syndromes consist only of recurrent seizures, and are not associated with identifiable structural brain lesions on MRI or abnormal neurological symptoms inter-ictally. The idiopathic generalised epilep-sies account for around a third of all epilepsies (Koutroumanidis, 2007). Box 30.2 lists the ILAE current classification of epileptic syndromes.

DIAGNOSIS

The diagnosis of epilepsy is usually dependent on a reli-able account of what occurs before, during and after a

---

> ### Box 30.2 Current ILAE classification of epilepsies and epileptic syndromes
>
> *Localisation-related (focal, local, partial) epilepsies and epileptic syndromes*
> - Idiopathic epilepsy with age-related onset:
>   ○ Benign childhood epilepsy with centrotemporal spikes
>   ○ Childhood epilepsy with occipital paroxysms
> - Symptomatic epilepsy e.g. temporal lobe epilepsy
> *Generalised epilepsies and syndromes*
> - Idiopathic epilepsy with age-related onset (listed in order of age at onset):
>   ○ Benign neonatal familial convulsions
>   ○ Benign neonatal non-familial convulsions
>   ○ Benign myoclonic epilepsy in infancy
>   ○ Childhood absence epilepsy
>   ○ Juvenile absence epilepsy
>   ○ Juvenile myoclonic epilepsy
>   ○ Epilepsy with generalised tonic clonic seizures on awakening
> - Other idiopathic epilepsies
> - Idiopathic or symptomatic epilepsy (listed in order of age at onset)
>   ○ West syndrome (infantile spasms)
>   ○ Lennox–Gastaut syndrome
>   ○ Epilepsy with myoclonic–astatic seizures
>   ○ Epilepsy with myoclonic absence seizures
> - Symptomatic epilepsy
> - Non-specific syndromes
>   ○ Early epileptic encephalopathy
>   ○ Early infantile epileptic encephalopathy
> - Specific syndromes (epileptic seizures as a complica-tion of a disease such as phenylketonuria, juvenile Gaucher's disease or Lundborg's progressive myo-clonic epilepsy)

---

seizure, from a witness to the event. The patient may also sometimes be able to recall relevant details. Where pos-sible, attempts are made to ascertain the cause of the epi-lepsy and establish syndromic classification. Investigations such as electroencephalogram (EEG) and MRI are usually undertaken. It is important for patients to understand that having a normal EEG and normal neuroimaging does not exclude epilepsy. This is because some epilepsies, such as idiopathic generalised epilepsies, are associated with normal imaging and a routine EEG is usually recorded for around 20 minutes, which is not always sufficient to capture any inter-ictal abnormalities if present.

Seizure observation/description

A detailed eyewitness account of the events occurring before, during and after a seizure is of great importance in the diagnosis of epilepsy. In the hospital setting, the ability to accurately describe and record the clinical manifestation of seizures is an important skill for nurses to develop. The clinical details of the seizure should be recorded on a seizure chart and the nurse should describe what occurred in detail during the event. In some specialist settings, nurses can be equipped with video cameras to record sei-zures as they occur, with the full informed consent of the person having been obtained in advance. Video records of seizures provided by handheld video cameras often provide invaluable objective data on the nature and sequence of events during a seizure (Samuel and Duncan, 1994). When seizures are not witnessed by nursing or medical person-nel, family members who may have witnessed the event can provide descriptions although these accounts can sometimes be inaccurate and provide misleading informa-tion (Rugg-Gunn *et al.*, 2001). It is also helpful to record the patient's recollection of what occurred before, during and after the seizure. Box 30.3 shows the points to con-sider when compiling a seizure description.

Differential diagnosis

Epilepsy can be a difficult condition to diagnose and the differential diagnoses include syncope, sleep disorders and dissociative seizures. Dissociative seizures, which are sometimes referred to as psychogenic non-epileptic sei-zures (pseudoseizures), are psychologically mediated epi-sodes of altered awareness and or behaviour which can be mistaken for epilepsy and treated with antiepileptic drugs for many years before a correct diagnosis is made. In terms of diagnosis, there is no single feature that dis-tinguishes dissociative seizures from epilepsy but whereas epileptic seizures are brief and stereotyped, dissociative seizures can have a gradual onset and are often prolonged.

Dissociative seizures include attacks of motionless collapse and attacks with motor activity which may wax and wane. The motor activity seen can include thrashing of limbs as opposed to the rhythmic jerking seen in convulsive epileptic seizures, pelvic thrusting movements and back arching.

MEDICAL MANAGEMENT

Antiepileptic drugs (AEDs)

The National Institute for Health and Clinical Excellence (NICE) guideline on the diagnosis and management of the epilepsies generally recommends treatment with an antiepileptic drug (AED) after a second epileptic seizure has occurred (NICE, 2004). Treatment after a single seizure may be considered if there is a high risk of recurrence due to the presence of a structural abnormality that may be responsible for the seizure or if an EEG shows epileptiform abnormalities. With effective management, around 70% of people with epilepsy will have their seizures controlled with AEDs (Sander, 2007). The NICE guideline on the diagnosis and management of epilepsies (2004) suggests that once a decision has been made to start treatment, the choice of AED should be individualised according to the seizure type, epilepsy syndrome, co-medication and co-morbidity, the individual's lifestyle, and the preferences of the individual and their family and/or carers as appropriate.

Until recently, the standard first line drugs used were carbamazepine for focal seizures and sodium valproate for generalised seizures. Over recent years, a number of newer AEDs have been licensed for the treatment of epilepsy. Two recent studies compared the newer drugs with the standard drugs (Marson *et al.*, 2007a,b). The findings suggested that lamotrigine may be preferable over carbamazepine for focal seizures. For generalised seizures, the findings suggested that sodium valproate should still be considered as the first option. However, several new AEDs have since been licensed which were not included in this study including levetiracetam, pregabalin, zonisamide, and lacosamide.

When AEDs are introduced, they are initiated at low doses with gradual increments at regular intervals to therapeutic levels. The aim of AED therapy is to maintain optimal seizure control on one drug if possible with minimal medication related adverse effects. If an AED causes adverse effects, it should be substituted with an alternative AED appropriate for the seizure type. Table 30.1 shows NICE guidance drug options by seizure type (NICE, 2004). Since the NICE guidance was produced pregabalin, zonisamide, and lacosamide have been licensed for the adjunctive treatment of focal seizures and rufinamide has been licensed for the adjunctive treatment of seizures in Lennox–Gastaut syndrome.

Surgery

For people whose epilepsy is not controlled with AEDs, surgery may be an option. Surgery for epilepsy can be categorised into resective and functional.

Some patients with focal epilepsy may be suitable for resective surgery. The aim of resective surgery is to remove an identified epileptogenic zone with the aim of preventing further seizures. Resective surgery is undertaken for lesions such as hippocampal sclerosis, tumours, vascular abnormalities and malformations of cortical development. A randomised controlled trial of surgery for mesial temporal lobe epilepsy found that 64% of those who had resective surgery were free of disabling seizures compared with 8% in the group randomised to continued medical therapy (Wiebe *et al.*, 2001).

Table 30.1 NICE guidance: drug options by seizure type.

Seizure type	First-line drugs	Second-line drugs	Other drugs that may be considered	Drugs to be avoided (may worsen seizures)
Generalised tonic–clonic	Carbamazepine Lamotrigine Sodium valproate Topiramate	Clobazam Levetiracetam Oxcarbazepine	Acetazolamide Clonazepam Phenobarbital Phenytoin Primidone	Tiagabine Vigabatrin
Absence	Ethosuximide Lamotrigine Sodium valproate	Clobazam Clonazepam Topiramate		Carbamazepine Gabapentin Oxcarbazepine Tiagabine Vigabatrin
Myoclonic	Sodium valproate (Topiramate)	Clobazam Clonazepam Lamotrigine Levetiracetam Piracetam Topiramate		Carbamazepine Gabapentin Oxcarbazepine Tiagabine Vigabatrin
Tonic	Lamotrigine Sodium valproate	Clobazam Clonazepam Levetiracetam Topiramate	Acetazolamide Phenobarbital Phenytoin Primidone	Carbamazepine Oxcarbazepine
Atonic	Lamotrigine Sodium valproate	Clobazam Clonazepam Levetiracetam Topiramate	Acetazolamide Phenobarbital Primidone	Carbamazepine Oxcarbazepine Phenytoin
Focal with/ without secondary generalization	Carbamazepine Lamotrigine Oxcarbazepine Sodium valproate Topiramate	Clobazam Gabapentin Levetiracetam Phenytoin Tiagabine	Acetazolamide Clonazepam Phenobarbital Primidone	

Source: National Institute for Health and Clinical Excellence, 2004.

Before resective surgery is undertaken, it must be established that AEDs have failed to achieve seizure control; seizures must be of sufficient frequency and severity to cause difficulties in everyday functioning and the surgery should offer an expected improvement in quality of life. Suitability for resective surgery is established by extensive pre-surgical investigation including:

- Assessment of the clinical course of the seizure semiology
- Neuropsychometry
- Neuroimaging (high resolution MRI)
- Video-EEG telemetry

In some cases further investigations may be required which may include positron emission tomography (PET), single photon emission computed tomography (SPECT), functional MRI and intracranial EEG monitoring (electrocorticography – ECOG), which can localise the seizure focus more accurately. The electrodes can be placed via a burr hole if they are being placed on the surface of the brain (subdural electrodes). A craniotomy is required if the

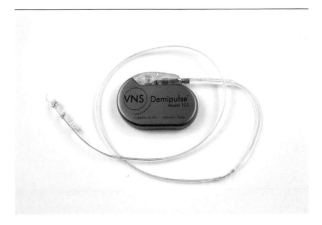

Figure 30.1 Vagal nerve stimulator.
© Cyberonics.

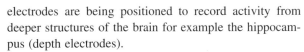

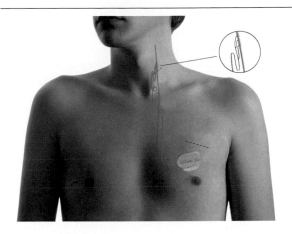

Figure 30.2 Position of vagal nerve stimulator.
© Cyberonics.

electrodes are being positioned to record activity from deeper structures of the brain for example the hippocampus (depth electrodes).

Functional surgical procedures are palliative rather than curative and aim to afford relief through reducing the frequency of seizures or reducing the occurrence of seizure types associated with injury. Functional surgery is considered if resective surgery is not possible, e.g. if the epileptic focus is not surgically amenable or if it is near to cortex associated with language, etc. Corpus callosotomy which disconnects the cerebral hemispheres through surgical division of the corpus callosum is one such procedure which is primarily used for atonic seizures.

Vagus nerve stimulation (VNS) is another functional surgical procedure which is used for drug refractory focal epilepsy with or without secondary generalisation. An electrical pulse generator (Figure 30.1) is implanted under the skin in the left side of the chest which connects to the left vagus nerve in the neck via a lead and electrode as shown in Figure 30.2. The generator is programmed to deliver stimulation at gradually increasing levels through a hand-held computer and programming wand. Extra stimulation can be delivered at the onset of seizures through swiping the device with a magnet with the aim of reducing the duration of the seizure, preventing clusters or quickening recovery times. Although VNS has been found to be an effective and well-tolerated treatment (Privitera *et al.*, 2002), it is extremely rare for seizure freedom to be attained. It is not known exactly how VNS modulates seizure activity. Around a third of patients will have a 50% or better reduction in the frequency of their seizures, a third will have a reduction of less than 50% in seizure frequency and a third

will show no response. Common side-effects include hoarseness, coughing and throat discomfort.

NURSING MANAGEMENT OF SEIZURES

Focal seizures

During a simple partial seizure, the person retains full awareness and may be anxious or upset as a result of the seizure. Giving gentle reassurance can be helpful. During complex partial seizures, the role of the nurse will depend on what occurs during the seizure. As there is at least a partial loss of awareness during a complex partial seizure, the person will not be completely aware of their surroundings and may appear confused. In this situation, it is preferable not to attempt restraint as this may increase confusion and result in an aggressive response. Where necessary the person should be gently guided from dangerous situations and be spoken to in a quiet and calm manner. When the seizure ends, the person should be supervised for the duration of any period of confusion and reoriented to time and place. If tired, they may need to sleep.

Non-convulsive status epilepticus

Status epilepticus is a prolonged seizure of any type (Walker, 2005). Non-convulsive status epilepticus can be difficult to diagnose and patients can present with confusion, personality change and psychosis with little evidence of ongoing seizures. When diagnosis is difficult, an EEG is required. Non-convulsive status epilepticus includes absence status, complex partial status and epilepsia partialis continua which consists of repetitive jerking of groups of muscles in the arm, leg or face. The aim of management is to stop the seizures and to identify and treat the cause.

Tonic clonic seizures

Most tonic clonic seizures are self limiting and do not require any specific medical intervention. The main role of the nurse attending a person having a tonic clonic seizure is to keep the person safe and to reduce the potential for injury by protecting the head and moving hazardous objects out of the immediate area. It is not advisable to attempt to move a person during a tonic clonic seizure unless absolutely necessary in order to maintain their safety. The seizure should be allowed to take its course and the person should not be restrained nor should objects be placed in the mouth as these may damage teeth and/or compromise the airway. If oxygen is available this can be given as there will be an increase in oxygen demand. When the clonic phase of the seizure passes, the person should be positioned in the recovery position and any oral secretions should be wiped away. Suctioning may be necessary if there has been excessive salivation or if there is bleeding from a bitten tongue. The airway should be checked and the person having the seizure should be under close observation until they have fully recovered, which may take some time. If the person is in a confused state, gentle reassurance may be necessary and the person's recovery can be assessed by asking simple questions such as, 'do you know where you are?' When they have recovered enough to be aware of their surroundings, it may be necessary to take steps to reduce embarrassment if the person has been incontinent during the seizure.

Tonic clonic status epilepticus

Tonic clonic seizures do not always resolve spontaneously and can become prolonged, or one seizure can be followed by another in quick succession without a period of recovery in between. When tonic clonic seizures continue in this way for a period of 30 minutes or more, this is known as tonic clonic status epilepticus (Shorvon, 1994), which is a life threatening condition.

Tonic clonic status epilepticus should be treated as a medical emergency as permanent neurological and cognitive impairment may result from delayed treatment. This is because sustained seizure activity increases the energy requirements of the neurones involved by up to 250% (Hickey, 1997). Systemic physiological changes associated with seizures include increased cerebral blood flow with increases in oxygen and glucose delivery to the brain to meet increased demands and to protect neurones against damage. After about 30 minutes these physiological mechanisms fail which leads to cerebral ischaemia and systemic injury. Treatment is indicated as soon as it is clear that the seizure is not resolving spontaneously. In practice this is

assumed when the seizure has persisted for two minutes longer than the usual seizure duration, or five minutes when the usual seizure duration is not known.

A series of progressive stages of tonic clonic status epilepticus are recognised and treatment can be planned accordingly around these stages (Walker and Shorvon, 2007):

Premonitory stage

In most people, the development of tonic clonic status epilepticus will be preceded by a period with more frequent, prolonged or more severe seizures. At this stage, prompt treatment can prevent the development of convulsive status epilepticus. Many patients or their carers carry 'rescue' medication in the form of benzodiazepines such as diazepam or midazolam with a plan to administer them promptly when necessary. The use of rescue medication is discussed later in this chapter.

Early status epilepticus (0–30 minutes)

When rescue medication has not been effective and it is clear that status epilepticus is developing, transfer to hospital for emergency treatment and care is necessary. First line treatment is usually undertaken with benzodiazepines; lorazepam is the preferred drug as it has a longer duration of action. Lorazepam is given intravenously at a dose of 4 mg for adults and this can be repeated after 10 minutes if needed.

Established status epilepticus (30–60/90 minutes)

At this stage, intubation should be considered and the patient should be managed in an intensive care unit. Treatment is usually given in the form of loading with intravenous phenytoin (15–20 mg/kg). Fosphenytoin has recently been licensed and may be used as an alternative; it is as effective as phenytoin and can be administered more rapidly. If seizures continue phenobarbitone is administered intravenously.

Refractory status epilepticus (after 60/90 minutes)

General anaesthesia, artificial mechanical ventilation and continuous monitoring is required at this stage. Prognosis will be much poorer for patients reaching this stage; the longer the duration, the higher the mortality and morbidity.

Nursing management of tonic clonic status epilepticus

Many A&E departments and neuroscience units have protocols in place for the management of tonic clonic status epilepticus which aim to: support the patient's airway, breathing and circulation; stop the seizure by administering intravenous medication, and identify and treat precipitating factors. Possible precipitants include withdrawal of antiepileptic drugs, intercurrent illness, metabolic disturbance and progress of the underlying disease which gives rise to the epilepsy.

Important nursing considerations during tonic clonic status epilepticus are as follows:

- The nurse will need to remain close to the patient at all times with working oxygen and suction available. There should also be an intubation tray available in case the patient requires intubation.
- The patient should be nursed on their side to help maintain a patent airway and prevent aspiration.
- Oxygen should be administered via a non-rebreath bag at 10 l/min (see Chapter 15)
- A safe environment should be maintained at all times and the use of cot sides with padding may be helpful but should be assessed in each case.
- Any seizure activity occurring should be observed and timed which will enable treatment to be given promptly if seizures are prolonged.
- All observed seizures should be documented and accurately described on a seizure chart together with any medication given.
- Administer any medication as prescribed with the aim of terminating seizures (see above). Patients will require cardiac monitoring as arrhythmias are not uncommon following administration of intravenous phenytoin. Also benzodiazepines can cause respiratory depression.
- Monitor and support vital functions. The level of consciousness should be closely monitored as well as respiratory and cardiac function. Blood sugar levels and temperature should be monitored regularly.

SEIZURE MANAGEMENT IN THE HOME

Prompt intervention in potential seizure emergencies is of great importance if the morbidity and mortality risks associated with status epilepticus are to be avoided. In order to minimise the risk of harm, family and carers need to be informed of what to do when a seizure occurs and when to seek urgent medical attention. Because of the dramatic nature of tonic clonic seizures, family members, carers and bystanders may be inclined to seek urgent medical attention every time a seizure occurs. As most seizures are self limiting, hospitalisation is usually not necessary and can result in inconvenience to the patient.

The nurse has an important role in educating family and carers about how to safely manage a seizure, which will include how to administer rescue medication to abort seizures. This is important as early administration of medication by paramedics to stop seizures has been found to be effective at terminating seizures prior to arrival at hospital and also to reduce the risk of being admitted to ITU (Alldredge *et al.*, 2001). This finding suggests that earlier treatment with rescue medication given at home may also be helpful at improving outcome when seizures are prolonged or recurrent (Pellock *et al.*, 2004).

In order to facilitate the administration of rescue medication in the home setting, families and carers need a detailed individualised plan about what medication to give and the circumstances in which it will be required as well as what to do after the medication has been administered (Joint Epilepsy Council, 2005).

Benzodiazepines are often given in the home setting for the purposes of terminating seizures and rectal diazepam has been the most commonly used medication for this purpose (Wilson *et al.*, 2004). However, the administration of rectal diazepam can be problematic as there are issues surrounding the intimate nature of giving medication by the rectal route. It may also be difficult to administer if the person is in a seated position and also during some seizure types. There may also be issues around the absorption of diazepam given rectally if the patient is constipated or if they open their bowels immediately following administration (Alldredge *et al.*, 1995).

In recent years, midazolam given via the buccal route has become available and this has obvious advantages over rectal diazepam; it is no less efficacious than rectal diazepam whilst being easier and less embarrassing to administer (Queally, 2007). The use of buccal midazolam has been limited though as it is not licensed for use in this way. However, its use is advocated by both NICE, for prolonged or continuous seizures, and the Joint Epilepsy Council (JEC), an umbrella group of 22 epilepsy organisations. The JEC has produced guidelines on training standards for the administration of buccal midazolam (JEC, 2005). When given via the buccal route, midazolam is usually given to adults in a dose of 5–10 mg. It is available in liquid form (10 mg in 1 ml). Using a syringe, half of the dose is administered between the lower gums and cheek on one side of the mouth and the remaining liquid between the lower gums and cheek on the other side of the mouth.

INFORMATION PROVISION
Epilepsy specialist nurses (ESNs)

The role of the nurse in epilepsy encompasses a range of activities and is not limited to managing patients during seizures. According to NICE guidance, epilepsy specialist nurses (ESNs) should be an integral part of the network of care of individuals with epilepsy. The key roles of the ESNs are to support both epilepsy specialists and general physicians, to ensure access to community and multi-agency services and to provide information, training and support to the individual, families and carers (NICE, 2004).

The provision of good quality relevant information about the condition is one of the most important roles that the nurse will undertake. Patients' information needs vary according to factors such as their gender, age, social situation and how long they have had the condition. They will require general and individualised information about the condition to enable them to make decisions to minimise the impact of their epilepsy on their lives. The provision of information is best viewed as an ongoing process and patients generally continue to require information at all stages of their lives. Use of information checklists can be helpful in identifying topics for discussion and ensuring that important topics are covered.

Passing information to patients takes time, which may be difficult to facilitate in acute settings and in outpatient departments. In the outpatient clinic setting, longer consultations may be required, which may not be easy to achieve in practice. ESNs can help meet the need for longer consultations to encourage frank and open discussion of important issues as well reviewing clinical issues. By ensuring that information has been understood, the potential for misunderstanding may be reduced. ESNs also are able to offer continuity of care allowing for a rapport to be established and trust to be developed (Scrambler *et al.*, 1996).

Many people with epilepsy will be under the care of a neurologist whom they will see at regular intervals with at least several months between appointments. If problems arise between appointments, it can be difficult to access specialist advice and GPs may not have the level of expertise in epilepsy to be able to resolve some of the difficult issues that may arise. Where they exist, ESNs are able to offer a point of access to the service through telephone or email advice lines and are able to respond to problems with the necessary expertise in a timely manner. In this way, patients can benefit from prompt appropriate advice which may prevent a worsening in their condition with all the potential negative consequences that may result from this (Hosking *et al.*, 2002).

Information needs of patients

The need for information is probably greatest at the point of diagnosis. This is because a diagnosis of epilepsy is often perceived as being life changing as the condition is stigmatising and associated with psychological problems, reduced social standing and employment difficulties (Jacoby *et al.*, 1996). A review of the literature around the information needs of patients with epilepsy identified the need amongst patients for information about almost every aspect of the condition. Patients wanted information about general epilepsy issues, diagnosis and treatment options, medication and adverse effects, seizures and seizure control, prevention of injury, psychological issues, benefits, driving and insurance, employment, prognosis, lifestyle and social issues. They were also found to have counselling needs in relation to anxiety, depression and expressed a need for emotional support (Couldridge *et al.*, 2001).

Employment and driving

Coming to terms with a diagnosis of epilepsy is made more difficult by the restrictions that such a diagnosis places on an individual's life. When there is a risk that seizures may occur, some people may avoid social situations to avoid any embarrassment. Despite legislation such as the Disability Discrimination Act, people with epilepsy do find it harder to find and remain in employment (Jacoby *et al.*, 1996). People with epilepsy are prohibited from driving by DVLA regulations until they have been free of seizures for a period of one year. The exception is, if there is a pattern of seizures arising from sleep only, with no seizures from wakefulness over a three year period. The driving regulations apply after a single seizure, even if the patient has not been diagnosed with epilepsy. It is the responsibility of the patient to inform the DVLA of their seizure activity. Failing to do so and continuing to drive is unlawful, invalidates insurance and poses an obvious safety risk. Health care professionals must inform the patient of their responsibilities and record this discussion in the patient's notes. Not being able to drive causes great difficulties for some people, particularly those in single parent families or those living in rural areas with poor public transport provision.

Mortality associated with epilepsy

People with epilepsy have a mortality rate two to three times higher than the general population (Sander and Bell, 2007). Death can occur as a consequence of seizure related injury, status epilepticus or sudden unexpected death in epilepsy (SUDEP) and is a topic that needs to be discussed sensitively with patients. SUDEP is defined as a sudden, unexpected, non-accidental death in an individual with epilepsy with or without evidence of a seizure having occurred (excluding documented status epilepticus) and where post-mortem does not reveal an anatomical or toxicological cause of death (Nashef, 1997). It is not fully understood why SUDEP occurs, centrally mediated cardiac and respiratory changes associated with seizures have been proposed.

Safety precautions

Information regarding issues such as safety in the home should be discussed. For example, drowning whilst bathing is an important avoidable cause of death in people with epilepsy (Spitz, 1998). Information about safer alternatives such as showering with the plug removed or taking supervised baths could clearly reduce the potential for harm. Where a person does not have access to a shower, a referral for an occupational therapy assessment can be helpful and funds can sometimes be accessed to remedy the situation.

Some patients who may experience seizures whilst they are out and about may find the use of identity cards or jewellery containing information about their condition useful. Although these items do not alleviate anxiety surrounding the unpredictability about when and where a seizure may occur, they do have practical benefit if a person is admitted to hospital as a result of seizures.

Support groups

Some people find it useful to meet with other people with epilepsy to discuss pertinent issues and share their experiences. Local and national support groups can facilitate this and details of such groups should be given to patients.

REDUCING SEIZURE OCCURRENCE

Adherence and concordance

It is essential that patients are made fully aware of the importance of taking antiepileptic medication (AEDs) regularly to prevent seizures from occurring. Poor adherence has been estimated to occur in 30–50% of patients with epilepsy (Leppik, 1990), despite the fact that this is associated with a deterioration in seizure control (Jones *et al.*, 2006) which is a major barrier to achieving optimal health (Eraker *et al.*, 1984)

Even when patients are aware of the importance of taking AEDs regularly, there are a number of factors which may influence whether or not a person is compliant. Patients with epilepsy are at increased risk of memory impairments (Thompson and O'Toole, 2007) which can interfere with remembering medication. Others may not take their medication because of concerns regarding adverse effects of the medication and some women may decide not to take their medication if they are considering pregnancy, due to concerns about teratogenicity (see: Factors affecting women/Pregnancy).

Taking medication becomes complicated when there are too many doses per day or if doses are changed at each outpatient visit, as is often the case in people with refractory epilepsy. If an AED is initiated in a busy A&E department whilst a patient is in a confused post-ictal state, explanations about taking AEDs may not be given or may not be retained by the patient following the acute stage. Subsequent abrupt withdrawal of the AED may later precipitate seizures leading to further acute admission to hospital.

The nurse has a crucial role in improving adherence through discussion and education and by making the patient aware of the consequences of not taking their medication as prescribed. When memory problems are present the use of pill boxes can be helpful to a limited extent. These are typically filled with a week's supply of AEDs and they can help to provide a visual reminder to take medication. Other interventions which can be considered include: scheduling medication to be taken once or twice daily, using mobile phone alarms or other alarm systems to remind that medication is due, fitting medication into the daily routine, and keeping medication in places where it is likely to be noticed such as with a toothbrush or teabags. Treatment plans can also be reinforced with written instruction.

Taking a collaborative approach through a process of concordance and involving patients in the decision making process with regards to their medication may also be helpful. The process of concordance changes the focus from whether or not patients take their medicines and instead focuses on a shared approach to the decision making process (Weiss and Britten, 2003). Whilst not all patients will want to be involved in discussions concerning their treatment and care, others do value the opportunity to be involved in making these decisions. Patients can also be assisted to develop their knowledge about epilepsy and encouraged to take greater responsibility for its management through initiatives such as the expert patient programme (DH, 2001).

Precipitating factors

Even when patients are compliant, there may be situations or lifestyle factors that make seizures more likely. Making patients aware of these factors allows the patient to make some alterations to their life with the aim of reducing seizures. Factors which may potentially precipitate seizures include:

- Sleep deprivation/excessive somnolence
- Fatigue
- Excessive alcohol
- Psychological stress and anxiety
- Menstrual cycle
- Systemic infection
- Poor concordance with AEDs
- Illicit drug use
- Overhydration
- Photosensitivity

When seizures occur, it is important to elicit whether they have been precipitated by potentially avoidable precipitants, as intervention may then be planned to moderate lifestyle factors before adjusting treatment.

Factors affecting women

Contraception

Women need to be aware that some AEDs impair the efficacy of the combined oral contraceptive pill (OCP) by inducing hepatic enzymes which speed up the metabolism of the oestrogen component of the OCP. These AEDs include: carbamazepine, oxcarbazepine, phenytoin, phenobarbitone, primidone and topiramate. In order to achieve effective contraception, women taking these medications will require an OCP containing at least 50 μg oestrogen. The presence of breakthrough bleeding mid-cycle may indicate that effective contraception has not been achieved although some women do not bleed mid-cycle and remain at risk of contraceptive failure.

Because there is a higher risk of contraceptive failure in women taking enzyme-inducing AEDs, it is recommended that additional barrier methods of contraception should be discussed (NICE, 2004). Other forms of contraception also affected by enzyme-inducing AEDs and not recommended for women taking these drugs include: the progesterone only pill and the three yearly progesterone implant. If the morning after pill (levonogestrel) is required a higher first dose of 1500 μg should be taken with the usual second dose at 12 hours of 750 μg (Guillebaud, 2004).The depot injection (e.g. Depot Provera) is not affected by enzyme-inducing AEDs, although a shorter interval between injections of 10 weeks is recommended.

Menstruation

In some women seizures cluster around the time of menstruation. This is known as catamenial epilepsy. In order to identify catamenial epilepsy, women with epilepsy should be supported to accurately document seizures as they occur, in a diary together with details of their men-

strual cycle. If catamenial epilepsy is identified, an additional AED such as clobazam taken peri-menstrually for several days may have a positive effect on seizures at this time.

Pregnancy

Whilst the majority of women with epilepsy will have a normal pregnancy and delivery with an unchanged seizure frequency and a higher than 90% chance of a healthy baby, pregnancies in women with epilepsy are considered high risk, requiring careful management by medical and obstetric services (Craig, 2007).

Young women should be reminded at regular intervals that, in advance of attempting to become pregnant, their AEDs should be reviewed as they have the potential to cause abnormalities in the unborn baby. Women should be aware that their risk of major congenital abnormality increases to two to three times the background risk of the general population of 1–2% (Morrow *et al.*, 2006). Polytherapy carries a greater risk of major congenital malformation than monotherapy and some AEDs have a lower risk profile than others.

There are particular concerns around the use of sodium valproate in pregnancy due to the higher risk of foetal abnormality and also due to emerging evidence that children born to mothers taking sodium valporate will have additional learning support needs at school (Adab *et al.*, 2004). Pregnant women with epilepsy should be encouraged to register with the UK Epilepsy and Pregnancy Register which continues to collect data on the outcome of pregnancies.

Some women may decide to temporarily discontinue their AEDs during the first trimester to minimise the risk to their foetus. Women in this situation should be counselled about the increased risk of harm to both themselves and their foetus which may result from subsequent worsening in seizure control.

Folic acid at a dose of 5 mg daily is recommended for all women with epilepsy to be taken pre-conceptually and until at least the end of the first trimester as it is thought to be protective against neural tube defects (NICE, 2004).

Delivery and post-partum management

During delivery and the immediate post-partum period the risk of seizures may be increased due to sleep deprivation and stress. Breastfeeding is encouraged for women with epilepsy as for any other woman. Small amounts of AEDs may be present in breast milk but these are thought to be less than the infant received *in utero* and are not believed to be harmful in the short term. If a woman has poorly controlled epilepsy there is a risk to the infant of harm resulting from seizures; for example, the infant may be dropped as a result of a seizure. Women must therefore be advised on safe handling, bathing and feeding.

Epilepsy: patient perspective

I have learnt to treat epilepsy like a demanding house-guest. He can be highly unpleasant and lash out unexpectedly, but for most of the time we grumble along together. When he hits out at me, I am always confused. I am often traumatised and invariably tired. I have a headache. I feel jittery and on edge. I need to stop and rest. Such episodes are horrid.

At the same time, this cantankerous old man and I have got used to living together and we have worked out different ways of relating to each other. His short sharp attacks come out of the blue and so I learn to appreciate periods of calm. With him in constant hovering attendance life will never be dulled enough to take the day-to-day rhythm of living for granted. A day without an epileptic act of violence is a gift.

I have the experience of piecing together my psyche once my equilibrium has been fractured. We are 'fearfully and wonderfully' made and this can be terrifying to do but marvellous to realise. I look at my wife and move from not knowing who she is to reconnecting with the fact that she is the woman I love. These are glimpses into life that are denied to people without epilepsy. Don't relegate my experience as deserving only of therapy or medical intervention. It is sometimes I who am the lucky one.

46-year-old man with temporal lobe epilepsy since the age of 30.

SUMMARY

Epilepsy is a common condition which affects not only the physical health of people with the condition but their psychological well-being too. Nurses can make a major contribution to the care of people with epilepsy in both inpatient and outpatient settings. In order to meet the needs of patients, nurses will need familiarity with the condition and to be aware of the various seizure types and how they are managed, as well as having an understanding of how the condition itself is treated.

The education of people with epilepsy and the provision of relevant information at appropriate times is just as important as managing seizure situations. Information can empower people with epilepsy and their significant others to participate in the management of their condition. This can lead to better outcomes through improved adherence and through the early administration of rescue medication by a trained carer which can prevent hospitalisation and the development of status epilepticus.

Whilst epilepsy may be a difficult condition for people to live with for various reasons, nurses can contribute in a meaningful way to help alleviate negative effects on daily life and allow people with the condition to achieve better outcomes.

REFERENCES

Adab N, Kini U, Vinten J *et al.* (2004) The longer term outcome of children born to mothers with epilepsy. *Journal of Neurology, Neurosurgery and Psychiatry* 75:1575–1583.

Alldredge BK, Gelb AM, Isaacs SM *et al.* (2001) A comparison of lorazepam, diazepam and placebo for the treatment of out of hospital status epilepticus. *New England Journal of Medicine* 345:631–637.

Alldredge BK, Wall DB, Ferriero DM (1995) Effect of prehospital treatment on the outcome of status epilepticus in children. *Paediatric Neurology* 12:213–216.

Couldridge L, Kendall S, March A (2001) A systematic overview – a decade of research. The information and counselling needs of people with epilepsy. *Seizure* 10:605–614.

Craig JJ (2007) Epilepsy and women. In: JW Sander, MC Walker, JE Smalls (eds). *Epilepsy 2007: From Cell to Community – a practical guide to epilepsy*. Crowborough: Meritus Communications.

Department of Health (2001) *The Expert Patient: a new approach to chronic disease management for the 21st century*. London: DH.

Duncan JS (2007) Temporal lobe epilepsy. In: JW Sander, MC Walker, JE Smalls (eds). *Epilepsy 2007: From Cell to Community – a practical guide to epilepsy*. Crowborough: Meritus Communications.

Engel J Jr (2001) A proposed diagnostic scheme for people with epileptic seizures and with epilepsy: Report of the ILAE Task Force on Classification and Terminology. *Epilepsia* 42:796–803.

Engel J (2006) Report of the ILAE Classification Core Group. *Epilepsia* 47(9):1558–1568.

Eraker SA, Kirscht JP, Becker MH (1984) Understanding and improving patient compliance. *Annals of Internal Medicine* 100(2):258–268.

Fisher RS, van Emde Boas W, Blume W *et al.* (2005) Epileptic seizures and epilepsy. Definitions proposed by the International League Against Epilepsy (ILAE) and the International Bureau for Epilepsy (IBE). *Epilepsia* 46:470–472.

Guillebaud J (2004). *Contraception: your questions answered.* (4th edition). Edinburgh: Churchill Livingstone.

Hanna NJ, Black M, Sander JW *et al.* (2002) *The National Sentinel Clinical Audit of Epilepsy-Related Death: Epilepsy–death in the shadows.* London: The Stationery Office.

Hauser WA, Kurland LT (1975) The epidemiology of epilepsy in Rochester, Minnesota, 1935 through 1967. *Epilepsia* 16(1):1–66.

Hauser WA, Annegers JF, Kurland LT (1991) Prevalence of epilepsy in Rochester, Minnesota: 1940–1980. *Epilepsia* 32(4):429–445.

Heaney DC, Macdonald BK, Everitt A *et al.* (2002) Socioeconomic variation in incidence of epilepsy: prospective community based study in south east England. *British Medical Journal* 235(7371):1013–1016.

Hickey J (1997) *The Clinical Practice of Neurological and Neurosurgical Nursing* (4th edition). Philadelphia: Lippincott-Raven Publishers.

Hosking PG, Duncan JS, Sander JW (2002) The epilepsy nurse specialist at a tertiary care hospital – improving the interface between primary and tertiary care. *Seizure* 11(8):494–499.

International League Against Epilepsy, Commission on Classification and Terminology (1981) Proposal for revised clinical and electroencephalographic classification of epileptic seizures. *Epilepsia* 22:489–501.

International League Against Epilepsy, Commission on Classification and Terminology (1989) Proposal for revised classification of epilepsies and epileptic syndromes. *Epilepsia*, 30:389–399.

International League Against Epilepsy, Commission on Epidemiology and Prognosis (1993) Guidelines for epidemiologic studies on epilepsy. *Epilepsia* 34:592–596.

Jacoby A, Baker GA, Steen N *et al.* (1996) The clinical course of epilepsy and its psychosocial correlates: findings from a UK community study. *Epilepsia* 37:148–161.

Joint Epilepsy Council (2005) *A Guideline on Training Standards for the Administration of Buccal Midazolam.* Leeds: JEC.

Jones RM, Butler JA, Thomas VA *et al.* (2006) Adherence to treatment in patients with epilepsy: associations with seizure control and illness beliefs. *Seizure* 15(7):504–508.

Koutroumanidis M (2007) Idiopathic generalised epilepsies. In: JW Sander, MC Walker, JE Smalls. (eds). *Epilepsy 2007: From Cell to Community – a practical guide to epilepsy.* Crowborough: Meritus Communications.

Leppik E (1990) How to get patients with epilepsy to take their medication: The problem of noncompliance. *Postgraduate Medicine* 88:253–256.

Macdonald BK, Cockerell OC, Sander JW, Shorvon SD (2000) The incidence and lifetime prevalence of neurological disorders in a prospective community-based study in the UK. *Brain* 123(4):665–676.

Manford M, Fish DR, Shorvon SD (1996) An analysis of clinical seizure patterns and their localising value in frontal and temporal lobe epilepsies. *Brain* 119:17–40.

Marson AG, Al-Kharusi AM, Alwaidh M *et al.* (2007a) on behalf of the SANAD Study Group. The SANAD study of effectiveness of carbamazepine, gabapentin, lamotrigine, oxcarbazepine, or topiramate for treatment of partial epilepsy: an unblinded randomized controlled trial. *Lancet* 369:1000–1015.

Marson AG, Al-Kharusi AM, Alwaidh M *et al.* (2007b) on behalf of the SANAD Study Group. The SANAD study of effectiveness of valproate, lamotrigine, or topiramate for generalised and unclassifiable epilepsy: an unblinded randomised controlled trial. *Lancet* 369:1016–1026.

Morrow J, Russell A, Guthrie E *et al.* (2006) Malformation risks of antiepileptic drugs in pregnancy: a prospective study from the UK Epilepsy and Pregnancy Register. *Journal of Neurology, Neurosurgery and Psychiatry* 77:193–198.

Nashef L (1997) Sudden unexpected death in epilepsy: terminology and definitions. *Epilepsia* 38:S6–S8.

National Institute for Health and Clinical Excellence (2004) *The Diagnosis and Management of the Epilepsies in Adults and Children in Primary and Secondary Care.* London: NICE. Available from: http://www.nice.org.uk/nicemedia/pdf/CG020NICEguideline.pdf Accessed July 2010.

Pellock JM, Mamarou A, De Lorenzon R (2004) Time to treatment in prolonged seizure episodes. *Epilepsy and Behaviour* 5:192–196.

Privitera MD, Welty TE, Ficker DM *et al.* (2002) Vagus nerve stimulation for partial seizures. *Cochrane Database*, CD002896.

Queally C (2007) The use of buccal midazolam in emergency seizure management in epilepsy. *British Journal of Neuroscience Nursing* 3(6):272–275.

Rugg-Gunn FJ, Harrison NA, Duncan JS (2001) Evaluation of the accuracy of seizure descriptions by the relatives of patients with epilepsy. *Epilepsy Research* 43:193–199.

Samuel D, Duncan JS (1994) Use of the hand held video camcorder in the evaluation of seizures. *Journal of Neurology, Neurosurgery and Psychiatry* 57:1417–1418.

Sander JW (2007) The prognosis of epilepsy. In JW Sander, MC Walker, JE Smalls (eds). *Epilepsy 2007: From Cell to Community – a practical guide to epilepsy.* Crowborough: Meritus Communications.

Sander JW, Bell GS (2007) The mortality of epilepsy. In: JW Sander, MC Walker, JE Smalls (eds). *Epilepsy 2007: From Cell to Community – a practical guide to epilepsy.* Crowborough: Meritus Communications.

Scrambler A, Scrambler G, Ridsale L *et al.* (1996) Towards an evaluation of the effectiveness of an epilepsy nurse in primary care. *Seizure* 5:255–258.

Shorvon SD (1994) *Status Epilepticus: its clinical features and treatment in children and adults.* Cambridge: Cambridge University Press.

Spitz MC (1998) Injuries and death as a consequence of seizures in people with epilepsy. *Epilepsia* 39:904–907.

Thompson P, O'Toole A (2007) Psychosocial outcome. In: JW Sander, MC Walker, JE Smalls (eds). *Epilepsy 2007: From Cell to Community – a practical guide to epilepsy.* Crowborough: Meritus Communications.

Walker MC (2005) Status epilepticus: an evidence based guide. *British Medical Journal* 331:673–677.

Walker MC, Shorvon SD (2007) Treatment of tonic clonic status epilepticus. In: JW Sander, MC Walker, JE Smalls (eds). *Epilepsy 2007: From Cell to Community – a practical guide to epilepsy.* Crowborough: Meritus Communications.

Weiss M, Britten N (2003) Concordance. *The Pharmaceutical Journal* 271(7270):493.

Wiebe S, Blume WT, Girvin JP *et al.* (2001) A randomised controlled trial of surgery for temporal lobe epilepsy. *New England Journal of Medicine* 345:311–318.

Wilson MT, Macleod S, O'Regan ME (2004) Nasal/buccal midazolam use in the community. *Archives of Disease in Childhood* 89:50–51.

31
Management of Patients with Myasthenia Gravis

Saiju Jacob

INTRODUCTION

Myasthenia gravis (MG) is the most common autoimmune disease affecting the neuromuscular junction, and causes painless weakness of voluntary muscle. The muscle is 'fatiguable' (i.e. it gets worse with increasing effort) and symptoms are usually due to antibodies against a post-synaptic muscle membrane protein, the acetylcholine receptor (AChR).

EPIDEMIOLOGY

Myasthenia gravis affects 80–125 patients per million population (Mantegazza *et al.*, 2003). With increasing awareness and improved diagnosis and survival, it is apparently becoming more common, especially in the elderly. Without treatment, MG has a spontaneous remission rate of about 5% per annum and the 10-year mortality rate is approximately 20–30% (Oosterhuis, 1989). MG can affect any age group, from infants to the elderly.

AETIOLOGY

Acetylcholine (ACh) is the key neurotransmitter at the neuromuscular junction (NMJ), (Figure 31.1). A nerve impulse triggers the release of ACh, which binds to the nicotinyl acetylcholine receptor (nAChR) on the muscle membrane, triggering the muscle contraction. The spare ACh is then destroyed by ACh esterase (AChE), which is present in the synaptic space.

Over 80% of patients with clinically typical generalised MG, and 50% of those with isolated ocular muscle involve-

Neuroscience Nursing: Evidence-Based Practice, 1st Edition.
Edited by Sue Woodward and Ann-Marie Mestecky
© 2011 Blackwell Publishing Ltd

ment (ocular myasthenia), have circulating auto-antibodies directed against the nAChR (AChR-Ab$^+$ MG) (Lindstrom *et al.*, 1976; Vincent and Newsom-Davis, 1985). Another 5–10% of the generalised MG (but very rarely the purely ocular form) have antibodies directed against muscle specific kinase (MuSK) (MuSK-Ab$^+$ MG) (Hoch *et al.*, 2001). MuSK is essential for the organisation and maintenance of the neuromuscular junction. The remaining patients are referred to as having seronegative myasthenia.

PATHOPHYSIOLOGY

The AChR antibodies are thought to cause: AChR degradation, complement mediated damage to the post-synaptic membrane, and reduced AChR numbers (Vincent, 2002). These mechanisms interfere with the effective triggering of muscle contraction and thereby cause muscle weakness, especially after prolonged use (hence the fatiguable weakness). The precise pathophysiological mechanism of MuSK-Abs is still unclear.

The thymus appears to have an important role in the pathogenesis of AChR-Ab$^+$ MG. In patients who present before the age of 40 years (early-onset disease) the thymus appears hyperplastic, whilst in older onset disease it is usually normal-for-age. In 10% of patients with AChR-Ab$^+$ MG, a thymoma may be present (Oosterhuis, 1989).

OTHER MYASTHENIC SYNDROMES

Lambert Eaton myasthenic syndrome (LEMS) is a rare neurological disease caused by antibodies against the voltage-gated calcium channels in the pre-synaptic membrane. The patients have predominant proximal limb muscle and autonomic involvement. Almost half of the patients may have an underlying lung tumour.

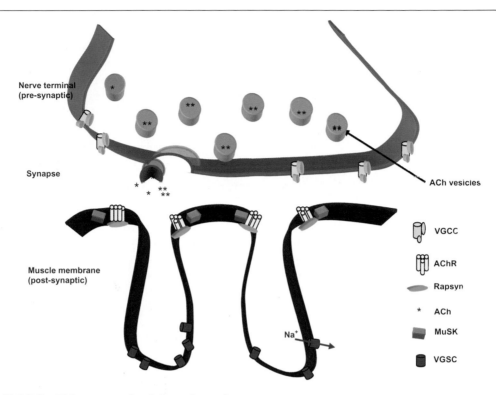

VGCC – Voltage gated calcium channel

AChR – Acetycholine receptor

Rapsyn – Cytoplasmic membrane-associated protein

ACh – Acetylcholine

MuSK – Muscle Specific Kinase

VGSC – Voltage gated sodium channel

Figure 31.1 Schematic representation of the neuromuscular junction.

Mutations affecting the number and structure of the neuromuscular proteins can cause congenital myasthenic syndromes. Infants may present with hypotonia and respiratory weakness. Some patients may not develop symptoms until childhood or even adult life, when they may present with symptoms very similar to MG.

CLINICAL FEATURES OF MYASTHENIA GRAVIS

Myasthenia gravis most commonly affects the ocular muscles, which results in drooping of eyelids (ptosis) and double vision (diplopia). In the majority of patients this is often the first manifestation and may go unnoticed (especially ptosis) for several months. Some patients never develop symptoms and signs elsewhere and are known to

have ocular myasthenia. Others develop generalised myasthenia with facial weakness (some patients complain of 'lack of smile'), swallowing, breathing and speech difficulties and weakness of the arms and legs. MuSK-Ab[+] patients tend to have predominant ocular, facial and bulbar involvement (Evoli *et al.*, 2003; Sanders *et al.*, 2003). Muscles develop weakness after sustained and prolonged use (fatiguability), which is the hall mark of myasthenia. Patients are often tested before and after a brief amount of muscle exertion to test for fatiguability.

It is important to understand that the symptoms fluctuate from time to time, often resulting in 'good' and 'bad' days. Symptoms could be exacerbated by a variety of factors, sometimes leading on to myasthenic crisis, e.g. infection, emotional and physical stress, a number of antibiotics and other medications. Medications for myasthenia can also exacerbate symptoms, i.e. the withdrawal of cholinesterase inhibitors (see: Myasthenic crisis; Cholinergic crisis) or the sudden initiation of cholinesterase inhibitors or steroids.

DIAGNOSIS

If MG is suspected by an experienced clinician, it may be confirmed by testing for AChR-Ab, which is positive in over 85% of patients. Patients suspected to have MG, but are negative for AChR-Ab should have their MuSK-Ab tested. In expert hands, detailed electromyographic (EMG) assessment, including repetitive nerve stimulation (RNS) and single fibre electromyography (SF-EMG), have high sensitivity. A tensilon test will often be performed. Edrophonium (Tensilon®) is a short-acting cholinesterase inhibitor which can be given intravenously to assess improvement in muscle strength. By inhibiting ACh esterase, more Ach will be available to bind to receptors, which will temporarily improve muscle strength. Significant objective improvement (e.g. ptosis or extra-ocular muscle weakness) is very characteristic of myasthenia. The heart rate may also slow temporarily, so resuscitation equipment and atropine should be readily available. When MG is suspected, a thymoma should be excluded by appropriate imaging of the mediastinum.

MEDICAL MANAGEMENT

Therapies used in myasthenia are summarised in Table 31.1.

Symptomatic relief

Patients are usually commenced on pyridostigmine (Mestinon®) which produces symptomatic relief by improving neuromuscular transmission, but does not treat the underlying autoimmune pathology. By inhibiting cholinesterase, it prolongs the lifetime of any ACh released and gives it a better chance of binding to the post-synaptic receptor. The maximum dosage of pyridostigmine should not exceed 450 mg daily, most patients requiring around 180 mg daily on average. Side-effects like abdominal cramps, diarrhoea, increased respiratory secretions and sweating are due to the muscarinic overactivity of ACh (see Chapter 5 for related physiology), but can be minimised by adding propantheline (antimuscurinic agent).

Immunosuppression

Since MG is an autoimmune disease, most patients (except those with very mild symptoms) would require some form of immunosuppression. Corticosteroids are the initial choice. The initial starting dose of prednisolone is usually 10–20 mg in the morning on alternate days, increased by 5–10 mg every week until the patient is on 1.5 mg/kg (or 100 mg, whichever is smaller) on alternate days, or until clinical remission. Once clinical remission is achieved, the dose is gradually reduced to the minimal maintenance level. The drug is usually given in the morning to mimic the body's natural cortisol production. Many experts use alternate day therapy to reduce the side-effects, and to minimise adrenal suppression. In some patients with generalised, bulbar or respiratory muscle weakness, steroids can increase the myasthenic weakness over the first one to two weeks, especially at high doses (Skeie *et al.*, 2006). For this reason, some specialists titrate steroid therapy over two to three weeks as an in-patient.

Commonly used immunosuppressants are summarised in Table 31.1. It should be noted that azathioprine does not achieve its full therapeutic benefits for at least 6 (often 12) months, so it is best started early, very soon after prednisolone. Hepatic failure and bone marrow suppression are amongst the possible adverse effects of immunsuppressive drugs which need to be monitored regularly (see Table 31.1).

Intravenous immunoglobulins (IVIg)

Acute exacerbations of myasthenia have been successfully and safely treated with IVIg (Gajdos *et al.*, 1997; Illa, 2005), which is thought to have a non-specific suppressive effect on the immune system. The usual dose is 0.4 g/kg/day for five days, but it can also be given as 1 g/kg/day for two days. The improvement, which may commence within a week or two, normally lasts only 6–12 weeks, and patients usually need oral maintenance immunosuppression afterwards.

Since IVIg is derived from pooled human plasma, there is a theoretical risk of transmission of blood-borne infections; though with strict screening, the risk is very low. Common complications include fever, chills, rigor, headache and skin rash. Some patients develop renal failure, so renal function has to be closely monitored. Anaphylaxis can usually be prevented by administering a small and slow test dose of IVIg prior to the main infusion. Because it increases the recipient's IgG concentration, very occasionally patients develop haemolysis, neutropenia or a rise in plasma viscosity (which may cause thrombotic complications).

Plasma exchange

Where facilities are available, plasma exchange is an extremely useful technique to treat myasthenic crisis or

Table 31.1 Therapies used in myasthenia gravis and related disorders.

Therapy	Usual adult oral dose	Common side-effects	Cautions/monitoring
Pyridostigmine	60–360 mg/day in 3–6 divided doses	Diarrhoea, abdominal cramps, nausea, increased salivation, bladder or bowel urgency	Asthma, recent MI, bradycardias
Corticosteroids	10 mg on alternate days increased by 5–10 mg/week, if necessary, up to 1.5 mg/kg or 100 mg on alternate days, or until clinical remission, whichever is earlier	Short term: sleep disturbance, mood changes, acne, weight gain, blurred vision, dyspepsia Long term: Peptic ulceration, osteoporosis, proximal myopathy, fluid retention, weight gain, diabetes mellitus and increased susceptibility to infections	Periodic bone density scans (Add bisphosphonates, vitamin D and calcium for bone protection, and proton pump inhibitors for gastric protection)
3,4 Diaminopyridine	10 mg 4 times/day increasing to a maximum of 20 mg 4–5 times/day	Peri-oral and distal paraesthesia (high doses rarely cause seizures)	Used only under specialist prescription
Azathioprine	Usually started at 25 mg/day gradually increased by 25–50 mg/week up to 2–2.5 mg/kg daily. May require up to 6–12 months for therapeutic effect	Nausea, vomiting, bone marrow suppression and liver dysfunction, late risk of cancer	Regular monitoring of full blood count and liver function (weekly for first 2 months and 3 monthly if blood results are stable)
Mycophenolate mofetil	1 g bd	Dyspepsia and bone marrow suppression. Late risk of cancer	Regular monitoring of blood pressure, full blood count, creatinine and liver function (weekly for first month, fortnightly for next 2 months and monthly thereafter)
Ciclosporin	Start at 25 mg twice daily increased by 50 mg every three days. Typically 2.5 mg/kg/day	Nausea, vomiting, excess body hair, hypertension and renal dysfunction. Late risk of cancer	Monitor renal function and blood pressure Some centres monitor blood levels
Tacrolimus	50 μg/kg/day. Trough level to be maintained at 5–10 ng/ml	Nausea, vomiting, hypertension, bone marrow suppression, glucose intolerance, renal and hepatic dysfunction. Late risk of cancer	Regular monitoring of full blood count, blood pressure, renal and liver function. Blood tacrolimus levels to be monitored regularly to adjust the dose

Table 31.1 *Continued*

Therapy	Usual adult oral dose	Common side-effects	Cautions/monitoring
Methotrexate	7.5 mg/week titrated up to a maximum of 20 mg/week as per response and side-effects	Nausea, vomiting, mouth ulcers, bone marrow suppression, respiratory and hepatic complications	Chest x-ray prior to starting treatment. Regular monitoring of full blood count and liver function (weekly for first 2 months and then 3 monthly) Add folic acid 5 mg weekly to prevent bone marrow suppression and GI side-effects
Cyclophosphamide	1–3 mg/kg/day	Nausea, vomiting, diarrhoea, fatigue, cystitis, haematuria, bone marrow suppression	Regular monitoring of full blood count, liver function and urine dip-stick for haematuria (weekly for first month, fortnightly for next 2 months and monthly thereafter)

severe exacerbation. Using venous access and a blood cell separating machine, the patient's plasma containing the antibodies is removed and replaced with either human albumin solution or fresh frozen plasma. Traditionally 2–3 litres of plasma (usually 5% of the body weight in litres) is exchanged daily or on alternate days for five sessions. Plasma exchange has been shown to be better (Stricker *et al.*, 1993) or comparable with IV immunoglobulins (Gajdos *et al.*, 1997) for patients in myasthenic crisis. The onset of improvement is quicker than with IVIg (often within a day or two) but, like IVIg, the effect is transient. There is little argument of the short-term benefit of plasma exchange (Gajdos *et al.*, 2002), but its long-term cumulative benefits are less promising (Newsom-Davis *et al.*, 1979).

Contraindications for plasma exchange include: severe sepsis, haemodynamic instability or abnormalities in haemostasis. Complications include transfusion reactions, catheter related venous thromboses, infection, bleeding, hypotension, cardiac arrhythmias, pneumothorax (when jugular venous access used), muscle cramps and paraesthesias.

Thymectomy

Thymectomy is usually recommended for patients with mild to moderate generalised AChR-Ab⁺ MG with onset before age 45 (Molnar and Szobor, 1990; Sanders and Scoppetta, 1994). Most post-operative complications are of pulmonary origin, the commonest being haemothorax and infections. The benefits of thymectomy are still not fully proven, but many European neurologists believe that, subsequently, the MG goes into remission in approximately 25% of patients, improves in another 50% and is unaffected in the final 25%. When a thymoma is suspected, thymectomy is indicated to prevent spread, but it rarely improves the myasthenia significantly (Crucitti *et al.*,1992; Masaoka *et al.*, 1996).

MYASTHENIC CRISIS

Myasthenic crisis is a medical emergency defined as severe muscle weakness leading to respiratory failure, requiring airway protection or ventilatory support (Berrouschot *et al.*, 1997). It affects 12–16% of myasthenia patients, usually within two to three years after diagnosis (Cohen and Younger, 1981; Thomas *et al.*, 1997), and especially in those with anti-MuSK antibodies. Some patients have multiple crises over the years, but this fortunately is rare.

Very rarely, myasthenic crisis could be the presenting manifestation of MG. Patients may have a history of increasing muscle weakness (e.g. double vision or swallowing difficulties) in the build-up to their current presentation. Tachypnoea, intercostal indrawing and nasal flaring may be early signs, although not necessarily in all patients. Subsequently there is reduced chest expansion and quieter breath sounds on auscultation, tachycardia and rise in arterial blood pressure.

In patients with myasthenia, the ventilation and perfusion capacity of the lungs are usually intact, so the oxygen saturation and arterial blood gases (ABG) are normal until quite late in the crisis. This is extremely important in an acute setting, since emergency physicians and nurses could be falsely reassured by a normal ABG or pulse oximeter reading. Regular assessments of vital capacity are essential to detect falling lung capacity (see: Nursing management). Fall in arterial oxygen saturation (PaO_2) and a rise in carbon dioxide ($PaCO_2$) with subsequent cyanosis occur very late into the crisis. Bulbar muscle weakness causes dysphagia, pooling of secretions and a significant risk of aspiration. A useful predictor of bulbar weakness is the development of neck flexor weakness (assessed by pushing the forehead against resistance applied by the examiner's hand). For patients already on the ward, subtle changes in speech, facial expression, ptosis and reduction in eye movements can be additional valuable warning signs. Although apprehension and fear are relatively common, weakness of facial muscles could mask the expression of these emotions.

CHOLINERGIC CRISIS

Cholinergic crisis occurs due to excess cholinesterase inhibitor medication and it can be confused with a myasthenic crisis. Symptoms and signs of cholinergic over activity (Hetherington and Losek, 2005) (sweating, lacrimation, salivation, diarrhoea, urinary incontinence, bradycardia or bronchospasm) usually distinguish this from myasthenic crisis (Jacob *et al.*, 2007).

Myasthenic crisis and cholinergic crisis require intensive respiratory management, preferably in an intensive care facility (Figure 31.2) (Jacob *et al.*, 2007).

NURSING MANAGEMENT

Patients suspected of having MG warrant referral to a neuroscience unit for specialist management. A detailed nursing assessment includes taking a full history to highlight any pre-existing problems and other medical conditions that may affect the patient.

By its nature MG, with its acute and chronic components, creates complex needs for both patients and their families (Kernich and Kaminski, 1995). Physical, emotional, psychological and social needs should be identified, and actions taken to address them. For a long-lasting clini-

cal stabilisation of MG symptoms, whether physical or psychological, a long-term close therapeutic relationship appears to be very important (Kohler, 2007). Ideally ongoing care will be managed by a neuroscience multidisciplinary team (MDT) specialised in the care of people with MG. Some neuroscience centres have clinical nurse specialists (CNS) whose role is dedicated to the care and support of patients with MG.

The role of the nurse caring for a patient with MG is to work in collaboration with the patient, family, neurologists and other members of the MDT in providing ongoing care, education and support. This involves assessing and monitoring the patient's muscle weakness, identifying potential problems, implementing appropriate interventions, establishing treatment goals, and monitoring the effects of treatment.

Initial management of newly diagnosed patients

Most patients with MG are diagnosed and managed in an out-patient setting. In newly diagnosed patients, education is essential for both patients and family, especially about the condition, its treatment, the support available and self-care strategies (see Box 31.1). This information should be reinforced at appropriate intervals, if necessary using leaflets. In the UK, patients, relatives, and carers can obtain further information and support from the Myasthenia Gravis Association (MGA) (Box 31.2), which also provides educational materials for health care professionals.

Patients should know that there is a very good chance that their symptoms will be greatly improved. With the current improved treatments, the majority become symptom-free and lead a full life, even though MG is a chronic disease, with fluctuating symptoms.

When the symptoms are well-controlled, pregnancy in a myasthenic patient is usually uncomplicated, although the patient should be informed of the risk of transient and usually benign myasthenic syndrome in the neonate (due to placental transfer of antibodies). Rarely, women having antibodies against the foetal AChR subunit may produce joint contractures in the offspring (Vincent *et al.*, 1995).

In-patient management

On occasions, in-patient care may be necessary, e.g. during relapses, crises, or when prednisolone therapy is started. For after-care post thymectomy, both neuroscience and cardio-thoracic nursing and surgical expertise may be needed.

Respiratory muscle weakness

Regular monitoring and reporting of increasing muscle weakness are key to preventing complications and treating

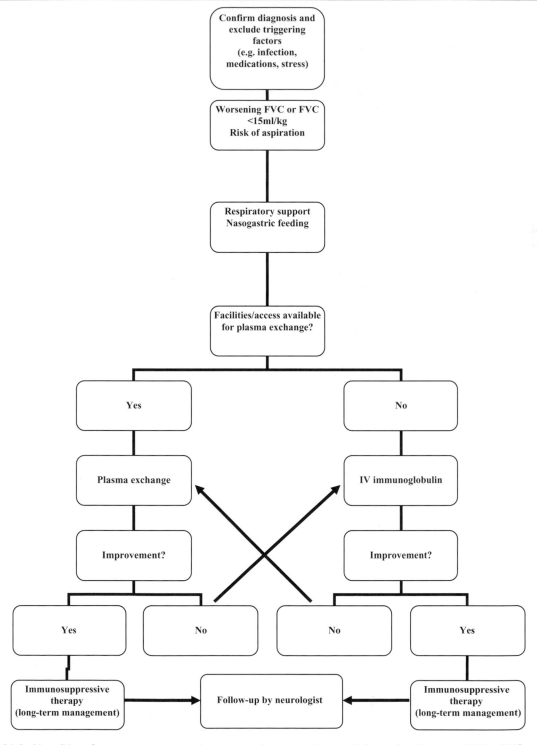

Figure 31.2 Algorithm for management of myasthenic crisis. Adapted from Jacob *et al.*, 2007. FVC – forced vital capacity.

Box 31.1   Information to be provided on initial diagnosis of myasthenia

Information about the following should be provided to patients:
- Disease mechanisms
- Natural history of the condition
- Treatment options
- Possible side-effects of therapy
- Self-care strategies to cope with their condition
- Community and social support available
- That infections often worsen or precipitate myasthenic weakness, and should therefore be treated promptly
- About other factors that could precipitate or exacerbate MG
- That patients should alert any health care professionals involved of the diagnosis, its specific effects, and of any medications being taken, as some may now be contraindicated
- To wear a MedicAlert® bracelet, in case they cannot communicate this information
- To seek urgent medical advice if their weakness is getting more severe or their breathing or swallowing is affected, as emergency treatment may be required

---

Box 31.2   Further information

Further information is available from The Myasthenia Gravis Association

Email: mg@mga-charity.org
Website: http://www.mga-charity.org/ or http://www.mgauk.org/

This is the official website of Myasthenia Gravis Association and contains a very comprehensive information pack about myasthenia gravis, Lambert Eaton myasthenic syndrome (LEMS) and congenital myasthenic syndrome (CMS). It also has general information leaflets about nutrition, fa tigue, psychosocial aspects, driving, accessing benefits, plasma exchange, etc.)

MG successfully. Weakness of the respiratory muscles may lead to an ineffective breathing pattern and respiratory failure. Early detection of deteriorating respiratory function is necessary and if the breathing pattern or respiratory function is ineffective, emergency respiratory management is required.

Patients with neuromuscular respiratory failure may not show some of the 'classic signs' of respiratory failure due to muscle weakness, i.e. breathing may not appear laboured, the use of accessory muscles may be absent, facial expression may not show anxiety or nasal flaring may be absent. It is therefore necessary to closely monitor for an increase in respiratory rate and a reduced vital capacity. Confusion and agitation may occur due to reduced cerebral oxygenation. Increasing neck weakness may be a sign of respiratory muscle involvement and bulbar muscle weakness.

The vital capacity (VC) should be measured three times (on each assessment) to assess respiratory muscle weakness (Litchfield and Noroian, 1989) and fatigue. If it falls below 1 litre or 15–20 ml/kg (or there is significant worsening of symptoms) elective respiratory support/ventilation is advised. It is important to ensure correct VC technique as false low readings can result from the patient's inability to close the lips around the instrument's mouthpiece or from air escaping from the nose (George, 1988). The use of a face mask attached to the spirometer may be necessary to obtain an accurate reading (see Chapter 15).

People with MG may be unable to produce an effective cough, therefore chest physiotherapy is recommended to prevent respiratory infections. This should include a programme of coughing, deep breathing and sighing after anti-cholinesterase medication when muscles are strongest (Litchfield and Noroian, (1989). Nurses should work collaboratively with the physiotherapist to optimise respiratory function. It is important that nurses know how to give assisted cough and to use intermittent positive pressure breathing IPPB (Bird) (see Chapter 15) to ensure continuity of care.

If the patient has a high risk of respiratory failure, it will be necessary to educate and instruct the family on resuscitation techniques and to supply equipment (e.g. Ambu bag, airway, suction) prior to discharge.

Bulbar muscle weakness

Weakness of the bulbar and jaw muscles may cause difficulty with swallowing and chewing, putting the patient at risk of choking, aspiration and inadequate hydration/nutrition. Anti-cholinesterase drugs should ideally be given 30–60 minutes before meals to maximise strength when eating. Physical activities should be minimised prior to eating and talking during meals should be avoided to conserve muscle strength and to reduce fatigue.

Assessment of swallowing and chewing should be performed before each meal. Signs of swallowing difficulties may include coughing when eating or drinking, pooling of saliva, food or fluids escaping from the nose, facial weakness, slow drinking, fatigue on chewing, an inability to cope with oral secretions and retained food in the mouth. If swallowing difficulties are suspected oral intake should be temporarily suspended; the medical team should be informed and the patient referred to the speech and language therapist for a thorough swallowing assessment, and to the dietician for nutritional advice (see Chapter 12 for further management of the patient with impaired swallowing). Safety measures should be in place i.e. suction equipment, O_2 and resuscitation equipment in case of aspiration or choking. A diet and fluid chart should be maintained and the patient should be assessed for early signs of dehydration and malnutrition (see Chapter 16). Nasogastric feeding should be considered in those patients with a clear risk of aspiration, where the daily fluid and nutritional intake is insufficient or where they are unable to swallow their medication safely.

Due to bulbar muscle weakness the voice may become quieter (dysphonic) and speech maybe more nasal and dysarthric. If speaking is difficult or tiring for the patient, long conversations should be avoided. See Chapter 12 for management of the patient with dysphonia and dysarthria.

Trunk, neck, limb muscle weakness

Weakness of these muscle groups may lead to reduced mobility, risk of injury, and an inability to conduct daily activities. Regular assessment of muscle strength (see Chapter 11) should be undertaken and signs of muscle weakness or further deterioration should be reported. Daily activities should be planned to be performed at times of optimum strength, i.e. when the effects of anticholinesterase medication are at their peak or in accordance with the patient's usual pattern of weakness. The level of assistance with mobilisation and daily activities such as bathing, dressing, etc., will be dependent on the severity of the patient's weakness which may change from day to day or during the course of the day. Adequate periods of rest should be planned throughout the day and a quiet, restful atmosphere should be promoted at night to enable good quality sleep and to minimise fatigue. Nurses should work collaboratively with the physiotherapist and occupational therapist to optimise the patient's independence.

Ocular muscle weakness

Weakness of the extraocular muscles can cause double vision (diplopia) and weakness of the muscles of the e yelid can cause drooping eyelids (ptosis). If ptosis and diplopia are causing significant problems the patient should be referred to an orthoptist for assessment and advice. Ocular muscles should be assessed regularly for increased weakness. Prism lenses may be prescribed to correct double vision or, for a temporary measure, an eye patch can be worn. A bar ptosis prop or 'Lundie Loop' (a spring-based support) can be fitted to glasses to support drooping eye lids.

Defects in the normal protective reflexes may confer a risk of damage to the cornea. Eye closure or blinking may be impaired, so it is important to check the eyes regularly for signs of dryness, corneal abrasion or infection. Hypromellose may be required hourly to moisten the eye and to reduce soreness. Long acting ointment is used to lubricate the eye at night to prevent frequent waking of the patient. A clear bubble shield is advocated for night wear to protect the cornea from abrasions. It must not be worn all the time as the warm moist environment that develops underneath can precipitate infections (BAO-HNS, 2002). The patient should receive education on eye care prior to discharge. Protective eye wear without prescription lenses will protect the eye from dust when outdoors.

PSYCHOSOCIAL ISSUES

Having to adjust to the fluctuating symptoms of MG, and its acute and chronic phases, may be draining not just physically but also emotionally and psychologically for patients and their families. A variety of psychological responses are experienced by patients and their families including: anxiety, frustration, anger, hostility, fear, regression, denial, guilt, depression, powerlessness, isolation and stigma. The physical effects of MG may cause: loss of independence, altered body image and changes in roles and inter-personal relationships. Key nursing interventions in the management of the emotional and psychosocial factors associated with MG are summarised in Box 31.3.

Since myasthenic syndromes produce variable and fluctuating symptoms, they are liable to several misdiagnoses (e.g. if patients are seen first thing in the morning, when at their strongest). In fact, several patients have been mislabelled as chronic fatigue syndrome or 'non-organic', partly due to lack of experience of the treating clinician. When a diagnosis is finally established, some patients feel relieved to find that they have a treatable, physical reason for their symptoms, while others may be shocked, and may feel unable to accept their illness. Gradually, with the support of their family and the neuroscience MDT, most patients show active coping strategies and usually have better compliance and more confidence in the treatment strategies than those with some of the other chronic diseases. Many patients and their families will find it helpful to have contact with others who are facing or have been

---

Box 31.3 Key nursing interventions in the management of emotional and psychosocial issues in MG

- Recognise and identify the reasons for the emotional and psychological responses experienced by the patient and implement appropriate actions to address and treat these responses
- Design a program to help the patient adjust to their illness and to take an active part in the day-to-day management of their symptoms and condition including symptom management, stress management, coping skills, and family communication
- Allow patients to express their thoughts and feelings, in a non-judgemental environment, using effective means of communication
- Recognise potential sources of anxiety, e.g. lack of information, increasing muscle weakness, changes in treatment, transfer to different departments or care facilities, or discharge home, and implement strategies to address these
- Ensure the patient and family receive appropriate information and verify that it has been understood. Supply written information where appropriate
- Involve the patient in the decision making and realistic goal setting
- Allow them to assume as much control and responsibility for themselves and their care as possible to promote independence
- Teach or suggest methods to reduce levels of anxiety and fatigue, e.g. relaxation techniques
- Offer support to help patient build their confidence and self-esteem
- Encourage the patient to be involved in pursuits he enjoys, and to maintain links with family and friends to prevent feelings of isolation
- Referral to the psychiatric team may be appropriate if the patient is exhibiting an extreme response to the emotional and psychological aspects of the illness or a reaction to prednisolone therapy
- Refer to social services for assessment of specific social needs
- Ensure patient and family know how to obtain further information and advice

---

through similar situations. The MGA provides information and forums for such support.

Patients may experience feelings of loss of independence due to muscle weakness which may affect normal body functions, basic life style, or self-concept. He may be unable to participate in activities that were once taken for granted. Difficulty with speech, chewing and swallowing may make social situations awkward and embarrassing. Visual problems have a major effect on day-to-day life and may affect the ability to drive. Patients are advised to notify the DVLA, once the diagnosis is confirmed. If patients can no longer work full-time, that will affect their financial independence and life-style and their role within the family or social group may change. It is important for the family to have a full understanding of MG and its variable and fatiguing effects on the patient.

The symptoms of MG and the side-effects, especially of steroid therapy, may well cause changes to the patient's body image. In particular, muscle weakness changes facial expressions so that even their best smile can look threatening. These effects can be embarrassing and demoralising, changing patients' self-concept and lowering self-esteem. In addition, long-term steroid therapy itself can result in changes in mood.

Fatigue is the most common and troublesome symptom reported by the myasthenic patient. Fatigue exists as a paradox, since it is both a symptom of the disease and an adaptive response for the maintenance of health. Activity restriction is the best predictor for fatigue severity (Kittiwatanapaisan *et al.*, 2003). Most MG patients self-manage fatigue using a combination of mental interventions (e.g. recognition of limits before becoming tired, avoidance of pushing to limits, avoidance of stress), physical interventions (e.g. most activity performed during peak energy time, organise home/work place to conserve energy), avoiding late hours, and regular rest (Grohar-Murray *et al.*, 1998). Reading and listening to music are constantly employed by most patients to divert themselves away from the feeling of fatigue.

Uncertainty and fear are common reactions of the patient and family whenever the patient experiences a myasthenic crisis (Kernich and Kaminski, 1995). Patients in myasthenic crisis may appear expressionless, mute and may have difficult keeping their eyes open. It should be borne in mind that their higher mental functions are completely intact. A calm and confident approach will help to reduce anxiety, and build the patient's confidence and morale. Psychotherapy is not required unless there are associated neurotic or reactive psychiatric symptoms (Doering *et al.*, 1993).

PROGNOSIS

With improving diagnosis and therapeutic options, myasthenia is being better managed in the community and the incidence of myasthenic crisis is falling. Most patients are well controlled with adequate immunosuppression. The mortality rate of myasthenic crisis has fallen dramatically from 80% in the 1960s (Osserman and Genkins, 1963) to less than 5% (Thomas *et al.*, 1997) with improved respiratory care. Patients with myasthenic crisis stay in hospital for an average of one month, half of which is likely to be with intensive respiratory support (Thomas *et al.*, 1997). Intubation for more than 2 weeks is known to increase the hospital stay up to threefold and to double the chances of functional dependence at discharge (Thomas *et al.*, 1997).

EMERGING TREATMENTS AND CLINICAL TRIALS

In addition to newer immunosuppressants, anti-CD20 B-cell monoclonal antibody, Rituximab has been recently described to be useful in resistant myasthenia, especially those associated with AChR or MuSK antibodies (Hain *et al.*, 2006). T-cell directed and antigen-specific immunogenetic therapies are in the experimental stages (Sieb, 2005). The role of thymectomy in non-thymomatous myasthenic patients is currently being evaluated in a multinational randomised control trial (NINDS, 2006).

SUMMARY

The management of myasthenia gravis has improved significantly in recent years. The majority of patients can now live normal lives but they are required to take immunosuppressive medication indefinitely. Hospital admission is required during relapses and crises. The sudden loss of function and independence can be very frightening so it is important to maintain a calm and supportive approach when managing the patient's care.

ACKNOWLEDGEMENTS

The author acknowledges the extensive help provided by Ms. Christina Goldsworthy, Myasthenia Specialist Nurse, Muscle and Nerve Centre, John Radcliffe Hospital, Oxford in the preparation of this manuscript. The author is also grateful for the valuable suggestions and critical reviews of this chapter by Prof. Nick Willcox, Dr. David Hilton-Jones and Dr. Maria Isabel Leite of the Department of Clinical Neurology, John Radcliffe Hospital, Oxford, United Kingdom.

SJ currently holds a neuromuscular research fellowship supported by the Muscular Dystrophy Campaign/Myasthenia Gravis Association.

REFERENCES

Berrouschot J, Baumann I, Kalischewski P *et al.* (1997) Therapy of myasthenic crisis. *Crit Care Med* 25(7):1228–1235.

British Association of Otorhinolaryngologists Head and Neck Surgeons (2002) *Acoustic Neuromas – Clinical Effectiveness Guidelines*. London: BAO-HNS Royal College of Surgeons.

Cohen MS, Younger D (1981) Aspects of the natural history of myasthenia gravis: crisis and death. *Ann N Y Acad Sci* 377:670–677.

Crucitti F, Dodlietto G, Bellantone R *et al.* (1992) Effects of surgical treatment in thymoma with myasthenia gravis: our experience in 103 patients. *J Surg Oncol* 50(1):43–46.

Doering S, Henze T, Schussler G (1993) Coping with myasthenia gravis and implications for psychotherapy. *Arch Neurol* 50(6):617–620.

Evoli A, Torali PA, Padua L *et al.* (2003) Clinical correlates with anti-MuSK antibodies in generalized seronegative myasthenia gravis. *Brain* 126(10):2304–2311.

Gajdos P, Chevret S, Clair B *et al.* (1997) Clinical trial of plasma exchange and high-dose intravenous immunoglobulin in myasthenia gravis. Myasthenia Gravis Clinical Study Group. *Ann Neurol* 41(6):789–796.

Gajdos P, Chevret S, Toyka K (2002) Plasma exchange for myasthenia gravis. *Cochrane Database Syst Rev* (4):CD002275.

George MR (1988) Neuromuscular respiratory failure: what the nurse knows may make the difference. *J Neurosci Nurs* 20(2):110–117.

Grohar-Murray ME *et al.* (1998) Self-care actions to manage fatigue among myasthenia gravis patients. *J Neurosci Nurs* 30(3):191–199.

Hain B *et al.* (2006) Successful treatment of MuSK antibody-positive myasthenia gravis with rituximab. *Muscle Nerve* 33(4):575–580.

Hetherington KA, Losek JD (2005) Myasthenia gravis: myasthenia vs. cholinergic crisis. *Pediatr Emerg Care* 21(8):546–548; quiz 549–551.

Hoch W *et al.* (2001) Auto-antibodies to the receptor tyrosine kinase MuSK in patients with myasthenia gravis without acetylcholine receptor antibodies. *Nat Med* 7(3):365–368.

Illa I (2005) IVIg in myasthenia gravis, Lambert Eaton myasthenic syndrome and inflammatory myopathies: current status. *J Neurol* 252(Suppl 1): I14–8.

Jacob S, Viegas S, Hilton-Jones D (2007) Assessment and management of myasthenic crisis: an evidence based approach. *Br J Neurosci Nurs* 3(5):198–204.

Kernich CA, Kaminski HJ (1995) Myasthenia gravis: pathophysiology, diagnosis and collaborative care. *J Neurosci Nurs* 27(4):207–215; quiz 216–218.

Kittiwatanapaisan W *et al.* (2003) Fatigue in myasthenia gravis patients. *J Neurosci Nurs* 35(2):87–93.

Kohler W (2007) Psychosocial aspects in patients with myasthenia gravis. *J Neurol* 254(Suppl 2): II90–II92.

Lindstrom JM *et al.* (1976) Antibody to acetylcholine receptor in myasthenia gravis. Prevalence, clinical correlates, and diagnostic value. *Neurology* 26(11):1054–1059.

Litchfield M, Noroian E (1989) Changes in selected pulmonary functions in patients diagnosed with myasthenia gravis. *J Neurosci Nurs* 21(6):375–381.

Mantegazza R, Bazzi E, Bernasconi P *et al.* (2003) Myasthenia gravis (MG): epidemiological data and prognostic factors. *Ann N Y Acad Sci* 998:413–423.

Masaoka A *et al.* (1996) Extended thymectomy for myasthenia gravis patients: a 20-year review. *Ann Thorac Surg* 62(3):853–859.

Molnar J, Szobor A (1990) Myasthenia gravis: effect of thymectomy in 425 patients. A 15-year experience. *Eur J Cardiothorac Surg* 4(1):8–14.

Newsom-Davis J *et al.* (1979) Long-term effects of repeated plasma exchange in myasthenia gravis. *Lancet* 1 (8114): 464–468.

NINDS (2006) *A multi-center, single-blind, randomized study comparing thymectomy to no thymectomy in non-thymomatous myasthenia gravis (MG) patients receiving prednisone.* Available from: http://www.clinicaltrials.gov/ct/show/NCT00294658 Accessed July 2010.

Oosterhuis HJ (1989) The natural course of myasthenia gravis: a long term follow up study. *J Neurol Neurosurg Psychiatry* 52(10):1121–1127.

Osserman KE, Genkins G (1963) Studies in myasthenia gravis: reduction in mortality rate after crisis. *JAMA* 183:97–101.

Sanders DB, Scoppetta C (1994) The treatment of patients with myasthenia gravis. *Neurol Clin* 12(2):343–368.

Sanders DB, El-Salem D, Massey JM *et al.* (2003) Clinical aspects of MuSK antibody positive seronegative MG. *Neurology* 60(12):1978–1980.

Sieb JP (2005) Myasthenia gravis: emerging new therapy options. *Curr Opin Pharmacol* 5(3):303–307.

Skeie GO, Apostolski S, Evoli A *et al.* (2006) Guidelines for the treatment of autoimmune neuromuscular transmission disorders. *Eur J Neurol* 13(7):691–699.

Stricker RB *et al.* (1993) Myasthenic crisis. Response to plasmapheresis following failure of intravenous gammaglobulin. *Arch Neurol* 50(8):837–840.

Thomas CE, Mayer SA, Gungor Y *et al.* (1997) Myasthenic crisis: clinical features, mortality, complications, and risk factors for prolonged intubation. *Neurology* 48(5):1253–1260.

Vincent A (2002) Unravelling the pathogenesis of myasthenia gravis. *Nat Rev Immunol* 2(10):797–804.

Vincent A, Newsom-Davis J (1985) Acetylcholine receptor antibody as a diagnostic test for myasthenia gravis: results in 153 validated cases and 2967 diagnostic assays. *J Neurol Neurosurg Psychiatry* 48(12):1246–1252.

Vincent A, Newland C, Brueton L *et al.* (1995) Arthrogryposis multiplex congenita with maternal autoantibodies specific for a fetal antigen. *Lancet* 346(8966):24–25.

Section VI
Management of Patients Following Head and Spinal Trauma

32
Management of Patients with Traumatic Brain Injury

Siobhan McLernon

INTRODUCTION

Traumatic brain injury (TBI) is an acquired brain injury (ABI) of sudden onset, which is caused by a significant impact to the cranium or sudden external force/s causing distortion to the brain within the cranium. It is considered to be a long term neurological condition (DH, 2005) as those who survive significant TBI often experience long-term physical disability, neurocognitive deficits and neuropsychiatric sequelae (NICE, 2007). TBI represents the leading cause of morbidity and mortality in young adults worldwide (Werner and Engelhard, 2007). It is associated with a high socio-economic cost both in terms of lost income potential and health care provision, as those that survive significant TBI would otherwise be socially and financially self-sufficient (NICE, 2007).

It is now widely accepted that not all the neurological damage following TBI occurs at the moment of impact (primary injury), but that it evolves over hours and days (secondary injury). Patient outcomes improve when secondary delayed insults are prevented or when they successfully respond to early treatment. The emphasis of care in this patient group is therefore: early diagnosis, appropriate assessment, and management aimed at preventing death and future neurological disability. Successful rehabilitation requires a multidisciplinary approach involving the family throughout the patient's journey.

There is currently a lack of level 1 evidence to support most treatments in the management of TBI. However, the Brain Trauma Foundation (BTF), in collaboration with the American Association of Neurological Surgeons (AANS) and other stakeholders, has developed recommendations for the management of severe traumatic brain injury (BTF, 2007) which are based on class II and class III evidence.

EPIDEMIOLOGY

Approximately 700, 000 patients per annum attend accident and emergency (A&E) departments throughout the UK with a head injury, 20% of whom will require hospitalisation (NICE, 2007). TBI most commonly occurs between the ages of 15 and 24 years and >75years (BSRM, 2003) with the majority of cases occurring in males (70–88%) (NICE, 2007).

The majority of head injuries are mild (Glasgow Coma Scale (GCS) 13–15) and therefore the mortality rate of the total TBI population is considered low, accounting for approximately 6–10 deaths per 100,000 of the population per year (Kay and Teasdale, 2001). The majority of fatal outcomes will be in the moderate (GCS 9–12) or severe (GCS ≤ 8) head injury groups, which account for 10% of all TBI attendees to A&E (Swann and Teasdale, 1999).

AETIOLOGY

The principle causes of head injury include road traffic accidents, falls, assaults, and injuries occurring at work, in the home and during sporting activities. The incidence of penetrating head trauma remains low (NICE, 2007). Assaults (30–50%) and falls (22–43%) are the most common cause of a mild head injury in the UK. Road traffic accidents are responsible for a large proportion of moderate–severe head injuries (NICE, 2007).

Neuroscience Nursing: Evidence-Based Practice, 1st Edition.
Edited by Sue Woodward and Ann-Marie Mestecky
© 2011 Blackwell Publishing Ltd

Alcohol may be involved in up to 65% of adult head injuries, either consumed by the injured person or by a person involved in the incident (NICE, 2007). There are marked regional variations in the causes of head injury particularly in relation to those caused by assaults and those involving alcohol (NICE, 2007).

CLASSIFICATION

Clinical severity of TBI may be classified based on the Glasgow Coma Scale (GCS) after initial resuscitation (Teasdale and Jennett, 1974) i.e. mild TBI (GCS 13–15), moderate (GCS 9–12) or severe (GCS 3–8). Mechanism of injury and computed tomography (CT) abnormalities are used as indicators of injury severity (Maas *et al.*, 2000). The severity of TBI is also determined by the duration of post-traumatic amnesia (PTA) (see: Post-traumatic amnesia).

The *damage* seen in head injury can be classified as focal and/or diffuse (Table 32.1); each will be presented below.

OVERVIEW OF PRIMARY AND SECONDARY INJURY

Head injury is a heterogeneous and complex pathobiological condition (Smith, 2003). It encompasses a wide range of pathologies including diffuse axonal injury (DAI), focal contusions and space occupying haematomas (Maas *et al.*, 2000). TBI is often described in terms of *primary* and *secondary* events.

Table 32.1 Patterns of damage in TBI.

Area	Type
Focal damage:	
Scalp	Lacerations
Skull	Fracture
Between skull and brain	Extradural (EDH), subdural (SDH)
Brain	Contusions and lacerations Intracerebral haemorrhage (ICH) Penetrating brain injury (PBI)
Diffuse damage:	
Brain (neuronal damage)	Diffuse axonal injury (DAI) Hypoxic–ischaemic damage Diffuse brain swelling (oedema)

Primary brain injury, originally defined as physical brain injury sustained at the moment of impact, leads to physical disruption of neurones, tearing of blood vessels and/or inadequate perfusion of brain tissue. Neurones are fragile and are vulnerable to acceleration and deceleration shearing forces which can tear their delicate axons. Blood vessels on the surface and within the brain may be torn causing haemorrhages. Brain tissue itself may be damaged by the bony protuberances of the skull during violent movements causing laceration to brain tissue and contusions. These injuries can be focal and/or diffuse and, when they coexist, contribute to morbidity (Povlishock and Katz, 2005).

During the first stages of cerebral injury there is impaired regulation of cerebral blood flow (CBF) and cell metabolism. This ultimately leads to the accumulation of lactic acid due to anaerobic glycolysis, increased membrane permeability, and consecutive oedema formation (Werner and Engelhard, 2007).

Primary injury was traditionally believed to be immediate and irreversible (Reilly *et al.*, 1975). It is now evident that a substantial component of cell death is not instantaneous but evolves over the ensuing hours and days and can overlap with secondary or additional injury processes (Reilly, 2001). These continuing effects of the impact are not all irreversible, but it may be possible with future therapies to halt the progression of the primary injury. Thus brain injury is viewed as a process beginning with an impact rather than a single event.

Secondary brain injury may be divided into two components: *damage* and *insults* (Maas *et al.*, 2000). Secondary *brain damage* occurs following activation by the primary injury and evolves over subsequent hours and days due to a complex array of intrinsic pathophysiological mechanisms which render the brain more susceptible to further secondary insults. The release of excitotoxic amino acids such as glutamate and aspartate, and increased production of lactate, hydrogen ions and oxygen free radicals are all implicated in the mechanisms of this ongoing damage (Obrenovitch and Urenjak, 1997). The end result of these cellular processes is the influx of calcium (Ca^{2+}) into cells which is thought to be responsible for the cascade of deleterious intracellular changes that lead to cell death (Kampfl *et al.*, 1997). Each of these processes associated with secondary brain damage is discussed in more detail in a following section.

Secondary *brain insults* exacerbate pathophysiological processes that further damage susceptible neurones and ultimately lead to a worse neurological outcome. These are largely preventable and treatable (Maas *et al.*, 1997). Secondary insults are common after TBI and have been reported to occur at some point in the patient's management in as many as 90% of patients requiring treatment in the neurocritical care unit (NCU) (Jones *et al.*, 1994). The two main extracranial causes, correlating with increased mortality and morbidity, are delay in appropriate surgical management and failure to correct systemic hypoxaemia and hypotension (RCS, 1999).

Hypotension (systolic blood pressure <90 mmHg) is the predominant contributing factor in secondary brain injury and has the highest correlation with morbidity and mortality (Chestnut, 1997). As the duration of hypotension lengthens, probability of a favourable outcome decreases. Hypoxia ($PaO_2 < 8\,kPa$) is the second most influential cause of secondary brain injury after hypotension and worsens outcome (Chestnut *et al.*, 1993).

Primary Brain Injuries

Extradural haematoma (EDH)

The incidence of EDH among TBI patients is approximately 2.7–4% and is most commonly seen between the ages of 20 and 30 years (Gupta *et al.*, 1992). Traffic–related accidents, falls and assaults account for 53% of all EDHs (Lee *et al.*, 1998). An EDH is an accumulation of blood in the extradural space between the inner surface of the skull and the dura mater. It is mainly associated with skull fracture and injury to the middle meningeal artery/vein, or one of the large venous sinuses. The meningeal artery lies beneath the pterion, part of the temporal bone where the skull is thinnest, and is relatively easily fractured by a blow to the head. Consequently EDH mainly affects the parieto-temporal areas (Maggi *et al.*, 1998). On CT it has a hyperdense (white) biconvex appearance (Figure 32.1).

A large percentage (22–56%) of patients with EDHs have a GCS<8 on admission or before surgery (Paterniti *et al.*, 1994). The patient may appear 'lucid' immediately after the injury and then deteriorate neurologically as the clot enlarges and begins to compress the brain, causing brain shift and raised intracranial pressure (ICP) (van den Brink *et al.*, 1999). Presenting symptoms can include: pupillary abnormalities, hemiparesis, decerebrate posturing and seizures. However, up to 27% of patients are neurologically intact on initial clinical presentation (Bullock *et al.*, 2006a,b). Deterioration in level of consciousness is an urgent clinical indicator that requires immediate action.

Acute subdural haematoma (ASDH)

ASDH is an accumulation of blood between the dura mater and the arachnoid mater due to tearing of cortical veins. It

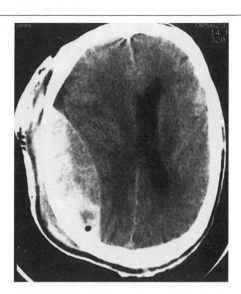

Figure 32.1 Extradural haematoma with the typical hyperdense biconvex appearance. Reproduced from Andrew Kaye, *Essential Neurosurgery*, Wiley-Blackwell, with permission.

occurs in approximately 30% of severe head injuries (Marik *et al.*, 2002). They are usually associated with motor vehicle accidents falls and assaults (Bullock *et al.*, 2006a,b). Most patients with ASDHs have some kind of accompanying brain injury, such as brain contusion at the frontal or temporal surface of the brain due to the forces involved, and are therefore associated with a poor outcome (Maas *et al.*, 2000). Those that present to hospital in a coma requiring surgery have a mortality rate between 57 and 68% (Servadei *et al.*, 1998). On CT an ASDH is hyperdense and concave towards the brain (see Figure 32.2). A poor outcome is more likely if a SDH is bilateral, accumulates rapidly, or there is >4 hours delay in the surgical management (Servadei *et al.*, 2000).

Chronic sub-dural haematoma (CSDH)

CSDH can present many weeks after head injury with progressive neurological deficits. The patient often does not remember a predisposing injury. The most common symptoms are headache, hemiparesis and fluctuating levels of consciousness that can vary with severity. Increasing ICP may lead to cognitive impairment causing confusion and a reduced level of consciousness. CSDHs are more common in older patients and those with a history of alcoholism, coagulopathy, epilepsy and with ventricular drains (Watkins, 2000)

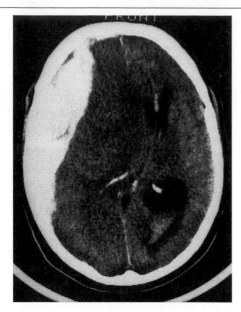

Figure 32.2 Acute subdural haematoma causing marked shift of the lateral ventricle. Reproduced from Andrew Kaye, *Essential Neurosurgery*, Wiley-Blackwell, with permission.

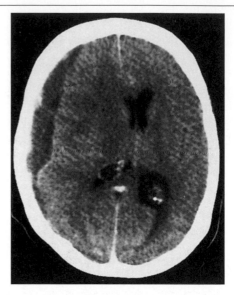

Figure 32.3 Chronic subdural haematoma. The fluid is hypodense compared with the adjacent brain. Reproduced from Andrew Kaye, *Essential Neurosurgery*, Wiley-Blackwell, with permission.

This lesion has a chronic progressive nature and it is thought that as the clot starts to breakdown the compounds that are released produce an irritative reaction (Watkins, 2000). A subdural membrane forms and fluid accumulates between the dura and the subdural membrane either by osmosis or by an inflammatory process. A CSDH will appear hypodense (dark) on CT (Figure 32.3). The treatment involves evacuation of the subdural collection by drilling burrholes and washing out the subdural space with warmed saline. A craniotomy may be required with resection of the subdural membranes in certain circumstances (Watkins, 2000).

Traumatic subarachnoid haemorrhage (tSAH)

tSAH is caused by bleeding from cortical arteries, veins and capillaries from the brain's surface. It is seen in 30–40% of patients following a moderate–severe TBI (Servadei *et al.*, 2002). The high mortality associated with tSAH is thought to be related to the severity of the primary injury rather than the effects of delayed vasospasm and secondary ischemic brain damage, i.e. it is an indicator of severity of brain damage (Servadei *et al.*, 2002). At the present time there is no specific treatment for tSAH.

Intracerebral haemorrhage (ICH)

ICHs occur commonly in moderate and severe TBI and often evolve over time to produce mass lesions. ICHs are a cause of delayed neurological deterioration in patients with severe TBI (Servadei *et al.*, 1995). Bleeding within the brain tissue can result from high velocity penetrating injuries, e.g. a bullet, or a low velocity focal impact in which bony fragments of the skull penetrate the brain tissue. In closed head injuries it results from acceleration/deceleration forces that tear the blood vessels. An ICH most commonly affects the frontal or temporal lobes (Marik *et al.*, 2002). ICHs are more commonly located within the white matter of the brain or sub-cortical structures such as the basal ganglia. Blood within brain parenchyma will be seen as hyperdense areas on the CT scan (Figure 32.4). Clinical deterioration or progressive uncontrolled ICP should prompt repeat CT scanning to detect any evidence of ICH. Small ICHs are managed conservatively. The surgical removal of large ICHs is controversial. The mortality rate for patients with large ICHs is high and there is increased morbidity in the majority of patients.

Haemorrhagic contusion

Post-traumatic cerebral contusions consist of areas of the brain with various degrees of haemorrhage, infarction,

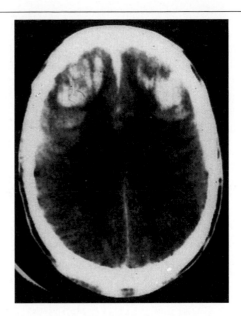

Figure 32.4 Traumatic frontal intracerebral haematomas resulting from contre-coup injury. Reproduced from Andrew Kaye, *Essential Neurosurgery*, Wiley-Blackwell, with permission.

necrosis and oedema (Maas *et al.*, 2000). They usually affect the cortex in the frontal and temporal lobes, and are sustained as the brain hits the bony protuberances of the skull due to the sudden acceleration/deceleration force.

They can occur at the site of impact (coup injury) and/ or on the side opposite the area that was impacted (contrecoup). The centre of the contusion is often irreversibly damaged (Raghupathi *et al.*, 2000). Local areas around the contusion, *the penumbra area*, have the potential to survive if blood flow to this region is optimised. Cerebral contusions frequently enlarge with time and are a significant cause of delayed neurological deterioration.

Penetrating brain injury (PBI)

PBI can be caused by bullets, shrapnel, and low velocity sharp objects such as knives (BTF, 2001).The factors that determine whether an object penetrates the intracranial space are:

- The energy and shape of the object
- The angle of approach
- The characteristics of intervening tissues (e.g. skull, muscle, mucosa)

(BTF, 2001)

In addition to destruction of tissue in the projectile's path, there is a transmission of kinetic energy which produces a temporary cavity larger than the size of the object (Neal *et al.*, 2007). Expansion and contraction of this cavity produces shearing forces that transect axons and blood vessels triggering secondary injury processes (Koszyca *et al.*, 1998). Cerebral oedema is a frequent cause of secondary injury following PBI (Neal *et al.*, 2007).

Some penetrating injuries such as a fall onto a sharp object or assault with a pointed weapon may at first appear insignificant, with only a small visible wound and a normal level of consciousness. However, if the object has penetrated deep into the cerebral tissues, delayed neurological deterioration can occur due to intracerebral bleeding along the penetration track (Watkins, 2000).

Skull fractures

Different types of skull fractures can occur depending on the type of trauma. Skull fractures indicate that the skull and brain have received a major impact and they are associated with a high incidence of intracranial haematomas (Watkins, 2000).

They often occur as a result of a blunt trauma and require admission for CT scanning to exclude any secondary complications such as intracranial haematoma or cerebral oedema (Mandrioli *et al.*, 2008).

Depressed skull fractures are usually a result of assault trauma (O'Shea, 2005). Bone fragments may lacerate the dura and brain with a risk of cortical damage and a subsequent risk of epilepsy; the fragments can also tear blood vessels resulting in intracranial haemorrhage. Surgical elevation, prophylactic antibiotics and tetanus immunisation/booster is the most common course of treatment.

Basal skull fractures account for 21% of all skull fractures and occur in 4% of all head injuries (Erol and Patchell, 2002). Clinical features may indicate the presence of a basal skull fracture that may not be evident on routine skull x-ray or even on specific views of the skull base. CSF rhinorrhoea, bilateral periorbital haematomas (panda or racoon eyes) and subconjunctival haemorrhage may indicate an *anterior fossa fracture*. Anosmia can result from injury to the olfactory nerve. Bleeding from the external auditory meatus, CSF otorrhoea and Battle's sign (bruising over the mastoid bone which may take 24–48 hours to develop) may indicate involvement of the temporal petrous bone (middle fossa fracture). Air and bacteria can enter the intracranial compartment causing bacterial meningitis or tension pneumocranium when brain swelling resolves (Mandrioli *et al.*, 2008). No studies have shown conclusive evidence regarding the efficacy of routine antibiotic prophylaxis in preventing the incidence of meningitis.

Concussion

Concussion is defined as any transient neurologic dysfunction resulting from a biomechanical force (Giza and Hovda, 2001). Mild traumatic brain injury (MTBI) is often referred to as concussion. Loss of consciousness may occur but is not required to make the diagnosis. Symptoms include: confusion, disorientation, unsteadiness, dizziness, headache and visual disturbances. While the symptoms of most concussions resolve within one week, many patients have persistent symptoms at three and seven months with some remaining symptomatic a year after the injury (Naunheim *et al.*, 2008) or even longer. These deficits can occur without any detectable anatomic pathology which suggests that they are based on temporary neuronal dysfunction rather than cell death (Giza and Hovda, 2001). For discussion of the management of mild traumatic brain injury see: Discharge of mild TBI patients.

Diffuse axonal injury (DAI)

DAI is a common pathologic feature present with any type of brain injury, focal or otherwise resulting from mechanical distortion of the brain (Smith *et al.*, 2003). It is a dynamic process at cellular level that begins hours after trauma and can continue for days post injury (Christman *et al.*, 1994). It is most commonly seen after high-speed motor vehicle accidents or falls (Reilly, 2001). Rotational forces cause the brain to twist within the skull resulting in torsion and shearing of neuronal tissue mainly at the boundary between neocortical grey and white matter. This sets in motion a chain of cellular events which results in the pathological changes evident in DAI (Smith *et al.*, 2003).

The pattern of axonal injury is often scattered and/or multifocal and occurs commonly in the corpus callosum and brain stem (Blumbergs *et al.*, 1995). Rapid stretch of axons can damage the axonal cytoskeleton and alter cell permeability resulting in progressive changes that affect axoplasmic transport (see Chapter 1). In severe DAI this course of evolving axonal pathology ultimately leads to progressive disorganisation of the axonal cytoskeleton with protein accumulations, which leads to disconnection of the axon (Povlishock and Katz, 2005) and the formation of the signature pathologic feature of a bulb formation at the terminal end of the axon (Buki *et al.*, 2000).

The progressive changes that occur after DAI to the neurones were traditionally believed to be an irretrievable event in which the neurone is unable to communicate with its targets (Smith *et al.*, 2003). Recent evidence has indicated that axonal damage and degeneration are not always associated with neuronal death. It may be possible for some functional recovery to take place as a result of localised plasticity in the grey matter or repair of damaged white matter neurones that did not result in disconnection (Lifshitz *et al.*, 2003).

Coma is the most common feature associated with severe DAI due to axonal damage in the reticular formation within the brain stem. Patients with minimal macroscopic injury can have extensive microscopic axonal changes but have normal CT scans and normal ICP (Mittl *et al.*, 1994). In those with severe DAI, some macroscopic changes may be evident on CT and MRI scans, which can illustrate small focal haemorrhages in the corpus callosum, around the third ventricle and brain stem. However these conventional imaging modalities are inadequate for the direct assessment of injured axons (MacDonald *et al.*, 2007).

PATHOPHYSIOLOGY

Altered cerebral haemodynamics and ischaemia

Cerebral ischaemia (see Chapter 6) is a dominant factor in determining outcome after severe TBI (Juul *et al.*, 2000). Regional and global cerebral ischaemia have been detected after TBI both during intensive care (Bouma *et al.*, 1992) and in 90% of patients at autopsy (Juul *et al.*, 2000). Cerebral haemodynamics alter following severe TBI with evidence indicating that cerebral blood flow (CBF) can be as low as 18 ml/100 g/min up to 48 hours post injury (Sioutos *et al.*, 1995). The mechanisms that maintain a constant CBF are impaired following TBI, with loss of autoregulation (see Chapter 6) in local areas of tissue damage and sometimes global loss. Therefore blood flow becomes dependent on systemic blood pressure and renders the brain more susceptible to ischaemia at lower blood pressures and to injury at higher pressures. As systemic hypotension is common in the early post-injury phase this contributes to CBF levels falling to critical levels that can lead to further cerebral ischaemic damage (Bouma *et al.*, 1992). This disordered haemodynamic state may last 72 hours or longer after the initial injury and may also be present in the chronic state (Eames *et al.*, 2002).

The penumbra

The penumbra is a vulnerable region of brain tissue that surrounds a core of severely ischaemic tissue. It is a moderately hypoperfused zone in which there is maintenance of homeostatic mechanisms in the cell membrane (Astrup *et al.*, 1981). This area of brain tissue is potentially salvageable tissue as it receives sufficient substrates for the cells to survive (adequate ATP production), but insufficient to maintain normal neuronal function.

Neuronal death by necrosis in the core is irreversible but in the penumbra, cell death is thought to be by the process of apoptosis in which there is a delayed onset of cellular deterioration. Experiments in ischaemia have demonstrated that neuronal cells under specific conditions of substrate deprivation could follow a pre-programmed pathway of controlled cell death known as apoptosis (Beilharz *et al.*, 1995). Unlike cells that die by necrosis, cells that undergo apoptosis die without membrane rupture and as a result elicit less inflammatory reactions (Tolias and Bullock, 2004). The time-lag associated with apoptosis has a clinical impact as it may be possible for cells in this area to re-establish normal function if the blood flow can be improved (reperfusion therapy). There may also be opportunities for future therapeutic anti-apoptotic interventions (Nortie and Menon, 2004). Hence this area has become a potential future target for management strategies in an attempt to preserve neuronal tissue and minimise the extent of secondary brain injury.

Excitotoxic cell damage

One of the metabolic changes that occurs following traumatic injury is a period of neuroexcitation which is caused by the excitatory neurotransmitter, glutamate. The cause for the increases in glutamate levels are potentially three-fold: disruption of the normal uptake mechanisms of glutamate from the synaptic junction; breakdown of the blood–brain barrier (BBB) which enables leakage of glutamate into the brain (concentrations of glutamate in blood are 1000 times that of the brain), and thirdly, leakage from the damaged axons into the interstitial space of the brain (Beaumont and Marmarou, 2000).

This excess in extracellular glutamate availability affects neurones as well as astrocytes and results in over stimulation of receptors which normally mediate excitatory synaptic transmission between neurones (i.e. N-methyl-D-aspartate NMDA receptors) (see Chapter 1 for more details on NMDA receptors). This abnormal agonist–receptor interaction ultimately leads to cell injury or death (Hillered *et al.*, 2005).

Excess glutamate damages neurones by excessively depolarising their membranes (terminal membrane depolarisation) leading to large fluxes of calcium (Ca^{2+}), sodium (Na^+) and potassium (K^+) ions. Critical processes are triggered due to Ca^{2+} overload, as the buffering systems of neurones, mitochondria and endoplasmic reticulum fail. The rise in internal Ca^{2+} levels triggers calcium

mediated neuronal disintegration (Xiong *et al.*, 1997; Vespa *et al.*, 1998).

Thus glutamate toxicity appears to be a prominent contributor to cell death in the acute phase of TBI. However despite compelling evidence, clinical trials utilising glutamate antagonists have not proved successful (Povlishock, 2000). This may be due to other excitatory and inhibitory neurotransmitters being involved in the traumatic episode (Povlishock and Katz, 2005). Future advances in microdialysis research in animals and in humans, combined with neuroimaging technology, may reveal the multifocal and global metabolic changes that occur following TBI. Pharmacological interventions that interrupt these processes may then follow.

Cerebral metabolic dysfunction

Disturbed metabolism of glucose in the brain has been demonstrated in positron emission tomography (PET) (Wu *et al.*, 2004) and microdialysis studies following TBI (Vespa *et al.*, 2003). In the first week post injury different brain regions, especially those that surround contusional brain, demonstrate increased glucose metabolism (hyperglycolysis) (Vespa *et al.*, 2003). Hyperglycolysis is thought to occur due to metabolic stress in an effort to maintain cellular homeostasis. This disturbed metabolic profile can occur in damaged brain regions interspersed with other brain tissue which shows a normal profile (Povlishock and Katz, 2005).

Post-traumatic vasospasm

Utilising transcranial Doppler (TCD) ultrasonography in clinical practice, haemodynamic evidence of brain vasospasm has been detected in patients following TBI. It occurs in 10–15% of patients with severe TBI on day 2–13 post injury (Bor-Seng-Shu *et al.*, 2006). Post-traumatic vasospasm has been found to occur in cases of focal contusion (Chan *et al.*, 1992) and in association with tSAH. The vasospasm differs in severity and distribution from the diffuse vasospasm observed in association with acute SAH (Fukuda *et al.*, 1998).

Patients with severe TBI are frequently sedated or in a coma making delayed neurological deficits associated with severe vasospasm difficult to detect. Diagnosis of brain vasospasm is often only possible by intracranial angiography or TCD (Bor-Seng-Shu and Teixcira, 2007).

Raised ICP

Raised ICP is common in the moderately and severely head injured population. Raised ICP may occur due to intracranial haematomas, inflammatory response to injury, cytotoxic and vasogenic oedema. The duration of ICP >20 mmHg has been found to strongly correlate with increased morbidity and mortality (Marmarou *et al.*, 1991). For further detail on ICP and cerebral oedema see Chapter 7.

DIAGNOSIS

Head computed tomography (CT) is the diagnostic technique of choice for the investigation of TBI and is recommended for all patients where there is suspicion of intracranial injury. Such imaging provides early assessment of the extent of the injury and is useful in identifying those individuals in whom deterioration is a result of a mass lesion. Regions of the brain damaged by DAI are best visualised using MRI as it is more sensitive at detecting white matter abnormalities than CT (Garnett *et al.*, 2001).

ASSESSMENT AND MANAGEMENT

There are a plethora of guidelines regarding assessment, treatment, and management decisions throughout the patient's journey with the aim of improving patient outcomes. These can be found at:

- Brain Trauma Foundation (BTF) 2001; 2003; 2007
- National Institute of Clinical Excellence (NICE) 2007
- British Society of Rehabilitation Medicine (BSRM) 2003
- Scottish Intercollegiate Guidelines Network (SIGN) 2009
- The Association of Anaesthetists of Great Britain and Ireland (AAGBI) 2006
- Intensive Care Society (ICS) 2002
- Royal College of Paediatrics and Child Health (RCPCH) 2001
- Royal College of Surgeons of England (RCS) 1999

Guidelines are not intended to replace clinical freedom of decision-making, but are intended for practitioners to use as a basis for their practice. Local resources, protocols and the needs of the individual patient all need to be considered.

Early management

There is universal agreement that initial management can influence the outcome of TBI patients. The key emphasis in the **early** management is based on three main principles:

- *Effective* resuscitation
- *Early* identification of significant head injury

- *Timely* transfer to a neurosurgical centre for those who need surgical intervention

At all stages of care, irrelevant of the environment, the priorities for this group of patients are based on the basic principles of:

- **A**irway
- **B**reathing
- **C**irculation
- **D**isability
- **E**xposure

Patients who have sustained a head injury should initially be managed and assessed according to clear principles and standard practice as set out by the advanced trauma life support (ATLS) principles (NICE, 2007). Prevention of secondary insults such as *hypoxia* and *hypotension* during initial resuscitation at the scene and during transfer can have a major impact on outcome (RCPCH, 2001).

Initial treatment priorities at the scene and within the A&E focus on:

Airway

Patients who have sustained a severe TBI have a reduced GCS ≤ 8 rendering them more susceptible to hypoxia and a risk of aspiration. An anaesthetist or critical care physician should be involved early to provide appropriate airway management (NICE, 2007).

Breathing

Once the airway is secured adequate oxygenation should be maintained either with high flow oxygen via facemask or with the aid of artificial ventilation. The aim is to maintain normocapnia, as hypercapnia and hypocapnia have been associated with poor outcome in intubated patients with TBI (Davis *et al.*, 2005) (refer to Chapter 7 for further detail).

Circulation

Hypotension should be treated promptly. Until ICP monitoring is *in situ*, one should aim to achieve a target MAP of 90 mmHg (NICE, 2007).

Disability

All patients with head injury should be assumed to have a cervical spine injury until proven otherwise. There is a 5% association of cervical spine injury, usually C1–C3, with severe head injury (O'Shea, 2005). Cervical immobilisation should be established unless the patient is fully conscious, cooperative and able to convince the examining doctor that he/she has:

- No neck pain or tenderness
- A full range of cervical movement
- No neurological deficits

A change in level of consciousness is the most useful clinical sign of deterioration. The risk of intracranial complications and the subsequent need for surgery increases as GCS score declines. Depressed level of consciousness should be ascribed to intoxication only after a significant brain injury has been excluded (NICE, 2007).

The assessment and classification of patients who have sustained a head injury should be guided primarily by the adult and paediatric versions of the Glasgow Coma Scale/score (GCS).

NICE (2007) has established clear guidelines on frequency of observations in A&E. The minimum frequency of observations for patients with GCS equal to 15 starting after the initial assessment in A&E are as follows:

- Half hourly for two hours
- One hourly for four hours
- Two hourly thereafter (NICE, 2007)

Should the patient with GCS equal to 15 deteriorate after the initial two hour period, observations should revert to half hourly and follow the frequency schedule outlined.

Pupil size and reactivity is a useful indicator of an expanding intracranial lesion. For more detail on signs and symptoms of raised ICP, please see Chapter 7.

If no abnormality is detected on CT scan, care should be taken to exclude metabolic and other causes of reduced level of consciousness. Once these have been excluded and the patient remains with a depressed level of consciousness, diffuse brain injury must be considered.

Exposure

The diagnosis and initial treatment of life threatening extracranial injuries always takes priority over intracranial injuries. Injuries can affect any part of the body and so during a secondary survey a complete examination of the body is required to look for evidence of any other trauma. Full body exposure with visualisation of the entire dorsal surface and a rectal examination are required (O'Shea, 2005).

Assessment

During the assessment process the following criteria should be determined:

- History and mechanism of injury
- Period of loss of consciousness
- Seizure activity
- GCS at the scene
- Pupillary response after resuscitation
- Period of hypoxia/hypotension
- Presence of headache and vomiting

Most departments incorporate guidelines (SIGN, 2009; NICE, 2007) into standard head injury proformas to aid documentation and to guide practice for all care professionals caring for TBI patients.

Discharge of mild TBI patients

In mild TBI a decision must be made as to whether the patient requires a skull radiograph and/or CT scan, as per NICE, (2007) criteria. Patients who have a GCS of 15, who have no history of loss of consciousness and have none of the criteria for CT scan/investigation may be considered for discharge according to local guidelines/policy. Patients who are discharged home should be under the supervision of a responsible adult, given verbal advice and a written head injury advice card (NICE, 2007).

Some patients who have had a MTBI and have concussion may be admitted for a period of neurological observation. Frequent neurological assessments are required to identify early any deterioration due to a possible underlying injury. Patients with MTBI should be given realistic expectations regarding recovery. Many patients do not recover quickly and have ongoing problems which can include: headaches, fatigue, emotional and behavioural problems and cognitive impairments (post-concussion syndrome) which may not be identified until the person has returned home. It is therefore essential for nurses to support and advise the patient and the next of kin about the potential for ongoing symptoms. See below for the management of specific problems following TBI.

Referral of patients to a specialist neurosurgical centre (moderate and severe head injury)

Indications for referral to a specialist neurosurgical unit or for specialist expert advice are listed in Boxes 32.1 and 32.2. In an attempt to improve the outcome for patients NICE, (2007) recommends an improvement in the rate of transfer of head injured patients to specialist units. They also recommend that all patients with isolated severe head injuries should ideally receive treatment in a neurosurgical unit irrelevant of the need for neurosurgery. Local and established national guidelines for the transfer of patients

Box 32.1   Indications for urgent referral to a neurosurgeon

- CT scan shows a recent intracranial haematoma and/or haemorrhage
- Patient fits the criteria for CT scan but cannot be performed locally
- Patient has concerning clinical features, irrespective of CT findings

Source: National Institute for Health and Clinical Excellence, 2007; Scottish Intercollegiate Guidelines Network, 2009.

Box 32.2   Clinical features to suggest that specialist neurosurgical management is appropriate and should be discussed with a neurosurgeon

- Persisting coma (GCS score <8/15) after resuscitation
- Confusion that persists for more than four hours
- Deterioration in level of consciousness after admission
- Progressive focal neurological signs
- A seizure without full recovery
- Depressed skull fracture
- Definite or suspected penetrating injury
- A CSF leak or other sign of a basal skull fracture

Source: National Institute for Health and Clinical Excellence, 2007; Scottish Intercollegiate Guidelines Network, 2009.

with head injuries to a specialist neuroscience centres must be adhered to when planning the transfer of TBI patients (ICS, 2002; AAGBI, 2006; NICE, 2007).

Emergency surgical decompression

The RCS (1999) recommends that life-saving decompressive surgery be available within four hours of injury. Rapid action is critical to the patient's outcome; the longer decompressive surgery is delayed after the injury the poorer the outcome will be.

The decision for surgical intervention is based on many factors including: clinical status and clinical deterioration, as well as CT parameters such as: size of lesion, amount of midline shift, cistern compression and the location of the lesion.

Intensive care

It is widely accepted that patients who are managed by neurointensivists in specialist units with protocol driven therapy have been found to have better outcomes (Patel *et al.*, 2002) and decreased mortality rates (Varelas *et al.*, 2006). Current medical management strategies are directed towards providing an optimal physiological environment to minimise secondary insults and maximise the body's own regenerative processes (Tisdall and Smith, 2007). The principles which underpin the nursing management of patients with severe TBI also relate to patients who are on a neuroscience ward and should be applied to all TBI patients regardless of their initial classification.

Neurology

Patients who are **not** sedated require a full neurological assessment as their condition demands. The minimum frequency of observations should be decided on an individual patient basis and reviewed regularly in consultation with medical colleagues. As discussed above, in the event of any deterioration in neurological status, senior nursing staff and medical staff should be informed and the observations should be performed more frequently. Undertaking a GCS assessment on patients who are sedated and ventilated is difficult but assessment of best motor score must be recorded (Maas *et al.*, 2000). Assessment of pupils (size, shape and reaction to light) should be conducted hourly, or more frequently if the condition requires, in order to detect raised ICP, irrespective of any paralysing agents or sedation being administered. Any change should be reported immediately.

It may be appropriate to conduct regular assessments of neurological function by temporarily reducing or discontinuing short acting sedation (Martin and Smith, 2004). This may not be appropriate for patients with unstable ICP who require adequate long acting sedation and who are fully ventilated. In such patients it is not possible to ascertain an accurate assessment of neurological functioning and usually more invasive monitoring is required (see: Multimodal neuromonitoring).

Systemic monitoring

Minimal monitoring requirements include electrocardiogram (ECG), pulse oximetry, invasive arterial blood pressure, central venous pressure (CVP), urine output, and end tidal carbon dioxide when appropriate. Femoral CVP lines are favourable in this group of patients during the acute phase, in order to avoid head down tilt for internal jugular line insertion which may exacerbate raised ICP. An oesophageal doppler may be inserted to check cardiac output, flow time velocity and systemic vascular resistance in order to guide inotropic and fluid requirements. Regular blood glucose, serum electrolytes and arterial blood gas analysis are required to optimise physiological parameters.

Intracranial pressure (ICP) and cerebral perfusion pressure (CPP) thresholds

Over the last two decades there has been a shift of emphasis from primary control of ICP to a multifaceted approach of maintaining an adequate CPP and oxygenation throughout the management period (see Chapter 7). BTF guidelines recommend instituting interventions to reduce ICP when ICP is above 20 mmHg. CPP of less than 50 mmHg is associated with critical reductions in brain tissue oxygen and an increase in mortality and morbidity (Changaris *et al.*, 1987) and should be avoided (BTF, 2007). Thus a low CPP may jeopardise regions of the brain with pre-existing ischemia (see Chapter 7 for more detail). The aim is to achieve a CPP of between 50 and 70 mmHg (BTF, 2007) through manipulation of mean arterial blood pressure (MAP) and reducing ICP.

ICP management

ICP monitoring allows for early detection of evolving mass lesions or increasing cerebral oedema in sedated patients as well as providing an essential parameter to optimise CPP and to guide treatment of ICP. Management strategies can therefore be targeted to the changing intracranial environment (see Chapter 7 for detailed management of raised ICP and ICP monitoring).

It is considered good practice to record and graph ICP and CPP as part of hourly observations and to document spontaneous rises in ICP as well as rises associated with nursing interventions. During acute rises in ICP >20 mmHg the nurse must:

- Check the pupillary response
- Check the position of the patient and ensure that he/she is in neutral alignment with head elevated at 30–45 degrees
- Ensure that endotracheal tapes or the cervical collar are not obstructing venous drainage
- Check sedation levels and increase if clinical signs of inadequate sedation are present. Evaluate the effect of a bolus and increase if required
- Check for noxious stimuli (e.g. urinary catheter)
- Reassure the patient, evaluate the effectiveness of family members' presence/absence

- Obtain an arterial blood gas (ABG) to ensure that carbon dioxide levels are within parameters
- If ICP remains elevated > 20 mmHg, the neurosurgical team should be informed as a CT scan may be required to exclude worsening intracranial pathology.

If the ICP remains elevated despite corrections to the above then interventions are gradually instituted to lower the ICP. Table 32.2 provides an overview of the interventions to treat raised ICP. For further rationale and evidence to support each intervention please refer to Chapter 7. Table 32.3 provides an overview of the Brain Trauma Foundation recommendations to manage severe TBI and the level of evidence to support each intervention (BTF, 2007). Each intervention is presented in more detail in Chapter 7.

Extracranial complications associated with TBI

Cardiovascular

Patients who sustain TBI are usually young and previously fit and do not suffer from underlying pre-morbid cardiovascular conditions. However ECG changes following injury are not uncommon, e.g. atrial and ventricular arrhythmias, abnormalities of the QRS complex, T wave and ST segment and QT prolongation, particularly in patients with diffuse injury, oedema and contusions (see Chapter 14 for further detail and management).

Careful observation of the continuous ECG is an important aspect of care in detecting the onset of any ECG changes, these must be reported immediately. A 12 lead ECG should be performed on admission and repeated daily if any subsequent changes are detected. Magnesium, potassium and phosphate levels should be regularly monitored and maintained within the normal range. Patients may also experience sympathetic storming, i.e. episodic increases in heart rate, blood pressure and temperature (see Chapter 14).

Hyperpyrexia

Temperature should be routinely monitored as elevations in temperature have been found to worsen outcome after TBI (Jones *et al.*, 1994). Systemic hyperpyrexia (>38°C) can develop 24 to 48 hours after injury and is a frequent cause of secondary brain injury in the intensive care setting (Maas *et al.*, 2000). Persistent hyperpyrexia unresponsive to any interventions may be a result of damage to the hypothalamus and must also be considered in severe TBI. Microbiological causes of infection must also be investigated.

Table 32.2 Overview of interventions used to manage intracranial pressure (ICP).

Intervention	Rationale	Nursing considerations
Sedation, analgesia	Facilitates invasive ventilation, minimises pain, agitation and anxiety	
Propofol	Short-acting anaesthetic with easy titration of sedation levels and rapid wake up. Causes a dose dependent reduction in cerebral metabolic rate of oxygen consumption ($CMRO_2$), CBF and ICP	Monitor for adverse effects of hypotension and propofol infusion syndrome (see Chapter 7)
Midazalam	Short acting benzodiazepine – aids long term sedation	Long term use has cumulative effects
Barbiturate coma	Control of intracranial hypertension unresponsive to other treatments. Lowers ICP by reducing $CMRO_2$ and CBF	Monitor for adverse effects of hypotension. Prolonged half-life makes clinical assessment difficult
Fentanyl, morphine and sufentanyl	Synthetic narcotics – used in conjunction with sedation to manage pain	Use with caution in haemodynamically unstable patients as may cause fall in MAP and an elevation in ICP
Neuromuscular blocking agents *Atracurium, vecuronium*	Used to minimise coughing and straining on the endotracheal tube which may increase ICP. May facilitate ventilation	Administer bolus first and evaluate its effect prior to commencement of infusion. Monitor for complications associated with its use, i.e. pneumonia, sepsis
Hyperventilation	Causes cerebral vasoconstriction, reducing cerebral blood volume and consequently ICP. Considered in patients with raised ICP and impending brain stem damage.	Should be instituted in a tailored way and under specific multimodality monitoring to ensure that oxygen delivery is not compromised
Positioning	Neutral position with moderate head up tilt (30–45°) to aid venous return and reduce ICP	Assess effect, i.e. MAP, ICP, CPP
Hyperosmolar therapy *Mannitol*	Increases osmolality of the blood which creates an osmotic gradient drawing fluid from the brain into the intravascular space – thereby reducing cerebral oedema and ICP	Potent diuretic which can cause hypotension and fluid electrolyte imbalance
Induced hypothermia	To control ICP (each degree above 37°C increases $CMRO_2$)	Consider the systemic side-effects of hypothermia (see Chapter 14)
Decompressive craniectomy	When all other measures have failed to reduce ICP	Avoid lying the patient on the operative site. Post-operative nursing management, see: Craniectomy Chapter 20

CBF – cerebral blood flow; $CMRO_2$– cerebral metabolic rate of oxygen consumption; CPP – cerebral perfusion pressure; ICP – intracranial pressure; MAP – mean arterial pressure.

Table 32.3 Recommendations for the management of severe traumatic brain injury (TBI).

Level I evidence (High degree of clinical certainty)	Level II evidence (Moderate clinical certainty)	Level III evidence (Unclear clinical certainty)
Administration of **steroids** does not improve outcome or reduce ICP.		
	Prophylactic and acute use of **hyperventilation** should be avoided. Parameters for $PaCO_2$: • If ICP <15 mmHg, then $PaCO_2$ 4.5–5.0 kPa • If ICP 15–25 mmHg, then $PaCO_2$ 4.0–4.5 kPa	**Hyperventilation** is only recommended as a temporary measure for the reduction of elevated ICP. Its use should be avoided in the first 24 hours after injury when CBF is reduced
	Systolic BP <90 mmHg avoided CPP >70 mmHg should be avoided	CPP of <50 mmHg should be avoided CPP target: 50–70 mmHg
	Indications for ICP monitoring: • GCS 3–8 with abnormal CT scan Or two or more of the following adverse features: • Age >40 years • Motor posturing • Systolic BP <90 mmHg	
	ICP thresholds Treatment should be initiated with ICP thresholds above 20 mmHg	A combination of ICP values, clinical findings and CT evidence of increased ICP (e.g. absent/compressed basal cisterns) should be used to determine the need for treatment
	Hyperosmolar therapy Mannitol is effective for control of raised ICP after severe TBI in doses ranging from 0.25 g/kg body weight to 1 g/kg body weight	Restrict mannitol use prior to ICP monitoring to patients with signs of transtentorial herniation or progressive neurological deterioration not attributable to extracranial causes
	High dose barbiturate therapy May be considered in haemodynamically stable patients to control elevated ICP refractory to maximal medical and surgical therapy Prophylactic administration of barbiturates to induce burst suppression EEG is not recommended	

Source: Brain Trauma Rating scheme for the strength of the evidence – Class I: Good quality randomised controlled trial (RCT); Class II: Moderate quality RCT, good quality cohort, or good quality case-control; Class III: Poor quality RCT, moderate or poor quality cohort, moderate or poor case-control, case series, databases, or registries.

Respiratory

Following injury hypoxaemia may be present due to factors such as direct pulmonary injury (e.g. pulmonary contusion, pneumothorax) aspiration of gastric contents, or neurogenic pulmonary oedema. Neurogenic pulmonary oedema is the most severe form of acute lung injury and is seen in patients with fatal or near fatal head injuries and after abrupt elevations of ICP. The exact mechanism of neurogenic pulmonary oedema is unclear, however the primary management requires reduction of ICP and appropriate ventilatory management to maximise oxygenation. The specific management of neurogenic pulmonary oedema is presented in Chapter 14. NICE recommends a PaO_2 of 13 kPa.

Electrolyte imbalance

Hyponatraemia (sodium less than 130 mmol/l) lowers seizure threshold and can exacerbate cerebral oedema. It can occur after TBI and the aetiology is complex with both cerebral salt wasting (CSW) and the syndrome of inappropriate antidiuretic hormone (SIADH) being implicated. The distinction between these two conditions is critical as the two require different treatment strategies. Serum and urinary electrolytes must be examined as well as a fluid and urinary assessment to help reach a definitive diagnosis (refer to Chapter 16 for specific management of CSW and SIADH).

Hypernatraemia, also common in TBI, may result from dehydration, the use of osmotic agents used in the acute phase, or diabetes insipidus (DI). DI occurs as a result of damage/dysfunction of the hypothalamic pituitary axis (HPA) (refer to Chapter 16 for management of hypernatraemia).

Deep vein thrombosis

The incidence of deep vein thrombosis (DVT) is related to the type and severity of the injury (Helmy *et al.*, 2007). Its incidence is as low as 3% in isolated head injury, rising to 23% in polytrauma patients (Rogers *et al.*, 2002). Graduated compression thigh length stockings with additional intermittent pneumatic compression devices have been recommended in the prophylaxis of DVT in TBI patients (BTF, 2007). Low dose unfractionated heparin should be used in combination with mechanical prophylaxis in the acute setting, and low molecular weight heparin used in the rehabilitation setting (Carlisle *et al.*, 2006). Cerebral contusions after TBI are at risk of expanding and this can be influenced by coagulopathy and anticoagulation (Oertel *et al.*, 2002). These factors influence the timing and commencement of venous thrombosis prophylaxis. Advice from the neurosurgeon in charge of the patient should be sought prior to commencing anticoagulation therapy and the risk/benefit ratio discussed.

Malnutrition

Patients who have sustained a severe TBI may develop a hypermetabolic, hypercatabolic and hyperglycaemic state in the acute stages following injury (Young *et al.*, 1996). The consequences of these metabolic events may be malnutrition resulting in reduced immunocompetence, accelerated visceral protein depletion and impaired healing (Young *et al.*, 1996). There can be an increase of up to 60% in basal metabolic rate (BMR) in the first 48 hrs following severe head injury and nitrogen losses can be significant in the acute phase resulting in the loss of muscle mass.

Factors such as reduced consciousness, swallowing and cognitive deficits should also be considered in TBI patients as these can affect the ability to maintain adequate nutritional support (Gentleman, 2001). Malnutrition is associated with a worse outcome and a slower neurological recovery (Yanagawa *et al.*, 2003). An orogastric tube should be utilised until a possible base of skull fracture has been excluded. For recommendations on enteral feeding refer to Chapter 16.

Hyperglycaemia

Blood glucose levels are frequently elevated following brain injury due to the stress response. The introduction of protocol driven glycaemic control to maintain glucose level of 4–7 mmol/litre has been found to reduce mortality in patients with severe TBI (Clayton *et al.*, 2004). There is also substantial evidence that highlights the adverse effects of hyperglycaemia in critically ill patients (van den Berghe *et al.*, 2001). Although the optimal target glycaemic range is yet to be determined for TBI patients in the acute phase, tight glycaemic control has become part of the routine management of patients.

Post-traumatic seizures (PTS)

Post-traumatic seizures may be classified according to their relationship to the time of injury, i.e. early (within 7 days) or late (after 7 days) (BSRM, 2003). Some neurosurgeons advocate the prophylactic use of antiepileptic drugs (AEDs) in certain high risk patients such as those with a depressed skull fracture (Temkin, 2003). Phenytoin is the AED of choice if patients have one or more seizures. The loading dose of 15–20 mg/kg is administered intravenously followed by a daily maintenance dose of 300 mg.

Serum levels should be checked regularly to ensure that they are within therapeutic range. Patients should be cardiac monitored when phenytoin is administered intravenously as side-effects include cardiac arrhythmias and hypotension. Protocols should be in place for the management of acute seizures (see Chapter 30).

General nursing care

The importance of basic nursing care cannot be underestimated. Bowel care is an important consideration, as constipation has implications for both ICP and respiratory management. Increased intra-abdominal pressure leads to increased intrathoracic pressure, which can in turn increase ICP and affect the management of ventilation. Bowel sounds should be assessed and recorded daily as part of the overall assessment as well as monitoring for any signs of abdominal distension. Aperients should be routinely administered and their effectiveness evaluated to avoid constipation.

Many nursing interventions may increase ICP and if carried out in succession can potentially have a cumulative effect on ICP (see Chapter 7 for further detail).

Multimodal neuromonitoring

The last decade has seen rapid developments in multimodality neuromonitoring techniques, which provide valuable data to the neurointensive care clinician. These techniques have been developed to guide TBI management in conjunction with conventional neuroimaging techniques to identify, or predict, the occurrence of secondary insults. Many of these monitoring techniques are still under investigation and to date are mainly used for research purposes. Future research may reveal their clinical potential and lead to a greater understanding of individual pathophysiology, allowing further development of individually targeted treatment strategies.

Jugular bulb venous oximetry (SjvO₂)

This technique is used to estimate cerebral oxygenation. A catheter is inserted into the dominant internal jugular vein and advanced to the jugular bulb (the bulbous dilatation of the jugular vein just below the base of the skull which carries only cerebral venous blood).

Jugular venous oxygen saturation (SjvO₂) can be measured continuously using a spectroscopic technique or intermittently by aspirating blood samples and using a co-oximeter. Normal SjvO₂ levels are approximately 60–80% and a reduction in SjvO₂ below physiological levels indicates that cerebral oxygen delivery is inadequate to meet demand (Tisdall and Smith, 2007). This may be due to reduced cerebral blood flow (CBF), secondary to decreased cerebral perfusion pressure (CPP) or hyperventilation-associated vasoconstriction following TBI. This may lead to cerebral ischemia if not corrected. Conversely, raised SjvO₂ may be caused by raised CBF or reduced oxygen demand secondary to mitochondrial dysfunction or cell death (Cruz, 1998). A reduction in SjvO₂ to less than 50–55% after TBI is associated with poor outcome (Robertson *et al.*, 1995) and it is recommended that a saturation below 50% is the threshold for treatment (BTF, 2007).

A limitation of jugular venous oximetry is its lack of sensitivity to focal areas of underperfused tissue. At present the widespread use of this technique is limited due to lack of expertise in its use and cost implications. However its use has been recommended in addition to ICP monitoring in the management of patients with severe TBI (BTF, 2007). Its widespread use in guiding therapy and its relationship to outcome is yet to be validated.

Microdialysis

Intracerebral microdialysis is a technique which monitors the chemistry of the brain's interstitial fluid. The microdialysis catheter is usually placed in at risk tissue such as the ischemic penumbra which allows biochemical changes to be measured in the area of brain most vulnerable to secondary insult (Tisdall and Smith, 2007). It is possible to measure dialysate concentrations of glucose, lactate/pyruvate ratio, glycerol and glutamate. Monitoring these values is an index of ongoing cell damage/death. Severe hypoxia/ischemia is associated with increases in the lactate/pyruvate ratio (LPR) (Stahl *et al.*, 2001). The measurement of metabolites via microdialysis may assist future clinical decision making, such as the management of CPP, guidance of hyperventilation, and the appropriateness of extensive surgical procedures (Tisdall and Smith, 2007).

Focal tissue oxygen tension (PbtO₂)

Measured PbtO₂ represents the balance between oxygen delivery and cellular oxygen consumption (Tisdall and Smith, 2007). PbtO₂ probes provide a highly focal measurement and offer the potential of selectively monitoring how well tissue is being perfused at a local level, reflecting CBF or oxygen extraction fraction (Scheufler *et al.*, 2002). This technique means that probe positioning is crucial and global changes may be missed. Normal PbtO₂ value using the Licox system (Integra Neurosciences) is in the range of 20–35 mmHg (Helliwell, 2009). Reduced $PbtO_2$ is associated with higher rates of mortality, and ischemic thresholds of between 5 and 20 mmHg for periods for greater than 30 minutes have been identified (Valadka *et al.*, 1998). It is therefore recommended that brain tissue oxygen tension of less than 15 mmHg is a threshold for treatment (BTF, 2007). Further investigation of this technique will reveal the clinical usefulness of $PbtO_2$ directed therapy.

Near infrared spectroscopy (NIRS)

NIRS is a non-invasive technique which measures the intensity of near infrared light passing through tissue. This allows measurement of absolute haemoglobin oxygen saturation and absolute concentrations of oxy and deoxy-haemoglobin in the tissue (Fantini *et al.*, 1999). This technique has the potential to provide continuous non-invasive measurement of cerebral haemodynamic and metabolic function in specific regions of the brain (Tisdall and Smith, 2007). It offers the potential to reflect the temporal change of cerebral blood volume (CBV) which may assist in the management of CPP.

Transcranial Dopplar ultrasonography (TCD)

TCD is a non–invasive technique which utilises ultrasound waves to derive cerebral blood flow velocity, usually of the middle cerebral artery (Tisdall and Smith, 2007). TCD is not able to provide absolute measurements of CBF but changes in blood flow velocities can reflect changes in blood vessel resistance which is helpful in the detection of vasospasm (refer to Chapter 23 for further detail).

Continuous electroencephalography (cEEG)

Seizures are a source of secondary insult to the injured brain and data from cEEG studies reveal that seizures occur in 20% of patients with TBI within the neurointensive care unit (Vespa *et al.*, 1999). Many of these seizures are of a non-convulsive variety and occur despite the use of phenytoin at adequate serum concentrations (Tisdall and Smith, 2007). cEEG also provides an objective estimate of the degree of electrical neuronal depression during barbiturate therapy (see Chapter 7 for further detail). External interference from monitors and ventilators can affect the reliability of this system.

NEURO-REHABILITATION: ACUTE PHASE

Early rehabilitation plays a crucial role in TBI management; maximising quality of life by reducing disability,

and helps to minimise costs of hospital and community care (BSRM, 2003). As soon as patients are clinically stable, even when altered conscious states persist, early sitting and standing is recommended to avoid problems such as osteopenia, loss of muscle bulk, and loss of normal cardiovascular and autonomic responses (Bloomfield, 1997). Early mobilisation also promotes normal postural tone, proprioceptive information, and helps to maintain range and alignment of joints. A graded programme in liaison with physiotherapists should be implemented to increase tolerance to sitting and standing with appropriately supportive equipment (BSRM, 2003). Although this requires a lot of time from the nurses and physiotherapist the benefits for the patient from a rehabilitative perspective are enormous.

The role of the physiotherapist in preventing long-term disability in patients with neurological dysfunction is crucial. Many patients develop abnormal posture, movement and spasticity due to upper motor neurone damage, and are at greater risk of developing structural deformity, e.g. contractures (see Chapter 11). Strategies must be initiated at the onset of neurological damage and continued on an ongoing basis throughout the patient's journey to prevent long-term physical disability. Passive movements of the limbs should be performed throughout the day to help maintain muscle tone and full range of joint movement. Nurses should work collaboratively with the physiotherapist and occupational therapist to ensure that the correct therapy is being maintained. Splinting of limbs is often required and nurses must carry out the regime prescribed by the physiotherapist as part of the patient's general care.

Ward environment

Patients with GCS 13–15 who appear well can deteriorate due to secondary injury processes during the acute period. Nurses, within all settings, therefore need to be vigilant and to deliver care that incorporates the principles discussed previously in an attempt to prevent secondary injury and further neurological deficits.

Individual need assessments are required, irrespective of the severity of injury to address issues of long-term morbidity. Awareness of particular problems will facilitate the assessment process with early involvement of the relevant personnel. Table 32.4 lists the wide range of problems that patients with TBI may experience, depending on the severity of the injury. The consequences of TBI can impede physical, emotional, social, marital and vocational functioning (Zasler and Martelli, 2003).

Some patients can experience a number of cognitive and/or behavioural symptoms within the immediate days

Table 32.4 Specific problems associated with TBI.

Physical	Cognitive	Behavioural/ emotional
• Paralysis	**Impairment of:**	• Emotional
• Abnormal	• Memory	lability
muscle tone	• Attention	• Poor
• Impaired	• Perception	initiation
coordination	• Problem	• Mood change,
• Incontinence	solving	e.g.
• Disorders of	• Insight	depression
speech	• Safety	• Apathy
• Visual	awareness	• Aggressive
disturbances	• Social	outbursts
• Dysphagia	judgement	• Disinhibition
• Seizures		• Inappropriate
• Headaches/		sexual
dizziness		behaviour
• Fatigue		• Poor
• Sleep		motivation
disturbances		• Anxiety
		• Irritability

Adapted from British Society of Rehabilitation Medicine, 2003.

following the injury whereas for others, these may not be apparent until the patient returns to their home environment.

Emotional and behavioural problems

Change in personality is not uncommon after TBI and is often reported by relatives to be the most difficult persisting change that they have to adjust to. Comments such as '… he is not the man I married …' or 'it's like living with a different person' are not uncommon (McMillan and Greenwood, 2002). Changes may or may not emphasise previous personality traits and include egocentricity, childishness, poor judgement, lack of initiation, reduced drive, lethargy, unconcern, lack of depth of feeling, irritability, aggressiveness, reduced tact and increased/or decreased sexual interest (McMillan and Greenwood, 2002). These changes can lead to marital break-up, social isolation and unemployment. Longitudinal studies suggest that planned behavioural modification programmes consistently applied are effective in preventing these undesired behaviours from becoming established (Eames and

Wood, 1985; BSRM, 2003) (see Chapter 10). Families should be given specific information and support to help them understand the nature of these problems and guidance on how to interact appropriately with the patient (BSRM, 2003).

Depression is a common emotional problem in the first year after TBI with estimates of post-traumatic depression ranging between 10 and 77% (O'Donnell *et al.*, 2004). This has many consequences as it increases the risk of developing other neuropsychiatric problems which can interfere with physical and cognitive rehabilitation (Alderfer *et al.*, 2005). Both neurobiological (i.e. injury related) and psychosocial factors contribute to the development and persistence of depression after TBI (Bay *et al.*, 2004). Psychosocial risk factors include: poor pre-injury occupational status, poor social functioning and poverty, alcohol abuse, female gender and a tendency to experience high levels of stress (Alderfer *et al.*, 2005). Depression is treated by clinical psychology techniques and/or with antidepressants.

Assessment of emotional state should be undertaken by clinical staff and referral for further assessment made if deemed necessary. Nurses should provide patients and their relatives with information and advice and the opportunity to talk about the impact of brain injury on their lives. Many patients and their families may need help from an expert in managing emotional issues after TBI and should be provided with access to individual and/or group psychological interventions where possible (BSRM, 2003).

Behavioural problems are a major challenge to ward staff and can put extreme pressure on time and morale. Behavioural management techniques should be utilised with advice from liaison psychiatry and/or clinical neuropsychology (see Chapter 10).

Agitation and aggression

Patients who have sustained a TBI have an increased risk of aggression and agitation during the first six months post injury (Tateno *et al.*, 2003). These are often the most troublesome changes for carers and patients (Fleminger *et al.*, 2006). Agitation and aggression on medical or surgical wards immediately following the injury can cause disruption to the normal running of the ward and cause distress for nursing staff and family members.

The terms agitation and aggression are difficult to define and are often treated interchangeably (Sandel and Mysiw, 1996). Agitation may be described as a disturbed behaviour as a result of overactivity and occurs frequently in the acute phase of recovery where it is usually related to features of post-traumatic amnesia (PTA) (Fleminger *et al.*, 2006) (see: Post-traumatic amnesia). Environmental intervention rather than drug therapy should be used initially to manage agitation in the acute phase as medication can adversely affect cognitive function and may exacerbate the problem. However, if the situation cannot be resolved through environmental strategies then a suitable drug treatment may be used (refer to Chapter 9 for supportive and environmental measures for managing agitation). Antidepressants are sometimes used; this is based on the observation that metabolites of noradrenaline and serotonin have been found to be reduced in CSF from agitated patients following acute brain injury (Arciniegas *et al.*, 2000). As most antidepressants potentiate noradrenaline and/or serotonin they may be useful considerations in TBI management (Fleminger *et al.*, 2006).

The symptoms of aggression include both verbal and physical aggression against self, objects and other people (Yudofsky, 1986). It may also include severe irritability, violent, hostile or assaultive behaviour. Antipsychotics are commonly used to manage aggression as a short term measure to quieten disturbed patients (Fleminger *et al.*, 2006). Sedating medications can cause confusion and may therefore exacerbate agitation. Refer to Chapter 10 regarding issues of restraint.

Current evidence suggests that the use of beta-blockers is the most effective in the management of agitation and/or aggression following acquired brain injury (Fleminger *et al.*, 2006). However more evidence is required as regards their efficacy.

Post-traumatic amnesia (PTA)

PTA is a period of confusion and amnesia following head injury. One of the hallmarks of PTA is anterograde amnesia which is the impaired ability to remember events after the onset of a condition, i.e. the head injury (Nakase-Thompson *et al.*, 2004). The patient may also suffer with retrograde amnesia. The duration of PTA may last for a number of hours, days, weeks or months and ends when the patient regains continuous day-to-day recall (BSRM, 2003). The duration of PTA is used as a measure of head injury severity. Although the exact pathophysiological mechanism of PTA is not known, damage to structures involved in memory, arousal and attention such as the brain stem, diencephalon and hippocampus may be implicated (Povlishock, 2000).

PTA represents a continuous measure of impaired cerebral function and is usually measured daily in the acute phase following injury. The two most commonly used scales for measuring PTA are the Revised Westmead PTA scale and the Galveston Orientation and Amnesia Test (GOAT).

Care of the patient emerging from coma and PTA

Patients who demonstrate confused and agitated behaviour after TBI should be assessed fully to establish the diagnosis and to rule out treatable causes such as drug and alcohol withdrawal (BSRM, 2003). Managing the patient in a quiet environment and avoiding over stimulation should be encouraged, with involvement of family members if effective. Drugs with sedative side-effects should be avoided where possible however in the presence of uncontrolled aggressive outbursts the use of medications such as carbamazepine or olanzepine should be considered in conjunction with psychiatric advice with regular review (BSRM, 2003).One to one supervision should be considered to ensure the safety of the patient and to help reassure and orientate them.

Cognitive problems

Cognitive problems are common after TBI and may be more problematic than physical disability. The nature of the cognitive deficit depends on the severity and location of injury and may include difficulties with attention, memory functions, perception, information processing, problem solving ability and executive function. These functions are necessary in order to plan, initiate, sequence, terminate and monitor a wide variety of tasks. Natural recovery from cognitive deficits is maximal in the first six months after injury, but the recovery can continue more slowly for up to two years (Gentleman, 2001). Different deficits recover at different speeds and progress is often episodic with the patient experiencing periods where function has reached a plateau. Appropriate clinical intervention can influence this process and enhance recovery (Millis *et al.*, 2001). An assessment by a clinical neuropsychologist is required to assess the type, extent and consequences of cognitive impairment (Gentleman, 2001).

Neuropsychological input to the rehabilitation team is essential to help identify clinical problems and to design coping strategies to reduce disability and support others within the multidisciplinary team. Memory disorders are an example of the cognitive sequelae of severe TBI and a wide range of treatment approaches can be tried in a structured rehabilitation programme to help reduce the handicapping effect of memory problems (e.g. a personal organiser with alarm systems, colour codes around the house, lists and diaries)(Gentleman, 2001). For further detail on the management of specific cognitive impairments see Chapter 9.

NEURO-REHABILITATION: ONGOING PHYSICAL PROBLEMS

Tracheostomy weaning (see Chapter 15)

Communication

Language deficits are common after TBI and in severe cases can affect the rehabilitation process as well as leading to frustration, increased behavioural problems and social isolation (BSRM, 2003). Various interventions can support the recovery of language function and patients should be assessed by speech and language therapists to delineate appropriate communication techniques and to optimise the patient's ability to express themselves.

Management of dysphagia (see Chapter 12)

Bladder and bowel management

During the acute stages, an indwelling urethral catheter may be used for assessing fluid balance accurately. However prolonged catheter use may be associated with infection and urethral stricture and should be avoided where possible (Rice–Oxley, 2000). The catheter should be removed as soon as possible and a toileting regime instituted as soon as the patient's condition allows. Following TBI patients may experience urge incontinence. For further detail of management refer to Chapter 18. Patients should have a regular bowel regime to avoid constipation and to manage faecal incontinence.

Spasticity and contractures

Therapeutic positioning should be employed during the acute phase and during ongoing care to avoid the development of abnormal postures, contractures, pain, skin breakdown and respiratory complications, all of which are associated with delayed discharge and poorer outcomes (BSRM, 2003). A suitable moving/handling programme for each patient should be implemented following a moving and handling risk assessment. Patients should have a clinical assessment for risk of pressure sores and should be provided with appropriate pressure relieving equipment. Assessment and evaluation of skin condition is ongoing to ensure that adequate protection is maintained.

Management of spasticity and prevention of contractures are essential in the care of TBI patients (BSRM, 2003). Where spasticity develops despite appropriate preventative positioning it may lead to the development of contractures. This will require advice from the interdisciplinary team and a coordinated plan for its management. Aggravating factors such as pain and infection should be considered and

managed accordingly. The treatment options include physical and occupational therapy, bracing/splinting, benzodiazepines, oral or intrathecal baclofen, tendon release and rhizotomy. The use of the microbial protein botulinum neurotoxin is also recommended in some cases as a treatment option (Simpson *et al.*, 2008). Refer to Chapter 11 for further detail on specific management.

Pain management

Pain is often underdiagnosed following TBI and patients with communication and cognitive deficits are often unable to describe sensory symptoms such as hypersensitivity and neurogenic pain (BSRM, 2003). Spasticity, contractures and deformity are causes of significant pain and distress to the individual. Shoulder pain arising from spasticity, malalignment or subluxation due to muscle imbalance or weakness or secondary damage to soft tissues can occur. Pain may be exacerbated by poor handling.

Pain assessment should be performed on a regular basis, paying particular attention to non-verbal cues in those with impaired communication and/or cognitive deficits (see Chapter 17).

Rehabilitation: A multidisciplinary approach

Successful rehabilitation programmes require carefully co-ordinated input from a variety of professionals with good verbal and written communication across disciplines. Rehabilitation should be goal orientated and planned on an individual basis, taking account of the patient's views, cultural background and pre-morbid lifestyle (BSRM, 2003). Early intensive specialist rehabilitation programmes are associated with better outcomes as well as being cost effective (Slade *et al.*, 2002). The effects of TBI can be long lasting and patients and their families require continued care and support. Rehabilitation must therefore be viewed as a continuum where ongoing support and supervision is available for those who require it. Vocational rehabilitation has been recognised as a quality requirement within the *National Service Framework for Long-term Conditions* (DH, 2005). The aim is that people with a long-term neurological condition can have access to appropriate vocational assessment, rehabilitation and ongoing support to work or engage in alternative occupational and educational opportunities.

Ongoing support for family and carers

Care of the family should be a multidisciplinary responsibility, however it is the nurse who spends most time with relatives. Information needs should be regularly assessed and information reiterated as required. Relatives who are shocked and/or distressed find it difficult to process and retain information therefore additional forms of communication should be provided, e.g. information booklets. Relevant support agencies should be considered and used where appropriate (e.g. Headway, Brain and Spine Association). Where in-house counselling services are available, family members should be offered the service to assist them in dealing with this traumatic period in their lives. The presence of family members at the bedside should be encouraged and where appropriate they should be encouraged to participate in basic care needs. This often makes the family feel less helpless and can help in meeting some of their psychological needs as well as those of the patient.

The need to support family and carers of people with a long-term neurological condition such as the consequences of TBI is highlighted as a quality requirement in the *National Service Framework for Long-term Conditions* (DH, 2005). Carers should have access to appropriate support and services that recognise their needs both in their role as carer and in their own right (BSRM, 2003). Families and/or carers need information, practical support, continued education and easy access to health and social care systems. Ongoing support is essential within the community to maximise independence and quality of life for the patient and his/her family. Family and carers should be involved in assessment and subsequent decisions about help that is required, and assessment to establish their own needs and to increase the sustainability of the caring role (BSRM, 2003). The assessment of carers' needs and the preparation for discharge home to the community is an important role of the nurse in the rehabilitation process. Good discharge planning can ensure that the transition from hospital to the community is safe and meets the needs of the patient and his/her family.

PROGNOSIS

It is not always possible to predict accurately the prognosis following TBI. The structural damage seen on imaging does not always reflect the severity of impairment /disability that the patient has sustained (BSRM, 2003). There are however a number of prognostic variables that are helpful in determining outcome. Older age, low GCS on admission, pupillary abnormalities (i.e. absent pupil reactivity) and the presence of major extracranial injury all predict poor prognosis in TBI (Pablo, 2008).

There is a significant increase in poor outcome in patients older than 60 years of age (Chestnut *et al.*, 2000),

possibly due to extracranial comorbidities or changes in brain plasticity. CT features such as absence of basal cisterns and obliteration of the third ventricle are associated with a poor prognosis. The independent prognostic value of tSAH has also been realised in recent years (Maas *et al.*, 2005).

The value of the admission GCS has changed over recent years. With the increased use of early sedation, intubation and ventilation in severe TBI the admission GCS has lost some predictive value (Balestreri *et al.*, 2004), however its use remains important in the assessment and classification of TBI. PTA duration is considered one of the best measures for predicting long-term functional and cognitive outcome. PTA represents a continuous measure of impaired cerebral function and, if it is measured daily in the acute period after injury, it can act as an important clinical marker of injury severity.

The oldest and most widely used tool to measure outcome is the Glasgow Outcome Scale (GOS) (Jennett and Bond, 1975). Although this scale has been used extensively it is not sensitive to the subtle deficits in cognition, mood and behaviour. However, it is useful for statistical comparisons particularly for the severe head injury group (Gentleman, 2001).

Outcome

Advances in monitoring, treatment and the effect of specialist neurointensive care units with protocol driven therapy has led to a reduction in severe TBI mortality (Lu *et al.*, 2005; Jose and Suarez, 2006). Despite the decrease in mortality the incidence of morbidity after TBI remains high (Thornhill *et al.*, 2000). Approximately 60% of those that survive moderate–severe TBI have some residual neurological deficit ranging from mild cognitive impairment to severe neurological deficit (Dikmen *et al.*, 2003). There is increasing awareness of the high level of disability as a consequence of MTBI. High morbidity results in long-term consequences for survivors, their families and health care systems.

THE FUTURE

In an attempt to improve the outcome for TBI patients the concept of 'neuroprotection' has evolved. This involves the development of pharmacological interventions that attempt to interrupt the complex neurochemical processes following injury (Tolias and Bullock, 2004). To date, none of these have been successful. Due to the complexity of TBI and the secondary injury cascades involved it may be necessary to administer combinations of neuroprotective agents.

There is extensive exploration of how to regenerate and repair central nervous system damage in experimental models. The use of gene therapy utilising neurotrophic and growth factors (e.g. nerve growth factor NGF) which stimulate the outgrowth of neurites may help in the repair and restoration of damaged neural pathways (Longhi *et al.*, 2004). The transplantation of adult stem cells may provide cures for the damaged nervous system after TBI, as may treatments which encourage endogenous stem cells to migrate to areas of damage (Harting *et al.*, 2008).

With ongoing advancements in molecular biology, stem cell therapy and a better understanding of the cellular cascades that occur following TBI it perhaps is only a matter of time before a combination of therapies is developed which can prevent or reverse neuronal damage.

SUMMARY

Enormous progress has been made in the treatment of patients with TBI. Advances in pre-hospital care, imaging, invasive monitoring, critical care and rehabilitation have all contributed to both a reduction in mortality and improved outcomes for this patient group. Outcome is dependent upon the severity of the primary injury, prompt diagnosis and adequate referral, together with limiting and treating the processes that lead to secondary brain injury.

Good clinical assessment skills are essential as the nurse plays a pivotal role in detecting early signs of neurological/systemic deterioration and alerting the appropriate medical personnel to such changes. Nurses need to be aware of current management strategies as well as possess specialist knowledge in order to optimise outcomes for this patient group. With continued advancements, good quality nursing, and medical care with protocol driven therapy, it is hoped that mortality and morbidity for this patient group will continue to improve.

REFERENCES

Alderfer B, Arciniegas D, Silver J (2005) Treatment of depression following traumatic brain injury. *The Journal of Head Trauma Rehabilitation* 20(6):544–562.

Arciniegas DB, Topkoff J, Silver JM (2000) Neuropsychiatric aspects of traumatic brain injury. *Current Treatment Options in Neurology* 2(2):169–186.

Association of Anaesthetists of Great Britain and Ireland (2006) *Recommendations for the Safe Transfer of Patients with Brain Injury*. London: The Association of Anaesthetists of Great Britain and Ireland.

Astrup, J, Siesjo BK, Symon L (1981) Thresholds in cerebral ischemia – the ischemic penumbra. *Stroke* 12(6):723–725.

Balestreri M, Czosnyka M, Chatfield D *et al.* (2004) Predictive value of Glasgow Coma Scale after brain trauma: change in trend over the past ten years. *Journal of Neurology, Neurosurgery and Psychiatry* 75:161–162.

Bay E, Kirsch N, Gillespie B (2004) Chronic stress conditions do explain post-traumatic brain injury depression. *Research Theory and Nursing Practice* 18(2–3):213–228.

Beaumont A, Marmarou A (2000) Responses of the brain to physical injury. In: Crockard A, Haywad R, Hoff J (eds). *Neurosurgery: The Scientific Basis of Clinical Practice* (3rd edition). Oxford: Blackwell Science.

Beilharz EJ, Williams CE, Dragunow M *et al.* (1995) Mechanisms of delayed cell death following hypoxic–ischemic injury in the immature rat: evidence for apoptosis during selective neuronal loss. *Molecular Brain Research* 29:1–14.

Bloomfield SA (1997) Changes in musculoskeletel structure and function with prolonged bedrest. *Medical Science Sports Exercise* 29(2):197–206.

Blumbergs PC, Scott G, Manavis J *et al.* (1995) Topography of axonal injury as defined by amyloid precursor protein and the sector scoring method in mild and severe closed head injury. *Journal of Neurotrauma* 12(4):565–572.

Bor-Seng–Shu E, Hirsch R, Teixeira MJ *et al.* (2006) Cerebral hemodynamic changes gauged by transcranial dopplar ultrasonography in patients with posttraumatic brain swelling treated by surgical decompression. *Journal of Neurosurgery* 104:93–100.

Bor-Seng–Shu E, Jacobsen Teixeira M (2007) Brain vasospasm after head injury. *Journal of Neurosurgery* 106(4):728–729.

Bouma GJ, Muizelaar JP, Stringer WA *et al.* (1992) Ultra early evaluation of regional cerebral blood flow in severely head injured patients using xenon enhanced computed tomography. *Journal of Neurosurgery* 77:360–368.

Brain Trauma Foundation (2001) The American Association of Neurological Surgeons. Guidelines for the management of penetrating brain injury. *Journal of Trauma, Injury, Infection and Critical Care* 51(2):Suppl S34–S40: S3–S6:S16–25:S41–S43:S53–S56.

Brain Trauma Foundation (2003) The American Association of Neurological Neurosurgeons and the Congress of Neurological Surgeons. Joint section on neurotrauma and critical care. *Guidelines for the Management of Severe Traumatic Brain Injury: Cerebral perfusion pressure*. New York: Brain Trauma Foundation.

Brain Trauma Foundation (2007) The American Association of Neurological Neurosurgeons and the Congress of Neurological Surgeons. Joint section on neurotrauma and critical care. *Guidelines for the Management of Severe Traumatic Brain Injury*. Available from: https://www.braintrauma.org/coma-guidelines/ Accessed July 2010.

British Society of Rehabilitation Medicine (2003) *Rehabilitation Following Acquired Brain Injury: National clinical guidelines*. London: Royal College of Physicians.

Buki A, Okonkwo D, Wang K *et al.* (2000) Cytochrome C release and caspase activation in traumatic axonal injury. *Journal of Neuroscience* 20(8):2825–2834.

Bullock M, Ross MD, Chestnut R *et al.* (2006a) Surgical management of acute epidural haematomas. *Congress of Neurological Surgeons* 58(3):Suppl PS2-7–S2-15.

Bullock M, Ross MD, Chestnut R *et al.* (2006b) Introduction. *Congress of Neurological Surgeons.* 58(3):Suppl S2-1–S2-3.

Carlisle MC, Yablon SA, Mysiw WJ *et al.* (2006) Deep venous thrombosis management following traumatic brain injury: a practice survey of the traumatic brain injury model systems. *Journal of Head Trauma Rehabilitation* 21(6):483–490.

Chan KH, Dearden NM, Millar JD (1992) The significance of posttraumatic increase in cerebral blood flow velocity: a transcranial dopplar ultrasound study. *Neurosurgery* 30:697–700.

Changaris DG, Mc Graw CP, Richardson JD *et al.* (1987) Correlation of cerebral perfusion pressure and Glasgow Coma Scale to outcome. *Journal of Trauma* 27:1007–1013.

Chestnut RM (1997) Avoidance of hypotension: conditiosine qua non of successful severe head–injury management. *Journal of Trauma* 42:S4–S9.

Chestnut RM, Ghajar J, Maas AR (2000) Guidelines for the management and prognosis of severe traumatic brain injury. Part 11: Early indicators of prognosis in severe traumatic brain injury. *Journal of Neurotrauma* 17:556–627.

Chestnut RM, Marshall LF, Klauber MR *et al.* (1993) The role of secondary brain injury in determining outcome from severe head injury. *Journal of Trauma* 34:216–222.

Christman CW, Grady MS, Walker SA *et al.* (1994) Ultrastructural studies of diffuse axonal injury in humans. *Journal of Neurotrauma* 11(2):173–186.

Clayton TJ, Nelson RJ, Manara AR (2004) Reduction in mortality from severe head injury following the introduction of a protocol for the intensive care management. *British Journal of Anaesthesia* 93(6):761–767.

Cruz J (1998) The first decade of continuous monitoring of jugular bulb oxyhemoglobin saturation: management strategies and clinical outcome. *Critical Care Medicine* 26:344–351.

Davis DP, Vadeboncoeur TF, Ochs M *et al.* (2005) The association between field Glasgow Coma Scale score and outcome in patients undergoing paramedic rapid sequence intubation. *Journal of Emergency Medicine* 29(4):391–397.

Department of Health (2005) *National Service Framework for Long-Term Conditions.* London: DH.

Dikmen SS, Machamer JE, Powell JE *et al.* (2003) Outcome 3–5 years after moderate–severe traumatic brain injury. *Archives Physiological Medical Rehabilitation* 84:1449–1457.

Eames P, Wood R (1985) Rehabilitation after severe brain injury: a follow up study of behavioural modification approach. *Journal of Neurology, Neurosurgery and Psychiatry* 48:613–619.

Eames PJ, Blake MJ, Dawson SL *et al.* (2002) Dynamic cerebral autoregulation and beat to beat blood pressure control are impaired in acute ischaemic stroke. *Journal of Neurology Neurosurgery and Psychiatry* 72:467–472.

Erol T, Patchell R (2002) Classification and management of skull base fractures. *Neurosurgery Quarterly* 12(1):42–62.

Fantini S, Hueber D, Franceschini MA *et al.* (1999) Non invasive optical monitoring of the newborn piglet brain using continuous–wave and frequency–domain spectroscopy. *Physics in Medicine and Biology* 44:1543–1563.

Fleminger S, Greenwood RJ, Oliver DL (2006) Pharmacological management for agitation and aggression in people with acquired brain injury. *Cochrane Database of Systematic Reviews.* Issue 4.Art No.,CD003299.

Fukuda T, Hasue M, Ito Hiroshi (1998) Does traumatic subarachnoid hemorrhage caused by diffuse brain injury cause delayed ischemic brain damage ? Comparison with subarachnoid hemorrhage caused by ruptured intracranial aneurysms. *Neurosurgery* 43(5):1040–1048.

Garnett MR, Cadoux-Hudson TA, Styles P (2001) How useful is magnetic resonance imaging in predicting severity and outcome in traumatic brain injury? *Current Opinion in Neurology* 14:753–757.

Gentleman D (2001) Rehabilitation after traumatic brain injury. *Trauma* 3:193–204.

Giza CC, Hovda DA (2001) The neurometabolic cascade of concussion. *Journal of Athletic Training* 36(3):228–235.

Gupta S, Tandon S, Mohanty S *et al.* (1992) Bilateral traumatic extradural haematomas: report of 12 cases with a review of the literature. *Clinical Neurology and Neurosurgery* 94:127–131.

Harting M, Baumgartner J, Worth L *et al.* (2008) Cell therapies for traumatic brain injury. *Journal of Neurosurgery* 24(3&4):E17.

Helliwell R (2009) Advances in brain tissue oxygen monitoring: using the Licox system in neurointensive care. *British Journal of Neuroscience Nursing* 5(1):22–24.

Helmy A, Vizaychipi M, Gupta AK (2007) Traumatic brain injury: intensive care management. *British Journal of Anaesthesia* 99(1)32–42.

Hillered L, Vespa PM, Hovda DA (2005) Translational neurochemical research in acute human brain injury: the current status and potential future for cerebral microdialysis. *Journal of Neurotrauma* 22(1):1–34.

Intensive Care Society (2002) *Guidelines for the Transport of the Critically Ill Adult.* London: ICS.

Jennett B, Bond M (1975) Assessment of outcome after severe brain damage: A practical Scale. *Journal of Neurosurgery* 4:673.

Jones PA, Andrews PJD, Midgley S *et al.* (1994) Measuring the burden of secondary insults in head–injured patients during intensive care. *Journal of Neurosurgical Anaesthesia* 6:4–14.

Jose I, Suarez MD (2006) Outcome in neurocritical care: advances in monitoring and treatment and effect of a specialised neurocritical care team. *Critical Care Medicine* 34(9):(Suppl)S232–S238.

Juul N, Gabrielle FM, Morris MN *et al.* (2000) Intracranial hypertension and cerebral perfusion pressure: influence on neurological deterioration and outcome in severe head injury. *Journal of Neurosurgery* 92(1):1–7.

Kampfl A, Postmantur RM, Zhao X *et al.* (1997) Mechanisms of calpain proteolysis following traumatic brain injury:implications for pathology and therapy: a review and update. *Journal of Neurotrauma* 14:121–134.

Kay A, Teasdale G (2001) Head injury in the United Kingdom. *World Journal of Surgery* 25(9):1210–1220.

Koszyca B, Blumbergs PC, Manavis J *et al.* (1998) Widespread axonal injury in gunshot wounds to the head using amyloid precursor protein as a marker. *Journal of Neurotrauma* 15:675–683.

Lee E, Hung Y, Wang L *et al.* (1998) Factors influencing the functional outcome of patients with acute epidural haematomas: analysis of 200 patients undergoing surgery. *Journal of Trauma* 45:946–952.

Lifshitz J, Friberg H, Neumar RW *et al.* (2003) Structural and functional damage sustained by mitochondria after traumatic brain injury in the rat: evidence for differentially sensitive populations in the cortex and hippocampus. *Journal of Cerebral Blood Flow Metabolism* 23:219–231.

Longhi L, Watson D, Saatman K *et al.* (2004) Ex vivo gene therapy using targeted engraftment of NGF-Expressing human NT2N neurons attenuates cognitive deficits following traumatic brain injury in mice. *Journal of Neurotrauma* 21(12):1723–1736.

Lu J, Marmarou A, Choi S *et al.* (2005) Mortality from traumatic brain injury. *Acta Neurochir Suppl* 95:281–285.

Maas AI, Dearden M, Servadei F *et al.* (2000) Current recommendations for neurotrauma. *Current Opinion in Critical Care* 6(4):281–292.

Maas AI, Dearden M, Teasdale GM *et al.* (1997) European Brain Injury Consortium–Guidelines for management of severe head injury in adults. *Aceta Neurochir (Wien)* 139:286–294.

Maas AI, Hukkelhoven CW, Marshall LF *et al.* (2005) Prediction of outcome in traumatic brain injury with computed tomographic characteristics: a comparison between the computed tomographic classification and combinations of computed tomographic predictors. *Neurosurgery* 57:1173–1182.

MacDonald CL, Dikranian K, Bayly P *et al.* (2007) Diffusion tensor imaging reliably detects experimental axonal injury and indicates approximate time of injury. *The Journal of Neuroscience* 27(44):11869–11876.

Maggi G, Aliberti F, Petrone G *et al.* (1998) Extradural hematomas in children. *Journal of Neurosurgery Science* 42:95–99.

Mandrioli S, Tieghi R, Galie M *et al.* (2008) Anterior skull base fractures: guidelines for treatment. *The Journal of Craniofacial Surgery* 19(3):713–717.

Marik P, Varon J, Trask T (2002) Management of head trauma. *Chest.* 122:699–711.

Marmarou A, Anderson RL, Ward JD, *et al.* (1991) Impact of ICP instability and hypotension on outcome in patients with severe head trauma. *Journal of Neurosurgery* 75:Suppl S59–S66.

Martin D, Smith M (2004) Medical management of severe traumatic brain injury. *Hospital Medicine* 65(11):674–680.

McMillan TM, Greenwood RJ (2002) *Handbook of Neurological Rehabilitation.* (2nd edition). London: Psychology Press Ltd.

Millis SR, Rosenthal M, Novack TA *et al.* (2001) Long-term neuropsychological outcome after traumatic brain injury. *Journal of Head Trauma Rehabilitation* 16:343–355.

Mittl RL, Grossman RI, Hiehle JF *et al.* (1994) Prevalence of MR evidence of diffuse axonal injury in patients with mild head injury and normal head CT findings. *American Journal of Neuroradiology* 15:1583–1589.

Nakase–Thompson R, Stuart MS, Yablon A *et al.* (2004) Acute confusion following traumatic brain injury. *Brain Injury* 18(2):131–142.

National Institute for Health and Clinical Excellence (2007) *Head Injury: triage, assessment, investigation and early management of head injury in infants, children and adults.* London: National Collaborating Centre for Acute Care. Royal College of Surgeons of England.

Naunheim R, Matero D, Fucetola R (2008) Assessment of patients with mild concussion in the emergency department. *The Journal of Head Trauma Rehabilitation* 23(2):116–122.

Neal CJ, Lee E, Gyorgy A *et al.* (2007) Effect of penetrating brain injury on aquaporin-4 expression using a rat model. *Journal of Neurotrauma* 24:1609–1617.

Nortie J, Menon D (2004) Traumatic brain injury: physiology, mechanisms and outcome. *Current Opinion in Neurology* 17(6):711–718.

Obrenovitch TP, Urenjak J (1997) Is high extracellular glutamate the key to excitotoxicity in traumatic brain injury. *Journal of Neurotrauma* 14:677–698.

O'Donnell ML, Creamer M, Pattison P *et al.* (2004) Psychiatric morbidity following injury. *American Journal of Psychiatry* 161(3):507–514.

Oertel M, Kelly DF, McArthur D *et al.* (2002) Progressive hemorrhage after head trauma: predictors and consequences of the evolving injury. *Journal of Neurosurgery* 96:109–116.

O'Shea RA (2005) *Principles and Practice of Trauma Nursing*. London: Churchill Livingstone.

Pablo PA (2008) Predicting outcome after traumatic brain injury: practical prognostic models based on large cohort of international patients. *British Medical Journal* 336:425–429.

Patel H, Menon DK, Tebbs S *et al.* (2002) Specialist neurocritical care and outcome from head injury. *Intensive Care Medicine* 28:547–553.

Paterniti S, Fiore P, Macri E *et al.* (1994) Extradural haematoma. Report of 37 consecutive cases with survival. *Acta Neurochir (Wien)* 131:207–210.

Povlishock JT (2000) Pathophysiology of neural injury: therapeutic opportunities and challenges. *Clinical Neurosurgery* 46:113–126.

Povlishock JT, Katz D (2005) Update of neuropathology and neurological recovery after traumatic brain injury. *Journal of Head Trauma Rehabilitation* 20(1):76–94.

Raghupathi R, Graham DI, Mc Intosh TK (2000) Apoptosis after traumatic brain injury. *Journal of Neurotrauma* 17(10):927–938.

Reilly PL (2001) Brain injury: the pathophysiology of the first hours. Talk and die revisited. *Journal of Clinical Neuroscience* 8:398–403.

Reilly P, Adams JH, Graham DI *et al.* (1975) Patients with head injury who talk and die. *Lancet* 11:375–377.

Rice-Oxley M (2000) Are we missing urethral stricture after acquired brain injury? *Clinical Rehabilitation* 14(5):548–550.

Robertson CS, Gopinath SP, Goodman JC *et al.* (1995) SjvO$_2$ monitoring in head injured patients. *Journal of Neurotrauma* 12:891–896.

Rogers FB, Cipolle MD, Velmahos G *et al.* (2002) Practice management guidelines for the prevention of venous thromboembolism in trauma patients: the EAST practice management work group. *Journal of Trauma* 53:142–164.

Royal College of Paediatrics and Child Health (2001) *Guidelines for Good Practice: Early management of patients with a head injury*. London: Royal College of Paediatrics and Child Health.

Royal College of Surgeons of England (1999) *Report of the Working Party on the Management of Patients with Head Injuries*. London: Royal College of Surgeons of England.

Sandel ME, Mysiw WJ (1996) The agitated brain injured patient. Part 1: Definitions, differential diagnosis and assessment. *Archives of Physical Medicine and Rehabilitation* 77(6):617–623.

Scheufler KM, Rohrborn HJ, Zentner J (2002) Does tissue oxygen tension reliably reflect cerebral oxygen delivery and consumption? *Anaesthesia and Analgesia* 95:1042–1048.

Scottish Intercollegiate Guidelines Network (2009) *Early Management of Patients with Head Injury: A national clinical guideline*. Edinburgh: Royal College of Physicians.

Servadei F, Murray GD, Penny K *et al.* (2000) The value of the worst computed tomographic scan in clinical studies of moderate and severe head injury. European Brain Injury Consortium. *Neurosurgery* 46:70–75.

Servadei F, Murray G, Teasdale G *et al.* (2002) Traumatic subarachnoid haemorrhage: demographic and clinical study of 750 patients from the European Brain Injury Consortium Survey of Head Injuries. *Neurosurgery* 50(2):261–269.

Servadei F, Nanni A, Nasi M *et al.* (1995) Evolving brain lesions in the first 12 hours after head injury. *Neurosurgery* 37:899–906.

Servadei F, Nasi M, Cremonini A *et al.* (1998) Importance of a reliable admission Glasgow Coma Score for determining the need for evacuation of posttraumatic subdural hematomas: a prospective study of 65 patients. *Journal of Trauma* 44:868–873.

Simpson D, Gracies JM, Graham H *et al.* (2008) Assessment of botulinum neurotoxin for the treatment of spasticity (an evidence based review): Report of the Therapeutics and Technology Assessment Subcommittee of the American Academy of Neurology SYMBOL. *Neurology* 70(19):1691–1698.

Sioutos PJ, Orozco JA, Carter LP *et al.* (1995) Continuous regional cerebral cortical blood flow monitoring in head-injured patients. *Neurosurgery* 36:943–949.

Slade A, Chamberlain MA, Tennant A (2002) A randomised control trial to determine the effect of intensity of therapy on length of stay in a neurological rehabilitation setting. *Journal of Rehabilitation Medicine* 34(6):260–266.

Smith M (2003) Diffuse axonal injury in adults. *Trauma* 5:1–8.

Smith D, Meaney D, Shull W (2003) Diffuse axonal injury in head trauma. *The Journal of Head Trauma Rehabilitation* 18(4):307–316.

Stahl N, Mellergard P, Hallstrom A *et al.* (2001) Intracerebral microdialysis and bedside biochemical analysis in patients with fatal traumatic brain lesions. *Acta Anaesthesiology Scandinavia* 45:977–985.

Swann IJ, Teasdale GM (1999) Current concepts in the management of patients with so-called minor or mild head injury. *Trauma* 1(2):143–155.

Tateno A, Jorge RE, Robinson RG (2003) Clinical correlates of aggressive behaviour after traumatic brain injury. *Journal of Neuropsychiatry and Clinical Neuroscience* 15(2):155–160.

Teasdale G, Jennett B (1974) Assessment of coma and impaired consciousness: a practical scale. *Lancet* 2:81–84.

Temkin NR (2003) Risk factors for posttraumatic seizures in adults. *Epilepsia* 44 (Suppl 10):18–20.

Thornhill S, Teasdale GM, Murray GD *et al.* (2000) Disability in young people and adults one year after head injury: prospective cohort study. *British Medical Journal* 320:1631–1635.

Tisdall M, Smith M (2007) Multimodal monitoring in traumatic brain injury: current status and future directions. *British Journal of Anaesthesia* 99:61–67.

Tolias CM, Bullock MR (2004) Critical appraisal of neuroprotection trials in head injury: what have we learned? *The Journal of the American Society for Experimental Neuro Therapeutics* 1:71–79.

Valadka AB, Gopinath SP, Contant CF *et al.* (1998) Relationship of brain tissue PO_2 to outcome after severe head injury. *Critical Care Medicine* 26:1576–1581.

van den Berghe G, Wouters P, Weekers F *et al.* (2001) Intensive insulin therapy in the critically ill patients. *New England Journal of Medicine* 345:1359–1367.

van den Brink WA, Zwienenberg M, Zandee SM *et al.* (1999) The prognostic importance of the volume of traumatic epidural and subdural haematomas revisited. *Acta Neurochir (Wien)* 141:509–514.

Varelas PN, Eastwood D, Yun HJ *et al.* (2006) Impact of a neurointensivist on outcomes in patients with head trauma in a neurosciences intensive care unit. *Journal of Neurosurgery* 104:713–719.

Vespa PM, McArthur D, O'Phelan K *et al.* (2003) Persistently low extracellular glucose correlates with poor outcome at 6 months after human traumatic brain injury despite a lack of increased lactate: A microdialysis study. *Journal of Cerebral Blood Flow and Metabolism* 23:865–877.

Vespa PM, Newer MR, Nenov V *et al.* (1999) Increased incidence and impact of nonconvulsive and convulsive seizures after traumatic brain injury as detected by continuous electroencephalographic monitoring. *Journal of Neurosurgery* 91:750–760.

Vespa P, Prins M, Ronne-Engstrom E *et al.* (1998) Increase in extracellular glutamate caused by reduced cerebral perfusion pressure and seizures after human traumatic brain injury: A microdialysis study. *Journal of Neurosurgery* 89:971–982.

Watkins L (2000) Head injuries: General principles and management. *Surgery* 18:219–224.

Werner C, Engelhard K (2007) Pathophysiology of traumatic brain injury. *British Journal of Anaesthesia* 99(1): 4–9.

Wu HM, Huang SC Hattori N *et al.* (2004) Selective metabolic reduction in grey matter acutely following human traumatic brain injury. *Journal of Neurotrauma* 21(2):149–161.

Xiong Y, Gu Q, Peterson PL *et al.* (1997) Mitochondrial dysfunction and calcium perturbation induced by traumatic brain injury. *Journal of Neurotrauma* 14:23–24.

Yanagawa T, Bunn F, Roberts I *et al.* (2003) Nutritional support for head injured patients. *Cochrane Review Cochrane Library* Issue 2.Oxford: Update software.

Young B, Ott L,Kasarskis E *et al.* (1996) Zinc supplementation is associated with improved neurologic recovery rate and visceral protein levels of patients with severe closed head injury. *Journal of Neurotrauma* 13:25–34.

Yudofsky SC, Silver JM, Jackson W *et al.* (1986) The overt aggression scale for the objective rating of verbal and physical aggression. *American Journal of Psychiatry* 143:35–39.

Zasler ND, Martelli MF (2003) Mild traumatic brain injury: impairment and disability assessment caveats. *Neuropsychological Rehabilitation* 13(1/2):31–32.

33
Management of Patients with Spinal Injury

Paul Harrison and David Ash

INTRODUCTION

Spinal cord injury (SCI) is a non-progressive neurological impairment which can result from a range of traumatic and non-traumatic causes. It predominates amongst adult males but could affect any one of us, or our children, at any time. Thanks to our modern understanding and management of this condition it has a low mortality and a reasonably good life expectancy. It is estimated that around 40,000 people are currently living in the UK with chronic spinal cord injuries. This chapter will consider the role of the nurse in the initial and continuing care of SCI patients within the hospital and community setting. NHS management of both traumatic and non-traumatic SCI includes referral to a specialist Spinal Cord Injury Centre (SCI centre) within 24 hours of diagnosis, although this is not necessary for every spinal cord injury patient. This chapter will emphasise the supporting role provided by the SCI centres and the Spinal Injuries Association (SIA – the national charity supporting spinal cord injured people) to nurses managing spinal cord injured people outside of specialist clinical environments and in the community.

EPIDEMIOLOGY

Spinal cord injury affects fewer than 1,000 UK citizens each year. Significant spinal column injuries can be present in up to 10% of all trauma admissions (Hu *et al.*, 1996) and up to 20% of severely injured patients (NCEPOD, 2007) whose injuries have the potential to result in damage

to the underlying spinal cord. 71% of spinal cord injuries are due to trauma (SIA, 2009). However, traumatic spinal cord injury is still a relatively rare event, representing approximately 2% of current trauma admissions (Banit *et al.*, 2000). There is a 7:3 male:female ratio amongst current new SCI centre admissions. SCI is not confined to any particular age group; acute admissions to SCI centres ranged between 3 and 103 years in 2007–2008, with 20% of new injuries occurring between 21 and 30 years of age (SIA, 2009).

The area of the spinal column most commonly involved in the incidence of traumatic SCI is the cervical spine (50% of all SCI centre admissions) (see Table 33.1). The most common levels of cervical trauma resulting in SCI are C5–C8 (26% of all SCI centre admissions) with 37% of SCI admissions involving the thoracic spinal cord (T1–T12) and 11% involve the lumbar spinal cord (L1–L5) (SIA, 2009).

Mortality amongst children and older people sustaining SCI is higher than other age groups as they are more susceptible to the effects of severe multi-trauma. Older people are much more vulnerable to cervical spinal cord compression resulting from minor trauma because of the presence of pre-existing age-related diseases such as ankylosing spondylitis and spinal stenosis (Roth *et al.*, 1992).

AETIOLOGY

Traumatic spinal cord injuries

The most common cause of spinal cord trauma in the UK is an incident involving sudden, unexpected, impact, collision or deceleration. Speed at impact or height of fall are unreliable in predicting the potential for spinal injury at the scene. Therefore, current UK trauma management

Neuroscience Nursing: Evidence-Based Practice, 1st Edition.
Edited by Sue Woodward and Ann-Marie Mestecky
© 2011 Blackwell Publishing Ltd

Table 33.1 Admissions to the UK Spinal Cord Injuries Centre by level of neurological Injury.

Level of injury	Percentage of admissions
C1–C4	21%
C5–C8	26%
T1–T12	37%
L1–L5	11%
S1–S5	0.1%
Not recorded	1.9%

Source: Spinal Injuries Association, 2009.

guidelines emphasise the need for rescuers to maintain a high index of suspicion of spinal injury within the initial management of most trauma scenarios along with the early implementation of appropriate spinal column protection strategies (BTS, 2003; Fisher *et al.*, 2006; ACS 2008).

Moving vehicle collisions (MVC) are the most common cause of SCI. In the majority of these cases, vehicle occupants were unsecured within the vehicle, or were ejected. Such casualties usually present with complex multi-system trauma in addition to SCI. Falls are the second most common cause of SCI centre admissions (SIA, 2009). However, the potential for a domestic fall to cause SCI is still poorly appreciated within most trauma care pathways (Helling *et al.*, 1999). Aquatic spinal cord injuries can often present as near-drowning episodes with accompanying respiratory compromise including cerebral anoxia. Equestrian injuries can also present with significant multi-trauma including head injury. Gunshot or penetration injuries often involve multiple organ trauma. A small percentage of SCIs are inflicted during failed attempts at suicide.

Non-traumatic spinal cord injuries

Not all spinal cord injuries are caused by trauma. Approximately 28% of all cases of spinal cord paralysis are due to non-traumatic causes resulting in a similar non-progressive neurological impairment (SIA, 2009). These include:

- Ischaemic vascular incidents such as a thrombosis or haemorrhage affecting the spinal cord blood supply
- Viral and bacterial infections and abscesses such as those associated with tuberculosis and meningitis
- Inflammatory conditions such as transverse myelitis

- Non-malignant growths resulting in spinal cord compression
- Congenital defects such as spina bifida

MECHANISMS OF INJURY

Forced flexion and flexion with rotation are the most common mechanisms of cervical injury. These occur in incidents such as when vehicle drivers are struck by unsecured rear-seat passengers or when a rugby scrum collapses. Hyperextension cervical injuries are common amongst vehicle occupants in rear-end collisions, especially where headrests are not in situ. They also occur frequently in domestic falls where the falling person most commonly falls forwards, striking their chin or head against furniture or a wall. Increased axial loading from being struck on the head by a falling object or diving into shallow water results in a burst compression fracture. Individuals falling from a height and landing on their feet or falling onto the base of their spine can present with multiple compression fractures in lumbar, thoracic or cervical zones. Crush fractures are common in industrial accidents where the person is trapped by moving machinery or a heavy vehicle. Penetration injuries to the spine can be due to gunshot or stabbing. High speed impact trauma such as ejection from a moving vehicle can result in gross disruption and distraction of the spinal column because all of the above mechanisms can occur.

PATHOPHYSIOLOGY

The traumatic displacement of one or more vertebral bodies results in compression of the underlying spinal cord (Iencean, 2003). Alternatively, the spinal cord may be stretched or 'concussed' without any visible disruption of the spinal column. The resulting post-traumatic inflammatory oedema and vascular disruption start a complex series of physiological and biochemical reactions within the spinal cord (Sapru, 2002). There is little room for swelling within the structural confines of the vertebral canal and the oedematous spinal cord is quickly compressed against the surrounding bone. Circulation of blood and oxygen within the spinal cord is disrupted and ischaemic tissue necrosis quickly follows. There is an almost immediate cessation of conductivity within the spinal cord neuones. This is termed 'spinal shock' (Nacimiento and Noth, 1999).

Spinal shock

Spinal shock is best described as the complete suppression of all autonomic, somatic, and reflex activity below the level of lesion. The term neurogenic shock refers specifically to the loss of sympathetic activity and the effects this has on the cardiovascular system. This is presented in Chapter 14. The effects of spinal shock are most profound in complete lesions above the level of T6.

The impact of spinal shock on specific systems of the body is presented in Table 33.2. On average, spinal shock usually resolves within 2–14 days of onset but can persist for up to 6 weeks (Nacimiento and Noth 1999; Ditunno *et al.*, 2004).

Although most patients with spinal shock will present at the scene of the accident with the loss of all voluntary movement and sensation in addition to loss of autonomic and reflex activity below the level of the injury, it is not uncommon for the onset of clinical symptoms to be delayed by up to 72 hours after the original incident. Even when symptoms are present immediately post trauma it is often difficult to be certain of the extent or permanence of the functional loss. The presence of paralysis or paraesthesia does not imply any finality to the process. In some instances, when spinal cord oedema and spinal shock resolve there can be a subsequent improvement in neurological function.

Further neurological deterioration, resulting from lesion extension after the initial SCI, can occur naturally in about 5% of trauma cases (Marshall *et al.*, 1987). A number of complications associated with the multisystem effects of SCI can lead to respiratory, cardiovascular or other system compromise which can further compromise the body's attempts to limit nerve tissue death and can further reduce any inherent potential for any degree of spinal cord recovery. Nursing and medical management is directed at limiting these potential problems.

Complete and incomplete lesions

Spinal cord injuries will result in either complete or incomplete loss of function below the level of the injury. A complete spinal cord lesion is when the cord is completely transected or when the ischaemia affects the entire width of the spinal cord. There is complete loss of all

Table 33.2 The impact of spinal shock on specific systems of the body.

Body system	Impact of spinal shock
Respiratory	Respirations compromised by flaccid skeletal muscles Inability to cough and expectorate Danger of vagal overstimulation during suctioning Nasal passages blocked due to vasodilation
Cardiovascular (see Chapter 14: Neurogenic shock)	Hypotension due to systemic vasodilation Bradycardia due to vagal domination Poikilothermia – adopting environmental temperature due to loss of vasodilation, vasoconstriction, sweating, shivering and piloerection (goose flesh)
Genitourinary	Poor renal perfusion due to hypotension Loss of ureteric peristalsis Atonic (flaccid) bladder and urethral sphincters Pseudopriapism in males due to passive vasodilation Amenorrhoea in females secondary to metabolic deficits
Gastrointestinal	Increased volume and concentration of gastric acid due to vagal domination Paralytic ileus due to loss of peristalsis (usually only for approximately 48 hours following injury) Atonic (flaccid) ano-rectum and sphincters
Skin	Increased pressure marking due to vasodilatation Reduced tissue density over bony prominences and weight-bearing areas due to redistribution of paralysed muscle bulk Dry skin as unable to sweat or produce sebum

Source: Ash and Harrison, 2007.

voluntary movement and sensation below the level of the injury. There is also a complete loss of autonomic nerve function throughout the same area. The majority of patients will have incomplete spinal cord lesions with varying degrees of impairment of sensory and/or motor function consistent with the extent of their lesion (see Box 33.1 for the clinical presentation of each of the incomplete syndromes and Figures 33.1a–d).

Tetraplegia (not quadriplegia) is the preferred medical term for documenting any spinal cord lesion affecting all four limbs. Paraplegia refers to a lesion affecting only the lower body and without any effect upon the upper limbs (see Figure 33.2).

Because of the dynamic nature of pathological processes that occur following the initial incident, the medium and long-term outcomes of any spinal cord lesion cannot be accurately predicted initially. However, detailed clinical assessments supported by diagnostic imaging during the first few days and weeks can often help an experienced clinician to predict what the most likely neurological and functional outcomes will be. MRI of the spinal cord can inform the clinical prognosis, as the extent of cord compression, swelling and bleeding are related to neurological outcome (Fehlings *et al.*, 2007).

PRIORITISING MEDICAL INTERVENTIONS

Medical management of traumatic SCI after admission to hospital follows established ATLS principles (BTS, 2003; ACS, 2008). During resuscitation, team members will endeavour to maintain spinal alignment as best as circumstances allow but life-threatening injuries take priority. Until the patient's condition has stabilised sufficiently to allow for medical imaging and detailed neurological assessment, the trauma team will assume the presence of a possible spinal injury. Early secondary complications that can occur include: lesion extension, respiratory insufficiency, cardiovascular insufficiency, hypothermia, pressure ulcers, urinary and faecal incontinence, and renal failure. Box 33.2 shows a summary of the immediate medical management and Box 33.3 gives guidance for patient transfer to a SCI centre.

Reduction and stabilisation of the spinal injury is the first priority in the stabilised SCI patient. In most instances, conservative methods will be exhausted first before considering surgical options.

Diagnostic imaging

Diagnostic imaging for potential spinal injury is directed by the accident history and clinical examination. It usually begins with a series of plain x-rays to provide anteropos-

terior and lateral views of the spinal column. Cervical views must include the odontoid peg and the C7–T1 junction. However, because of the difficulty in adequately imaging the spine in this way, many emergency departments now prefer to routinely CT the whole spine instead.

CT of the spine is essential for any patient who presents with a neurological deficit following trauma. MRI of the spine should follow at the earliest opportunity, especially if surgical stabilisation is being planned.

When head injured or multi-trauma patients are sent for CT scanning, every opportunity should be sought to extend the scan to include the whole spine to avoid the need to return later after admission (NICE, 2007).

Neurological examination

Neurological examination for both sensory and motor impairment should progress from head to toe. Ideally all clothing should be removed before or during the examination. Because of the danger of hypothermia, only the actual area of the body being examined should be exposed.

Both sides of the body should be examined separately as variation can occur. Sensation should be compared with an area of the body known to be unaffected by paralysis such as the face of a tetraplegic. Motor power should be assessed against age and any established pre-injury impairment. Refer to Chapter 11 for how to assess sensory and motor level and also see: Neurological systems.

The level of spinal cord injury is the level at which sensation is noted to be absent or altered or at which absence or weakness of movement is noted.

Steroid use

Evidence to support the administration of short-term, high-dose steroids such as methylprednisolone as a definitive strategy for reducing the impact of a traumatic SCI is extremely limited. The accumulated studies have been critically appraised within the framework of evidence-based practice (Short, 2001) and the routine administration of high-dose methylprednisolone can no longer be justified within current medical practice as a standard treatment for acute spinal cord injury (Ravichandran and El-Masri, 2005; BOA, 2006; Consortium for Spinal Cord Medicine, 2008; ACS, 2008). High dose methylprednisolone can prove hazardous for the patient and is associated with a significant increase in the incidence of unexpected sepsis and pneumonia leading to ventilation and admission to intensive care (McCutcheon *et al.* 2004). Nursing and medical staff facing requests to undertake or assist in the administration of high-dose methyprednisolone to traumatic SCI patients should consider their professional

Box 33.1 Incomplete spinal cord lesions

Anterior cord syndrome

This is the most common form of incomplete lesion after a high-velocity impact trauma. Flexion-rotation results in pressure against the anterior grey horn (contains cell bodies of motor neurones) of the spinal cord, the anterior spinal artery, and the anterior columns (contain the spinothalamic and corticospinal tracts). The spinal cord lesion develops through a combination of physical trauma, bony compression and ischaemia. Anterior cord lesions result in loss of motor function and the sensations of pain and temperature below the level of the lesion. The senses of crude touch, position (proprioception) and vibration are preserved below the level of the lesion

Posterior cord syndrome

Posterior impact injuries or hyperextension forces compress or traumatise the posterior column and posterior grey horns (sensory) of the spinal cord. Posterior lesions present with the loss of deep touch, position and vibration below the level of the lesion, with preservation of motor function and sensations of pain and temperature. Unfortunately, the sense of proprioception (the unconscious awareness of a limb's position in space) is lost, which can limit the patient's potential for developing a functional gait

Brown-Séquard syndrome

This lesion presents as a hemisection of the spinal cord. It is most commonly associated with stabbing/penetration injuries, but it may also occur from gross lateral flexion injuries. Motor power is absent or reduced on the same side as the lesion, but pain and temperature sensation are preserved. This presentation is reversed on the uninjured side which has good power but absent or reduced pain and temperature sensation. This results from the fact that the spinothalamic tracts cross over within the spinal cord, enabling sensory signals to travel up the side opposite to that where the origin of the sensation is perceived to be

Central cord syndrome

Usually occurs in elderly or spondylotic patients after minor hyperextension trauma to the neck. Vertebrae, discs and ligaments, which have become stiffened or thickened with age, focus compression forces and ischaemia towards the central portion of the cord, where the cervical nerve tracts originate. Patients present with significant loss of function in their upper limbs and hands, and partial preservation of function in their lower limbs, usually with retained sacral sensation and partially preserved bladder and bowel function

Adapted from: Gall and Harrison, 2007.

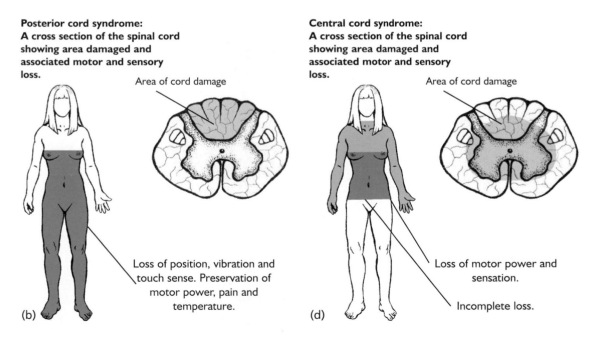

Figure 33.1 (a) Anterior cord syndrome; (b) posterior cord syndrome; (c) Brown-Séquard syndrome; (d) central cord syndrome. Reproduced from Ash D, Harrison P (2007) Understanding spinal shock. In: Harrison P (ed) *Managing Spinal Cord Injury: The First 48 Hours*. Milton Keynes: Spinal Injuries Association (SIA), with permission.

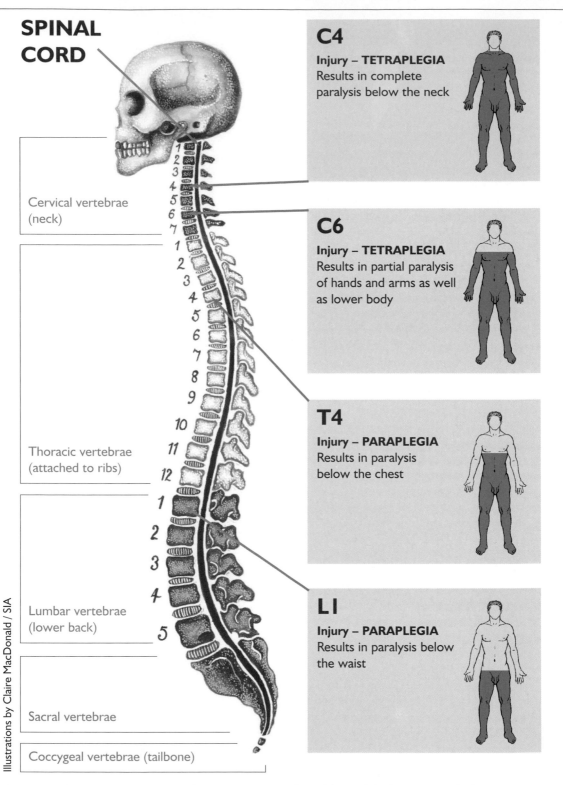

SPINAL CORD

Cervical vertebrae (neck)

Thoracic vertebrae (attached to ribs)

Lumbar vertebrae (lower back)

Sacral vertebrae

Coccygeal vertebrae (tailbone)

Illustrations by Claire MacDonald / SIA

C4

Injury – TETRAPLEGIA
Results in complete paralysis below the neck

C6

Injury – TETRAPLEGIA
Results in partial paralysis of hands and arms as well as lower body

T4

Injury – PARAPLEGIA
Results in paralysis below the chest

L1

Injury – PARAPLEGIA
Results in paralysis below the waist

Figure 33.2 Level of injury and extent of paralysis. Reproduced from Ash D, Harrison P (2007) Understanding spinal shock. In: Harrison P (ed). *Managing Spinal Cord Injury: The First 48 Hours*. Milton Keynes: Spinal Injuries Association (SIA), with permission.

Box 33.2   Medical management of acute spinal cord injury

Early recognition of actual or potential spinal cord injury utilising:
- Accident history and mechanism of Injury
- Patient history and presenting symptoms
- Clinical survey including neurophysiological examination (including sacral nerve pathways)
- Diagnostic Imaging

Implement initial management of patient in accordance with local trauma protocols:
- Prioritise interventions according to ATLS guidelines. Ensure the judicious administration of fluid and pharmaceutical resuscitation protocols in accordance with the diagnosis of actual or potential spinal cord injury as there is a significant potential for substantial over-infusion and subsequent pulmonary oedema if neurogenic hypotension is confused with hypovolaemia (see Chapter 14 for the management of neurogenic shock)
- Management of spinal shock may include the adaptation of local hospital early warning score indicators to incorporate the physiological impact of spinal shock to avoid inappropriate 'triggering' of unnecessary medical alerts or treatment interventions

Ensure accurate documentation of findings and actions undertaken:
- American Spinal Injury Association Standard Neurological Classification of Spinal Cord Injury Worksheet (available in publications section of www.asia-spinalinjury.org)

Telephone referral of actual or suspected spinal cord injured patient to spinal cord injury consultant at locally nominated spinal cord injury centre within 24 hours of diagnosis being made. Additional information sent by fax and/or electronic data transfer as soon as possible after referral.

Maintain close collaboration with spinal cord injury consultant regarding the options for surgical management of spinal trauma and the initial medical and multi-professional management of spinal shock until transfer or further case discussion. This may include seeking advice regarding the way in which the paralysis may mask the normal symptoms of underlying soft tissue trauma or visceral complications.

Inform patient's next-of-kin accurately of the diagnosis and tentative prognosis (if appropriate) as advised by expert clinical peer. Where patient has been accepted for transfer, include within this discussion the need to eventually transfer their relative to a tertiary specialist centre which may be some distance away.

Where available, ensure referral has been made to local hospital SCI link-workers for additional advice and assistance in managing this patient until transfer.

Source: British Trauma Society, 2003; Ravichandran and El Masri 2005; British Orthopaedic Association, 2006; Harrison 2007; American College of Surgeons, 2008.

Box 33.3   Guidelines for transferring acute spinal cord injured patients

- The expected total journey time should usually not exceed 2.5 hours. If the journey is likely to exceed 2.5 hours, consider aeromedical transfer or consult with the receiving SCI centre regarding the possibility of delaying the transfer
- Inform the receiving SCI centre of the time that the patient left and their expected time of arrival at the SCI centre
- All relevant medical, nursing and therapy notes, diagnostic imaging files and laboratory reports must accompany the patient as either copies or originals
- An experienced and informed member of medical and/or nursing staff, who is familiar with the care that the patient has received before transfer to the SCI centre, is an essential requirement as an escort. An anaesthetist must escort the SCI patient at risk of respiratory difficulties

- It is possible for the SCI patient to vomit while being transferred, so their stomach should be emptied before transfer. Other potential complications that may be encountered en route are hypothermia, pressure ulcers, respiratory compromise, further neurological deterioration and autonomic dysreflexia. Additional patient distress may occur if the level of pain control is inadequately maintained during transportation
- Transferring a SCI patient on a spinal board is not always required and the planned use of any spinal protective devices during transfer should always be discussed in advance with SCI centre staff

Source: Ravichandran and El Masri, 2005; British Orthopaedic Association, 2006; Sarhan and Harrison, 2007.

obligation to protect patients from the effects of inappropriate prescribing or administration of medicines.

Spinal surgery in the presence of SCI

The role of surgery in the management of acute traumatic SCI is controversial. The systemic impact of spinal shock means that patients in the acute phase of SCI management are at grave risk of neurological deterioration if oxygenation and blood pressure are not properly maintained during anaesthesia, surgery and post-operative recovery. In addition, post-operative oedema and swelling increases the potential for additional insult to the already traumatised spinal cord. Therefore, wherever possible, surgery (where intended) should be delayed to allow for better systemic stabilisation of the patient prior to surgery. Given the implications of wound infection, delayed healing and failed instrumentation for SCI patients, and their vulnerability to acquiring 'preventable' complications post-operatively such as pressure ulcers and chest infections, it is preferable for spinal surgery to be undertaken within, or in close association with, a specialist SCI centre (Ravichandran and El-Masri, 2005; BOA, 2006; Consortium for Spinal Cord Medicine, 2008; NHSSCGHSS, 2009; Spinal Task Force, 2010).

Cervical traction is the preferred method for the initial reduction and/or stabilisation of cervical dislocations and fractures. However, proper insertion of traction devices and regular neurological assessment by experienced practitioners are vital as the injured cord is particularly vulnerable to distraction (BOA, 2006). Also it is not unknown for traction tongs to be displaced and re-dislocation to occur during turning or repositioning of patients and transferring patients between surfaces.

Conservative reduction of thoraco-lumbar injuries is less likely to achieve satisfactory alignment and therefore surgical reduction and stabilisation is performed when the patient is stable.

There is no clear evidence to suggest that routine early surgical interventions such as surgical decompression are beneficial to patient outcomes and, if undertaken inappropriately, they have the potential to reduce a patient's rehabilitation potential (Boerger *et al.*, 2000). Early surgical intervention is usually only undertaken for the following: extradural lesions such as epidural haematomas, cauda equina syndrome, acute neurological deterioration, and specific injuries which cannot be resolved by conservative methods such as bilateral locked cervical facet joints (Kishan *et al.*, 2005; BOA, 2006; Consortium for Spinal Cord Medicine, 2008).

Spinal cord protection programmes

The perception that a patient with an actual or suspected spinal or spinal cord injury can be completely 'immobilised' is a fallacy. An individualised spinal protection programme utilising a range of devices designed to reduce the impact of spinal column movement and weightloading through the length of the spinal column is implemented for all patients suspected of having a SCI. Failure to implement or maintain appropriate spinal protection or to deliver appropriately informed care in the presence of apparent or suspected neurological impairment can compound what is already 'one of the worst disasters that can ever befall an individual' (Ravichandran, 1989). There are three main scenarios in which hospital-based health care professionals may encounter the need for a spinal cord protection programme: acute, potential and uncleared spinal cord injury.

Actual spinal cord injury

Where symptomatic spinal cord trauma is present, it must be considered when undertaking all aspects of patient care and therapeutic interventions to prevent any deterioration in the patient's neurological or physiological status. This patient scenario will form the basis for most of the following discussion on nursing management.

Potential spinal cord injury

The management of the conscious, orientated and cooperative patient who presents with an actual spinal column injury but without any symptoms of accompanying spinal cord trauma is well established in most trauma departments. However, each patient is still at risk of delayed onset of SCI symptoms or secondary neurological deterioration due to inappropriate management.

Uncleared spinal cord injury

Where doubt exists over the presence of spinal column or spinal cord trauma, experience has proved time and again that it is better to err on the side of caution. In the presence of multi-system trauma or traumatic brain injury, SCI should continue to be suspected until consciousness returns or a later tertiary review is concluded (Harrison, 2000; BTS, 2003; NICE, 2007). In the unconscious or sedated patient, a cervical collar often acts as a 'flag' to alert staff to the possibility of an uncleared cervical spine.

Concomitant injury in the presence of traumatic SCI usually necessitates a significant delay in transfer to the specialist SCI centre until the patient's condition has been stabilised and the receiving centre can provide the appropriate level of care required. Such delays in transfer are associated with an increase in the potential for complications such as bowel impaction, pressure ulcers and joint contractures. Pre-transfer complications such as these result in an extended period of hospitalisation, protracted rehabilitation programmes, delayed discharge and, potentially, a reduced quality of life post discharge including early readmission to hospital (Carvell and Grundy 1994; Tator *et al.*, 1995; Aung and El Masry, 1997). The additional impact of concomitant trauma upon morbidity and mortality after SCI has yet to be comprehensively audited and evaluated. It is therefore essential that local trauma teams refer such patients quickly in order to avail themselves of the additional clinical support available within a SCI centre.

Practical issues for nurses in the use and maintenance of spinal protective devices and cervical traction

The routine but uninformed use of spinal protective devices such as head restraints, cervical collars, cervical traction and halo bracing systems can prove disastrous for individuals with pre-existing spinal disorders or diseases. Age-related spinal diseases such as ankylosing spondylitis cause increased rigidity and deformity of the spinal column and it is well documented that trying to force an ageing spinal column into an inappropriate position during the fitting of a rigid cervical collar, or supine positioning on a spinal board, scanner couch or theatre table can result in spinal cord injury (Moreau *et al.*, 2003). Where evidence or history of any such condition is available alternative methods of positioning the patient and protecting the spine, must be utilised.

Cervical traction and halo devices

Cervical traction is a non-invasive method for the reduction and stabilisation of spinal fractures and dislocations. It is the method of choice for patients unsuitable for surgery or for whom surgery is not a priority. Guidelines for the appropriate application and maintenance of cervical traction and halo brace systems are well established in most trauma and critical care environments.

Nursing management is orientated towards monitoring the patient after application for any discernible change in neurology and maintaining the condition and security of the traction cord, knots, weights and runners. The position of the traction tongs or halo ring should be checked for any signs of slipping from the original position. Pin-sites should be inspected daily for signs of excessive encrustation, pain, bleeding, swelling or obvious infection. Cleaning, dressing and swabbing of pin sites is undertaken in accordance with local policy, but normal saline usually suffices for routine cleaning.

Gardner–Wells traction tongs have an indicator pin situated within a pin head. Secure pressure is indicated whenever the pin stands proud of its base and set on insertion. The traction should be tightened whenever the pin is noted to be receding from this position. A compatible torque screwdriver is needed for checking and tightening halo pins as required. A suitably sized spanner, key or wrench, should always be available at the patient's bedside in the event that the traction needs to be removed in an emergency.

During reduction of a cervical dislocation, traction weights are applied under x-ray guidance. These are increased in stages and weight in excess of 60 lb can be required before a successful reduction is achieved. During this time, the consultant may manually adjust the angle of the patient's neck between extension and flexion. He may also request changes in the foot down angle of the patient's bed to alter the amount of counter traction provided by the patient's body. With so many staff circulating around the patient's bed, care must be taken not to dislodge a traction weight onto a foot.

After reduction of the dislocation, the traction weight and bed angle will be reduced to support a minimum maintenance weight of only a few pounds. This weight must never be removed during turning unless it is first replaced by manual traction and/or a suitably prescribed cervical collar. In addition, the consultant will indicate the degree of neck flexion/extension required to maintain cervical alignment. This must be maintained during logrolling. Similar precautions should be applied during transfers between flat surfaces. When moving a patient in bed between departments, ensure the traction weight does not pendulum too much.

If a halo jacket is being used, check to ensure that the jacket has been fitted with the hinged access panel facing uppermost, for use in the event of cardiac arrest to provide chest compressions. Check fastenings for security and wear and tear daily. Also ensure that an appropriate wrench or hexagonal key to unfasten the frame struts is available (usually kept taped to the jacket) in the event of an emergency. The cutaway panels in modern jackets usually allow sufficient access for checking underlying skin condition. Skin under the jacket can be washed with a damp cloth and dried. To maintain the underlying skin and jacket lining in best condition, moisturising creams should be used sparingly and talcum powder should not be used. If necessary, with the patient supine, the lining of most jackets can be replaced or laundered as appropriate. Never use any part of the halo, jacket or framework as a handhold during turning or transferring between surfaces.

Cervical collars

The management of cervical collars for patients with SCI during an extensive period of supine bedrest continues to present nurses with many challenges (Hogan *et al.*, 1997; Harrison, 2000). The decision to discontinue spinal precautions is a medical decision and the clinical and radiological investigations necessary to inform such a decision may take some time to complete. Therefore, the decision to discontinue spinal precautions should not be unduly influenced by the pressures and constraints that such a device places upon the delivery of nursing care procedures. Nursing staff, as much as doctors, need to understand that radiological clearance alone is insufficient to discontinue the use of spinal protective devices. The doctor authorising removal of a cervical collar must document this decision in the patient's medical notes, citing the screening process which was followed before it is removed.

The two most commonly reported nursing concerns are the development of pressure ulcers beneath the collar and the potential for increasing intracranial pressure (ICP) in patients with accompanying or suspected traumatic brain injury (TBI) (Ho *et al.*, 2002).

Reducing pressure ulcer incidence in cervical collar use

It is important for nurses to know how to measure and size a cervical collar and to be aware of the different types available. SCI patients are usually admitted wearing a rigid extraction collar that was measured and fitted at the accident scene or in A&E. These collars are often applied whilst a patient is sitting and need to be adjusted or replaced with a collar of a different size or type to accommodate supine-lying pressures, for greater security and patient comfort. Aspen and Philadelphia collars have been evaluated as having the lowest potential for causing pressure ulcers in longer-term use (Hogan *et al.*, 1997) and should replace the hard extraction collars within 48 hours of admission. Most collars contain pre-cut access panels for observation of the position of the trachea, accessing the blood vessels of the neck and positioning tracheostomy tubes. Most pressure ulcers related to the wearing of cervical collars during supine bed rest can be prevented through a programme of regular turning and observation of the underlying skin, good skin hygiene and, where permitted, periods spent without the collar *in situ* (Harrison, 2000). Strict attention must also be paid to collar hygiene. The inner surface of the collar should be washed and dried, or its inner lining changed, every day.

Managing cervical collars in the presence of actual or suspected raised ICP

Collars should not be routinely discarded just because of the presence of actual brain injury. Any new or problematic increase in ICP or symptomatic neurological deterioration must first be identified as being related to the cervical collar in use. In such instances, close and regular liaison with local specialists enables staff to adapt their care provision over time, and to provide appropriate levels of spinal protection throughout the patient's admission.

First establish that the collar has been sized and fitted appropriately. If loosening or adjusting the collar does not improve ICP within 15 minutes then the collar is not a contributing factor and should be re-secured appropriately (Ho *et al.*, 2002). If ICP does improve following loosening of the collar then re-sizing the collar or changing it to a different type of collar may provide cervical support without compromising ICP.

Moving and handling patients with SCI

Wherever there is a reasonable suspicion of acute SCI, the aim is to maintain full spinal alignment during any moving and handling activity. Careful handling, positioning and turning, on every occasion, can reduce the potential for secondary spinal cord trauma during patient transfers and movements. Maintaining full spinal protection during logrolling involves at least four members of staff to maintain spinal alignment throughout the procedure. Additional staff will be required to undertake examination or care associated with the logroll such as washing and checking of skin, placement of pillows, insertion or removal of transfer devices, etc. Nurses required to undertake the turning or transferring of actual or potential SCI patients during the acute period must have supreme confidence in their ability to work as a team, especially when other health service staff are involved. It is essential that all moving and handling is coordinated by a nominated team leader.

Routine two-hourly turning and repositioning of SCI patients during the initial period of spinal shock can reduce the incidence of multi-system complications of acute bedrest by reducing the extent and duration of pressure on weight-bearing areas and also the duration of fluid stasis in the body (Hawkins *et al.*, 1999). As spinal shock resolves and the patient's systemic condition improves, a three to four hourly turning regime can be implemented until transfer to a SCI centre or specialist rehabilitation unit.

Logrolling

Four nurses are needed to log-roll an acute tetraplegic patient and this does not vary in the acute SCI patient even following surgery. Three nurses suffice for paraplegic patients as the head does not need to be held. All commands will come from the team leader who is always the nurse holding or nearest to, the patient's head.

Logrolling patients with cervical SCI

After explaining how the turn is to be accomplished, the team leader positions their hands to support the patient's head and cervical spine. Hands should be positioned to support the whole of the patient's neck. The left hand of the second nurse is positioned at the patient's shoulder and the right hand on the upper pelvis. The left hand of the third nurse is positioned on the patient's upper hip and the right hand is under the patient's upper (left) thigh. The fourth nurse supports the lower portion of the patient's upper leg (see Figure 33.3a). When members of the turning team are of different heights, the bed height should benefit all and should be negotiated on each occasion.

The logroll is undertaken using the commands: 'Ready, Steady, Roll'. The patient is logrolled in unison by the turning team to a 90° side-lying position (see Figure 33.3b) Spinal alignment during logrolling includes maintaining lateral alignment, therefore the upper leg should always be held so that the outer malleolus of the heel is aligned with the trochanter of the upper hip. The nurse holding the head experiences a degree of lateral flexion during the maneouvre but adjusts to a more comfortable posture at the end

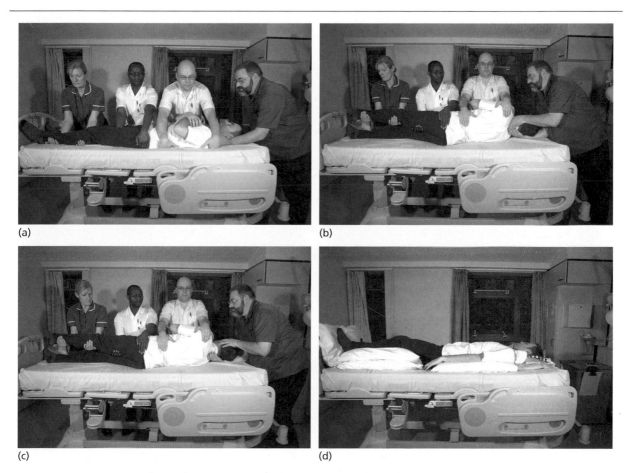

(a)

(b)

(c)

(d)

Figure 33.3 (a) Position of hands for a log-roll; (b) turn to 90° side lying position; (c) posture of the nurse holding the head at the end of the log roll; (d) 30° side lying position.

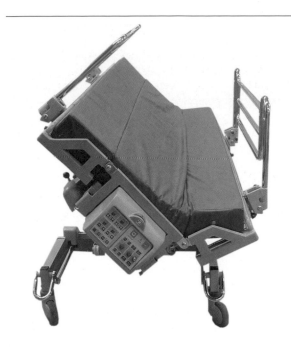

Figure 33.4 Electric turning bed.

of the logroll (Figure 33.3c). When the next turn is due it is imperative that staff members occupy a different position in the turning team to avoid repetitive strain injury. This is particularly so for the nurse holding the head.

After full examination of the underlying skin for signs of pressure damage, pillows or foam wedges can now be placed *in situ*, sufficient to maintain the patient in a 30° lateral position (see Figure 33.3d). Lateral positioning can vary between 30° and 90° dependent upon skin condition, comfort and clinical need, although a position between 20° and 30° is preferred in order to prevent excessive pressure being exerted upon the lower (right) trochanter of the hip.

Where staffing numbers make manual turning difficult, or where a patient presents with injuries to both the cervical and thoracolumbar spine, or with multiple injuries, which make lateral positioning difficult or painful, an electric turning bed such as Huntleigh's Atlas (see Figure 33.4) can be used.

NURSING MANAGEMENT OF THE ACUTE SCI PATIENT

Respiratory system

The impact of SCI upon the respiratory system creates the greatest potential for morbid complications. Complete traumatic paralysis above the level of C3 usually results

in death for many before paramedic intervention or hospitalisation can occur. Survival at this level requires lifetime ventilator support following an extended period of rehabilitation. This requires the patient to adapt not only to depending on personal carers to maintain their activities of daily living, but also to their chronic dependency on a medical device to provide for their basic respiratory need – to breathe (North, 1999). However, the non-progressive nature of SCI coupled with advances in both respiratory medicine and medical device technology means that most ultra-high level SCI patients can realise a longevity and quality of life after discharge.

For those with lesions at C4 and below, the respiratory impact of SCI is relative to the extent of respiratory muscle paralysis. Most of the initial respiratory problems are due to accompanying trauma or pulmonary contamination at the scene. Careful monitoring of respiratory effort is required as patients can fatigue quickly, In addition to regular comprehensive respiratory assessments, forced vital capacity (FVC) should be measured (see Chapter 15 for respiratory assessment). Inspiratory effort in tetraplegics is usually better than expiration, therefore monitoring for carbon dioxide retention is essential to avoid hypercapnia.

During bedrest, the diaphragmatic excursion is enhanced if the patient is nursed supine; therefore, any need to nurse the patient in a semi-recumbent or sitting position should first be discussed with an SCI specialist as this can increase the risk of lower lobe consolidation. Regular side-to-side turning also improves the movement of pulmonary secretions, preventing pooling and the stasis of fluid which can increase the risk of bacterial growth.

Tetraplegics and high paraplegics are unable to cough effectively due to their non-functional abdominal muscles. Clearing secretions often requires the use of manual 'assisted coughing' techniques, intermittent positive pressure breathing (IPPB) and the use of suction equipment (see Chapter 15). During tracheal and pharyngeal suctioning the patient's pulse should be closely monitored as tetraplegics are prone to vasovagal stimulation resulting in excessive bradycardia and cardiac syncope (refer to Neurogenic shock in Chapter 14).

Cardiovascular system

Much has already been said of the impact of neurogenic shock (see Chapter 14) on the cardiovascular system. Nurses must ensure that the new parameters established for 'acceptable' blood pressure, pulse and urinary output as well as 'triggers' prompting intervention are well documented and communicated at every handover and between disciplines. This should also be emphasised whenever the patient is transferred to another ward or department.

Hypotension and persistent bradycardia are prevalent in higher levels of SCI but after resuscitation and stabilisation of the patient, they remain relatively stable during the initial period of bedrest. However, blood pressure can still drop due to orthostatic hypotension during periods of sitting and/or standing necessitating a programme of gradual mobilisation which may include the use of recliner wheelchairs, abdominal binders and prophylactic vasoconstrictor drugs. Orthostatic hypotension usually resolves within the first month of mobilisation but severe orthostatic hypotension can both delay and extend the initial mobilisation and rehabilitation of SCI patients, and if ignored or overlooked can even lead to neurological deterioration in previously stable patients (El-Masry, 1993).

Due to loss of sympathetic activity temperature control will be significantly compromised. The patient's temperature will be dependent on that of the environment (poikilothermia – see Chapter 14). It is therefore imperative for nurses to protect the patient from adverse environmental temperature, i.e. too hot or too cold. During bedbathing and neurophysiological examination, the minimum amount of flesh should be exposed in turn. During diagnostic imaging and surgery, extra layers of protection may be needed to protect against the effects of air conditioning. Heating coils and warm-air devices should be used cautiously and only if properly distanced or insulated from contact with any paralysed skin. In contrast, during hot spells the patient will need to be cooled.

Even in the presence of appropriate prophylaxis, enforced bedrest and systemic paralysis increase the risk of venous thromboembolism (VTE). Unexplained fever is often the first indicator of deep vein thrombosis (DVT) as the patient will not experience pain in the affected limb. A general feeling of malaise, sweating, confusion or bizarre speech or behaviour may be early indicators of pulmonary or fat embolism.

Prophylactic anticoagulation (unless contraindicated) and the application of properly sized thigh length thromboembolic device (TED) stockings, or the application of pneumatic compression devices, and passive movements are well established preventative strategies for SCI patients. Often overlooked however are the benefits of regular turning and repositioning of limbs by nursing staff throughout the day. Frequent turning during the day has a beneficial effect on circulation throughout the body. In addition, frequent handling of lower limbs enables earliest detection of 'suspect' areas of heat, swelling or discolouration. TEDs should be removed at least twice every day to

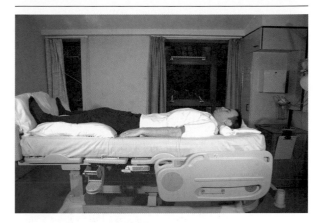

Figure 33.5 Tetraplegic in flat supine with legs supported.

check for pressure marking and should be resized regularly. The repositioning of lower limbs on pillows during turning and when the patient is supine also encourages venous drainage (see Figure 33.5). Remember that the patient also has a role to play in the prevention of VTE by complying wherever possible with active respiratory and limb exercises as outlined by the physiotherapist.

VTE is not just a risk for the patient in bed. Thromboprophylaxis continues into the early mobilisation programme as the paralysed body adapts to new pressures during sitting. Proximal rather than distal vessels become the most prevalent site of DVT. As with turning in bed, the graduated mobilisation and/or standing programme incorporating regular position changes and pressure relief are also beneficial to the circulatory system.

Neurological system

The frequency at which neurological observations are performed is based upon the patient's neuro-physiological presentation at admission, but generally they are recorded at fifteen minute intervals for the first two hours following admission and at less frequent intervals as the patient's condition stabilises. Sensation is assessed at and around the point at which the patient says sensation has changed (see Chapter 11). This point should be clearly indicated on a dermatome chart to enable detection of deterioration in function between nurse observers. Motor power is assessed by asking the patient to demonstrate strength and range of movement in muscle groups at and above the level of paralysis. Patient effort is graded and recorded on a myotome chart. Inter-rater reliability between nurse observers is enhanced by asking the patient to demonstrate best motor effort during handover. Any noticeable degree of deterioration or improvement in neurophysiology should be reported immediately to a senior colleague or doctor for further evaluation.

Spasticity can occur during the acute period of SCI (see Chapter 11). It is most prevalent in patients with sensory incomplete lesions. Reflex spasms can be triggered by cuticular stimulation during daily patient care such as turning and bedbathing. The spasms can prove an additional challenge to maintaining spinal alignment and staff safety during turns and transfers. Spasms can also occur in response to a patient's physical and emotional discomfort and thus can serve as a useful indicator of complications causing visceral discomfort below the level of lesion, such as bladder and bowel distension. The onset of spasticity should be anticipated and the patient and family educated about the cause and informed that it is not a sign of restoration of normal motor function. Spasm can prove useful to many SCI patients who can use it to assist in standing and transferring between sitting surfaces.

The initial management is usually focused upon correct positioning in bed, stretching and exercising of limbs by physiotherapists and small doses of antispasmodic medicines such as baclofen until such time that the potential benefits have been fully explored by the rehabilitation team.

Neuropathic pain

Pain is common following spinal cord injury; it is discussed in more detail in Chapter 17. Pain originating above the level of spinal cord injury can be managed in accordance with standard local pain management guidelines with the proviso that opiate use is initially avoided in non-ventilated tetraplegic patients for fear of suppressing voluntary respiratory effort. In addition, early opiate use may mask the initial detection of cervical lesion extension, which can also present as respiratory distress.

Pain perceived by the patient at or below the level of spinal cord lesion may arise from a local tissue injury or may have been referred from another region of the body or a visceral organ. Any complaint of pain below the level of lesion should first be investigated in order to exclude any pathology before a diagnosis of chronic neuropathic pain is made.

The guiding principle for pharmacological treatment of neuropathic pain after SCI is to first use those treatments that are simply administered and less likely to cause untoward side-effects. However, a variety of alternative treatment methods are available and a multi-faceted approach often proves more effective. All treatments tried, whether pharmacologically based or not, should be given an adequate trial and withdrawn appropriately if ineffective. Multidisciplinary teamwork is the cornerstone of effective pain management and the contributions of individual team members often overlap. Careful handling and correct positioning of the patient by nurses may make lying in bed more comfortable for the patient thereby potentially increasing the effect of current analgesia and possibly even reducing prescribed dose or frequency. Patient engagement in physical therapy may be enabled by timing exercise programmes to match the achievement of therapeutic levels of analgesia in the patient's body. The formulation of a comprehensive treatment plan which is appropriately discussed with SCI centre staff and agreed to by the patient is essential if neuropathic pain is not to become a barrier to rehabilitation.

Gentitourinary system

The SCI patient initially will present with a flaccid bladder, which will require an indwelling catheter to protect the bladder and upper urinary tracts from the effects of over-distension, in addition to enabling close monitoring of urine output. A wider than usual bore of catheter (FG14–16) is required as the flaccid bladder is prone to accumulating sedimentation debris that will cause catheter obstruction. A programme of planned catheter changes is based on the patient's catheter history as a prophylactic measure against obstruction. When spinal shock resolves and the patient's condition is stable bladder training will begin (see: Bladder management following SCI).

Gastrointestinal system

The immediate impact of spinal shock is to temporarily suspend gut peristalsis for approximately the first 48 hours after onset. In the presence of this paralytic ileus, the SCI patient is kept nil enterally for this period. When bowel sounds return, fluids are gradually introduced leading to eventual restoration of normal diet and fluids. Failure to follow this guideline can result in abdominal distension, diaphragmatic splinting and aspiration pneumonia. As with suction catheters, nasogastric tubes should be passed cautiously in tetraplegic patients as they can cause vasovagal stimulation.

Prophylactic gastric protection medication should commence within 24 hours of diagnosis and continue until transfer to a SCI centre or specialist rehabilitation centre. Gastric ulceration is a long-term complication of SCI and prophylactic medicines should not be discontinued on commencement of diet or enteral feeding, even in critical care environments.

A daily per rectum (PR) check is required during the spinal shock period to check for the presence of faeces and to monitor the return of any reflex activity. Any faeces present must be removed to prevent overdistension of the bowel. (See: Bowel management following SCI).

Musculoskeletal system

During the initial period of bedrest it is necessary to protect the patient's joints during handling as the joints of flaccid limbs are at risk of overextension. The use of foot-drop splints is discouraged due to the high risk of causing pressure ulcers. Rather feet should be 'blocked' with pillows against a footboard during bedrest. Wrist splints should only be applied on the advice of a SCI centre occupational therapist to ensure the use of an appropriate type or design. Wherever splints are used for SCI patients, nurses must ensure that they apply and remove them as indicated in the patient's therapy notes. Nurses should work collaboratively with physiotherapists to ensure correct positioning of the patient.

Integumentary system

At least a third of new SCI patients develop a pressure ulcer prior to being admitted to a SCI centre (Ash, 2002). These individuals are therefore required to enter rehabilitation with skin that has already been compromised. Pressure ulcers on admission cause significant delay and disruption to mobilisation and rehabilitation programmes, extend length of initial hospitalisation, increase the potential for readmission and increase hospital care costs (NICE, 2005). The prevention of pressure ulcers requires the careful management and rigorous monitoring of both intrinsic and extrinsic factors in tandem. During acute care and initial rehabilitation, the SCI patient is dependent upon nursing staff to provide regular pressure relief.

Manual turning and repositioning in bed, initially two hourly and progressing to three to four hourly intervals when spinal shock resolves (see: Moving and handling patients with SCI), is the principal method of relieving skin pressure in acute SCI patients. Mechanical turning beds are an alternative but still require the patient to be repositioned on the mattress between turns. Pneumatic alternating pressure mattresses should NEVER be used for acute SCI patients. Thermal contouring foam mattresses are appropriate but require careful monitoring of the patient's heels to ensure that they are generating enough body heat to transform the underlying foam to its gel state.

Discolouration of the skin is often the first indicator of skin suffering under physical pressures (NICE, 2005). In hospital environments, whenever a pressure ulcer is detected in the early stages of its development, it usually resolves quickly if the patient is able to be positioned in bed in such a way as to avoid placing any further pressure on the affected area. Pressure ulcers occurring after patient mobilisation most often occur in those parts of the body which are under constant pressure during sitting. Therefore effective treatment requires the patient to stay out of their wheelchair until the damage is resolved and skin integrity is restored. This requires both the patient and the care team to accept and accommodate a temporary loss of mobility and the suspension of key rehabilitation activities.

Psychological and emotional support during acute care

The initial impact of spinal cord injury (SCI) on an individual is sudden and unexpected. Reactions will vary enormously, depending on the individual's personality, coping style, personal circumstances and their beliefs about the future. Age, gender and previous background/experiences will have an important impact (Royle and Glass, 2007). In addition to struggling to cope with the impact of their own paralysis they may also have concerns regarding the loss of, or injuries to partners and family members involved in the same accident. Guilt and self-blame regarding the circumstances surrounding their own injury can also be present at this time.

It is not unusual for the patient and family to imagine a complete cure or recovery is possible. Media coverage of developments in research into possible cures is often exaggerated giving patients false hope of recovery. Sensitive and informed handling of this topic is essential.

Nursing staff can also feel overwhelmed and may feel inadequately prepared or supported to provide sufficient information about such a complex diagnosis (North, 1999). Experienced nursing staff may be able to support their patient with greater confidence based upon learned experience in their field of practice, but the low incidence of SCI means that outside of specialist centres such experience is often lacking. Psychological management and support of the SCI patient at this time should therefore aim to orientate both the patient and their family to the immediate hospital environment and to inform them regarding the immediate diagnosis, but sufficient only to gain their cooperation (Royle and Glass, 2007). Many patients report post-traumatic amnesia, especially in multi-trauma scenarios, so the initial information provided regarding their injury and initial impairment needs to be frequently reiterated by nursing and medical staff.

There is no established pattern or predictability of response to SCI (Trieschmann, 1988; Webster and

Kennedy, 2007). The young age of many of these individuals can mean a lack of developed coping mechanisms. Therefore an initial withdrawal from or reluctance to engage in any discussion of their condition is a common defense mechanism, as is a declaration of wishing they had not survived the accident. Crying, shouting and swearing are normal responses to the frustration of immobility and the prospect of prolonged hospitalisation. Patients who perceive that their condition engenders fear and anxiety in nursing staff can also direct the same behaviours at staff because they feel threatened.

Unlike in specialist centres, where staff have chosen to work with SCI patients, nurses and medical staff unfamiliar with the post-discharge potential for quality of life after SCI may, quite reasonably, struggle to maintain a consistently informed and positive attitude in front of their patient. However difficult it may seem, nurses need to display a competence and confidence in their own abilities so that the patient feels safe in their hands. This is particularly important because the physical contact and movement experienced by the patient during turning and routine nursing care is an effective means for reducing sensory deprivation caused by the loss of touch and positional awareness.

It is important to ensure that information given to the patient and family is consistent. All SCI centres provide outreach clinical support and education. The Spinal Injuries Association website (www.spinal.co.uk) is an appropriate means of support for patients and families. Nurses should anticipate relatives 'Googling' 'spinal cord injury' and provide details of the association at admission.

Effective support requires a higher degree of understanding of both the human and social impact of the disability than is usually found in general hospital environments. Enabling patients with SCI to gain early access to specialist staff and environments is the only strategy available to reduce the potential for long-term psychological problems after injury (Trieschmann, 1988).

Autonomic dysreflexia

Autonomic dysreflexia (see Chapter 14) can occur at any time following the onset of spinal cord paralysis although its occurrence is usually observed after the period of spinal shock has resolved (Consortium for Spinal Cord Medicine, 2001). It occurs in patients with both complete and incomplete lesions. Up to 90% of people with tetraplegia or high paraplegia will experience it at some time in their lives (Braddom and Rocco, 1991). Following

the first occurrence, the 'expert' patient becomes intimately familiar with the symptoms of AD. Autonomic dysreflexia alert cards are available from the SIA for patients at risk.

NURSING ROLE AND RESPONSIBILITIES WITHIN SCI REHABILITATION PROGRAMMES

Inpatient rehabilitation and education following SCI involves a lot more than simply re-learning new skills. People with newly acquired SCI will experience a series of challenges during their initial coping and adjustment phase. Aside from addressing the acute psychological dimension, life skills such as empowerment, self-efficacy and problem solving abilities are crucial if the patient is to be autonomous, confident and capable of dealing with day to day minor issues, or prepared to tackle major life issues such as further education, returning to work, managing finances and exploring personal and social relationships (Webster and Kennedy, 2007). The development of appropriate coping skills is known to contribute to positive mood, social integration and life satisfaction (Elliott and Warren, 2007). Individuals who are able to adjust to their new disability status, will have less dependency behaviour and this correlates positively with quality of life, while individuals with poor emotional adjustment tend to demonstrate negative coping styles (Elfstrom *et al.*, 2005).

Elliott *et al.* (2006) suggest that individuals with poor problem solving abilities are more at risk of developing additional health problems and complications. Since the incidence of health problems increases with the ageing process, the more information and advice available to the individual, the better prepared they will be to cope with them.

During the initial rehabilitation phase, information needs to be delivered in a format that is relevant and appropriate to the individual. The nurse should always bear in mind the volume of information that the patient needs to digest at this time, and so information regarding changes to their status or disability as a consequence of ageing may not be appropriate or a priority. Expanding the individual's knowledge base in such a direction should be saved for a more appropriate time (Elliott and Warren, 2007). Whilst health care professionals would like to explore with the patient the potential for future complications and problems and to some degree these are touched upon, the initial focus is much more on immediate concerns and initial post-discharge care issues and not what will happen as they age.

As an organisation predominantly run by people with SCI, the Spinal Injuries Association shares a commitment with other SCI service providers to deliver continuous and long term support, and their peer support scheme bears testament to this. Peer support officers are positive role models, whose unique insight enables newly paralysed individuals to acquire a more informed opinion of their future potential in the world after discharge. Unlike health care professionals, peer support officers are in a unique position to engage in facilitating problem-solving approaches with other spinal cord injured individuals and, because their role and relationship with them extends beyond the initial hospital experience, they can continue to provide their peer support 'lifeline' to the individual after hospital discharge.

Community Peer Support can include introducing the newly discharged individual to a more extensive peer network that can enable wider access to a range of vocational and non-vocational opportunities. Peer networks are an excellent source of post-discharge support and community integration, all of which are known to contribute to positive well-being (Beedie and Kennedy, 2002).

Bladder management following SCI

The change to bladder function after SCI is caused by the disruption of nerve supply and is therefore termed neurogenic bladder dysfunction. Some patients with incomplete lesions (e.g. Brown-Séquard), may have normal or near-normal bladder function. If the sacral segments of the spinal cord have been destroyed the bladder is totally disconnected from nervous control. People with complete sacral SCI effectively have an areflexic bladder, although the bladder muscle may recover some tone and therefore fail to relax during filling which results in high bladder pressures, kidney damage and infection. The urethral sphincter is weak, causing stress incontinence (leakage on coughing, straining, etc).

A typical patient with an areflexic bladder will have a lesion below T12/L1 level (Fulford *et al.*, 2004). If the sacral segments survive, the bladder detrusor muscle and urethral sphincter maintain a nerve supply from the sacral micturition centre, but their actions are not coordinated by the pontine micturition centre because of the disruption in communication caused by the intervening SCI. If the bladder emptying process is not perfectly coordinated, detrusor–sphincter dyssynergia (DSD) can occur. This is where the detrusor may contract against a tight sphincter resulting in abnormally high bladder pressures which damage the upper tract. A further consequence of DSD is incomplete emptying of the bladder which can lead to retention of 'stale' urine and urinary tract infection (UTI) (Reynard *et al.*, 2003). A typical patient with a reflex bladder potential will have a lesion above T12/L1 (Fulford *et al.*, 2004).

There are a number of other patterns of bladder dysfunction. Many people with incomplete SCI may have some degree of sensory sparing or even voluntary control of the urethral sphincter. Urge incontinence (see Chapter 18) is common in central cord syndrome (Fulford *et al.*, 2004). Others may have a degree of voluntary control over voiding but be unable to use a toilet or urinal independently because of a lack of hand function or reduced mobility. Yet others may experience unpleasant or painful sensations as the bladder fills. Those with partial damage to the sacral spinal cord may have a reflex bladder but a weak urethral sphincter causing both urge and stress incontinence (Fulford *et al.*, 2004).

The primary aims of bladder management after SCI are to:

- Achieve a system of management that is safe and acceptable, arising from a process of negotiation with the patient
- Protect the upper tract by preserving a low-pressure system and ensuring adequate emptying
- Minimise the risk of renal and ureteric stone formation and chronic infection
- Preserve the capacity of the bladder.

Box 33.4 shows a summary of the methods available for managing neurogenic bladder.

Catheters (intermittent or indwelling) may cause urethral stricture. Erosion of the penile urethra is possible if indwelling catheters or external urinary collection devices are poorly managed. Bladder stones are common in patients with indwelling catheters (Fulford *et al.*, 2004).

Management of urinary incontinence and bladder dysfunction is discussed further in Chapter 18.

Bowel management following SCI

As voluntary control is mainly conferred via the sacral nerves (S2–S4), any SCI is likely to affect neurological communication between the brain and the anorectal structures (Fulford *et al.*, 2004). Lesions above T12/LI principally affect upper motor neurones, leaving the reflex pathways that utilise the lower motor neurones intact. In this type of dysfunction, the reflex functions of the anorectum are preserved, but sensation and voluntary control

---

Box 33.4   Methods for managing the neurogenic bladder

Intermittent self-catheterisation

- Preferred method for areflexic bladder
- Allows the bladder to fill and completely empty periodically
- Reduces risk of UTI
- May need to take anticholinergic drugs (oxybutynin, tolterodine, propantheline) to stay dry between catheterisations
- May lead to urethral stricture formation

Indwelling urethral catheters

- Least satisfactory option
- Increased risk of infection, trauma, encrustation and autonomic dysreflexia

Suprapubic catheterisation (SPC)

- Advantages over indwelling urethral catheters, e.g.
  - Improved quality of life
  - Easier to manage for wheelchair users
  - Easier if sexually active
  - More comfortable and reduced urethral trauma
- Patient may still void urethrally – this can be reduced by anticholinergics

External urinary collection devices (e.g. penile sheath, bioderm)

- Take advantage of the return of detrusor voiding reflexes in suitable SCI males
- May need to try range of products to identify most suitable equipment for the individual
- May still be at risk of kidney damage due to the dysfunctional bladder
- Regular monitoring of renal function is required (Reynard *et al.*, 2003; Fulford *et al.*, 2004)

Voiding with voluntary control

- Some neurologically incomplete patients may achieve voluntary control
- Monitor long-term for upper tract damage

For further detail see Chapter 18.

---

are abolished (Fulford *et al.*, 2004). Areflexic dysfunction typically affects patients with neurologically complete lesions at L1 and below. As with reflex dysfunction, voluntary control and sensation are disrupted, but in addition, there is an absence of reflex function. This restricts the options for management (Fulford *et al* 2004). Some individuals with incomplete lesions may have a degree of preserved sensation or residual voluntary control. However this may not be sufficient to enable reliable bowel control (Consortium for Spinal Cord Medicine, 1998).

The primary aims of bowel management after SCI are to:

- Achieve a system or programme of management that is both safe and acceptable to the individual
- Prevent incontinence in order to enable social and recreational activities including employment and educational opportunities
- Enable sexual activity and other intimate human behaviours

- Protect skin integrity
- Enable the patient to complete a routine bowel management episode within a maximum of one hour from commencement

Involvement of community nurses is best avoided wherever possible because of the restrictions this places on the lifestyle of the individual. The capacity of local community nursing services to assist with bowel care in accordance with an established programme should always be confirmed beforehand and the alternative option of employing personal carers explored where available.

The components of a bowel management programme are as follows:

- Maintain continence, avoid constipation, and facilitate regularity of evacuation, by maintaining an appropriate

consistency of stool through careful attention to diet, fluid intake and physical activity as well as the use of oral laxatives and rectal stimulants (Coggrave *et al.*, 2006)
- Gentle abdominal massage can be used as a precursor to the insertion of rectal stimulants, and before and after digital stimulation, in order to aid evacuation (Coggrave, 2005)
- Most individuals with reflex bowel dysfunction can be established on an alternate day routine, while those with areflexic bowel dysfunction usually need, or prefer, to evacuate at least once a day

Box 33.5 shows a summary of the management of neurogenic bowel.

There are comprehensive guidelines for neurogenic bowel management on the Multidisciplinary Association

---

Box 33.5   Evacuation techniques for managing the neurogenic bowel

Areflexic bowel management
Because the bowel will not respond to rectal stimulants, as there is no reflex activity, the principal evacuation technique in areflexic bowel dysfunction is digital removal of faeces (DRF) This is an established form of bowel management and there is no evidence that it is harmful if performed properly. For most patients there is no satisfactory alternative

Reflex bowel management
The nursing care strategy for long-term reflex bowel management is to achieve complete *and timely* evacuation by using the mildest form of a proprietary chemical stimulant initially (usually suppositories or microenemas), reserving stronger stimulants for future occasions when problems may arise

- Place patient in a left lateral position on the bed and undertake digital rectal examination (DRE) by inserting a single gloved and lubricated finger into the rectum
- Any faeces present in the rectum can be digitally removed using a circling and 'beckoning' motion with the finger. This action is repeated until the rectum is empty
- Since areflexic dysfunction mainly occurs in lesions below T12/L1, the patient will often have reasonable hand function and during rehabilitation will learn how to perform DRF independently on the toilet

- Place patient in a left lateral position on the bed and undertake DRE as above
- If faeces already present in the rectum, digitally remove some of this until sufficient space is created to accommodate the rectal stimulant and to achieve maximum contact with the rectal wall for best effect
- Insert the prescribed rectal stimulant and leave *in situ* for an appropriate period of time to deliver effective stimulation
- Following reflex bowel evacuation, undertake DRE to confirm that the rectum is completely empty
- In the event of incomplete emptying, perform DRS by circling a finger within the rectum two or three times maintaining gentle contact with the rectal wall throughout. Do not repeat DRS more than three times within each bowel management episode, allowing five minutes rest between stimulations

Consortium for Spinal Cord Medicine, 1998; Multidisciplinary Association of Spinal Cord Injury Professionals, 2009.

of Spinal Cord Injury Professionals (MASCIP) and SIA websites (MASCIP, 2009). Professional guidelines are also available from the Royal College of Nursing (RCN, 2005; RCN, 2008). The National Patient Safety Agency recommends that every hospital and community NHS trust has a policy in place which meets the need to provide digital rectal evacuation procedures for patients with established spinal cord injuries (NPSA, 2004). Failure by a nurse to provide for this fundamental patient care requirement may precipitate autonomic dysreflexia (see: Autonomic dysreflexia) and would constitute both professional and clinical negligence.

SCI people requiring continuing assistance with bowel care should have a discharge care plan which outlines:

- The specific interventions to be used
- The regularity and timing of interventions
- Who is going to perform interventions
- Where bowel evacuation will take place
- Equipment and any adaptations required

Any changes that are made to the bowel management programme need to be assessed for effectiveness, so it is best to adopt a systematic approach: change only one element of the programme at a time, and allow at least a week between each change. Problems are generally grouped under three headings:

- Incontinence (unplanned evacuations)
- Constipation
- Prolonged management episodes

Management of constipation and fecal incontinence is discussed further in Chapter 18.

Changes in bowel habit or stool formation (loose stools, constipation or the unexpected presence of blood) that have persisted for six weeks or have resisted three separate changes to the established bowel management programme may be indicative of bowel cancer and should be investigated without further delay (www.cancerscreening.nhs.uk). Persisting in the belief that symptoms are solely related to neurogenic bowel dysfunction can have serious implications for the SCI individual (Poduri and Schnitzer, 2001).

Other options for managing the neurogenic bowel

For a minority of individuals with SCI a conservative bowel management programme may fail to meet the aims outlined above. In this case, the suitability of transanal irrigation should be considered (Christensen *et al.*, 2006).

The Peristeen device for transanal irrigation (Coloplast UK) can improve bowel management and independence with bowel care in many SCI patients. However, its suitability for an individual should be carefully assessed by an experienced professional (MASCIP, 2009). Otherwise, the formation of a stoma may be required to maintain the individual's personal comfort and holistic health. Stoma formation may be considered in the following cases:

- Intractable faecal leakage
- Pressure sores caused by prolonged toilet routine
- To deliver a continent solution that can be independently managed by an individual with limited hand function

Whenever a stoma is considered, it is essential that the SCI centre or rehabilitation team are consulted to ensure that the full implications of SCI, such as the impact of ageing on the neurogenic bowel and active wheelchair living with a stoma, have been appropriately considered to enable the SCI person to give his fully informed consent to surgery (Consortium for Spinal Cord Medicine, 1998).

Sexual issues and sexual dysfunction after SCI

Sexual function is highly complex, involving a continuous combination of psychological, hormonal, vascular and neurological factors (Frohman, 2002). The neurological changes following injury undoubtedly have the most profound and permanent effect on sexual function for individuals with a SCI. Possible concerns that they may have are listed in Box 33.6.

Addressing the totality of the impact of SCI on the sexual function and sexuality of individuals is challenging, as many of the effects emerge relatively slowly as individuals readjust and reintegrate after initial hospitalisation. It is difficult to prepare a newly paralysed individual for what to expect, especially as the focus for professionals and SCI people alike is frequently on the more basic functional aspects of SCI rehabilitation (bowel and bladder care, self-care skills, etc.). In addition, many professionals feel that they do not have sufficient interpersonal skills or specialist knowledge to deal with such intimate and complex issues (Herson *et al.*, 1999).

Initiating discussions about sexual issues, should, as far as is possible, be directed by the SCI person who should be enabled to choose someone they trust, at a time they feel appropriate and in a setting they feel suitable. For their part, professionals should be able and willing to respond to direct or indirect cues that the patient is ready to talk, and should find ways to let them know that it is acceptable

Box 33.6 Possible sexual and sexuality concerns of SCI people

* Projecting a confident and sexually attractive body image
* Maintaining relationships with existing sexual partners
* Finding new sexual partners and forming new relationships
* Loss of libido (sex drive)
* Perceived or actual loss of spontaneity
* Difficulties as a result of changing roles and expectations within relationships as a consequence of SCI
* Ability to achieve erections (erectile dysfunction) in men, or vaginal lubrication in women, as a response to sexual arousal
* The pleasurable sensations arising from diverse sexual activity
* The experience of orgasm
* The ability to ejaculate as a result of sexual activity (ejaculatory dysfunction) in men
* Reproductive ability and contraception
* Managing menstruation
* The ability to self-stimulate or masturbate
* The ability to adopt different sexual positions
* Maintaining continence during sexual activity
* Maintaining intact skin
* Pain and spasm during sexual activity
* Autonomic dysreflexia triggered by sexual stimulation

Source: Lobley, 2002.

to start talking about these intimate concerns (Herson *et al.*, 1999). They should also be aware of sources of additional support and specialist knowledge and expertise either locally or nationally, such as that provided by the SIA.

Most SCI males have some degree of erectile dysfunction and in addition, any SCI is likely to disrupt ejaculatory function. However, there have been many advances in treatment over the past 20 years (Hatzichristou and Pescatori 2001) and it is now possible to treat most erectile and ejaculatory dysfunction in SCI men. Specialist clinics now exist in many hospitals to supplement the services provided by SCI centres. Skilled patient education and

follow-up is essential for all of these treatments and can have a marked impact upon effectiveness.

After an initial period of amenorrhoea, which is a normal reaction to the severe metabolic disturbance that occurs immediately post injury, women with SCI usually regain their full reproductive abilities within their first post-injury year (Charlifue *et al.*, 1992) although there is a slight chance that in some vulnerable mature women, the trauma of SCI may induce an early menopause. The same neurological pathways (both reflexogenic and psychogenic) that govern erectile function in men produce clitoral and vulval engorgement and vaginal lubrication in women in response to arousal (psychogenic) or cutaneous genital stimulation (reflex). The degree of dysfunction will depend on the level and degree of completeness of the SCI.

This emphasis on dysfunctions and their treatment may give SCI people and their partners the impression that sexual activity is no longer about having fun or sharing sensual pleasure, and can no longer be spontaneous. On the other hand, once the initial psychological and emotional impact of SCI subsides, arousal and desire are often fully restored. Though genital sensation is often absent, greatly diminished or altered, most spinal cord injured people report a magnification of the pleasurable sensations in erogenous zones above the level of injury. Individuals should be encouraged to explore the possibilities of such changes in sensation. Most spinal cord injured people also discover that a huge part of the pleasure of sexual activity comes from giving pleasure to their partner, and that this does not necessarily require penetrative sex or genital sensation.

The prevention and management of pressure ulcers

The risk of pressure ulcer development increases with age and 80% of people with a chronic SCI will experience at least one pressure ulcer of significance within their lifetime (Byrne and Salzberg, 1996). Pressure ulcers form at least 30% of SCI centre readmissions (Rodriguez and Garber, 1994; Krause, 1998) and up to 8% of spinal cord injured individuals will die as a direct consequence of developing a pressure ulcer (Byrne and Salzberg, 1996). For this reason, the education of patients and their carers in the care and protection of those areas of skin presenting with lost or reduced sensation is a fundamental and heavily promoted component of SCI rehabilitation programmes. Pre-discharge education programmes within SCI centres benefit from their ability to utilise peer support to enable patients to develop a more realistic appreciation of the true impact of developing a pressure ulcer. The true potential for pressure ulcer development after discharge is based upon the individual's self-perception of risk (Arnold, 1994). Those who are able to establish and maintain a responsible attitude towards active living cannot avoid pressure ulcers but, by acting appropriately when one does occur, will experience fewer days adversely affected by them. In the initial period following discharge, compliance with precautionary skin care procedures is usually high as the perceptible risk increases with the return of the patient to a new environment. However, following discharge the routine monitoring of skin using a hand mirror may soon become perceived as an avoidable chore. To sustain this task over time requires a level of belief, motivation and discipline that may prove difficult to maintain in the face of the distractions which present after discharge.

In the community, the development of a pressure ulcer means that a previously independent paraplegic may find himself reliant upon family, friends, community professionals and home care services for a wide range of personal care tasks. It may be no different for tetraplegic individuals being nursed in bed at home with subsequent disruption of established care packages and family routines. Many SCI people express a distinct lack of confidence in community services and local general hospitals (Gibson, 2002). This is because they need to be convinced that nurses outside of specialist centres can demonstrate an appropriate knowledge of SCI in general and of the management of pressure ulcers in people with SCI in particular. As a consequence, most spinal cord injured people expect their pressure sore to be managed by SCI centre community liaison teams and to be readmitted to a SCI centre if hospitalisation is necessary. This additional reliance upon the SCI centre is in fact proving detrimental, resulting in an increased workload which should be the remit of community services (Gibson, 2002).

FUTURE RESEARCH

At this time, spinal cord injury results in a permanent loss of neurological function because, although the embryonic spinal cord can repair itself, the adult spinal cord does not regenerate spontaneously after injury. Research has identified a number of factors which currently influence our ability to repair or regenerate the spinal cord after injury. These include:

• The presence of inhibitory substances in the tissue that surrounds the damaged nerve fibres

• Changes inside adult nerve fibres that make them unable to respond well to growth-inducing signals that are effective in embryonic fibres
• The formation of cysts (cavities) within the injury site, that growing fibres cannot cross
• The lack of molecules (called nerve growth factors) in the surrounding area that stimulate nerve fibres to grow
• The formation of scar tissue at the injury site that forms a physical barrier to regrowth as well as containing additional inhibitory substances

Neuroprotective research is exploring the use of pharmaceutical agents or tissue factors administered very soon after the initial injury to limit the extent of cell damage, or to reduce the amount of scarring. The benefits of particular surgical techniques to stabilise or reduce pressure on the cord due to the column fracture are also being examined. Research into the repair or regrowth of the spinal cord is exploring the introduction of embryonic tissue, and attempting to transform nerve fibres in the adult spinal cord to a state that more resembles embryonic nerve fibres. Attempts are also being made to increase the growth of new nerve fibres into and around spinal cord lesion sites by overcoming the inhibitory factors described above. The current scientific consensus believes that combining individual treatments into a form that is appropriate clinically is the next step in developing an effective therapy for spinal cord repair (Adams and Cavanagh, 2004).

The core aim of most of this research is to protect or restore spinal cord functions for the benefit of a future population. Research intended to benefit chronically injured individuals is still in the early stages of development. A realistic expectation for this population is that small advances in the primary research projects outlined above will enable a similar level of discrete clinical opportunities such as regaining upper limb dexterity in tetraplegia, improving bladder, bowel or sexual function, or the relief of chronic pain (Adams *et al.*, 2007). Individuals seeking further insight into this research are best directed to the websites of the International Spinal Research Trust (www.spinalresearch.org) and The International Campaign for Cures in Spinal Cord Injury Paralysis (ICCP) (www.campaignforcure.org) as the two most credible authorities on this subject.

In addition to these attempts to repair or regrow the spinal cord we should not overlook the efforts of other researchers whose intentions are to bypass the effects of a spinal cord lesion through the use of implantable computerised nerve stimulators.

Spinal cord injury: patient perspective

Spinal cord injury (SCI) is a complex lifetime condition, it is rarely fully understood by clinicians working outside its field, although in my experience many find it hard or refuse to admit this.

As a SCI patient of over 40 years I have both experienced and seen, through my peers, what happens when our condition is managed badly. Not through intent or neglect, rather through lack of knowledge, understanding and expertise, and often through a lack of willingness on the part of the treating clinicians, at all levels, to liaise with and consult with expert peer clinicians (within a SCI centre), who fully understand the condition and the serious (life-threatening) consequences that can and do arise from inappropriate treatment. Perhaps you could call that neglect, or perhaps professional pride being put before the welfare of the patient. Whatever label you give, the consequences for someone with SCI can be devastating. I am fortunate in having a GP who despite being extremely capable recognises my expertise in my condition. He listens to me. He listens to my SCI centre.

That is not to say I would want all my acute treatments to be carried out in my SCI centre, only those that directly relate to my SCI. For instance, if I were to suffer a heart attack I would want my treatment to be in a coronary unit. But I would want my care whilst I was in that unit to be managed under the guidance of my SCI centre, particularly my nursing care. Similarly, if a member of my family were to suffer a suspected SCI, I would want/expect the A&E unit they were taken to, to contact the nearest SCI centre immediately, and be guided by them, setting up a programme of care to manage their condition, a condition that may include trauma incidences other than SCI, until such times as they could be safely transferred to a specialist SCI centre.

In my 40 years of being SCI I have, like many of my peers, retrained, gone back to full employment, married, integrated fully into my community, travelled the world, lived an ordinary life under extraordinary circumstances. Being comfortable in the knowledge that I have the constant support of a SCI centre, that knew me and my condition was, and still is, a major factor in allowing me to live a relatively normal life.

Written by a C5 tetraplegic

SUMMARY

A spinal cord injury is a life changing event because it impacts on every aspect of the individual's life. The challenges the individual faces are numerous and are often complex, requiring skilled and experienced professionals to manage them. The support of a specialist multidisciplinary team is essential to give the individual the best possible chance to reach their full potential and to equip them with the necessary skills to enable them to be autonomous and confident in dealing with day to day challenges that they will face.

USEFUL WEBSITES

www.iscos.org.uk	The International Spinal Cord Society (ISCoS) is an international association whose purpose is to study all problems relating to traumatic and non-traumatic lesions of the spinal cord and to support health care professionals involved in SCI patient care throughout the world.
Spinal Cord Injury UK (website pending in 2010)	A new consortium of the core professional associations and charities outlined below intended to develop and promote a national consensus regarding core issues for government, professionals and the public.
www.mascip.co.uk	The Multidisciplinary Association of Spinal Cord Injury Professionals provides peer support and consensus guidelines for multi-professional teams caring for spinal cord injured individuals both within and outside of UK and Irish SCI centres.
www.bascis.pwp.blueyonder.co.uk	The British Association of Spinal Cord Injury Specialists incorporates UK and Irish SCI centre consultants and clinicians associated with SCI medicine and rehabilitation. BASCIS provides peer support and consensus guidelines for the medical and surgical management of spinal cord injured individuals.

www.spinal-research.org	Spinal Research is the UK's leading charity funding medical research around the world to develop reliable treatments for paralysis following spinal injury.
www.campaignforacure.org	The International Campaign for Cures of SCI Paralysis (ICCP) is a body of affiliate nonprofit organisations, working to fund research into cures for paralysis caused by spinal cord injury. The ICCP coalition mission is 'to expedite the discovery of cures for SCI paralysis.'
www.escif.org	The European SCI Federation represents a federation of national self-help SCI organisations working to safeguard and promote the interests of spinal cord injured people.
www.spinal.co.uk	The website of the Spinal Injuries Association, the UK charity for people living with spinal cord injury. An excellent resource for patients and families.
www.sisonline.org	Spinal Injuries Scotland is a charity supporting people living with spinal cord injury in Scotland.
www.aspire.org.uk	Aspire is a charity which offers practical support to the people living with SCI in the UK so that they can lead fulfilled and independent lives in their homes, with their families, in work-places and leisure time.
www.backuptrust.org.uk	The Back-Up Trust is a charity which provides a range of activity-based services for people with SCI as well as their friends, family and volunteers to encourage independence, self-confidence and motivation following a life changing injury.

REFERENCES

Adams M, Cavanagh JFR (2004) International campaign for cures of spinal cord injury paralysis (ICCP): another step forward for spinal cord injury research. *Spinal Cord* 42:273–280.

Adams M, Carlstedt T, Cavanagh J et al. (2007) International Spinal Research Trust research strategy III: A discussion document. *Spinal Cord* 45:2–14.

American College of Surgeons' Committee on Trauma (ACS) (2008) *Advanced Trauma Life Support Manual for Physicians*. (8th edition). Chicago: ACS.

Aung S, El-Masry WS (1997) Audit of a British centre for spinal injury. *Spinal Cord* 35:147–150.

Arnold N (1994) Clinical study: the relationship between patient perceived risk and actual risk of for the development of pressure sores. *Ostomy Wound Management* 40(3):36–45.

Ash D (2002) An exploration of the occurrence of pressure ulcers in a British spinal injuries unit. *Journal of Clinical Nursing* 11:470–478.

Ash D, Harrison P (2007) Understanding spinal shock. In: Harrison P (ed). *Managing Spinal Cord Injury: The first 48 hours*. Milton Keynes: Spinal Injuries Association.

Banit DM, Grau G, Fisher JR (2000) Evaluation of the acute cervical spine: A management algorithm. *Journal of Trauma: Injury, Infection and Critical Care* 49:450–456.

Beedie A, Kennedy P (2002) Quality of social support predicts hopelessness and depression post spinal cord injury.

Journal of Clinical Psychology in Medical Settings 9:227–234.

Braddom RL, Rocco JF (1991) Autonomic dysreflexia: A survey of current treatment. *American Journal of Physical Medicine and Rehabilitation* 70:234–241.

Boerger TO, Limb D, Dickson RA (2000) Does 'canal clearance' affect neurological outcome after thoracolumbar burst fractures? *Journal of Bone and Joint Surgery (Br)* 82-B:629–635.

British Orthopaedic Association (BOA) (2006) *The Initial Care and Transfer of Patients with Spinal Cord Injuries*. London: BOA.

British Trauma Society (2003) Guidelines for the initial management of spinal injury. *Injury* 34:405-425.

Byrne DW, Salzberg CA (1996) Major risk factors for pressure ulcers in the spinal cord disabled: a literature review. *Spinal Cord* 34:255–263.

Carvell J, Grundy, D (1994) Complications of spinal surgery in acute SCI patients. *Paraplegia* 32:1389–1395.

Charlifue SW, Gerhart KA, Menter RR et al. (1992) Sexual issues of women with spinal cord injuries. *Paraplegia* 30:192–199.

Christensen P, Bazocchi G, Coggrave M et al. (2006) A randomized, controlled trial of transanal irrigation versus conservative bowel management in spinal cord-injured patients. *Gastroenterology* 131(3):738–747.

Coggrave M (2005) Management of the neurogenic bowel. *British Journal of Neuroscience Nursing*. 1(1): 6–13.

Coggrave M, Wiesel PH, Norton C (2006) Management of faecal incontinence and constipation in adults with central neurological diseases. *Cochrane Database of Systematic Reviews* Issue 1. Art. No.: CD002115. DOI: 10.1002/14651858.CD002115.pub3

Consortium for Spinal Cord Medicine (1998) *Neurogenic Bowel Management in Adults with SCI: Clinical practice guidelines*. Washington DC: Paralyzed Veterans of America.

Consortium for Spinal Cord Medicine (2001) *Acute Management of Autonomic Dysreflexia: Individuals with spinal cord injury presenting to health care facilities*. Washington DC: Paralyzed Veterans of America.

Consortium for Spinal Cord Medicine (2008) *Early Acute Management in Adults with Spinal Cord Injury*. Washington DC: Paralysed Veterans of America.

Ditunno JF, Little JW, Tessler A *et al.* (2004) Spinal shock revisited: a four-phase model. *Spinal Cord* 42:383–395.

El-Masry WS (1993) Physiological instability of the spinal cord following injury. *Paraplegia* 31:273–275.

Elliott T, Warren AM (2007) Why psychology is important in rehabilitation. In: Kennedy P (ed). *Psychological Management of Physical Disabilities*. London: Brunner-Rutledge Press.

Elliott T, Bush B, Chen Y (2006) Social problem solving abilities predict pressure sore occurrence in the first three years of spinal cord injury. *Rehabilitation Psychology* 51:69–77.

Elfstrom M, Ryden A, Kreuter M *et al.* (2005) Relations between coping strategies and health-related quality of life in patients with spinal cord lesion. *Journal of Rehabilitation Medicine* 37(1):1650–1677.

Fehlings MG, Miyanji F, Furlan JC *et al.* (2007) Acute cervical traumatic spinal cord injury: MR imaging findings correlated with neurologic outcome – prospective study with 100 consecutive patients. *Radiology* 243:820–827.

Fisher JD, Brown SN, Cooke MW (eds) (2006) *UK Ambulance Service: Clinical practice guidelines*. Joint Royal Colleges Ambulance Liaison Committee and the Ambulance Services Association: London. Available from (http://www.jrcalc.org.uk). Accessed July 2010.

Frohman EM. (2002) Sexual dysfunction in neurologic disease. *Clinical Neuropharmacology* 25:126–132.

Fulford S, Coggrave M, Wright L (2004) *Bladder and Bowel Management for People with Spinal Cord Injury*. London: Spinal Injuries Association.

Gall A, Harrison P (2007) The process of spinal cord lesion formation. In: Harrison P (ed) *Managing Spinal Cord Injury: The First 48 Hours*. Milton Keynes: Spinal Injuries Association.

Gibson L (2002) Perceptions of pressure ulcers among young men with a spinal injury. *British Journal of Community Nursing* 7:451–460.

Harrison P (2000) *Spinal Injury: Critical care*. London: Spinal Injuries Association.

Harrison P (2007) (ed) *Managing Spinal Cord Injury: The first 48 hours*. Milton Keynes: Spinal Injuries Association.

Hatzichristou DG, Pescatori ES (2001) Current treatments and emerging therapeutic approaches in male erectile dysfunction. *British Journal of Urology International* 88 (Suppl 3):11–17.

Hawkins S, Stone K, Plummer L (1999) An holistic approach to turning patients. *Nursing Standard* 14:(3)52–56.

Helling TS, Watkins M, Evans LL *et al.* (1999) Low falls: an underappreciated mechanism of injury. *Journal of Trauma* 46:453–456.

Herson L, Hart KA, Gordon MJ (1999) Identifying and overcoming barriers to providing sexuality information in the clinical setting. *Rehabilitation Nursing* 24:148–151.

Ho M, Fung KY, Joynt GM *et al.* (2002) Rigid collar and intracranial pressure of patients with severe head injury. *Journal of Trauma: Injury, Infection and Critical Care* 53:1185–1188.

Hogan BJ, Blaylock B, Tobian TL (1997) Trauma multidisciplinary QI project: evaluation of cervical spine clearance, collar selection and skin care. *Journal of Trauma Nursing* 4:60–67.

Hu R, Mustard CA, Burns C (1996) Epidemiology of incident spinal fracture in a complete population. *Spine* 21:492–499.

Iencean SM (2003) Classification of spinal injuries based on the essential traumatic spinal mechanisms. *Spinal Cord* 41:385–396.

Kishan S, Vives MJ, Reiter MF (2005) Timing of surgery following spinal cord injury. *Journal of Spinal Cord Medicine* 28:11–19.

Krause JS (1998) Skin sores after spinal cord injury: relationship to life adjustment. *Spinal Cord* 36:51–56.

Lobley K (2002) *Sex Matters*. Milton Keynes: Spinal Injuries Association.

Marshall LF, Knowlton S, Garfin SR *et al.* (1987) Deterioration following spinal cord injury. A multicenter study. *Journal of Neurosurgery* 66:400–404.

Multidisciplinary Association of Spinal Cord Injury Professionals (2009) *Guidelines for Management of Neurogenic Bowel Dysfunction after Spinal Cord Injury*. Peterborough: Coloplast Ltd. (see also http://www.mascip.co.uk/)

McCutcheon EP, Selassie AW, Gu JK *et al.* (2004) Acute traumatic spinal cord injury, 1993–2000. A population-based assessment of methylprednisolone administration and hospitalization. *Journal of Trauma: Injury, Infection and Critical Care* 56:1076–1083.

Moreau APM, Willcox N, Brown MF (2003) Immobilisation of spinal fractures in patients with ankylosing spondylitis: two case reports. *Injury* 34:372–373.

Nacimiento W, Noth J (1999) What, if anything, is spinal shock? *Archives of Neurology* 56:1033–1035.

National Confidential Enquiry into Patient Outcome and Death (2007) *Trauma: Who Cares? A report of the National Confidential Enquiry into Patient Outcome and Death*. London: NCEPOD.

National Institute for Health and Clinical Excellence (2005) *The Management of Pressure Ulcers in Primary and Secondary Care*. London: NICE.

National Institute for Health and Clinical Excellence (2007) *Head Injury: triage, assessment, investigation and early management of head injury in infants, children and adults*. London: NICE.

National Patient Safety Agency (2004) *Improving the Safety of Patients with Established Spinal Injuries in Hospital*. Patient Safety Information Bulletin. London: NPSA. Available from: http://www.npsa.nhs.uk

NHS National Commissioning Group for Highly Specialised Services (NHSSCGHSS) (2009) *Specialised Services: National definitions set* (3rd edition). *Definition No 6: Specialised spinal services (all ages)*. London: Department of Health. Available from: www.specialisedcommissioning. nhs.uk Accessed July 2010.

North NT (1999) The psychological effects of spinal cord injury: a review. *Spinal Cord* 37:671–679.

Poduri KR, Schnitzer EM (2001) Carcinoid tumour mistaken for persistent neurogenic bowel symptoms in a patient with paraplegia: a case report. *Archives of Physical Medicine and Rehabilitation* 82:996–999.

Ravichandran G, El-Masri WS (2005) *Management of Individuals with Spinal Cord Injury in General Hospitals: Good practice guide*. Oswestry: British Association of Spinal Cord Injury Specialists.

Ravichandran G (1989) Errors and omissions in the acute management of spinal cord injury. *Journal of the Medical Defence Union* 5:14–16.

Reynard JM, Vass J, Sullivan ME *et al*. (2003) Sphincterotomy and the treatment of detrusor-sphincter dyssynergia: current status, future prospects. *Spinal Cord* 41:1–11.

Rodriguez GP, Garber SL (1994) Prospective study of pressure ulcer risk in spinal cord injury patients. *Paraplegia* 32 (3):150–158.

Roth EJ, Lovell L, Heinemann AW *et al*. (1992) The older adult with a spinal cord injury. *Paraplegia* 30:520–526.

Royle J, Glass C (2007) Psychological and emotional support. In: Harrison P (Ed) *Managing Spinal Cord Injury: The first 48 hours*. Milton Keynes: Spinal Injuries Association.

Royal College of Nursing (2005) *The Procedure for Digital Removal of Faeces*. London: RCN.

Royal College of Nursing (2008) *Bowel Care: Including digital rectal examination and manual removal of faeces*. London: RCN.

Sapru H (2002) Spinal cord: anatomy, physiology and pathophysiology. In: Kirschblum S *et al*. (eds). *Spinal Cord Medicine*. Philadelphia: Lippincott, Williams and Wilkins.

Sarhan F, Harrison P (2007) Transferring patients to SCI centres. In: Harrison P (ed). *Managing Spinal Cord Injury: The first 48 hours*. Milton Keynes: Spinal Injuries Association.

Short D (2001) Is the role of steroids in acute spinal cord injury now resolved? *Current Opinion in Neurology* 14:759–763.

Spinal Injuries Association (2009) *Preserving and Developing the National Spinal Cord Injury Service: Phase 2 – seeking the evidence*. Milton Keynes: Spinal Injuries Association.

Spinal Task Force (2010) *Organising Quality and Effective Spinal Services for Patients: A report for local health communities by the Spinal Taskforce*. London: Department of Health. Available from: http://www.dh.gov.uk/en/ Publicationsandstatistics/Publications/ PublicationsPolicyAndGuidance/DH_114528 Accessed July 2010.

Tator CH, Duncan EG, Edmonds VE *et al*. (1995) Neurological recovery, mortality and length of stay after acute spinal cord injury associated with changes in management. *Paraplegia* 33:254–262.

Trieschmann RB (1988) *Spinal Cord Injuries: Psychological, social and vocational rehabilitation*. New York: Demos.

Webster G, Kennedy P (2007) Spinal cord injuries. In: Kennedy P. (Ed) *Psychological Management of Physical Disabilities*. London: Brunner-Rutledge Press.

Section VII
Management of Patients with Neuropathies and Spinal Disorders and Disease

34

Management of Patients with Disorders of the Vertebral Column and Spinal Cord

Cath Waterhouse and Glynis Pellatt

INTRODUCTION

This chapter will discuss the diagnosis and management of patients that present with signs and symptoms of spinal cord and or nerve root compression, focusing on the surgical management and nursing care. Every year it has been estimated that 80% of the population has experienced some degree of back pain, accounting for the loss of 81 million working days (Backcare, 2008). The cost of back pain to the individual, to the economy and the NHS is considerable and the true cost to industry is difficult to define, but Millar (2005) suggests that the cost to the economy is £5 billion. In nine out of ten cases the pain will have gone or be much better within six weeks, so very few will require surgical intervention (PatientUK, 2006).

Patients with diseases and disorders of the vertebral column that compromise the functioning of the spinal cord and nerve roots not only suffer pain and limitations in movement and mobility that adversely affect all aspects of their daily living, but may also experience neurogenic bowel, bladder and sexual dysfunction (Skyrme *et al.*, 2005). Management options depend on assessing the patient from a holistic perspective, taking into consideration their presenting symptoms, the diagnosis and the potential for the patient to make a good recovery following appropriate treatment.

AETIOLOGY AND PATHOPHYSIOLOGY

Degenerative disorders of the vertebral column

Non traumatic causes of vertebral column disease are mostly the result of degenerative changes that occur as a result of the normal ageing process. The spine essentially stiffens and loses its flexibility due to thinning of the disc spaces, thickening of the bone and ligaments, and restriction of the facet joints due to the development of osteophytes (bony spurs). The most common degenerative conditions of the vertebral column are spondylosis and intervertebral disc disease.

Spondylosis

The natural process of ageing causes the intervertebral discs to degenerate. As the discs degenerate more pressure is put on the articulating facet joints. The body's response is to attempt to overcome the problem by trying to fuse together the vertebra above and below the affected disc. The bony outgrowths (osteophytes) can reduce the available space for the spinal cord and spinal nerves (spinal canal stenosis) resulting in compression of the spinal cord and or spinal nerve roots.

The cervical and lumbar areas are particularly vulnerable to wear and tear, so it is not surprising that these are the sites where most damage occurs. Although most of the population over 50 years of age has cervical spondylosis, only a small number become symptomatic due to nerve root or spinal cord compression. The amount of pain experienced by the patient does not always correlate with the degree of degeneration.

Neuroscience Nursing: Evidence-Based Practice, 1st Edition.
Edited by Sue Woodward and Ann-Marie Mestecky
© 2011 Blackwell Publishing Ltd

Spondylolisthesis

Spondylolisthesis refers to the forward displacement of one vertebra over another caused by trauma, neoplasms, degenerative changes or congenital mechanical defects (Guiot and Mendel, 2005). It most frequently affects the lumbosacral joint at L5 – S1, but may occur at any spinal level. The degree of stability is measured by the severity of slippage from the posterior edge of the superior vertebral body to the posterior edge of the inferior vertebral body. Spondylolisthesis will result in the narrowing of the spinal canal, which may or may not be symptomatic. It is recommended that patients with symptomatic spondylolisthesis of more than 25% slippage are referred for a surgical opinion (Skyrme *et al.*, 2005).

Intervertebral disc disease

Intervertebral disc prolapse occurs when there is a weakness or a tear in the annulus fibrosus allowing the nucleus pulposus to push through into the spinal canal. Herniated discs may be found in people who are asymptomatic without any history of back problems (Boden *et al.*, 1996), emphasising the importance of treating the patient rather than the radiological images. A prolapse may occur suddenly or more insidiously, initially presenting as a mild protrusion and extending to a prolapse. Symptoms deteriorate as the disc extrudes into the spinal canal, finally becoming displaced (sequestrated) beyond the outer annulus (Figure 34.1). Many acute symptoms of herniation improve significantly after 6–8 weeks following conservative management with physiotherapy and exercise, but can continue as a chronic nerve irritation due to ongoing disc degeneration (Skyrme *et al.*, 2005).

Each spinal level affected produces specific symptoms and peculiarities depending on the degree of herniation. The lumbar spine is by far the most common site for disc prolapse, principally affecting L4/5, L5/S1 nerve roots. The typical symptoms include sciatica, muscle wasting, weakness and parastheasia in the toes or feet.

Spinal canal stenosis

Spinal canal stenosis is the narrowing of the spinal canal. Spondylosis, herniated disc, spondylolysthesis and ossification of the posterior longitudinal ligament are the common causes; it can also be congenitally narrowed. Narrowing of the canal causes nerve root compression and less often cord compression. It usually affects the cervical and lumbar areas. Most people over the age of seventy have some degree of spinal stenosis although the majority are asymptomatic (Sinikallio et al., 2006).

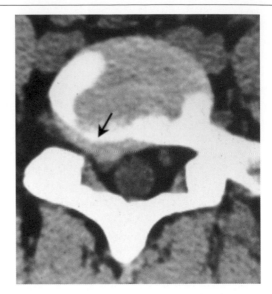

Figure 34.1 Prolapsed lumbar intervertebral disc. CT scan showing lateral disc protrusion (arrowed). The patient presented with sciatica due to nerve root compression. Reproduced from L. Ginsberg, *Lecture Notes: Neurology*, Wiley-Blackwell, with permission.

Infections

Spinal epidural abscess may develop as a primary infection following any of the following: lumbar puncture, epidural anaesthesia, penetrating back injury or spinal surgery. Staphylococcus aureus is the causative organism in 90% of cases (Lindsey and Bone, 2004). Seeding of the spinal epidural space with micro-organisms can also occur secondary to a bacteraemia from a focus of infection elsewhere in the body, e.g. respiratory tract infection, dental abscess, urinary tract infection, endocarditis or vertebral osteomyelitis, although in many cases no underlying pathology can be determined. While staphylococcus aureus accounts for the majority of the infections, other infective organisms include streptococcus, pseudomonas, escherichia coli and mycobacterium tuberculosis (Weinstein and Eismont, 2005). Any patient who presents with persistent back pain plus anorexia, weight loss and fever should be investigated for spinal infection (Skyrme *et al.*, 2005). Abscesses and localised oedema cause compression of the spinal cord, and distortion of nerve roots and blood vessels, which then produce neurological deficits.

Onset of symptoms is often insidious and referred pain extending across the shoulder and down the arm may be attributed to cardiac or abdominal conditions, contributing to delays in diagnosis. Risk factors include: IV drug misuse, alcoholism, diabetes mellitus or human immunodeficiency virus (Weinstein and Eismont, 2005). Prompt diagnosis and intervention is essential to avoid permanent sequelae.

Haematomas

Arterio-venous malformations (AVMs) are congenital malformations caused by developmental abnormalities in the spinal vascular network (see Chapter 23). A tangled knot of abnormal arteries and veins are connected by weak fistulae and can cause cord compression directly, but may also burst and haemorrhage. The haematoma will compress the cord with subsequent ischeamia or infarction (Ho *et al.*, 2007). Spinal AVMs are very rare and difficult to diagnose. They can produce pressure symptoms, but when they bleed they will often cause catastrophic disability.

Spinal epidural haematomas (bleeding in the spinal epidural space) can be caused by extradural AVMs, epidural anesthesia, lumbar puncture in patients with a bleeding diathesis, or following spinal or thoracic surgery (Vacca, 2007).

Spinal column tumours

Spinal cord tumours may present as extradural (outside of the dura), intradural-extramedullary (within the dura, but outside of the spinal cord) or intramedullary (within the spinal neural tissue) lesions (Ho *et al.*, 2007, Wolcott *et al.*, 2005).

Extradural tumours are usually malignant or metastatic arising from the spread from lymphomas or melanomas of prostate, breast, lungs, bowels or kidney (Patchell *et al.*, 2005). 60% of metastatic lesions occur in the thoracic spine where bone density is highest, 30% in the lumbosacral spine and the remaining 10% in the cervical spine (Abraham, 2004). For some patients, malignant spinal cord compression (MSCC) is the first indication that there is a further undiagnosed malignancy (Loblaw *et al.*, 2005; Purdue, 2003).

Intradural extramedullary tumours originate from the meninges or nerve roots. These tumours are principally benign meningiomas and neurofibromas and are nearly three times more common than intramedullary lesions (Huff, 2007). Meningiomas can occur anywhere along the cord and are the most common intradural tumour. They typically compress and displace the cord. Considerable displacement and flattening of the cord can occur before the patient is symptomatic. Nerve root tumours arise from the nerve sheath and can be either a schwannoma or neurofibroma. These tumours compress the root of the affected spinal nerve.

Intramedullary tumours are very rare and, like their intracranial counterparts, originate from the glial tissues of the spinal cord. Spinal cord tumours of each particular type are identical to those of the brain, e.g. a spinal astrocytoma has the same pathological features as a brain astrocytoma.

Astrocytomas and ependymomas are the most common primary intramedullary tumours. Astrocytomas most commonly affect the cervical and thoracic cord. Ependymomas typically occur around the counus medullaris.

Damage to the cord may be caused by: tumour invasion and infiltration displacing and destroying neural tissues, bone collapse, ischaemia or infarction arising from occlusion of spinal arteries and obstruction to venous outflow, or as a consequence of vasogenic cord swelling (Abraham, 2004).

Chiari malformation

Previously referred to as Arnold Chiari malformation (ACM), Chiari malformation describes a spectrum of structural abnormalities in the brain and spinal cord, resulting in the cerebellar tonsils herniating through the foramen magnum into the cervical spinal canal, blocking the flow of CSF and producing variable signs and symptoms of sensory loss, motor deficits, quadriparesis, spasticity and ataxia (Wellons *et al.*, 2005). The deformity usually presents as a congenital malformation at birth or, rarely, it may be acquired secondary to trauma or infections (Sun, 2001). The precise incidence is unknown as many patients with type I and type II Chiari malformation are asymptomatic until their adolescence.

There are four primary classifications that describe Chiari malformation:

- Type I: the cerebellar tonsils extend into the cervical spinal canal. In most cases this is asymptomatic, however hydrocephalus can occur in approximately 10% of cases (see Chapter 25).
- Type II: involves caudal descent of the cerebellum and lower brain stem into the cervical spinal canal. It is associated with spina bifida. Meningomyelocele and hydrocephalus are invariably present (see Chapter 25).
- Type III: generates serious neurological deficits due to cerebellum and brain stem herniation through the foramen magnum. It is rarely compatible with post-natal life.
- Type IV: a very rare form of CM. There is gross underdevelopment of the cerebellum, and defects in the posterior fossa. It is associated with high morbidity.

Syringomyelia

Syringomyelia is a rare, chronic, progressive degenerative condition occurring in approximately 8 in 100,000 predominantly younger people (Leon, 2007). It refers to a cavity or syrinx that forms in the spinal cord and fills with CSF, destroying neural tissue and leading to severe neurological deficits. A syrinx may form at any level of the spinal cord and can occur in isolation or in multiple loculated areas. Syringomyelia often develops secondary to other conditions such as spinal tumours, acute spinal cord injury, neurological infections, haemorrhage, hydrocephalus or prolapsed disc (Yuras, 2000). It is commonly present in cases of Chiari malformation type I and II. Symptoms can vary; they include headache, limb weakness, pain and parasthaesia (exacerbated by coughing and sneezing), bladder and bowel dysfunction and loss of proprioception. The syrinx may also disrupt parasympathetic and sympathetic nerve pathways leading to atypical body temperatures and sweating.

Spinal infarcts

Spinal cord infarction (sometimes called spinal stroke) is not common. There is an acute onset of paralysis and sensory disturbance caused most commonly by occlusion of an artery by thrombosis or embolus. The anterior spinal artery is the most commonly affected.

The anterior spinal artery supplies the anterior two thirds of the cord. The posterior spinal artery supplies the posterior columns. The anterior spinal artery originates from the branches of the intracranial vertebral arteries in the upper cervical region and passes down the anterior surface of the cord. Below the level of T4 it receives further blood flow from the intercostal radicular arteries arising from the aorta. The thoracic region has the largest space between radicular arteries in comparison to other spinal segments. This means that there is a watershed of increased ischemic vulnerability in the distribution of the anterior spinal artery. The most vulnerable level is T4 (Millichip *et al.*, 2006).

As 95% of infarcts occur in the anterior two thirds of the spinal cord the presentation is one of anterior cord syndrome, i.e. the same clinical manifestations as an acute spinal cord injury affecting the anterior cord (see Chapter 33).

Spina bifida

Spina bifida is a congenital malformation where there is a defect in the closure of the vertebral arches. It is caused by failure of the neural tube to close, 21 to 28 days following conception, and is estimated to occur in 1–2 people per 1,000 of the population. Spina bifida can present with differing severity.

Spina bifida occulta is the most common type of spina bifida. The majority remain asymptomatic and many people are unaware that they have the condition. Those that do become symptomatic usually do so in childhood or adolescence because of tethering of the spinal cord. In such cases the conus medullaris is attached to one or more lumbar vertebrae which prevents it from ascending to follow its normal course; the nerve roots become stretched resulting in neurological dysfunction. There is often a small dimple or small patch of hair on the skin over the area of defect.

Meningocele is the result of the meninges, but not the spinal cord, protruding through the defect in the vertebral arch which creates a cystic CSF fluid filled sac. The sac may be felt on the surface of the skin. A *myelomeningocele* is the result of the meninges and cord protruding through the defect in the vertebral arch; the neural tissue and meninges are contained within a dural sac. A myelomeningocele will cause significant neurological dysfunction below the level of the lesion.

The cause of spina bifida is still unclear but genetic defects in the LPP1 gene have been identified (Wolcott *et al.*, 2005). Risk factors such low folic acid levels due to abnormal metabolism or insufficient dietary intake are thought to interfere with the formation of genetic material. Diabetes, obesity and anti-convulsant medications, such as sodium valporate and carbemazipine, have been shown to increase the incidence of the condition. Pre-natal testing measuring the levels of serum alpha-fetoprotein (AFP), amniocentesis and ultrasound has increased detection of spina bifida and other neural tube defects (Huff, 2007).

The causes of spinal cord and nerve compression are summarised in Table 34.1. Traumatic injury to the spinal cord is presented in Chapter 33.

SIGNS AND SYMPTOMS

Whilst specific signs of symptoms of each pathological cause are presented above, the general signs and symptoms of root and cord compression are discussed in the following section. Signs and symptoms will depend on the level and location of the disease or lesion and the speed with which the pathology develops.

Level and location

When a nerve root is compressed or damaged the function of the nerve is impaired. Radiculopathy is the term commonly used to denote a disorder of the spinal nerve root.

Table 34.1 Causes of spinal cord and spinal nerve root compression and back pain.

Cord and or nerve compression	Other causes of back pain
Trauma: (see Chapter 33)	Muscular strain
• Crush or compression fractures	Repetitive and
• Subluxation	cumulative
• Spinal abscess (*Staphylococcus aureus*, tuberculosis)	strain
	Referred pain:
• Discitis	• Gall bladder
• Osteomyelitis	• Kidneys
Tumours:	• Viscera
• Metastatic disease (from breast, kidney, lung and prostate)	
• Meningioma	
• Myeloma	
• Neurofibroma	
• Ependymoma	
• Schwannoma	
Degenerative disease:	
• Prolapsed intervertebral disc	
• Spondylosis	
• Spondylolisthesis	
Haematoma:	
• AVM	
• trauma	
Syringomyelia ± Chiari malformation	
Vascular disorders:	
• Infarcts	

The power and tone of the muscles innervated by the specific nerve root/s are decreased. The deep tendon reflexes are also decreased but are rarely absent because the muscles involved are innervated by two or more spinal nerves. There is dermatomal sensory loss (see Chapter 33) or pain. The predominant complaint of pain correlates with a specific dermatome, this often becomes worse when the patient coughs, sneezes or exercises (Rodts, 2002). The clinical findings of a radiculopathy caused by cervical spondylosis of C5 and C6 nerve roots would therefore most commonly be: weakness of the deltoid and bicep muscles, pain or less commonly sensory loss in the sensory nerve root distribution, i.e. about the shoulder and outer aspects of the arm and forearm, and reduced bicep reflexes. See Chapter 4 for the muscles that each main nerve root innervates (myotomes) and the sensory area that each supplies (dermatomes).

A myelopathy occurs when there is direct compression of the spinal cord creating segmental compression, rather than compression of a single nerve root (Strayer, 2005). There will be sensory and/or motor impairment below the level of the lesion due to interruption of the ascending and/or descending tracts. There may also be sphincter disturbance. Disturbance to the cord below T1 will only affect the lower limbs whereas above this level there will be involvement of all four limbs. Involvement of the cord below C5 to T1 will result in only partial impairment of the upper limbs.

Speed of onset

The onset of myelopathy and radiculopathy can be insidious or it can be sudden depending on the pathology. An acute compression of the cord, e.g. due to a haemorrhage, will result in spinal shock with flaccid muscle tone and areflexia (i.e. the same clinical manifestations as an acute spinal cord injury (see Chapter 33).

Pain and spinal tumours

The most common presenting symptom of spinal tumours is back pain, which may be intense, progressive and is sometimes described as a tight band around the body that tends to worsen on coughing, straining or lying flat (Haas, 2003). This can be accompanied by stiffness, tingling, numbness and ataxia. Later symptoms include autonomic dysfunction, urinary incontinence or retention, altered bowel function, impotence and loss of mobility (Fallon and Hanks, 2006).

What are now referred to as 'red flag' signs of spinal cord compression (Box 34.1) are triggers for early referral to appropriate specialist consultants and early surgery (Rodts, 2002).

Cauda equina syndrome

Cauda equina syndrome involves compression of the nerve roots below L1–3 vertebrae by a tumour, infection, central disc prolapse, haematoma or fracture. Symptoms usually arise acutely, but onset can be more insidious for patients with progressive spinal tumours (Devlin, 2003). Whilst the development of significant neurological motor deficits is the principle concern, cauda equina syndrome may produce a range of symptoms that frequently demands urgent surgical decompression to prevent permanent paraplegia (Box 34.2) (Fehlings *et al.*, 2005).

Box 34.1   Red flag signs

- Previous history of malignancy
- Significant trauma, e.g. fall from a height
- Minor trauma in immunosuppressed patients or patients diagnosed with osteoporosis
- Unexpected weight loss
- Pre-existing infection – urinary tract, respiratory or skin infection
- Exposure to infection, e.g. tuberculosis
- Enlarged or tender cervical lymph nodes
- Underlying renal disease if pain unilateral in the lower back
- Complaints of pain that is worse when lying down or is particularly severe during the night
- Bilateral leg pain below knee level
- Evidence of cauda equina syndrome – urinary retention

Adapted from Rodts, 2002.

Box 34.2   Symptoms necessitating urgent surgical decompression

- Progressive paralysis
- Difficulty initiating micturition
- Retention or incontinence of urine
- Altered bowel function
- Saddle area anaesthesia
- Loss of sphincter control
- Impotence

Box 34.3   History taking and assessment

- Previous medical history
- Degree to which pain interferes with lifestyle
- Paraesthesia or focal neurological signs
- Complaints of continued pain, unresponsive to conservative measures
- Signs of infection – pyrexia, malaise or headache
- Bladder or bowel involvement
- Neurological assessment – straight leg raise, dorsiflexion of foot, ankle and knee reflexes, sensory changes, muscle wasting
- Assessment of normal movement – flexion, extension, rotation
- Mechanical factors – scoliosis, leg length disparities.

Box 34.4   Twelve points to back pain assessment

- Site – local tenderness on palpation
- Severity and level of incapacity
- Onset (sudden or insidious)
- Progression
- Precipitating factors
- Character and intensity
- Radiation across dermatomes
- Alleviating measures
- Duration – acute, sub-acute, chronic
- Exacerbating factors – posture, exercise
- Course of pain
- Previous episodes of pain

DIAGNOSIS

Accurate diagnosis relies on a good clinical history (Box 34.3) and a comprehensive neurological examination with evaluation of the full range of clinical signs, including detailed pain assessment, presentation of symptoms (Box 34.4) and results from CT and MRI scanning. One of the most important points in diagnosis and management of patients presenting with back pain and other neurological signs must be to identify those patients who have a serious underlying pathology. Diagnosis of spinal disorders can be complicated because of referred pain from other organs or because of local pathology such as aneurysms or malignancy (Tan, 2002).

Neurological testing should include: testing of reflexes, assessment of the myotomes and dermatomes to determine areas of motor weakness, parasthaesia and sensory involvement, and muscle power measurement (Strayer, 2005) (see Chapter 11). The patient's gait, posture and general movements should be observed. A thorough pain assessment should be performed noting aggravating factors such as coughing or sneezing which may indicate nerve root compression or muscle and ligament damage.

INVESTIGATIONS

Specific patient preparation or care relating to each of these investigations is detailed in Chapter 19.

Plain x-rays

Anterior/posterior lateral and oblique views can highlight structural problems such as stenosis, bony spurs, spondylosis, curvature of the spine and spondylolisthesis. 90% of patients with spinal metastases will show abnormalities on plain x-rays, particularly in the vertebral body and bony pedicles, with vertebral collapse, wedge fractures or dislocation being particularly evident (Ecker *et al.*, 2005).

CT scanning

Computer tomography (CT) is particularly useful for identifying the location and extent of metastasis, fractures or collapse of the vertebral body and identifying signs of spondylosis or spondylolisthesis (Arce *et al.*, 2001).

MRI

Magnetic resonance imaging (MRI) produces good quality imaging across sagittal and axial plains. It is used to examine soft tissue including the spinal cord, nerves and disc integrity and is able to distinguish between extradural, intradural, or intramedullary lesions such as abscesses, tumours and non-traumatic vascular lesions (Arce *et al.*, 2001). MRI has superseded myelography as the investigation of choice to identify nerve root compression.

Myelogram

A myelogram is rarely performed, but may be helpful when patients are especially claustrophobic or if MRI is contra-indicated (Huff, 2007). It involves an intrathecal injection of radiopaque water soluble contrast medium into the subarachnoid space and is able to identify root compression caused by stenosis, disc prolapse or tumours. Although complications are rare following myelography, they include focal neurological deterioration, mechanical or adverse reactions following the lumbar puncture or introduction of the dye (Skyrme *et al.*, 2005).

EMG studies

Electromyography measures nerve conduction to the muscles and can differentiate between muscle disease and local nerve root involvement. It is also useful to detect level of damage or multiple levels of disease not identified by CT or MRI scanning. EMG can clarify whether a lesion seen on imaging is the cause of nerve root pathology (Baron and Young, 2007).

Bone density scanning

Bone density scans use injectable radio-isotopes to identify changes in the bone, and are more sensitive than a plain x-ray.

MEDICAL MANAGEMENT
Conservative treatment options

The majority of people with an acute episode of back pain, without acute cord or nerve compression recover, within a few weeks, irrespective of the treatment regimen. Conservative management includes a short period of rest, muscle relaxants, analgesia and non-steroidal anti-inflammatory drugs (NSAIDs). NSAIDs block prostaglandin production, reduce inflammation and pain, are usually effective, and enable the patient to resume gentle exercise and activity (PatientUK, 2006). The small proportion of patients that fail to respond to conservative measures will require a hospital consultation. Most general practitioners will recommend a plain x-ray if the back pain persists for longer than two weeks to exclude a more complex pathology. Prompt hospital referrals should reduce the amount of time spent by many back pain sufferers applying self-help remedies and remedial action that only add to a patient's physical and psychological distress (Devlin, 2003).

Surgical treatment options

The management of acute spinal problems has undergone a radical transition over recent years. Only a few years ago patients following a laminectomy were rarely allowed home until their wound had healed and their sutures were removed; mobilisation was a more gradual process following assessment by the physiotherapists. Payment by results (Lewis and Appleby, 2006) has been hugely influential in changing management pathways. The majority of patients requiring uncomplicated spinal surgery, such as a microdiscectomy, will now only receive in-patient care for a couple of days following surgery, and the introduction of day-case surgery is already a reality. With good pre-assessment and adequate pre-operative preparation, studies have identified no significant differences in post-operative complications following early discharge (DH, 2002; Ansell and Montgomery, 2004).

The choice of surgical procedure depends on the disease process, the location within the spine and the results from radiological findings. Cauda equina compression (Box 34.3) either from disc prolapse or tumour expansion is the only absolute indication for surgical treatment (Todd, 2005). Only a small percentage of patients will gain long term benefit from surgery. These may include patients with:

* Severe, persistent pain that interferes with their quality of life or ability to continue working

- Focal neurological signs
- Failed conservative measures
- Positive radiological findings that support the clinical symptoms

Operations to surgically decompress the cord or nerve roots

Laminectomy

Laminectomy is an established procedure for the management of spinal disorders where cord or nerve root compression is involved, for example spinal canal stenosis and degenerative conditions of the vertebral column. It is the most commonly employed operation to facilitate the excision of tumours and to drain abscesses. A laminectomy may be performed at any point along the spinal column. The total portion of the lamina and the spinous processes are removed. Once decompression around each nerve has been achieved, metal plates or screws can be used to replace the laminar arch to maintain stability of the spine (Rodts, 2002). Once this has been completed and bleeding secured, the muscle layers and skin are closed with sutures or staples.

Each spinal level presents specific technical difficulties and different approaches lend themselves better to particular underlying pathologies (Abraham, 2004). Depending on the position and underlying aetiology, anterior or posterior approaches may be indicated. A laminectomy performed from a posterior approach with the patient positioned prone removes the lamina with the spinous process, allowing decompression of bony spurs, prolapsed disc or tumours. In order to reduce the risk of spinal instability post-operatively, a spinal fusion or a laminoplasty (the lamina is hinged on one side and replaced at the end of the procedure) will be needed. The development of an anterior surgical approach either through the peritoneum or retroperiteum (with the patient lying supine) is particularly useful when two or three vertebral levels are involved and provides greater accessibility to correct deformities such as scoliosis or remove tumours or infection involving the vertebral body (Carragee *et al.*, 2003). For more complex cases, a combined approach (anterior and posterior) is sometimes required necessitating turning the patient over during the procedure.

Cervical laminectomy

Cervical vertebrae are particularly mobile and vulnerable to damage because of the extensive range of movement. Disc prolapse and arthritic changes with subsequent spinal stenosis are frequently identified on x-ray. Cervical laminectomy often requires removal of the transverse pro-

cesses and complete removal of the disc, which invariably produces a degree of instability necessitating fusion to stabilise the joint. This is commonly referred to as anterior cervical decompression and fusion (ACDF) (Abraham, 2004).

Thoracic laminectomy

A thoracic laminectomy from T1 – T12 may be performed to remove extradural, intradural extramedullary, or intradural intramedullary tumours. Infections, trauma, degenerative changes and disc herniations causing spinal stenosis are less common indications for a laminectomy. Although the procedure may be performed using a posterior approach, a thoracotomy, trans-sternal approach and removal of a portion of a rib to gain access to the higher thoracic or lower cervical levels may be required (Winter *et al.*, 1995). Occasionally a combined approach is indicated when there are multi-level problems or in the presence of gross kyphotic deformities (Swezey and Calin, 2003).

Lumbar laminectomy

Lumbar laminectomy surgically removes part or all of the posterior vertebral elements including laminae, ligamentum flavum and facet joints. It is performed to relieve cord or nerve root compression arising from degenerative conditions such as spinal stenosis caused by protruding osteophytes (Best, 2002), infection or tumour infiltration. The procedure is frequently performed with a discectomy to remove herniated portions of disc material.

Hemi-laminectomy

Hemi-laminectomy is commonly performed to treat severe sciatica caused by degenerative changes in the lumbar spine. This is a slightly less invasive procedure that minimises the amount of bone removed from the lamina and posterior facet joints. It can also be performed bilaterally ensuring that the spinous process remains intact (Miers, 2002).

Foraminectomy

Foraminectomy removes bone and tissue surrounding the nerve root as it emerges from the intervertebral foramina. It is commonly performed to treat spinal stenosis, lateral disc herniation or arthritic changes (Miers, 2002).

Discectomy

Discectomy involves removing the extruding portion of the nucleus pulposus that has herniated through the annulus compressing the spinal nerve root. Removal of the entire disc is rarely indicated due to the position of the blood vessels on the anterior surface. Patients must appreciate that removal of a herniated disc does not prevent the possibility of recurrence either at the same level or at a different level (Wolfa, 2005). It is frequently performed using endoscopic or micro surgical techniques that maintain the lamina and spinous processes and limits muscle dissection from the spinal fasciae thereby reducing the perioperative risks of sustaining a dural tear, local trauma to surrounding blood vessels, or infection. Post-operatively, patients are able to mobilise much earlier as muscle spasm and pain is reduced in comparison to more invasive spinal procedures (Ehni *et al.*, 2005).

Spinal fusion

Spinal fusion is performed when there is evidence of instability, for example in patients with congenital spinal deformities, fractures or tumours, or if degenerative changes or the surgical procedure is likely to cause instability particularly with multi-level laminectomy. Suitable patients for surgery must be carefully assessed as many patients will continue to experience a degree of back pain following the fusion and a small proportion could actually be made worse (Chuang *et al.*, 2005). Cervical fusions in particular can result in up to 25% symptomatic deterioration within 10 years of the original fusion (Devlin, 2003). It is important that patients have realistic expectations of recovery and appreciate that they will have a degree of stiffness and limited spinal mobility following the procedure.

The process of fusion has benefited from improvements in technology and choice of materials that can be applied. Metal instrumentation such as steel rods, wires and pedicle screws provide a structural framework to support the bony structures. Further arthrodesis (a method of promoting ossification between two bones) is promoted by using bone grafts from the patient (autograft), from a donor (allograft) or from a synthetic material that can be applied to remaining laminae, facet joints or spinous processes. These will fuse over a period of time to restrict movement and biomechanical stress between adjacent segments, providing long-term stability (Rodts, 2002).

Patients with significant spinal instability may require a short period of cervical traction to restore alignment of the vertebrae prior to surgery. This may be associated with some degree of discomfort and can be distressing, especially for elderly patients who will need considerable supporting nursing care tailored to meet the needs of individual patients (Zychowicz, 2003). See Chapter 33 for discussion regarding the care and management of a patient with spinal traction.

Corpectomy

Corpectomy is a procedure that is frequently used to treat unstable fractures and to relieve anterior root compression cause by degenerative changes. It involves removing a 'wedge shaped' portion of the vertebral body as well as the adjoining discs (Swezey and Calin, 2003). The resulting defect is then replaced with a bone graft or fusion cage.

Vertebrectomy

Vertebrectomy is a complex procedure to relieve compression from bony fragments that have extended into the spinal cord, or from metastatic tumours that compromise the structural integrity of the whole of the vertebral body. Surgery involves removal of the whole body of the vertebra (Miers, 2002) (Figure 34.2). Stability has to be recon-

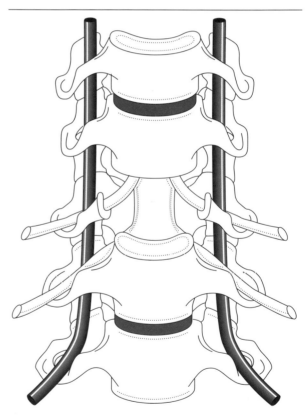

Figure 34.2 For resection of the vertebral body, the intervertebral disc is excised above and below the affected segment, which is then removed with curettes, drill and suction. The posterior longitudinal ligament is removed to ensure thorough decompression of the dural sac and root sleeves. This illustration was published in *Principles of Neurosurgery*, Rengachary & Ellenbogen, p670, Copyright Elsevier (2005).

structed by the insertion of an intervertebral titanium mesh cage, implanted with either autogenous bone material or bone cement such as methacrylate (Figure 34.3).

Trans-oral surgery

Trans-oral surgery provides access through the oropharynx to gain clear access and visualisation of the C1 occipito-cervical junction. Using a mandible splitting (maxillotomy) anterior approach through the posterior pharynx, access is gained to the cranio-cervical junction and the base of skull facilitating resection of the odontoid peg, decompression and stablisation of C1–2 vertebrae with graft material (Govender, 2005). Patients usually have an elective tracheostomy and will require high dependency or intensive care post-operatively (see Chapter 20).

Prosthetic disc replacement

One of the major complications following spinal surgery for degenerative disc disease is the subsequent loss of disc height and loss of mobility that can precipitate further problems at adjacent vertebral levels. Prosthetic disc replacement is a relatively new technique that may be used for patients with persistent pain following initial disc surgery, as an alternative to spinal fusion surgery, or used in the initial management for a herniated disc prolapse. The prosthesis is inserted via an anterior approach and resembles two metallic endplates separated by a rubber polyethylene inner core that replicates the role of the nucleus pulposus. Similar prostheses are able to replace the inner disc nucleus (Figure 34.4). Potential complications are associated with breakage of the metal disc plate,

dislocation of the implant and infection. As a relatively new procedure, data evaluating the long term effectiveness of the procedure are limited. Current results are demonstrating better functional outcomes for younger patients having single level disc replacement. Preserving mobility between each vertebral segment appears to reduce potential complications associated with adjacent disc degenerations following spinal fusion (Kowalski *et al.*, 2005).

Management of spinal tumours and spinal metastasis

Surgery is not always the first choice of treatment and depends on the site of the lesion, whether it is a primary or metastatic lesion and the degree of co-morbidity. Surgery is indicated when the patient is medically fit, when there is single site of cord compression, evidence of spinal instability or cauda equina compression, or when there is acute neurological deterioration during or following radiotherapy (Loblaw *et al.*, 2005; Fallon and Hanks, 2006). A prospective randomised trial for spinal cord compression caused by metastatic cancer showed that patients treated with direct decompressive surgery followed by post-operative radiotherapy, retained the ability to walk for longer and regained a degree of mobility more often than patients treated with radiotherapy alone (Patchell *et al.*, 2005). Less commonly, chemotherapy may be given when the patient has a cancer that is responsive to chemotherapy such as a germ cell tumour or lymphoma (Purdue, 2003).

Treatment options can vary from a recommendation for radical treatment including extensive surgery and radiotherapy or palliative treatment, steroid therapy and sup-

(a)   (b)

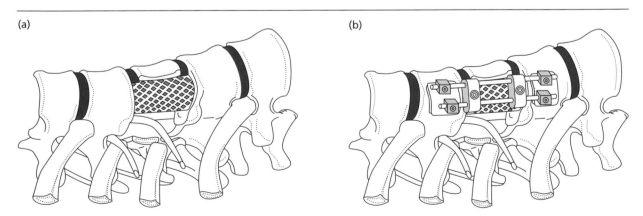

Figure 34.3 Titanium mesh cage in the thoracic spine (a), anchored with Kaneda instrumentation (b). This illustration was published in *Principles of Neurosurgery*, Rengachary & Ellenbogen, p670, Copyright Elsevier (2005).

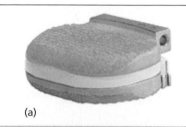

(a)

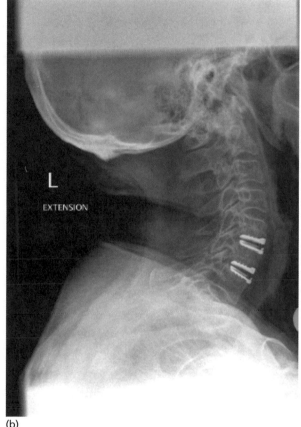

(b)

Figure 34.4 (a) Photograph of artificial cervical disc implant. (b) Lateral cervical spine x-ray showing artificial disc implants at two levels. Reproduced from C. Clarke *et al.*, *Neurology: A Queen Square Textbook*, Wiley-Blackwell, with permission.

portive care. Neurological status at the start of treatment is the most important factor to influence the choice of treatment and the eventual prognosis (Hardy and Huddart, 2002) and up to 50% of patients will already have developed deterioration in motor function and neurological status at presentation. Many of these patients are unable to walk and will have significant bowel and bladder dys-

function that is not improved by treatment (Cowap *et al.*, 2000; McLinton and Hutchinson 2006).

Unfortunately, delays in diagnosis and investigations may be attributed to referred pain from visceral or musculoskeletal back pain. Tan (2002) notes that attention to back pain in patients already diagnosed with cancer and subsequent rapid intervention when subtle neurological changes occur, can lead to earlier diagnosis before function is lost. It is important to target patient information at this group of patients to raise awareness of the signs and symptoms of malignant spinal cord compression (MSCC), and to decrease the numbers of patients who present with advanced neurological deterioration. Table 34.2 summarises the treatment of the most commonly occurring spinal tumours. See Chapter 21 for the care and management of patients undergoing radiotherapy.

The management of spinal metastatic tumours is often palliative to relieve intractable pain and to maintain function for as long as possible (Ecker *et al.*, 2005). There is some controversy regarding the optimal dose of dexamethasone, but a bolus dose of up to 100 mg IV followed by 16–96 mg in divided doses over several days is commonly prescribed. 16 mg is thought to be as effective as a high dose (96 mg) and avoids toxicity (Drudge-Coates and Rajbabu, 2008).

Surgical management of spina bifida

In the early stages, surgical management is required to close the myelomeningocele and may sometimes be performed in utero. Correction of other spinal and limb deformities or un-tethering of the spinal cord may be planned for a later date and may help to reduce the level of disability (Zychowicz, 2003). Management uses a multidisciplinary approach to address complex urodynamic and bowel problems, physiotherapy and occupational therapy to optimise mobility and independence.

Surgical management of syringomyelia

The aim of treatment is to alleviate the symptoms, and to prevent further deterioration by treating the primary problem or by inserting a syringo-peritoneal shunt. However, the procedure does carry risks such as injury to the spinal cord and blockages, and it does not work for everyone (NINDS, 2008). Some experts advise against surgery in asymptomatic patients (Pringle, 2000).

Surgical management of infections

Decompressive laminectomy, verterbrectomy and drainage of abscess are often required although some patients

Table 34.2 Causes Treatment of the most commonly occurring spinal tumours.

Location	Tumour type	Treatment
Extradural	Metastasis	High-dose corticosteroids for acute neurological presentation If primary known then immediate radiotherapy If no known primary and full screen does not identify a primary then biopsy is undertaken Treatment is often palliative to relieve intractable pain and maintain function for as long as possible. Decompression and stabilisation for unremitting pain followed by radiotherapy
Intradural	Meningioma	Usually complete surgical excision is possible Recurrence is possible but is rare
	Schwannoma/neurofibroma	Complete excision is usually possible but the nerve root has to be sacrificed
Intramedullary	Astrocytoma (low grade)	Biopsy followed by complete or partial surgical excision. Radiotherapy following partial excision
	Astrocytoma (high grade)	Biopsy followed by radiotherapy with or without partial excision
	Ependymoma	Biopsy. Usually complete surgical excision is possible. Radiotherapy following partial excision

will respond to long term antibiotic therapy (Sorenson, 2003).

Surgical management of spinal arterio-venous malformations (AVM)

Direct surgical excision can remove the AVM but embolisation or radiosurgery, whereby high energy beams are focused on the internal diameter of the malformation causing it to produce scar tissue to gradually obliterate the blood flow to the lesion, may be used (see Chapter 23).

NURSING MANAGEMENT

Pre-assessment for elective patients

Once a diagnosis has been made and it has been determined that the patient is an appropriate candidate for surgery, elective admission to hospital generally occurs 2–4 weeks following their pre-assessment. Pre-operative assessment and evaluation is of major importance for spinal surgery to reduce surgical complications and morbidity and to return the patient to their optimal functioning as soon as possible following the procedure.

Given the shortened length of hospital stay for some procedures, patient education and information is essential to ensure pre and post-operative concordance with treatment regimes. Giving sufficient information pre-

operatively has been shown to significantly decrease anxiety, reduce post-operative complications and ultimately leads to shortened length of hospital stay (Gammon and Mulholland, 1996).

Discharge planning begins at the pre-assessment stage by ensuring that the patient has some awareness of their diagnosis, treatment, pain control and personal responsibilities for exercise regimes, future employment or possible changes in lifestyle to optimise their recovery (Beck, 2007). In addition to ascertaining whether the patient is a suitable candidate for anaesthetic, highlighting any major risk factors, it is also an opportunity for the nurse to perform a holistic assessment of the patient's condition, assessing their general medical status and providing health education guidance on any issues related to smoking, alcohol or substance misuse, weight loss and nutrition.

Neurological assessment

Baseline vital signs and spinal observations, including assessment of power and sensation, are a useful asset to the ward nurses who will later use them to make comparisons post-operatively, identifying changes, improvements or possible signs of further deterioration (Miers, 2002).

Cardiovascular assessment

General medical clearance and investigation of potential problems is a vital component of the pre-operative plan (Rodts, 2002). A history of existing cardiac problems, transient ischaemic attacks, vascular disease and claudication will not necessarily preclude an anaesthetic, but the patient will require more intensive monitoring peri- and post-operatively. Spinal surgery is associated with an increased risk of developing a deep vein thrombosis (DVT) or pulmonary embolus (PE), largely due to immobility and venous stasis during the procedure. The patient should be measured for thigh-length, sequestrated, anti-embolic stockings (Walker and Lamont, 2008) and advised to continue to wear them for six weeks post-operatively.

Respiratory assessment

Patients are advised to stop smoking prior to admission to reduce anaesthetic complications. While there is limited literature on the relationship between smoking and spinal surgery outcome, there is some evidence to suggest that smokers are significantly less likely to achieve a good outcome from spinal surgery (Block *et al.*, 2003). Older adults may have physiological changes in the pulmonary system that may affect respiration. Chest x-ray is usually a mandatory requirement for patients over 50 years, where there is a history of hypertension or respiratory problems. Patients who already have high risk factors such as emphysema, chronic obstructive airways disease or asthma, may need further assessment by the anaesthetist, respiratory function team or physiotherapist. Any anatomical oral or dental problems relating to potentially difficult intubations are also noted (Miers, 2002).

Haematological assessment

Many patients take low-dose aspirin, warfarin or non-steroidal analgesia that must be discontinued pre-operatively. Routine bloods should include electrolytes, full blood count, coagulation, group and save, ESR, C-reactive protein, calcium and liver function tests (Gibson, 2006).

Endocrine assessment

Insulin dependent diabetic patients must be admitted to the ward at a slightly earlier date to stabilise and actively manage glucose levels pre-operatively.

Nutritional assessment

The patient's weight, height and body mass index (BMI) are measured to optimise drug and anaesthetic dosages. Nutritional status and dietary preferences are recorded in the nursing documentation.

Family support

Early discharge from hospital necessitates good home support structures and this may be problematic, particularly for older patients who may need to remain in hospital until they are more independent and mobile. The patient and their family need to have a thorough understanding of the proposed plan of care and the time frame for that plan to be completed (Rodts, 2002).

For the majority of patients, the prospect of major surgery is associated with considerable anxiety and apprehension (Gibson, 2006). Patients undergoing any invasive procedure must sign a consent form, effectively giving the doctor permission to proceed with the surgery; failure to obtain 'informed consent' can be construed as assault and battery, trespass or actual bodily harm (Baxter *et al.*, 2002). The doctor must ensure that the patient understands the extent of the surgery, the associated risks of anaesthetic or possible complications such as haemorrhage, permanent disability, loss of function and independence. Finally, the risks associated with hospital acquired infections are well known and an MRSA screen is an important prerequisite prior to admission.

As well as the routine pre-operative preparation, patients that are going to be admitted on the morning of surgery are advised to take no solids for six hours or water for two hours prior to their surgery (O'Callaghan, 2002). On arrival on the ward, reassessment by the anaesthetist and pre-operative checks, including consent and completion of documentation, are performed. Routine oral medication should still be administered irrespective of fasting (omitting any angiotensin converting enzyme inhibitor tablets).

COMPLICATIONS FOLLOWING SPINAL SURGERY

There are risks inherent in any surgical procedure that involves a general anaesthetic and complications may develop perioperatively or immediately post-operatively including: haematoma formation, CSF leak, infection, adhesions and neurological deficits.

Haematoma formation

Minor local wound haemorrhage is of little concern and usually resolves spontaneously, however a haematoma can develop and cause pressure symptoms on the spinal cord and nerve roots. Patients will usually complain of increasing pain and exacerbation of neurological symptoms. Delays in diagnosis will adversely affect both sensory and motor function and may result in permanent neurological deficits (Miers, 2002). The development of a haematoma following cervical laminectomy is particularly hazardous and demands urgent medical intervention; local swelling will compress the trachea, compromising the airway and making intubation difficult. Clip removers should be readily available in the clinical area and most patients will require an emergency exploratory procedure to secure the bleeding and evacuate the haematoma.

Cerebrospinal fluid (CSF) leak

A CSF leak can occur due to a dural tear or durotomy resulting from debridement of bone and or disc fragments close to the dural sac. Signs and symptoms are severe headache, especially on sitting or standing, and clear drainage on the dressing that is positive to glucose. The majority of CSF leaks will heal spontaneously with conservative management, including flat bed rest for 7–10 days, that allows the tear to heal. Rarely, surgery may be required for some patients if the tear does not heal (Harvey 2005; McCormack *et al.*, 2005).

Infection

Any infections of the wound or around the surgical area can significantly delay the patient's recovery. Superficial wound infections must be identified early to reduce the likelihood of an infection leading to an epidural abscess. More serious infections may demand removal of any graft material or metal prosthesis, effectively compromising spinal stability and requiring spinal traction or application of halo apparatus with fitted vest (Bhagat *et al.*, 2007).

Discitis is an infection of the disc space that can develop into an abscess, spondylodiscitis or osteomyelitis and cause a return of neurological symptoms. During pre-assessment and again prior to discharge, the patient must be informed of the presenting signs and symptoms including: recurrence of original symptoms, localised back or neck pain, pyrexia, focal neurological signs, bladder or bowel disturbance and general malaise.

Progression of the infection depends on the presence of co-morbidities such as diabetes, malignancy, substance misuse and the strain and virulence of the organism (Williams and Leaper, 1998). Staphylococcus aureus is the most common organism, although in some cases no growth is isolated and symptoms may be the result of an inflammatory response triggered by other low grade infections. Treatment is more effective if the organism can be isolated and appropriate antibiotics administered. Long-term antibiotic therapy is often required for six weeks intravenously followed by six weeks of oral therapy with monitoring of inflammatory markers (Skyrme *et al.*, 2005). Ideally this should be administered via a peripherally inserted central catheter (PICC) that is more comfortable and convenient for the patient and means that in some cases the antibiotics can be administered at home via a domiciliary service.

Persistent neurological deficits

Following spinal decompression it is important that patients recognise that they are unlikely to experience immediate relief from the symptoms, which may take weeks if not months to resolve. The degree of recovery will be variable and dependent on the duration and cause of the original compression. Sustained nerve root damage may leave the patient with some degree of disability that requires an intensive programme of physiotherapy to optimise recovery. From the patient's perspective, a procedure that fails to resolve their symptoms or pain, e.g. failed back syndrome (Hickey and Rodta, 2001), must be overwhelmingly disappointing and repeated laminectomies are not unusual. The efficacy of laminectomy and discectomy versus conservative management (Peul *et al.*, 2007), and decompressive laminectomy versus physiotherapy (Critchley *et al.*, 2007, Weinstein *et al.*, 2007) have been evaluated. The authors concluded that patients most likely to benefit from lumbar spinal surgery are generally young, positively motivated, with a short history, where leg pain is the predominant feature and unequivocal imaging supports the diagnosis. Whilst some patients treated surgically experienced greater improvement in pain and return to normal function during the first two years, after four years the improvements were no longer statistically significant.

POST-OPERATIVE NURSING MANAGEMENT

Immediately post-operatively, the major role of the neurosurgical nurse is continual assessment and observation of the patient and prompt notification of changes in vital signs, sensory or motor function. Subsequent management will again depend on the complexity of the procedure and the underlying pathology. Acute in-patient care for a patient following a single level laminectomy and discectomy is usually straightforward and discharge from hospital within –two to three days is the norm, but an in-patient stay may be as short as 24 hours. It is important that the nurse does not underestimate the importance of their role in managing not only the physical effects of surgery, but supporting the patient psychologically. It is important to try and appreciate the significance of the experience of surgery from the patient's perspective particularly when faced with nursing pressures to optimise bed occupancy and maintain patient throughput (Lewis and Appleby, 2006). Patient education and preparation for discharge must be a high priority supplemented with written discharge instructions addressing wound care, mobility, elimination disturbance, management of ongoing pain and anticipated recovery regime.

GENERAL NURSING MEASURES

Spinal and other observations

Once the patient returns to the ward from theatre, post-operative observations of vital signs and spinal observations must be performed half hourly for the first two hours, every hour thereafter for twenty four hours, and every four hours after that period if the patient's condition is stable.

Intra-operative spinal cord injury can occur due to direct trauma, ischemia, stretch or hypothermia (Rao *et al.*, 2006). Essential post-operative nursing management therefore includes spinal observations and close monitoring of motor and sensory function (Hilton and Henderson, 2003) (see Chapter 11 for how to conduct an assessment of motor and sensory function). Rapid detection of changing patterns and trends can be important in identifying early signs of deterioration, such as motor weakness or paraesthesia, and must be reported to the medical staff as soon as possible. As the patient improves, observations can be reassessed and the nursing intervention adjusted accordingly.

Bed rest, reduced mobility and mobilising

Initially the patient will most likely be positioned supine in bed. Following major spinal fusion 'log rolling' (see Chapter 33) with at least four nurses may be required to change the patient's position (Harvey, 2005). Patients who have had multiple level surgery, re-exploration, or who have had significant mobility problems pre-operatively will need to remain on flat bed rest until reviewed by medical and therapy staff.

Depending on the procedure and whether spinal stability is still in question, patients should be encouraged to alter their position whilst maintaining spinal alignment. A post-operative x-ray may be requested prior to mobilisation to verify the position and placement of spinal grafts or prosthesis. An assessment of the patient's pressure area risk should be recorded in the patient's records and pressure areas should be assessed regularly. Appropriate pressure relieving surfaces should be provided (Miers, 2002, Harvey, 2005).

Patients will be more comfortable following a cervical laminectomy if the bed head is raised and their head supported on a soft pillow. Soft collars are rarely advocated, but a fitted hard collar (i.e. Aspen or Philadelphia) may be prescribed to prevent excessive flexion, extension, or neck rotation following multi-level fusion or when there are continuing concerns over stability (Miers, 2002). The nurse must teach the patient how to manage hygiene needs by removing the collar and carefully washing the skin to prevent pressure symptoms and skin excoriation (see Chapter 33).

Most patients following a single level discectomy or lumbar laminectomy will be allowed to gently mobilise once they have recovered from the anaesthetic. Patients are instructed to roll to the edge of the bed, swing their legs to the floor and stand up in one smooth action, preventing twisting, flexion, or tension to the surgical site (Figure 34.5) (Rodts, 2002). Nursing care pathways should incorporate gentle exercises and a range of movements to maintain function, limit development of contractures and prevent muscle wastage. Physiotherapy assessment is often brief for short stay patients and the therapist has

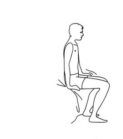

Down
Feel the edge of the bed with the backs of your legs. Place your more comfortable leg backward under the edge of the bed. Use your hands to help support you. Use your arms and hands to lift your buttocks and move back into a comfortable seated position on the bed.

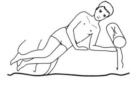

Place both hands on the bed, on the side toward the head of the bed. Slide your hands toward the pillow to support your body as you gently swing your legs onto the bed. You should now be lying on your side.

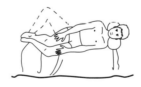

Keeping your knees bent, place your hands on your thighs, do a pelvic pinch and roll onto your back, moving your shoulders, trunk and knees together as one unit – a "log roll". Adjust your legs one at a time for comfort.

Up
Lying on your back with your knees bent, do a pelvic pinch and hold. Holding the pelvic pinch, do a log roll to the side. Raise your shoulders by pushing off the bed with your hand and elbow, at the same time, gently swing both legs over the side of the bed. Use your arms and hands to help lift and slide your buttocks to the edge of the bed. Place one foot slightly in front of the other with your rear foot (your more comfortable foot) under the bed if possible. Keeping your buttocks tucked under (with a pelvic pinch) and your back straight, use your arms and legs to push up to a standing position.

Figure 34.5 Lying down and getting up from bed.

limited time to identify any immediate problems that might hinder the patient's recovery. Written guidance with various exercises is handed to the patient before discharge and out-patient physiotherapy may be arranged locally (Danielson *et al.*, 2000, Ostelo *et al.*, 2002). The hospital orthotist will supply and fit limb splints as clinically indicated to promote mobility, e.g. for foot drop.

Patients diagnosed with malignant spinal cord compression are often nursed on complete bed rest until spinal stability is assured or radiotherapy has been completed (Dougherty and Lister, 2004; Pease *et al.*, 2004;). However, given the limited life expectancy for many of these patients, which is 3 to 12 months from diagnosis of MSCC (Guo *et al.*, 2003; McLinton and Hutchinson, 2006,), the potential complications associated with prolonged bed rest (e.g. increased dependence, low mood and anxiety) (Purdue, 2003) may be reduced through early mobilisation where it is safe to do so. Close collaboration with medical staff is required to ensure that unambiguous guidelines are in place for this aspect of care, including early referral pathways to the physiotherapist.

Fluid and electrolyte balance

Disturbance in body fluids and electrolytes accompany many surgical procedures largely due to the underlying pathology and the physiological effects of perioperative stress. Elevated levels of anti-diuretic hormone (ADH) and high aldosterone levels can increase water reabsorption and effectively increase extracellular fluid volume and reduce urine output. Consequently, a well hydrated patient can retain fluid and have a high positive balance immediately post-operatively. It is important to regularly assess the patient's hydration status in the immediate post-operative period (see Chapter 16). Intravenous fluid replacement should be maintained until the patient is able to tolerate oral fluids.

Urine volume and concentration should be carefully recorded (ideal output > 0.5 ml/kg body weight). Fluid balance measurements for routine spinal surgery patients are usually discontinued in the immediate post-operative period once it has been confirmed that they have passed urine and they are tolerating oral fluids. However, the syndrome of inappropriate secretion of antidiuretic hormone (SIADH) (see Chapter 16) is a potential problem following spinal fusion. The combination of decreased blood volume, the physical and emotional stress response and the use of anaesthesia and analgesia stimulates the release of ADH so that fluids are retained. Fluids are remobilised into the vascular system so the patient is in a relative state of fluid overload. Additionally, large amounts of fluid are delivered intra and post-operatively. The patient becomes hyponatraemic and urinary output is reduced. The syndrome usually resolves within 24 hours as anaesthetic agents are metabolised and stress reduces (Harvey, 2005). Further detail of fluid and electrolyte management is given in Chapter 16.

Swallowing

Special caution should be taken for patients following anterior cervical laminectomy as dysphagia is a common and transient problem. A combination of localised oedema, manipulation of the oesophagus and damage to the laryngeal nerve (a branch of the vagus nerve) or glossopharyngeal nerve during surgery can affect the swallow reflex and produce a hoarse voice (Rao *et al.*, 2006). A swallowing assessment should be undertaken (see Chapter 12) if the patient exhibits any signs of dysphagia.

Respiratory assessment

Some patients will require humidified oxygen therapy until their oxygen saturation levels return to their baseline values (> 95%). All patients who have received a general anaesthetic are at risk of developing a chest infection, but early mobilisation and deep breathing exercises will help to mitigate any adverse effects. Following major spinal surgery, patients are particularly at risk of developing chest infection due to enforced flat lying, which makes full lung expansion more difficult. Some patients may need incentive spirometry with at least ten deep breaths an hour (Harvey, 2005). Respiratory management is discussed further in Chapter 15.

Cardiovascular assessment

Spinal surgery is associated with a high risk of developing a DVT. Without prophylaxis the incidence can be as high as 25% (Auter, 1998). NICE (2007) recommends that all patients undergoing neurosurgery (which includes spinal surgery) have a mechanical method of prophylaxis (i.e. graduated compression stockings, intermittent pneumatic compression devices or foot impulse devices). Mechanical prophylaxis plus low molecular weight heparin (LMWH) is recommended for patients at increased risk of venous thromboembolism. Patients with spinal vascular malformations should not have LMWH until the lesion is secured (NICE, 2007). LMWH should not be administered until wound drains have been removed (NICE, 2007).

Nutrition

There is growing evidence of the importance of early nutrition following trauma and surgery (see Chapter 16).

Bed rest results in protein loss of about 8 mg per day, and calcium loss of up to 1.54 g per week, which can delay wound healing and reduce muscle mass. This is particularly significant in patients diagnosed with malignant spinal cord lesions and those patients who have a generally poor health status (Block *et al.*, 2003). Referral to a dietician is indicated if feeding is delayed for what ever reason.

Pain control

Nurses play a key role in alleviating post-operative pain and regular assessment is fundamental to pain management. Bupivacaine and fentanyl infusions directly into the epidural space are useful analgesia following extensive spinal procedures. Giving opioids and anaesthetic agents together into the epidural space can provide a synergistic effect on pain relief (Duke, 2005). Opioids are more commonly the basis for immediate post-operative analgesia and are usually administered as patient controlled analgesia (PCA) which offers greater pain relief than intermittent injections (Macintyre and Ready, 2001). Anti-emetics should be administered regularly to reduce associated nausea and vomiting.

The nurse must monitor the patient's response to analgesia using appropriate rating scales (see Chapter 17) (Macintyre and Ready, 2001). Unfortunately, pain is often exacerbated for hospitalised patients due to lack of sleep caused by the constant disturbance from frequent observations, ward noise and alarms. In elderly patients this can lead to development of delirium (Bowman, 1997) (see Chapter 9).

Uncontrolled post-operative pain can develop into a chronic condition (Mitchell, 2003), but effective pain control can be challenging in the case of short-stay patients who will experience pain from local swelling to nerve roots or severe muscle spasms across the back, shoulders or neck. Patients must be instructed to take medication at the first indication of discomfort and not to wait until it becomes too severe.

Use of non-steroidal, anti-inflammatory drugs (NSAIDs), such as diclofenac sodium or ibuprofen may be useful in the initial stages, and addition of NSAIDs to opiate analgesic has been shown to provide better pain relief than opiates alone (Jirarattanaphochai and Jung, 2008). Later many patients find effective pain relief with paracetamol, sometimes used in combination with low dose benzodiazepines to relax muscle spasm. Patients with chronic or neuropathic pain may benefit from gabapentin and tricyclic anti-depressants to manage their persistent pain (Duke, 2005) (see Chapter 17).

Wound care

There are many factors that can interfere with the natural healing process including the type of surgery, obesity, immunosuppression, previous radiotherapy, poor nutritional state and diabetes. Prevention of infection begins pre-operatively ensuring that the patient has been screened for possible MRSA or other remote infections. During surgery good tissue perfusion around the wound is recognised as an important factor that can influence wound healing (Buggy, 2000). Wound drainage must be monitored and recorded to assess the degree of seepage through the dressing. It is important not to disturb the dressing until haemostasis is assured, usually 48 hours post-operatively. When there are obvious signs of excess drainage medical staff should be informed to ensure that the wound does not require any additional sutures or clips. The dressing must then be changed immediately and not repadded, maintaining aseptic principles (Harvey, 2005).

Wound drains are inserted to drain blood or exudates and prevent haematoma formation that may precipitate infection. They give a clear indication of the amount of blood loss and are usually removed after 24 hours or when there is no further drainage (Harvey, 2005).

Donor sites can be particularly painful and they must be observed for signs of bleeding, excess drainage or infection. Iliac crest wounds are easily irritated because of clothing or pyjamas brushing against the wound and they must be protected (Miers, 2002). The first indication of an infection is usually pyrexia and general malaise followed by increased complaints of pain, inflammation, swelling, exudate and a raised white cell count (Harvey, 2005). In-patients are carefully monitored and nurses maintain strict aseptic techniques when changing the dressing. Patients discharged early need to be able to recognise the signs and symptoms of infection and contact their GP or ward for further advice. The decision when to remove skin closures depends on the site, for example, most sutures/clips can be removed after 7–10 days in the lumbar or thoracic spine and 5 days in the cervical region. Other factors such as previous radiotherapy to that region, ageing or diabetes also need to be taken into account (Thompson and Jones, 2005).

CSF leak and spinal drains

Evidence of CSF fluid leak can usually be identified as yellow staining or a 'halo effect' on the dressing. Doctors must be notified immediately as the wound may require some additional sutures or in rare instances the patient may require insertion of a spinal drain for a few days to allow the dural tear to heal and prophylactic antibiotic cover.

Bowel management

Constipation is a common problem post-operatively, occurring as a consequence of the anaesthetic agents, immobility and the side-effects of opioid analgesia. It is also difficult for patients on flat bed-rest to use a bedpan; this is not a good functional position in which to defecate, coupled with post-operative pain and the embarrassment of defecating with little privacy afforded by a curtain round the bed (Baillie and Arrowsmith, 2005). Patients should be reassured that it can take a while for bowel function to return to normal. The frequency and consistency of bowel movements must be monitored, initially ensuring that bowel sounds are present. Occasionally, stool softeners or laxatives may help to re-establish usual bowel routines, but should not be prescribed long-term (Harvey, 2005).

Patients with neurogenic bowel dysfunction either occurring as a pre-operative symptom or arising as a post-operative complication will require a more comprehensive bowel regime. The type of bowel complications that patients can experience will vary, for example, patients with MSCC can have reflex, flaccid or mixed neurogenic bowel dysfunction depending on the location and degree of compression (Ash, 2005; Coggrave, 2005) (see Chapter 18). Constipation in patients with neurological spinal problems above T6 can trigger autonomic dysreflexia (see Chapter 14).

The approach to bowel management for an individual patient needs to be appropriate to the type of bowel dysfunction they are experiencing (see Chapter 18). Failure to institute adequate bowel care constitutes clinical negligence (NPSA, 2004; RCN, 2008) and is a serious nursing failure. Finally, to ensure consistency and continuity of care, documentation is as important as the assessment and management of bowel dysfunction, otherwise it becomes impossible to establish an effective bowel management regime.

Bladder management

Urinary retention is not uncommon during periods of immobility, increased anxiety or severe post-operative pain. Following laminectomy surgery, sympathetic nerve fibres, particularly around the L5/S1 nerve root may become irritated, triggering an acute retention response. Some of the problems are postural, with men in particular finding it difficult to void urine in a horizontal position. The majority of male spinal surgery patients are allowed to stand out of bed to use a urinal once they have recovered from the anaesthetic; medical staff normally leave instruction when this is contra-indicated (Harvey, 2005). Once the patient's privacy and dignity has been assured, most patients will normally manage to pass urine given the

necessary patience, support and encouragement. Obviously the use of urinary catheters should be avoided whenever possible due to the associated risks of infection (Gibson, 2006) (see Chapter 18). Catheterisation must not be undertaken without consultation with medical staff who should perform a neurological assessment to exclude neurological deterioration. Catheterisation is indicated for patients unable to void urine, who have a palpable, distended or painful bladder. The decision to remove the catheter following drainage of a residual volume of urine or to leave the catheter in place, is based on bladder function pre-operatively and the complexity and level of surgery. Intermittent catheterisation under these circumstances is preferred (Harvey, 2005) (see Chapter 18).

Effects on sexual function

Spinal cord or local nerve damage can diminish perineal sensation or cause erectile dysfunction that will have a negative effect on a patient's self-esteem and body image (White and Getliffe, 2003). Patients are often unaware of the implications of their deficits whilst in hospital or they may be reluctant to address the issues. The neurosurgical nurse has a responsibility to introduce the subject prior to discharge, however the follow-up out-patient appointment might be a more realistic time to discuss concerns and seek referral for specialist assessment from a continence advisor or urologist. Miers (2002) suggests that sexual activity can be resumed when the patient feels comfortable to do so.

REHABILITATION

Discharge planning has even greater significance with the increase in day case surgery (Mitchell, 2003). Decreased length of hospital stay often has a negative effect on the ability of ward staff to formulate effective discharge arrangements. Prior to discharge the patient must receive clear instructions about their medication, wound management, exercise regime, when they may recommence driving, sexual intercourse, as well as emergency contact details. There should be a seamless transition from hospital care to the community to decrease the risk of readmission due to inability to manage self-care (Maramba *et al.*, 2004). In some cases a home assessment may be required by the occupational therapist and primary health care team, particularly if the patient is still unable to mobilise independently. In some circumstances the patient's role within the family will change. Loss of health or independence may mean that a return to their original employment may be impossible. Although most patients who have undergone simple spinal procedures should be able to return to work after 8–12 weeks (Strayer, 2005), it can be a significant financial burden for the family, particularly for self-employed patients.

Realistic goal setting must be a priority as the rehabilitation process may take several weeks or months. Most patients are able to return to normal activities within two to three months although for those who have had spinal fusion it may take six to twelve months (Harvey, 2005). Referral to a spinal injury unit may be appropriate for patients with continuing motor dysfunction and or problems with bladder or bowel function. Patients with nontraumatic spinal cord injury may have worse outcomes, such as more preventable complications, if they are not cared for in a specialised unit (New, 2006). Other patients will require physiotherapy on an out-patient basis. The essential components of any rehabilitation programme should focus on the consequences of immobilisation, the long term prognosis and the effect of therapeutic interventions on both the physical and emotional responses to the injury or disease process. This would be a continuous assessment and evaluation process, changing the programme to accommodate recent or perhaps increasing disability with initial efforts directed towards ambulatory self-care or assisting the patient to living with a wheelchair. Any exercise programme needs to be tailored to the individual to enable them to achieve their goals (Rodts, 2002).

Palliative care is no longer considered an 'end of life' treatment and is instituted for patients undergoing rehabilitation for MSCC as part of the management plan. The aim is to stabilise or improve quality of life and minimise physical discomfort such as pain, and to enable patients to find alternative activities to promote their self esteem and independence.

SPECIAL CONSIDERATIONS IN NURSING PATIENTS WITH MALIGNANT SPINAL CORD COMPRESSION (MSCC)

It is difficult to comprehend or explain the overwhelming effect that a malignant tumour diagnosis evokes on the whole family. Many patients present with severe, yet sudden onset of functional impairment, 'they suffer from greater dependency and hopelessness than any other cancer patients' (Taillibert *et al.*, 2004). Patients often face the challenge of coping with sudden and unexpected disability alongside a diagnosis of advanced cancer. The realisation that the disease has spread, perhaps after being symptom free for a while, may cause considerable psychological distress. Nurses have a vital role in assessing patients' psychological, emotional and support needs so that they can provide information and referral to appropriate agencies (Pellatt, 2008). Referral for supportive counseling may sometimes be beneficial in providing a forum to learn more effective coping skills or to teach relaxation techniques to help control anxiety and stressors on the patient's support network.

A holistic approach to address the family's need for emotional and practical support is paramount, particularly if the spinal cord compression is the initial sign of a cancer diagnosis. The neuro-oncology nurse is pivotal to facilitating a seamless journey along the cancer pathway and plays a key role in supporting the patient and their family through this devastating period in their lives. Refer to Chapter 21 for how to mange the supportive care needs of patients diagnosed with cancer.

SUMMARY

The nursing management of patients following spinal surgery is challenging and goals will vary and change over the period of the patient's illness, requiring on-going assessment, evaluation and review. Having a good understanding of the disease processes, the pre and post-operative management for common spinal surgical procedures, and the physical and psychological effects of spinal disease on the patient is necessary to provide effective care and to assist patients to cope and come to terms with what they are likely to face. Meeting these complex needs requires the involvement of the full range of expertise represented in the multi-disciplinary team.

Disorders of the vertebral column and spinal cord: patient perspective

It's over five years since my first laminectomy and since then I have needed a further two procedures. Although I am pain free (most of the time), my life has changed significantly as a consequence of the first injury.

I have worked as a sister on a neurosurgical ward for over thirty years. In the early days we didn't have access to the movement and handling equipment, training or electronic beds that are available today. Every day we lifted heavily dependent patients out of bed, what we locally referred to as the 'Harry Holmes technique' which was really just a modified 'top and tail' procedure. Years of abuse and chronic back pain eventually resulted in a sudden acute episode that changed the course of my career. At the time, the pain was excruciating, and I experienced some bladder problems for a short period postoperatively. It took a further three months of intensive physiotherapy before I could return to my original job. Unfortunately within a year I had a further disc prolapse occurring at the same level. I found that I was unable to return to patient handling, but even sitting at a computer or anything that involved adopting static postures exacerbated my back problem. Finally, my last laminectomy occurred as a result of sitting on an aeroplane on a long haul flight returning from holiday. It affected the next level above the original surgery and although I recovered very quickly and returned to work it continues to affect all aspects of my life. Back injury doesn't just affect your work life but all aspects of everyday living – shopping, gardening, socialising and even swimming is difficult. A flexible, healthy back is precious and I believe that good back care should begin in school.

REFERENCES

Abraham JL (2004) Assessment and treatment of patients with malignant spinal cord compression. *Journal of Support Oncology* 2:377–401.

Ansell GL, Montgomery JE (2004) Outcome of ASA III patients undergoing day case surgery. *British Journal of Anaesthesia* 92(1):71–74.

Arce D, Sass P, Abdul-Khoudoud H (2001) Recognising spinal cord emergencies. *American Family Physician* 64(4):631–638.

Ash D (2005) Sustaining safe and acceptable bowel care in spinal cord injured patients. *Nursing Standard* 20(8):55–64.

Auter R (1998) Calculating patients' risk of deep vein thrombosis. *British Journal of Nursing* 7:7–12.

BackCare – The Charity for Healthier Backs (2008). http://www.backcare.org.uk/

Baillie L, Arrowsmith V (2005) Meeting elimination needs. In: Baillie L (ed) *Developing Practical Nursing Skills* (2nd edition). London: Arnold.

Baron E, Young W (2007) *Cervical Spondylosis: diagnosis and management.* Available from: http://www.emedicine.com/neuro/topic564.htm Accessed July 2010.

Baxter CM, Brennan MG, Caldicott YG (2002) *The Practical Guide to Medical Ethics and Law.* Bodmin: MPG Books.

Beck A (2007) Nurse led pre-operative assessment for elective surgical patients. *Nursing Standard* 21(51):35–38.

Best JT (2002) Understanding spinal stenosis. *Orthopaedic Nursing* 21(3):48–55.

Bhagat S, Mathieson R, Jandhyala R *et al.* (2007) Spondylodiscitis (disc space infection) associated with negative microbiological tests: comparison of outcome of suspected disc space infections to documented non-tuberculous pyogenic discitis. *British Journal of Neurosurgery* 21(5):473–477.

Block A, Gatchel R, Deardoff W *et al.* (2003) *The Psychology of Spine Surgery.* Washington DC: American Psychological Association.

Boden SD, Davis DO, Dina TS *et al.* (1996) Abnormal magnetic resonance scans of the lumbar spine in asymptomatic subjects. A prospective investigation. *Journal of Bone and Joint Surgery Am* 78:403–411.

Bowman AM (1997). Sleep satisfaction, perceived pain and acute confusion in the elderly clients undergoing orthopaedic procedures. *Journal of Advanced Nursing* 26(3):550–564.

Buggy D (2000) Can anaesthetic management influence surgical wound healing? *Lancet* 356(9227):355–357.

Carragee EJ, Han MY, Suen PW (2003) Clinical outcomes after lumbar discectomy for sciatica: The effects of fragment type and anular competence. *Journal of Bone and Joint Surgery Am* 85(1):102–108.

Coggrave M 2005 Management of neurogenic bowel. *British Journal of Neuroscience Nursing* 1(1):6–13.

Cowap J, Hardy J, A'Hern R (2000) Outcome of malignant spinal cord compression at a cancer centre: Implications for palliative care services. *Journal of Pain and Symptom Management* 19(4):257–264.

Chuang H, Cho DY, Chang CS *et al.* (2005) Efficacy and safety of the use of titanium mesh cages and anterior cervical plates for interbody fusion after anterior cervical corpectomy. *Surgical Neurology* 65:464–471.

Critchley DJ, Ratcliffe J, Noonan S *et al.* (2007) Effectiveness and cost-effectiveness of three types of physiotherapy: results. *Spine* 2(14):1474–1481.

Danielson J, Johnson R, Kibsgaard S *et al.* (2000) Early aggressive exercise for postoperative rehabilitation after discectomy. *Spine* 25(8):1015–1029.

Department of Health (2002) *Day Surgery: Operational guide. Waiting, booking and choice.* London: DH.

Devlin V (2003) *Spine Secrets.* Philadelphia: Hanley and Belfus.

Dougherty L, Lister S (2004) *The Royal Marsden Manual of Clinical Nursing Procedures* (6th edition). Oxford: Blackwell Publishing.

Drudge-Coates L, Rajbabu K (2008) Diagnosis and management of malignant spinal cord compression: part 1. *International Journal of Palliative Nursing* 14(3):110–116.

Duke S (2005) Pain. In: *Alexander M, Fawcett J, Runciman PJ Nursing Practice. Hospital and Home. The Adult* (3rd edition). Edinburgh: Churchill Livingstone.

Ecker R, Endo T, Wetjen N *et al*. (2005) Diagnosis and treatment of vertebral column metasteses. *Mayo Clinic Proceedings* 80(9):1177–1186.

Ehni B, Benzel E, Biscup R (2005) Lumbar discectomy. In: Benzel C (ed). *Spine Surgery: Techniques, complication avoidance and management*. (2nd edition). Edinburgh: Elsevier, Churchill Livingstone.

Fallon M, Hanks G (2006) *ABC of Palliative Medicine*. Oxford: BMJ Books, Blackwell Publishing.

Fehlings M, Zeidman S, Rampersaud Y (2005) Cauda equina syndrome. In: Benzel C (ed). *Spine Surgery: Techniques, complication avoidance and management*. (2nd edition). Edinburgh: Elsevier, Churchill Livingstone.

Gammon J, Mulholland CW (1996) Effect of preparatory information prior to elective total hip replacement on physical coping outcomes. *International Journal of Nursing Studies* 33(6):589–604.

Gibson C (2006) The patient facing surgery. In: Alexander M, Fawcett J, Runciman P (eds). *Nursing Practice: Hospital and home. The adult*. (3rd edition). Edinburgh: Churchill Livingstone.

Govender S (2005) Outcome of transoral surgery. *Journal of Bone and Joint Surgery* 87(111):283.

Guiot B, Mendel,E (2005) Degenerative spondylolisthesis. In: Rengachary S, Ellenbogen R (eds). *Principles of Neurosurgery*. (2nd edition). Oxford: Elsevier Mosby.

Guo Y, Young B, Palmer J *et al*. (2003) Prognostic factors for survival in metastatic spinal cord compression. *American Journal of Physical Medicine and Rehabilitation* 82:665–668.

Hardy J, Huddart R (2002) Spinal cord compression – what are the treatment standards? *Clinical Oncology* 14:132–134.

Harvey C (2005) Spinal surgery patient care. *Orthopaedic Essentials* 24(6):426–440.

Haas F (2003) Management of malignant spinal cord compression *Nursing Times* 99(15):32–34.

Hickey M, Rodta MF (2001) The spine. In: DC Schoen (ed). *National Association of Orthopaedic Nursing: Core curriculum for orthopaedic nursing*. (4th edition). New Jersey: Pitman.

Hilton E, Henderson L (2003) Neurosurgical considerations in posttraumatic syringomyelia. *AORN Online* 77(1) 135–156.

Ho CH, Wuermser LA, Priebe MM *et al*. (2007) Spinal cord injury medicine 1: Epidemiology and classification. *Archives of Physical Medicine and Rehabilitation* 88(Suppl 1):S49–54.

Huff JS (2007) *Neoplasms: spinal cord*. Available from: http://emedicine.medscape.com/article/779872-overview Accessed July 2010.

Jirarattanaphochai K, Jung S (2008) Nonsteroidal antiinflammatory drugs for postoperative pain management after lumbar spine surgery: a meta-analysis of randomized controlled trials. *Journal of Neurosurgery: Spine* 9:22–31.

Kowalski R, Ferrara L, Benzel E (2005) Biomechanics of mechanical motion preservation strategies. In: Benzel E (ed). *Spine Surgery: Techniques, complication avoidance and management*. Edinburgh: Elsevier, Churchill Livingstone.

Leon K (2007) The diseases less reported. *Paraplegic News* 61(3):18–21.

Lewis R, Appleby J (2006) Can the English NHS meet the 18-week waiting list target? *Journal of the Royal Society of Medicine*. 99:10–13.

Lindsey KW, Bone I (2004) *Neurology and Neurosurgery Illustrated* (4th edition). Edinburgh: Churchill Livingstone.

Loblaw DS, Perry J, Chambers A *et al*. (2005) Systematic review of the diagnosis and management of malignant extradural spinal cord compression. *Journal of Clinical Oncology* 23:2028–2037.

Macintyre PE, Ready LB (2001) *Acute Pain Management: A practical guide*. London: Saunders.

Maramba PJ, Richards S, Larrabee JH (2004) Discharge planning process: applying a model of evidence based practice. *Journal of Nursing Care Quality* 19(2):123–129.

McCormack B, Zide B, Kalfas I (2005) Cerebral fluid fistuila and pseudomeningocele after spine surgery. In: Benzil E (ed). *Spine Surgery: Techniques, complication avoidance and management*. (2nd edition). Edinburgh: Elsevier, Churchill Livingstone.

McLinton A, Hutchinson C (2006) Malignant spinal cord compression: a retrospective audit of clinical practice at a UK regional cancer centre. *British Journal of Cancer* 94:486–491.

Miers A (2002) Nontraumatic disorders of the spine. In: Barker E (ed). *Neuroscience Nursing: A spectrum of care*. (2nd edition). St Louis: Mosby.

Millar M (2005) *Back care costs UK business £5 billion*. Available from: http://www.personneltoday.com/articles/2005/06/03/30163/back-pain-costs-uk-business-5bn.html Accessed July 2010.

Millichip J, Sy B, Leacock R (2006) Spinal cord infarction with multiple etiologic factors. *Society of General Internal Medicine* 22(1):151–154.

Mitchell M (2003) Impact on discharge from day surgery on patients and carers. *Journal of Advanced Nursing* 12(7):402–407.

National Institute for Health and Clinical Excellence (2007) *Reducing the Risk of Venous Thromboembolism (deep vein thrombosis and pulmonary embolism) in Patients Undergoing Surgery*. London: NICE.

National Institute of Neurological Disorders and Stroke (2008) *Syringomyelia fact sheet*. Available from: http://www.ninds.nih.gov/disorders/syringomyelia/detail_syringomyelia.htm Accessed July 2010.

National Patient Safety Agency (2004) *Improving the Safety of Patients with Established Spinal Injuries in Hospital.* London: NPSA.

New P (2006) Non-traumatic spinal cord injury: what is the ideal setting for rehabilitation? *Australian Health Review* 30(3):353–361.

O'Callaghan N (2002) Pre-operative fasting. *Nursing Standard* 16(36):33–37.

Ostelo R, Waddell G, Leffers P (2002) Rehabilitation after lumbar disc surgery. *The Cochrane Database of Systematic Reviews* Vol 4.

Patchell R, Tibb PA, Regine WF *et al.* (2005) Direct decompressive surgical resection in the treatment of spinal cord compression caused by metastatic cancer: a randomised trial. *Lancet* 366(20):643–648.

PatientUK (2006) *Low back pain in adults.* Available from: http://www.patient.co.uk/printer.asp?doc=23068686 Accessed July 2010.

Pease N, Harris R, Finlay I (2004) Development and audit of a care pathway for the management of patients with suspected malignant spinal cord compression. *Physiotherapy* 90(1):27–34.

Pellatt G (2008) Non-traumatic spinal cord injury part 3: care for spinal cord compression. *British Journal of Neuroscience Nursing* 4(11):549–553.

Peul W, Van Houwelingen H, Wilbert B *et al.* (2007) Surgery versus prolonged conservative treatment for sciatica. The Hague Spine Intervention Prognostic Study. *New England Journal of Medicine* 22(356):2245–2256.

Pringle R (2000) Post traumatic syringomyelia. *Spinal Cord* 38(3):199.

Purdue C (2003) Diagnosis and treatment of malignant spinal cord compression. *Nursing Times* 11(38):38–41.

Rao R, Gourab K, David K (2006) Operative treatment of cervical spondylotic myelopathy. *Journal of Bone and Joint Surgery* 88A(7):1619–1640.

Rodts M (2002) Disorders of the spine. In: Maher A, Salmond S, Pellino F (eds). *Orthopaedic Nursing* (3rd edition). Philadelphia: WB Saunders.

Royal College of Nursing (2008) *Bowel care: including digital rectal examination and the manual removal of faeces. Guidance for nurses.* London: RCN.

Sinikallio S, Aalto T, Airaksinen O *et al.* (2006) Depression and associated factors in patients with lumbar spinal stenosis. *Disability and Rehabilitation* 28:415–422.

Skyrme A, Selmon G, Apthorp L (2005) *Common Spinal Disorders Explained.* Chicago: Remedica.

Sorenson P (2003) Spinal epidural abscesses: conservative treatment for selected subgroups of patients. *British Journal of Neurosurgery* 17(6):513–518.

Strayer A (2005) Lumbar spine: common pathology and interventions. *Journal of Neuroscience Nursing* 37(4): 181–193.

Sun P (2001) Complete spontaneous resolution of childhood Chiari 1 malformation and associated syringomyelia. *Paediatrics* 107(1):182–185.

Swezey R, Calin A (2003) *Low Back Pain.* Oxford: FastFacts Health Press.

Taillibert S, Laigle-Donadey F, Sanson M (2004) Palliative care in patients with primary brain tumours. *Current Opinion in Oncology* 16(6):587–592.

Tan S (2002) Recognition and treatment of oncologic emergencies. *Journal of Infusion Nursing* 25(3):182–188.

Thompson D, Jones J (2005) Principles of wound care. In: Baillie L (ed). *Developing Practical Nursing Skills.* (2nd edition). London: Arnold.

Todd NV (2005) Cauda equina syndrome: the timing of surgery probably does influence outcome. *British Journal of Neurosurgery* 19(4):301–306.

Vacca VM Jr (2007) Acute paraplegia. *Nursing* 37(6):64.

Walker L, Lamont S (2008) Graduated compression stockings to prevent deep vein thrombosis. *Nursing Standard* 22(40):35–43.

Weinstein MA, Eismont FJ (2005) Infections of the spine in patients with human immunodeficiency virus. *Journal of Bone and Joint Surgery Am* 87(3):604–609.

Weinstein JN, Lurie JD, Tosteson T *et al.* (2007) Surgical versus nonsurgical treatment for lumbar degenerative spondylolisthesis. *New England Journal of Medicine* 356(22):2257–2270.

Wellons J, Tubbs S, Oakes J (2005) Chiari malformations and syringohydromyelia. In: Rengachary S, Ellenbogen R (eds). *Principles of Neurosurgery.* (2nd edition). Oxford: Elsevier Mosby.

White H, Getliffe K (2003) *Incontinence in perspective.* In: Getkliffe KA, Dolman M (eds). *Promoting Continence.* London: Balliere Tindall.

Williams NA, Leaper DJ (1998) Infection. In: Leaper DJ, Harding KG (eds). *Wounds: Biology and management.* Oxford: Oxford Medical Publications.

Winter R, Longstein J, Denis F *et al.* (1995). *Atlas of Spine Surgery.* Oxford: WB Saunders Company.

Wolcott W, Malik M, Shaffrey C *et al.* (2005) Differential diagnosis of surgical disorders of the spine. In: Benzel E (ed). *Spine Surgery: Techniques, complication avoidance and management.* Edinburgh: Elsevier, Churchill Livingstone.

Wolfa C (2005) Lumbar disc herniation. In: Rengachary S, Ellenboden RG, *Principles of Neurosurgery.* (2nd edition). Oxford: Elsevier Mosby.

Yuras S (2000) Syringomyelia: an expanding problem. *Journal of the American Academy of Nurse Practitioners* 12(8):322–324.

Zychowicz M (2003) *Orthopaedic Nursing Secrets.* Philadelphia: Hanley and Belfus Inc.

35

Management of Patients with Guillain–Barré Syndrome and Other Peripheral Neuropathies

Sue Woodward

INTRODUCTION

Neuropathy means nerve damage and there are four main types of peripheral neuropathies: mononeuropathy, polyneuropathy, mononeuritis multiplex and autonomic neuropathy. Each different type of neuropathy has unique epidemiology, aetiologies and management, although the cause may never be identified. Mononeuropathy affects a single peripheral nerve, while polyneuropathies affect multiple peripheral nerves, usually symmetrically. Mononeuritis multiplex affects many individual peripheral nerves asymmetrically either concurrently or sequentially. Autonomic neuropathy is a form of polyneuropathy that specifically affects the autonomic nervous system. Neuropathies can cause motor, sensory or autonomic dysfunction (e.g. altered sensation, pain, muscle weakness and fatigue), depending on the nerves affected (White *et al.*, 2004). This chapter will present some details of different neuropathies, but will focus in the main on the care and management of patients with the acute polyneuropathy: Guillain–Barré syndrome.

Guillain–Barré syndrome (GBS) is a relatively rare acute post-infective disorder that causes damage to the peripheral and cranial nerves (peripheral neuropathy). GBS was first described in 1916 by two French neurologists when the syndrome became apparent among soldiers during World War I. GBS is now thought to encompass a collection of different sub-types of the disorder, possibly

each with a different pathological process underlying the neurological damage. It is the most common form of acute neuromuscular paralysis in the western world (Pritchard, 2008). It can occur in children, but is more prevalent among adults and can result in significant morbidity for some affected individuals and a mortality rate of approximately 2–3% (van Doorn, 2009). While most people affected by GBS make a full neurological recovery, up to 20% of affected individuals die or remain disabled and dependent two years following diagnosis (Forsberg *et al.*, 2005; Hughes *et al.*, 2007). GBS is normally a monophasic illness, but recurrent episodes of worsening can occur in approximately 7–16% of patients following initial improvement (Vucic *et al.*, 2009).

EPIDEMIOLOGY

The annual incidence of GBS is approximately 1–2 per 100,000 and varies slightly between countries and ages. The highest incidences have been reported in young and older adults, with most studies of the incidence and prevalence being undertaken within Europe and North America (McGrogan *et al.*, 2009). The lifetime risk of developing GBS is approximately 1:1000 (Lunn and Willison, 2009). Among older adults (over 75) the annual incidence of GBS is estimated at 4 per 100,000 (Haber *et al.*, 2009). GBS is also thought to affect more men than women (Haber *et al.*, 2009), but the difference is not large.

AETIOLOGY

The aetiology of the four main types of neuropathies is presented in Table 35.1. The aetiology and pathophysiol-

Neuroscience Nursing: Evidence-Based Practice, 1st Edition.
Edited by Sue Woodward and Ann-Marie Mestecky
© 2011 Blackwell Publishing Ltd

Table 35.1 Aetiology of different neuropathies.

Type of neuropathy	Possible aetiology
Mononeuropathy	• Trauma • Localised infection • Compression (e.g. carpal tunnel syndrome) • Localised ischaemia • Localised inflammation
Mononeuritis multiplex	• Diabetes • Systemic lupus (SLE) • Sarcoidosis • HIV • Lyme disease • Amyloidosis
Polyneuropathy	• Diabetes • Motor neurone disease • Guillain–Barré syndrome • Demyelination • Inflammatory disease • Vitamin (e.g. B12) deficiencies • Toxic effects of drugs and alcohol
Autonomic neuropathy	• Diabetes • Guillain–Barré syndrome

ogy of GBS is not completely understood, but a number of potential factors that impact on the immune system are implicated in the development of the disease including both infections and vaccines (Haber *et al.*, 2009). Other potential causative triggers have been suggested, including some cancers (e.g. Hodgkin's disease and lymphomas), because of the temporal relationship between the malignancy and the onset of symptoms of GBS, surgery and head trauma (Haber *et al.*, 2009; Vucic *et al.*, 2009).

Infections

An upper respiratory or gastrointestinal infection precedes the development of GBS in approximately two thirds of cases (McGrogan *et al.*, 2009) and different causative organisms predominate in different countries. The most commonly cited causative organisms include the Epstein–Barr virus, mycoplasma pneumoniae, campylobacter jejuni, cytomegalovirus and HIV (Vucic *et al.*, 2009).

Campylobacter jejuni is the causative organism in approximately 30–35% of cases and predominates in China.

Vaccines

Some vaccines have been implicated in the aetiology of GBS due to the immune stimulation induced by the vaccine (Haber *et al.*, 2009). The mechanism by which vaccines result in GBS is unclear, but it has been suggested that this could be due to the initiation of antibodies that cross-react with myelin, the destruction of the myelin directly by the vaccine virus or virus-related products, or the individual may have a genetic susceptibility to development of GBS (Haber *et al.*, 2009). There is clear evidence of vaccine causing GBS following a swine flu immunisation programme in the United States in 1976, which led to over 500 recorded cases of GBS, 25 deaths and the suspension of the vaccination programme.

Other vaccines that have been suggested to cause GBS include: rabies vaccine, other influenza vaccines, oral polio vaccine, diphtheria and tetanus vaccines, measles and mumps vaccines, hepatitis vaccines and smallpox vaccine, but there is little evidence to support the causation of GBS from these (Haber *et al.*, 2009). Numerous studies of the influence of vaccines on development of GBS have been undertaken which have shown low risk and non-significant associations (Vucic *et al.*, 2009).

PATHOPHYSIOLOGY

GBS is generally accepted to be an immune-mediated disorder that occurs following the production of autoimmune antibodies (Haber *et al.*, 2009), but it is unclear why some patients develop GBS following an infection or why some have more severe disease than others (van Doorn, 2009).

Macrophages have been shown to invade myelin and to cause demyelination (Vucic *et al.*, 2009), although again the reason for this is unclear. It has been suggested that this may be due to activated T-cells against specific antigens on the myelin sheath directing the macrophages, which release inflammatory mediators that ultimately cause the damage to the myelin sheath and the axon (Vucic *et al.*, 2009). It is also possible that antibodies attack specific epitopes on the surface of the Schwann cell and cause destruction of the myelin prior to invasion by macrophages (Vucic *et al.*, 2009). An epitope is a macromolecule on the surface of a cell, the shape of which is recognised by antibodies, B cells and T cells.

Many patients have been shown to develop antibodies against gangliosides (part of the cell membranes), which are thought to have a role in neuroprotection (Mocchetti, 2005). There are many different gangliosides and development of antibodies to different gangliosides has been demonstrated in different forms of GBS, e.g. Miller Fisher Syndrome (Kuijf *et al.*, 2007). It has also been shown in animal studies that antibodies can cause disruption to sodium channels (van Doorn, 2009). There is now increasing evidence that it is antibodies to specific gangliosides at the nodes of Ranvier that cause reversible dysfunction of the voltage-activated sodium channels (Vucic *et al.*, 2009) and therefore prevent conduction of impulses, leading to the muscle weakness. It is the blocking of these sodium channels, as well as the demyelination, that produces the symptoms in GBS and may account for the rapid improvement of some patients following treatment, which occurs much too quickly to be caused by remyelination (Vucic *et al.*, 2009).

The pathophysiology of acute motor axonal neuropathy (AMAN, see below) is slightly different, in that the macrophages invade the space between the Schwann cell and the axon and leave the myelin sheath intact (Vucic *et al.*, 2009). The pathophysiology of Miller Fisher syndrome (see below) is unclear, but there is evidence of segmental demyelination of motor and sensory spinal nerve roots and the 3rd, 7th, 10th and 11th cranial nerves (Vucic *et al.*, 2009).

SUB-TYPES OF GUILLAIN–BARRÉ SYNDROME

Four main sub-types of GBS exist and are now discussed.

Acute inflammatory demyelinating polyradiculoneuropathy (AIDP)

AIDP is the predominant form of GBS within the developed world (Lunn and Willison, 2009) and accounts for 90% of cases in North America and Europe (Vucic *et al.*, 2009). The main features of AIDP include generalised muscle weakness, normally ascending from the lower to the upper limbs and torso (Vucic *et al.*, 2009). Sensory symptoms are less common, but bilateral facial weakness is a feature in approximately half of patients.

Acute motor axonal neuropathy (AMAN) and acute motor and sensory axonal neuropathy (AMSAN)

The axonal variants of GBS (AMAN and AMSAN) account for approximately 3–5% of cases within the developed world (Lunn and Willison, 2009), but are more common in China, Japan and Mexico, accounting for 30–47% of cases in Asia and Central and South America (Vucic *et al.*, 2009), secondary to infection with campylobacter jejuni. Generally speaking these axonal forms of GBS have a more rapid onset and severity, frequently lead to neuromuscular respiratory failure and ventilator dependence and cranial nerve

involvement (Pritchard, 2008). Although these two variants may present in very similar ways to AIDP, they can be distinguished by nerve conduction studies. AMAN involves purely motor symptoms, while AMSAN encompasses both motor and sensory features.

Miller Fisher syndrome

The main symptoms of Miller Fisher syndrome are oculomotor dysfunction, ataxia and absent reflexes (McGrogan *et al.*, 2009) and it accounts for approximately 5% of all cases of GBS. The annual incidence of this syndrome is much lower than other forms of GBS at 0.1 per 100,000. While Miller Fisher syndrome is self-limiting, patients often develop facial and bulbar palsies and a few will require mechanical ventilation (Vucic *et al.*, 2009).

Chronic idiopathic demyelinating polyradiculoneuropathy (CIDP)

Whereas GBS is a syndrome of acute demyelination, CIDP presents with chronic progressive or relapsing weakness, sensory loss and paraesthesia, absent reflexes and/or cranial nerve dysfunction (Lunn and Willison, 2009). The symptoms and presentation of CIDP are similar to GBS, but the progressive or remitting and relapsing nature of the disease distinguishes it from GBS, which does not normally recur. The prevalence of CIDP is approximately 3–4 per 100,000 (Mahdi-Rogers *et al.*, 2008) and it affects men and women equally. Neuromuscular respiratory failure and cranial nerve dysfunction can occur, although these symptoms are less common in CIDP than AIDP (Lunn and Willison, 2009).

SIGNS AND SYMPTOMS

The onset of symptoms normally occurs over a period of a few days to weeks, with the nadir (lowest point or worst symptoms) being reached after no more than four weeks (Pritchard, 2008), although the symptoms are usually at their worst within two weeks. Symptoms include progressive ascending and normally symmetrical loss of motor function leading to flaccid paralysis and absence of reflexes. Skeletal muscle weakness may ascend to involve the diaphragm and intercostal muscles. Cranial nerves may also become involved, but sensory symptoms are usually thought to be mild (McGrogan *et al.*, 2009).

Acute complications
Neuromuscular respiratory failure

Respiratory muscle weakness necessitates ventilation in approximately 25% of patients who present with AIDP (Vucic *et al.*, 2009) and GBS is the most common cause of neuromuscular respiratory failure (Mukerji *et al.*, 2009). For those patients admitted to an intensive care unit the mean length of stay has been shown to be three weeks, with 80% of patients admitted requiring mechanical ventilation (Dhar *et al.*, 2008). Facial weakness and bulbar palsy are prognostic indicators of the need for mechanical ventilation (Lawn *et al.*, 2001).

Cardiac and autonomic sequelae

Autonomic dysfunction occurs in approximately 15% of patients with AIDP and includes cardiac arrhythmias, labile blood pressure and postural hypotension, paralytic ileus and urinary retention (Vucic *et al.*, 2009). Significant morbidity and mortality from GBS are associated with cardiovascular complications such as blood pressure changes, tachyarrhythmias, bradyarrhythmias and myocarditis (Mukerji *et al.*, 2009) and affect up to two thirds of patients (see Box 35.1). Some of the cardiac complications are due to the impact of GBS on the autonomic nervous system, but the heart also contains similar gangliosides to those within the nervous system and this has been suggested as a possible mechanism. There is evidence that autonomic involvement results in sympathetic overactivity as opposed to parasympathetic underactivity (Pfeiffer *et al.*, 1999).

Box 35.1   Common cardiovascular complications

Rhythm abnormalities
- Sinus tachycardia
- Atrial and ventricular arrhythmias
- Sinus bradycardia
- Atrioventricular block
- Asystole

Blood pressure changes
- Transient or persistent hypotension
- Hypertension

Myocardial involvement
- Asymptomatic myocarditis
- Myocardial infarction

ECG changes
- Giant T-waves
- Prolonged Q-T intervals
- U waves
- AV block

Source: Mukerji *et al.*, 2009.

Syndrome of inappropriate ADH secretion (SIADH)

SIADH (see Chapter 16) can occur in GBS and may be severe (Lunn and Willison, 2009). Electrolytes should therefore be monitored carefully throughout the acute phase of the illness.

Prognosis and mortality

The highest numbers of people developing GBS are among older adults (>50 years) and this group is also likely to have a poorer prognosis (Haber *et al.*, 2009). Other predictors of poor prognosis apart from age include: the need for mechanical ventilation, severe weakness and rapid onset of weakness, co-morbidity, cardiac complications and sepsis, infection with *Campylobacter jejuni* or cytomegalovirus (van Doorn, 2009; Vucic *et al.*, 2009).

An outcome score for predicting outcomes from GBS has been developed recently: the Erasmus GBS Outcome Scale (EGOS) has shown that the ability to walk unaided after six months can be predicted on the basis of age, preceding diarrhoea and GBS disability score within 2 weeks from onset (van Koningsveld *et al.*, 2007). Approximately one third of patients will need to change their employment, hobbies or social activities as a result of residual disability following GBS (Vucic *et al.*, 2009).

DIAGNOSIS

Diagnosis of GBS remains mainly clinical, but investigations are used both to confirm the suspected diagnosis and to differentiate the different sub-types of the disease. Investigations include lumbar puncture, to enable examination of CSF, and nerve conduction studies (NCS) (see Chapter 19), with nerve conduction abnormalities occurring in 85% of patients (Lunn and Willison, 2009). NCS normally reveal delayed conduction velocities and motor conduction block suggestive of demyelination. Sensory nerve conduction studies can differentiate AMAN from AMSAN (Vucic *et al.*, 2009). Electromyography (EMG) can assist in excluding muscular causes for symptoms and later in GBS can assess the degree of axonal loss (Vucic *et al.*, 2009).

Lumbar puncture should be performed to exclude other possible diagnoses before IVIg is commenced as this treatment can cause aseptic meningitis (Pritchard, 2008). CSF protein levels are raised in 80% of patients (Vucic *et al.*, 2009) but may be normal within the first week of the disease. White cell counts are not normally raised and, while higher white cell counts within the CSF do not rule out GBS, they can be suggestive of an infective cause for the symptoms (Pritchard, 2008).

MEDICAL MANAGEMENT

Plasma exchange

Plasma exchange was originally the mainstay of treatment of GBS and has been utilised for over 30 years. Plasma exchange involves the removal of the patient's plasma, containing circulating immune complexes, and replacing this with fresh frozen plasma or similar fluid (e.g. albumin). In many trials the beneficial effects of plasma exchange are equivalent to the benefits from IVIg (Raphaël *et al.*, 2008), although plasma exchange is more complex to administer, more expensive and not as widely available. It has been demonstrated that in mild disease two exchanges are better than none and in moderate disease four exchanges are more effective than two, but no incremental benefit is achieved beyond this, even in severe disease (Raphaël *et al.*, 2008).

Plasma exchange has been shown to be beneficial in treatment of CIDP in the short-term, but deterioration occurs rapidly once the treatment is stopped (Mehndiratta *et al.*, 2004) and no long-term studies of the effectiveness of the treatment have been undertaken. Plasma exchange was also shown to be associated with significant adverse events, such as haemodynamic effects, in 3–17% of exchanges (Mehndiratta *et al.*, 2004).

Intravenous immunoglobulin (IVIg)

IVIg has been shown to have similar efficacy to plasma exchange, but has fewer side-effects (Hughes *et al.*, 2006; Elovaara *et al.*, 2008) and the shift from using plasma exchange to IVIg has led to a reduction in the need for inter-hospital transfers and in-patient rehabilitation (van Doorn, 2009). IVIg has been recommended for the treatment of GBS (DH, 2008). There are few randomised trials in adults comparing IVIg with placebo, but there are trials comparing the treatment against plasma exchange, which was known to be effective. It would be unethical not to treat a patient, by giving them a placebo, in a trial of an intervention for a potentially life threatening disease, so it is right that trials compare a new intervention against the current gold standard. It has been shown that IVIg administered within two weeks from the onset of GBS is as effective as plasma exchange, which is known to be more effective than supportive care (Hughes *et al.*, 2006). However, adding IVIg following plasma exchange has not been shown to add any significant incremental benefit.

IVIg has also been used successfully to treat CIDP in both the short and long-term (Elovaara *et al.*, 2008; Lunn and Willison, 2009). IVIg has been shown to improve symptoms for at least two to six weeks following adminis-

tration (Eftimov *et al.*, 2009) and may have longer term benefits. Efficacy is comparable to that of steroids and plasma exchange. Those patients requiring only small doses to keep their disease under control may receive their immunoglobulin via a sub-cutaneous route (Lunn and Willison, 2009), which has been shown to improve patient satisfaction with treatment and reduce in-patient costs (Lee *et al.*, 2009). IVIg is the most expensive treatment for CIDP, but has fewer side-effects compared to other treatments and, given the similar efficacy of all the treatments for this condition, IVIg may be preferred (Lunn and Willison, 2009).

Steroids

Both high dose oral steroid (prednisolone) and intravenous steroids (methylprednisolone) have been tried in the treatment of AIDP as the disorder is thought to be the result of an auto-immune inflammatory process. It is therefore logical that the anti-inflammatory and immunosuppressant effects of steroids may be effective. However, there is no evidence of benefit from steroids and they may even delay recovery, so should not be used (Hughes *et al.*, 2010).

Steroids are effective for the management of CIDP, however, and are often thought of as the first-line management for this condition (Lunn and Willison, 2009). Many of the studies investigating the effectiveness of steroids have methodological flaws, but there is still convincing evidence of benefit from large non-randomised studies (Mehndiratta and Hughes, 2002). Steroids have considerable undesirable side-effects and cannot be used long-term, so other treatments (e.g. immunosuppressants, IVIg or plasma exchange) may be considered.

Immunosuppressants and interferons

CIDP is treated with immunosuppressants (Lunn and Willison, 2009), although these will usually be added after initial treatment with either steroids, IVIg or plasma exchange. A number of different immunosuppressants may be used (Box 35.2). While some trials of different cytotoxics and interferons have been published, most of these are either too small or non-randomised studies so it has not been possible to make evidence-based recommendations and further research is required (Hughes *et al.*, 2009).

NURSING MANAGEMENT

Care and management of patients with GBS is by necessity multi-disciplinary and nurses have a crucial role to play, particularly in the acute stages of the disease, but also throughout the patient's rehabilitation. Priorities of care will change depending on the stage of the illness and in the acute stages the nursing priorities are to prevent or detect

---

Box 35.2   Commonly used immunosuppressants for chronic idiopathic demyelinating polyradiculoneuropathy (CIDP)

- Azathioprine
- Cyclophosphamide
- Methotrexate
- Ciclosporin
- Rituximab
- Alemtuzumab
- Enteracept

Box 35.3   Signs of respiratory failure

- Tachypnoea
- Flaring of nostrils
- Use of accessory muscles
- Shallow breathing
- Paradoxical abdominal movements
- Inability to clear secretions
- Anxiety/exhaustion
- Reduced forced vital capacity (FVC)
- Hypoxia and hypercarbia (late signs)

Source: Garner and Amin, 2006.

---

life-threatening complications. Nursing care throughout the illness is both supportive and symptomatic.

NURSING MANAGEMENT IN THE ACUTE PHASE

Respiratory monitoring

Signs of neuromuscular respiratory failure are detailed in Box 35.3. Forced vital capacity (FVC – the maximum volume expired slowly after maximal inspiration) must be monitored regularly. If patients have facial weakness and cannot form a good lip seal around a mouthpiece, the FVC must be measured using a face mask as accurately as possible. Normally the FVC should be 70–75 ml/kg (Garner and Amin, 2006). Elective invasive mechanical ventilation will be considered if this falls below 20 ml/kg (Vucic *et al.*, 2009) or if it drops by more than 30% (Garner and Amin, 2006), so that intubation can be planned and the need for emergency intubation if the patient has a respiratory arrest can be eliminated. At this point the patient should be transferred to an intensive care setting for observation and respiratory management (Rabinstein and Wijdicks, 2003).

These patients will often require long-term mechanical ventilation and a tracheostomy will normally be required. The mean duration of ventilation is normally between 15 and 43 days (Hughes *et al.*, 2005). Although early tracheostomy can lead to increased patient safety and comfort and can assist weaning from ventilation, the decision may be delayed for up to two weeks. Respiratory monitoring and management is discussed further in Chapter 15.

Bulbar dysfunction can cause difficulty with clearing secretions and may compromise gas exchange (Hughes *et al.*, 2005). Patients are also at risk of developing aspiration pneumonia due to dysphagia, so careful assessment of swallowing and signs of aspiration are necessary (see Chapter 12).

Cardiac and other haemodynamic monitoring

Careful monitoring and control of cardiovascular function (heart rate and blood pressure) is essential, given that up to 61% of patients can develop cardiac dysrhythmias due to autonomic involvement (Vucic *et al.*, 2009). Nurses must also ensure that continuous cardiac monitoring is maintained and must remain vigilant for the abnormal rhythms discussed below. Tracheal suctioning is often necessary, but care must be taken during the procedure as this may also trigger arrhythmias (Mukerji *et al.*, 2009). It is recommended that patients with labile blood pressure undergo prolonged cardiac and intra-arterial blood pressure monitoring within an intensive care unit as they are at high risk of developing arrhythmias (Mukerji *et al.*, 2009). Cardiac and haemodynamic monitoring are discussed further in Chapter 14.

Sinus tachycardia is the most common abnormality seen on cardiac monitoring and does not normally require treatment, as beta-blockers and anti-hypertensives may exacerbate other cardiac complications (Mukerji *et al.*, 2009). However, treatment may become necessary in older patients with a history of coronary artery disease (Pfeiffer *et al.*, 1999). Bradycardia may also become evident due to vagal overactivity in up to 50% of patients and may require treatment with either temporary transcutaneous pacing or atropine (Mukerji *et al.*, 2009).

Regular blood pressure monitoring is required, the frequency of which will be determined by the patient's condition. If the blood pressure is labile or a sustained hypo or hypertension is evident, this will need to be assessed more frequently. Blood pressure variability can occur due to: disturbances in the baroreceptor reflex pathway, changes in catecholamine levels and alterations in vasomotor tone and peripheral vascular resistance (Mukerji *et al.*, 2009) (see Chapter 14). This variability can be more prevalent among ventilated patients. If patients develop hypotension a fluid challenge is advocated, while patients with hypertension (mean arterial pressure >125 mmHg) may require treatment with anti-hypertensives (Mukerji *et al.*, 2009).

DVT prophylaxis

Patients with GBS are particularly at risk of developing venous thromboembolism due to the flaccid nature of the paralysis (Hughes *et al.*, 2005) and they are often expected to have significantly reduced mobility for three days or longer (NICE, 2010). Patients should not be allowed to become dehydrated. Oral fluids should be encouraged if the patient is able to swallow safely, but intravenous fluid administration may be required. DVT prophylaxis will be required for non-ambulant patients, having assessed the patient's risk of bleeding, with both pharmacological (e.g. low molecular weight heparin) and/or mechanical (e.g. anti-embolic stockings or pneumatic compression) interventions according to NICE guidelines (NICE, 2010). Prophylaxis will be required until patients are able to walk independently (Hughes *et al.*, 2005).

Administration of IVIg

IVIg is a blood derivative and its administration is not without risk. It is now the most widely used plasma component in health care settings (DH, 2008) and is a sterile preparation of concentrated antibodies. Guidelines for administration of IVIg for people with neurological conditions have been produced by the Association of British Neurologists (2005), the Department of Health (2008) and the European Federation of Neurological Societies (Elovaara *et al.*, 2008). Nursing administration of IVIg is also the subject of a national benchmark (National Neuroscience Benchmarking Group, 2007).

The recommended dose of IVIg is 2 g/kg (DH, 2008) rounded down to the nearest whole vial, but may be divided into five doses of 0.4 g/kg/day for five days (Elovaara *et al.*, 2008), so the patient's weight must be documented prior to administration to facilitate dosage calculations. IVIg must always be prepared and administered using an aseptic technique and universal precautions (RCN, 2003) and once prepared it cannot be stored and needs to be administered within a few hours, according to manufacturer's instructions. These products do not contain any additives to prevent bacterial contamination and should therefore be used immediately the cap is removed. IVIg must be administered via a dedicated cannula, using an infusion pump and a 15 micron filtered giving set (RCN, 2003) and always in accordance with the manufacturer's instructions detailed on the 'summary of product characteristics' that comes with the product. Using the 15 micron filtered giving set will prevent infusion of any undissolved immunoglobulin or other foreign particles, but any solutions that are cloudy or contain obvious particulates should not be used. The infusion should be allowed to warm to room temperature prior to administration and should be protected from light.

When beginning an infusion of IVIg for the first time the nurse must ensure that the rate of administration is increased in incremental steps when starting the infusion to ensure that the patient is able to tolerate the infusion (RCN, 2003). This reduces the side-effects. Subsequent infusions can be started at the full rate. The same procedure should be followed if the brand of IVIg is changed or if there is a gap of eight weeks between infusions, e.g. if the patient is receiving IVIg for CIDP. Infusion rates are product specific so should be titrated according to the manufacturer's guidelines. For every infusion the batch number, timing, product details and procedure followed must be documented in the patient's records (RCN, 2003). Ideally the product given should not be altered and different brands should not be used interchangeably due to the differences in the manufacturing process (DH, 2008).

Management of side-effects

Side-effects of IVIg are detailed in Box 35.4. As IVIg is a blood product, one of the most significant associated risks is an allergic or anaphylactic reaction, although this

---

Box 35.4   Side-effects of IVIg

Mild
- Headaches
- Nausea and vomiting
- Dizziness
- Fatigue
- Flu-like symptoms (muscle aches, shivering, low grade pyrexia)
- Rashes and urticaria

Moderate
- Severe headaches
- Chest pain
- Wheezing

Severe
- Dysphagia
- Severe breathlessness or wheezing
- Severe dizziness/fainting
- Collapse

is a comparatively rare complication. The risk of an allergic reaction occurs when administering the initial infusion or if the product or brand is changed at any time (RCN, 2003), so the nurse should ensure that oxygen and an emergency trolley are available at this time. Vital signs (temperature, pulse, respiratory rate and blood pressure) must be recorded at baseline, with each increase in infusion rate and four hourly thereafter for the remainder of the infusion (RCN, 2003). Should an allergic reaction occur the infusion must be stopped immediately and medical staff informed urgently. The patient may require treatment with adrenaline (e.g. 0.5–1 mg IM), corticosteroids or anti-histamines, so the nurse should change the giving set and replace the IVIg infusion with normal saline to maintain patency of the IV cannula.

Other side-effects that might occur with IVIg administration include headache and flu-like symptoms, mild hypertension and post-infusion headaches accompanied by nausea and vomiting due to aseptic meningitis. Headaches and hypertension that occur during the infusion may be alleviated by reducing the infusion rate (e.g. to 0.25 ml/minute) (Schleis, 2000) and if the symptoms have resolved after approximately 30 minutes the infusion rate can be increased again slowly. If symptoms are more severe or persistent, the infusion should be stopped and medical staff informed. Flu-like symptoms can usually be treated effectively with either paracetamol or NSAIDs (RCN, 2003). If the patient develops symptoms of an aseptic meningitis, they may require treatment with anti-histamines or corticosteroids. It may be possible to reduce the onset of these symptoms by ensuring that the patient is well hydrated before beginning the infusion, or by administering the infusion over a 24 hour period (RCN, 2003).

Pain management

Both somatic and neuropathic pain can be problematic during the acute stages of GBS (Pritchard, 2008) and can affect between 33 and 71% of patients (Hughes *et al.*, 2005). Pain is often experienced in the back, buttocks and thighs and described as cramping or muscular tenderness (Tripathi and Kaushik, 2000). Treatment with paracetamol, NSAIDs and/or opioids may be required following careful pain assessment by nursing staff (see Chapter 17). Simple analgesia often proves insufficient (Hughes *et al.*, 2005) and it has been shown that up to 70% of patients will require oral or intravenous opioid administration, with careful monitoring for side-effects.

Neuropathic pain can be successfully treated with anti-epileptic drugs in most cases (such as carbamazepine or gabapentin) or anti-depressants (such as amitriptyline)

(Pritchard, 2008). Administration of carbamazepine has been shown to reduce requirements for opioid analgesia in patients in intensive care (Tripathi and Kaushik, 2000) and has been recommended as an adjuvant treatment (Hughes *et al.*, 2005).

Simple supportive measures such as careful patient positioning can also help with pain management. Knee pain can become problematic – as the muscles around the joint become weaker, hyperextension can occur and cause pain (see Chapter 11). Nursing the patient on a profiling bed with an element of knee flexion can help to support the joints. Neuropathic pain can also develop during the rehabilitative phase of GBS as axonal and myelin regeneration occurs – paraesthesia (such as pins and needles) may be experienced and can be exacerbated by clothing and bedclothes touching the skin.

Bladder and bowel dysfunction

Detrusor areflexia and reduced bladder sensation has been demonstrated in GBS (Sakakibara *et al.*, 1997). Nurses need to be vigilant for the development of urinary retention. Urine output must be monitored and, if signs of retention develop (e.g. frequency, post-micturition dribbling, difficulty passing urine or a feeling of incomplete emptying), a bladder scan must be performed to assess the post-void residual urine measurement. If retention develops the patient will need to be catheterised; management of urinary retention is discussed further in Chapter 18.

Patients are at risk of developing constipation due to reduced mobility, but nurses should also be vigilant for the development of a paralytic ileus due to the involvement of the 10th cranial nerve (vagus), which can affect up to 50% of patients (Hughes *et al.*, 2005). Assessment and management of constipation is discussed further in Chapter 18.

Nutrition

Dysphagia is common due to bulbar palsy and involvement of cranial nerves. Swallowing assessment is therefore necessary and may need to be reviewed regularly as the patient's condition progresses (see Chapter 12). If dysphagia occurs enteral feeding may be required to maintain fluid and nutritional intake, but this may be complicated if there is any ileus and the gut cannot be used. In this case the patient will need to have parenteral feeding. Nutrition management is discussed further in Chapter 16.

Communication and psychological support

Consciousness is unimpaired with GBS and careful communication is vital, particularly with patients receiving mechanical ventilation. Patients may also experience facial weakness due to 7th cranial nerve involvement, which can cause dysarthria. Patients with GBS experience anxiety and are often fearful, needing constant reassurance and psychological support. Communication is a vital component of nursing these patients and is discussed further in Chapter 12.

Facial palsy

Facial palsy can occur in GBS due to the effect of the disease on the 7th cranial nerve. If severe and bilateral the patient is at risk of corneal damage and eye care is essential. This is discussed in detail in Chapter 13.

REHABILITATION

Most patients with GBS will require rehabilitation, but it has been identified that there have been very few long-term studies of rehabilitation outcomes (Hughes *et al.*, 2005). It is recommended that rehabilitation focuses around careful limb positioning, posture, use of orthotics and nutritional support (Hughes *et al.*, 2005).

Fatigue

Fatigue can be persistent during recovery from GBS, possibly due to axonal loss (Vucic *et al.*, 2009). Severe fatigue has been found in up to 80% of patients, but is not related to disease severity or duration (Hughes *et al.*, 2005). Fatigue may be helped by a structured exercise programme and is discussed further in Chapter 28.

Recovery of motor function

Early referral to a physiotherapist during the acute stage of the illness is required and physiotherapy input will continue throughout the patient's rehabilitation. Exercise programmes that do not over-fatigue affected muscles are required as this can impede recovery and has been shown to cause paradoxical weakening (Hughes *et al.*, 2005).

Flaccidity can continue for some time and foot drop can occur. Management of flaccidity and prevention of foot drop is discussed in Chapter 11. Shortening of the soft tissues and contractures can also occur (Hughes *et al.*, 2005), so careful positioning of the limbs and joints is required (see Chapter 11).

Ongoing support

Nurses should ensure that patients and their families are given the details of the GBS support group (www.gbs.org.uk), who will be able to provide details of local support groups. The GBS support group provides both support and information for patients affected by GBS and CIDP throughout Britain and Ireland.

SUMMARY

GBS is a potentially life-threatening neurological disease that can result in residual disability, but one from which most patients will make a full neurological recovery. The variable severity means that it is impossible to predict who will recover and who will be adversely affected in the long-term. Patients require considerable psychological support from nursing staff throughout their illness trajectory and may become completely dependent for all activities of living. Management of these patients is mainly symptomatic and requires involvement of all members of the multidisciplinary team.

Guillain–Barré syndrome: patient perspective

It's over three years since I spent nearly eighteen months on the neurosurgical intensive care unit and the rehabilitation ward. It was a horrendous time in my life and I genuinely believed on many occasions that I was going to die. I can't remember the earliest few weeks, I just remember the complete helplessness, the pain when being moved, when they did suction down my tracheostomy tube, the lack of control and frustration over my lack of communication and feeling frightened when I couldn't see the nurses. For months I didn't seem to be getting any better and I suffered from chest infections, a paralysed gut and I needed TPN feeding for several weeks. I hated that line in my neck – it was always pulling and the tape was always tugging on my skin. As much as I hated the tracheostomy tube, the thought of having it removed terrified me. I kept suffering from stridor whenever the tube was removed and it took several attempts before it eventually came out.

If I thought the time that I was on a ventilator was bad, the recovery was really hard. I spent nine months as an in-patient and I still attend out-patient physiotherapy. Even now I become easily tired and I haven't been able to return to work yet.

I am grateful to all the nurses who cared for me and I enjoy calling on the ward when I return for my out-patient appointments. I don't think I will ever forget the support, encouragement, cajoling and hard work that contributed to my eventual recovery. The nurses often ask me to speak to other patients suffering from the same condition on the unit and whilst I'm glad to help and it is a practical way of saying thank-you, I find it difficult recounting my experiences, knowing what they are going through, it's important that they know that it won't last forever.

REFERENCES

Association of British Neurologists (2005) *Intravenous Immunoglobulin in Neurological Disease*. London: ABN.

Department of Health (2008) *Clinical Guidelines for Immunoglobulin Use* (2nd edition). London: DH.

Dhar R, Stitt L, Hahn AF (2008) The morbidity and outcome of patients with Guillain-Barré syndrome admitted to the intensive care unit. *Journal of Neurological Science* 264:121–128.

Eftimov F, Winer JR, Vermeulen M *et al.* (2009) Intravenous immunoglobulin for chronic inflammatory demyelinating polyradiculoneuropathy. *Cochrane Database of Systematic Reviews* Issue 1. Art. No.: CD001797.

Elovaara I, Apostolski S, van Doorn P *et al.* (2008) EFNS guidelines for the use of intravenous immunoglobulin in treatment of neurological diseases. *European Journal of Neurology* 15:893–908.

Forsberg A, Press R, Einarsson U *et al.* (2005) Disability and health-related quality of life in Guillain-Barré syndrome during the first two years after onset: a prospective study. *Clinical Rehabilitation* 19:900–909.

Garner A, Amin Y (2006) The management of neuromuscular respiratory failure: a review. *British Journal of Neuroscience Nursing* 2(8):394–398.

Haber P, Sejvar J, Mikaeloff Y *et al.* (2009) Vaccines and Guillain-Barré syndrome. *Drug Safety* 32(4):309–323.

Hughes RAC, Raphaël JC, Swan AV *et al.* (2006) Intravenous immunoglobulin for Guillain-Barré syndrome. *Cochrane Database of Systematic Reviews* Issue 1. Art. No.: CD002063.

Hughes RA, Swan AV, Raphael JC *et al.* (2007) Immunotherapy for Guillain-Barré syndrome: a systematic review. *Brain* 130:2245–2257.

Hughes RAC, Swan AV, van Doorn PA (2009) Cytotoxic drugs and interferons for chronic inflammatory demyelinating polyradiculoneuropathy. *Cochrane Database of Systematic Reviews* Issue 4. Art. No.: CD003280.

Hughes RAC, Swan AV, vanDoorn PA (2010) Corticosteroids for Guillain-Barré syndrome. *Cochrane Database of Systematic Reviews* Issue 2. Art. No.: CD001446.

Hughes RAC, Wijdicks EFM, Benson E *et al.* (2005) Supportive care for patients with Guillain-Barré syndrome. *Archives of Neurology* 62:1194–1198.

Kuijf ML, Godschalk PC, Gilbert M *et al.* (2007) Origin of ganglioside complex antibodies in Guillain-Barré syndrome. *Journal of Neuroimmunology* 188:69–73.

Lawn ND, Fletcher DD, Henderson RD *et al.* (2001) Anticipating mechanical ventilation in Guillain-Barre syndrome. *Archives of Neurology* 58:893–898.

Lee DH, Linker RA, Paulus W *et al.* (2009) Subcutaneous immunoglobulin infusion: a new therapeutic option in chronic inflammatory demyelinating polyneuropathy. *Muscle and Nerve* 37:406–409.

Lunn MPT, Willison HJ (2009) Diagnosis and treatment in inflammatory neuropathies. *Journal of Neurology, Neurosurgery and Psychiatry* 80:249–258.

Mahdi-Rogers M, Al-Chalabi A, Hughes RAC (2008) Prevalence and morbidity of chronic inflammatory neuropathies in South East England. *Journal of the Peripheral Nervous System* 13(Suppl 1):176.

McGrogan A, Madle GC, Seaman HE *et al.* (2009) The epidemiology of Guillain-Barré syndrome worldwide. *Neuroepidemiology* 32:150–163.

Mehndiratta MM, Hughes RAC (2002) Corticosteroids for chronic inflammatory demyelinating polyradiculoneuropathy. *Cochrane Database of Systematic Reviews* Issue 1. Art. No.: CD002062.

Mehndiratta MM, Hughes RAC, Agarwal P (2004) Plasma exchange for chronic inflammatory demyelinating polyradiculoneuropathy. *Cochrane Database of Systematic Reviews* Issue 3. Art. No.: CD003906.

Mocchetti I (2005). Exogenous gangliosides, neuronal plasticity and repair, and the neurotrophins. *Cellular and Molecular Life Sciences* 62(19–20):2283–2294.

Mukerji S, Aloka F, Farouq MU *et al.* (2009) Cardiovascular complications of the Guillain-Barré syndrome. *American Journal of Cardiology* 104:1452–1455.

National Institute for Health and Clinical Excellence (2010) *Venous Thromboembolism. Reducing the risk: full guideline*. London: National Clinical Guideline Centre.

National Neuroscience Benchmarking Group (2007) *Benchmark no 8: Administration of Immunoglobulins*. Salford: NNBG.

Pfeiffer G, Schiller H, Kruse J *et al.* (1999) Indicators of dysautonomia in severe Guillain-Barré syndrome. *Journal of Neurology* 246:1015–1022.

Pritchard J (2008) What's new in Guillain-Barré syndrome? *Postgraduate Medical Journal* 84:532–538.

Rabinstein AA, Wijdicks EFM (2003) Warning signs of imminent respiratory failure in neurological patients. *Seminars in Neurology* 23(1):97–104.

Raphaël JC, Chevret S, Hughes RAC *et al.* (2008). Plasma exchange for Guillain-Barré syndrome. *Cochrane Database of Systematic Reviews* Issue 2. Art. No.: CD001798.

Royal College of Nursing (2003) *Standards for Infusion Therapy*. London: RCN.

Sakakibara R, Hattori T, Kuwabara S *et al.* (1997) Micturitional disturbance in patients with Guillain-Barré syndrome. *Journal of Neurology, Neurosurgery and Psychiatry* 63:649–653.

Schleis T (2000) The financial, operational and clinical management of intravenous immunoglobulin administration. *Journal of Intravenous Nursing* 23(5S):S23–S31.

Tripathi M, Kaushik S (2000) Carbemazepine for pain management in Guillain-Barré syndrome patients in the intensive care unit. *Critical Care Medicine* 28(3):655–658.

van Doorn PA (2009) What's new in Guillain-Barré syndrome in 2007–2008? *Journal of the Peripheral Nervous System* 14:72–74.

van Koningsveld R, Steyerberg EW, Hughes RAC *et al.* (2007) A clinical prognostic scoring system for Guillain-Barré syndrome. *Lancet Neurology* 6:589–594.

Vucic S, Kiernan MC, Cornblath DR (2009) Guillain-Barré syndrome: An update. *Journal of Clinical Neuroscience* 16:733–741.

White CM, Pritchard J, Turner-Stokes L (2004) Exercise for people with peripheral neuropathy. *Cochrane Database of Systematic Reviews* Issue 4. Art. No CD003904.

Section VIII
Fundamental Concepts of Neuroscience Nursing

36
Ethical and Legal Issues

Stephen Leyshon and Alison Hobden

INTRODUCTION

An understanding of the application of law and ethics to health care is an essential element of any nurse's or other health professional's knowledge. This chapter provides an overview of relevant aspects of law and ethics and their application to neuroscience nursing. By no means exhaustive, it gives an insight into how law and ethics have an impact on practice. In achieving this, it focuses on five exemplar areas (human rights, consent, risk management, resource allocation and end of life care) to draw out issues for further consideration. Nurses who proactively incorporate ethico-legal issues into reflection can improve the quality of care to patients.

ETHICS

Most health care professionals can think of a situation in which they have struggled to make the 'right' decision. Neuroscience and other health care disciplines are increasingly complex. With daily advancements in medical science decisions regarding patient care can become overloaded with uncertainty. In the light of this, an awareness of health care ethics has become increasingly important.

Broadly speaking, ethical principles are concerned with attempts to guide us in what we should or should not do, what is right or wrong, good or bad. An understanding of ethical theories and principles will not provide us with the 'right answer', but they can offer a structure to facilitate the discussion of available options in an attempt to ensure robust and fair decision making. A number of ethical theories have been applied to health care (Figure 36.1). Perhaps the most commonly used are deontology, utilitarianism, virtue theory and principalism.

Deontology has its roots in the work of Immanuel Kant and is concerned with understanding our duties. According to Kant (1948), our actions ought to be motivated by our moral obligation towards someone rather than for any personal gain. It supposes that we treat people as we would want every person to be treated and so an act is good if it can be applied to all people.

Jeremy Bentham (2000) and John Stuart Mill (1991) are seen as the founders of utilitarianism, which is a form of consequentialism that focuses on the outcomes (or consequences) of our actions. It takes the view that an action is good if it produces a positive outcome (specifically happiness) for the greatest number of people.

Virtue theory takes a different approach in that it does not consider an act itself, but looks at the character and nature of the person carrying out that act. This means that the merit of the act is dependent on the person undertaking the act and their motivation: the same act can be carried out by two different people and produce two different outcomes.

Arguably the dominant ethical theory in health care today is principalism. Developed by Beauchamp and Childress (2009) in the USA and Gillon (1986) in the UK, this takes the approach that there are four ethical principles that should be applied to health care:

- Respect for autonomy
- Non-maleficence (to do no harm)
- Beneficence (to do good)
- Justice (fairness and equality)

Neuroscience Nursing: Evidence-Based Practice, 1st Edition.
Edited by Sue Woodward and Ann-Marie Mestecky
© 2011 Blackwell Publishing Ltd

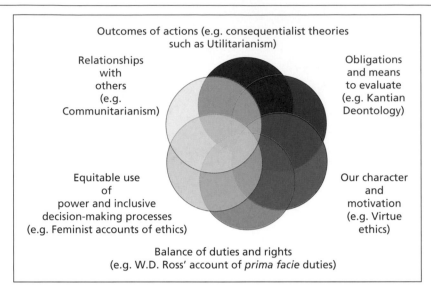

Figure 36.1 Key ethical theories and their focus.

It is suggested that the application of these principles to health care problems frees workers from agreeing with a particular moral philosophy and yet still provides a framework to ensure that health care practice is undertaken in a systematic and considerate way (Gillon, 1986). The weakness with this approach lies in deciding which principle has the final say, for example should our desire to do good overrule patient choice in health care? This is not a question that the authors of the principles answer, but instead leave to our own professional judgement to decide. Box 36.1 provides an example of a framework for ethical decision making (adapted from Thomson, 1999) that tries to place the principles within the context of particular decisions that individuals have to make.

LAW

The law gives a formal guide to our conduct by setting minimum standards of behaviour. It differs from ethics in that the law also stipulates the punishments or remedies for failing to meet such standards. Law, put simply, is about the rules that govern society and the institutions that enforce them. The law has significance throughout all areas of life and health care is no exception. Broadly speaking, the law arises from three key sources:

- Statute (i.e. laws passed by parliament)
- Case law (i.e. precedent or 'judge-made' law)
- International sources (e.g. the European Community)

Box 36.1 Framework for ethical decision making

- Consider why a decision is needed (is it needed at this time?)
- List the options (i.e. the various possible courses of action). Think about whether any options have been ruled out on ethical or legal grounds. If so, is this justified?
- For each option:
  - (a) List the consequences – make sure that implications for autonomy, non-maleficence, beneficence and justice have been included. Include also any legal consequences that may arise (remember the different sources of law)
  - (b) Consider how likely are any consequences identified under (a) – take account of any evidence and assess its validity and reliability (how robust and applicable to your particular practice setting is it?)
  - (c) Consider how important the consequences are (rate them on a scale of 0 to 10 – 0 being 'not important' and 10 being 'extremely important')
  - (d) Decide whether each of the listed consequences counts for or against the option
- Make a choice between the options in light of your comments under (a)–(d)

Adapted from Thomson, 1999.

Health care law, however, is not a single, easily defined entity. It is made up of:

> *'bits from a large number of different branches of law: criminal law, human rights law, tort law, contract law, property law, family law and public law'*
>
> Herring, 2006 p2

This is made more complicated by the fact that there is not a single, unified legal system: each country differs in important ways. In the United Kingdom, for example, England and Wales have one system, Scotland another, and Northern Ireland a third.

LAW AND ETHICS IN NURSING

It would be unreasonable to expect nurses to know everything about all laws and ethical issues. Instead, practitioners must have an understanding of laws that have a direct impact on their role (e.g. the Mental Capacity Act 2005 and Human Rights Act 1998 in the United Kingdom) as well as an appreciation of what is right and wrong and how to resolve conflicting demands or dilemmas (NMC, 2008). The incorporation of ethical and legal issues into everyday practice is important because it goes to the heart of being an accountable practitioner (Marks-Maran, 1996). The need to be able to provide such justification is clear when one remembers the multiple ways in which registered nurses can be called to account (Figure 36.2).

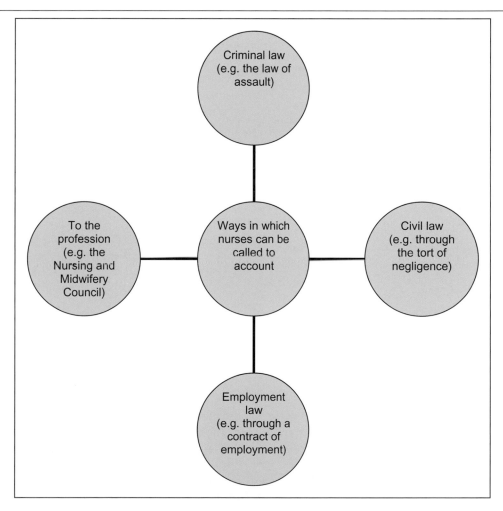

Figure 36.2 Ways in which nurses can be called to account.

CONSENT AND MENTAL CAPACITY

Gillon defines consent as:

'A voluntary un-coerced decision made by a sufficiently auton-omous person, on the basis of adequate information to accept or reject some proposed course of action which will affect him or her.'

(Gillon, 1986 p113)

In western society, the moral foundation for seeking consent is based on three ethical approaches:

* Utilitarianism
* Kantian deontology
* Principalism

Each of these approaches emphasises the importance of respecting individual autonomy in different ways. In utilitarianism, it is considered part of maximising happiness. Kantian deontology, in contrast, argues that respect for autonomy is not simply a means to happiness, but is also something that can be justified through reason and, therefore, is important for its own sake. These two viewpoints have supported principalist approaches that see the principle of respect for autonomy as part of a common morality (Beauchamp and Childress, 2009).

Seeking consent, and thereby promoting autonomy, is a critical element of ethical nursing practice. Obtaining consent, or abiding by its refusal, recognises the intrinsic value of individuals and fosters patients' trust and confidence in their carers. This is reflected in both the Nursing and Midwifery Council's *Code of Professional Conduct* (NMC, 2008) and English law.

English law has long respected the right of individual, competent adults to give or withhold consent. Lord Reid made this clear in S *v* S; W *v* Official Solicitor [1972]:

'There is no doubt that a person of full age and capacity cannot be ordered to undergo a [medical test or treatment] against his will. The . . . reason is that English law goes to great lengths to protect a person of full age and capacity from interference with personal liberty.'

Consent should be thought of as a process, rather than a one-off act and ought to be sought at each stage of an individual's care, investigation and treatment. Practitioners should think in terms of legally valid consent, which needs to be voluntary, appropriately informed, and made by a competent person.

Consent is voluntary if it is given without undue pressure or coercion. This does not mean that nurses and others (e.g. carers and relatives) cannot influence a patient's decision. Most patients expect to receive support and advice when they are determining a course of treatment or investigation but any influence must not be so forceful that it prevents the person from thinking for him/herself (Centre for Reproductive Medicine *v* U [2002]). The role of nurses and other professionals is arguably to help patients by outlining the treatment options, explaining the known risks and supporting the individual as they evaluate the options and the risks they are prepared to accept.

Clients with a neurological disorder can pose a particular challenge if the person has limited independence from relatives or carers. The way in which care is organised inevitably influences the behaviour and expectations of people who find themselves located within those systems (Weber, 1947). Nurses who are working alongside carers and relatives who are used to caring in a way that offers limited opportunities for clients to be independent, may find it challenging to gain consent from the client that is truly voluntary. In such circumstances, nurses have an important role to act as advocates for the individual, giving that person the chance to consider what he/she would like to happen and providing support to make that choice known (NMC, 2008).

Patients should receive appropriate information and in such a way that they are able to understand the proposed investigation or treatment, alternative options and the associated risks. In practice, this means nurses and other health professionals have a duty to explain in broad terms what a procedure involves. Failing to provide such an explanation will mean that the consent is invalid and the professional is liable to an action for trespass (Chatterton *v* Gerson and another [1981]) and/or negligence (Sidaway *v* Board of Governors of the Bethlem Royal Hospital and the Maudsley Hospital and others [1985]; Pearce and another *v* United Bristol Healthcare NHS Trust [1998]; Chester *v* Afshar [2004]).

Communication difficulties

The provision of information in an appropriate form can be problematic when caring for patients with a neurological disorder. The nature of such disorders means that some clients may have a reduced ability to understand information or to communicate about a decision to be made. Such a diminished ability, however, does not, in itself, mean that the person is unable to consent. In formulating the Mental Capacity Act 2005 the government took on board the Law Commission's (1995 paragraph 3.18) recommendation that:

'A person should not be regarded as unable to understand the information relevant to a decision if he or she is able to understand an explanation of that information in broad terms and simple language.'

Nurses have an obligation, therefore, to provide information about proposed investigations or treatments in a manner that is easily understood. This should be tailored to the needs and circumstances of the individual (Kennedy and Grubb, 2000) and is likely to require a team approach involving close working with specialist neurology teams, psychological services, occupational therapy, and speech and language therapy services. Guidance on how to produce accessible information is available from organisations such as MENCAP (2002).

Competency and mental capacity

Competency is the capacity to give or refuse consent. English law presupposes that each adult has such capacity, but that assumption can be challenged and rebutted. This is shown in the Mental Capacity Act 2005 (MCA – HMSO 2005), which applies in England and Wales to adults aged 16 and over, and was written specifically to promote patients' autonomy and to make clear the processes for caring adults with diminished capacity. The Act sets out key principles that should guide the care and treatment of adults (Box 36.2).

The threshold for competency depends on the risk associated with the decision. Professionals must think about

---

Box 36.2   Key principles of the Mental Capacity Act, 2005

- A person must be assumed to have capacity unless it is established that he lacks capacity
- A person is not to be treated as unable to make a decision unless all practicable steps to help him to do so have been taken without success
- A person is not to be treated as unable to make a decision merely because he makes an unwise decision
- An act done, or decision made, under this Act for or on behalf of a person who lacks capacity must be done, or made, in his best interests
- Before the act is done, or the decision is made, regard must be had to whether the purpose for which it is needed can be as effectively achieved in a way that is less restrictive of the person's rights and freedom of action

---

whether, at the time of making the decision, the individual has capacity commensurate with the seriousness of the decision he/she is being asked to make. A patient may have the competency to consent to some investigations or treatment (e.g. a CT scan) but lack the ability to consent to more serious ones (e.g. a craniotomy) as they are unable to understand the gravity or weigh up the risks and benefits associated with the intervention. This does not mean that patients who make seemingly 'unwise' medical choices (e.g. Jehovah's Witnesses who refuse blood transfusion) are incompetent. Rather, such choices (and the capacity underpinning them) should be seen within the individual's wider social, cultural and religious beliefs.

Temporary factors such as fear, pain, drugs or shock may also erode competency if they overwhelm the person's ability to take other issues into consideration when reaching a decision (Re: MB [1997]), but such factors do not in themselves amount to incompetence (Hendrick, 2000). Fear of the pain of a procedure may, for example, be a rational reason for refusing such a procedure.

As noted above, the MCA was written with the aim of promoting autonomy. Its first principle is that adults should be assumed to have capacity unless it is proven otherwise. The burden to demonstrate that a person lacks capacity lies with the health professional. According to the MCA lack of capacity exists when a person is:

'unable to make a decision for himself in relation to the matter [at hand] because of an impairment of, or a disturbance of the functioning of, the mind or brain'.

Mental Capacity Act 2005 (part 1, s.2, para.1)

The criteria for determining an inability to make decisions are detailed in Box 36.3.

The MCA specifies that when a decision is made or an action is undertaken on behalf of an incapacitated adult, the decision or action must be in their best interests. 'Best interests' should be thought of in the wider sense and not just 'best medical' or 'best physical' interests. Discussions of best interests should not include the age of the patient, their appearance, or aspects of their behaviour that might lead others to make unjust assumptions about what their best interests would be. It must also be considered whether the person will at some time have capacity in relation to the matter in question. It may be possible to delay making a decision until the patient is able to do so for themselves (e.g. once consciousness is regained). If the patient remains unable to make a decision, he or she must be encouraged to participate in any decision affecting him so far as is possible. If determination of best interests relates to

---

Box 36.3   Criteria for determining lack of capacity

The person must have an inability to:
- Understand the information relevant to the decision
- Retain that information
- Use or weigh that information as part of the process of making the decision
- Communicate a decision (whether by talking, using sign language or any other means)

Information relevant to making a decision includes information about the reasonably foreseeable consequences of deciding one way or another or failing to make the decision.

   The ability to retain the information relevant to a decision for only a short period does not prevent an individual from being regarded as able to make the decision (so-called 'consent in the moment').

Source: Mental Capacity Act, 2005.

Box 36.4   Main powers of the Mental Capacity Act, 2005

- Establish a revised Court of Protection, which will have the power to make declarations as to whether a person has capacity and the power to declare if an act or proposed act is or would be lawful
- The court will be able to make decisions about the personal welfare of a person lacking capacity or to appoint a deputy to do so instead
- Advance decisions will be given statutory recognition together with a presumption that valid advance decisions will be binding on those made aware of their contents
- Lasting powers of attorney will replace enduring powers of attorney and extend powers beyond financial and property matters into health and welfare decisions. Lasting powers of attorney will enable a person to nominate another to act on their behalf should they become incapacitated at a future date
- Court appointed deputies may be appointed by the Court of Protection to decide on matters of health, welfare and finance for incapable adults who have not appointed a lasting power of attorney prior to their incapacity
- Creates a new offence of ill-treatment or neglect of a person who lacks capacity

---

life-sustaining treatment, decisions must not be motivated by a desire to bring about the patient's death.

   Where possible the person's past and present wishes and feelings (especially any relevant written statement or advance decision made by him when he had capacity), his beliefs and values, and any other factors that the patient would be likely to consider if he were able to do so, must be taken into account. In addition, the views of anyone named by the person as someone to be consulted on matters of that kind, who is caring for the person or interested in his welfare, who has been granted lasting power of attorney, or who has been appointed by a court to act as a deputy in making decisions about 'best interests' should be sought if appropriate or practicable.

   The MCA contains formal measures for dealing with situations when a nurse or other health professional is providing care, treatment or investigations to adults who are incapable of consenting (Box 36.4). These include the creation of a revised Court of Protection, statutory recognition of advance decisions, the development of lasting powers of attorney, and the creation of court appointed deputies. NHS bodies will have to seek the advice of a consultee in making decisions relating to providing, withholding or withdrawing serious medical treatment or where it is proposed to move a person to a different care establishment or into long-term care in a hospital or care home.

HUMAN RIGHTS

Respect for human rights is core to nursing practice. Showing such respect enables nurses to treat people as individuals, to support them in making choices and to have appropriate regard for their wishes. Human rights rest on three key principles (Smith and van der Anker, 2005):

- Universal inherence (every person holds certain rights, which exist in them by virtue of their humanity alone)
- Inalienability (a person cannot be deprived of those rights by another or by their own acts)
- The rule of law

In the United Kingdom, the Human Rights Act (HRA) (HMSO, 1998) came into full force in October 2000. It incorporates into domestic UK law the bulk of rights from the European Convention for the Protection of Human Rights and Fundamental Freedoms (ECHR) – see Table 36.1.

Table 36.1 Articles and rights and freedoms incorporated in the Human Rights Act, 1998.

Article	Rights and freedoms
2	Right to life
3	Prohibition of torture
4	Prohibition of slavery and enforced labour
5	Right to liberty and security
6	Right to a fair trial
7	No punishment without law
8	Right to respect for private and family life
9	Freedom of thought, conscience and religion
10	Freedom of expression
11	Freedom of assembly and association
12	Right to marry
14	Prohibition of discrimination (NB this relates to enjoyment of the rights and freedoms set forth in the HRA)
16	Restrictions on political activity of aliens
17	Prohibition of abuse of rights
18	Limitation on use of restrictions on rights

The HRA regulates the relationship between the state and its citizens. It creates positive and negative obligations on the state and its public authorities (e.g. NHS hospital trusts, the courts and tribunals and public regulatory bodies such as the NMC). Positive obligations require the state (and its public authorities) to ensure that laws and policies are in place to protect citizens so that they may enjoy the rights and freedoms contained within the HRA. Negative obligations, by contrast, require the state and public authorities to refrain from breaching these rights.

The rights and freedoms contained within the HRA and ECHR are not all of equal weight. A distinction exists between absolute, limited and qualified rights. Examples of absolute rights include:

- Article 2 (the right to life)
- Article 3 (the prohibition of torture)
- Article 4 (the prohibition of slavery)

Absolute rights may not be breached in any circumstances.

Limited rights, such as Article 5 (the right to liberty and security) contain limited explicit exceptions which are set out in the ECHR itself. For example, Article 5 (1) (a) allows for the lawful detention of someone convicted of a crime by a legitimate court.

Finally, qualified rights may be derogated (i.e. partially relaxed) where such derogation has a basis in law (Griffiths, 2005).

Although none of the rights and freedoms set out in the HRA is specifically health related, a number of cases that link health care decisions to the ECHR have already been presented before the courts (e.g. R v MHRT, North and East London, ex p. H 2001; R v MHRT, ex p. KB 2002).

Deprivation of liberty and restraint

A case involving a client living in the community who was transferred to an in-patient facility, is that of HL v United Kingdom (45508/99) (2004) (also known as the Bournewood case, after the Community and Mental Health NHS Trust involved). This centred on a man (HL) living in the community with severe autism and a history of self-harming, who lacked the capacity to give or withhold consent to treatment. HL became disturbed whilst at a day centre, hitting himself on the head with his fists and banging his head against a wall. He was assessed as needing in-patient treatment but was not admitted to the in-patient facility under a section of the Mental Health Act 1983 because he did not resist admission. HL's carers asked for his discharge, but the psychiatrist in charge of HL's care considered that this would not be in his best interests. The carers, acting on HL's behalf, challenged this decision and sought a review of its legality, which was eventually heard before the European Court of Human Rights.

Nurses coping with this type of scenario are faced with tensions between a desire to respect the freedom and autonomy of individuals to live in a place of their choosing and the need to protect vulnerable people from harm. In Bournewood, the court criticised the UK for failing to demonstrate adequate procedures to safeguard individuals against arbitrary deprivation of liberty. The court held that, because there was no procedure prescribed by law for authorising an admission in HL's circumstances, this was a breach of Article 5 (1) of the ECHR (the right to liberty) and Article 5 (4) (the right to have the lawfulness of detention decided speedily by a court). In response, the UK government has developed Deprivation of Liberty Safeguards (DoLS), which came into force in 2009 and provide transparent processes that can be challenged.

Box 36.5   Factors that contribute to deprivation of liberty

* Staff exercised complete and effective control over care and movement for a significant period
* A decision has been taken that the person would be prevented from leaving if they made a meaningful attempt to do so
* A request by carers for the person to be discharged to their care was refused
* The person was unable to maintain social contacts because of restrictions placed on access to other people and
* The person lost autonomy because they were under continuous supervision and control

Adapted from: *Deprivation of liberty safeguards code of practice* (Department of Health, 2008).

The code of practice for the DoLS (DH, 2008) states that there is no simple definition of what constitutes deprivation of liberty, but lists factors that courts have, to date, found to contribute to deprivations of liberty (Box 36.5). Many practices carried out 'in the patient's best interests' such as holding their hands or removing mobility aids, using boxing gloves or electronic tagging/locked ward doors, and all forms of restraint, could be considered to be breaching the patient's right to liberty. Legal and ethical issues relating to restraint are discussed further in Chapter 10.

The DoLS legislation requires that whenever a hospital or care home identifies a person who lacks capacity is being (or risks being) deprived of their liberty they must apply to the 'supervisory body' for permission to provide care in that way. For people in care homes the supervisory body will be the local authority, whilst for people in hospitals this will be the PCT (in England).

RESOURCE ALLOCATION

It is not uncommon for practitioners and managers to be faced with competing (but equally worthy) sets of patient demands. Neurological conditions are common and their clinical significance for patients and carers is recognised in government policy (DH, 2005). As an overarching group, diseases of the nervous system 'represent the greatest – and still increasing – public health burden that western societies are facing' (Illes and Racine, 2007).

A consequence of this clinical significance has been 20 years of investment and advancement in neuroscience research and development (Blank, 2007). The end of the last century and the beginning of the current one have seen a rapid increase of knowledge into how the brain and nervous system work, supported by a growth of technology in areas such as neuroimaging, neurophysiology and neuroembryology (Kandel *et al.*, 2000). As such, neuroscience represents an area of supercomplexity.

Part of this supercomplexity is the tension between the growing potential to treat illnesses, levels of demand or need (as above), and the limited financial resources that are available for governments to spend. While health care receives a large amount of funding (£105 billion in the UK in 2007/08), decisions on which work to undertake within the allocated budget have to be made every day. Decisions are made at many levels, but those of most relevance to nursing are made at an organisational (meso) level (e.g. which services to fund) or at an individual (micro) level (e.g. health care teams deciding which patients to see and what care to provide). The NHS Act (OPSI, 2006) requires the provision of health services to meet all *reasonable* requirements (e.g. hospital services, medical, dental, nursing and ambulance services, maternity services, primary care services). The Act does not require *all* demands to be met and this has been recognised in case law.

Frameworks have been devised to outline steps for the fair allocation of scarce health care resources (Daniels, 2000; Pencheon *et al.*, 2001). These frameworks rely heavily on providing care and treatment that are both evidence-based and cost-effective. For England and Wales the National Institute for Health and Clinical Excellence (NICE) will often make decisions about the provision of treatment on the basis of systematic reviews of the evidence, such as NHS funding of drugs for dementia. While their decisions are not always popular with all concerned, the decision making process is transparent and nurses, patients and other stakeholders are able to present their views during public consultation.

One developing mechanism whereby nurses can get directly involved with the allocation of resources is through commissioning. Commissioning is simply a set of planned activities undertaken with the aim of achieving measurable improvements in the health and well-being of a population (Drennan and Goodman, 2007). It uses processes of change management to ensure the most effective and efficient use of resources (Drennan and Goodman, 2007; LNNM, 2007).

RISK MANAGEMENT

Health care is not automatically a benign activity and the interventions that we use in nursing care can cause harm in themselves. There are approximately 850,000 adverse events in hospital each year: a rate of 10% of all hospital admissions (DH, 2000). Restraint, for example, is a risky intervention because it is associated with poor patient outcomes including higher mortality rates, increases in hospitalisation, health care acquired infections, pressure sores and worsening levels of confusion (Waterhouse, 2007) (see Chapter 10). There is a clear need, therefore, for nurses to play an active role in risk management.

Risk management (RM) is a process involving the identification, selection and evaluation of measures to reduce hazards to human health (i.e. an attempt to prevent harm befalling patients (non-maleficence), staff and others). In the UK, the Health and Safety at Work Act (HMSO, 1974) and the Management of Health and Safety at Work Regulations (HMSO, 1999) place a statutory duty on employers and employees to make sure that all reasonable steps have been taken to ensure the safety of staff, patients, visitors and the general public.

In order for a risk to be managed it must first be identified, including both estimation and evaluation of potential hazards. Statistics about past events are collated (e.g. previous complaints and critical incident forms) and can be used to make judgements about the likelihood of future adverse occurrences. In addition, nurses and other health professionals should consider factors that influence practice and identify areas of concern in the clinical setting that may lead to untoward outcomes before they happen (see Table 36.2).

Once risks have been recognised, the next stage is to prioritise and determine the possible options for handling the risk. Risk strategies incorporate risk control, risk acceptance and risk avoidance, all of which can be used individually or in combination to suit the needs of the situation at hand (Wilson, 2003). It is not always possible to eliminate a risk completely, so control measures are used to lessen the probability of an adverse occurrence (e.g. moving and handling training; protocols and guidelines).

Table 36.2 A framework of factors that can influence risk in clinical practice.

Factor type	Influencing and contributory factors	Examples
Institutional context	Economic and regulatory context, central government policies	Inconsistent policies, funding problems
Organisational and management factors	Financial resources and constraints, organisational structure, policy standards and aims, safety culture (or lack thereof) and priorities	Lacking senior management involvement and support for risk reduction
Work environment	Staffing levels and skill mix, workload and shift patterns, design of buildings and units/wards, design, availability of maintenance for resources; administrative and managerial support	High workload, inadequate staffing, limited access to essential equipment
Team factors	Communication (verbal and written), supervision and seeking help, competency and use of information and communication technology, team structures (consistency and leadership)	Poor communication between staff
Individual staff factors	Knowledge and skills, understanding, attitude, physical and mental health	Lack of knowledge or experience of specific staff
Task factors	Task design and clarity of structures, availability and use of protocols (such as in the use of restraint), availability and use of results	Non-availability of test results or protocols
Patient factors	Condition (complexity, seriousness, presence of challenging behaviour); language and communication, personality and social factors	Distressed patients or family, language barriers, poor social circumstances (such as inadequate housing)

Adapted from Vincent *et al.*, 2000.

Risk acceptance is used in situations when it is not possible to control or avoid the risk. In particular, it is employed when the probability of a risk is high but the possible consequences of the hazard are within the organisation's and individual's level of acceptability. It is important to note, however, that judgements of acceptability may differ for health care organisations and individual patients or staff. Organisations are likely to view an acceptable risk as one that is within their financial ability to meet the cost incurred, whereas individuals may focus more on the emotional burden associated with the harm.

Risk avoidance occurs when a particularly serious threat exists that cannot be otherwise controlled or reduced. In such situations, the cost likely to be incurred (financial or otherwise) is so high as to make the perceived risk unacceptable. The only option available then is to change the way practice is delivered in order to avoid the risk happening at all.

Resources to support the development of effective risk management and quality care are available through the National Patient Safety Agency (NPSA) in England and Wales. The NPSA was set up as part of the clinical governance agenda and includes a means to report patient safety incidents as well as data on incidents (at a national and organisational level), guidance to overcome identified risks (including alerts and rapid response reports), and tools to promote an open culture within teams. Further details can be found on the NPSA website: www.npsa.nhs.uk.

END OF LIFE CARE

Perhaps one of the most difficult ethical and clinical areas to consider is that of end of life care. This is a highly emotive subject area that is sometimes complicated by the reality that many health care professionals regard death as a failure of their treatment (Montgomery, 2003). From a physiological point of view, death is regarded as the ending of the biological functions necessary to sustain life. However, is it difficult to view death as a moment in isolation and instead it should be considered in light of the continuum from the beginning of life to its end.

In order to facilitate any discussion on end of life care, it is necessary to first reflect on what it means to be alive and, therefore, if death can ever be considered a good option. It has been argued that sometimes the mere state of being alive is always better than not, though this view will then lead on to discussions regarding quality of life and when quality of life begins to take precedent over quantity.

If we consider the case of someone on a ventilator with no expectation of recovery; whilst in one sense they are

being kept 'alive' and could be said to be experiencing life, this cannot be equated to their experience of life prior to this illness. The same may hold for a person with severe dementia whose quality of life may have so deteriorated that death (i.e. non-existence) could be viewed as good or preferable. Here it is possible to begin to see how levels of functioning need to be added into considerations of what it means to be alive or to living a good life.

The philosopher Aristotle (2003) discusses this in terms of flourishing or doing that which you are designed to do and Foot (1978) takes the view that there is a level of basic human life someone should be functioning at, including concepts of freedom of choice and safety. From an ethical point of view both argue that merely being alive is not necessarily good in itself but that there are higher levels of being (associated with fulfilling your purpose or meaning) that make life good. It is often in consideration of this that we gain some understanding of when suicide or assisted suicide might be the right choice to be made from an ethical point of view and so discussions regarding euthanasia begin.

Euthanasia

When thinking about end of life care and euthanasia it is important to distinguish between the different terms used. Harris (1985 p82) defines euthanasia as 'the implementation of a decision that the life of a particular individual will come to an end before it need do so'. Although true, this definition fails to acknowledge that the motivation underpinning the decision is to bring about a 'good' death (however 'good' may be defined): this is shown by the prefix 'eu', meaning well or easily. It is also important to differentiate between the types of euthanasia that might be enacted (see Box 36.6). Unfortunately, there is no clear agreement within the literature on how these terms are used and one can often find them employed synonymously, which adds to confusion (Herring, 2006).

A distinction can be made in end of life care regarding the voluntariness of the act (see Box 36.6), i.e. if the action is in line with the patient's wishes or not. Reflecting on the principle of respect for autonomy (Beauchamp and Childress, 2009) if a competent patient does not wish treatment, it would be unethical to overrule their decision as that would mean placing greater weight on the decisions of health care professionals over that of the patient. With this in mind, voluntary passive euthanasia (whereby treatment might be withdrawn at a patient's request, even though the end result is death) is entirely within the law and ethical. This relies on having an understanding of what the patient would choose and increasingly patients are

---

Box 36.6   Definitions

Assisted suicide (often referred to as physician-assisted suicide):

Providing the means for someone to end their own life (e.g. a physician prescribing a drug, which the patient then administers to themselves or gets a third-party to administer)

This upholds the principle of autonomy, enabling the patient to fulfil their own wishes regarding their treatment.

Active euthanasia:

Committing a positive act (such as administering a drug) with the primary intention of causing death

If voluntary, this upholds the principle of autonomy, allowing the patient to fulfil their own wishes regarding their treatment. However there is tension if death is not viewed as a good outcome, you would not be carrying out a beneficent act and would also be maleficent as you would be causing a person harm. This is often seen to clearly be the case with involuntary active euthanasia.

Passive euthanasia:

Withdrawing or withholding treatment with the primary intention of causing death (i.e. 'allowing someone to die')

Again the perceived rightness of the act is based on whether the outcome is deemed to be good or bad, and therefore if we appear to be causing harm to the patient or not.

Active and passive can be further subdivided as follows (e.g. voluntary active, involuntary active and so on):

Voluntary euthanasia:

Behaviour to cause the patient's death at the express wish of a competent patient

Once more this upholds the principle of autonomy, allowing the patient to fulfil their own wishes regarding their treatment.

Non-voluntary euthanasia:

An act to cause the patient's death where the patient is unable to consent or object (e.g. due to unconsciousness)

The principles of non-maleficence and beneficence are used here to determine the merit of the act.

Involuntary euthanasia:

Behaviour to cause a competent patient to die against their expressed wishes – some argue that this should not be classed euthanasia as it goes against the notion of a 'good' death

This could only be upheld ethically if the death of the person is in some way deemed to be a greater good than their right to stay alive.

Adapted from Montgomery, 2003; Herring, 2006.

---

choosing to write advance decisions or 'living wills' to outline what interventions they would want in certain predetermined circumstances if they lose decision making capacity at a later date. When practitioners do not know what a patient wants then the patient should be treated in their best interests (NMC, 2008; GMC, 2006).

This concept is founded upon upholding the principles of beneficence and non-maleficence and so our intervention should aim to do good, but if we cannot guarantee that, at the very least our intervention should not harm our patient. Again, this still leads us to make a decision founded upon our own views of good in terms of health outcomes and this increases the risk that the intervention (or non intervention) might not be what the patient would have chosen.

In recognition of the growing use of advance decisions, the Mental Capacity Act 2005 in England and Wales is an example of legislatures tightening up the legal standing of such documents, and also allows a person to appoint someone as proxy to make decisions regarding their health if they are incapable of doing so. Any such documentation must be regarded as legal and valid, and the wishes of a proxy must also be adhered to, so it is vital to ascertain if any such documentation has been completed.

Withdrawing and withholding treatment

The different categories of euthanasia are used to frame discussions around withdrawing or withholding treatment. The GMC (2006) has produced guidance on decision making in this area, ensuring appropriate treatment is given to dying patients, whilst making sure that actions remain within the law. They highlight the concern of either over or under-treating dying patients. It is undesirable to continue to treat patients or initiate new therapies which are unlikely to benefit the patient. In doing so, it would be difficult to argue that we were doing good for that patient, and it could be argued that we were harming the patient by unnecessarily prolonging the natural process of death. Conversely, we do not want to withdraw treatment too soon, and any decision to withdraw care also has to be made in light of the process of weighing up any likely benefit of continuation of therapy.

Physician assisted suicide

When considering euthanasia, it is important to remember that whilst we might ethically be able to defend our actions, they might not be legal. Physician assisted suicide is illegal in the UK. However care may be provided that falls under the bracket of passive euthanasia, i.e. when there might be treatment that we could give to prolong life, however it is not seen to be in the patient's best interests to do this and so the natural dying process is facilitated.

Physician assisted suicide is permissible in Switzerland and there have been a number of high profile cases of British citizens travelling to Dignitas to end their life. Patients cannot legally be prevented from travelling to Switzerland to take advantage of this service, but anyone supporting someone to do this could be found guilty of aiding or abetting suicide under the 1961 Suicide Act, a crime punishable by imprisonment for up to fourteen years. Famously in 2001 Dianne Pretty, a 42-year-old woman with motor neurone disease, fought for the right for her husband to help her end her life, and not be prosecuted (Pretty v. Director of Public Prosecutions and Secretary of State for Home Department [2001]). Whilst the judge stated that this was a very sad case, it was felt that the 1961 Suicide Act would have to be followed if her husband was found to assist her to end her life.

This ruling was challenged in 2008 where Debbie Purdy, a 41-year-old woman with multiple sclerosis wanted to travel to make use of Dignitas, but did not want her husband to be prosecuted on his return to England (R (on the application of Purdy) v Director of Public Prosecutions [2008]). Again the judge upheld the principles of the 1961 Suicide Act and said that only a change in legislation from Parliament would allow them to judge differently. Just prior to this ruling, Daniel James, a 23-year-old man with spinal injuries, flew to Switzerland to end his life at the Dignitas clinic. Every such case is

investigated by the Crown Prosecution Service, but as yet no relative who has helped someone die in this way has been prosecuted. In the light of this, there is increasing debate and calls to change the law, which has resulted in new guidelines being issued.

Care pathways

When planning for end of life care, patient involvement is paramount and it is essential that health care professionals work with the patient to explain the options available throughout the progression of a disease. Any planning should take place with family members or carers, especially if someone has been appointed as a proxy. It is not always possible for patients to plan for their death (for example, if someone was brought in to hospital unconscious after sustaining a head injury), but the same principles apply and health care staff should seek to understand what the patient would want if they were able to speak.

Protocols such as the Liverpool Care Pathway (LCP) for the Dying Patient (Marie Curie Palliative Care Institute, 2009) and Gold Standards Framework (NHS End of Life Care Programme, 2005) are increasingly being utilised to ensure that appropriate care is given. With their roots in the philosophy of care founded by the hospice movement, these pathways are designed to ensure that patients receive appropriate end of life care, regardless of the cause of illness or the care environment. Although designed to focus primarily on the last days and hours of life for cancer patients, the LCP has already been modified to cover the care of the dying patient in the intensive care setting. Both pathways aim to ensure that patients are involved in their care and are able to state what they want to happen to themselves when they are no longer able to speak for themselves. Through the process of advance care planning, decisions regarding end of life care can be made in a timely manner within a supportive environment (NHS National End of Life Care Programme, 2009). Although end of life care may remain a difficult area to work within, when faced with uncertainty the application of legal and ethical principles can provide frameworks to ensure that care is planned in a suitable manner.

SUMMARY

At its core, nursing is about making decisions: choices over what resources to use, what treatments to give or withhold, when to intervene in someone's life and when not to. This chapter has explored some of the decisions neuroscience nurses can be faced with on a day to day basis.

REFERENCES

Aristotle (2003) *Ethics Translated*. In: JAK Thomson, H Tredennick and J Barnes (eds). London: Penguin Classics.

Beauchamp TL, Childress (2009) *Principles of Biomedical Ethics* (9th edition). Oxford: Oxford University Press.

Bentham J (2000) *Selected Writings on Utilitarianism*. Chatham: Wordsworth Editions Limited.

Blank RH (2007) Policy implications of the new neuroscience. *Cambridge Quarterly of Healthcare Ethics* 16:169–180.

Centre for Reproductive Medicine *v* U [2002] EWCA 565.

Chatterton *v* Gerson and another [1981] QB 432.

Chester *v* Afshar [2004] UKHL 41.

Daniels N (2000) Accountability for reasonableness in private and public health insurance. In: Coulter A, Ham C (eds). *The Global Challenge of Health Care Rationing*. Buckingham: Open University Press.

Department of Health (2000) *An Organisation with a Memory*. London: The Stationery Office.

Department of Health (2005) *National Service Framework for Long Term Conditions*. London: DH.

Department of Health (2008) *Deprivation of Liberty Safeguards Code of Practice*. London: The Stationery Office. Available from: www.dh.gov.uk/prod_consum_dh/groups/dh_digitalassets/@dh/@en/documents/digitalasset/dh_087309.pdf (Accessed July 2010).

Drennan V, Goodman C (eds) (2007) *Oxford Handbook of Primary Care and Community Nursing*. Oxford: Oxford University Press.

Foot P (1978) *Virtue and Vices and other Essays in Moral Philosophy*. Oxford: Basil.

General Medical Council (2006) *Withholding and Withdrawing Life-prolonging Treatments: Good practice in decision-making*. London: GMC. Available from: http://www.gmc-uk.org/guidance/ethical_guidance/witholding_lifeprolonging_guidance.asp Accessed July 2010.

Gillon R (1986) *Philosophical Medical Ethics*. Chichester: Wiley.

Griffiths R (2005) Human rights and district nursing practice. *British Journal of Community Nursing* 10(2):86–91.

Harris J (1985) *The Value of Life*. London: Routledge.

Hendrick J (2000) *Law and Ethics in Nursing and Health Care*. Cheltenham: Stanley Thornes.

Her Majesty's Stationery Office (1974) *Health and Safety at Work Act*. London: HMSO.

Her Majesty's Stationery Office (1998) *Human Rights Act*. London: HMSO. Available from: http://www.opsi.gov.uk/ACTS/acts1998/ukpga_19980042_en_1 Accessed July 2010.

Her Majesty's Stationery Office (1999) *Management of Health and Safety at Work Regulations*. London: HMSO.

Her Majesty's Stationery Office (2005) *Mental Capacity Act*. Available from: www.opsi.gov.uk/acts/acts2005 Accessed July 2010.

Herring J (2006) *Medical Law and Ethics*. Oxford: Oxford University Press.

HL *v* United Kingdom (2004) European Court of Human Rights (Application number: 45508/99)

Illes J, Racine E (2007) Guest editorial: neuroethics – from neurotechnology to healthcare. *Cambridge Quarterly of Healthcare Ethics* 16:125–127.

Kandel ER, Schwartz JH, Jessell TM (2000) *Principles of Neural Science* (4th edition). London: McGraw-Hill Publishing.

Kant I (1948) *The Moral Law: The groundwork of the metaphysics of morals*. Translated: HJ Patton. London: Routledge.

Kennedy I, Grubb A (2000) *Medical Law: Text and materials*. Oxford: Oxford University Press.

Law Commission (1995) *Mental Incapacity*. Law Commission report 231. London: Law Commission.

London Network for Nurses and Midwives (2007) *Commissioning a Patient-Led NHS: A toolkit for nurses*. London: LNNM PCG. Available from: http://www.rcn.org.uk/newsevents/news/article/london/primary_care_toolkit_from_the_london_network_for_nurses_and_midwives (Accessed July 2010).

Marie Curie Palliative Care Institute (2009) *Liverpool Care Pathway for the dying patient (LCP)*. Liverpool: MCPCIL. Available from: http://www.liv.ac.uk/mcpcil/liverpool-care-pathway/ (Accessed July 2010).

Marks-Maran D (1996) Accountability. In: V Tschudin (ed). *Ethics: Nurses and patients*. London: Bailliere-Tindall.

MENCAP (2002) *Am I Making Myself Clear? Mencap's guidelines for accessible writing*. London: MENCAP.

Mill JS (1991) *On Liberty and Other Essays*. J Gray (ed). Oxford: Oxford University Press.

Montgomery J (2003) *Health Care Law*. (2nd edition). Padstow: Oxford University Press.

NHS National End of Life Care Programme (2005) *The Gold Standards Framework*. Available from: http://www.goldstandardsframework.nhs.uk/ Accessed July 2010.

NHS National End of Life Care Programme (2009) *Advance care planning* Available from: http://www.endoflifecareforadults.nhs.uk/publications/advance-care-planning-national-guideline Accessed July 2010.

Nursing and Midwifery Council (2008) *Code of Professional Conduct*. London: NMC.

Office of Public Sector Information (2006) *NHS Act*. Available from: http://www.opsi.gov.uk/acts/acts2006/ukpga_20060041_en_2#pt1-pb1-l1g1 Accessed July 2010.

Pearce and another *v* United Bristol Healthcare NHS Trust [1998] AC 48

Pencheon D, Guest C, Melzer D, Muir Gray JA (2001) *Oxford Handbook of Public Health Practice*. Oxford: Oxford University Press.

Pretty *v* Director of Public Prosecutions and Secretary of State for Home Department [2001] EWHC Admin 788.

R *v* MHRT, North and East London, ex p. H (2001) EWCA Civ 415.

R *v* MHRT, ex p. KB (2002) EWHC Admin 639.

R (on the application of Purdy) *v* Director of Public Prosecutions [2008] EWHC 2565 and [2008] WLR (D) 337. Re: MB [1997] 2 FLR 426.

S *v* S; W *v* Official Solicitor [1972] AC 24

Sidaway *v* Board of Governors of the Bethlem Royal Hospital and the Maudsley Hospital and others [1985] AC 871.

Smith RKM, van der Anker C (2005) *The Essentials of Human Rights*. London: Hodder Arnold.

Thomson A (1999) *Critical Reasoning in Ethics: A Practical Introduction*. London: Routledge.

Vincent C, Taylor-Adams S, Chapman EJ *et al.* (2000) How to investigate and analyse clinical incidents: Clinical Risk Unit and Association of Litigation and Risk Management protocol. *British Medical Journal* 320:777–781.

Waterhouse C (2007) Development of a tool for risk assessment to facilitate safety and appropriate restraint. *British Journal of Neuroscience Nursing* 3(9):421–426.

Weber M (1947) *The Theory of Social and Economic Organizations*. Trans. AM Henderson and T Parsons. London: Oxford University Press.

Wilson J (2003) Risk reviews and using risk management strategy. In: Wilson J, Tingle J (eds). *Clinical Risk Modification: A route to clinical governance?* Edinburgh: Butterworth Heinemann.

37

The History and Development of Neuroscience Nursing

Thom Aird

'Whether your work lies in medical or surgical nursing, you will hear constant reference made to the nervous system; and the more you read about its functions, the more you will be struck by the wonderful results which are achieved by the nerve centres and nerve cords, which have been often compared to a set of telegraph wires between the galvanic centre and the various distant points to which they are distributed.'

(Norris 1891 p63)

THE BACKGROUND TO A DEVELOPING SPECIALISM

Until the mid seventeenth century medical practices were based predominantly on the Hippocratic theory that health and illness represented a balance or imbalance of body fluids or humours. These fluids, generated in different parts of the body and circulated as needed, were considered to be of far greater importance than the solid, hollow organs within the body cavities. Bile and phlegm were only visible when secreted during illness. Seasonal attachments were also made, with winter colds ascribed to phlegm, and summer dysentery and vomiting to bile. National characteristics were often ascribed to the effects of humours. Inhabitants of the north were described as white, flabby, cold and phlegmatic, in contrast to the swarthy hot, dry, bilious inhabitants of the south. Both were considered inferior to the Greeks who lived in a well-balanced harmonious climate.

Blood was viewed with a sense of ambiguity but was recognised to be of importance to life; it was however, a fluid that was visibly ejected from the body during menstruation, nose bleeds, and piles. This observation formed the basis of a treatment which remained in practice for centuries – blood letting. In terms of nervous disorders, epilepsy was thought to be caused by phlegm generated in the head which formed a thick barrier to the passage of air. In mania or melancholy, bile was 'boiling in the brain' (Nutton, 1995). Galen, for example, practicing Hippocratic medicine in the second century, advocated blood letting. He was:

'convinced that nature prevented disease by discharging excess blood'

pointing out that:

'menstruation spared women many diseases – gout, epilepsy and apoplexy.'

(Porter, 1999 p77)

Holmes (1954) acknowledges that Hippocrates recognised that paralysis and convulsions, delirium and other disturbances of mind may result from cerebral disease. He also recognised that injury to one side of the head could result in paralysis of the opposite side of the body. This, however, he linked to the all important circulation and distribution of fluid. Aristotle believed the heart to be the organ of mental activities. He argued that since the brain was insensitive to direct stimulation such as cutting or burning, the brain could not be the organ of sensory perception.

The term 'neurology' was defined by Thomas Willis in 1664 as meaning 'the doctrine (or teaching) of the nerves' (Feindel 1999). In 1664 his book *Cerebri Anatome*

Neuroscience Nursing: Evidence-Based Practice, 1st Edition.
Edited by Sue Woodward and Ann-Marie Mestecky
© 2011 Blackwell Publishing Ltd

(anatomy of the brain) was published. Willis traced and classified the cranial nerves and importantly located functions of the brain to the solid parts of the cerebrum and cerebellum. This differed from existing theories based on the movement of fluids which had placed the emphasis on the 'hollow parts' of the brain, the ventricular system, because:

> 'they stored, processed and distributed the important juices.'
> (Martensen, 1999 p19).

During the nineteenth century psychiatric illnesses were classified into two major groups: organic illness and functional illness (Kandel, 2006). The classifications emerged from post-mortem examinations of the brains of mental patients. The methods available for examining the brain at that time were too limited to detect subtle anatomical changes. As a result, only mental disorders that entailed significant loss of nerve cells and brain tissue, such as Alzheimer's disease and Huntington's disease were classified as organic, or based in biology. Schizophrenia, the various forms of depression and anxiety states produced no loss of nerve cells or other obvious changes in brain anatomy and therefore were classified as functional, or not based in biology. Shorter puts it succinctly and says that:

> 'what Nissl and Alzheimer could find under their microscopes they declared 'neurology'. What they couldn't find was psychiatry.'
>
> (Shorter, 1997 p109)

Youngson and Schott (1996) believe that, while waiting for the 'mental diseases' to be discovered, neurologists resorted to various nonsensical forms of pseudo-diagnostic terminology. Patients were suffering from '*nervous prostration, nervous disintegration and neurasthenia*'. Indeed the two most common conditions often referred to in the literature are hysteria and neurasthenia. Shepherd refers to an American neurologist who suggested that:

> 'finding the patient lachrymose and emotional (the doctor) calls the disorder hysteria; if depressed and inert he calls it neurasthenia.'
>
> (see Shepherd, 2002 p9)

During the nineteenth century one of the most significant figures in the new emerging field of neurology was Jean Martin Charcot. As chief physician at the Saltpetriere in Paris he developed an interest in neurological illness. Charcot had a particular interest in hysteria believing it to be:

> 'a real organic disease transmitted genetically and associated with presumptive but unidentified changes in nervous tissue.'
> (see Shorter 1997 p85)

Indeed Caplan (2001) makes reference to the concept of '*hidden organicity*.' Charcot is remembered for his use of hypnosis in both diagnosis and developing his ideas on the aetiology of hysteria.

Youngson and Schott (1996) suggest that half the patients being treated by psychiatrists were suffering from a condition with a recognised organic origin, e.g. syphilis or arteriosclerosis, while:

> 'neurologists, armed with their reflex hammers, their tuning forks and their ophthalmoscopes for peering into eyes and their pins kept trying to tell people whose complaints were entirely psychological that they had a disease.'
>
> (see Youngson and Schott, 1996 p293)

When following the work of Gall phrenology, Youngson and Schott believe that 'feeling the bumps on peoples heads gave them something to do with their hands.' Shorter suggests however that by the second half of the nineteenth century multiple sclerosis could be distinguished from hysteria, or general paralysis from hypochondria.

> 'If patients toppled over after you asked them to stand up straight with their eyes closed (Romberg's sign), they probably had neurosyphilis not nerves.'
>
> (see Shorter, 1997 p129)

BIRTH OF A SPECIALISM

The first General Court of the Governors and Subscribers of the Hospital for the Paralysed and Epileptic, London, met on March 19th 1860 and Rubin (1960) indicates that on that day a resolution was passed that the hospital be opened and start receiving patients (Rubin, 1960). This was the first hospital in the world established for the treatment of neurological disease and acts as a reference point for the origins of neuroscience nursing. The prime movers in the foundation of the hospital were Johanna, Louisa and Edward Chandler, who were faced with caring for their paralysed grandmother. Although their grandmother died, the family became aware of the problems encountered by others with such problems.

To establish such a hospital at this time was risky. Specialist hospitals were frowned upon by those in general medicine and surgery. Granshaw (1989) estimates that by 1860 London alone was served by at least 66 special hospitals, ranging from hospitals for eyes, to consumption and cancer. Specialist hospitals were relatively easy to establish, the practitioner usually renting a house or just a couple of rooms and installing a few beds in the care of a residential matron and perhaps a house surgeon. Maida Vale Hospital, for example, was founded in 1866 as the London Infirmary for Epilepsy and Paralysis. It initially functioned on an outpatient basis only, admitting patients from 1868. In 1873 it was renamed the Hospital for Epilepsy and Paralysis. In 1948 it was amalgamated with the National Hospital to form the National Hospital for Nervous Diseases (Feiling, 1958).

During the 1850s the British Medical Journal ran a campaign against the establishment of specialist hospitals, suggesting that they serve no useful purpose. They held the opinion that such institutions starved the general hospitals of the kind of cases which were so instructive to medical students stating that they:

'will never furnish great surgeons or advance the art beyond mere manipulative smartness.'

(see Abel-Smith, 1963 p163)

The resentment towards specialist hospitals was also expressed by Queen Victoria who, upon the founding of the London Cancer Hospital in 1851, refused patronage declining to:

'contribute to a hospital devoted exclusively to a single malady when those who suffered from it were not excluded from general hospitals.'

(see Weinreb 1983 p676)

Between 1870 and 1880 30–40% of indoor patients suffered from epilepsy. By 1929 the proportion had fallen to less than 5%. This simply reflected a change in the approach to the management of such patients, and especially drug regimes. By the 1930s it was widely recognised that drug therapy alone was not the solution. MacFarlane advocated the attendance at school or work believing that:

'enforced idleness has a deleterious effect on the individual, and mental boredom is almost as potent a precipitory factor as intellectual or emotional excitement.'

(MacFarlane, 1930 p614)

The social implications of neurological disease are, however, addressed within appeals to the press. Highlighting that paralysis 'spares neither age nor class' the National Hospital presented a case for donations to allow extension to the existing research in cause and treatment. More important is the acknowledgement that a number of diseases are still incurable and that the hospital committee would like to:

'provide small pensions for some of the more destitute sufferers.'

(Gower, 1960 p6)

In 1909 King Edward VII opened a new wing of the National Hospital. In a letter to the secretary of the board of management which was sent following the opening, he praised the work of the hospital stating:

'The remarkable growth in the number of attendances and the increase in the accommodation required both for in and out patients is evidence of the utility of your work and of the zeal and energy with which it is carried on. While I consider the nature of the maladies for which provision is made in your hospital I do not wonder that it should have aroused the charitable instincts of the benevolent and called forth the enthusiastic service and devotion of your medical and nursing staff. Sufferers from paralysis and epilepsy are as helpless, so utterly dependent for their very existence on the exertions of others, that without such institutions as the National Hospital many of the poor, who can afford no general appliances and no efficient medical attendance, must inevitably be reduced, with their families, to the greatest of miseries.'

(National Hospital, 1909)

Holmes (1954) writes that, in the first fifty years of the hospital's existence, a number of patients were admitted who had given a history of consumption and typhoid. A number were classed as insane, but probably were suffering from some form of organic neurological disorder. One patient, a girl of fourteen, was admitted with polyneuritis. She gave a history of having been sent out to work as a dressmaker, got very wet and cold and sat in her clothes all day. Soon after the exposure to damp the peripheral sensation in her hands and feet diminished, and two days later she became paralysed. The average length of stay for in-patients was three to six months and comments reflect the limited treatments available: *'same condition'*, *'discharge in status quo'*.

From a nursing perspective, Domville writes a slightly cautionary note, describing paralysis as:

'very troublesome and wearying for the nurse as well as for the patient, their course being usually from bad to worse and there seems to be little chance of any credit being obtained for the management of them.'

(Domville, 1907 p86)

It was not until the cessation of the Second World War (1939–1945), however that the specialism would substantially grow. Rivett (1998) points out that the developments in descriptive neurology and neurosurgery largely preceded the National Health Service. He describes the specialism as being centred on the accuracy of diagnosis, with very little treatment being available. The general nursing treatment of nervous diseases is described by Down as:

> *'consisting namely of rest, fresh air, and healthy interests or occupations. Nourishing food in abundance is more essential in these cases than in almost any others. The diet should be generous unless sickness is present.'*
>
> (Down 1922, p297)

In the period prior to the commencement of the National Health Service, the Royal College of Physicians committee on neurology, seeing a need to develop the speciality outside London, recommended the development of active neurological centres in all medical teaching centres, in which neurology, neurosurgery and psychiatry could work together (Rivett, 1998). Subsequent developments in biochemistry, immunology, radiography, genetics, pharmacology and surgical techniques, to name a few, have all had a major impact on the on-going development of the specialism.

EPILEPSY

The stigma and plight of patients suffering from epilepsy was highlighted in a pamphlet *Notes on Epileptics in Workhouses*, published in 1867 by the Committee of the Lady Samaritan Society of the hospital. Epileptic patients were described as 'the pariahs of benevolence'. This refers to the limited opportunities for employment of any sort for such patients and the 'peculiar nature of their affliction'. More importantly, however, is the danger facing such patients when almost all hospitals and convalescent hospitals refuse entry to such patients. The pamphlet warns that:

> *'the larger proportion become absorbed by the workhouse, or swell the numbers who crowd the asylums for the insane.'*
>
> (see Mostyn Bird, 1953)

During the first half of the nineteenth century it was common practice to incarcerate epileptic patients in lunatic asylums. The stigma so often attached to epileptic seizures reflects the physical manifestations, described in 1823 as:

> *'a horribly wild, and, as some fancy, supernatural expression, as if the wretched patient were possessed.'*
>
> (see Beck, 1997 p38)

An attempt was made to change the approach to the management of such patients. The National Hospital, in 1876, established a convalescent home for 25 women and children at East Finchley, London. This convalescent home was to be a forerunner of the epileptic colony established at Chalfont, Middlesex, which was to provide long-term care, education and employment for individuals suffering from epilepsy. This was a starting point for change, but it could also be argued that no attempt was made to change public perception of the illness. East Finchley at that time lay outside the boundary of London. Hughlings Jackson, physician to the hospital in the early 1880s, proposed a neurological basis for epilepsy.

This, alongside developments in neurosurgery, offered new hope to some patients with epilepsy. In 1886, Sir Victor Horsley, surgeon to the hospital, successfully performed his first brain operation on a young Scotsman who suffered with frequent attacks of local epilepsy as a result of a head injury at the age of 7. His seizures began at age 15. Some dulling of his mental processes was noted along with a partial paralysis of the right arm and leg. Seizure activity amounted to 2,870 attacks during the first 13 days of admission (Paget, 1919).

THE NEED FOR EDUCATION

The National Hospital implemented a training programme for nurses in 1890. Bendall and Raybould say that:

> *'specialist hospitals developed their own nurse training schemes but had problems with recruitment, nurses trained in these hospitals having difficulty in finding employment outside their own speciality.'*
>
> (Bendall and Raybould, 1969 p69)

They emphasise that to have trained at a larger teaching hospital would have placed the nurse in a much better position. Not only would the experience be wider, the social network would have been larger. This point is highlighted by Cassell in the following statement (their emphasis) arguing that:

> *'unless age prevents it, it may be laid down as a sound rule that* **general training should always precede all special training.***'*
>
> (Cassell, 1913 p9)

Prior to the First World War (1914–1919), two different pre-registration nurse training routes were available at the National Hospital. Probationers could obtain a certificate for two or three years training. Another option existing for trained nurses was to pay a fee of three guineas for a three-month course; this effectively reflects one of the first post-qualifying education opportunities (Ling, 1960).

In 1949 the National Hospital instituted the first programme for registered nurses who wished to specialise in neuroscience nursing. The course essentially started as an experiment, no guidelines were available setting out the content or structure of such a course. Chritsine Rubin who established the course writes that one of the main reasons for drawing up the curriculum was her deep interest in the speciality and her concern regarding the lack of opportunity for post-qualifying studies (Rubin, 1969).

The General Nursing Council, at this time, had no control over post-registration nursing programmes. During the passage of the Nurses Act 1949, the General Nursing Council had proposed amendments which would have increased the scope of their power. The key impetus, however, for the government of the day was the provision of the new National Health Service, and the belief that the creation of a 'generalist nurse' who could nurse all types of cases in hospital, trained through a broad pre-registration curriculum was preferable to additional specialist post-registration training.

During the 1950s, in line with developments in medicine and surgery, more hospitals provided specialist post-registration courses. White suggests that this increase in specialised courses resulted because:

> 'the former general physicians and general surgeons found themselves overtaken by colleagues who dealt only with a particular body system. These consultants demanded specialist nurses who developed their own particular fields of narrow expertise.'
>
> (White, 1985 p51)

In 1963 the Ministry of Health addressed the increasing need for standardising post-registration nursing courses. It was estimated that there were at least 121 post-registration courses available at non-psychiatric hospitals in England and Wales (Ministry of Health, 1966). A sub committee of the standing Nursing Advisory Committee was set up, publishing its report in 1966: *The Post-Certificate Training and Education of Nurses*. This report confined itself to the requirements of registered nurses in general hospitals up to the grade of ward sister. It acknowledged that additional training was necessary upon completion of pre-registration

training. Its review of the clinical courses existing at the time stated:

> 'They are run as in-service training from matron's office. The primary purpose of some seems to be the recruitment of staff by attracting nurses into temporary employment and the instruction given is limited.'
>
> (Ministry of Health, 1966 p3)

The report considered that the deficiencies associated with these hospital run courses lay with their strong emphasis on recruitment and the geographical distribution of courses. The sub-committee considered that there were advantages in a system whereby a national body could co-ordinate a number of functions, including the duration, content and learning resources.

As a result of the 1966 report, the Joint Board of Clinical Nursing Studies (JBCNS) was established in March 1970. The joint board effectively centralised post-registration courses by laying down national standards to be met by hospital authorities providing courses. These were: co-ordination of the planning and provision of courses, control of the syllabuses, prescribing the methods of assessing the proficiency of students, and arranging the award of nationally recognised certificates to successful students (JBCNS, 1972).

The joint board placed a strong emphasis on the need for a continuation of basic training which should continue throughout the nurse's career. They stated that the overall aim for post-basic clinical education was to give better service to the patients, and that the courses should be directed to this end (JBCNS, 1972). Castledine (1998) suggests that the considerable range of JBCNS courses available reflected a tendency for them to follow medical specialities, and in some instances they emphasised the medical treatment. This central control of course provision was further enhanced by the implementation in 1983 of the United Kingdom Central Council for Nursing, Midwifery and Health Visiting (UKCC), and the four national nursing boards for nursing, midwifery and health visiting, to ensure that post-registration courses were all based on a national curriculum.

In 2002 the UKCC was disbanded along with the national boards and replaced with the Nursing and Midwifery Council (NMC). The progressive move of post-registration courses into higher education during the 1990s required close working relationships between the national boards and higher education providers. The demise of the national boards, however, meant that course providers, in association with the purchasers of the course, had greater flexibility in the development of courses.

A CONTINUALLY DEVELOPING SPECIALISM

In 1988 the Royal College of Nursing published a report *Specialities in Nursing*. Within this report they differentiate between nurse specialists and nurses working within a specialism. Nursing specialism is defined as:

> '*a component of the whole field of nursing, usually identified by being concerned with an age, sex or population group (for example midwifery or paediatric nursing), a body system, a health or status situation, a method of investigation or another aspect of nursing.*'
>
> (RCN, 1988 p5)

In an attempt to differentiate between terminology the RCN defined clinical nurse specialists as:

> '*experts in a particular aspect of nursing care ... they demonstrate refined clinical practice, either as a result of significant experience or advanced expertise.*'
>
> (RCN, 1988 p6)

The creation of nurse specialist and consultant nurse roles within the field of neuroscience nursing has expanded over the last decade to cover almost all areas within the specialism. Some of the key drivers for the development of multiple specialist roles include diagnostic and treatment regimes, increased medical specialisation and policy initiatives, such as the *National Service Framework for Long Term Conditions* (DH, 2005).

Service users and related charities, such as the Parkinson's Disease Society, the Multiple Sclerosis Society, the Multiple Sclerosis Trust, the Stroke Association, etc., have supported the development of specialist nursing roles. The futures of such roles, however, are vulnerable to changes in government initiatives and priorities and the availability of funding. In 2007 Baroness Masham of Ilton raised concern in a House of Lords debate on reduced spending on specialist nursing services for long term conditions. She makes reference during the debate to multiple sclerosis, epilepsy, spinal cord injury, progressive supranuclear palsy, and stroke, stating that:

> '*Being a specialist nurse is almost generic because any chronic condition that you care to name has its own specialist nurse. Whatever they specialise in, they are key to successful management of long-term conditions ... the findings also prove that they are cost-effective.*'
>
> (Hansard, 2006)

SUMMARY

Neuroscience nursing in the United Kingdom evolved from a philanthropic concern for patients with neurological disease who were excluded from admission to general hospitals. Techniques in diagnosis and treatment, and the increasing development of surgery presented challenges to nursing practice. This required the development and provision of specialist education programmes. The development of nursing practice within the neurosciences continues to present challenges to nurses and all health care specialists working within the specialism, as pharmacological interventions, imaging techniques and surgical interventions continue to develop.

REFERENCES

Abel-Smith B (1963) *The Hospitals 1800–1948*. London: Heinemann.

Beck SV (1997) Epilepsy the falling evil. In: KF Kiple *Plague, Pox and Pestilence*. London: Weidenfeld and Nicolson.

Bendall ERD, Raybould E (1969) *A History of the General Nursing Council for England and Wales 1919–1969*. London: HK Lewis and Co Ltd.

Caplan E (2001) Trains and trauma in the American gilded age. In: Micale MS, Lerner P (eds.) *Traumatic Pasts: History, psychiatry and trauma in the modern age, 1870–1930*. Cambridge: Cambridge University Press.

Cassell (1913) *Cassell's Peoples Physician: a book of medicine and of health for everybody*. London: Cassell.

Castledine G (1998) Clinical specialists in nursing in the UK: the early years. In: Castledine G, McGee P (eds). *Advanced and Specialist Nursing Practice*. Oxford: Blackwell Science.

Department of Health (2005) *The National Service Framework for Long-term Conditions*. London: Department of Health.

Domville EJ (1907) *A Manual for Hospital Nurses and Others Engaged in Attending the Sick*. (9th edition). London: J and A Churchill.

Down A (1922) *A Complete System of Nursing*. London: Waverley Book Co.

Feiling A (1958) *A History of the Maida Vale Hospital for Nervous Diseases*. London: Butterworth.

Feindel W (1999) The beginnings of neurology: Thomas Willis and his circle of friends. In: Clifford Rose F *A Short History of Neurology: The British contribution 1660–1910*. Oxford: Butterworth Heinemann.

Gower E (1960) *Queen Square and the National Hospital 1860–1960*. London: Edward Arnold.

Granshaw L (1989) Fame and fortune by means of bricks and mortar: the medical profession and specialist hospitals in Britain 1800–1948. In: Granshaw L, Porter R (eds). *The Hospital in History*. London: Routledge.

Hansard (2006) *Official Reports. Parliamentary debates (Hansard)*. 29 November Available from: http://www.publications.parliament.uk/pa/ld200607/ldhansrd/text/61129-0001.htm#061129102000303 Accessed July 2010.

Holmes G (1954) *The National Hospital, Queen Square 1860–1948*. London: E and S Livingstone Ltd.

Joint Board of Clinical Nursing Studies (1972) *First Report*. London: JBCNS.

Kandel ER (2006) *In Search of Memory*. London: WW Norton and Co.

Ling M (1960) The National Hospital: 100 Years at Queen Square, Bloomsbury. *Nursing Times* December 16th.

MacFarlane RM (1930) Treatment of organic nervous disorders. In: Arbuthbot Lane W (ed). *The Golden Health Library*. Vol 2. London: William Collins.

Martensen R (1999) When the brain came out of the skull: Thomas Willis (1621–1675). Anatomical technique and the formation of the 'cerebral body' in 17th century England. In: Clifford Rose F *A Short History of Neurology: The British contribution 1660–1910*. Oxford: Butterworth Heinemann.

Ministry of Health (1966) *Post Certificate Training and Education of Nurses*. London: HMSO.

Mostyn Bird M (1953) *The Ladies Samaritan Society of the National Hospital for Nervous Diseases: A short history of its foundation and development*. London: National Hospital.

National Hospital, Queen Square (1909) *Letter from King Edward VII to the Secretary of the Board of Management*. Buckingham Palace 4th November.

Norris R (1891) *Norris's Notes Being a Manual of Medical and Surgical Information*. London: Sampson Low, Masterton and Co.

Nutton V (1995) Medicine in the Greek world, 800–50BC. In: Conrad LI et al. (eds). *The Western Medical Tradition 800 BC to AD 1800*. Cambridge: Cambridge University Press.

Paget S (1919) *Sir Victor Horsley: A study of his life and work*. London: Constable.

Porter R (1999) *The Greatest Benefit to Mankind*. London: Fontana Press.

Rivett G (1998) *From Cradle to Grave: Fifty years of the NHS*. London: Kings Fund.

Royal College of Nursing (1988) *Specialities in Nursing: A report of the working party investigating the development of specialities within the nursing profession*. London: Royal College of Nursing.

Rubin C (1960) Century's background to nursing. *Nursing Mirror* July 19th.

Rubin C (1969) Advanced teaching in neurological and neurosurgical nursing at the National Hospital London. *Nursing Clinics of North America* 4(2):285–291.

Shepherd B (2002) *A War of Nerves: Soldiers and psychiatrists 1914–1994*. London: Pimlico.

Shorter E (1997) *A History of Psychiatry: From the era of the asylum to the age of prozac*. Chichester: John Wiley and Sons.

Weinreb B (1983) *The London Encyclopaedia*. London: Papermac.

White R (1985) *The Effects of the NHS on the Nursing Profession 1948–1961*. London: Kings Fund.

Youngson R, Schott I (1996) *Medical Blunders*. London: Robinson.

Index

Page numbers in *italics* represent figures, those in **bold** represent tables.

Neuroscience Nursing: Evidence-Based Practice, 1st Edition. Edited by Sue Woodward and Ann-Marie Mestecky
© 2011 Blackwell Publishing Ltd